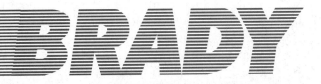

SIXTH EDITION

Emergency Care

Harvey D. Grant
Robert H. Murray, Jr.
J. David Bergeron

Contributing Editors
Gloria Bizjak
Bob Elling
Erik S. Gaull
Daniel Limmer

Medical Advisor
Edward T. Dickinson, M.D.

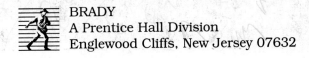
BRADY
A Prentice Hall Division
Englewood Cliffs, New Jersey 07632

Library of Congress Cataloging-in-Publication Data

Grant, Harvey D., (date)
    Emergency care/Harvey D. Grant, Robert H. Murray, Jr., J. David Bergeron;
contributing editors, Gloria J. Bizjak . . . [et al.]; medical advisor, Edward
Dickinson. — 6th ed.
        p.   cm.
    Includes bibliographical references and index.
    ISBN 0-89303-155-0
    1. Emergency medicine.   2. First aid in illness and injury.   3. Rescue
work.   4. Emergency medical personnel.   I. Murray, Robert H., 1934-.   II.
Bergeron, J. David, 1944- .   III. Title.   IV. Title: Emergency care.
    [DNLM: 1. Emergencies.   2. Emergency Medical Services.   3. Emer-
gency Medical Technicians.   4. First Aid.   WX 215 G762b 1994]
RC86.7.G7   1994
616.02.'5—dc20
DNLM/DLC
for Library of Congress   93–5576

Editorial/production supervision: Barbara Marttine
Page layout: Laura Ierardi
Acquisitions editor: Natalie Anderson
Marketing manager: Ann Elizabeth Hendrix
Developmental managing editor: Lois Berlowitz
Development editor: Sandra Breuer
Editorial assistant: Wendy Rivers
Interior design: Lorraine Mullaney
Cover design: Pakhaus Design Group
Cover art: Photography by Manny Akis, Akis Productions—Illustration
    by Paul Pullara, Pakhaus Design Group
Frontispiece: Liaison © Craig Wells
Photography: George Dodson
Photography editor: Michal Heron
Prepress buyer: Ilene Levy Sanford
Manufacturing buyer: Ed O'Dougherty

ELECTRONIC PUBLISHING

The Sixth Edition of EMERGENCY CARE was entirely produced and
illustrated by members of the Brady/Prentice Hall editorial, production, and design teams. Quark XPress® 3.1 and Adobe Illustrator®
were used on MacIntosh® II computers.

Permissions and Photo Acknowledgments may be found following the
Index.

Printed in the United States of America
10 9 8 7 6 5 4 3 2 1

ISBN: 0-89303-155-0
        0-89303-185-2 (IE)

Prentice-Hall International (UK) Limited, London
Prentice-Hall of Australia Pty. Limited, Sydney
Prentice-Hall Canada Inc., Toronto
Prentice-Hall Hispanoamericana, S.A., Mexico
Prentice-Hall of India Private Limited, New Delhi
Prentice-Hall of Japan, Inc., Tokyo
Prentice-Hall of Southeast Asia Pte. Ltd., Singapore
Editora Prentice-Hall do Brasil, Ltda., Rio de Janeiro

NOTE ON CARE PROCEDURES

It is the intent of the authors and publishers that this textbook be
used as part of a formal Emergency Medical Technician course taught
by a qualified instructor. The care procedures presented here represent accepted practices in the United States. They are not offered as a
standard of care. EMT-level emergency care is to be performed under
the authority and guidance of a licensed physician. It is the reader's
responsibility to know and follow local care protocols as provided by
the medical advisors directing the system to which he or she belongs.
Also, it is the reader's responsibility to stay informed of emergency
care procedure changes.

NOTE ON GENDER USAGE

Past attitudes have allowed our language to develop with the pro-
nouns "he" and "his" being used in general to signify persons of either
gender. For example, when describing the care for an injury to the
upper limb, most people will say "his arm" even though 50% of the
patients will probably be females. Our editors tell us that the repeated use of "he" or "she" is not proper in a long manuscript and the use
of (s)he is incorrect in all cases.

Authorities in both professional journals and popular publications have stated that the "quick fix" approach should be discouraged. They recommend different sentence structures when
appropriate and the traditional use of "he" and "his" when necessary.
This is why you will find "he" often used when referring to the actions
taken by an EMT. It is not the intent of the authors or the publisher
to imply that women should not be EMTs or that they are any less
professional than men in carrying out EMT-level care.

CREDITS

Elling, R. and R. Guerin, *Ambulance Accident Prevention Seminar Student Workbook,* New York State EMS Program, 1988
    Information on defensive driving in Chapter 24

*Guidelines for Cardiopulmonary Resuscitation and Emergency Cardiac
Care,* Emergency Cardiac Care Committee and Subcommittees, American Heart Association, JAMA, October 28, 1992 Vol. 268 No. 16,
2172-2298
    Guidelines on adult and pediatric basic and advanced life support,
    rescue breathing, and CPR in Chapters 4, 5, 17, and elsewhere

Epilepsy Education, Department of Neurology, University of Minnesota,
Minneapolis, Minnesota
    Information on seizure disorders in Chapter 16

New York State EMS Critical Trauma Care Course
    CUPS and "Platinum 10 Minutes" concepts in Chapter 3 and else-
    where

Russ M. Richards, EMI-I, I/C
Doña Ana Branch Community College
Las Cruces, New Mexico
    Review of information on snakebites in Chapter 16

Brief Contents

Detailed Table of Contents

Basic Life Support

CHAPTER 4

The Airway and Rescue Breathing 100

CHAPTER 5

CPR—Cardiopulmonary Resuscitation 134

CHAPTER 11

Lower Extremities 290

CHAPTER 12

The Skull and Spine 324

CHAPTER 13

Soft Tissues of the Head and Neck 360

CHAPTER 14

The Chest, Abdomen, and Genitalia 388

Medical Emergencies

CHAPTER 15

Cardiovascular and Respiratory Emergencies 412

Reference Section

Patient Assessment Highlights

Preface

You are about to begin your training to become an emergency medical technician (EMT). EMT courses range from 110 to 150 hours in length, with the typical EMT course being 110 hours long. Regardless of the hours you spend in class, your course is most likely based on guidelines set by the U.S. Department of Transportation (DOT). This is not to say that there is one universal EMT course. Using the DOT curriculum as a foundation, physicians and instructors in your local Emergency Medical Services System have designed your course to meet specific needs of your community. The basic training is the same, but there are differences in each state as to what materials are presented.

This textbook takes into account some of the variations in emergency care procedures used in different states. That is why you will find alternative methods cited throughout the text. There are some procedures that vary so much that only the most common methods in use are discussed. For such cases, you will be directed to follow local protocols.

Why is there no one method of providing care for certain illnesses and injuries? First of all, there are cases where more than one procedure works. Your EMS System may have tested only one procedure and decided that it was efficient, easy to learn, and simple to use. A different EMS System may have tested a second method and had the same results. This means that you will be trained to use the methods in which your local EMS System has confidence based upon its own rigorous testing.

One thing is certain: Not all the methods you learn in your training will stay the same during your career as an EMT. You must keep up-to-date with local procedures. Your instructor will tell you how continuing education programs for EMTs are presented in your locality, the prehospital emergency care journals and videos recommended by your EMS System, and any state- or locally-produced newsletters that are available to help the EMT stay current.

RECOMMENDATIONS OF INSTRUCTORS AND REVIEWERS

We at Brady are proud to present the Sixth Edition of **Emergency Care**. We asked many instructors and reviewers—many of you—how to improve the textbook. You told us to expand Patient Assessment. We did. You asked us to include the most current information on CPR and infection control. We did. Based on input from you and hundreds of other users and reviewers of **Emergency Care**, we have expanded, updated, and reorganized the text in the following additional ways:

- The information on Communicable Diseases and Infection Control has been updated and expanded according to OSHA and CDC guidelines and has been moved forward to Chapter 1. OSHA and CDC guidelines were used to update the material on cleaning the ambulance and disposing of hazardous wastes in Chapters 23 and 28.

- The information on Patient Assessment in Chapter 3 has been revised to include the Expanded Primary Survey (the ABCDEs) and the Status Decision based on CUPS categories (Critical, Unstable, Potentially Unstable, Stable). The entire chapter has been reorganized for clarity and still contains the popular illustrated Head-to-Toe Survey.

- Chapters 4, 5, 6, and 17, as well as the text in general, have been revised in accordance with the latest American Heart Association guidelines for BLS and CPR.

- Information on Defibrillation with AEDs has been added as an optional skill to Chapter 5 on CPR.

- In Chapter 6, the information on Oxygen Therapy and Oxygen Delivery Devices has been clarified and updated.

• Bleeding and Shock have been divided into two chapters (Chapters 7 and 8).

• Information on Anti-Shock Garments in Chapter 8 has been updated.

• Information on Trauma Procedures, including traction splinting and head immobilization, has been updated and reorganized for clarity in Chapters 9 through 14.

• New material on Normal and Rapid Extrication Procedures for removal of a patient from a vehicle onto a spine board is included in Chapters 12 and 29.

• Medical Emergencies have been divided into two chapters (Chapters 15 and 16).

• In Chapters 16, the material on Diabetes has been revised, in accordance with the advice of medical reviewers, to place emphasis on hyperglycemia and hypoglycemia. The material on Epilepsy and Other Seizure Disorders has been updated, according to Epilepsy Foundation of America guidelines, to include new classifications and terminology for types of seizures and recommendations on information EMTs should gather and report.

• Chapter 17 on Pediatrics has been expanded and rewritten for more complete and updated coverage of Pediatric Medical Emergencies and Pediatric Trauma.

• Chapter 19 on Burns and Hazardous Materials has been rewritten and the hazardous materials segment, in particular, updated.

• A chapter on Multiple-Casualty Incidents and Disaster Management, including Triage, has been updated (Chapter 22).

• Information on The Ambulance Run in Chapters 23 through 28 has been revised for clarity and updated.

• Chapter 27 on Communications and Reports has been completely rewritten, expanded, and updated.

• In Chapter 29, a new, streamlined, three-step procedure for vehicle extrication is presented.

LEARNING MADE EASIER

The Sixth Edition of **Emergency Care** has also been reorganized for easier learning. To make teaching, studying, and testing easier, the relationship among objectives, chapter text, bold-faced key terms, and review material has been clarified and strengthened.

The following features are part of chapter instruction.

On the Scene Each chapter opens with a realistic "you-are-there" scenario in which EMTs arrive on the scene to encounter a patient suffering from an injury or a medical or emotional problem. The real-world setting is intended to promote your interest and to help you relate what you are reading to what you are likely to encounter in the field.

Chapter Overview The Chapter Overview gives you a preview of the key content and concepts of the chapter you are about to read.

Expected Outcome A single, overall chapter objective is stated.

Infection Exposure Warning In every chapter that presents situations in which EMTs may be exposed to infection or communicable diseases, an infection-control warning and advice on protective barrier devices appears at the beginning of the chapter. (Additional warnings appear, as warranted, throughout the textbook.)

Chapter Outline An outline of major chapter headings appears at the beginning of each chapter to help you preview the chapter and to help guide reading and studying.

Objectives The Objectives are presented as Knowledge Objectives and Skills Objectives. You should be able to master the Knowledge Objectives by reading the chapter. To make these especially useful, they are page-referenced. Skills Objectives refer to key hands-on skills that are also covered in the chapter but that will require instructor-guided practice to master.

Patient Assessment Patient Assessment information is highlighted and featured for 130 injuries and medical problems. *Signs and Symp-*

toms are frequently presented as bulleted lists within this feature.

Patient Care Patient Care information is highlighted and featured for 130 injuries and medical problems. *Emergency Care Steps* are frequently presented as numbered lists within this feature.

Scans Key information and step-by-step procedures are summarized and presented for easy reference in illustrated Scans. The number of Scans has been increased to 84 in this edition.

Chapter Review Every chapter concludes with a Chapter Review, which consists of Key Terms and Summary. Key Terms lists all terms that appear in bold type in the chapter with their definitions. The Summary is a concise section-by-section review of important information.

Together, Key Terms and Summary provide a review of each chapter's objectives.

IMPROVING FUTURE TRAINING

Some of the best ideas for better training methods come from students who can tell us what areas of study caused them the most trouble. Other sound ideas come from practicing EMTs who let us know what problems they face in the field.

Any student, practicing EMT, or EMS instructor who has an idea on how to improve EMT training or the emergency care provided to patients should write to the authors at

The Brady Telesales Department
c/o Judy Stamm
Prentice Hall
113 Sylvan Avenue
Englewood Cliffs, NJ 07632

Acknowledgments

This is the Sixth Edition of the "yellow book." The development of this edition was greatly enhanced by the assistance of our contributing editors: Gloria Bizjak, Bob Elling, Erik Gaull, and Dan Limmer. Individually, they each worked with extraordinary commitment on this revision. Together, they form a team of highly dedicated professionals who have upheld the highest standards of current EMT instruction.

Contributing Editors
Gloria Bizjak, EMT-A has been a faculty member of the Maryland Fire and Rescue Institute (MFRI), University of Maryland, for 13 years, developing, teaching, evaluating, and coordinating emergency care, instructor training, and professional development programs. She was formerly with the West Lanham Hills Volunteer Rescue Squad in Prince George's County, Maryland, holding the positions of training officer and rescue chief. She has collaborated on several editions of Brady **Emergency Care** as well as on Brady's **First Responder**. Gloria is an EMT instructor, evaluator, and instructor trainer for the State of Maryland. She holds a Bachelor of Science degree in Health Education and a Master's degree in Education.

Bob Elling, MPA, NREMT-P has been active in EMS instruction since 1975. He has published numerous articles in *JEMS, Emergency, EMS, Annals of Emergency Medicine, Firehouse, Fire Command*, and other publications. He is the co-author of continuing education courses in Trauma, Pediatrics, and Ambulance Driving and has served as a State EMS Training Coordinator. Bob is the Education Coordinator for *Emergency Medical Update*, a monthly video service, as well as an EMS education consultant for Synergism Associates, Ltd. He is also an active paramedic for the Town of Colonie (NY) EMS Department and a firefighter for the Verdoy Fire Department.

Erik Gaull, NREMT-P became an EMT when he was in high school. He has served as New Mexico State Training Coordinator and writes regularly for EMS publications. He is a paramedic and firefighter with the Cabin John Park Volunteer Fire Department in Maryland.

Daniel Limmer, EMT-P is a New York State Certified EMT-Paramedic and EMS instructor. He serves as an instructor and Internship Coordinator for the Hudson Valley Community College

EMS Programs in Troy, New York. Additionally, he is a consultant and frequent speaker on EMS safety and survival issues. Dan has been an active paramedic, instructor, and police officer for over ten years.

Medical Advisor

Edward T. Dickinson, M.D., NREMT-P We would like to express special appreciation to our medical advisor, Dr. Edward T. Dickinson. Dr. Dickinson reviewed the entire text to ensure currency and accuracy in prehospital emergency care procedures. He is committed to the highest levels of excellence. Dr. Edward T. Dickinson is an attending physician and Director of EMS for the Department of Emergency Medicine at the Albany Medical Center and is Medical Director for the Town of Colonie (NY) Department of EMS. He was first certified as an EMT in 1979 and remains active as an instructor, paramedic, and firefighter. He is the recipient of *Firehouse Magazine*'s National Award for Heroism and Community Service.

Organizations

We also wish to thank the following organizations for their assistance in developing the Sixth Edition.

Annapolis City Fire Department, especially Chief Edward P. Sherlock, Sr.

Anne Arundel County Fire Department, especially Paul C. Haigley, Jr., Fire Administrator

Claymont Fire Company, Claymont, Delaware

Lincoln Fire Company, Whitemarsh, Pennsylvania

Maryland Fire and Rescue Institute. Steven T. Edwards, Director, and other MFRI staff and faculty who gave so generously of their time.

Prince George's County Fire Department, especially Chief Marion H. Estepp

Prince George's Hospital Center Emergency Department personnel, especially Mark Arsenault

Swedeland Fire Company, Upper Merion, Pennsylvania

Thanks also to Doug LaPerche and Charlene Larkin of County EMS/Nyack Hospital EMS for their technical assistance in creating the front cover image.

Reviewers

The following reviewers on the Sixth Edition provided invaluable feedback and suggestions. We wish to thank each of these highly motivated EMS professionals for their input.

Susan Barnes
Ohio Department of Highway Safety
Division of EMS
Columbus, OH

James L. Brother
Hartford Hospital—School of Allied Health
Hartford, CT

Rick Buell
EMS—Department of Health
Olympia, WA

Bill Cheatwood
Campbell County Volunteer Rescue Squad
Lynchburg, VA

Paul H. Coffee
Office of EMS
Department of Public Health
Boston, MA

Patrick Coonan
Center for Emergency Training
North Shore University Hospital
Manhasset, NY

John C. Davanzo
Life Star Associates
Detroit, MI

Gail Dubs
State EMS Training Coordinator
Harrisburg, PA

Brian P. Dunmyer
EMT/Paramedic Program
Tallahassee Community College
Tallahassee, FL

Dolly Fernandes
Washington Department of Health
Olympia, WA

Donna Ferracone
Crafton Hills College
Yucaipa, CA

Jacquelyn Francesconi, MS
EMT/Paramedic Program Director
Rockland Community College
Suffern, NY

John K. Gaffney
Division of Emergency Medicine
University of New Mexico
Albuquerque, NM

Grant Goold
Center for Prehospital Research and Training
UCSF Medical Center
San Francisco, CA

David M. Habben
State EMS Training Coordinator
State of Idaho EMS Bureau
Boise, ID

K. C. Jones
Delta Tech
Jonesboro, AK

Lou Jordan
Emergency Training Associates
Baltimore, MD

Gregory Juersivich
North Canton Emergency Medical Services
North Canton, OH

Laura Lloyd
City of Portsmouth EMS
Suffolk, VA

Fred Matthes
Great Oaks Vocational School
Cincinnati, OH

Phil Petty
Georgia Board of Education
Post-Secondary Vocational
Atlanta, GA

Monte Posner
Training Institute for Medical Emergency
Staten Island, NY

Joseph R. Russo, Jr.
South Windsor Ambulance Corps
South Windsor, CT

James L. Smith
Dothan Police Department
Dothan, AL

Louis Souder
Apollo Career Center
Lima, OH

Doug Stevenson
Houston Community College
Houston, TX

Mary Jo Vincent
Department of Health
Santa Ana, CA

Jason White
Former State EMS Training Coordinator
Missouri Department of Health
Jefferson City, MO

Richard Wiederhold
Brevard County Public Safety
Melbourne, FL

To
Harvey Grant
June 24, 1934–January 24, 1993
৵

Through his work
in Emergency Medical Services
and through the
editions of this book,
Harvey helped create and
keep alive a movement that
influences the lives of
thousands of people each year.

Harvey's spirit and
his message live on.
৵

He will be missed.

On the Scene

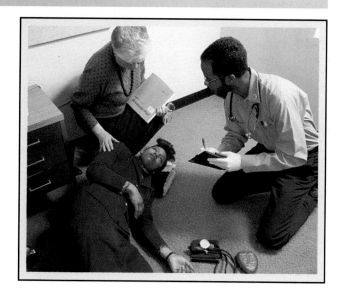

You: Mrs. York, I'm Joe Henry. I'm an Emergency Medical Technician from the Oakview Ambulance Service. Can you tell me what happened?

Mrs. York: I just got a little dizzy, that's all. If I can just get up, I'll be O.K.

You: Before you move, I'd like to check you over. May I?

Mrs. York: No, don't bother. I just haven't been feeling right lately.

As an EMT you will sometimes encounter people who call an ambulance when they don't need one. Mrs. York is the opposite. She needs the ambulance but does not want it. Mrs. York had passed out, which may indicate an underlying condition that requires medical care. Also, she might have sustained injuries when she fell. Even though she does not want help, she may need it.

Your Emergency Medical Services unit is called to the workplace of a 30-year-old woman. The woman, Mrs. York, left her desk to get a cup of coffee and passed out. Concerned co-workers immediately called 911 for help and insisted that Mrs. York not try to get up.

When you arrive, Mrs. York is lying on the floor. Although conscious and talking coherently, your patient appears shaky. Co-workers tell you that Mrs. York has been working long hours recently.

Two important topics in Chapter 1 are consent and negligence. When Mrs. York says no to your offer of help, she is withholding her consent and you may not treat her without it. However, if you leave Mrs. York on the floor without attempting additional care, including a trip to the emergency department, you will be guilty of negligence. Often patients need information, coaxing, and time to convince them that they need your help.

The Emergency Medical Technician

Chapter Overview

Years ago, an ambulance crew's job was to lift the victim into the ambulance and deliver him to a hospital. The only qualifications were strength and a driver's license. Today, the ambulance attendant has been replaced by the Emergency Medical Technician (EMT), who serves as an extension of the hospital emergency department. From the moment of arrival at the emergency scene, the EMT is responsible for providing an unbroken chain of prehospital medical care: at the scene, during the ambulance ride, and until the hospital emergency department staff takes over. Today's EMT is a trained and skilled medical professional. The EMT's job carries serious responsibilities and legal implications.

Expected Outcome, Chapter 1: *You will understand and be able to describe the basic roles and responsibilities of an EMT.*

THE EMERGENCY MEDICAL SERVICES SYSTEM
    How It Began
    Elements of the System

THE EMERGENCY MEDICAL TECHNICIAN
    Roles and Responsibilities
    Background, Training, and Experience
    Traits of a Good EMT

THE EMT AND THE LAW
    Duty to Act
    Negligence
    The Standard of Care
    Abandonment
    Patient Rights—Consent
    Patient Rights—Confidentiality
    Immunities
    Other Legal Aspects

EQUIPMENT
    The Ambulance
    Equipment and Supplies

INFECTION CONTROL AND THE EMT
    The Need for Infection Control
    Preventing Infection
    Infection Control and the Law

Knowledge *After reading this chapter, you should be able to*

1. Define *Emergency Medical Services (EMS) System.* (pp. 4-5)
2. Define *emergency care.* (p. 5)
3. Define *Emergency Medical Technician (EMT).* (pp. 5, 11-12)
4. List the NINE major duties of an EMT. (p. 12; Scan 1-1)
5. Describe the traits of a good EMT. (pp. 14-15)
6. Define *duty to act.* (p. 16)
7. State how the concept of *negligence* applies to EMT-level emergency care. (pp. 16-17)
8. Define *standard of care.* (p. 17)
9. Define *abandonment.* (p. 17)
10. Define *informed consent*, and distinguish between *actual consent* and *implied consent.* (pp. 18-19)
11. Distinguish between *voluntary consent* and *involuntary consent.* (p. 18)
12. Relate the laws governing patient consent and refusal of care to the child, or minor, patient. (pp. 18-19)
13. Relate EMT responsibilities and standard of care to Good Samaritan laws. (p. 19)
14. List at least SIX emergencies that may require you to file special reports. (p. 19)
15. Describe the role and actions of an EMT when caring for a deceased person and for a terminally ill person. (pp. 20-21)
16. Describe the THREE types of ambulances. (pp. 21-22)
17. Name categories of medical equipment, basic tools, and supplies used by the EMT. (pp. 22-23)
18. Define infectious disease and communicable disease. (p. 23)
19. Describe the major ways in which infectious diseases are communicated. (pp. 24-25)
20. List the primary means of carrying out universal precautions and body substance isolation. (pp. 25-26)

Skills *As an EMT you should be able to*

1. Develop and display the desirable traits of an EMT.
2. Provide EMT-level care as defined by law and regulations
3. Exercise methods of infection control under your EMS system's infection exposure control plan.

As an Emergency Medical Technician (EMT), you will be part of an Emergency Medical Services (EMS) System. EMS Systems are a fairly recent development in the history of medical care. Modern EMS Systems began in the 1960s, but the idea of emergency medical service started almost two hundred years earlier.

THE EMERGENCY MEDICAL SERVICES SYSTEM

How It Began

In the 1790s the French began to transport wounded soldiers so they could be cared for by physicians away from the scene of battle. This is the earliest documented emergency medical service. No medical care was provided for the wounded on the battlefield. The idea was simply to carry the victim from the scene to a place where medical care was available.

Other wars inspired similar emergency services. Clara Barton, a nurse, began such a service for the wounded during the American Civil War and later helped establish the American Red Cross. During World War I, many volunteers joined battlefield ambulance corps.

Nonmilitary ambulance services began in some major American cities in the early 1900s—again as transport services only, offering little or no emergency care. Smaller areas did not begin to develop ambulance services until the late

1940s, after World War II. Often the local undertaker provided a hearse for ambulance transport. Where services developed to offer emergency care along with transport to the hospital, the fire service was often the responsible agency.

During the Korean Conflict in the 1950s and the Vietnam War in the 1960s and '70s, medical teams produced advances in field care for injuries (trauma). Parallel advances in the civilian sector led to the first specialized emergency medical centers devoted to the treatment of trauma, for example the Shock Trauma Unit at University Hospital in Baltimore.

The importance of extending hospital-quality care to the sick and injured at the emergency scene—of beginning care at the scene and continuing it, uninterrupted, during transport to the hospital—was recognized, as was the need to organize systems for such emergency prehospital care and to train personnel to provide it.

During the mid 1960s, the National Academy of Sciences' National Research Council studied the problem of emergency care. Its intent was to establish standards for prehospital care. The concept of modern emergency medical services was first stated in 1968 when the National Research Council issued the following statement.

Employees or volunteer members of public and private organizations having a responsibility for the delivery of health services must be trained in and held accountable for administration of specialized care and delivery of the victims of acute illness or injury to a medical facility. This category of lay persons includes ambulance personnel, rescue squad workers, policemen, firemen, lifeguards, workers in first aid or health facilities of public buildings and industrial plants, attendants at sports events, civil defense workers, paramedic personnel, and employees of public or private health service agencies. Specialized training, retraining and accreditation of such persons necessitate development of training courses, manuals and training aids adequate to provide instruction in all emergency care short of that rendered by physicians or by paramedic personnel under their direct supervision.

Ambulance personnel are responsible for all lay emergency care from the time they first see the victim through transportation and delivery to care of a physician. They must therefore be able not only to appraise the extent of first aid rendered by others, but also to carry out what additional measures will make it safe to move the victim and minimize morbidity and mortality. They must operate the vehicle safely and efficiently; maintain communication between the scene of the emergency, traffic authorities, dispatchers, and emergency departments; render necessary additional care en route; and transmit records and reports to medical and other authorities. Although the emphasis on certain subjects will vary with the nature of employment of those who are not ambulance personnel but who have a responsibility for delivery of health services, they should be equally trained so that minimum care can be assured, whether they transfer responsibility to the ambulance attendant, or, in his absence, carry out the functions required of him.

Training of Ambulance Personnel and Others Responsible for Emergency Care of the Sick and Injured at the Scene and During Transportation. Division of Medical Services, National Academy of Sciences' National Research Council, March, 1968.

The above may not have much meaning so early in your training. However, once you become an EMT, come back to this quotation. You will note that it is the framework on which this course is based.

Keep in mind what emergency care must have been like in many areas of the country before medical direction, standards, and a national commitment were developed. With the preceding statement, the long-held concept of ambulance service as a means merely for transporting the sick and injured passed into oblivion. No longer could ambulance personnel be viewed as people with little more than the physical strength required to lift a victim in and out of an ambulance.

Victims now became patients, receiving prehospital emergency care from highly trained professional personnel. **Emergency care** began to include treating both the sick and injured at the emergency scene and during transport, with the providers of this care being trained to consider the physical and emotional needs of the patient. The hospital emergency department was extended, through the **Emergency Medical Services (EMS) system**, to reach the sick and injured at the emergency scene and begin immediate care. The ambulance attendant was replaced by the **Emergency Medical Technician (EMT).**

Other landmarks in the development of EMS Systems and care included

1966—The National Highway Safety Act charged the United States Department of Transportation (DOT) with developing Emergency Medical Services (EMS) standards and assisting the states to upgrade the quality of their prehospital emergency care. Most EMT courses today are based on models developed by the DOT.

1966—The American Heart Association (AHA) developed training programs for cardiopulmonary resuscitation (CPR) and basic life support aimed at emergency care for airway obstruction, cessation of breathing, and heart attack. A program for public education from AHA and the National Academy of Sciences' National Research Council was started in 1973. As a result, millions of private citizens and thousands of EMTs were, and continue to be, trained in CPR and basic life support.

1970—The National Registry of Emergency Medical Technicians was founded to establish professional standards and provide services to local EMS Systems. Other organizations to improve prehospital care were also established.

1973—Congress passed the National Emergency Medical Services Systems Act. This act was the cornerstone of a federal effort to implement and improve EMS systems across the United States. Funding was provided for EMS system development. States were encouraged to define EMS regions and to create "state-lead agencies" to foster that development.

1974—The National Health Planning and Resources Development Act increased planning activities and services to help the states develop their EMS Systems. Today, most states have their own quality EMS System, offering basic, advanced, and continuing education programs to most providers of prehospital emergency care.

1974 to Present—During the 1980s the federal government relinquished more power over EMS systems to the states. The standards, training, equipment, and organization of EMS systems nationwide has continued to develop, as does community reliance on this essential service. Members of the nation's EMS Systems are proud of their history and what they have been able to accomplish in the ongoing effort to improve prehospital emergency care.

Elements of the System

The EMS System is more than EMTs and emergency department personnel. It is a chain of human and physical resources linked together to provide total patient care. To better understand this chain of resources, consider an event in the life of Mr. Tom Henderson. Note how all the links of the chain of resources joined to carry Tom through an unfortunate experience (Figures 1-1 through 1-15).

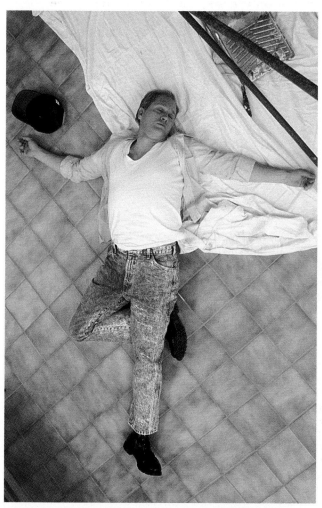

Figure 1-1 Wednesday, June 21, 11:50 A.M. Tom is working on scaffolding in the warehouse of the Acme Paper Products Company. While painting, he leans too far over the scaffold and falls nearly 8 feet to the floor. He lands on his right leg and falls backward, striking his upper back and shoulders on the floor.

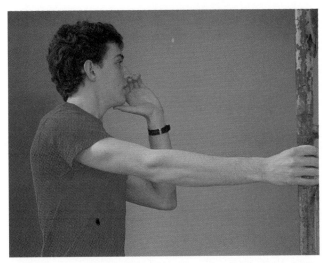

Figure 1-2 11:51 A.M. A co-worker nearby sees Tom fall. Before going to Tom's assistance, he quickly calls out to the floor supervisor, who, in turn, notifies the nurse on duty in the plant infirmary. Before she leaves the infirmary, the nurse dials 911 and requests assistance from the local EMS System.

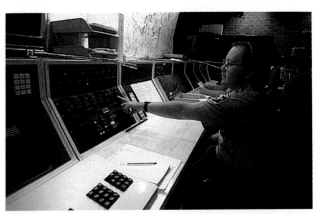

Figure 1-3 11:51 A.M. The local emergency communications center dispatcher receives the call from the plant nurse. He gathers as much information about the accident as he can and passes this information on as he alerts the ambulance and rescue squad. In some areas of the country, if the caller had been a lay person without emergency care training or trained personnel at the scene, the dispatcher would have offered basic care instructions to be carried out until trained professionals arrived.

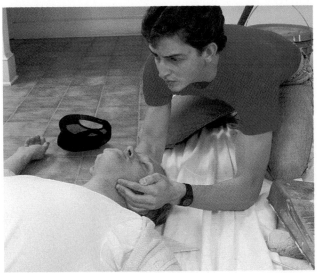

Figure 1-4 11:52 A.M. The co-worker who witnessed the accident reaches Tom's side. It is obvious that Tom has been injured. A quick assessment shows him that Tom is unconscious and is having difficulty breathing. He quickly positions himself at Tom's head and opens Tom's airway by using a jaw-thrust maneuver that he learned in a plant-sponsored First Responder course. He is careful not to move Tom's head any more than absolutely necessary because of the possibility of spinal injuries. This simple maneuver reduces Tom's breathing problems. The co-worker does not move Tom; instead, he closely watches Tom's breathing efforts. He is ready to assist Tom in the event that respirations stop.

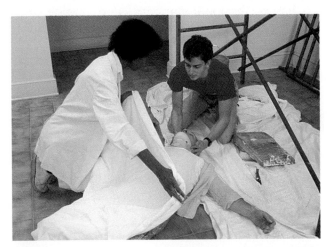

Figure 1-5 11:56 A.M. The plant nurse arrives with a first aid kit and blankets. Tom's co-worker describes the breathing problem he noticed and the results of the jaw-thrust. The nurse determines that Tom is no longer having difficulty with his breathing. She makes a quick assessment and, based on her observation of the mechanism of injury, has the First Responder stabilize Tom's head and neck while she secures a rigid cervical collar (extrication collar) around Tom's neck. She has the co-worker continue to stabilize Tom's head after the collar is applied. Knowing that EMTs will soon arrive, she does not move Tom. However, she does cover him to help conserve body heat.

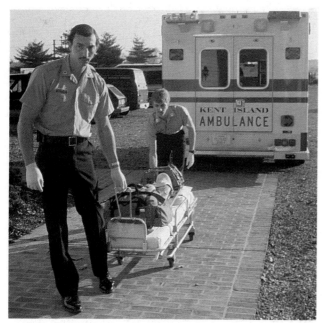

Figure 1-6 12:01 P.M. The ambulance arrives on the scene. The EMTs enter the building, bringing with them a wheeled stretcher, a long spine board, a portable oxygen delivery system, and a trauma kit.

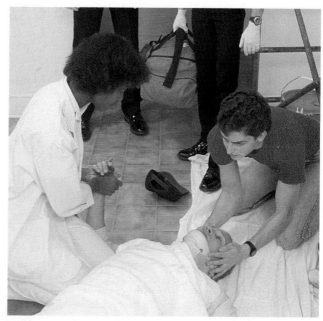

Figure 1-7 12:03 P.M. The EMTs reach the site of Tom's accident. A quick primary survey shows that Tom is now alert, is breathing, has a full and regular pulse, and has no serious bleeding wounds. There are no indications that Tom is going into shock.

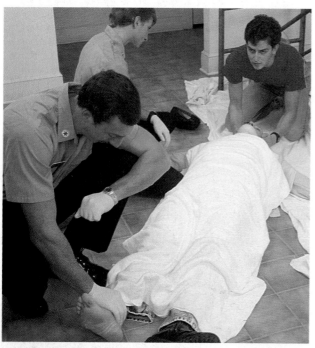

Figure 1-8 The EMTs conduct a complete body survey and find that Tom has a possible fracture of the right femur (thigh bone). He does not have any field-test indications of spinal injury. Nonetheless, they elect to leave the cervical (extrication) collar in place, knowing that spinal injuries are possible in this type of accident. To further protect Tom from additional injury, the EMTs plan to immobilize him on a long spine board after a traction splint is applied to the injured leg. Checking the pulse in the injured leg completes the EMT's survey.

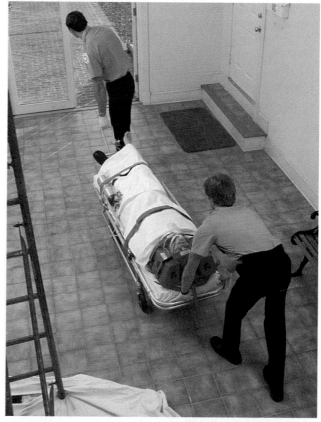

Figure 1-9 12:09 P.M. The EMTs begin to administer oxygen to help lessen any complications should Tom develop shock. Properly splinted and immobilized, placed on a stretcher, covered, secured, and receiving oxygen, Tom is wheeled from the accident site.

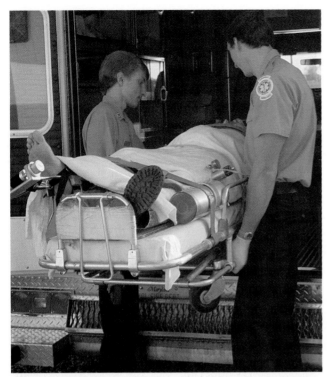

Figure 1-10 12:13 P.M. Only ten minutes have passed since the EMTs reached the patient's side. Tom is loaded into the ambulance and transported to the hospital. He is attended by an EMT during transport in case additional emergency care is required. During transport, concise radio communications inform the emergency department staff of the circumstances of Tom's accident, the possible extent of his injuries, his condition, the care provided, and the estimated time of arrival. The emergency department staff will be alerted if there is any change in Tom's condition during transport.

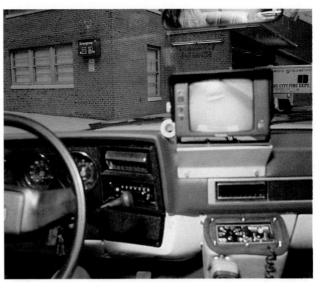

Figure 1-11 12:30 P.M. The ambulance arrives at the medical facility. The EMTs stay with Tom until they are able to personally transfer his care to the emergency department staff. As they make the transfer, they present an oral report about the accident and Tom's condition and the emergency care they have provided. Then they complete their written prehospital care report and leave a copy with the emergency department staff. The EMTs have removed Tom's wallet and watch and now turn these effects over to the nurse at the emergency department desk, receiving a written receipt for them. They check with the emergency department physician to be sure that their services are no longer needed and, having received their release, depart to ready the ambulance for the next call. They feel confident that there has been no break in the chain of care for their patient and that Tom will receive excellent hospital care.

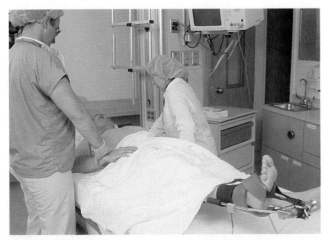

Figure 1-12 Tom's immediate needs are cared for by the emergency department staff. Tests are performed and x-rays are taken. The emergency department physician finds that Tom does not have any spinal injuries. The required care for Tom's injuries is determined, and he is wheeled to an operating room where an orthopedic surgeon cares for Tom's fracture.

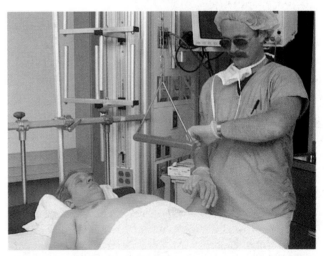

Figure 1-13 Tom is moved to a recovery room and placed in traction. A nurse closely observes him until he is completely recovered from the anesthesia. When appropriate, he will be moved to a room in an area of the hospital where the staff specializes in the care of patients who have orthopedic injuries.

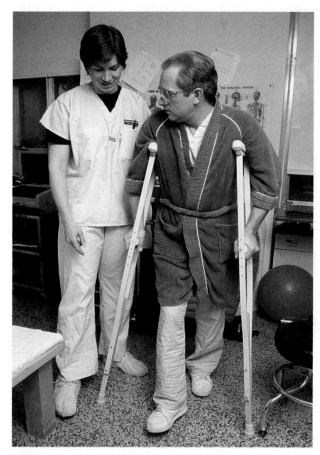

Figure 1-14 Saturday, June 24. A physical therapist begins working with Tom, providing him with patient education and a program on exercises to prevent muscle wasting in his uninjured extremity. On Monday, August 14, Tom begins a program of rehabilitation for his injured leg under the supervision of a physical therapist.

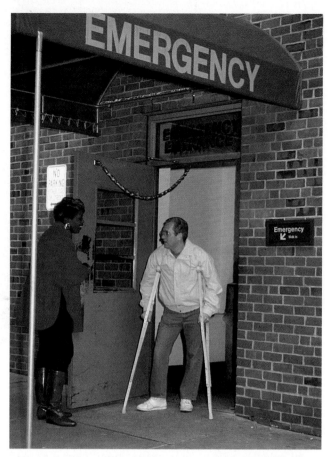

Figure 1-15 Sunday, August 20. Tom has received total patient care while he was in the hospital and has been discharged. He will be away from work for some time, and he will have to return to the hospital periodically for therapy. But . . . he is alive, and he can walk!

Having read of Tom's experience, consider how many different persons were involved with his care from accident through recovery. AT ANY POINT, TOM COULD HAVE SUSTAINED IRREVERSIBLE INJURY IF ANY ONE OF THESE PERSONS HAD FAILED TO ACT OR HAD PROVIDED IMPROPER CARE. The chain of human and physical resources, the EMS System in Tom's community, held together because none of the links in the chain failed. This chain of resources is reviewed in Figure 1-16.

Some parts of the EMS System were not visible in the preceding example. An advisory council and medical director for EMS decided how the system was to respond and what care procedures were to be used. Public information officers had provided the citizens with the knowledge of what the EMS System is, what it could do, and how to seek assistance. The EMS System certified instruc-

tors, who then trained the EMTs who responded to help Tom. Many other persons, including those involved with personnel, record keeping, and equipment and supplies were important parts of the EMS System being able to help Tom.

A person who has an accident, or a person who suddenly becomes ill, is called a **victim**. Once the person enters into the EMS System, he becomes a **patient**.

As an EMT, you will be part of the EMS System. More specifically, you will carry out your duties as a part of a prehospital emergency care delivery subsystem. Components of this subsystem are

- The EMT
- The ambulance
- The supplies and equipment carried on the ambulance

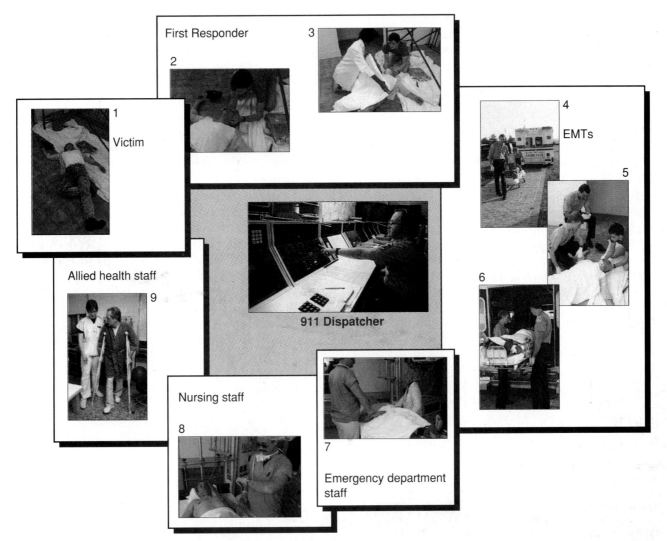

Figure 1-16 The chain of human and physical resources of the EMS System.

THE EMERGENCY MEDICAL TECHNICIAN

The EMT is a professional provider of emergency care. Both the volunteer and career EMT are considered to be professional members of the EMS System. The term *professional* does not imply payment for services. It refers to training, dedication, desire to perform to the best of one's abilities, and willingness to continue with formal training. Working within the EMS System, the EMT is a team member helping to provide total patient care. Trained and appropriately certified, the EMT is capable of providing emergency care at the scene and en route to the hospital.

There is more than one level of EMT. In this book, we will use the term to mean the EMT-Basic unless otherwise stated. The levels of EMTs include

- EMT-Basic—a person who has successfully completed the DOT EMT National Standard Training Program or its equivalent and has been certified as an EMT by a state emergency medical services program or other authorized agency.
- EMT-Intermediate—a basic-level EMT who has passed specific training programs in order to provide some level of advanced life support, for example the initiation of IV (intravenous) lines and administration of some medications. In some states, this level includes those EMTs who are given the title of Cardiac Technician, Cardiac Rescue Technician, Shock-Trauma Technician, and Critical Care Technician.
- EMT-Paramedic—a person who has successfully completed paramedic training including or equal to the DOT National Standard Paramedic Curriculum and has

received the appropriate certification. Paramedics can generally perform relatively invasive field care, including insertion of endotracheal tubes, initiation of intravenous lines, administration of medications, interpretation of electrocardiograms, and cardiac defibrillation (electric shock to restart an arrested heart).

The EMT deals with both injury and illness and the emotional problems that result from such emergencies. You will have to provide basic life support for patients if they cannot breathe adequately, have stopped breathing, have developed cardiac arrest, or have developed shock. You will have to provide care for patients having cuts, bruises, fractures, gunshots, burns, and internal injuries. You will be called on to deal with heart attacks, strokes, respiratory illnesses, seizures, diabetic emergencies, childbirth, poisoning, drug abuse, and problems due to excessive heat and cold. In addition, you will have to provide care for patients suffering emotional or psychiatric emergencies. Some problems will be simple, while others will be life threatening. All will require professional emergency care.

Roles and Responsibilities

At an emergency scene, the primary concern is the patient, but your first concern must be your own personal safety. You must never allow your desire to help the patient make you overlook the potential hazards at the scene.

As an EMT, you will have nine main duties (Scan 1-1). They are

1. Preparation—Be prepared to respond.
2. Response—Respond to the scene swiftly, but safely.
3. Scene Control—Make certain that the scene is safe, and when called on to do so, assist in the control of the activities at the scene (e.g., traffic- or multiple-casualty incident command.).
4. Access—Gain access to patients, using special tools when necessary.
5. Assessment and Care—Determine, to the level of your training, what may be wrong with the patient and provide the appropriate level of emergency care. This includes recognizing the need for, and requesting, specialized personnel to be sent to the scene (e.g., advanced life support personnel). Care and assessments must be done

with personal safety in mind. The scene must be safe and you must be protected from injury and disease.
6. Disentanglement—Free, lift, and move the patient, when required, and do so without causing additional injury to the patient or to yourself. These procedures are also called disentanglement, extrication, and transfer.
7. Transfer—Prepare and properly transfer the patient to the ambulance.
8. Transport—Transport the patient safely to the appropriate medical facility, providing the needed care and en route communications and transferring the patient and patient information to the staff at the medical facility. This involves both an oral report to the nurse or physician and completing the prehospital care report.
9. Termination of Activities—Return safely from the run, complete any other records and reports, disinfect the ambulance, equipment, and yourself, restock the vehicle, and prepare yourself for the next response.

Some of the EMT's duties, such as resuscitating a patient whose heart has stopped, are dramatic. Report writing and taking inventory are far less glamorous. All duties are important.

Note: Duties and skills may vary among localities. Within any given area, specific policies, laws, and regulations determine the duties each member of an EMT team has. Usually, all basic-level EMTs are equally trained in all duties and responsibilities so that they may function independently or interchangeably.

Background, Training, and Experience

Many areas of the nation use a job description for the EMT based on one that was prepared by the United States Department of Transportation and supported by the National Highway Traffic Safety Administration. In most localities, the minimum levels of training and experience required for the EMT include

- Age 18 or older
- Training to the level recognized as the DOT National Standard Curriculum for EMT-Basic personnel
- Practical experience in the care and use of emergency care equipment commonly used by EMTs (e.g., suction devices, installed and portable oxygen delivery systems, anti-

Scan 1-1
Nine Main Duties of the EMT

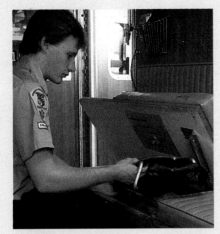

1. Preparation

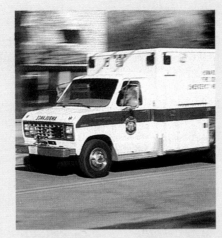

2. Response

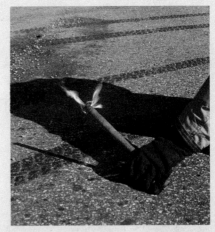

3. Scene control

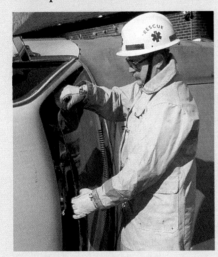

4. Gaining access

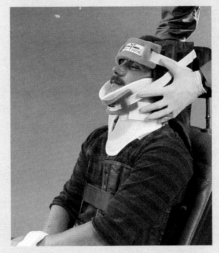

5. Assessment and emergency care

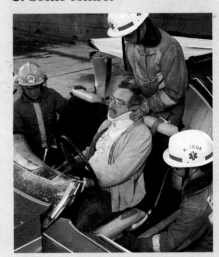

6. Disentanglement

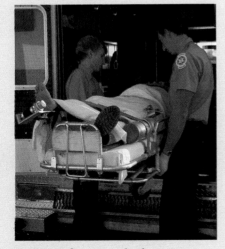

7. Transfer to ambulance

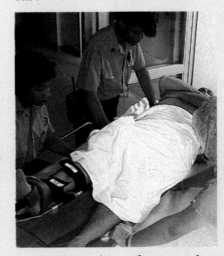

8. Transport/transfer to medical facility

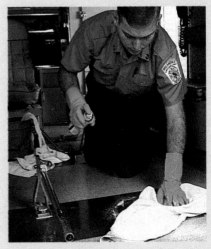

9. Termination of activities

shock garments, splints and immobilization equipment, emergency medical kits, obstetric kits, patient transfer devices, and basic rescue tools)

- Practical experience in sanitizing and disinfecting procedures for all equipment, including the ambulance; knowledge of infection control procedures
- Knowledge of safety and security procedures to allow for duties to be carried out in certain hostile environments
- Knowledge of the territory within the EMT's service area
- A valid driver's license, an acceptable driving record, and any professional certificate or license as required by law indicating that you know the motor vehicle codes and that you as a vehicle operator can skillfully and safely operate an ambulance. Some localities do not require all EMTs to be ambulance operators
- Ability to use communications equipment
- Certification from your state or an appropriate agency that is responsible for EMT certification within a specific jurisdiction

Traits of a Good EMT

There are certain physical traits and aspects of personality that are desirable for an EMT.

Physical Traits Physically, you should be in good health and fit to carry out your duties. If you are unable to provide needed care because you cannot bend over or catch your breath, then all your training may be worthless to the patient who is in need of your help.

You should be able to lift and carry up to 100 pounds. Practice with other EMTs is essential so that you can learn how to carry your share of the combined weight of patient, stretcher, linens, blankets, and portable oxygen equipment. For such moves, coordination and dexterity are needed, as well as strength. You will have to perform basic rescue procedures, lower stretcher patients from upper levels, and negotiate fire escapes and stairways while carrying patients.

Your eyesight is very important in performing your EMT duties. Make certain that you can clearly see distant objects as well as those close at hand. Both types of vision are needed for patient assessment, reading labels, driving tasks, and controlling emergency scenes. Should you have any eyesight problems, they must be corrected with prescription eye glasses or contact lenses.

Be aware of any problems you may have with color vision. Not only is this important to driving, but it could also be critical for patient assessment. Colors seen on the patient's skin, lips, nailbeds, ear lobes, and eyelids often provide valuable clues to a patient's condition.

You should be able to give and receive oral and written instructions and communicate with the patient, bystanders, and EMS and emergency department personnel. Eyesight, hearing, and speech are important to the EMT; thus any significant problems must be corrected if you are to be an EMT.

Personal Traits Good personality traits are very important to the EMT. You should be

- Pleasant—to inspire confidence and help to calm the sick and injured
- Sincere—able to convey an understanding of the situation and the patient's feelings
- Cooperative—to allow for faster and better care, establish better coordination with other members of the EMS System, and bolster the confidence of patients and bystanders
- Resourceful—able to adapt a tool or technique to fit an unusual situation
- A self-starter—to show initiative and accomplish what must be done without having to depend on someone else to start procedures
- Emotionally stable—to help overcome the unpleasant aspects of an emergency so that needed care may be rendered and any uneasy feelings that exist after care has been provided may be resolved
- Able to lead—to take the steps necessary to control a scene, to organize bystanders, to deliver care, and, when necessary, to take complete charge of an emergency.
- Neat and clean—to promote confidence in both patients and bystanders and to reduce the possibility of contamination
- Of good moral character, having respect for others—to allow for trust in situations when the patient cannot protect his own body or valuables and so that all information relayed is considered to be truthful and reliable
- In control of personal habits—to reduce the possibility of rendering improper care and to prevent discomfort to the patient. This would include not smoking when providing

care (REMEMBER: smoking may contaminate wounds and is a danger around oxygen delivery systems) and never consuming alcohol within 8 hours of duty

- Controlled in conversation—able to communicate properly, to inspire confidence, and to avoid inappropriate conversation that may upset or anger the patient or bystanders or violate patient confidentiality
- Able to listen to others—to be compassionate and empathetic, to be accurate with interviews, and to inspire confidence

All of this is part of developing a CALM, PROFESSIONAL MANNER that will result in better patient care.

At first, some people do not see the importance of these personality traits. They believe that all that an EMT needs to worry about is how to efficiently provide the correct care procedure. Experience has shown that all of the traits listed are relevant to the complex world of emergency care.

For example, consider leadership ability. In many cases, others will be in charge at the scene. However, YOU may have to take control of an accident scene. YOU may have to initiate rescue efforts. YOU may have to direct the sorting and removal of multiple casualties from the scene. YOU may have to deal with distraught relatives. YOU may have to cope with spectators who are disrupting an otherwise smooth-running operation. YOU may have to make unpleasant decisions. In short, at one time or another, YOU will be in charge and there will be no one else to take over. In those instances you must be able to lead calmly, decisively, and firmly.

EMS Systems place a strong emphasis on a neat, clean appearance and good personal grooming (Figure 1-17). Put yourself in the place of an injured but conscious patient. If one EMT arrives in a clean uniform and another arrives in greasy overalls and if you know nothing of their capabilities, which one would you want to help you? You would probably pick the uniformed EMT, if for no other reason than he looks the part. Be it a full uniform, a jacket, or simply a shirt with a patch, it helps to put the patient at ease and to gain the cooperation of bystanders.

Neatness and good personal grooming not only inspire confidence, they also protect the patient from contamination from a rescuer's dirty clothing, hands, fingernails, or unkempt hair.

One of the biggest mistakes made by new EMTs is inappropriate conversation. Saying the

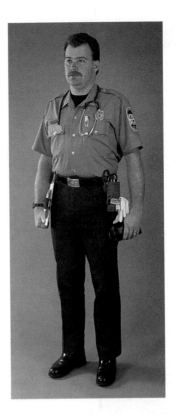

Figure 1-17 A professional appearance inspires confidence.

wrong thing or using the wrong words may upset a patient and worsen his condition. It may also upset relatives or bystanders. Remember, it is not only what you say but how you say it. Shouting only leads to confusion. A harsh voice may make others uncooperative or reluctant to accept your help. The tone of your voice may be the key that allows you to provide proper care.

People who are not trained to deal with emergencies often use phrases such as, "Don't worry, everything is all right" when dealing with the sick and injured. As an EMT, you must discipline yourself to avoid these types of statements. A patient knows that everything is not all right. An inappropriate statement, even if said in an effort to show concern, will not gain confidence or cooperation.

Learning to use appropriate, calm, neutral conversation is part of becoming a professional EMT. Conversation can help a patient relax, especially if you are calm and honest. Telling the patient that you are trained in emergency care, that you are there to help, and what you are planning to do inspires confidence.

As you can see, good patient care requires more than merely applying the correct treatment procedures. The best EMTs are capable of doing the right thing for the patient in a caring, dignified, and humane manner. Model EMTs believe that patients are people first.

THE EMT AND THE LAW

When it comes to the law, a textbook can only offer you general guidelines. Each state has its own laws that govern emergency care provided by the nonphysician. This text covers some of the basics, using layperson's terms, but the legal advisors for your EMS System will have to provide you with the specifics that apply in your state. The information presented here is not intended as legal advice. When you are in doubt about the law and how it applies to your duties as an EMT, seek the advice of an attorney familiar with the EMS System in your state.

Most individuals involved in providing emergency care are concerned with the legal aspects of care. Occasionally, they are concerned with being sued. No one will tell you to think lightly of this issue. You can be sued; however, you will probably be able to defend yourself if you have provided proper care to the level of your training, within the laws of your state. You can be sued and held liable for many different acts, including (but not limited to)

- Not providing care—Whether you are a paid EMT or a volunteer who is voluntarily responding to a call, you have a duty to the patient to provide care to your level of training.
- Rendering improper care when what was needed should have been obvious to a trained EMT.
- Abusing or mistreating a patient—This includes assault (e.g., threatening to physically hurt someone), battery (e.g., touching someone who does not wish to be touched), or violating the patient's civil rights (e.g., denying care because of the patient's national origin).
- Providing care above the level of your certification—You cannot be sued for this unless there is resulting harm to the patient, but it is cause for decertification in most states.
- Causing injury or mental anguish or allowing a correctable condition to worsen and cause damage.
- Forcing care on a competent adult who has refused your care—This may result in a charge of battery.
- Abandoning a patient before the completion of care or before being relieved by someone of equal or higher training.
- Irresponsible or reckless driving or violating other laws that apply to emergency driving.

There are other activities that can lead to your being sued. Your instructor can inform you of recent problems in your own state. Keep in mind that the laws have been written to help you carry out your duties and provide emergency care. If you know the law and you act professionally, you should have little to worry about in terms of successful lawsuits. Your worry should not be so great that it prevents you from caring for sick and injured patients.

Note: Learn to protect yourself by keeping accurate, detailed records on the prehospital care reports, sometimes called "run sheets," provided by your EMS System.

Duty to Act

Laws vary from state to state as to the responsibility an individual has to attempt to help someone in an emergency, known as the **duty to act**. As an EMT, more is expected of you than of the general public, but these expectations may only apply to you when you are on duty. In your state you may be required to respond and to provide care. Usually, these laws have been written to take into consideration the level of your training and your emergency care skills. The safety of the rescuer may also be considered. Your instructor can inform you of the laws concerning the duty to act that apply to your locality. In most cases, if an agency is given the responsibility to provide care, and you are an EMT in that agency, you will have a responsibility to provide care at emergencies, perhaps even when off duty.

If you have a duty to act and fail to do so, you can be held liable.

Negligence

To the layperson, **negligence** means that something that should have been done was not done or was done incorrectly. The legal concept of negligence in emergency care is not this simple. A finding of negligence requires that ALL of the following circumstances be proved.

- The EMT had a duty to the patient (duty to act).
- The EMT did not provide the standard of care (breach of duty). This may include the **failure to act**, that is, not providing needed care as would be expected of an EMT in your locality. Failure to act is the major cause of legal actions against EMS systems or EMTs.
- The actions of the EMT in not providing the

standard of care caused harm to the patient. This harm can be physical or psychological.

Negligence is the basis for a large number of lawsuits involving prehospital emergency care. If the above circumstances are proved, the EMT may be required to pay damages if the harm to the patient is considered by the court to be a loss that requires reimbursement (compensable). The negligent EMT may be required to pay for medical expenses, lost wages (possibly including future earnings), pain and suffering, and various other factors as determined by the court.

The Standard of Care

Each state has a **standard of care** that must be observed. This is the minimum acceptable care based on sources such as state laws and judicial decisions, administrative orders, local protocols and locally accepted guidelines published by emergency care organizations and societies, and what has been found to be acceptable in the past (precedent). This standard of care allows you to be judged based on what is expected of someone with your training and experience acting in the same or a similar situation.

A textbook does not set the standard of care. Your course is based on the guidelines originally proposed by the DOT and other authorities who have studied what training, skills, and equipment are required for an EMT to provide the standard of care at the EMT level. You will be trained so you can provide this standard of care. Training and continuing education are your best ways to ensure that you will be able to provide the standard of care required in your state.

Abandonment

Once you begin to help someone having a medical emergency or someone who is injured, you have legally initiated care. Leaving this patient before completing care or transferring care to someone who has less training, constitutes **abandonment** of the patient, and you may be subject to legal action for negligence. This concept exists to ensure that required care is completed and to avoid situations in which someone else does not stop to provide care, thinking that you are taking responsibility for the patient and will stay with him.

Some states view as abandonment a situation in which you leave a medical facility after bringing in a patient but have failed to turn over the information you had about the patient's problem and the care you provided. There are also states where abandonment may apply if you do not respond to a call or fail to complete a run. Abandonment may even apply if equipment failure or your own health prevents you from completing a response and you do not immediately report this failure.

Serious problems can occur when you decide that a patient does not need emergency care or transport. This may be viewed as abandonment if later it is shown that the patient did require care or transport. Do not make these decisions lightly. Interview all potential patients at the scene and conduct proper examinations. When in doubt, call the emergency department physician for assistance in care and transport decision making; otherwise, transport all patients.

Patient Rights—Consent

Note: Your state has specific laws as to when you can and cannot provide care. You must follow your local protocols (the accepted standard of care as defined by the local medical community). The following sections on consent are provided to inform you of some of the problems that exist in regard to consent and some of the solutions to these problems that have been created in various EMS Systems.

Adults who are mentally and physically able to make judgments are assumed to be competent and cannot be forced by the EMT to accept emergency care. Adults, when conscious and mentally competent, have the RIGHT TO REFUSE CARE.* This must be *informed* refusal, given after the person knows that assessment and care are recommended by a trained professional, the EMT (see *informed consent* in the next section). The reasons for refusal may be based on any number of things, including religious beliefs or a lack of trust. In some cases, you may believe their reasoning to be senseless. For whatever reasons, a competent adult can refuse care. You may not treat such patients, nor may you restrain them.

The law recognizes *implied* refusal of care. If a patient pulls away from you, holds up a hand in a "universal" gesture to signal you to stop, or shakes his head to indicate "no," then you have received refusal for care. The sign of refusal

---

* Persons who are intoxicated, under the influence of drugs, or suicidal are not considered to be able to make a rational decision concerning care. At times, it may be very difficult to determine if a patient belongs in one of these categories. Some states have laws that give the medical provider a margin of error in such decisions (e.g., an index of suspicion).

should be reasonably clear to the average individual, legally termed a "reasonable person."

If the patient is fearful or lacks confidence in your abilities, conversation may help you gain trust and approval for care. Do not argue with a patient, particularly if his reasons are based on religious belief. To do so will add stress that may intensify the patient's problem.

When a patient refuses your care, you should document this with the patient's signature on a **release form**. In such cases, be certain to inform the patient of what may be wrong with him, what you think should be done, and why you believe such actions are necessary. Ask the patient to confirm that he has understood what you have told him. In rare cases a patient may refuse your care and also refuse to sign the form. You will have to rely on eyewitnesses to verify that the patient has refused care. This information should also appear on the release form or incident report.

In all cases of refusal of care, have a witness to your offer of care, your explanations, the refusal, and the signing of any forms. Obtain the signatures and addresses of the witnesses, making certain that they have documentation to prove their identity.

Note: Law enforcement officers make excellent witnesses to the refusal of care.

Report any refusal of care to the dispatcher, immediately. Be certain to fill out all necessary forms, including a description of the patient's problem, his condition, the number of times you asked for the patient's consent, how you stated this request for consent, and how the patient refused care (when possible, quote the patient's exact words).

Parents or legal guardians can refuse to let you treat their child. Once again, if fear or lack of confidence is the apparent reason, try to explain the situation to them using simple conversation. Do not try to make the adult feel guilty of wrongdoing, particularly if religious reasons are the basis for the decision. Obtain the necessary signatures and identifications. In some states you must immediately report any case in which a parent or legal guardian refuses emergency care for a minor. These states have special laws governing the welfare of children. The information you provide may be passed on quickly to the courts so that care may be ordered or to find out if the child received proper care or is still in need of care.

Actual Consent An adult patient, when conscious and mentally competent, can give you **actual consent** to provide care. Oral consent is considered to be valid; however, a signed consent form provides you with more protection. Unfortunately, written consent is not practical for most emergency situations.

This consent must be **informed consent**. Most of the laws dealing with informed consent were created to cover surgical procedures being performed by physicians. These laws required that the physician must make known the risk of treatment and nontreatment and the alternatives to this treatment. These requirements cannot be applied in an emergency situation. At best, you may only be able to tell the patient who you are, the level of your training, and what you are going to do.

Actual consent for the adult patient can be **voluntary consent** as stated above, or it can be **involuntary consent**, as would occur with a court order.

The laws on *actual consent for a minor*, as well as the definition of a minor, vary widely from state to state. Usually, a parent, guardian, or a close adult relative (when the parents cannot be reached) can give you actual consent to care for the child. When this is done, actual consent exists, even if the child does not wish to be treated. In certain situations, the minor may be able to give you consent or refuse care. For example, a married minor is considered "emancipated" and may give you actual consent in your state. The same may hold true for a pregnant minor. In some states the minor who claims to be the victim of child abuse may be able to give you voluntary actual consent. You MUST follow the guidelines established in your state.

Involuntary consent for a minor may be issued by court order, a law enforcement officer who has taken custody of the minor, or a child welfare officer (in some states). A law enforcement officer may be able to place the minor in protective custody. This would make the minor a ward of the court and would allow for the officer to grant consent.

Implied Consent In cases in which a person is unconscious or for some other reason unable to give actual consent, and you believe a life-threatening illness or injury exists, the law assumes that the patient, if able to do so, would want to receive treatment. This is known as **implied consent**. Typically, the law requires an emergency in which there is a significant risk of death, but it also may recognize situations in which there is the possibility of the patient developing serious problems or a disability if care is not rendered immediately.

The law assumes that the parents or guardians would want care to be provided for their child. When they cannot be reached, and the child has a life-threatening condition, implied consent may be used to allow for care to begin.

The same may hold true in your state for patients who are mentally ill, emotionally disturbed, or developmentally disabled (e.g., mentally retarded) who have a life-threatening problem. If this is not the case in your state and if the patient will not or cannot give voluntary actual consent, you may have to seek involuntary consent. Since the EMT is not able to determine if a patient has any of these disorders, it is wise, when time allows, to seek advice from your medical director or emergency department physician and have a law enforcement officer place the patient in protective custody or seek a court order to begin care.

Patient Rights—Confidentiality

Many jurisdictions have yet to write specific laws about the confidentiality due a patient receiving emergency care from an EMT. Laws do exist that prevent the intentional invasion of a person's privacy. These may be applied to cases involving emergency care. In many states, the deliberate invasion of a patient's privacy by an EMT may lead to the loss of certification and could lead to legal actions being taken.

Individuals in emergency care usually feel very strongly about protecting the patient's right to privacy. You must not provide care for a patient and then speak to the press, your family, friends, or other members of the public about the details of the care. If you speak of the emergency, you must not relate specifics about what a patient may have said, who he was or was with, anything unusual about his behavior, or any descriptions of personal appearance. The same holds true if you receive this information from another member of the EMS System. Confidentiality applies not only to cases of physical injury, but also to cases involving possible infectious diseases, illnesses, and emotional and psychological emergencies.

Immunities

Each state has its own laws regarding the **immunity** granted to those who provide emergency care. Such laws spell out when you are exempt from legal liability in cases in which you rendered care or were unable to render care. It is your responsibility to know the laws for your state. Note, too, that there is also governmental immunity provided to some government and military agencies.

Good Samaritan laws have been developed in most states to provide immunity to individuals trying to help people in emergencies. Most of these laws will grant immunity from liability if the rescuer acts in good faith to provide care to the level of his training, to the best of his ability. These laws do not prevent someone from initiating a lawsuit, nor will they protect the rescuer from being found liable for acts of gross negligence and other violations of the law. These laws are strongly tied to the standard of care laws.

You must familiarize yourself with the laws that govern your state. Good Samaritan laws may not apply to EMTs in your locality. In some states, the Good Samaritan laws only apply to volunteers. If you are a paid EMT, different laws and regulations may apply.

Some states have specific EMT statutes that authorize, regulate, and protect EMTs (also the physicians and other health care professionals who give instructions to these individuals by radio or telephone). To be protected by such laws, you must be recognized as an EMT in the state where care has been provided. Some states have specific licensing and certification requirements that must be met and that obligate the holder to the standard of care recognized in the state.

Other Legal Aspects

Responsibility for Possessions Some care procedures require you to remove articles of the patient's clothing and jewelry. When you do, you are legally responsible for these articles. Record what articles were removed from the patient and safeguard them until you transfer the patient at the medical facility. At such time, hand the possessions over to the emergency department staff and receive a signed receipt for the articles.

Records and Reporting Requirements The information you gather when assessing and monitoring a patient is to be written down on the prehospital care report. This form will become part of the patient's medical records. It is a legal document that must be complete and accurate.

There are situations that may require you to file a special report with the medical facility, the police, or a government agency. This varies from state to state. You may be required to report child abuse, rape, assault, drug-related injuries, injury received during the commission of a crime, gunshot wounds, attempted suicide, communicable diseases, or animal bites. The failure to make such reports carries legal penalties in some states.

Legal Implications in Special Patient Situations There are special patients and special care situations in which specific laws may apply. Some of these are described below.

- **Mentally Disturbed Patients**—Care is usually provided under the laws of implied consent. If the patient is violent and likely to hurt himself or others, then restraint may be necessary. The law does not expect an EMT to risk personal safety to care for any patient. Typically, local laws will not allow an EMT to apply restraints unless ordered to do so by a physician or by the police. In some cases, a court order may be required. The restraints must be applied so as not to harm the patient (police handcuffs may injure a person who is violent—wide strips of cloth or leather are usually recommended). Once restraints are in place, they must be kept in place until the patient is handed over to more highly trained personnel at a medical facility. See Chapter 21 for more information concerning these patients.
- **Alcohol and Substance Abuse Patients**—You must, when possible, carry out a complete patient assessment and provide needed care for patients who are under the influence of alcohol or drugs or who have been injured while under such influence. Since medical practice views both alcohol and drug abuse as illnesses and not crimes, you should know if your state requires you to report cases of alcohol and drug abuse to legal authorities. See Chapter 16 for more information on the care of these patients.
- **Attempted Suicides**—Specific care for patients who have attempted suicide is covered in Chapter 21. You are not required to endanger yourself to reach and care for patients attempting suicide (unless your agency spells out such a responsibility). If you believe an injury or poisoning was due to an attempted suicide, your state may require you to report your suspicions to the emergency department staff or the police.
- **Crime-Related Cases**—If you have any reason to believe that the patient is the victim of a crime or was injured during the commission of a crime, then you may be required to report this suspicion to the police. This may hold true for possible cases of assault, rape, child abuse or neglect, gunshot wounds, knife wounds,

and any other suspicious wound or injury. Your best course of action is to report to the emergency department staff and/or the police any cases in which you believe a possible crime is related to the patient's problem. EMT actions at the crime scene will be covered in Chapter 21.

- **Animal Bites**—Such cases are usually required to be reported to the hospital personnel or to the police. If the animal is dead, you should protect the carcass so that it can be examined by medical authorities. If the live animal is at the scene, you should protect yourself first, then the patient and bystanders. Do not try to capture the animal unless you are specifically trained to do so and such action is part of your duties.
- **Care for the Deceased**—In most states, an EMT does not have the authority to pronounce a patient dead. Therefore, unless local protocols direct otherwise, you must provide basic life support measures even if you believe that the patient is deceased. (In cold water drowning, for example, the patient may be successfully resuscitated an hour or more after he has stopped breathing.) There are cases of obvious death, as when a person is decapitated, his body is severed, or he is virtually cremated. It is recommended, and may be legally required, that you do not move such bodies so as not to hinder possible police investigations.

  In some states, you can contact the coroner or medical examiner and receive permission to declare a patient dead. There are even localities that allow EMTs to independently declare death. You will have to follow your local guidelines on these matters.
- **Resuscitation of the Terminally Ill**—A major problem may exist when terminally ill patients are being cared for at home. The patient may have requested and the physician may have ordered that no resuscitative measures be taken when the patient's lungs and heart cease to function (so-called DNR, or "Do Not Resuscitate," orders). Originally, this approach was designed to allow specific physician's orders to be on file at the patient's hospital or nursing home. Obtaining legal proof of this request and order may prove to be a difficult task, forcing you to initiate CPR as you would for any patient. Unless proof can be obtained and relayed to you immediately, resuscitative measures have to be initiated. Many states have implemented DNR programs that help to solve this

problem by having terminally ill patients formally register their DNR orders. Such registrations let the EMTs know that they are not to initiate resuscitative procedures. If available in your area, an effective hospice program for the terminally ill, with instructions on resuscitation understood by all parties, will also greatly alleviate this problem.

Malpractice Insurance Having adequate malpractice insurance does not reduce your chances of being sued. The purpose of the insurance is to reduce your financial risk when providing care. Even though you believe that you will be the best EMT you can be, the unforeseen can occur. You cannot be certain how the courts will view your actions. Too many laws concerning emergency care are still in question.

As an EMT, you may be able to obtain malpractice insurance through a program offered to members of various EMT societies and organizations, from your own insurance company (most are highly selective if they offer such a service), or from your EMS System or employer. Legal advice as to how much coverage for each patient incident is desirable should be sought.

EQUIPMENT

This section provides just an overview of the kinds of equipment used by EMTs. Your instructor will introduce the equipment he or she thinks is important for you to know about this early in your course.

The Ambulance

An ambulance is a vehicle for emergency care that provides an operator's compartment and a patient compartment that usually can accommodate two EMTs and two litter patients. At least one of these patients must be able to be positioned so that intensive life-support measures can be provided during transport. The vehicle must be able to carry, at the same time, the equipment and supplies needed to provide optimum EMT-level emergency care at the scene and during transport. Equipment for light rescue procedures is recommended. Two-way radio communication with dispatch should be provided.

A good ambulance must be designed and constructed to provide maximum safety and comfort to patients and EMTs. A well-designed ambulance will also prevent aggravation of the patient's condition and exposure to any factors

that may complicate the patient's condition or threaten his survival.

According to federal specifications for emergency care vehicles (KKK-A-1822C) there are three types of ambulances. These are shown and described in Figure 1-18. The vehicle that meets these specifications is identified by "the Star of Life." The word "AMBULANCE" should appear in mirror image on the front so that the drivers of other vehicles can identify the unit as seen in

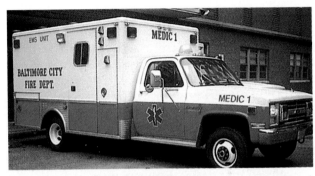

Figure 1-18a A type-I ambulance has a conventional cab and chassis, on which is mounted a modular ambulance body. There is no passageway between the operator's and patient compartments.

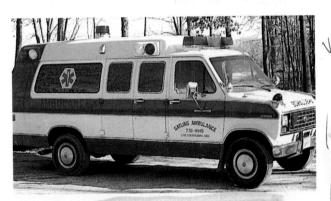

Figure 1-18b A type-II ambulance is commonly called a van-type ambulance. The body and cab form an integral unit, and most models have a raised roof.

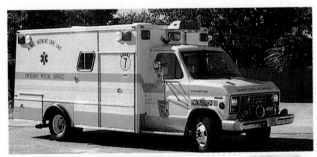

Figure 1-18c A type-III ambulance is commonly called a specialty van ambulance. It has a forward cab and an integral body that is generally larger than that of a type-II ambulance. There is a walk-through compartment.

CHAPTER 1 The Emergency Medical Technician

their rear-view mirrors. The vehicle is to have warning lights, including flashing roof lights in the upper corners of the vehicle body (this often varies according to local laws and regulations).

Because of infection control procedures, ambulances in which there is access between the operator's compartment and the patient compartment are no longer recommended.

Equipment and Supplies

Federal specifications were set when federal funding was used in the purchasing of EMS System supplies. However, most ambulances and supplies are now purchased without federal funding. For this reason, the lists of equipment and supplies are presented as those items that should be carried and not those items that must be carried. Many systems base their equipment list on recommendations made in the American College of Surgeons' Essential Equipment List. Your instructor will be able to tell you what is considered mandatory for your area.

The equipment and supplies carried (Figure 1-19) may be categorized as follows:

- Basic Supplies—those items carried to protect the patient (linens, pillows, blankets), to provide for patient needs (emesis bags, tissues, bedpans, towels), and to monitor the patient (stethoscope, penlight, and blood pressure measuring devices)
- Equipment for Patient Transfer—including wheeled stretchers, folding stretchers, stair chairs, and scoop-style stretchers
- Equipment for Ventilation and Resuscitation—including oropharyngeal airways, artificial ventilation devices, fixed and portable oxygen delivery systems, fixed and portable suction equipment, and spine or CPR boards for chest compression
- Supplies for Immobilizing Extremity and Spinal Fractures—including lower extremity traction splints, padded board splints for upper and lower extremities, air-inflatable splints (where required), rigid collars, spine boards, and triangular bandages for slings and swathes
- Supplies for Wound Care—including sterile gauze pads, sterile universal or multi-trauma dressings, self-adhering roller bandages, sterile nonporous occlusive dressings, and sterile burn sheets, as well as adhesive tape, safety pins, and bandage shears

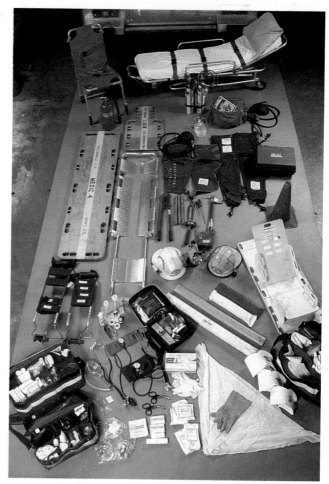

Figure 1-19 The well-equipped ambulance.

- Supplies for Care of Shock—anti-shock garments, where local protocols recommend their use
- Supplies for Childbirth—a sterile childbirth (OB) kit, including all necessary gloves, towels, baby blankets, bags, sanitary napkins, gauze pads, surgical scissors, cord tape or clamps, and rubber bulb syringes
- Supplies for Poisonings and Substance Abuse—including activated charcoal, drinking water, and syrup of ipecac (where local protocols recommend its use; may be for advanced personnel use in some areas)
- Intermediate-level Care Supplies—mainly for the treatment of shock, including intravenous agents, sterile intravenous administration kits, and esophageal obturator airways (EOAs)
- Physician and Paramedic Supplies (when carried)—including endotracheal intubation kits, pleural decompression kits, drug administration kits, monitor/defibrillator

(may also be for intermediate personnel in some areas), and a surgical kit (for some units).

- Equipment for Gaining Access and Disentanglement—including hand tools, power tools, and required rope, blocks, wedges, chains, and straps
- Equipment for Safeguarding Ambulance Personnel—including disposable gloves, gowns, caps, masks, work gloves, safety goggles, helmets, reflective protective gear, and raingear
- Equipment for Warning and Signaling—including flares, battery-powered hand lights, and floodlights
- Equipment to Extinguish Fires—including the fire extinguishers required by local ordinance
- Communications Equipment—including fixed and portable two-way radios

Remember that an EMT must be able to do more than carry out emergency care procedures. Gaining access, disentanglement and extrication, moving patients, and transferring patients are all part of the duties rendered.

INFECTION CONTROL AND THE EMT

As an EMT you will come into close contact with a wide variety of people, some of whom may be carrying infectious or communicable diseases. While these two terms are often interchanged, they do not mean exactly the same thing. An **infectious disease** is one that is caused by an organism entering the body. A **communicable disease** is one that can be passed from one person to another. Some diseases, such as tuberculosis, are both infectious and communicable. Some, such as tetanus, are infectious but not communicable.

As an EMT working in the prehospital setting, you need to be concerned with preventing the spread of communicable diseases to yourself and others. Practices aimed at these ends are called infection control.

You will be learning more about infection control procedures as you go through this book and your EMT course, but the following is an introduction to this topic.

The Need for Infection Control

Only a few years ago, infection control was basically limited to washing hands and sterilizing equipment between patients. However, the epidemic spread of HIV (human immunodeficiency virus), the virus that causes AIDS (acquired immune deficiency syndrome) has brought infection control concerns to the forefront. All EMTs must understand the variety of communicable diseases they may come in contact with, as well as the things that must be done to prevent acquiring each type of infection.

Although there are many infectious diseases, three that are of particular concern are hepatitis, tuberculosis, and HIV/AIDS.

- **Hepatitis** is an infection that causes an inflammation of the liver. Hepatitis comes in at least four forms: A, B, C, and non-A/non-B. Once infected, a person remains infected for life. The disease is acquired through contact with blood, stool, or other body fluids. The virus that causes hepatitis is especially hardy. Hepatitis B has been found to live up to seven days in dried blood spills, so it poses a risk of transmission long after many other viruses would have died. For this reason, it is critical that any body fluid in any form, dried or otherwise, should be assumed to be infectious until proven otherwise. Hepatitis can be deadly. Hepatitis B (HBV) kills approximately 200 health care workers every year in the United States—more than any other infectious disease.
- **Tuberculosis** (TB) is an infection of the lungs that can be fatal. It was thought to be largely eradicated, but since the late 1980s it has been making a steady comeback. TB is highly contagious. Unlike many other infectious diseases, TB can be spread easily through the air. Health care workers and others can become infected even without any direct contact with a carrier of TB. Compounding the problem is that some new strains of TB are proving to be resistant to the drugs previously used to combat this disease. Because TB can be so easily spread in forms that are untreatable, EMTs need to assume that any person with a cough may have TB and to be aware that certain locations, such as shelters for the homeless, often have a high incidence of TB.
- **AIDS** is the name for a set of conditions that result when the immune system (the body's infection-fighting system) has been rendered unable to combat infections adequately. Referring to AIDS as a disease is technically inaccurate since the term refers

to a whole range of illnesses the body is vulnerable to when the immune system begins to fail as a result of HIV infection. For simplicity, however, we often think of AIDS as a disease and refer to it as such.

AIDS has captured the attention of the news media and the public as a "deadly epidemic" because it is always fatal (no cure for AIDS has been discovered at the time of publication of this text). In reality it presents far less risk to health care workers than hepatitis and TB. This is because HIV, the virus that causes AIDS, does not survive well outside the human body. This limits the routes of exposure to those that involve direct exposure to blood: intravenous drug use, unprotected sexual contact, or blood transfusions. Puncture wounds into which HIV is introduced, such as with an accidental needle stick, have been shown to be extremely poor methods of infection; less than half of one percent of such incidents result in infection, according to the U.S. Occupational Safety and Health Administration (OSHA), compared to 30 percent for

HBV. The difference is due to the quantity and strength of HBV compared to HIV.

Table 1-1 lists common communicable diseases, their modes of transmission, and their incubation periods (the time between infection and first appearance of symptoms). EMTs faced with patients who have or are suspected of having any of these diseases need to understand how they are transmitted (Figure 1-20) in order to understand how to isolate themselves from infection. In addition, knowing the incubation period of a disease will assist the EMT in determining whether a patient presents a risk of disease transmission and will also help an EMT who has developed disease symptoms to trace their possible cause.

Preventing Infection

The chief method of infection control is the use of *barriers* to transmission of **pathogens** (the organisms that cause infection). *Human skin is a particularly effective barrier when it is intact (not broken).* Infectious pathogens will not cross intact

TABLE 1-1 Communicable Diseases

Disease	Mode of Transmission	Incubation Period
Acquired immune deficiency syndrome (AIDS)	Sexual contact, blood or body fluids from someone with AIDS or carrying the virus, drug abusers sharing needles with someone who has or is carrying the virus, infected mothers passing the virus to their unborn children	Unknown
Chickenpox (varicella)	Direct contact. Note: moist crusts are infectious	14 to 16 days
Diphtheria	Person to person by respiratory droplets, or indirectly from contaminated objects	2 to 5 days
German measles (rubella)	Airborne droplets	14 to 21 days
Infectious hepatitis	Contact with objects contaminated by person's feces (including their hands), blood or body fluids	25 to 30 days
Measles (rubeola)	Airborne droplets and secretions from the mouth, nose, and eyes	10 to 12 days
Meningitis (bacterial)	Oral and nasal secretions	2 to 10 days
Mumps	Droplets of saliva or objects contaminated by saliva	14 to 21 days
Pneumonia (bacterial and viral)	Droplets and secretions from mouth and nose	Several days
Scarlet fever (scarlatina)	Nose and throat secretions; pus from ears	Several days
Staphylococcal skin infections	Direct contact with sore, its discharge, or contaminated objects	Several days
Syphilis	Venereal contact; saliva, semen, vaginal discharge, and blood can carry the organism into open cuts	10 days to several months
Tuberculosis (TB)	Respiratory secretions, contaminated objects, organisms on patient's hands	4 to 6 weeks
Typhoid fever	Feces, urine, and contaminated objects	7 to 21 days
Whooping cough (pertussis)	Respiratory secretions and airborne droplets	5 to 21 days

METHODS OF TRANSMISSION

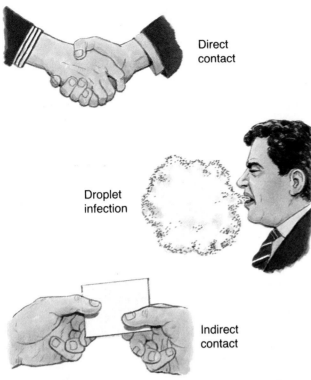

Direct contact

Droplet infection

Indirect contact

Figure 1-20 How communicable diseases may be transmitted.

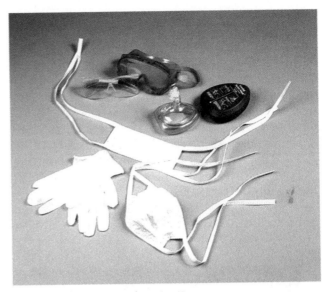

Figure 1-21 Personal protection.

skin; however, they will enter through cuts and will cross mucus membranes quite easily.

To prevent pathogens from entering the body, the EMT should use barrier protection such as disposable gloves, masks, eyewear, and gowns (Figure 1-21). This does not mean that an EMT needs to wear all of these items on every call, but rather as appropriate. Generally, gloves will be all that is required; however, procedures such as suctioning may cause splashing, which would be a good reason to use more protection.

The EMT should also use extreme caution around sharp blood-covered objects such as knives and intravenous needles, as wounds made with these objects may provide a route of infection.

EMTs responding to emergencies should never have to perform direct mouth-to-mouth rescue breathing. Ample equipment is available on an ambulance to provide breaths for a patient through a pocket mask or other device designed to prevent cross infection (infection passing from you to the patient or from the patient to you). Many EMTs even carry rescue masks in their cars while off duty.

The oldest recognized method of infection

control, hand washing, is still an effective means of reducing or preventing cross-infection. The EMT should always wash between calls and before food preparation or consumption.

Finally, EMTs must realize that equipment and supplies that have been contaminated with body fluids must not be left either on the scene of an emergency, in the ambulance, or around the station. This may expose other people to infection. Responsible EMTs will ensure that contaminated equipment and supplies are properly decontaminated or disposed of in accordance with local protocols or operating procedures (see Chapter 28).

Infection Control and the Law

During the 1980s, scientists identified the main culprits in the transmission of deadly infectious diseases as blood and body fluids. EMTs and other health care workers were recognized as having a higher than usual exposure to blood and body fluids, and therefore a higher risk of contracting these unwanted infections. The federal government responded by taking several steps to ensure the safety of people who were in such high-risk positions.

Original guidelines issued by the Centers for Disease Control (CDC) identified a practice called **universal precautions** as the means that should be employed to prevent infection by bloodborne pathogens such as HBV and HIV. Under the universal precautions concept, the blood and *certain* body fluids of all patients were to be considered potentially infectious and precautions taken to protect against them.

As part of more recent efforts, CDC in 1989 issued a document titled "Guidelines for Prevention of Transmission of Human Immunodeficiency Virus and Hepatitis B Virus to Health Care and Public Safety Workers." This report set the standard that in emergency situations, *all* body fluids should be considered potentially infectious. This means that emergency workers must practice a stricter form of infection control called **body substance isolation**.

The primary infection control methods recommended as universal precautions and for body substance isolation are

- Use of personal protective equipment and clothing (gloves, masks, eyewear, gowns)
- Taking care with contaminated sharps (needles, knives, broken glass)
- Use of masks and/or ventilation bags for rescue breathing
- Hand washing
- Proper decontamination of surfaces, equipment, and clothing

On March 6, 1992, the U.S. Occupational Safety and Health Administration (OSHA) regulation on bloodborne pathogens became effective and was summarized in a booklet titled "Occupational Exposure to Bloodborne Pathogens: Precautions for Emergency Responders."

The OSHA regulation sets forth certain standards to protect employees who are likely to be exposed to blood and other body fluids. One of the basic principles behind the regulation is that infection control is a joint responsibility between employer and employee. The employer must provide training, protective equipment, and vaccinations to employees who are subject to exposure in their jobs. In return, employees must participate in an infection exposure control plan that includes training and proper workplace practices. Without the active participation of both the employer and the employee, any workplace infection control program is destined to fail. Your responsibility as an EMT is to be sure that your system has an active and up-to-date infection exposure control plan and that you and your fellow EMTs follow it carefully at all times.

CHAPTER REVIEW

KEY TERMS

You may find it helpful to review the following terms.

abandonment—to leave an injured or ill patient before the responsibility for care is properly transferred to someone of equal or superior training. Leaving the hospital without giving essential patient information to the staff is viewed by some courts as a form of abandonment.

actual consent—consent given by the rational adult patient, usually in oral form, accepting emergency care. This must be informed consent.

AIDS—acquired immune deficiency syndrome; a set of conditions that result from infection by HIV (human immunodeficiency virus). AIDS is fatal.

body substance isolation—a form of infection control that assumes that all body fluids should be considered potentially infectious.

communicable disease—a disease that can be passed from one person to another.

duty to act—the legal responsibility to provide emergency care. Typically a local law identifies which agencies have this responsibility. If an EMT is a member of such an agency, he or she has a legal responsibility to render emergency care while on duty.

emergency care—at the EMT level this is usually the prehospital assessment and treatment of the sick or injured patient. This care is initiated at the emergency scene and is continued through transport and transfer to a medical facility.

Emergency Medical Services (EMS) system—the complete chain of human and physical resources that provides patient care in cases of sudden illness or injury.

Emergency Medical Technician (EMT)—a professional-level provider of emergency care. This individual has received formal training and is appropriately certified. An EMT can be a paid career or a volunteer professional.

failure to act—not providing needed care as would be expected in your locality.

Good Samaritan laws—a series of laws, varying in each state, designed to provide limited legal protection for citizens and some health care personnel when they are administering emergency care.

hepatitis—an infection that causes inflammation of the liver, communicated through blood, stool, and other body fluids, even when dried. Hepatitis can be fatal.

HIV—human immunodeficiency virus. See *AIDS*.

immunity—in the law, exemption from legal liability.

implied consent—a legal concept that assumes an unconscious patient (or one so badly injured or ill that he cannot respond) would consent to receiving emergency care if he or she could do so. In some states, implied consent may apply to children when parents or guardians are not at the scene, to the developmentally disabled (e.g., mentally retarded), and to the mentally or emotionally disturbed.

infectious disease—a disease caused by an organism entering the body.

informed consent—agreement by a rational adult patient to accept emergency care, after having been informed of what you believe the patient's condition to be and what you plan to do. In many cases, informed consent does not exist unless the patient also knows the risks and the alternatives.

involuntary consent—consent for care obtained by court order when the adult patient or the child patient's parent or guardian refuses care.

negligence—at the EMT level this is the failure to provide the expected care at the standard of care, leading to the injury or death of the patient.

pathogens—the organisms that cause infection.

patient—the victim of an accident or illness who has entered the EMS system or other professional medical care.

release form—a document signed by a patient or witnesses indicating that the patient has refused care.

standard of care—the minimum acceptable level of emergency care to be provided.

tuberculosis (TB)—an infection of the lungs communicable through skin contact and through the air. TB can be fatal.

universal precautions—a form of infection control that assumes that blood and certain body fluids of all patients are potentially infectious.

victim—a person who has had an accident or has suddenly become ill. (See also *patient*.)

voluntary consent—consent for care given by an adult patient or by a child patient's parent or guardian of his or her own accord.

SUMMARY

The Emergency Medical Services System

The Emergency Medical Services System is a chain of human and physical resources established to provide complete emergency care. As an EMT your duties are performed as part of an emergency care delivery subsystem that includes EMTs, ambulances, and equipment and supplies.

The Emergency Medical Technician

The Emergency Medical Technician is trained and certified or licensed to provide professional emergency care at the scene and during transport to a medical facility. The first concern of the EMT is personal safety.

To provide proper care, the EMT must carry out nine main duties. These duties include

1. Preparing to respond,
2. Responding,
3. Making certain that the scene is safe,
4. Gaining access to the patient,
5. Finding out what is wrong with the patient and providing emergency care,
6. Freeing and moving the patient,
7. Transferring the patient to the ambulance,
8. Transporting and handing over the patient and patient information, and
9. Terminating activities by returning to quarters and preparing for the next run.

As an EMT, you are a health care professional, required to be pleasant, sincere, cooperative, resourceful, emotionally stable, and of good moral character. You must have leadership abilities and be a self-starter. You must be concerned with your personal appearance, your personal habits, and your conversation at the scene. All these traits help you to develop the calm, professional manner needed to provide proper emergency care.

The EMT and the Law

Laws regarding your responsibility, or duty to act, vary from state to state. Negligence means that something that should have been done was not done. Each state has a standard of care, or minimum accepted care. This means that your performance will be judged based on what is expected of someone with your training and experience.

When you begin to care for a patient, you have the responsibility to continue care until you are relieved by equally or more highly trained personnel or until you have transferred the patient and patient information to the staff of a medical facility. If you start care and then stop, or if you leave the scene, you may be charged with abandonment.

Some patients can refuse your care. You must have actual consent from a conscious, clear-thinking adult patient. It must be informed consent, with the patient knowing your level of training and what you are planning to do.

Actual consent may be voluntary or involuntary. A court order or the order of a law enforcement officer may be needed to assume involuntary consent.

There are cases in some states in which a minor can give actual consent (e.g., married minor). Usually, if voluntary consent is given it must come from a parent, legal guardian, or close adult relative (only when parents or guardians cannot be contacted). Involuntary consent requires a court order, an order from a law enforcement officer, or orders from a child welfare officer (in some states).

In cases in which the patient is unable to give consent, and has life-threatening problems, you may care for the patient under the doctrine of implied consent.

In some localities, implied consent also may apply to children, to the mentally disturbed, and to developmentally disabled patients when their parents or legal guardians are not present.

Patients have a right to privacy. EMTs must respect and protect patient confidentiality.

In most states, specific laws have been written to allow you to provide emergency care. Good Samaritan laws may provide you with limited immunity from civil liability. You may be protected if you act in good faith, providing the EMT standard of care, to your level of training and to the best of your abilities.

You are legally responsible for possessions you remove from the patient. The standard forms on which you record information are legal documents. In certain states you may be required to file special reports for child abuse, rape, assault, drug- or crime-related injuries gunshot wounds, attempted suicide, communicable diseases, or animal bites

Special laws or local protocols may apply to the care of certain patients. For example, you must continue to provide basic life support even when you believe a person to be deceased until an authorized person pronounces the patient dead. You must follow state laws or local protocols with regard to terminally ill patients who have requested that no resuscitation measures be taken. Malpractice insurance may help to reduce your financial risk if you are sued.

Equipment

The ambulance includes a patient compartment with emergency care equipment. A wide variety of equipment and supplies can be carried on the ambulance.

Infection Control and the EMT

EMTs must be concerned with preventing the spread of communicable diseases. Of the many communicable diseases, three are of special concern: hepatitis, a potentially fatal liver infection acquired through contact with blood, stool, and other body fluids; tuberculosis (TB), a highly contagious and potentially fatal liver infection spread through direct contact or through the air; and acquired immune deficiency syndrome (AIDS), a set of conditions that result from failure of the body's immune system, caused by the human immunodeficiency virus (HIV) that is acquired through direct exposure to body fluids, primarily blood. AIDS is not highly contagious but, once acquired, is eventually fatal.

Barriers to infection are the chief method of infection control. Intact skin is an effective barrier, but pathogens (infectious organisms) will pass through mucus membranes and cuts. Use of protective clothing such as disposable gloves, masks, eyewear, and gowns is recommended.

Guidelines for universal precautions and body substance isolation have been issued by the Centers for Disease Control. This means that the blood and all body fluids of all persons should be regarded as potentially infectious. The primary methods for guarding against infection are

1. Use of protective equipment and clothing,
2. Taking care with contaminated sharps,
3. Use of masks and/or ventilation bags for rescue breathing,
4. Hand washing, and
5. Proper decontamination of surfaces, equipment, and clothing.

The U.S. Occupational Safety and Health Administration (OSHA) has issued regulations for occupations in which exposure to infection is likely. These regulations require employers and employees to work together to develop and follow an exposure control plan designed to protect employees and the public from infection.

CHAPTER 2

On the Scene

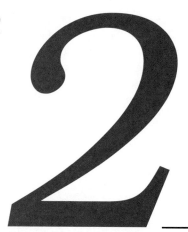

You are called to a street near a school playground. You arrive to find 10-year-old Janey lying in the street. She is crying and appears to be in pain. You notice that her left thigh appears oddly bent.

You: Hi, I'm Ken from the ambulance. What's your name?

Janey: (through tears) Janey.

You: Okay, Janey, we're going to take real good care of you. I want you to lie still while we see where you're hurt. I'll make sure someone calls your parents. Tell me what happened.

Janey: I ran into the street to get my ball and a car hit me.

You: Can you tell me where you hurt?

Janey: My leg hurts. And my belly hurts.

You: Can you point to where it hurts? (She does.)

At the hospital you report to the triage nurse: "Janey was struck by a car. It does not appear as if she lost consciousness. She complains of pain in her left upper quadrant which radiates to her shoulder, and she has a possible left midshaft femur fracture. Her last vital signs were . . ."

Why did you use terms like "left upper quadrant"? Couldn't you just have said "She has a pain in her belly"? In this chapter you will learn the importance of knowing the human body and being able to use correct terminology to describe the body so that you can communicate clearly and accurately with other medical professionals.

The Human Body

As an EMT you will usually arrive at the emergency scene to find a fully dressed patient who may complain of pain in, or may have an obvious injury to, some part of his or her body. You can't see through the patient's clothes, and even if the clothes are removed, you can't see through the skin. So how do you know what organs or structures inside the body may be malfunctioning or injured?

This is where study of the human body—anatomy and physiology—comes in. You must learn to visualize where the organs and structures of the body are and what functions of the body may be affected by illnesses and injuries. You also need to learn to use professional medical terminology to describe the body and its functions.

In this chapter you will be introduced to the anatomy and physiology of the human body at a level that will help you to function effectively as an EMT.

Expected Outcome, Chapter 2: *You will be able to name, locate, and describe (using correct terminology) the major organs, structures, and systems of the human body.*

THE STUDY OF ANATOMY AND PHYSIOLOGY

THE LANGUAGE OF ANATOMY AND PHYSIOLOGY
     Directional Terms
     Anatomical Postures
     Directions of Movement

AN INTRODUCTION TO ANATOMY
     Body Regions
     The Spine
     Body Cavities
     Abdominal Quadrants
     Locating Body Structures

AN INTRODUCTION TO PHYSIOLOGY
     Body Systems

Objectives

Knowledge *After reading this chapter, you should be able to*

1. Describe the anatomical position. (p. 33)
2. Define and apply the terms *anterior, posterior, superior, inferior, midline, medial, lateral, proximal, distal, patient's left,* and *patient's right.* (pp. 33-34)
3. Identify FOUR anatomical postures. (p. 34)
4. Correctly use SEVEN terms that relate to direction of movement. (pp. 34-35)
5. List the FIVE major regions of the body and the subdivisions of each region. (pp. 35-36)
6. Label the FIVE divisions of the spine. (pp. 36-37)
7. Name and locate the FOUR major body cavities. (pp. 37)
8. Name and identify the FOUR abdominal quadrants. (pp. 37-38)
9. Locate, on your own body, the position of the diaphragm, heart, lungs, stomach, liver, spleen, pancreas, gallbladder, small intestine, large intestine, kidneys, and urinary bladder. (Scan 2-1; pp. 42-45)
10. Name the body systems and describe their functions. (p. 45)

Skills *As an EMT you should be able to*

1. Apply the knowledge gained in this chapter so that you can look at a patient's body and mentally determine the positions of the major organs of the chest and abdomen.
2. Use correct terminology when communicating with other members of the patient care team.

Two terms appear early and often in an EMT training program. They are **anatomy** and **physiology**. Anatomy is the study of body structure, while physiology is the study of body function. As an EMT you will have to know the major body structures and systems and how these parts function. You will need a working knowledge of the body in order to determine the nature of the patient's illness or injury (the patient assessment) and to provide the appropriate care.

THE STUDY OF ANATOMY AND PHYSIOLOGY

You won't—and can't—learn all about human anatomy and human physiology in a basic EMT course. Nursing students average 180 classroom hours of study in anatomy and physiology: more than you will have for your entire EMT course. However you will learn enough to understand and be able to perform EMT assessment and care. You will also gain a good foundation for further study, your EMT continuing education.

This chapter is just a start. It does not contain all the anatomy and physiology that is in this textbook or in the EMT course; it does provide some basic information. Later chapters contain more information on anatomy and physiology as it relates to the assessment and care of specific injuries and medical problems.

At the end of this book is a reference section containing Anatomy and Physiology Plates that illustrate the major body systems and an Atlas of Injuries that illustrates major types of body injuries. As with any reference sources, these are not intended to be studied and learned all at once but rather to be referred to as learning aids throughout the course.

As you begin learning anatomy and physiology, first learn to visualize where organs and structures are located as you view a person who is fully clothed, since this is the way you will find most patients. Then learn landmarks of the unclothed body that will help you locate organs and structures within the body. Keep in mind that the patient's problem may be internal, but all you will be able to see is the external body.

THE LANGUAGE OF ANATOMY AND PHYSIOLOGY

You must learn to use correct medical terminology, the language of your profession, so that you can communicate accurately with other emergency and medical personnel and in your written reports. In this chapter we will introduce some basic medical terminology. If you want to learn more, "Medical Terminology" in the reference section at the end of this book defines and explains many medical terms and also contains a section on formation of medical terms. The Glossary is useful if you need to look up the meaning of a term you hear or read.

Directional Terms

The following is a set of basic terms to use when referring to the human body (Figure 2-1):

- **Anatomical** (AN-a-TOM-i-kal) **Position**—Consider the human body, standing erect, facing you. The arms are down at the sides *with the palms of the hands facing forward.* Unless otherwise indicated, all references to body structures are made when the body is in the anatomical position. This is very important when considering anatomical structures.
- **Right** and **Left**—As you face the patient, his left is on your right. When you assess the patient and note or report your findings, always make reference to the *patient's* right and *patient's* left.
- **Anterior** and **Posterior**—*Anterior* means the front and *posterior* means the back of the body. For the head, the face and top are considered anterior while all of the remaining structures are posterior. The rest of the body can be easily divided into anterior and posterior by following the side seams of your clothing.

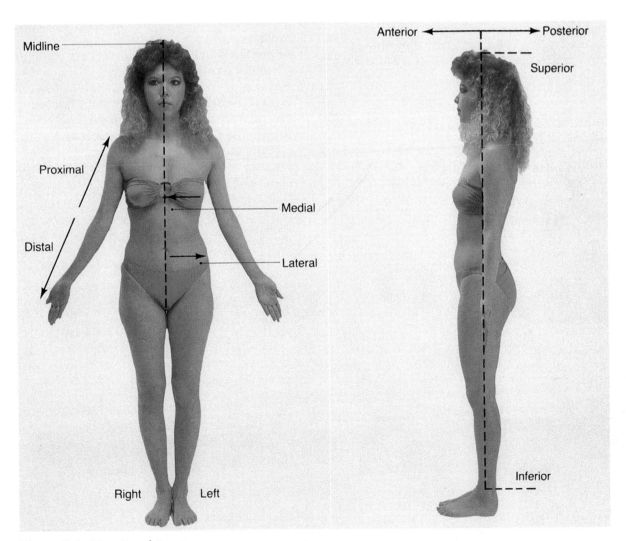

Figure 2-1 Directional terms.

- **Midline**—This is an imaginary vertical line that divides the body into right and left halves. Anything toward the midline is said to be **medial**, while anything away from the midline is said to be **lateral**. Remember the anatomical position, with the thumb on the lateral side of the hand and the little finger on the medial side of the hand.
- **Superior** and **Inferior**—*Superior* means toward the top or toward the head, as in *The eyes are superior to the nose. Inferior* means toward the bottom or toward the feet, as in *The mouth is inferior to the nose.* (**NOTE:** You cannot correctly say something is superior or inferior unless you are comparing it with another structure or location. For example, the heart is not superior by itself, it is superior to the stomach.)
- **Proximal** and **Distal**—*Proximal* means closer to a point of reference, *distal* means farther away from a point of reference. These terms are used primarily for the upper and lower extremities, with the shoulder and the hip as the points of reference. The knee is proximal when compared with the ankle. The fingernails are on the distal ends of the fingers.

Anatomical Postures

Terms for anatomical postures (Figure 2-2) are used frequently in communications between EMTs and the hospital emergency department to describe the patient's position, either the position he is already in or the position in which he has been or will be placed. The anatomical postures are

- **Erect**—the upright position
- **Supine**—lying on the back, face up
- **Prone**—lying on the stomach, face down
- **Lateral Recumbent**—lying on the side (*lateral* means "side," *recumbent* means "lying down"), specifically *right lateral recumbent* (on the right side) or *left lateral recumbent* (on the left side)

Directions of Movement

Terms used to describe directions of movement (Figure 2-3) are

- **Abduction**—movement away from the midline of the body. (One way to remember this is to recall that *abduction* is also used to mean "kidnapping," or carrying someone *away*.)
- **Adduction**—movement toward the midline. (Think of ADDing to the body.)
- **Rotation**—turning or twisting on an axis. A **lateral rotation** of the leg twists the leg so that the foot is turned outward, away from the midline. A **medial rotation** turns the foot inward, toward the midline.
- **Flexion**—the act of bending, usually a joint such as a knee or elbow

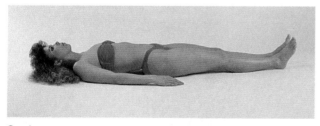

Supine

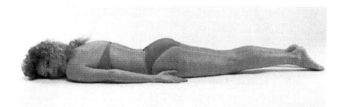

Prone

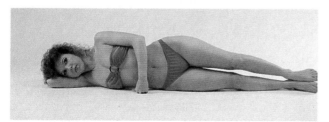

Right lateral recumbent

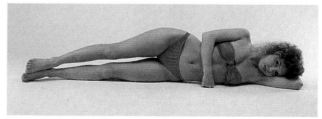

Left lateral recumbent

Figure 2-2 Anatomical postures.

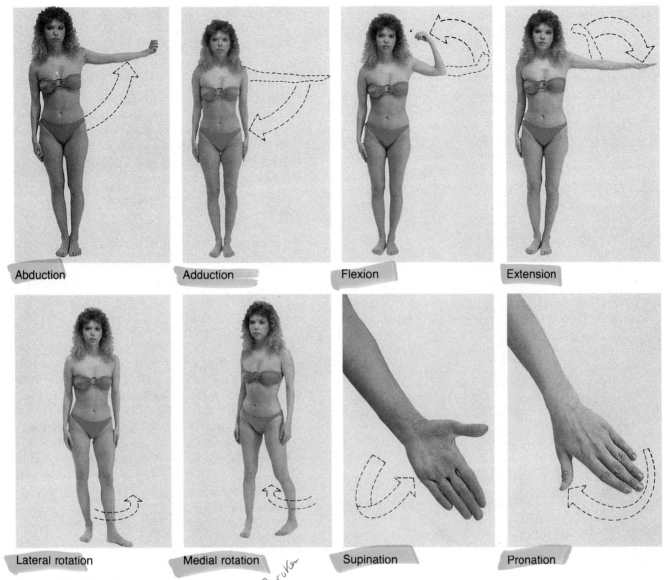

Abduction	Adduction	Flexion	Extension
Lateral rotation	Medial rotation	Supination	Pronation

Figure 2-3 Directions of movement.

- **Extension**—the act of straightening, usually a joint such as a knee or elbow
- **Supination**—related to the term *supine* (above). A supination of the forearm is a rotation into the anatomical position so that the back of the hand is down, the palm facing up.
- **Pronation**—related to the term *prone* (above). A pronation of the forearm turns the palm down.

AN INTRODUCTION TO ANATOMY

When beginning to study anatomy, it is important not only to know what the organs and structures of the body are but also to get a sense of where they are located within the body. The following segments on body regions, the spine, body cavities, abdominal quadrants, and locating body structures will help you begin to develop this "organizational" sense of the body.

Body Regions

The human body can be divided into five regions (Figure 2-4): (1) the head, (2) neck, (3) trunk, (4) upper extremities (shoulders to tips of fingers), and (5) lower extremities (pelvis and hips to tips of toes). Later in this text you will study specific areas within each of these regions. We will start with the simplest subdivisions.

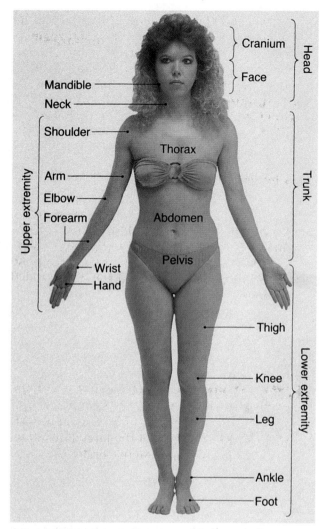

Figure 2-4 Body regions.

- Pelvis—formed and protected by the bones of the pelvic girdle (the pelvic bones are part of the lower extremities)

Upper Extremities (as found on each side)

- Shoulder girdle and joint—composed of the scapula (SKAP-u-lah, shoulder blade) posteriorly, the clavicle (KLAV-i-kul, collarbone) anteriorly, and the joint formed by the head of the humerus (HU-mer-us, arm bone) and the scapula
- Arm—sometimes referred to as the upper arm
- Elbow
- Forearm—sometimes referred to as the lower arm
- Wrist
- Hand
- Fingers

Lower Extremities

- Pelvic girdle and joint—composed of the fused bones of the pelvis and lower spine and the joint made with the femur (FE-mur, thigh bone)
- Thigh—from the hip to the knee. Sometimes it is referred to as the upper leg.
- Knee
- Leg—also called the lower leg or shin and calf
- Ankle
- Foot
- Toes

Head

- Cranium (KRAY-ne-um)—housing the brain. Many people use the term *skull* for *cranium*. (The skull includes cranium and face.)
- Face
- Mandible (MAN-di-b'l)—the lower jaw, considered separately because its joints allow for movement

Neck

Trunk—from the neck to the groin (anteriorly) and the buttocks (posteriorly); also called the torso

- Thorax (THO-raks)—the chest
- Abdomen—extending from the lower ribs to the pelvis

The Spine

The spine is divided into five regions (Figure 2-5).

- **Cervical** (SER-ve-kal) **Spine**—the section of the spine in the neck.
- **Thoracic** (tho-RAS-ik) **Spine**—the section of the spine in the upper back. The ribs attach to the bones (vertebrae) of the thoracic spine.
- **Lumbar** (LUM-bar) **Spine**—the section of the spine in the midback.
- **Sacrum** (SA-krum)—the section of the spine in the lower back.
- **Coccyx** (KOK-six)—the inferior end of the spine. Some laypersons call this the tailbone.

These divisions can be used as points of reference to locate other structures and injuries.

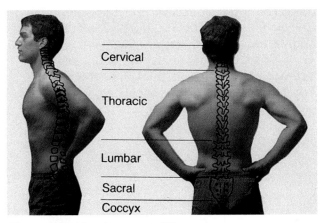

Figure 2-5 The divisions of the spine.

A puncture wound to the back just above the waist would be reported as a wound to the lumbar region of the back. In Chapter 12 you will study the spinal column in detail.

Body Cavities

There are four major body cavities, two anterior and two posterior (Figure 2-6). Housed in these cavities are the vital organs, glands, blood vessels, and nerves.

Anterior Cavities The anterior body cavities are

- **Thoracic** (tho-RAS-ik) **Cavity**—the entire chest cavity, enclosed by the rib cage, protecting the lungs, heart, great blood vessels, part of the trachea (windpipe), and most of the esophagus (the tube connecting the

throat and the stomach). The lower border of the thoracic cavity is the **diaphragm**, a dome-shaped muscle used in breathing. The diaphragm separates the thoracic cavity from the abdominopelvic cavity.

- **Abdominopelvic** (ab-DOM-i-no-PEL-vik) **Cavity**—the anterior body cavity below the diaphragm. There are two portions of the abdominopelvic cavity: abdominal and pelvic.

  Abdominal Cavity—extending between the diaphragm and the pelvis, containing all the abdominal organs, including the liver, stomach, gallbladder, pancreas, spleen, small intestine, and most of the large intestine. Most of the abdominal cavity, unlike the other body cavities, is not surrounded by bones. Only the upper portion of the cavity is protected by the lower ribs. If you consider all the organs in this cavity and the lack of bony protection, it is easy to see why blows to the abdomen are so potentially harmful.

  Pelvic Cavity—protects a portion of the lower anterior cavity with bones of the pelvic girdle. This cavity contains the urinary bladder, portions of the large intestine, and the internal reproductive organs.

Posterior Cavities The posterior body cavities are

- **Cranial Cavity**—This is the portion of the skull housing the brain and its specialized membranes.
- **Spinal Cavity**—This cavity runs through the center of the backbone, protecting the spinal cord and its specialized membranes.

Abdominal Quadrants

The abdomen is a large body region, and the abdominal cavity contains many vital organs. In other body regions, bones may be used for reference, such as counting the ribs or feeling a bump or notch on a bone. This is not the case when trying to be specific about references to the areas of the abdomen. The navel or **umbilicus** (um-BIL-i-kus) is the only quick point of reference available for the beginning student. To improve this situation, the abdominal wall is divided into four quadrants, called the **abdominal quadrants** (Figure 2-7) .

- **Right Upper Quadrant** (RUQ)—containing

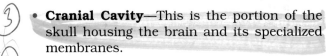

Figure 2-6 Body cavities.

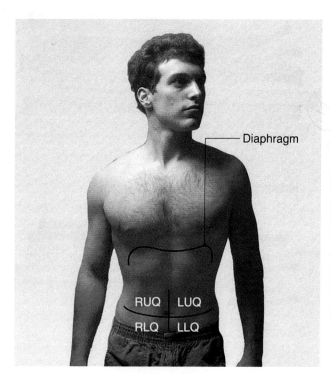

Figure 2-7 Abdominal quadrants.

most of the liver, the gallbladder, and part of the large intestine.
- **Left Upper Quadrant** (LUQ)—containing most of the stomach, the spleen, the pancreas, and part of the large intestine.
- **Right Lower Quadrant** (RLQ)—containing the appendix and part of the large intestine.
- **Left Lower Quadrant** (LLQ)—containing part of the large intestine.

Some organs and glands are located in more than one quadrant. As you can see from the previous list, the large intestine is found, in part, in all four quadrants. The same is true for the small intestine. Most of the stomach is in the left upper quadrant, but part of it can be found in the right upper quadrant. The bulk of the liver is found in the right upper quadrant; however, the left lobe of the liver extends into the left upper quadrant.

These quadrants also are used to help locate the pelvic organs. For example, the right ovary is located in the right lower quadrant and the left ovary is in the left lower quadrant. The uterus (womb) and the urinary bladder are assigned to both lower quadrants.

The kidneys are a special case. They are not within the abdominal cavity but located behind the cavity's membrane lining, the peritoneum (per-i-to-NE-um). Consider one kidney to be in

the right upper quadrant and the other to be in the left upper quadrant. However, do not let this abdominal classification make you forget that the kidneys are behind the abdominal cavity and subject to injury from blows to the mid-back. Any pain or ache in the back may be caused by problems with the kidneys.

The pancreas also is located behind the peritoneum (retroperitoneal); however, most general anatomy textbooks classify it along with the abdominal organs.

Locating Body Structures

Above, you learned four ways to locate body structures or the sites of injuries. You can refer to

- Body regions
- Divisions of the spine
- Body cavities
- Abdominal quadrants

Here we will discuss two additional ways to locate body structures.

- Visualizing—being able to picture organs and structures inside the body as you look at the external body (a kind of mental "x-ray vision")
- Topography—learning external landmarks: specific structures, notches, joints, and "bumps" on bones. Some are obvious (navel, nipples); some you know by other names but will have to learn the medical terms (Adam's apple = thyroid cartilage); and some will probably be new to you (xiphoid process). It is important to learn where internal organs and structures are in relation to these landmarks that you can easily see or feel from outside the body.

Scans 2-1, Major Body Organs, and 2-2, Topography and Skeleton, can help you begin to visualize and use body typography to locate body structures. You will also need to practice—by looking at other people, working with a partner, or looking at your own body in a mirror. Then, in the press of activities at an emergency scene, you will be able to locate and communicate about body organs, structures, or injuries swiftly, confidently, and accurately.

Here are some things to note as you study Scan 2-1 and Figures 2-8 to 2-13.

Major Body Organs

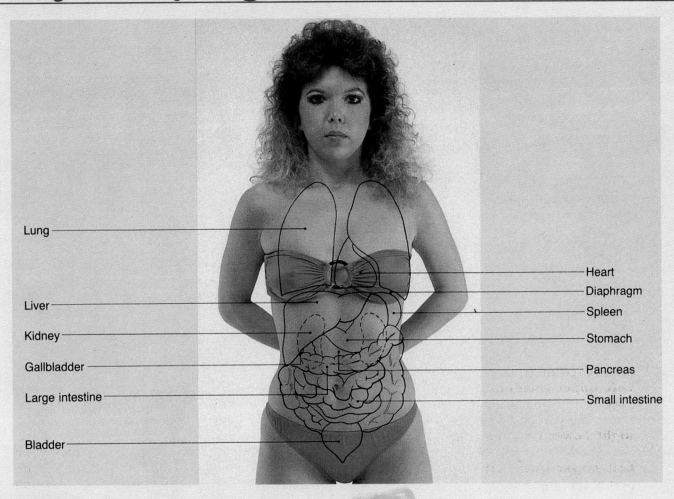

Lung — Heart
— Diaphragm
Liver — Spleen
Kidney — Stomach
Gallbladder — Pancreas
Large intestine — Small intestine
Bladder

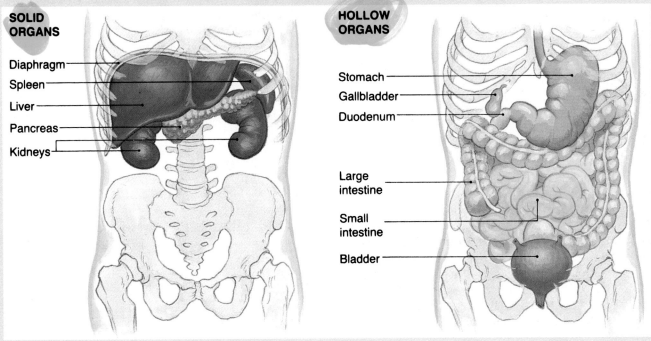

SOLID ORGANS

Diaphragm
Spleen
Liver
Pancreas
Kidneys

HOLLOW ORGANS

Stomach
Gallbladder
Duodenum

Large intestine

Small intestine

Bladder

39

Topography and Skeleton

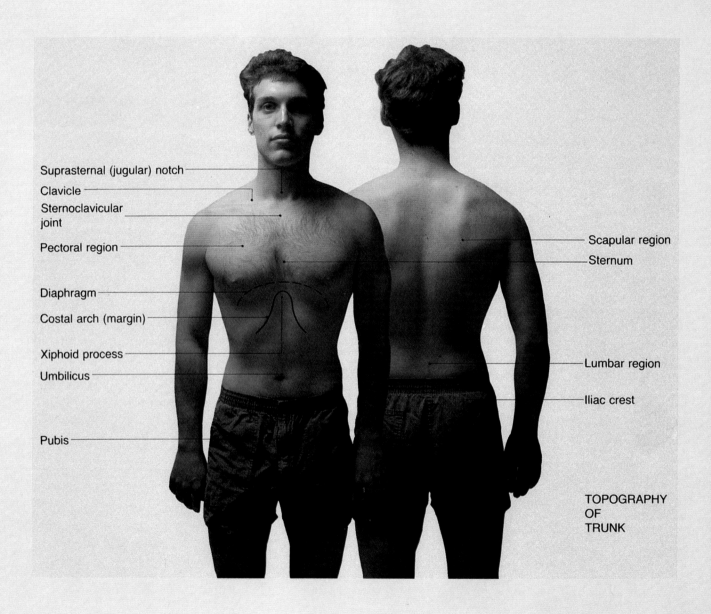

Suprasternal (jugular) notch

Clavicle

Sternoclavicular joint

Pectoral region

Diaphragm

Costal arch (margin)

Xiphoid process

Umbilicus

Pubis

Scapular region

Sternum

Lumbar region

Iliac crest

TOPOGRAPHY OF TRUNK

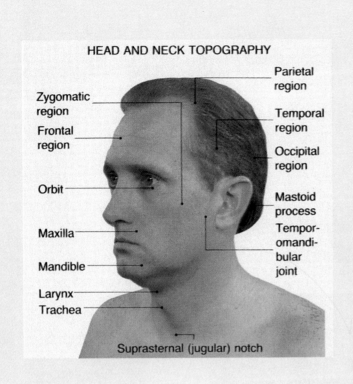

HEAD AND NECK TOPOGRAPHY

Parietal region

Zygomatic region

Temporal region

Frontal region

Occipital region

Orbit

Mastoid process

Maxilla

Temporomandibular joint

Mandible

Larynx

Trachea

Suprasternal (jugular) notch

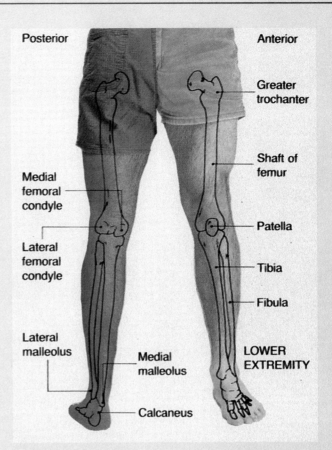

Posterior

Anterior

Greater trochanter

Shaft of femur

Medial femoral condyle

Lateral femoral condyle

Patella

Tibia

Fibula

Lateral malleolus

Medial malleolus

LOWER EXTREMITY

Calcaneus

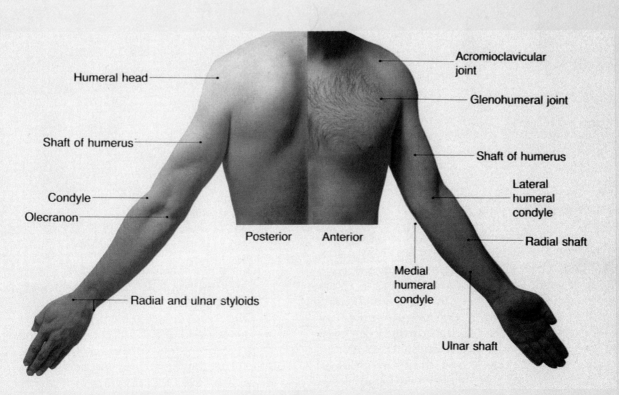

Humeral head

Acromioclavicular joint

Glenohumeral joint

Shaft of humerus

Shaft of humerus

Lateral humeral condyle

Condyle

Olecranon

Posterior   Anterior

Radial shaft

Medial humeral condyle

Radial and ulnar styloids

Ulnar shaft

41

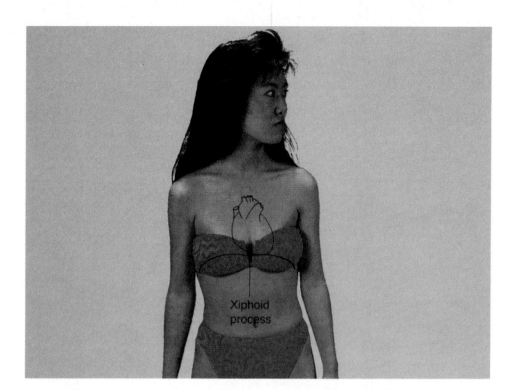

Figure 2-8 Position of the heart.

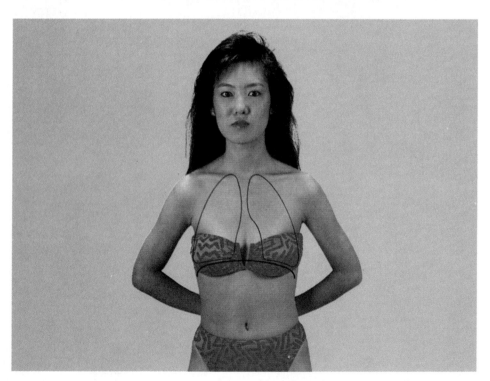

Figure 2-9 Position of the lungs.

- *The position of the heart in the thoracic cavity* (Figure 2-8)—As a quick point of reference, use your fingers to find a small hard spot at the inferior end of your sternum (breastbone). This is the **xiphoid** (ZI-foyd) **process**, a major body landmark. You can find a point directly over the heart by measuring two to three finger widths up from this point. Look at yourself in a mirror and find this point. Each time you look in the mirror during your training, try to visualize where your heart is located.

- *The position of the lungs in the thoracic cavity* (Figure 2-9)—Notice that the lungs do not extend downward as far as the bottom of the rib cage. The *diaphragm* forms the infe-

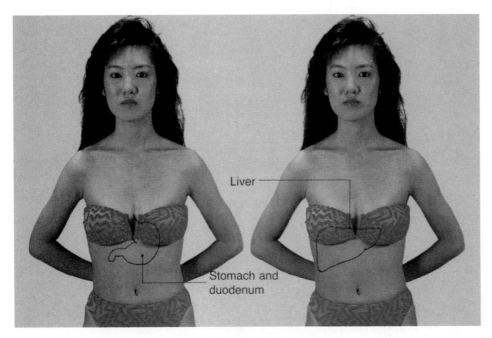

Figure 2-10 Position of the liver, stomach, and duodenum.

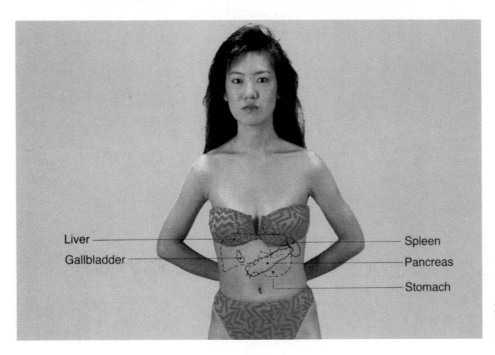

Figure 2-11 Position of the liver, gallbladder, spleen, pancreas, and stomach.

rior border of the lungs. By studying Scan 2-1, you will have a very good idea of the size, shape, and position of the lungs.

- *The positions of the organs in the abdominal cavity* (Figures 2-10 and 2-11)—Notice the positioning of the *stomach*, *liver*, and the first portion of the small intestine called the *duodenum* (du-o-DE-num). Before leaving this region of the abdomen, you can quickly learn the positions of three other structures close to the stomach and the liver. The *gallbladder* is below the liver, the *pancreas* is

behind the lower part of the stomach, and the *spleen* is lateral to the left side of the stomach. The point at which the *esophagus* enters the stomach, immediately after passing through the diaphragm, is at the level of the xiphoid process. Notice how the lower ribs partially protect the stomach, spleen, pancreas, duodenum, and liver.

Notice the space occupied by the *small intestine*. As you can see, most of the abdominal cavity is filled with this structure. The illustration shows the space occu-

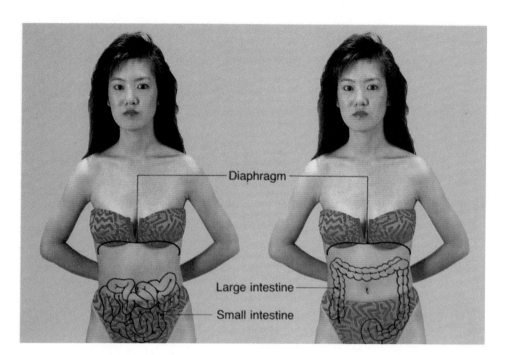

Figure 2-12 Position of the small and large intestine.

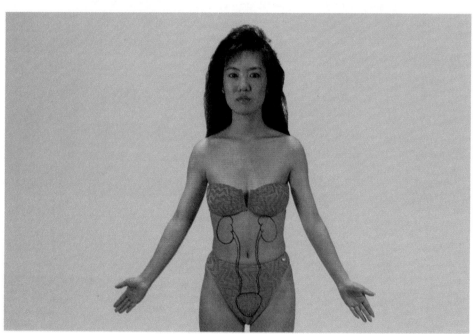

Figure 2-13 The urinary system.

pied by the *large intestine*. Note how it passes through each of the four abdominal quadrants (Figure 2-12).

As you study Scan 2-1, keep in mind that the abdomen is rich in blood vessels, nerves, and membranes. Punctures and blunt trauma can rupture blood vessels and hollow organs. Blood loss may quickly prove to be life threatening. The blood and body fluids released may cause the rapid inflammation of membranes and other body tissues, causing intense pain and adding to the patient's decline.

The duodenum is held in a more rigid position than the rest of the small intestine. Forceful blows to the abdomen, such as those often received in motor vehicle accidents, may damage the duodenum without causing any immediate significant damage to the rest of the intestine.

- *The positions of the kidneys and the urinary bladder* (Figure 2-13)—Remember that the kidneys are behind the abdominal cavity and the bladder is in the pelvic cavity.

AN INTRODUCTION TO PHYSIOLOGY

As mentioned earlier in this chapter, anatomy is the study of body structures, physiology the study of body functions. When you begin to learn about body systems (below), you are starting your study of physiology.

Body Systems

A body system is a group of organs that carry out specific functions. Learning as much as you can about the body systems and their functions will prove to be of great value when you begin to provide emergency care. Remembering the different body functions can be useful when trying to determine the extent of injury or the nature of a medical emergency. The following is a list of the major body systems and their primary functions.

- **Musculoskeletal System**—bones provide protection and support, and skeletal muscles act with the bones to permit body movement. Skeletal muscles are voluntary muscles. This means that we can consciously direct these muscles to contract and relax. (Not all the body's muscles are part of the musculoskeletal system. The heart is made of cardiac muscle that keeps the heart functioning automatically. The walls of organs are made up of smooth, involuntary muscles that contract and relax without our conscious control.)
- **Nervous System**—controls movement, interprets sensations, regulates and coordinates body activities, and generates memory and thought
- **Circulatory (Cardiovascular) System**—the heart and vessels that move blood, carrying oxygen and food to the body's cells and removing wastes and carbon dioxide from these cells
- **Respiratory System**—exchanges air to bring in oxygen and expel carbon dioxide. Oxygen is placed into the bloodstream as carbon dioxide is being removed to be expelled into the atmosphere.
- **Digestive System**—enables us to eat, digest, and absorb foods and provides for the removal of wastes
- **Urinary System**—involved in the removal of chemical wastes from the blood and helps balance water and salt levels of the blood
- **Reproductive System**—the structures of the body involved with sexual reproduction. Sometimes this is classified with the urinary system as the genitourinary (JEN-i-to-U-ri-nair-e) system.
- **Integumentary** (in-TEG-u-MEN-ta-re) **System**—the skin and its accessories (hair, oil glands, sweat glands, and nails). The skin is the body's largest organ. It is also often classified as a membrane. For more on membranes see "Integumentary System and Membranes" in the Anatomy and Physiology Plates at the end of this book.
- **Special Senses**—various organs that link with the nervous system to provide sight, hearing, taste, smell, and the sensations of pain, cold, heat, and tactile (touch) responses
- **Endocrine** (EN-do-krin) **System**—produces chemicals called hormones that help regulate most body activities and functions (e.g., growth)
- **Immune System**—a network of specialized cells found in the bloodstream, lymphatic system, liver, spleen, thyroid, and throughout the body's connective tissues. These cells function mainly to kill, or otherwise render harmless, microorganisms (germs).

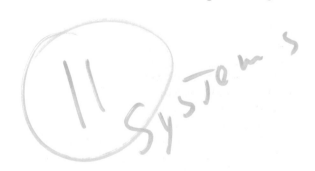

CHAPTER REVIEW

KEY TERMS

You may find it helpful to review the following terms.

abduction—movement away from the vertical midline of the body.

abdominal quadrants—the four zones of the abdominal wall, used for quick reference: the *right upper quadrant, left upper quadrant, right lower quadrant,* and *left lower quadrant.*

abdominopelvic (AB-dom-i-no-PEL-vik) **cavity**—the anterior cavity below the diaphragm, made up of the *abdominal cavity* and the *pelvic cavity.*

adduction—movement toward the vertical midline of the body.

anatomical position—the standard reference position for the body in the study of anatomy. The body is standing erect, facing the observer. The arms are down at the sides and the palms of the hands face forward.

anatomy—the study of body structure.

anterior—the front of the body or body part.

cervical (SER-ve-kal) **spine**—the section of the spine in the neck.

circulatory (cardiovascular) system—the system of heart and blood vessels that circulate blood throughout the body.

coccyx (KOK-siks)—the lower end of the spine. It is sometimes referred to by the layperson as the tailbone.

cranial (KRAY-ne-al) **cavity**—the area within the skull that houses the brain.

diaphragm (DI-ah-fram)—the dome-shaped muscle of respiration that separates the chest from the abdomen.

digestive (di-JES-tiv) **system**—the system of esophagus, stomach, and intestines that enables the taking in and digesting of food.

distal—away from a point of reference or attachment (e.g., the shoulder or hip joint); used as a comparison with *proximal.*

endocrine (EN-do-krin) **system**—the system that produces the hormones that regulate body functions.

erect—the upright position.

extension—to straighten a joint.

flexion—to bend a joint.

immune (im-YOON) **system**—the network of specialized cells that help prevent disease by killing germs or rendering them harmless.

inferior—away from the head; usually compared with another structure that is closer to the head (e.g., the lips are inferior when compared with the nose).

integumentary (in TEG-u-MEN-ta re) **system**—the skin and its accessories (hair, oil glands, sweat glands, nails).

lateral—to the side, away from the vertical midline of the body; used only in reference to another body part. Thus, there is a lateral side to the arm.

lateral recumbent—lying on the side.

lateral rotation—to turn the foot or hand outward away from the midline.

lumbar (LUM-bar) **spine**—the section of the spine in the midback.

medial—toward the vertical midline of the body; used only in reference to another body part. Thus, you can have a medial side to the arm.

medial rotation—to turn the foot or hand inward toward the midline.

midline—an imaginary line drawn down the center of the body, dividing it into right and left halves.

musculoskeletal (MUS-ku-lo-SKEL-e-tal) **system**—the system of bones and skeletal muscles that support and protect the body and permit movement.

nervous system—the system of brain, spinal cord, and nerves that govern sensation, movement, and thought.

physiology—the study of body function.

posterior—the back of the body or body part.

pronation—A rotation of the forearm so that the back of the hand is facing forward.

prone—lying face down.

reproductive system—the male and female organs involved in sexual reproduction.

respiratory (RES-pir-a-tor-e) **system**—the system of nose, mouth, throat, and lungs that brings oxygen into the body and expels carbon dioxide.

proximal—close to a point of reference or attachment (e.g., the shoulder or hip joint); used as a comparison with *distal.*

sacrum (SA-krum)—the section of the spine in the lower back.

senses—sight, hearing, taste, smell, and sensations of pain, cold, heat, and touch.

spinal cavity—the area within the spinal column that contains the spinal cord.

superior—toward the head; often used in reference with inferior.

supination—A rotation of the forearm so that the palm is facing forward.
supine—lying on the back.
thoracic (tho-RAS-ik) **cavity**—the anterior body cavity above the diaphragm, containing the heart and its great vessels, part of the trachea, and most of the esophagus.
thoracic (tho-RAS-ik) **spine**—the section of the spine in the upper back, to which the ribs attach.
umbilicus (um-BIL-i-kus)—the navel.
urinary (U-rin-air-e) **system**—the system of kidneys, bladder, and urethra that remove wastes from the blood and excrete them as urine.
xiphoid (ZI-foyd) **process**—the lower (inferior) extension of the sternum (breastbone).

SUMMARY

The Study of Anatomy and Physiology

It is important to know some basic anatomy (the study of body structure) and physiology (the study of body function) to work effectively as an EMT. You also must learn and use correct medical terminology.

The Language of Anatomy and Physiology

All references made to body structures consider the body to be in the anatomical position (facing you, arms at sides, palms forward). Always use *patient right* and *patient left*. Also remember that

- Anterior = front
- Posterior = back
- Medial = toward the midline
- Lateral = away from the midline
- Superior = top, higher, or toward the head
- Inferior = bottom, lower, or away from the head
- Proximal = closest to the point of origin or reference
- Distal = farthest from the point of origin or reference

The anatomical postures are

- Erect—standing
- Supine—on the back, face up
- Prone—on the stomach, face down
- Lateral Recumbent—on the side

Terms that describe directions of movement are

- Abduction—moving away
- Adduction—moving toward
- Flexion—bending
- Extension—straightening
- Supination—rotation of the forearm so the palm faces forward
- Pronation—rotation of the forearm so the back of the hand faces forward

An Introduction to Anatomy

Four ways to locate or organize body organs and structures are by

- Body regions—head (cranium, face, mandible), neck, trunk (thorax, abdomen, pelvis), upper extremities (shoulder, arm, elbow, forearm, wrist, hand, fingers), lower extremities (pelvis, thigh, knee, leg, ankle, foot, toes)
- Divisions of the spine—cervical, thoracic, lumbar, sacrum, coccyx
- Body cavities—anterior (thoracic, abdomino-pelvic), posterior (cranial, spinal)
- Abdominal quadrants—right upper, left upper, right lower, left lower

Visualizing internal organs and structures and using topographical landmarks are also useful ways of locating body organs and structures.

An Introduction to Physiology

There are major body systems, or groups of organs, that carry out specific body functions: musculoskeletal, nervous, circulatory (cardiovascular), respiratory, digestive, urinary, reproductive, integumentary (and membranes), special senses, endocrine, and immune.

Work with a partner or look in a mirror. Use Scans 2-1 and 2-2 and the Anatomy and Physiology Plates at the end of this book to practice locating organs and structures of the body. Practice using the correct directional terms and terms for body postures, body regions, spine divisions, body cavities, and abdominal quadrants to identify positions and locations.

On the Scene

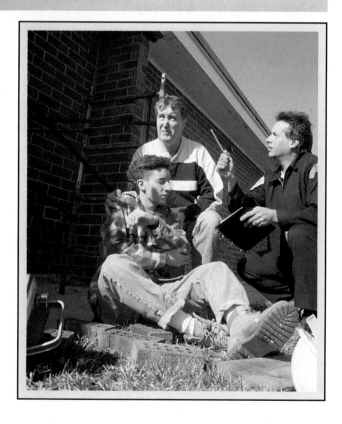

You: Can you tell me what happened, Mr. Stangle?

Mr. Stangle: I fell off that roof. (He points upward.)

You: OK, Mr. Stangle. Tell me where you hurt.

Mr. Stangle: My arm. I hit the ground pretty hard. I'm sure it's broken.

You: Is there any place else you hurt?

Mr. Stangle: No. My arm . . . What did you say? (Obviously getting confused.)

Your assessment of a patient begins as you arrive on the scene, before you even speak to the patient. What signs did the scene give you as to the probable severity of Bill Stangle's injuries? Mr. Stangle's arm does appear to be broken. Do the signs he exhibits lead you to suspect additional, more serious problems? Why?

Experienced EMTs often use the "look test." Mr. Stangle shows signs of shock (pale, gray and sweaty skin with rapid respirations). He looks bad. He is unable to concentrate. He exhibits signs of being in shock and of having injuries more serious than the obvious fractured arm. He has failed the "look test."

You categorize Bill Stangle's status as unstable, realizing that severe shock can lead to death within minutes. You decide to immobilize his spine, provide a high concentration of oxygen by a nonrebreather face mask, and to then transport him to the hospital at once, without completing a full assessment. You will provide additional treatment for shock en route.

Your EMS unit is dispatched to a construction site for a "fall." The patient, Bill Stangle, was working on the roof of a building when he lost his footing and fell to the ground. You arrive to find Mr. Stangle sitting on the ground holding his left elbow. He appears to be in great pain. As you approach Mr. Stangle, you notice that his skin is a pale gray color. He is sweaty and breathing rapidly. You introduce yourself and begin talking with him. As you listen, you notice that he has trouble concentrating.

Patient Assessment

Once you, the EMT, arrive at the emergency scene, the *victim* of injury or illness becomes your *patient*. What do you do for this patient—and in what order? There are two parts to your job: (1) patient assessment—gathering information so you can determine what is wrong with the patient—and (2) patient care—giving the patient emergency medical treatment.

This chapter is about the first part of your job: figuring out what is wrong.

Expected Outcome, Chapter 3: *You will be able to assess the scene for safety and the patient in order to determine appropriate care and transport priority.*

Warning: Protect yourself from infectious diseases by using appropriate barrier devices such as a pocket face mask with one-way valve, face shield, or bag-valve mask; goggles or other eye shield; and disposable gloves. Always conform to your local EMS system's infection exposure control plan.

Knowledge *After reading this chapter, you should be able to*

1. Describe the procedures involved in sizing up the situation when you are en route to and upon arrival at the emergency scene. (pp. 51-57)

2. Define *primary survey*, stating its purpose and indicating when it is done during the patient assessment. (pp. 50, 57)

3. State how you should identify yourself on arrival at the emergency scene. (p. 51)

4. List SIX quick sources of patient information. (p. 53)

5. Define *mechanism of injury* and relate types of accidents to types of injuries. (pp. 54-57)

6. Describe how to determine patient responsiveness. (p. 59)

7. Describe how to ensure an open airway and check a patient for adequate breathing. (pp. 60-61)

8. Describe how to detect a carotid pulse. (p. 61)

9. Indicate how you can assess a patient's level of consciousness. (pp. 57, 62, 68; Figure 3-19)

10. List the equipment an EMT should have to perform the primary and secondary surveys. (pp. 62-63, 63-64)

11. Define *status decision* and explain its purpose. (p. 63)

12. Define *secondary survey*, stating its purpose and when it is done during the patient assessment. (pp. 50, 63)

13. Define *subjective interview* and *objective examination*. (pp. 64, 67)

14. List the types of information that should be sought during your interviews of patients and bystanders. (pp. 64-66)

15. Define *sign, symptom,* and *vital sign.* (p. 67)

16. State the THREE rules you must consider

P atient assessment is the gathering of information needed to help determine what is wrong with the patient. The assessment that you, as an EMT, conduct in the field—that is, at the emergency scene and, perhaps, during transport—is known as a *field assessment.*

THE FIELD ASSESSMENT

Throughout the entire process of patient assessment, your goal is to **DO NO HARM**. *Your first responsibility is always to protect yourself,* then to protect the patient from additional injury and stress, as you gather the information needed to allow for proper and efficient care.

The field assessment is a *systematic* procedure; that is, there is a definite order of steps to follow. Later, you will learn circumstances in which the assessment steps may be varied; but first you should learn the basic sequence.

The Sequence of Patient Assessment

The first part of your job—that you can learn to accomplish en route to the scene and within a few seconds after arrival—is

• Sizing up the situation

Immediately after or even simultaneously with your size-up, you will begin the formal processes known as the primary survey and the secondary survey.

I. **The primary survey** is a rapid initial assessment to detect and treat life-threatening conditions that require immediate care, followed by a status decision about the patient's stability and priority for immediate transport to a medical facility.

II. **The secondary survey** is a complete and detailed assessment consisting of
   A. Subjective interview
   B. Objective examination
      1. Vital signs
      2. Head-to-Toe Survey

when conducting the patient examination. (pp. 67-68)

17. State the FOUR observations it is important to make during the objective examination. (p. 68)

18. Describe the procedures used by an EMT in the gathering of vital signs. (pp. 68-74)

19. List the head-to-toe survey steps in the correct order. (pp. 75-90)

20. List the ONE concern for yourself and the FOUR major concerns you have for the patient as you gather information. (p. 92)

21. List at least FIVE problems at the emergency scene that can complicate the information gathering process. (pp. 92-93)

Skills   *As an EMT you should be able to*

1. Determine level of consciousness.

2. Ensure an open airway.

3. Take a carotid pulse, radial pulse, and distal lower extremity pulse (both dorsalis pedis and posterior tibial) and determine rate, rhythm, and character of a radial pulse.

4. Determine respiratory rate and character.

5. Measure blood pressure by auscultation and palpation.

6. Determine relative skin temperature.

7. Gather information and conduct a primary survey and a secondary survey at an emergency scene.

8. Make a status decision on patient stability and transport priority.

9. Use a stethoscope to assess breathing sounds.

10. Record and communicate the information gained from the patient assessment.

11. Use the Glasgow Coma Scale (or other similar scales) if required in your EMS System.

This chapter provides considerable detail about assessment procedures. To keep from getting lost in the details, you may want to refer to the above outline from time to time to remind yourself where the details you are studying fit into the assessment sequence.

Think of this outline as a road map to the rest of the chapter.

Sizing Up the Situation

If you receive your calls from a properly trained emergency medical dispatcher, you may learn something of a person's illness or injury before leaving quarters. Even though this information may later prove to be erroneous, you can at least be thinking of what equipment you will have to remove from the ambulance and what special procedures may be required immediately on arrival.

Arrival at the Scene   When you arrive at the scene (Scan 3-1), be alert and begin to gath-

er information—first on scene safety, for your own protection, then on the patient or patients. Do not allow the dispatcher's report or information given to you by untrained bystanders to be the basis of a quick conclusion. You will have to consider many factors before you will know what is wrong with a patient and what course of emergency care you will take.

On arrival, you must

1. State your name (and rank or classification and the organization you represent).
2. Identify yourself as an Emergency Medical Technician (not everyone knows what "EMT" means).
3. Ask the patient if you may help.

While doing the above, remember to be looking for any obvious life-threatening problems.

Identifying yourself is very important, even if you believe the patient is unconscious. If you are in uniform, most patients and bystanders

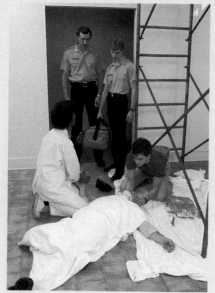

1. Stay alert.

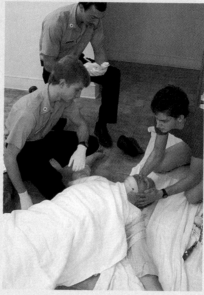

2. Identify yourself and ask to help.

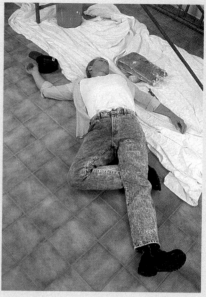

3. Quickly look for mechanisms of injury.

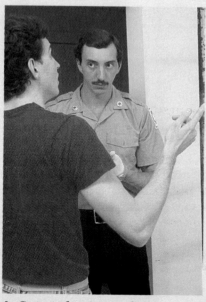

4. Gain information from patient and bystanders.

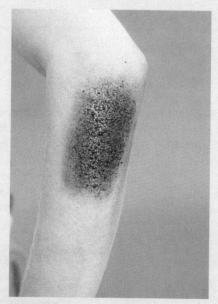

5. Note minor injuries.

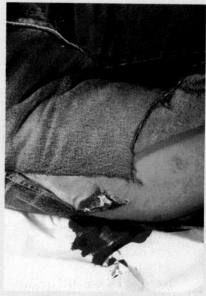

6. Note major injuries.

will respond to the uniform and let you take charge. When out of uniform, identifying yourself may be the only way you will be allowed to provide care. State your name and the name of your organization, and then the following: "I am an Emergency Medical Technician. I have been trained to provide emergency care."

Even if you believe the patient to be unconscious, your next words should be, "May I help you?" Keep in mind that some patients who appear to be unconscious may respond to your voice. Many patients maintain a functional sense of hearing, even when near death.

Surprisingly, some patients will say "no" to your offer of help. Usually, their fear is so great that they are confused. Simple conversation works best in gaining confidence. Even if the patient says "no" to your offer of help, continue to talk to him quietly, offering reassurance. His first refusal may be due to an initial lack of trust, denial that anything is wrong, confusion, or fear. In the vast majority of cases, the patient will allow you to help.

Quick Sources of Information In a few seconds, you can gain valuable information as to what may be wrong with a patient. Observe and listen as you quickly, but safely, reach the patient as soon as possible. You must not delay the detection of life-threatening problems. At this point you are doing a *quick* assessment and must rely on clues that are obvious or quickly provided to you by others. Some immediate sources of information may come from the following:

- The Scene—Is it safe or hazardous? Does the patient have to be moved? Is the weather harsh? Are there crowds to control? More than one patient may indicate the presence of a hazardous substance such as carbon monoxide.
- The Patient—Is he conscious, trying to tell you something, or pointing to a part of his body?
- Bystanders—Are they trying to tell you something? Listen. They might be saying, "He's had a bad heart for years," "He was having chest pains before he fell," "He fell off that ladder," "He is lying on a live wire."
- Mechanisms of Injury—Has something fallen on the patient? Was there a fire? Has the patient been thrown against the steering column? Is the steering wheel bent, the dashboard dented, or does the windshield have a spider web crack from the patient's

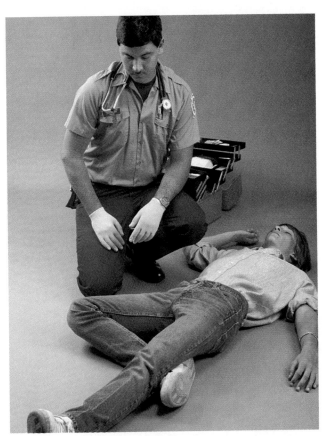

Figure 3-1 Obvious deformities and injuries may provide clues as to the extent of a patient's problem.

head? Did another patient die in the same vehicle?

- Deformities or Injuries—Does the patient's body appear to be lying in a strange position? Is there blood around the patient? Are there burns, crushed limbs, or any other obvious wounds (Figure 3-1)?
- Signs—What do you quickly see, hear, or smell when approaching the patient? Is there blood around the patient? Has he vomited? Is the patient having convulsions? Is there obvious pain? Are his clothes torn?

You must be highly observant as you approach the patient. What you see before you even touch the patient may indicate that there are life-threatening problems or that the patient's condition will probably worsen rapidly. At the scene of a motor vehicle collision, these observations are part of what is sometimes called the "windshield survey," that is, what you see walking up to and looking into the vehicle (Figure 3-2). These early observations can be critical factors in how you initiate care.

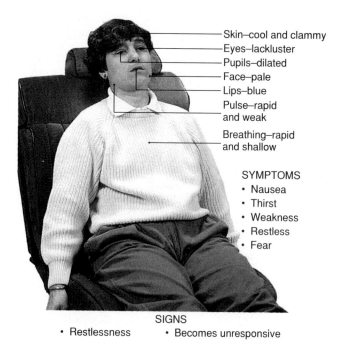

Skin–cool and clammy
Eyes–lackluster
Pupils–dilated
Face–pale
Lips–blue
Pulse–rapid and weak
Breathing–rapid and shallow

SYMPTOMS
• Nausea
• Thirst
• Weakness
• Restless
• Fear

SIGNS
• Restlessness   • Becomes unresponsive

Figure 3-2 Windshield survey.

First Responders Anyone who arrives at the scene before the EMTs and has training in first aid, basic life support, or elementary emergency care—or even a person with allied health training such as a nurse or physician's assistant—is known as a first responder. Many police officers, firefighters, and industrial health personnel are trained in the U.S. Department of Transportation curriculum and are state-certified **First Responders**. A first responder is trained to a level below that of the EMT.

As a member of the EMS system, respect the work that first responders have done before you arrive. They can provide valuable information about how the emergency came about, how the patient was acting when they arrived, what they found to be wrong with the patient, perhaps some baseline vital signs so that you can compare your findings, and what care procedures have been started. Recognize that the first responders may already have stabilized or improved the patient's condition. You will have to do your own assessment and evaluate the care already provided, but the information the first responders give you along with your own assessment may alert you to the fact that the patient is improving or deteriorating.

When you arrive tactfully assume medical command or responsibility for the patient, thank the first responders, and give them credit for any prompt and efficient care they provided for the patient. Allow first responders to help when you need assistance.

If you discover any errors made by the first responders, do not confront them about it at the scene. Alert them and their training officers after the run so that future care can be improved.

Mechanisms of Injury The **mechanism of injury** is what caused the injury (e.g. a rapid deceleration causing the knees to strike the dash of a car; a fall on ice causing a twisting force to the ankle) (Scan 3-2).

Certain injuries are considered "common" to particular accident situations. Fractured bones are usually associated with falls and vehicle collisions (Figure 3-3); burns are common to fires and explosions; penetrating soft tissue injuries can be associated with gunshot wounds, and so on.

Even if you cannot determine what injury the patient has sustained, knowing the mechanism of injury allows you to predict various injury patterns. For example, in many situations you will immobilize the patient's spine because the mechanism of injury is a frequent cause of spinal injury. You do not need to know that the patient's spine is actually injured; you assume it is and treat accordingly. Knowing that the patient has fallen, you check for signs and symptoms of fracture and perhaps splint the

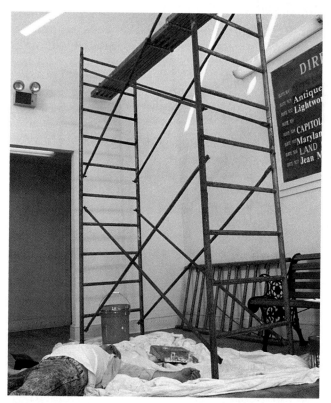

Figure 3-3 Mechanisms of injury may provide valuable clues to the nature of a patient's injury.

54 Patient Assessment

Mechanisms of Injury and Affected Areas of the Body

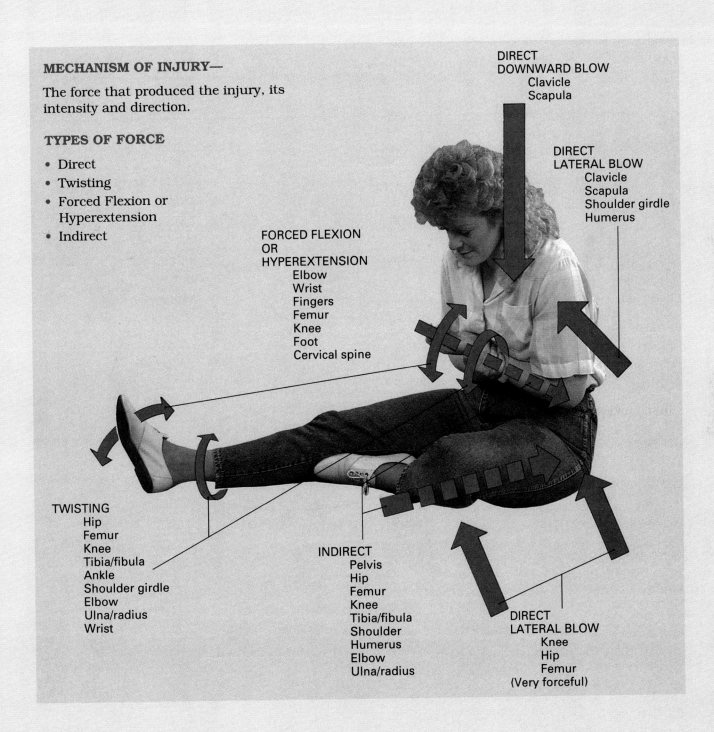

MECHANISM OF INJURY—

The force that produced the injury, its intensity and direction.

TYPES OF FORCE

- Direct
- Twisting
- Forced Flexion or Hyperextension
- Indirect

FORCED FLEXION OR HYPEREXTENSION
Elbow
Wrist
Fingers
Femur
Knee
Foot
Cervical spine

DIRECT DOWNWARD BLOW
Clavicle
Scapula

DIRECT LATERAL BLOW
Clavicle
Scapula
Shoulder girdle
Humerus

TWISTING
Hip
Femur
Knee
Tibia/fibula
Ankle
Shoulder girdle
Elbow
Ulna/radius
Wrist

INDIRECT
Pelvis
Hip
Femur
Knee
Tibia/fibula
Shoulder
Humerus
Elbow
Ulna/radius

DIRECT LATERAL BLOW
Knee
Hip
Femur
(Very forceful)

55

affected limb even if you can't be sure it has been fractured.

There are many systems for classifying injuries. One system considers the type of tissue or structure that has been injured: soft tissue injuries, fractures, dislocations, and internal organ injuries. (For example, Table 3-1 shows mechanisms of injury classified by types of fracture.) Another system uses the force causing the damage: blunt trauma, penetrating trauma, deceleration injury, thermal injury, and so on. The National Safety Council categorizes injuries by types of accidents: motor vehicle collisions, falls, fires and explosions, assaults (e.g. beatings, knife wounds, gunshot wounds), swimming and boating accidents, firearms accidents, poisonings, machinery accidents, and accidents involving electricity (including lightning).

TABLE 3-1 Examples of Mechanisms of Injuries for Fractures

| Upper Extremities | | Lower Extremities | |
Structure	Mechanism	Structure	Mechanism
SHOULDER		PELVIS	Fall (landing on the buttocks), fall (more common with elderly), forceful direct blow, crush injury, strenuous activity (young patients)
• Clavicle (collarbone)	Fall on lateral shoulder direct blow, blow to upper back and posterior shoulder, downward blow striking the bone		
• Scapula (shoulder blade)	Direct blow, severe downward blow to the shoulder (e.g., falling objects), fall on the lateral shoulder (very rare)	HIP	Direct blow to knees (e.g., striking dashboard), direct blow (e.g., vehicle strikes pedestrian's hip), posterior dislocation
• Proximal humerus (arm bone near shoulder)	Direct blow to the lateral arm (falls or striking vehicle compartment wall in crash)	FEMUR (thigh bone)	
HUMERUS (arm bone)—shaft	Direct blow from striking an object (motor vehicle collisions), direct blow from a fall, fall on the elbow, fall on the hand of an outstretched arm	• Femoral head	Direct blow, anterior dislocation
		• Proximal shaft	Fall on hip, fall on hip with twisting forces
ELBOW		• Shaft	Severe blow to thigh, severe blow to knees
• Distal humerus	Direct blow to flexed elbow, indirect force of landing on outstretched arm, forceful hyperextension of elbow	KNEE	
		• Distal femur	Direct blow (usually motor vehicle collisions or falls), hyperextension or severe twist of the knee
• Proximal forearm bones	Direct blow to elbow, indirect force from fall on outstretched arm, elbow dislocation		
FOREARM BONES		• Proximal leg (lower leg bones)	Direct force from a fall, transfer of force from falling and landing on the feet, object strikes leg (e.g., vehicle strikes pedestrian)
• Shaft	Direct blow (often to forearm while raised to protect face), compression occurring from a fall (usually to children)		
• Distal forearm	Fall on hand, forced flexion or extension of hand	• Patella (kneecap)	Direct blow (e.g., falls, knee strikes dashboard), severe muscle contractions (e.g., from the force of a fall)
WRIST	Forced flexion or hyperextension, direct blow, indirect force from falling on an outstretched hand, crush injury, force of thumb being driven back into its joint with the wrist	LEG (lower leg bones)	Direct blow, twisting forces, blow to the side of the knee
		ANKLE	Twisting forces, crush injury, falls (landing on the feet)
HAND	Direct blows (falls), objects striking the distal fingers, falling objects striking the hand, forced flexion or hyperextension of fingers, twisting force to the fingers, impact to the fist	FOOT	Heel strikes ground during fall, forced extreme flexion or hyperextension of foot, severe ankle twist, direct blow to the toes (falling objects or kicking an object)

Knowing the mechanism of injury is very important when dealing with motor vehicle collisions. A collapsed or bent steering column suggests that the driver has suffered a chest wall injury with possible lung damage and perhaps damage to the heart and its great blood vessels. A bent steering wheel also tells of the possibility of fractured ribs. A shattered, blood-spattered windshield points to the likelihood of a forehead or scalp laceration (cut) and possibly a severe blow to the head that may have caused a head or spinal injury.

Maintain a high index of suspicion based on the mechanism of injury.

THE PRIMARY SURVEY

The information gained as you sized up the situation (above) provides you with a starting point for the primary survey. As stated earlier, the primary survey is a process carried out to detect and treat life-threatening problems. As these problems are detected, lifesaving measures are taken immediately (Scan 3-3), and early transport—within 10 minutes of arrival at the scene—may be initiated.

The ABCDEs

During the primary survey you are concerned with the **ABCDEs** of emergency care: Airway, Breathing, Circulation, Disability, and Expose. For many years, EMTs have learned that the primary survey involves the ABCs of emergency care. Most EMS systems now teach the *expanded* primary survey with D and E steps added and treatment of any life threatening problems initiated as soon as they are uncovered during the survey. It is the expanded primary survey that is described here.

First recall that the purpose of the primary survey is to discover and treat conditions from which the patient will otherwise quickly die, conditions that cannot wait for the complete secondary survey with its systematic interview, vital sign assessment, and thorough head-to-toe survey (which will be discussed later in this chapter). For this reason, the primary survey is a "treat-as-you-go" process. As each major problem is detected, it is treated *immediately*, before moving on to the next since it doesn't matter what "C" is if you don't have "A."

As soon as the ABCDE process is concluded, the EMT or EMT team must make a **status**

decision, a judgment about the degree of severity of the patient's condition and whether the patient requires immediate transport to a medical facility without undertaking a secondary survey at the scene.

All EMS personnel should be aware of the concept of the "Golden Hour." Survival rates will fall drastically for victims of trauma who do not receive specialized hospital care within one hour of injury. But patients with the immediately life-threatening conditions the primary survey is intended to reveal may have only minutes to live. That is why EMTs at the scene must strive to complete the entire process—ABCDE steps, status, and transport decisions—within the "Platinum 10 Minutes" after their arrival on the scene.

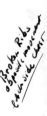

- A = Airway. An obstructed **airway** (the path from nose and mouth to lungs) may quickly lead to respiratory arrest or compromise and death. Assess responsiveness and, when necessary, open the airway.
- B = Breathing. Respiratory arrest will quickly cause cardiac arrest. Assess breathing and, when necessary, provide rescue breathing. Look for and treat problems that may compromise breathing such as flail segments or penetrating trauma to the chest.
- C = Circulation. If the patient's heart is not beating, carrying blood and oxygen to the brain, irreversible changes will begin to occur in the brain in 4 to 6 minutes; cell death will usually occur within 10 minutes of cardiac arrest. Assess circulation and, when necessary, provide cardiopulmonary resuscitation (CPR). Also check for profuse bleeding that can be controlled. Assess and begin care for severe shock or the potential for severe shock.
- D = Disability. Serious central nervous system (brain and spinal column) disability can lead to death. Assess the patient's level of consciousness and, if you suspect head or neck injury, apply a rigid extrication collar if you have not already done so. Observe the neck before you cover it up. Also do a quick assessment of the patient's ability to move all extremities.
- E = Expose. You cannot treat conditions you haven't discovered. Remove clothing, especially if the patient is not alert and communicating with you, to see if you missed any life-threatening injuries. Protect the patient's privacy and keep him warm with a blanket if necessary.

Primary Survey

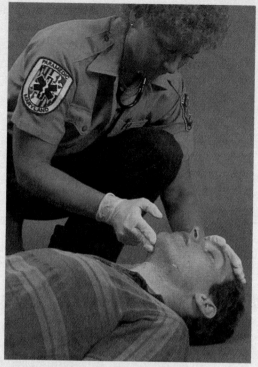

1. Open airway

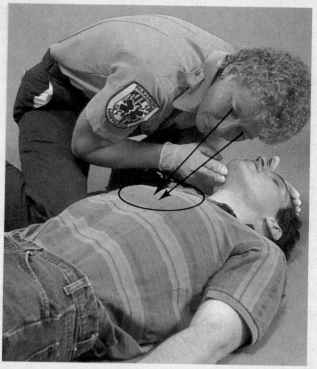

2. Check breathing

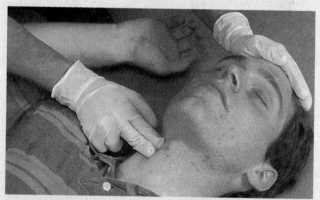

3. Check circulation: pulse, bleeding, shock

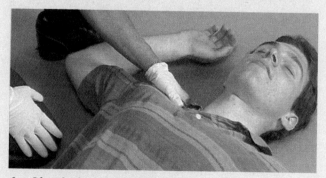

4. Check disability (level of consciousness)

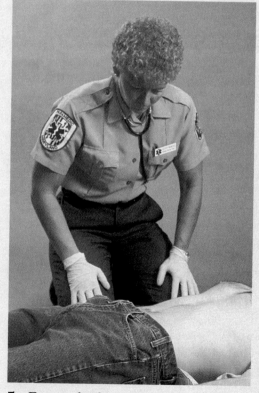

5. Expose body

Note: Your course and local requirements may state that you should look for medical identification devices while you are doing the primary survey and check the patient's pupils during the D step. Your instructor is the authority on such matters. It is understood, however, that these tasks are *not* to delay lifesaving care.

The primary survey procedures you should follow to assess and care for the ABCDE are detailed below.

Note: It is very important to protect the patient's spine throughout the patient assessment.

1. **Check for responsiveness** (Figure 3-4). Consciousness indicates breathing and circulation. Breathing may not be adequate and you may have to clear the airway, but if the patient is conscious, you know that he is breathing and has circulation. Keep in mind that consciousness may be lost quick-ly, breathing may change, and circulation may stop. To check for responsiveness, *gently* tap the patient's shoulder and say: "Are you okay?"

2. **Reposition the patient if necessary**. You will find it difficult to determine if an unconscious patient in the prone position has an open airway and adequate breathing. Even though you have not surveyed the patient for possible spinal and other serious injuries you will have to place him in a supine position (Figure 3-5; see also Chapter 4). If the patient is not breathing, or you cannot tell if he is breathing, use a simple **log-roll** maneuver to move the patient from a prone to a supine position. Kneel at his side, leaving enough room so that the patient will not roll into your lap. Gently straighten his legs and position the arm that is closest to you as shown in Figure 3-6. Place one of your hands so that it cradles the head and neck from behind. Place your other hand under the patient's distant shoulder, at the armpit. Move the patient as a unit onto his side and then onto his back.

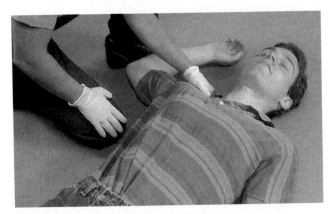

Figure 3-4 Establish responsiveness.

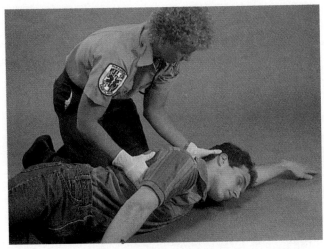

Figure 3-5 Placing a patient in the supine position.

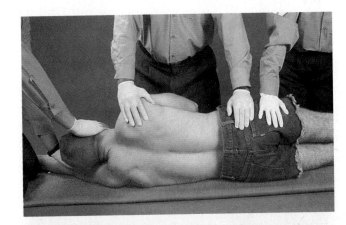

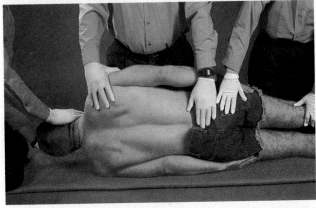

Figure 3-6 Log rolling the patient (A) with arm raised or (B) with arm at side.

You must move his head, neck, and torso as a unit to reduce the chances of aggravation to spinal injuries.

Note: The log roll is best done by two or more rescuers with one rescuer responsible for stabilizing the head and neck and directing the actual repositioning of the patient (see Chapter 12). The one-rescuer log roll is to be used only when basic life support may be needed and adequate personnel are not immediately on hand to assist.

3. **Check for an open airway.** If the patient is unresponsive, always ensure an open airway (Figure 3-7). For cases in which you do not suspect spinal injury, position yourself at the patient's side. Perform a head-tilt, chin-lift maneuver (see Chapter 4). Use the fingers of your hand that is closest to the patient's chest to support the lower jaw. Place these fingers under the jaw at the chin. Your fingers should rest on the bony part of the jaw, avoiding the soft tissue that is found under the chin. Lift to move the jaw forward.

For patients with possible spinal injury, you should use the jaw-thrust (see Chapter 4). Manage all unconscious trauma

patients as if they have spinal injuries. Do finger sweeps with a gloved finger to remove debris from the mouth. Consider suctioning the mouth and placing an oral or nasal airway to help you keep the airway open. (See Chapters 4 and 6.) You can't move on in your survey if the airway is not open.

4. **Determine that breathing quantity and quality are appropriate.** You must check to ensure that there is sufficient air exchange. Position the side of your head close to the patient's face, then *Look*, *Listen*, and *Feel* (Figure 3-8).

LOOK for chest movements that are associated with breathing. (Note: Males often show the most pronounced respiratory movement at the level of the diaphragm; females tend to show more pronounced movement at the clavicles.)

LISTEN for air moving at the patient's mouth and nose.

FEEL for air being expired through the patient's nose and mouth.

Take no more than 3 to 5 seconds to establish breathlessness.

If the patient is not breathing, or if there is an airway obstruction, or if the patient is suffering severe respiratory distress, YOU MUST TAKE IMMEDIATE ACTION. Also, some patients with very erratic chest movements may not be exchanging air and may develop cardiac arrest. Administer rescue breathing as necessary. If your patient's breathing rate is over 28 or under 10 breaths per minute, you should supplement rescue breathing with a bag-valve mask and a reservoir sys-

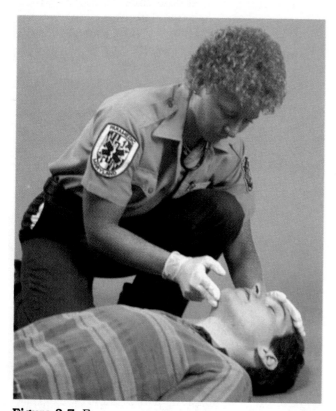

Figure 3-7 Ensure an open airway.

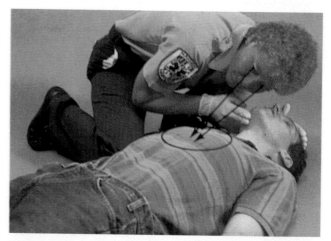

Figure 3-8 LOOK, LISTEN, and FEEL for adequate breathing.

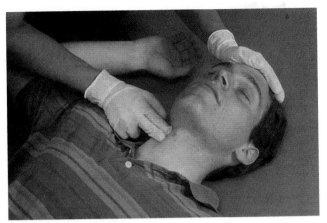

Figure 3-9 A quick check of the carotid pulse confirms circulation.

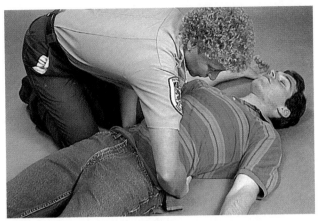

Figure 3-10 Locate and control all profuse bleeding.

tem or an oxygen delivery device (mask) that provides a high concentration of oxygen. To protect yourself from infectious diseases, use a pocket mask with a one-way valve, a bag-valve mask, or other barrier device (see Chapter 4). If the patient is breathing adequately through an open airway, continue the primary survey.

Note: During the primary survey, if you notice breathing problems, you should quickly check to see if the patient has a chest wound that has opened the thoracic cavity or an object impaled in the chest. The same holds true if you notice that a section of ribs or the sternum has broken free from the rib cage (flail chest). These types of injury will need immediate care. Seal holes in the chest wall with an air-occlusive dressing, stabilize but do not remove impaled objects, stabilize flail segments, and administer a high concentration of oxygen (see Chapter 14).

5. **Check for circulation.** If the patient has been in respiratory arrest for a few minutes, he may have developed cardiac arrest as well. Determine if there is heart action and blood circulation by palpating (feeling for) a **carotid** (kah-ROT-id) **pulse** (Figure 3-9).

While stabilizing the patient's head and maintaining the proper head-tilt by keeping one hand on the patient's forehead, use your hand that is closest to the patient's neck to locate his "Adam's apple" (the most prominent part of the thyroid cartilage). Place the tips of your index and middle fingers directly over the midline of this structure. (Do not use your thumb. It has a pulse that you may feel instead of the patient's carotid pulse.) Slide your fingertips to the side of the patient's neck closest to you. Keep the palm side of your fingertips against the patient's neck. *Do not* slide your fingertips to the opposite side of the patient's neck.* Feel for a groove between the Adam's apple (larynx) and the muscles located along the side of the neck.

Very little pressure need be applied to the neck to feel the carotid pulse. Precise pulse rate is not important; however, you should note the strength and regularity of the pulse. You should take no more than 5 to 10 seconds to establish pulselessness.†

If there is no carotid pulse, cardiopulmonary resuscitation (KAR-de-o-PUL-mo-ner-e re-SUS-ci-TA-shun) or CPR and application of an automated external defibrillator (AED), if so trained, will have to be initiated (see Chapter 5). If there is a pulse, but no breathing, continue your efforts at artificial ventilation with periodic checking for a carotid pulse. If the patient is breathing and has a carotid pulse, then count the pulse rate to see if it is fast (greater than 100) or slow (less than 60), strong, or weak.

Control profuse bleeding (Figure 3-10). Only *profuse* bleeding is considered during the primary survey. Look and feel for bleed-

---

*To do so may place your fingers on the patient's windpipe, reducing your ability to palpate the pulse and possibly causing you to apply incorrect pressure that may interfere with the patient's airway or reduce the proper head-tilt. Also, this will keep you from having your thumb on one side of the neck and your fingers on the other side. You should never try to feel for a pulse on both sides of the neck at the same time. To do so may cause you to interrupt circulation to the brain.

†Up to 1 minute is recommended for cases of hypothermia (see Chapter 20).

ing with extreme care. Keep in mind that the patient may have spinal injuries and other serious injuries requiring him to be kept still. Bleeding wounds are not always as severe as they may first appear, so be certain that you are dealing with bleeding that requires immediate action. Look for wounds from which blood is spurting or flowing freely and for signs of internal bleeding. Methods for estimating the severity of and controlling such bleeding will be covered in Chapter 7.

Note: There are special cases in which you find a patient who is not bleeding profusely, but who has been bleeding slowly for a long period of time, having lost a significant amount of blood. Such cases may require you to consider any additional bleeding as life threatening. In this case control bleeding and begin to treat for shock immediately following the primary survey.

Note: In situations in which you immediately notice profuse bleeding, you may have to begin to control it while, at the same time, you begin to check for respiration. Keep in mind that severe bleeding, with blood spurting from a wound, indicates some heart action (circulation). Remember, even though bleeding is occurring, assessment of airway and breathing cannot be ignored.

Check for shock. If the patient is likely to develop shock, or if he exhibits signs of severe shock, you should carefully begin your care for shock before moving on to the next step of the assessment. Remember that the best treatment for shock is prevention. Methods of detecting and treating for shock will be covered in Chapter 8.

6. **Check for disability.** Quickly assess the patient's **level of consciousness** (LOC). An alert person is aware of what is going on around him. He is oriented if he knows who he is, where he is, and the day of the week and can respond quickly to both vocal and physical stimuli. A confused, disoriented person usually has trouble answering questions and responding to specific instructions. Experience will soon allow you to determine easily a person's level of consciousness.

Some EMS systems use a simple form for assessing the level of consciousness.

This form uses the **AVPU** method, which stands for

A Alert—The patient is aware of what is happening around him. He knows (1) his name, (2) the day of the week, and (3) where he is. If he answers these questions appropriately, we say that he is "alert and oriented times 3."

V Verbal—The patient is not alert (x 3) but may be talking and responds to your voice.

P Painful response—The patient will not obey your commands or may not respond at all to your voice. He does respond to painful stimuli (e.g., being pinched) by (1) withdrawing from the pain source (2) pushing into the pain source, or by (3) flexion, or (4) extension of the extremities (with 1 being the "best" response and 4 being the"worst" response to pain).

U Unresponsive—The patient does not respond to any stimuli.

Check pupils if local protocols require it, apply a rigid collar, and check all four extremities to make sure there is sensory and motor function.

7. **Expose the patient's body.** Remove clothing, as necessary, to check for any other serious injuries, especially if the patient is unconscious or uncommunicative. Protect the patient's privacy to the extent possible.

Performing the ABCDEs of the expanded primary survey (clearing the airway, initiating artificial ventilation or CPR if necessary, assessing level of consciousness, exposing the body) can best be accomplished if you reach the patient's side carrying the following initial equipment and supplies.

- Disposable gloves and goggles or eye shield
- Suction unit
- Oral and nasal airways
- Stethoscope
- Oxygen tank literflow regulator and non-rebreather mask
- Pocket face mask with one-way valve or bag-valve mask with a reservoir
- Assortment of dressings, bandages, wide tape, and occlusive dressings
- Blood pressure cuff
- Anti-shock garment as local protocol recommends

- Rigid collars (full set)
- Scissors
- Penlight or flashlight
- An assessment card

Making a Status Decision

Once the ABCDEs are completed, you must immediately make a decision about the patient's status. Is the patient stable enough to continue with the secondary survey, or does he need continuing resuscitation and immediate transport to a medical facility? Base your decision on the **CUPS** categories.

C Critical—a patient in cardiac arrest (requiring CPR) or respiratory arrest (requiring rescue breathing)

U Unstable—a patient with an airway that cannot be opened or sustained, serious chest injuries or breathing difficulties, uncontrollable bleeding, obvious signs of shock, serious head injury, or crushing chest pain

P Potentially Unstable—a patient who is not unstable but has signs or symptoms of serious injury requiring secondary assessment for better identification. For example, early vital signs with normal values may suggest compensated shock (see Chapter 8), mechanisms of injury (e.g. cracked windshield or broken steering wheel) suggest hidden injury, there are major isolated injuries, or there are extremity injuries with nerve or circulatory damage (see Chapters 10 and 11).

S Stable—a patient with a minor isolated injury without major blood loss, without nerve or circulatory damage, with no signs of shock or other complications

If a patient is categorized C or U, begin transport immediately, providing only resuscitative measures, and do the secondary survey en route to the hospital if time or personnel permit. If the patient is categorized P or S, conduct a secondary survey at the scene, remaining alert for changes indicating deterioration into a C or U category during the secondary survey.

Be aware that only about 10% of all the patients you encounter will be categorized as C or U patients whose conditions are so serious that you will bypass a secondary survey at the scene. These patients need a total commitment to resuscitation. Their problems cannot get much worse. They are in grave danger of death without aggressive resuscitative treatment at a medical facility.

Most patients—90% or more—will need a more thorough on-the-scene assessment, emergency treatment, and stabilization. For the majority of patients, after completing the primary survey, you should proceed to the next phase, the secondary survey.

Warning: Many patients who are stable enough to undergo the secondary survey will nevertheless have conditions that require early administration of oxygen, both before and during the secondary survey. Provision of oxygen is a key early treatment that, if needed, must not be delayed.

THE SECONDARY SURVEY

The objective of the secondary survey is to discover medical and injury-related problems that do not pose an immediate threat to survival but may do so if allowed to go untreated. Unlike the primary survey, the secondary survey is *not* a "treat-as-you-go" process. Rather, as you complete the survey in a systematic manner, you mentally note injuries and problems and formulate priorities and a plan for treatment once the survey is completed.

Note: The secondary survey for a patient who presents with medical illness will differ somewhat from that for a patient who has sustained an injury. Usually the trauma survey is about 20% patient interview and 80% physical exam, whereas the medical assessment is 80% patient interview and 20% physical exam. Both physical exam and patient interview should always be done for all medical and trauma patients.

Remember: If the patient has a life-threatening illness or injury, or deteriorates into a C or U status, it may not be possible to complete the secondary survey before starting to transport the patient.

The following are basic items you will need for the secondary survey.

- A blood pressure cuff, or **sphygmomanometer** (SFIG-mo-mah-NOM-e-ter),—used to measure and monitor blood pressure
- A stethoscope—used in conjunction with a blood pressure cuff in the determination of

blood pressure. A stethoscope can also be used for listening to the sounds of air entering and leaving the lungs.

- A penlight—used for examining the patient's mouth, nose, ears, and pupils. It is also useful in poor lighting.
- Heavy-duty bandage scissors—to cut away clothing and footwear that may obscure an injury site or prevent access to a pulse or blood pressure site
- An assessment card and pen—to record survey results and prompt the EMT on relevant questions to ask
- A watch with either a sweep second hand or digital seconds counter—to measure pulse and respiration rates
- Protective equipment—disposable gloves, goggles, pocket face mask, or other barriers for rescue breathing

Several examination instruments can be carried in a belt holster.

You will also need a survey form or assessment card—whatever prehospital care report form is required by your EMS system—for recording information obtained during the survey. There is more about forms at the end of this chapter.

Keep in mind that you will have to reconsider and re-evaluate some of the things you did on arrival at the scene. Also, you may have missed something during the primary survey or something may have changed since you did it. Before starting the secondary survey, always

- *Look over the scene.* Is it still safe? Did you overlook a mechanism of injury? Are there any other patients in need of attention?
- *Look over your patient.* Are there obvious injuries or indications of illness? Is his condition deteriorating? Is the patient wearing a medical identification necklace or bracelet you can read without moving him?

Now you are ready to begin the two parts of the secondary survey: the interview and the examination. The results of these two inquiries will be combined and related to allow you to make an overall assessment of your patient's condition and to form a plan of emergency care.

Be realistic as you conduct the secondary survey. If you are too systematic, you may find the patient getting upset about answering a lot of questions when he just wants you to look at his leg. So you may begin the examination while you are still asking questions. Be flexible enough

to tailor your activities to the situation—without letting the patient dictate your job!

The Subjective Interview

The **subjective interview** is not unlike the interview a physician conducts prior to a physical examination. It is a conversational, information-gathering effort. Not only will you gain needed information from the interview, but you will also reduce the patient's fear and promote cooperation.

Time is to be used wisely at the emergency scene. As you become an experienced EMT, you will find that it is possible to begin the physical examination of a patient while you are interviewing him.

Relatives and bystanders also may serve as sources of information; however, do not interrupt interviewing the patient to gather information from a bystander. When a patient is unconscious, you may gain information from bystanders and medical identification devices while you are conducting the physical examination.

Interviewing the Patient When conducting a patient interview, you should

1. *Position yourself close to the patient.* Depending on the patient's situation, kneel or stand close to him. If possible, position yourself so that the sun or bright lights are not at your back. When practical, position yourself so the patient can see your face.
2. *Identify yourself and reassure the patient.* It is important that the patient know he is in competent hands. Maintain eye contact with the patient and state your name, that you are an Emergency Medical Technician, and the organization you represent.

   Speak in your normal voice. If you ask a question, wait for a reply. Remember, at first the patient may not want you to help. Work to gain his confidence through calm conversation. Avoid inappropriate remarks like "Don't worry," and "Everything is all right," because the patient knows everything is not all right, and false assurances should not be offered.

   If you believe it to be appropriate, gently touch the patient's shoulder or rest your hand over his. A simple touch is comforting to most people. Keep in mind that a sign of caring for the sick and injured is to momentarily place the back of your hand on a person's forehead. This gesture will not only help to reassure the patient, it will also provide some information about his skin temperature.

3. *Learn your patient's name.* Once you know it, use it in the rest of your conversations. Children will expect you to use their first names. For adults, use the appropriate "Mr.," "Mrs.," "Miss," or "Ms." unless they introduce themselves by their first name.

   You need the patient's name for completion of your forms and to give a personal touch that is often very reassuring to the patient. Having the patient's name could prove to be of great importance should he become unconscious and not be carrying any identification.

4. *Learn your patient's age.* This may be needed for reports and communications with the medical facility. If you cannot judge your patient's general age (early adulthood, middle adulthood, late adulthood), always ask his age. D.O.B.

   Children expect to be asked their age. To do so will help keep a "normal" tone to the conversation. You should ask adolescents their age to be certain that you are dealing with a minor.

   It is a good idea at this time to ask minors how you can contact their parent or guardian. Sometime, this question upsets children because it intensifies the fear they are having about being sick or hurt without their parent being there to help. Be prepared to offer comfort and assure the child that someone will contact his parent or guardian.

5. *Seek out what is wrong.* In this part of the interview you are seeking information about the patient's **symptoms**, things the patient feels or senses, such as pain or nausea. What is the patient's primary (chief) complaint (the reason the ambulance was called)? Be certain to record this complaint even if you suspect several more significant problems. Encourage the patient to elaborate. Ask him what is wrong. If he tells you several things, ask what is bothering him the most. Find out if the patient is in pain and where he hurts. Unless the pain of one injury or medical problem masks that of another, or unless a spinal injury has interrupted nerve pathways, most injured people will be able to tell you of painful areas. A sick person will be able to tell you of pain or discomfort.

When your patient has been injured in an accident, try to ask open-ended questions, that is, questions that do not limit the response because they are too specific. Start by asking if anything feels wrong. Then, if necessary, become more specific to direct the patient's responses. For example, if the patient says that everything feels fine or if he appears to be confused by your broad questions, you could ask if his arms and legs feel OK. If he says that there is a problem and does not offer a description of that problem, you may have to ask more specific questions. You may have to ask if there is numbness, tingling, burning, or any other unusual sensations in his arms or legs. Such sensations in the extremities suggest damage to the spinal cord and warn you against moving the patient any more than necessary during the remainder of the survey.

As you learn more about various illnesses and injuries, you will see what additional questions can be asked to develop specific responses.

6. *If the patient is experiencing pain or breathing difficulties, ask the PQRST questions.*
   - P Provocation—What brought this on?
   - Q Quality—What does it feel like?
   - R Region—Where is it?
   - R Referral—Does it go anywhere (e.g. "into my left shoulder")?
   - R Recurrence—Has this happened before?
   - R Relief—Does anything make it feel better?
   - S Severity—How bad is it on a scale of 1 to 10?
   - T Time—When did it begin?

7. *To obtain the patient's history, ask the AMPLE questions.*
   - A Allergies—Are you allergic to any medication—or anything else?
   - M Medication—What medications are you currently taking (prescription, over the counter, or recreational)?
   - P Previous Medical History—Have you been having any medical problems? Have you been feeling ill? Have you been seeing a doctor? What is your doctor's name (so the emergency medical dispatcher can contact the doctor and learn what may be critical in helping the patient)?
   - L Last meal—When did you eat last? What did you eat? (Remember that

food could cause the symptoms or aggravate a medical condition. Also, if a patient will need to go to surgery, the hospital staff must know when he has eaten last.)

E Events—What sequence of events led up to today's problem (passed out then got into car crash versus got into car crash and then passed out)?

If you feel uncomfortable and unsure what to ask when conducting your first few patient interviews, just ask the questions that will enable you to fill out your patient assessment card. It takes only a few minutes to conduct the interview and the brief history obtained may provide information that is essential to patient care. This is especially true if the patient loses consciousness before he can be interviewed by the emergency department staff.

Remember, stay in control by conducting the interview in a calm, professional manner. Avoid inappropriate conversation. Record information as it is gathered on an assessment card.

Interviewing Bystanders When interviewing bystanders, determine if any are relatives or friends of the patient. They usually have more information to provide about past problems. See which of the bystanders saw what happened. When questioning bystanders, you should ask

1. *The patient's name.* If the patient is obviously a minor, you should ask if the parent or guardian is present or if he or she has been contacted.

2. *What happened?* You may be told that the patient fell off a ladder, appeared to faint, fell to the ground and began convulsing, was hit on the head by a falling object, or other possible clues.

3. *Did they see anything else?* For example, was the patient clutching his chest or head before he fell?

4. *Did the patient complain of anything before this happened?* You may learn of chest pains, nausea, concern about odors where he was working, or other clues to the problem.

5. *Did the patient have any known illnesses or problems?* This may provide you with information about heart problems, alcohol abuse, or other problems that could cause a change in the patient's condition.

6. *Do they know if the patient was taking any medications?* Be sure to use the words

"medications" or "medicines." If you say "drugs" or some other term, bystanders may not answer you, thinking that you are asking questions as part of a criminal investigation. In rare cases, you may feel that the bystanders are holding back information because the patient was abusing drugs. Remind them that you are an EMT and you need all the information they can give you so proper care can begin.

If your patient is the victim of a motor vehicle collision and was taken from the wreckage prior to your arrival, ask if he was the driver or a passenger and if he was wearing a seat belt. You can often associate the mechanism of injury with where a person was sitting in a vehicle, (e.g. a lateral collision should always lead the EMT to question the patient who sat on the side of the collision). Also ask if the person was conscious when he was taken from the wreckage and if he has lost consciousness, even for a brief moment.

Document the removal of the patient before your arrival at the scene.

Do not ask these questions as an isolated part of the secondary survey. You can be active, beginning the examination while you ask questions and listen to bystanders' answers.

Medical ID Devices Medical identification devices can provide needed information. One of the most commonly used medical-alerting devices is the Medic Alert emblem shown in Figure 3-11. Over one million people wear a medical identification device in the form of a necklace or wrist or ankle bracelet. One side of the device

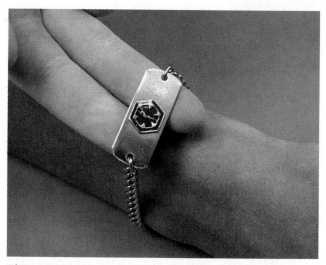

Figure 3-11 A medical identification device.

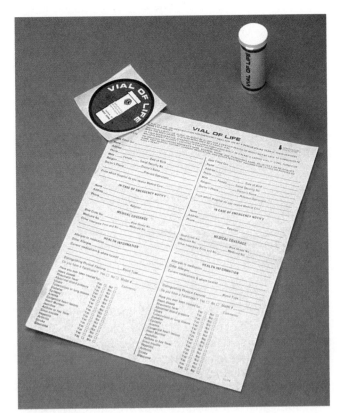

Figure 3-12 A "Vial of Life" sticker.

has a Star of Life emblem. The patient's medical problem is engraved on the reverse side, along with a telephone number to call for additional information.

Look for necklaces and bracelets. Never assume you know the form of every medical identification device. Check carefully any necklace or bracelet, taking usual care when moving the patient or any of his extremities. You should alert the emergency department staff (usually by radio or cellular phone transmission) that the patient is wearing a medical identification device. Give the staff the wearer's identification number, the nature of the problem, and the telephone number they are to call. If you are in a patient's residence, see if there is a "Vial of Life" (Figure 3-12) or similar type of sticker on the main outside door, closest window to the main door, or the refrigerator door. Patient information and medications can be found in the refrigerator. There is more information on patients subject to anaphylactic shock (severe allergic reactions) and the "Vial of Life" in Chapter 8.

Do not move the patient to reach for his wallet in order to find a medical alert card. You should not check his wallet unless you are directed to do so on the bracelet or necklace. If

there is any chance of spinal injury, you should not move the patient to gain access to his wallet. To do so may cause severe injury to the patient.

The Objective Examination

The **objective examination** is a comprehensive, hands-on survey of the patient's body. During the objective examination you check for vital signs and for very specific signs and symptoms of less-than-obvious injuries or the effects of illness. Before going on, make certain you understand the following terms:

- **Signs**—What you see, hear, feel, and smell when examining the patient. Since you will use these signs to try to determine what is wrong with the patient, they are sometimes called diagnostic signs.
- **Symptoms**—What the patient tells you is wrong. Such things as chest pains, dizziness, and nausea are considered symptoms. Many of these may have been gathered through the interview with the patient. Others can be gained by continuing to ask questions during the examination.
- **Vital Signs**—Pulse, respiration, blood pressure, and skin temperature. Many localities also use level of consciousness, pupils, and skin color which can be gathered at the same time as vital signs.

There are three rules to bear in mind as you begin your examination of the patient.

- *Tell the patient what you are going to do.* Fully explain what you will be doing during the examination. Let the patient know if there may be pain or discomfort. Always let the patient know if you must lift, rearrange, or remove any article of his clothing. Do all you can to ensure privacy for the patient. Stress the importance of the examination and work to build the patient's confidence. Ask the patient if he understands what you are doing, seeking his response. Try to maintain eye contact whenever possible, and never turn away while you are talking or while the patient is answering your questions.
- *Obtain consent.* When the patient is alert, be certain to obtain actual consent before starting to determine vital signs or to conduct the head-to-toe survey.
- *Assume spinal injury.* Unless you are cer-

tain that you are dealing with a patient free from spinal injury (e.g., a medical patient with no trauma), assume the patient has such injuries. *Always* assume that the unconscious trauma patient has a spinal injury.

Spinal injuries can occur even in apparently minor accidents. Keep in mind that a patient with a medical emergency may have fallen and hurt his spine. You must conduct the physical examination without aggravating spinal injuries.

Observations It is important to observe and re-observe the patient, not only to determine his condition when you first see him but to pick up on any changes. Observe the patient for the following:

- Anything That Looks Wrong—Before you begin, TAKE A GOOD LOOK AT YOUR PATIENT. Note whatever you can that is *obvious* about his condition. Note *anything* that looks wrong. Quickly look for obvious wound sites, burns, fractures and any obvious deformities, swellings and puffiness, ulcers and blotches on the skin, and any blood-soaked areas.
- Level of Consciousness (LOC) and orientation—During the primary survey you did a quick check of the level of consciousness using the AVPU method. Now re-assess the LOC. Your EMS system may use the **Glasgow Coma Scale** during the secondary survey (see Table 3-8 and Figure 3-19 and "The Survey Form" later in this chapter). You should stay aware of the patient's level of consciousness until he is turned over to the emergency department staff. More specifics on measuring the level of consciousness will be presented in Chapter 12.
- Changes—Even patients who appear to be stable may worsen rapidly. An EMT must always be aware of changes in a patient's condition. Constant monitoring of patients is an essential part of emergency care.

Look for change as you continue the survey. Be on the alert for loss of awareness, failing respiration, distress due to pain, new bleeding, and indications of the onset of shock, such as restlessness, anxiety, and profuse sweating. Remember that patient improvement is also a change to be noted.
- Skin Condition—Observe the patient's skin. Cool, clammy skin is a key sign of shock.

TABLE 3-2 Medical Significance of Changes in Skin Color

Skin Color	Possible Cause of Abnormality
Red	High blood pressure, stroke, heart attack, alcohol abuse, sunburn, infectious disease, carbon monoxide poisoning, simple blushing
White	Shock, heart attack, fright, anemia, simple fainting, emotional distress
Blue	Asphyxia (suffocation), hypoxia (lack of oxygen), heart attack, poisoning
Yellow	Liver disease
Black and blue	Seepage of blood under skin surface

Skin color may suggest a variety of medical problems and is a good indicator of heart and lung function (Table 3-2).

You need to note any odd colorations of the patient's skin and stay alert for changes. When a person has deeply pigmented or dark skin it may be necessary to look for color changes in his lips, nailbeds, palms, ear lobes, whites of the eye, inner surface of lower eyelid, gums, or tongue.

These observations can and should be made simultaneously with taking the vital signs and conducting the head-to-toe survey as well as during emergency care and transport to the hospital.

Taking Vital Signs

Vital signs include pulse, respiration, blood pressure, and temperature. In basic EMT-level emergency care, relative skin temperature is usually measured. In some localities, level of consciousness and pupil size and reactivity are recorded with vital signs. Even though they are not technically vital signs, they can be conveniently observed when vital signs are being taken. It is also very convenient to determine other skin characteristics (e.g., color, dry, moist) when assessing skin temperature.

Your EMS System may have you always take vital signs *after* the head-to-toe survey, thus having an assessment protocol of (1) primary survey, (2) interview, (3) head-to-toe survey, and (4) vital signs. In some areas of the country, vital signs are taken after the head-to-toe survey for unconscious patients (to reduce the risk of aggravating spinal injuries, fractures, or dislocations), but *before* the head-to-toe survey for conscious patients; thus: (1) primary survey, (2) interview, (3) vital signs, and (4) head-to-toe survey. Variations in the approach to patient assessment followed by EMS systems are discussed later in this chapter under "Approaches to Assessment and Care."

Warning: Don't forget for any patient who is critical or unstable—or who deteriorates into such a status during assessment—assessment must give way to immediate treatment and transport.

Determining vital signs will take you about 2 minutes. You will have to develop a smooth, efficient method of determining vital signs. Most patients will have to have their vital signs taken more than once. In some cases, when the patient is unstable and the transport is short, you may find yourself completing the determination of vital signs only to begin the next determination.

Note: The vital sign values discussed in this chapter are for adults. For information about the vital signs of infants and children see Chapter 17.

Pulse The pumping action of the heart is normally rhythmic, causing blood to move through the arteries in waves, not smoothly and continuously at the same pressure like water flowing through a pipe. A fingertip held over an artery where it lies close to the body's surface and crosses over a bone can easily feel characteristic "beats" as the surging blood causes the artery to expand. What you feel is called the **pulse**. When "taking a patient's pulse," you are concerned with two factors: rate and character (Figure 3-13).

- Pulse Rate—For **pulse rate**, you will have to determine the number of beats per minute. This will allow you to decide if the patient's pulse rate is *normal*, *rapid*, or *slow* (Table 3-3).

    Pulse rate varies among individuals. Factors such as age, sex, physical condition, degree of exercise just completed, medications or substances being taken, blood loss, and stress all have an influence on the rate. The *normal* rate for an *adult at rest* is between 60 and 80 beats per minute. Any pulse rate above 100 beats per minute is *rapid* (tachycardia), while a rate below 60 beats per minute is *slow* (bradycardia). An athlete may have a normal at-rest pulse

rate between 40 and 50 beats per minute. This is a slow pulse rate, but it is certainly not an indication of poor health. As an

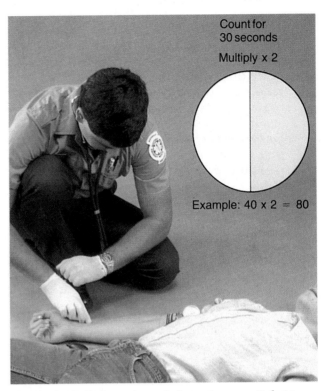

Figure 3-13 Pulse rate and character are vital signs.

TABLE 3-3 Pulse Variations and Medical Conditions

Pulse Rates (beats per minute, at rest)		
Adult	60 to 80	Normal
	100+	Rapid
	Below 60	Slow

Pulse	Possible Cause of Abnormality
Rapid, regular and full	May be caused by nothing more than exertion; may also be caused by fright, fever, hypertension (high blood pressure), or first stage of blood loss
Rapid, regular and thready	Reliable sign of shock; often evident in later stage of blood loss
Slow	Head injury, drug use (barbiturates and narcotics), some poisons, certain cardiac (heart) problems
No pulse	Cardiac arrest leading to death

EMT, you are concerned with the typical adult whose pulse rate stays above 100 or below 60 beats per minute.

In an emergency it is not unusual for this rate to be between 100 and 150 beats per minute. An adult patient must see a physician as soon as possible whenever the pulse rate *stays* above 150 beats per minute. If you take a patient's pulse several times during care at the scene and find him holding a pulse rate above 120 beats or below 50 beats per minute, you must consider this to be a sign that something may be seriously wrong with the patient and that he should be transported as soon as possible.

- Pulse Character—The rhythm and force of the pulse are considered for **pulse character**.

   Pulse rhythm relates to regularity. A pulse is said to be *regular* when intervals between beats are constant. When the intervals are not constant, the pulse is *irregular*. You should report irregular pulse rhythm and if you felt what seemed to be a skipping of a beat or beats.

   Pulse force refers to the pressure of the pulse wave as it expands the artery. Normally, the pulse should feel as if a strong wave has passed under your fingertips. This is a *full* pulse. When the pulse feels weak and thin, the patient has a *thready* pulse.

   Many disorders can be related to variations in pulse rate, rhythm, and force (Table 3-3).

   Pulse rate and character can be determined at a number of points throughout the body. During the determination of vital signs, a **radial pulse** is measured. This is the wrist pulse, named for the radial artery found in the lateral portion of the forearm (remember the anatomical position). If you cannot measure one radial pulse, try the radial pulse of the other arm. When you cannot measure either radial pulse, use the carotid pulse, as described earlier in this chapter under "The Primary Survey."

- Measuring Radial Pulse—In order to measure a radial pulse, find the pulse site by placing your first three fingers on the thumb side of the patient's wrist just above the crease (toward the proximal end). Do not use your thumb. It has its own pulse that may cause you to measure your own pulse

rate. Slide your fingertips toward the lateral (thumb) side of the patient's wrist, keeping one finger over the crease. Apply moderate pressure to feel the pulse beats. A weak pulse may require applying greater pressure. But take care—if you press too hard you may press the artery shut. If you experience difficulty, try the patient's other arm.

Count the pulsations for 30 seconds and multiply by 2 to determine the beats per minute. While you are counting, judge the rhythm and force. Record the information: for example, "Pulse 72, regular and full," and the time of determination. It is best to wait until you also have determined respiratory rate and character before recording pulse information (see below). When recording the pulse rate and character, also record the time of the determination.

If the pulse rate, rhythm, or character is not normal, continue with your count and observations for a full 60 seconds. The number counted is the rate in beats per minute.

Respiration The act of breathing is called **respiration**. A single breath is considered to be the complete process of breathing in (inhalation or inspiration) followed by breathing out (exhalation or expiration). For the determination of vital signs, you are concerned with two factors: rate and character (Figure 3-14).

- Respiratory Rate—**Respiratory rate** is the number of breaths a patient takes in one minute (Table 3-4). The rate of respiration is classified as *normal*, *rapid*, or *slow*. The normal respiration rate for an adult at rest is between 12 and 20 breaths per minute. Keep in mind that age, sex, size, physical conditioning, and emotional state can influence breathing rates. Fear and other emotions experienced during an emergency can cause an increase in respiratory rate. However, if you have an adult patient maintaining a rate above 28 or below 10 breaths per minute, you must consider this to be a serious emergency.

- Respiratory Character—**Respiratory character** includes *rhythm*, *depth*, *ease of breathing*, and *sound* (Table 3-4).

   Respiratory rhythm refers to the manner in which a person breathes. Breathing is considered *regular* when the interval between breaths is constant and *irregular* when the interval varies.

Respiratory depth relates to the amount of air moved with each breath. Normal is something you will have to judge for yourself by watching people breathe when at rest. Then you will be able to differentiate between *deep* and *shallow* respirations.

Ease of breathing can be judged while you are judging depth. Does the patient exhibit *labored* breathing, *difficult* breathing, or *painful* breathing? If the patient shows pronounced movement of his shoulder and neck and/or abdominal muscles while breathing, report this as the use of accessory muscles.

Sounds of respiration include *snoring*, *wheezing*, *crowing*, and *gurgling*. (See Step 14 of the Head-to-Toe Survey and Scan 3-4 later in this chapter. There will be more information on breathing sounds in Chapter 4.)

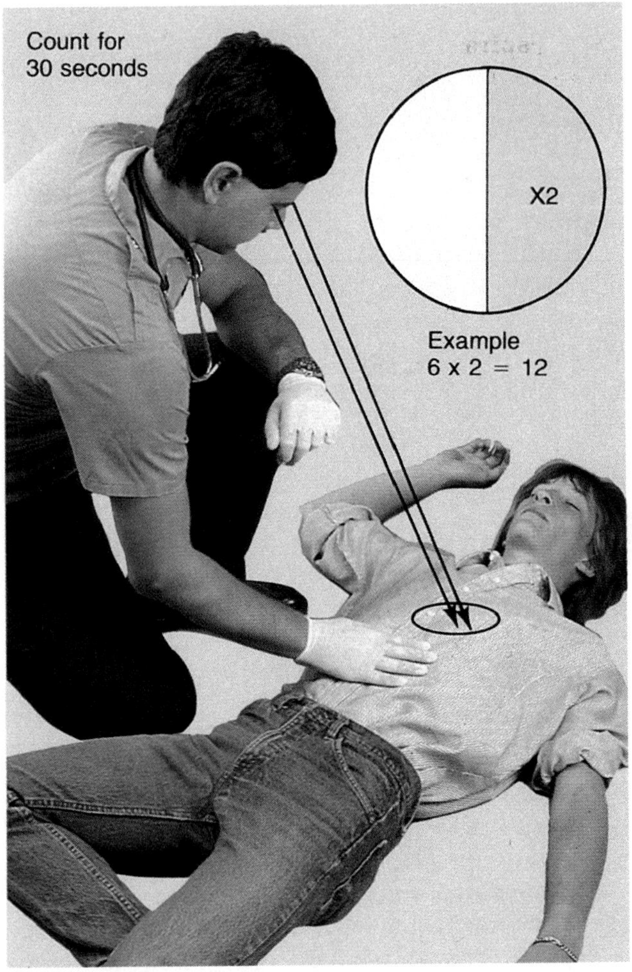

Start counting respirations as soon as you have determined the pulse rate. Many individuals change their breathing rate if they know someone is watching them breathe. For this reason, do not move your hand from the patient's wrist. After you have counted pulse beats, immediately begin to watch the patient's chest for breathing movements. Count the number of breaths taken by the patient during 30 seconds and multiply by 2 to obtain the breaths per minute. While counting, note rhythm, depth, ease, and sounds of respiration. Record your results. For example. "Respirations are 16, regular and normal." Record the time of the assessment.

Figure 3-14 Breathing rate and character are vital signs.

Count for 30 seconds

X2

Example
6 x 2 = 12

TABLE 3-4 Respiration Variations and Medical Conditions

Respiration Rates (breaths per minute, at rest)		
Adult	12 to 20	Normal
	Above 28	Very serious
	Below 10	Very serious

Respirations	Possible Cause of Abnormality
Deep, gasping, labored	Airway obstruction, heart failure, asthma
Rapid, deep	Diabetic coma, hyperventilation
Rapid, shallow	Shock, cardiac problems, chest injury
Painful, difficult, labored	Respiratory distress, lung disease, pulmonary embolus, heart problems
Difficulty in breathing while lying down	Heart failure, lung infection, asthma
Snoring	Stroke, fractured skull, drug influence and alcohol intoxication
Wheezing	Asthma, allergic reaction, upper airway obstruction
Gurgling (as though the breaths are passing through water)	Foreign matter in throat, pulmonary edema (accumulation of fluid in lungs)
Crowing (birdlike sounds)	Spasms of the larynx, upper airway obstruction
Temporary cessation of respirations	Hypoxia (lack of oxygen), congestive heart failure, head injuries
Slowed breathing	Stroke, head injury, chest injury, certain drugs (e.g., narcotics)
No respirations	Respiratory arrest, airway obstruction

Blood Pressure The pressure blood exerts against the walls of blood vessels is known as **blood pressure**. Usually, it is arterial blood pressure (pressure in an artery) that is measured. To prepare to measure blood pressure, first place the stethoscope around your neck with the earpieces pointing forward (in the direction of your ear canals). Position yourself at the patient's side and place the blood pressure cuff on his arm (Figure 3-15). Be certain that there are no suspected or obvious injuries to this arm. There must be no clothing under the cuff. If you can expose the arm sufficiently by rolling the sleeve up, do so, but make sure that this roll of clothing does not become a constricting band.

Wrap the cuff around the patient's upper arm so that the lower edge of the cuff is about one inch above the anterior crease of the elbow. Know the equipment that you are using. The center of the bladder must be placed over the **brachial** (BRAY-key-al) **artery**. The marker on the cuff (if provided) should indicate where you place the cuff in relation to the artery, but many cuffs do not have markers in the correct location. Tubes entering the bladder are not always in the right location either. The American Heart Association states that the only accurate method is finding the bladder center. If you know your equipment, then you will know if the markers are correct, if you can use the tubes entering the bladder, or if you will have to find the center of the bladder. Always apply the cuff securely but not overly tight. You should be able to place one finger easily under the bottom edge of the cuff. You are now ready to begin your determination of the patient's blood pressure.

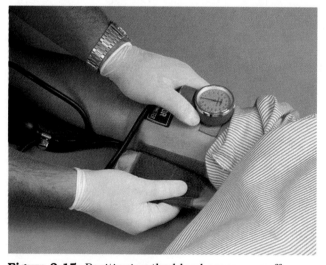

Figure 3-15 Positioning the blood pressure cuff.

Keep in mind that you have no way of knowing the patient's normal blood pressure unless the patient is alert and knows this information (his information must be current). For this reason, one reading of blood pressure may not be very meaningful. You will have to make several readings over a period of time while care is provided at the scene and during transport. Remember that changes in blood pressure are very significant. The patient's blood pressure may be normal in the early stages of some very serious problems, only to change rapidly in a matter of minutes.

Each time the lower chamber of the left side of the heart contracts it forces blood out into circulation. The pressure created in the arteries by this blood is called the **systolic** (sis-TOL-ik) **blood pressure**. When the lower left chamber of the heart is relaxed and refilling, the pressure remaining in the arteries is called the **diastolic** (di-as-TOL-ik) **blood pressure**. The systolic pressure is reported first, the diastolic second, as in 120 over 80.

Just as pulse and respiratory rates vary among individuals so does blood pressure. There is a generally accepted rule for estimating blood pressure of adults up to the age of 40. For an adult male at rest, add his age to 100 to estimate his systolic pressure. For an adult female at rest, add her age to 90 to estimate her systolic pressure. Thus, using this formula, a 36-year-old man would have an estimated normal systolic blood pressure of 136 millimeters of mercury (mmHg). *Millimeters of mercury* refers to the units of the blood pressure gauge. A 36-year-old woman would have an estimated normal systolic pressure of 126 mmHg. Normal diastolic pressures usually range from 60 to 90 mmHg.

Serious low blood pressure (hypotension) is generally considered to exist when the systolic pressure falls below 90 mmHg. High blood pressure (hypertension) exists once the pressure rises above 150/90. Keep in mind that many individuals in emergency situations will exhibit a temporary rise in blood pressure. More than one reading will be necessary to decide if a high or low reading is only temporary. If your patient's blood pressure drops, the patient may be developing shock (other signs are usually more important early indicators of shock). Report any major changes in blood pressure to emergency department personnel without delay.

In adults, consider any systolic reading above 180 or below 90 mmHg to be very serious. A diastolic reading above 104 or below 60 mmHg must also be considered to be very serious (see Table 3-5).

There are two common techniques used to measure blood pressure with a sphygmomanometer: (1) **auscultation** (os-skul-TAY-shun), when a stethoscope is used to listen for characteristic sounds (Figure 3-16); and (2) **palpation**, when the radial pulse or brachial pulse is palpated (felt) with the finger tips (Figure 3-17).

TABLE 3-5 Blood Pressure—Indications of Very Serious Problems

Patient	Systolic (mmHg)	Diastolic (mmHg)
Adult	Above 180 Below 90	Above 104 Below 60

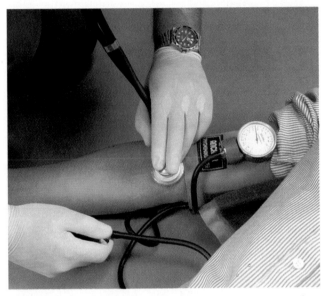

Figure 3-16 Measuring blood pressure by auscultation.

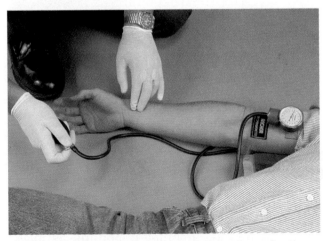

Figure 3-17 Measuring blood pressure by palpation.

- *Determining blood pressure by auscultation*—Begin by placing the tips of the stethoscope arms in your ears (the earpieces should be pointing forward). The patient should be seated or lying down. If the patient has not been injured, support his arm at the level of his heart. With your fingertips, palpate the brachial artery at the crease of the elbow. Position the diaphragm of the stethoscope directly over the brachial pulse site or over the medial anterior elbow if no brachial pulse site can be determined. Do not place the head of the stethoscope underneath the cuff, since this will give you false readings.

With the bulb valve (thumb valve) closed, inflate the cuff. As you do so, you soon will be able to hear pulse sounds. Inflate the cuff, watching the gauge. At a certain point, you will no longer hear the brachial pulse. Continue to inflate the cuff until the gauge reads 30 mmHg higher than the point where the pulse sound disappeared.

Slowly release air from the cuff by opening the bulb valve, allowing the pressure to fall smoothly at the rate of approximately 2 mmHg per second.

Listen for the start of clicking or tapping sounds. When you hear the beginning of these sounds, note the reading on the gauge. This is the systolic pressure. Continue to deflate the cuff, listening for the point at which these distinctive sounds fade (not when they disappear*). When the sounds turn to dull, muffled thuds, the reading on the gauge is the diastolic pressure. After obtaining the diastolic pressure, let the cuff deflate rapidly. If you are not certain of a reading, repeat the procedure. You should use the other arm or wait one minute before re-inflating the cuff. Otherwise, you will tend to obtain an erroneously high reading.

Record the measurements and the time of determination. For example, "B.P. is 140/90." Blood pressure is reported in even numbers. If a reading falls between two lines on the gauge, use the higher number.

If you are not sure of the reading you are getting, try again or get some help. Never make up vital signs!

Some patients who have high systolic blood pressures will have the pulse sounds *disappear* as you deflate the cuff, only to have these sounds *reappear* as you contin-

*This may be just the opposite in your state.

ue with the deflation. When this happens, *false* systolic and diastolic readings may be obtained. If you determine a high diastolic reading, wait from 1 to 2 minutes and take another reading. As you inflate the cuff, feel for the disappearance of the radial pulse to ensure that you are not measuring a false diastolic pressure. Listen as you deflate the cuff down into the normal range. The diastolic pressure is the reading at which the last fade of sound takes place.

- *Determining blood pressure by palpation*— This method is not as accurate as the auscultation method, since only an *approximate* systolic pressure can be determined. The technique is used when there is too much noise around a patient to allow the use of the stethoscope or when the situation involves many patients and too few persons to deliver care.

    Begin by finding the radial pulse site on the limb to which the blood pressure cuff has been applied. Make certain that the adjustable valve is closed on the bulb and inflate the cuff to a point where you can no longer feel the radial pulse. Note this point on the gauge and continue to inflate the cuff 30 mmHg beyond this point.

    Slowly deflate the cuff, noting the reading at which the radial pulse returns. This reading is the patient's systolic pressure. Record your findings as, for example, "Blood pressure 140 by palpation" or "140/P." and the time of the determination. (You cannot determine a diastolic reading by palpation.)

Relative Skin Temperature Some areas have EMTs measure oral, axillary (armpit), or rectal temperatures for a determination of body temperature for certain patients. However, most area guidelines for basic EMT-level care call for a measurement of relative skin temperature. This is not a true vital sign in higher levels of care, but in the field it is useful to find abnormally high and low temperatures.

Note: While determining relative skin temperature you also should note skin color and condition.

To determine skin temperature and condition, feel the patient's forehead with the back of your hand (Figure 3-18). Note if his skin feels *normal, warm, hot, cool,* or *cold.* At the same time, notice if his skin is *dry, moist,* or *clammy.*

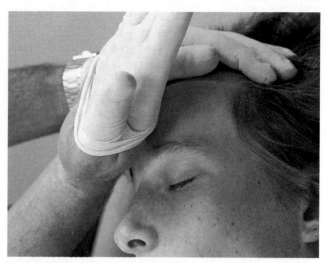

Figure 3-18 Determining relative skin temperature.

TABLE 3-6 Temperature Variations and Relevant Medical Conditions

Skin Temperature	Possible Cause of Abnormality
Cool, clammy	Usual sign of shock, anxiety
Cold, moist	Body is losing heat
Cold, dry	Body has been exposed to cold and has lost considerable heat
Hot, dry	Excessive body heat (as in heatstroke and high fever)
Hot, moist	High fever, heat exhaustion
"Goose pimples" accompanied by shivering, chattering teeth, blue lips, and pale skin	Chills, communicable disease, exposure to cold, pain, or fear

Look for "goose pimples," which are often associated with chills. Many patient problems are exhibited by changes in skin temperature and condition. As you continue with the assessment and care of the patient, be alert for major *temperature differences* on various parts of the body. For example, you may note that the patient's trunk is warm but his left arm feels cold. Such a finding can direct you to detecting problems with circulation (Table 3-6).

The Head-to-Toe Survey

The head-to-toe procedure (a toe-to-head sequence is less frightening for children 6 years or younger) is a systematic approach designed to prevent your missing anything important, as might happen if you "skipped around" during the physical exam. The head-to-toe survey may cause the patient some pain and discomfort. Warn the patient of these possibilities. Ask the patient to let you know when anything that you do causes pain. The more systematic you are in your approach and the better you know how to conduct each aspect of the examination, the less likely you are to cause pain and discomfort. As an EMT, you MUST know the head-to-toe procedures and be able to perform each move without any hesitation.

All of the survey does not have to be performed on every patient. The survey is geared to the patient's chief complaint, the nature of the accident or illness, and the seriousness of his condition. A commonsense approach should be taken.

Take care not to contaminate wounds and aggravate injuries. If bleeding has obviously stopped, *do not* pull the clothing or skin around the site. *Do not* probe into the site.

Readjust, remove, or cut away only those articles of patient clothing that interfere with your ability to examine the patient. *Do not* try to pull clothing off the limbs of a patient. Such procedures could increase bleeding and worsen existing injuries.

Be certain to tell the patient that you have to rearrange his clothing and explain why this must be done. Do all you can to ensure the patient's privacy, even if it means asking bystanders to face away from the patient or to hold up a blanket to serve as a shield.

Some authorities recommend having a woman EMT present during the examination of a female patient by a male EMT. However, no one recommends delaying the examination or care of a patient of the opposite sex. As a professional EMT, your intentions should be respected.

During the head-to-toe survey
- LOOK—for discolorations, deformities, penetrations, wounds, openings in the neck, and any unusual chest movements.
- FEEL—for deformities, tenderness, pulsations, abnormal hardness or softness, spasms, and skin temperature.
- LISTEN—for changes in breathing patterns, unusual breathing sounds, and any grating noises made by the ends of broken bones (do not ask the patient to move or move his limbs so that you can confirm grating sounds).
- SMELL—for any unusual odors coming from the patient's body, breath, or clothing.

The head-to-toe survey appears to be a long process, but as you practice the procedure you will find that it can be done in a few minutes.

Conducting the Head-to-Toe Survey

Conduct a head-to-toe survey, wearing all necessary protective equipment. If anything looks, feels, sounds, or smells strange to you, assume that there is something seriously wrong with the patient.

There may be some variation in the head-to-toe survey depending on local guidelines. Traditionally, the examination started with the head. However, most medical authorities now recommend that the neck be examined first in an effort to detect possible spinal injuries and any serious injury to the trachea (windpipe) that may lead to airway obstruction. When such injuries are detected, the head and neck can be immobilized to reduce chances of aggravating spinal or airway injury during the rest of the survey.

Begin your head-to-toe survey by placing yourself in a full kneeling position at the side of the patient's head. Take a quick overview of the patient's body. You should then perform the 26 steps described in the following section. (See also Scan 3-4.)

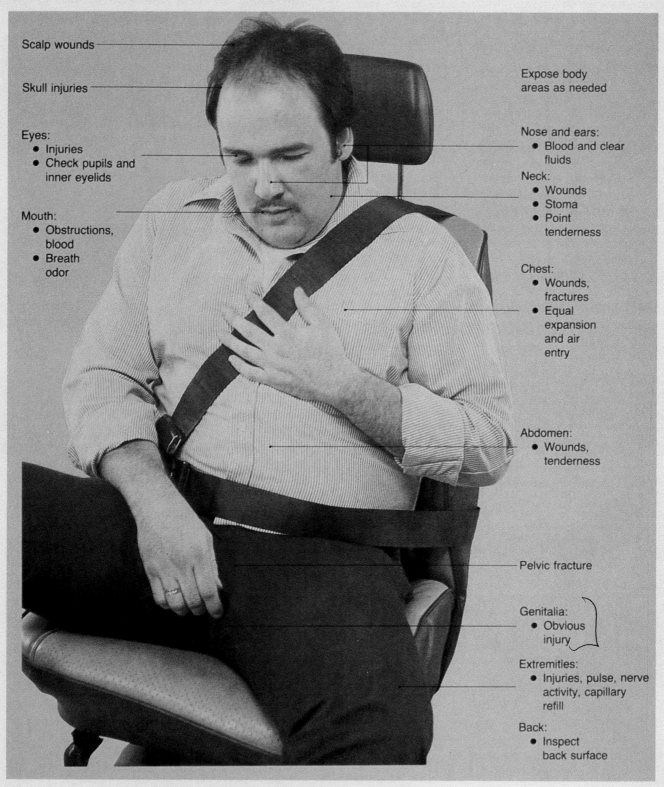

Scalp wounds

Skull injuries

Eyes:
- Injuries
- Check pupils and inner eyelids

Mouth:
- Obstructions, blood
- Breath odor

Expose body areas as needed

Nose and ears:
- Blood and clear fluids

Neck:
- Wounds
- Stoma
- Point tenderness

Chest:
- Wounds, fractures
- Equal expansion and air entry

Abdomen:
- Wounds, tenderness

Pelvic fracture

Genitalia:
- Obvious injury

Extremities:
- Injuries, pulse, nerve activity, capillary refill

Back:
- Inspect back surface

Note: Examine the neck first to detect possible cervical spine injury.

Head-to-Toe Survey

1. CHECK THE CERVICAL SPINE FOR POINT TENDERNESS AND DEFORMITY.

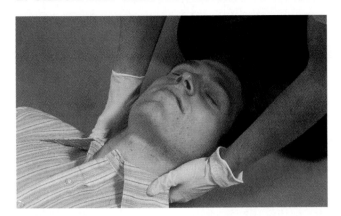

PROCEDURE: The portion of the spinal column that runs through the neck is called the **cervical** (SER-ve-kal) **spine**. Prepare the patient for possible pain. With the palms up, *gently* slide your hands under the sides of the patient's neck, moving your fingertips toward the cervical midline. Check the back of the neck from the shoulders to the base of the skull. Apply gentle finger pressure. A painful response to this pressure is **point tenderness**.

POSSIBLE FINDINGS: Midline deformities, point tenderness, or muscle spasms indicate possible cervical spinal injury. You cannot rule out, or exclude, cervical spine injury if there is no point tenderness.

Note: If there are signs of possible spinal injury, stop the survey and provide stabilization of the head and neck. This can be done manually by another EMT.

Warning: If the patient is seated or in an unusual position, stabilize the head with one hand on his chin while you inspect with your other hand. If possible, have another EMT stabilize the head. If a rigid collar is to be applied, make certain that you have examined the posterior, anterior, and sides of the neck before its application.

2. INSPECT THE ANTERIOR NECK FOR INDICATIONS OF INJURY AND NECK BREATHING.

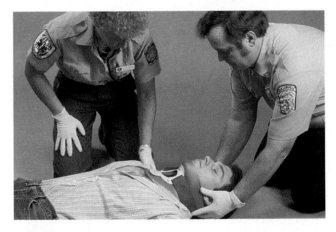

PROCEDURE: The anterior neck must be exposed so that you can check for surgical openings or a metal or plastic tube that indicates the patient is a "neck breather." See if the patient has a **stoma** (STO-mah), or permanent surgical opening in the neck through which he breathes. He may have a **tracheostomy** (TRA-ke-OS-to-me). This is a surgical incision held open by a metal or plastic tube or tubes. In either case, the patient will breathe through the opening. This probably would have been discovered during the primary survey, especially if the patient's chest is rising but he has no air exchange from nose or mouth.

Look for signs of injury. Does the larynx (voice box) or trachea (windpipe) appear to be deviated from the midline of the neck? Are there bruises or deformities? Penetrating injuries? Is there distention of the jugular vein (the large vein in the side of the neck)? If so, the patient may have an obstructed airway (determined during the primary survey), a cervical spine injury, damage to the trachea, or a serious chest injury.

Look for a medical identification necklace if you did not already find one during the primary survey. Note the information provided, but *do not* remove the necklace.

After the anterior neck has been examined, a rigid cervical or extrication collar should be applied if spinal injury is suspected (see Chapter 12). If the patient is unconscious, assume that there is spinal injury.

POSSIBLE FINDINGS: Cuts, bruises, discolorations, deformities, or signs of airway deviation may be seen. Bruises or deformities directly over the trachea may indicate that if a serious airway obstruction does not already exist, it will soon occur owing to tissue swelling or a ruptured trachea (immediate care is needed). The patient may have a stoma. There may be a medical identification necklace.

3. INSPECT THE SCALP FOR WOUNDS.

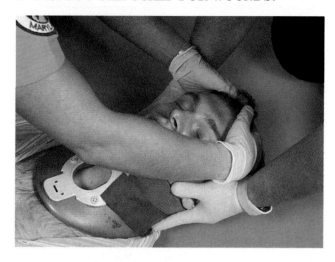

PROCEDURE: Extreme care must be exercised so as not to move the patient's head, aggravating possible spinal injuries. Move to the top of the patient's head and run your gloved fingers gently through the patient's hair, feeling the scalp. If you believe you have found an injury site, *do not* separate strands of hair matted over the site. To do so may restart bleeding. When the patient is found lying on his back, check the hidden part of his scalp by placing your fingers behind his neck. Slide them upward toward the top of his head. Check your fingers for blood. If you have any reason to believe there are spinal or neck injuries, *delay* this procedure until the head and neck are immobilized. Also, *do not* lift the head

off the ground to bandage it if you suspect neck injury.

POSSIBLE FINDINGS: Blood, cuts, puncture wounds, swellings or hematomas ("goose eggs"), deformities, and any other indications of injury may be found.

Note: You may find the patient is wearing a hairpiece or wig. If so, you will feel the netting of the hairpiece or the border where the piece or wig joins the patient's natural hairline. *Do not* try to remove the hairpiece. It may be held in place by adhesive, tape, or permanent glue. To attempt removal may aggravate injuries or restart bleeding. Some wigs remove easily; others may have to be cut away. This may prove to be a difficult procedure, forcing you to combine cutting and sliding to remove the wig, which may cause undesired movement of the head and neck. Proper immobilization of the head and neck must be done before attempting wig removal. Unless you suspect profuse bleeding, it is best to leave the wig in place. It is probably acting as an effective dressing. If the patient is wearing a hairpiece, gently feel through the netting for bleeding or deformity. *Do not* reach under a wig to inspect the scalp.

Warning: Take great care not to drive bone fragments or force dirt into any scalp wound while examining or pressing the scalp with your fingers.

4. CHECK THE SKULL AND FACE FOR DEFORMITIES AND DEPRESSIONS.

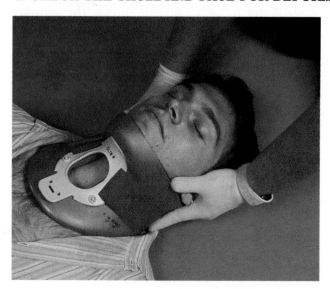

PROCEDURE: While feeling the scalp, note any depressions or bony projections that would indicate possible injury to the skull. Visually check the facial bones for any signs of fractures. Gently palpate the cheekbones, forehead, and lower jaw unless there are obvious signs of injury.

POSSIBLE FINDINGS: Depressions, bony projections, obvious breaks in the bones, swellings, heavy discolorations, or the obvious crushing of bones.

5. EXAMINE THE PATIENT'S EYES.

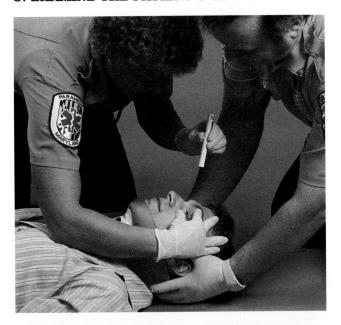

PROCEDURE: Return to a side position. Begin by looking at the patient's eyelids. Have the patient open his eyes. With unresponsive patients, gently open their eyes by sliding back the upper eyelids. Visually check the globe of each eye. Do not apply pressure on the eyeballs.

POSSIBLE FINDINGS: Cuts, foreign objects, impaled objects, bruising or discoloration around the eyes, and signs of burns may be noted.

Warning: Do not attempt to open the eyelids of a patient with burns, cuts, or other injuries to the eyelids. Assume there is damage to the eye and treat accordingly (See Chapter 13).

6. CHECK THE PUPILS FOR SIZE, EQUALITY, AND REACTIVITY.

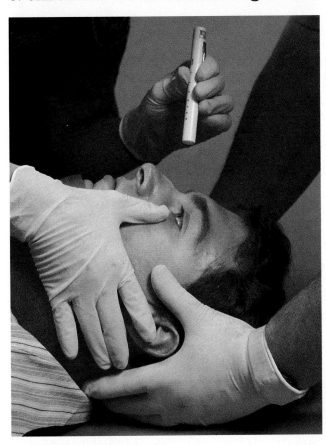

PROCEDURE: Use your penlight to examine both eyes. Note pupil size and if both pupils are equal in size. See if the pupils react to the beam of light. Note if the pupils are slow to react. Note

any eye movements. Both eyes should move as a pair when they track persons or objects.

POSSIBLE FINDINGS: Pupils are *normal*, *constricted* (small), or *dilated* (large). Pupils are either *equal* or *unequal* in size. Pupils react to the beam of light, or one or both are fixed. The eyes may appear *lackluster* (dull). Tracking (movement of the eyes to follow a moving object) may be *normal* or *abnormal*.

Pupil Size	*Possible Cause of Abnormality*
Dilated, unresponsive	Cardiac arrest, influence of drugs such as LSD and amphetamines, unconsciousness from numerous causes
Constricted, unresponsive	Central nervous system disease or disorder, influence of narcotic such as heroin, morphine, or codeine
Unequal	Stroke, head injury
Lackluster, pupils do not appear to focus	Shock, coma

Note: Check the unconscious patient for contact lenses. Many EMS Systems' guidelines recommend prompt removal of these lenses to help prevent damage to the patient's eyes. Contact lens removal procedures are described in Chapter 13. If possible, close the eyes of unconscious patients so they remain lubricated.

7. INSPECT THE INNER SURFACES OF THE EYELIDS.

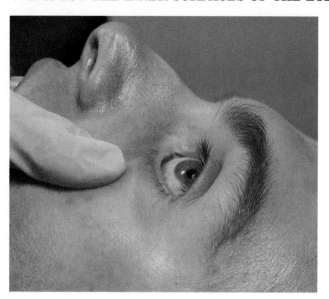

PROCEDURE: Gently pull down either lower eyelid and check the color of the inner surface.

POSSIBLE FINDINGS: Normally these surfaces should be pink. However, with blood loss they become pale or with jaundice, they become yellow. This is an excellent place to see cyanosis (blue color), especially in patients with dark skin pigmentation.

Warning: *Do not* attempt to open the eyelid of a patient with obvious eye injury.

8. INSPECT THE EARS AND NOSE FOR INJURY AND BLOOD OR CLEAR FLUIDS.

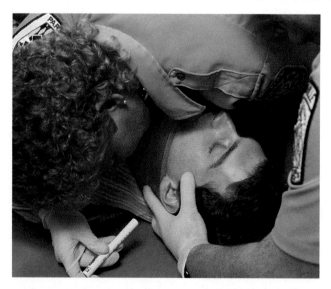

PROCEDURE: Observe the ears and nose for cuts, tears, and burns. Look carefully in the ears and nose for blood, clear fluids, or bloody fluids. Carefully look for bruises behind the ears, commonly called "Battle's sign" (a late finding).

POSSIBLE FINDINGS: Blood in the nose may be the result of simple nasal tissue injury (a bloody nose). It could also indicate a skull fracture. Blood in the ears and clear fluids in the ears or nose are strong indicators of skull fracture. This clear fluid may be **cerebrospinal** (ser-e-bro-SPI-nal) **fluid (CSF)**, a watery substance that surrounds the brain and spinal cord. If the patient is sitting, the CSF may drain into the throat and taste salty to the patient. Bruises behind the ears are strong indicators of possible skull and cervical spine injury. Burned or singed nasal hairs indicate possible burns to the airway.

Warning: *Do not* rotate the patient's head to inspect the ears.

9. INSPECT THE MOUTH.

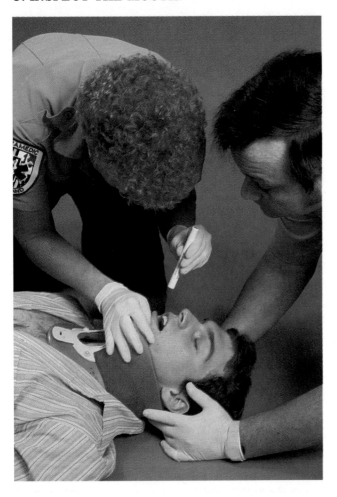

PROCEDURE: Look for anything that may have been missed during the primary survey that may be causing or could become an AIRWAY OBSTRUCTION. Take care not to move the patient's head during this inspection. Look for chemical burns or soot from smoke around the mouth.

POSSIBLE FINDINGS: Foreign objects, broken teeth, broken dentures, blood, or vomitus may be found. The tongue may be swollen, discolored, injured, or obstructing the airway. Chemical burns suggest that the patient may have ingested a poison.

10. SNIFF FOR AN ODD BREATH ODOR.

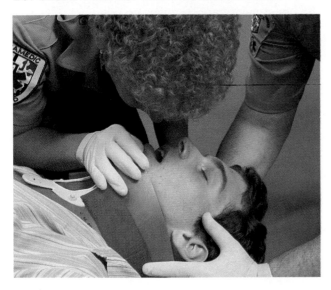

PROCEDURE: Position your face close to the patient's mouth and nose and note any unusual odors.

POSSIBLE FINDINGS: A fruity smell (diabetic coma or prolonged vomiting and diarrhea), petroleum odor (ingested poisoning), or alcohol (alcohol intoxication) may be noted.

Note: You will need to expose the examination areas. The lower chest and abdomen must be exposed to observe chest movements. Listen for equal air entry, check for penetrations, and palpate the abdomen for tenderness. Be certain to protect the patient from the stares of onlookers. Remember, clothing that cannot be easily rearranged should be cut away.

11. INSPECT THE CHEST FOR WOUNDS.

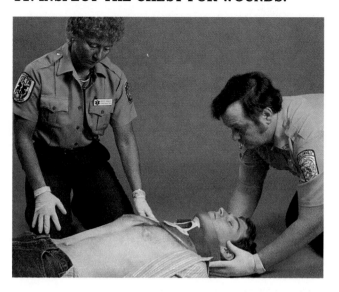

PROCEDURE: Look for obvious injuries. Follow local protocol in regard to baring the patient's chest. It is best to bare the chest of an unconscious patient or trauma patient. If there are any indications of chest injury or the patient has breathing problems (a respiratory rate less than 10 or greater than 28 in an adult patient), completely bare the chest.

POSSIBLE FINDINGS: Cuts, bruises, penetrations, impaled objects, deformities, burns, or rashes. If puncture wounds are found, they may indicate that an object has passed through the chest. You will have to feel or look for exit wounds when inspecting the back.

12. EXAMINE THE CHEST FOR POSSIBLE FRACTURES.

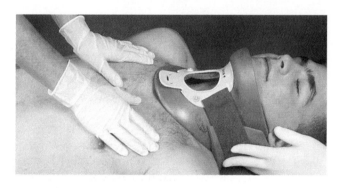

PROCEDURE: Warn the patient of possible pain and gently feel the clavicles (KLAV-i-kulz). These are the collarbones. Next, gently feel the sternum (STER-num). This is the breastbone. Feel the entire rib cage for deformities. Use your hands to apply gentle pressure to the sides of the rib cage. This process, known as compression, usually produces pain in cases of fractured ribs. When applying compression, position your forearms as shown. Finally, gently slide your hands under the patient's scapulae (SKAP-u-le). These are the shoulder blades. Feel for deformity and tenderness.

POSSIBLE FINDINGS: Point tenderness, painful reaction to compression, deformity, or grating sounds may occur. If air is felt (like crunching popcorn) or heard (crackling sounds) under the skin, this indicates that at least one rib has been fractured or that there is a pneumothorax (punctured lung; see Chapter 14). Air is escaping into the chest cavity and the wound.

13. CHECK FOR EQUAL EXPANSION OF THE CHEST.

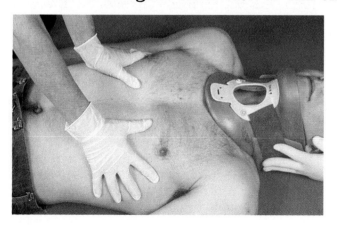

PROCEDURE: Look for chest movements and feel for equal expansion. Be on the alert for sections of the chest that seem to be "floating" or moving in opposite directions to the rest of the chest during respirations.

POSSIBLE FINDINGS: Deformed chest, loss of chest symmetry, or floating (flail) sections may be found.

14. LISTEN FOR SOUNDS OF EQUAL AIR ENTRY.

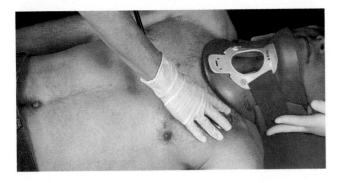

PROCEDURE: Most EMS Systems have their EMTs perform breathing sound assessment using a stethoscope. Most EMTs are trained to assess equal entry and breathing sounds for the supine and the seated patient (anterior and lateral assessment). The majority of EMS Systems have been training their EMTs to increase their level of skills in this assessment.

Use your stethoscope to listen to both sides of the anterior and lateral chest. The sounds of air entry will usually be clearly present or clearly absent. See Scan 3-5.

POSSIBLE FINDINGS: The absence of air movement indicates injury or illness to the internal chest or lungs. Bubbling, wheezing, rubbing, or crackling sounds may indicate a medical problem or injury from trauma.

15. INSPECT THE ABDOMEN FOR WOUNDS.

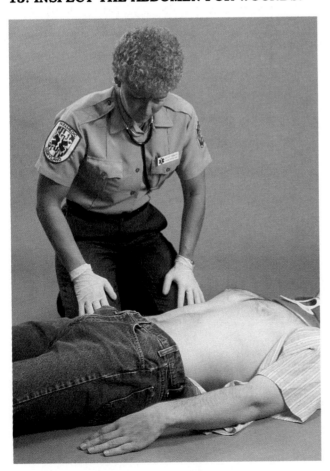

PROCEDURE: Look for obvious signs of injury in all quadrants or sides.

POSSIBLE FINDINGS: Cuts, bruises, penetrations, impaled objects, open wounds with protruding organs (evisceration), rashes, or burns may be seen. The patient may have his legs drawn up to help guard his abdomen.

Note: The patient may have had a **colostomy** (ko-LOS-to-me) or **ileostomy** (il-e-OS-to-me). You will see a surgical opening in the abdominal wall and a bag in place to receive excretions from the digestive tract. Do not remove the bag. Having this bag exposed may be embarrassing to the patient. If you note this bag when rearranging or cutting away clothing, make every effort to keep it covered by clothing or other suitable materials. Be careful when cutting clothing in this area not to cut such a bag that may be hidden by the clothing.

16. PALPATE THE ABDOMEN FOR TENDERNESS.

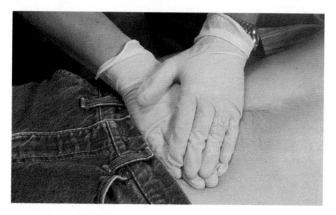

PROCEDURE: Look for any attempts by the patient to protect the abdomen (e.g., knees pulled up). Prepare the patient for possible pain and then gently palpate his entire abdomen (all four quadrants). If the patient tells you he has pain limited to a specific area of the abdomen, palpate this site last. When practical, make sure your hands are warm. Press in on the abdomen with the palm side of your fingers, depressing the surface about one inch. Many rescuers prefer to use two hands, one on top of the other at the fingertips. Do not palpate over an obvious injury site or where the patient is having severe pain. Always start away from an area of pain. Note any painful response. Ask the conscious patient. "Does this hurt?" "Can you feel this?" The patient may show tensing of the abdominal muscles. While palpating the abdomen for tenderness, note any tight (rigid) or swollen (distended) areas. Stay alert for any lumps (masses) that may be felt through the abdominal wall. Palpating for injuries is important because if an area is tender it usually does not hurt until palpated.

POSSIBLE FINDINGS: If the pain is confined to one spot, it is said to be *localized*. Should it be spread over the entire abdomen, it is classified as *general* or *diffuse*. Relate painful responses to the abdominal quadrants. Specifically note guarding, rigidity, distention, masses, tenderness, spasms, or pulsations. Pain types as reported by the patient may be *sharp*, *tearing*, *colicky*, *crampy*, or *dull* in nature.

17. FEEL THE LOWER BACK FOR POINT TENDERNESS AND DEFORMITY.

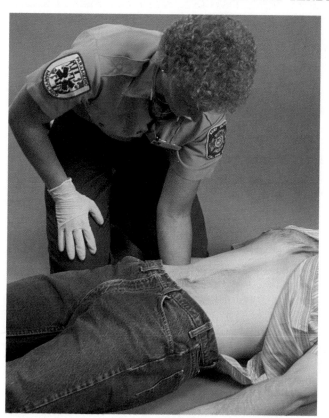

PROCEDURE: Prepare the patient for possible pain and gently slide your hand under the void (space) created by the curve of the spine. Apply gentle finger pressure to detect both point tenderness and deformity. (Sometimes this area is saved for last, for when the patient is ready to be log rolled onto a backboard. Palpate the void space, prepare to log roll the patient onto the board, and when back is exposed visually examine and palpate the back as described in Step 26.)

POSSIBLE FINDINGS: Point tenderness or deformity suggests possible spinal injury and may require you to immobilize the patient's spine before continuing the survey.

Warning: *Do not* attempt to inspect the upper back of the patient at this time. To do so will require you to lift the patient slightly. You have yet to rule out spinal damage and damage to the upper extremities that could be aggravated by such a procedure.

18. EXAMINE THE PELVIS FOR INJURIES AND POSSIBLE FRACTURES.

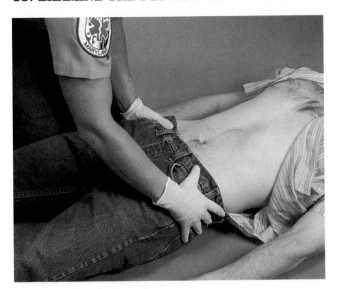

PROCEDURE: Evaluate the pelvic area for obvious injuries. Next, gently slide your hands from the small of the patient's back to the lateral wings of the pelvis and gently apply compression downward and then inward to check the stability of the pelvic girdle. Again, warn the patient of possible pain, then lightly apply compression to the pelvis, noting any painful response and pelvic deformities. Do not place your hands over any obvious injury site.

POSSIBLE FINDINGS: Penetrating wounds, impaled objects, deformity, and compression pain or pain upon the release of compression may be found. There may be grating sounds if the injury also involves the hip joint or if the pelvis is fractured.

19. NOTE ANY OBVIOUS INJURY TO THE GENITAL (GROIN) REGION.

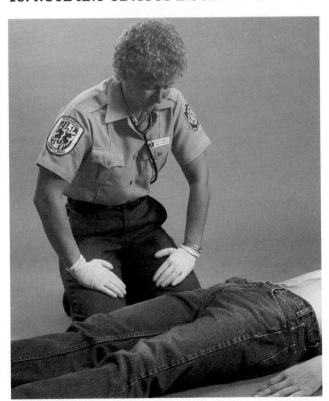

Look for **priapism** (PRE-ah-pizm) in male patients. This is a persistent erection of the penis often brought about by spinal injury or certain medical problems (e.g., sickle cell crisis). Usually, there are other signs of spinal injury or the mechanism of injury requires you to assume that there is spinal injury. Noting this sign by touching the patient will not provide you with any information that will change the care to be rendered.

POSSIBLE FINDINGS: Bleeding wounds and impaled objects, burns, and the spinal injury sign of priapism.

Note: When examining the lower limbs and feet, it may be necessary to rearrange or cut away clothing. Injury to the lower limb is best observed with little additional aggravation if pants legs are cut away from the site. Cutting is best done along the seams. If there is a painful response when you feel the patient's foot, or there is no sign of injury, you may not need to remove the patient's shoes (follow local protocol). A pulse can be taken without removing low-cut shoes. If the patient is wearing gym shoes, high-top dress shoes, or boots, it may be necessary to cut the laces or to cut away the footwear if unlacing and removal might aggravate an injury. *Do not* attempt to remove ski boots unless you are specifically trained in the procedure.

PROCEDURE: Look for bleeding and impaled objects, but *do not* expose the area unless you are reasonably sure that an injury has been sustained.

20. EXAMINE THE LOWER LIMBS AND FEET.

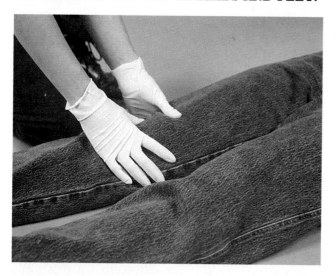

PROCEDURE: Inspect each limb, one at a time, from hip to foot, looking for signs of injury. Look for any abnormal inward or outward rotation of the lower limbs. Gently feel along the front and sides of each limb. Unless the injury is obvious, carefully palpate any suspected fracture site for point tenderness, warning the patient beforehand.

POSSIBLE FINDINGS: Deformities, bleeding, bone protrusions, swellings, and discolorations may occur. One or both limbs may be rotated inward or outward.

Warning: *Do not* move or lift the patient's lower limbs. Do not change the positions of the limbs or feet from the position they were in at the beginning of the examination.

21. CHECK FOR A DISTAL PULSE AND CAPILLARY REFILL.

Note: A **distal pulse** is a pulse taken at the foot or the wrist. It is called a *distal* pulse because it is at the distal end of the limb. Absence of a distal pulse indicates that a major artery supplying

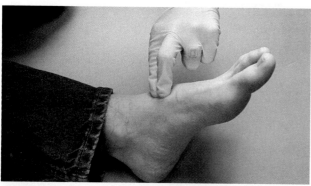

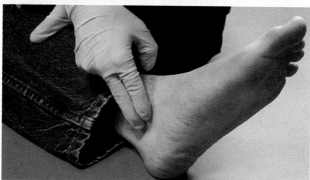

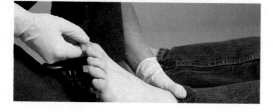

the limb has been pinched or severed, usually by a broken or displaced bone end or a blood clot. Absence or weakness of a distal pulse after a limb has been splinted or bandaged may indicate that the bandage is too tight.

Note: Most EMS systems have the EMT check for capillary refilling. (See Chapter 8 for more information.) This is done by squeezing the toe or finger or palm of the hand and then letting go. The extremity should blanch of blood under your finger (whiten as blood is squeezed out), then rapidly return to its original color. Capillary refill is said to be delayed if the return of color takes more than 2 seconds.

PROCEDURE: You need to know if circulation to both feet is impaired or interrupted. Palpate the distal pulse of each foot, called a **pedal pulse**, either behind the medial ankle (**posterior tibial pulse**) or on the anterior surface of the foot, lateral to the large tendon of the great toe (**dorsalis pedis pulse**). You must bare the patient's foot to palpate the dorsalis pedis pulse. The posterior tibial pulse is not as reliable as the dorsalis pedis pulse because in many healthy, uninjured people this pulse cannot be felt.

Compare the quality of the pulses in each lower limb.

POSSIBLE FINDINGS: Presence of a pulse indicates that circulation is intact, while no pulse suggests shock or that a major artery supplying the limb has been pinched, severed, or blocked.

Note: if you are unable to feel a pulse, check for skin color and capillary refill. (See Chapter 8.)

22. CHECK FOR NERVE FUNCTION AND POSSIBLE PARALYSIS OF THE LOWER EXTREMITIES—CONSCIOUS PATIENT.

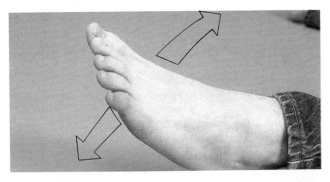

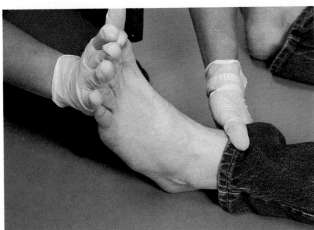

PROCEDURE: Touch a toe and ask the patient to identify which toe you touched. Do this for each foot. If the patient cannot feel your touch or the touch sensations for each foot are not the same, assume nerve damage in the limb or spinal damage (it is best to assume spinal damage). If sensation appears normal, have the patient wave his feet. Finally, ask the patient to press the sole of his foot gently against the palm of your hand. Do this for each foot if there are no signs of injury to the limbs.

POSSIBLE FINDINGS: Failure by the patient to accomplish any of these tasks or any difference in sensations for either limb indicates the possibility of injury to nerve pathways. At this point, ASSUME SPINAL INJURY.

CHECK FOR NERVE FUNCTION AND POSSIBLE PARALYSIS OF THE LOWER EXTREMITIES—UNCONSCIOUS PATIENT. (This may be optional since other signs and the mechanism of injury are more useful. Follow your local protocol.)

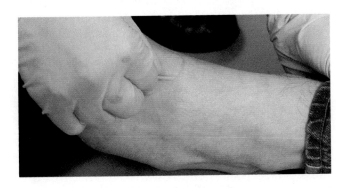

PROCEDURE: To test the unconscious patient for nerve function, grasp the patient's limb at or near the ankle and pinch an accessible distal area that appears free of injury.

POSSIBLE FINDINGS: The patient, even though unconscious, may show a reflex action by pulling the leg away or by making a pronounced upward or downward toe movement. There should be a reaction to pain. Failure to do so MUST be assumed to be the result of spinal injury; however, movement by the patient does not allow you to rule out possible spinal injury.

23. EXAMINE THE UPPER EXTREMITIES FOR INJURY.

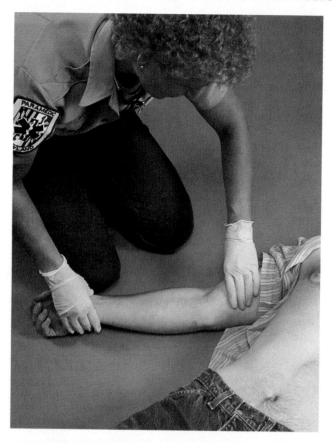

PROCEDURE: Check the patient from clavicles (collarbones) to fingertips. Look for signs of injury. Check for point tenderness at the site of possible fractures. Look for a medical identification bracelet.

POSSIBLE FINDINGS: Note any deformities, bleeding, bone protrusions, swellings, discolorations, rashes, or burns. Assume point tenderness to mean possible fracture. A medical identification bracelet may be found.

24. CHECK FOR A DISTAL PULSE.

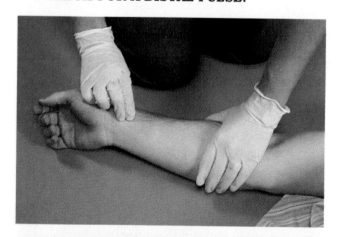

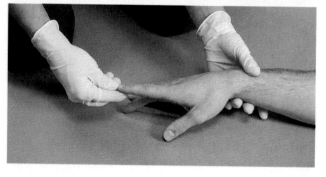

PROCEDURE: Confirm a radial pulse for each limb. (The procedure for taking a radial pulse is given under "Vital Signs" earlier in this chapter.) *Do not* measure pulse rate. Instead, compare the quality of each pulse. If the pulse is not palpable, check skin color and capillary return.

Note: Most EMS systems have the EMT check for capillary refilling. (See Chapter 8 for more information.) This is done by squeezing the toe or finger or palm of the hand and then letting go. The extremity should blanch of blood under your finger (whiten as blood is squeezed out), then rapidly return to its original color. Capillary refill is said to be delayed if the return of color takes more than 2 seconds.

POSSIBLE FINDINGS: Presence of a pulse indicates circulation is intact. The absence of a pulse suggests shock or that a major artery has been pinched, severed, or blocked by a clot. Most often, this is the result of a fracture to a bone in the limb.

25. CHECK FOR NERVE FUNCTION AND POSSIBLE PARALYSIS OF THE UPPER EXTREMITIES—CONSCIOUS PATIENT.

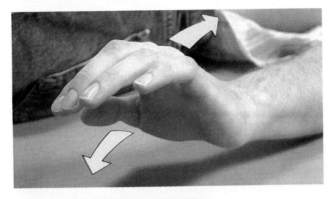

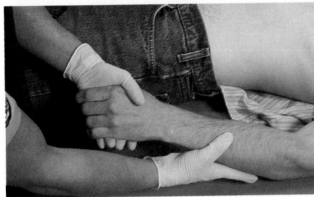

PROCEDURE: Have the conscious, responsive patient identify the finger you touch, wave his hand, and grasp your hand. Do this for each upper limb, only if the extremity is apparently uninjured.

POSSIBLE FINDINGS: If the patient fails to accomplish any of these tasks, there is possible injury to the nerve pathways. At this point, ASSUME SPINAL INJURY.

Warning: If an awake, alert patient cannot move his hands or arms, be on the alert for the rapid onset of difficult breathing or respiratory arrest due to a very high cervical injury. The patient's breathing will have to be constantly monitored.

CHECK FOR NERVE FUNCTION AND POSSIBLE PARALYSIS OF THE UPPER EXTREMITIES—UNCONSCIOUS PATIENT.

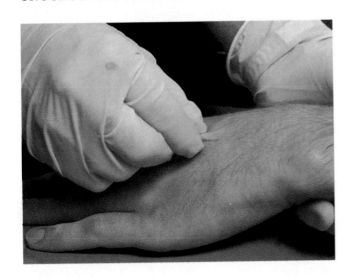

PROCEDURE: If the patient is unconscious or unresponsive, grasp his limb at or near the wrist and pinch an accessible distal area. Do this for each limb. The patient may try to pull his hand away or show some other reaction to the pain. If the patient is deeply unconscious, he will not move his hand. This test must be considered to be fairly unreliable under field conditions.

POSSIBLE FINDINGS: Failure of the patient to react to the pain stimulus must be considered to be a sign of possible spinal injury. You would do well to assume that all unconscious trauma patients have possible spinal injury.

Note: If a patient fails to respond properly on any test for upper or lower extremity nerve function, *you must consider this to be a sign of spinal injury.*

26. INSPECT THE BACK AND BUTTOCKS FOR INJURY.

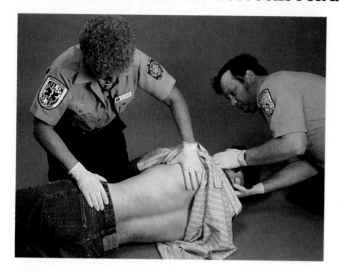

PROCEDURE: Provided there are no indications of injuries to the skull, neck, spine, or extremities, and you have no evidence of severe injury to the chest or abdomen, gently roll the conscious patient as a unit toward your knees and inspect the back surfaces for bleeding and obvious injuries.

The back surface can be inspected prior to positioning the patient for transport or delayed until the patient is transferred to a spine board or other immobilizing device.

POSSIBLE FINDINGS: Cuts, puncture wounds, impaled objects, and burns may be noted.

Note: Since possible neck and spinal injuries are difficult to detect in some unconscious patients, your local guidelines may state that this procedure should not be done unless you need to control profuse bleeding or it can be done while repositioning or immobilizing the patient.

Assessing Breathing Sounds

BREATHING SOUNDS

- Rales—heard during inspiration. Air is passing through secretions or fluids in lower airways. Sounds range from crackling or powdery to gravelly or gurgling.
- Rhonchi—coarse "popping" or snoring noises heard during expiration (exception: asthma— also may be heard during inspiration). Sounds indicate a narrowing of larger lower airways.
- Wheezing—heard on expiration (or inspiration in more severe cases). A high-pitched, whistling sound associated with a narrowing of or an obstruction in the lower airways.

SIMPLE ASSESSMENT

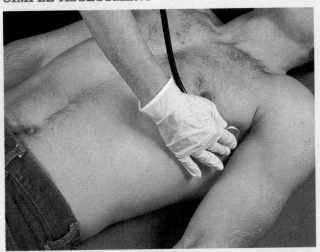

Listen for equal air entry on both sides of the chest.

MIDCLAVICULAR
(center of each clavicle, just below the bone)

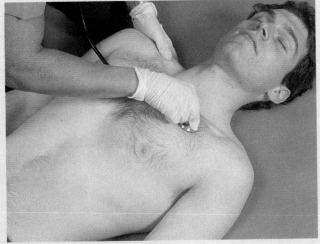

Listen for entry and sounds. For medical patients, assess supine and seated. Compare left side to right side.

MIDAXILLARY
(nipple level under the arm)

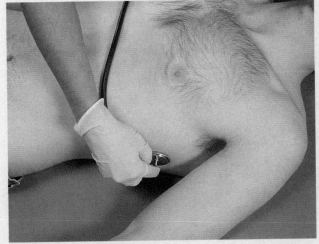

Listen for entry and sounds. For medical patients, assess supine and seated. Compare left side to right side.

SPECIAL ASSESSMENT CONCERNS

Patient assessment is the gathering of the information needed to help determine what is wrong with the patient. During this process, the first concern is to identify and correct any life-threatening problems. Always keep this in mind. It is foolish to be gathering information from bystanders while the patient is in cardiac arrest (his heart has stopped beating) or has some other life-threatening problem.

The patient assessment is a *systematic* procedure, but it is not always done in the same step-by-step order. Different types of patients will require different types of assessment. A patient who has been injured in an accident will need to be assessed differently than one who is having breathing problems related to a known illness. A serious injury to a patient's chest may require care that cannot wait until a complete survey is performed.

As an EMT you will have to assess

- Medical Patients—those who have problems related to infections, the failure of a body organ or system, a psychological problem, certain environmental factors (e.g., excessive cold), drugs or other chemical substances, or childbirth.
- Trauma Patients—those who have suffered trauma, that is, they have been injured or have a problem that has developed as a result of injury.*

You *must* always do as complete a survey as possible. Medical patients who are clearly free of injury can be assessed to obtain information relating directly to their medical problem. However, some medical patients suffer falls or other types of accidents and will require assessments that consider possible injury. Trauma patients will need to be assessed so that you may determine the nature and extent of their injuries and, when possible, any medical problems. This is done because trauma patients may have pre-existing medical problems that need attention, may have caused an accident to take place because of medical problems, or may have medical problems surface because of an accident (e.g., a heart attack).

A patient's condition must be considered as a *dynamic process*. Something may change, requiring you to stop in the middle of an assessment and repeat a procedure you completed only seconds after you arrived. Also, the gathering of information does not end after the initial assessment. You will have to keep re-assessing the patient, gathering new information. This is called *monitoring* the patient.

No matter where you are in the information-gathering process, you must remember that as an EMT, your overriding concern at all times is your own safety. For the patient

- *Your First Concern* is to identify and attempt to correct life-threatening problems.
- *Your Second Concern* is to make a status decision about whether immediate transport is or is not needed on the basis of the patient's C (Critical), U (Unstable), P (Potentially Unstable), or S (Stable) status.
- *Your Third Concern* is to identify any other injuries or medical problems and to provide basic EMT-level care in an effort to stabilize the patient and, when possible, to reduce the severity of his problem.
- *Your Fourth Concern* is to try to keep the patient stable and to continue reassessing the patient in case his condition worsens or improves.

Problems with Assessment

As an EMT, you may face many problems that interfere with patient assessment. You will have to overcome other problems that may be unique to the emergency scene. Problems with assessment can include

- Dangerous scenes (e.g., fires, collapsing buildings, hazardous materials)
- Harsh environments (including unfavorable weather conditions)
- Unfavorable conditions (e.g., too much noise, darkness, no privacy for the patient)
- Unfavorable location (e.g., the bottom of a hill, around a blind curve, in water)
- Uncooperative bystanders and motorists
- Uncooperative patients
- Special patients (children, elderly, blind, deaf, non-English speaking, chronically ill, handicapped, and those affected by drugs, including alcohol)
- More than one patient (multi-casualty incident)
- Severe injury (especially spinal or head injury)
- Patients with more than one serious injury (multitrauma)

* The word trauma is often used in prehospital emergency care to refer to injury brought about by an accident or act of aggression. Note that the word also may be used to refer to psychological injury or the injury to tissues brought about by disease (e.g., traumatized heart muscle).

- Grotesque injuries that tax your emotional stability

Each of these problems will be considered at various points throughout this text. Many are covered in Chapters 21, 22, 24, and 29. As part of your complete training you will study traffic, crowd control, fire, and other dangers and problems at the scene. Some special problems (e.g., spinal injury) have been mentioned in this chapter, but we will delay in-depth studies of these problems until later.

Note: Assessment and care are meant to be done without risk to the rescuer. Keep in mind that direct contact with the patient's blood and body fluids may expose you to a dangerous infectious disease. Make certain that you wear the assigned protective equipment needed for assessment and care of all patients. The minimum protective equipment to be worn is disposable gloves. Eye protection (goggles or face shield), gowns, and masks should be worn as required by your agency's exposure control plan.

Approaches to Assessment and Care

As noted earlier, not every person requiring emergency care will have to be surveyed to the same depth. Some examples of assessment approaches are shown in Table 3-7. Every unconscious patient should be thoroughly examined, regardless of whether the emergency is due to illness or injury. Of course, if a life-threatening problem is found it is to be cared for immediately. Never delay basic life support in order to conduct a complete hands-on examination.

The Survey Form An assessment card provides a quick, positive means of recording information obtained during the interview and examination. In your system, this may be an individual form or it may be part of a prehospital care report. This form is a legal document and made part of the patient's medical records. If practical to do so, findings should be recorded as they are found. The survey procedure can be speeded up if one EMT conducts the survey while another records the findings. (For more information see Chapter 27 on communications and reports.)

Many EMS Systems are now including in the secondary survey a trauma score that includes a coma scale such as the Glasgow Coma Scale. An example of one such form in common use is shown in Figure 3-19. Table 3-8 shows the coded values for the revised trauma score that is used in some EMS Systems. More will be said about using the coma scale in Chapter 12.

TABLE 3-7 Examples of Approaches to Patient Assessment

Medical Problem (No Injuries)	
Conscious Patient	*Unconscious patient*
• Begin an interview, continuing to maintain verbal contact through the rest of assessment and care. Assess airway and if breathing is adequate during interview. • Determine vital signs (pulse, respirations, blood pressure, and relative skin temperature) and continue to determine level of consciousness. • Examine the patient as required, directed by the information obtained during the interview.	• Make certain that the patient has an open airway, adequate breathing, and a carotid pulse. Look for and control profuse bleeding or potential shock. Assess level of consciousness. Care for any life-threatening problems as they are detected. • Determine vital signs. • Examine the patient, but at the same time . . . • Begin to formally interview bystanders.
Trauma	
Conscious Patient	*Unconscious patient*
• Look for mechanism of injury. • Begin to interview the patient and check for adequate breathing and profuse bleeding. Stop the interview and care for any life-threatening problems as they are found. • Determine vital signs if the patient appears to be unstable. • Do a complete examination of the patient. • Determine the patient's vital signs.	• Look for mechanism of injury. • Assess patient for airway, breathing, carotid pulse, and profuse bleeding or signs of shock. Expose the body to look for other life threatening injuries. Correct life-threatening problems as they are found. (Status critical or unstable: load and go!). • Take vital signs. • Conduct a complete examination of the patient, but at the same time . . . • Begin to formally interview bystanders. • Determine the patient's vital signs.

THE CHAMPION SACCO TRAUMA SCORE

The Trauma Score is used to give each injured patient a numerical score that can be used to estimate the severity of injury. The patient is graded in terms of cardiopulmonary and neurologic functions. Each category receives a numerical score. A high number indicates normal function, while a low number signifies impaired function. The numbers are totaled to give a Trauma Score. The lowest possible score is 1 (severe impairment). The highest possible score is 16 (normal for all categories).

The use of the Trauma Score can help to determine the order of care and transport, the level of care required, and if transport to a special facility is needed

Each patient should be scored during the initial assessment and each time that vital signs are taken.

The following is based on the Trauma Score developed by Champion and Sacco. For additional information, see: Champion HR, Sacco WJ, Carnazzo AJ, et al: Trauma Score. *Critical Care Medicine* 9 (9): 672-676, 1981. Note that variations of this procedure have been adopted by some EMS Systems.

WARNING: Follow local guidelines if you are allowed to apply painful stimuli to a patient. Your local protocol should include what actions you may take when the mechanism of injury or state of consciousness indicates possible spinal injury.

TRAUMA SCORE

Respiratory Rate	10-24/min	4	
	24-35/min	3	
	36/min or greater	2	
	1-9/min	1	
	None	0	
Respiratory Expansion	Normal	1	
	Retractive	0	
Systolic Blood Pressure	90 mmHg or greater	4	
	70-89 mmHg	3	
	50-69 mmHg	2	
	0-49 mmHg	1	
	No Pulse	0	
Capillary Refill	Normal	2	
	Delayed	1	
	None	0	
Cardiopulmonary Assessment			

GLASGOW COMA SCALE

Eye Opening	Spontaneous	4	
	To Voice	3	
	To Pain	2	
	None	1	
Verbal Response	Oriented	5	
	Confused	4	
	Inappropriate Words	3	
	Incomprehensible Words	2	
	None	1	
Motor Response	Obeys Command	6	
	Localizes Pain	5	
	Withdraw (pain)	4	
	Flexion (pain)	3	
	Extension (pain)	2	
	None	1	
Glasgow Coma Score Total			

TOTAL GLASGOW COMA SCALE POINTS

14-15=5
11-13=4
8-10=3
5-7=2
3-4=1

CONVERSION = APPROXIMATELY ONE-THIRD TOTAL VALUE

Neurologic Assessment

Total Trauma Score = Cardiopulmonary + Neurologic ⟶

Figure 3-19 The Champion Sacco Trauma Score.

SCORING THE PATIENT

There are four elements to the cardiopulmonary assessment. The numerical values are added together to produce a cardiopulmonary score.

There are three elements to the neurological assessment. These are derived from the Glasgow Coma Score. Each category of the Glasgow Coma Score is given a numerical value. These numerical values are added together to produce a subtotal. This number is then reduced by approximately one-third its value to produce the neurologic assessment score.

The cardiopulmonary assessment and the neurologic assessment scores are added together to give the Trauma Score.

For example, a patient has a respiratory rate of 30 breaths per minute (3), retractive chest movements (0), a systolic blood pressure of 80 mmHg (3), and delayed capillary refill (1). The total score for cardiopulmonary function is 3+0+3+1=7.

This same patient shows no eye opening (1), no verbal response (1), and an extension reaction to pain (2). Added together, the total is 4. Approximately one-third of this number is 1. The cardiopulmonary and neurologic scores are added together (7+1) to give a Trauma Score of 8.

TRAUMA SCORE DEFINITIONS

RESPIRATION RATE
The number of respirations (1 inspiration and 1 expiration) in 30 seconds, multiplied by two.

RESPIRATION EXPANSION
NORMAL – clearly visible chest wall movements that are associated with breathing.
RETRACTIVE – the use of accessory muscles (neck and abdominal muscles) to assist with breathing.

SYSTOLIC BLOOD PRESSURE
The systolic pressure recorded by auscultation or palpation.

CAPILLARY REFILL
This is determined by pressing a nail bed, the skin on the forehead, or the lining of the mouth (oral mucosa) until there is a loss of normal color (blanching or turning white). The pressure is released and the time for color to return is measured. Normal return of color will take place in approximately two seconds (about the time it takes to say to yourself, "capillary refill").
NORMAL REFILL – the color returns within two seconds.
DELAYED REFILL – the color returns sometime after two seconds.
NONE – there is no indication of capillary refill.

GLASGOW COMA SCALE DEFINITIONS

EYE OPENING
This test is valid only if there is no injury or swelling that prevents the patient from opening the eyes.
SPONTANEOUS – the patient opens his or her eyes without any stimulation.
TO VOICE – the patient will open his or her eyes in response to your request. Say, "Open your eyes." If the patient's eyes remain unopened, shout the command.
TO PAIN – if the patient does not open his or her eyes in response to your voice command, pinch the back of his or her hand or the skin at the ankles (apply the stimulus to an uninjured limb).

VERBAL RESPONSE
ORIENTED – an aroused patient should be able to tell you his or her name, where he or she is, and the date in terms of the year and month.
CONFUSED – the patient cannot give accurate responses, but he or she is able to say phrases or sentences and perhaps take part in a conversation.
INAPPROPRIATE WORDS – the patient says one or several inappropriate words, usually in response to a physical stimulus. Often, the patient will curse or call for a specific person. This may happen without any stimulus.
INCOMPREHENSIBLE SOUNDS – the patient mumbles, groans, or moans in response to stimuli.
NO VERBAL RESPONSE – repeated stimulation will not cause the patient to make any sounds.

MOTOR RESPONSE
OBEYS COMMANDS – this is limited by the apparent nature of the patient's injuries and the injuries that can be associated with the mechanism of injury. The patient is asked to perform a simple task such as moving a specific finger or holding up two fingers.

If the patient does not carry out the command, painful stimuli can be utilized by applying firm pressure to an uninjured nail bed for five seconds or pinching the skin on the back of an uninjured hand or at an uninjured ankle.

LOCALIZES PAIN – the patient reaches to the source of the pain. Often, the patient will try to remove your hand from the pain site.
WITHDRAWS – the patient moves the limb rapidly away from the source of the pain. The arm may be moved away from the trunk.
FLEXION – the patient slowly bends the joint (elbow or knee) in an attempt to move away from the pain. The forearm and hand may be held against the trunk.
EXTENSION – the patient will straighten a limb in an effort to escape the pain. The movement appears slow and "stiff." There may be an internal rotation of the shoulder and forearm.
NONE – the patient does not respond to the repeated application of the stimulus.

Note: A special thanks is given to the people at Emergency Health Services, Department of Health, Commonwealth of Pennsylvania for their help in supplying information for this figure.

TABLE 3-8 Revised Trauma Score Breakpoints (> means greater than)

Glasgow Coma Scale	Systolic Blood Pressure	Respiratory Rate	Coded Value
13–15	>89	10–29	4
9–12	76–89	>29	3
6–8	50–75	6–9	2
4–5	1–49	1–5	1
3	0	0	0

The Priority of Care You must know more than how to conduct a primary and secondary survey. You must understand the *significance* of the information you have gathered in order to provide the proper care for the patient.

After completing the patient examination you will consider all the signs and symptoms recorded and how the combinations of these signs and symptoms may point the way to specific illness or injury. A *lack* of certain findings may also prove to be important. For example, if the patient has a severe obvious injury, but shows no reactions to indicate pain, you will have to consider problems such as spinal injury, brain damage, shock, or drug abuse. You will learn more about the significance of various signs and symptoms as you progress through this text.

The information you have gathered in the field assessment will be used to establish a *priority of care*. This priority changes somewhat depending on the stability of the patient, what other injuries are present, how many patients and rescuers there are, how long it will take to transport the patient, and factors that may be unique to a particular emergency. Each EMS System has established a definite order of care, stating what you should do first for any particular patient. In Chapter 22, we will consider patient assessment and the order of care if there is more than one patient.

TABLE 3-9 Priority of Care Example—One-Patient Incident

The following example is meant to serve as a guide as you learn your EMS System's order of care. Note that some of these problems overlap and that care for one often provides partial care for another. Note, too, that the care for shock is a part of the required treatment for most illness and injury.

1. Determine responsiveness.
2. Maintain an open airway, while protecting spine throughout.
3. Make certain the patient is breathing or receiving rescue breathing (artificial ventilations). Provide oxygen if status is critical or unstable.
4. Make certain there is circulation or CPR is provided. Check for and control profuse bleeding. Treat for shock or potential shock.
5. Determine level of consciousness.
6. Remove clothing to look for any additional life-threatening injuries.
7. Treat chest wounds that have opened the thoracic cavity and flail chest that compromises breathing.
8. Provide care for severe to moderate breathing distress.
9. Care for spinal injuries (cervical collar, etc).
10. Treat possible heart attack (patient unstable).
11. Determine severe head injuries and expedite transport.
12. Care for severe injuries of the chest, abdomen, and pelvis.
13. Treat severe medical problems or drug overdose.
14. Provide care for severe burns.
15. Control moderate bleeding.
16. Care for moderate medical problems.
17. Splint fractures.
18. Care for minor burns.
19. Care for minor cuts and bruises.

An example of an order of care is provided in Table 3-9. As you learn about a specific type of injury or illness, check to see where the care fits into this list. Modify the list as necessary to comply with your EMS System's order of care. Do not try to memorize this table. You will have learned and applied all the procedures by the end of your course.

CHAPTER REVIEW

KEY TERMS

You may find it helpful to review the following terms.

ABCDEs—the steps of the expanded primary survey: Airway, Breathing, Circulation, Disability, Expose.

airway—the pathway from nose and mouth that carries air to the gas exchange levels of the lungs.

auscultation (os-skul-TAY-shun)—the process of listening to sounds that occur within the body. An example is the procedure that uses a blood pressure cuff and a stethoscope to determine blood pressure. This method requires you to listen for certain sounds and changes in sound that correspond to systolic and diastolic blood pressures.

AVPU—stands for alert, verbally responsive, painful response, unresponsive; an index for quickly determining the level of consciousness.

blood pressure—the pressure caused by blood exerting force against the walls of blood vessels. Usually arterial blood pressure (the pressure in an artery) is measured.

brachial (BRAY-key-al) **artery**—the major artery supplying blood to the arm.

carotid (kah-ROT-id) **pulse**—the pulse that can be felt on each side of the patient's neck, over top of the carotid arteries.

cerebrospinal (ser-e-bro-SPI-nal) **fluid (CSF)**—the clear, watery fluid that surrounds and protects the brain and spinal cord.

cervical (SER-vi-kal)—in reference to the neck. The **cervical spine** is that portion of the spine that passes through the neck.

colostomy (ko-LOS-to-me)—A colostomy, like an ileostomy, is a surgical opening in the abdominal wall with an external bag in place to receive digestive excretions.

CUPS—stands for critical, unstable, potentially unstable, stable; an index of patient status used in deciding priority for transport to a medical facility.

diastolic (di-as-TOL-ik) **blood pressure**—the pressure in the arteries when the lower left chamber of the heart (left ventricle) is refilling.

distal pulse—a pulse taken at the foot or wrist. It is called *distal* because it is at the distal end of the limb.

First Responder—a person who is part of the EMS System, having been trained in a First Responder course and, where it is policy, having the appropriate certification. Such an individual is trained below the level of the basic EMT.

Glasgow Coma Scale—a detailed measurement of level of consciousness.

ileostomy (il-e-OS-to-me)—See *colostomy*.

level of consciousness (LOC)—degree of alertness (awareness and orientation). There are several methods of estimating level of consciousness in use by EMS systems such as the Glasgow Coma Scale or AVPU: Alert and oriented (patient is aware of what is happening), Verbal (patient talks and/or responds to voice), Painful stimuli (patient withdraws from a painful stimulus such as a pinch), Unresponsive (patient does not respond to any stimuli).

log roll—a maneuver for changing a patient's position by rolling him as a unit, keeping head, neck, and torso aligned.

mechanisms of injury—what forces caused the injury, allowing you to relate types of accidents to certain types of injuries. You must consider the kind of force, its intensity and direction, and the area of the body that is affected.

objective examination—a part of the secondary survey. This is a hands-on survey of the patient in which you determine vital signs and perform a head-to-toe survey.

palpate, palpation—to feel any part of the body, as to palpate the radial pulse; also, to use the blood pressure cuff and the feeling of the radial pulse to determine approximate patient systolic blood pressure.

pedal (PEED-al) **pulse**—a foot pulse. There are two locations used in field emergency care: the **dorsalis pedis** (lateral to the large tendon of the big toe) and the **posterior tibial** (behind the medial ankle).

point tenderness—a painful response to pressure.

priapism (PRE-ah-pizm)—persistent erection of the penis often associated with spinal injury and some medical problems.

primary survey—a patient assessment process carried out to detect and treat life-threatening problems. Basic life support is provided as needed during the primary survey.

pulse—the rhythmic beats caused as waves of blood move through and expand the arteries.

pulse character—the **rhythm** (regular or irregular) and **force** (full or thready) of the pulse.

pulse rate—the number of pulse beats per minute.

radial pulse—a pulse found in the lateral wrist.

respiration (res-pi-RAY-shun)—the act of breathing in (inhaling) and breathing out (exhaling).

respiratory (RES-pi-ra-tor-e) **character**—the **rhythm** (regular or irregular), **depth** (deep or shallow), **ease** (easy, labored, difficult, or painful), and **sounds** (such as snoring, wheezing, crowing, or gurgling) of breathing.

respiratory rate—the number of breaths per minute.

secondary survey—a patient assessment process that includes the subjective interview, the head-to-toe survey of the patient, and the taking of vital signs.

signs—what you see, hear, feel, and smell in relation to a patient's problem.

sphygmomanometer (SFIG-mo-mah-NOM-e-ter)—the cuff and gauge used in blood pressure determination.

status (STAY-tus or STAT-us) **decision**—a decision about whether immediate transport is or is not needed on the basis of assigning the patient to a C (Critical), U (Unstable), P (Potentially Unstable), or S (Stable) category of stability.

stoma (STO-mah)—a permanent opening surgically made in the body. A "neck breather" breathes through a stoma in the anterior neck.

subjective interview—a part of the secondary survey that uses the patient and bystanders as sources of information by having them answer specific questions.

symptoms—what the patient tells you about his problem.

systolic (sis-TOL-ik) **blood pressure**—the pressure created in the arteries when the lower left chamber of the heart (left ventricle) contracts and forces blood out into circulation.

tracheostomy (TRAY-ke-OS-to-me)—a surgical opening made through the anterior neck entering into the windpipe (trachea).

vital signs—the patient's pulse rate, rhythm and character, respiratory rate and character, blood pressure, and temperature. Some approaches consider level of consciousness and appearance of the pupils of the eyes to be part of the vital signs.

SUMMARY

The Field Assessment

The first rule of patient assessment and care is **DO NO HARM**—to yourself or to the patient.

The sequence of patient assessment is

- Sizing up the situation
- Primary survey—to detect and control life-threatening emergencies
- Status decision
- Secondary survey—a detailed assessment
    —Subjective interview
    —Objective examination
        Vital signs
        Head-to-toe survey

The thoroughness and order of these steps may vary according to local protocols and the situation.

On arrival at the scene, size up the situation and identify yourself. Use the information gained from the dispatcher. Gain information quickly from the scene, patient, bystanders, first responders, mechanisms of injury, and obvious deformities and signs of injury or illness.

The Primary Survey

The primary survey involves assessment of and emergency care for, life-threatening condition. The expanded primary survey involves the ABCDEs of emergency care—Airway, Breathing, Circulation, Disability, and Expose—and also profuse bleeding and severe shock.

The steps to follow are (1) check for responsiveness, (2) reposition the patient if necessary, (3) check for an open airway, (4) determine breathing quantity and quality, (5) check for circulation (feel for carotid pulse) and check for severe bleeding and signs of shock, (6) check for disability (determine level of consciousness using the AVPU method), (7) expose the patient's body to check for additional injuries. *Provide immediate emergency care as needed at each step.*

At the conclusion of the primary survey, make a status decision as to whether immediate transport is needed based on assigning the patient to a C (Critical), U (Unstable), P (Potentially Unstable), or S (Stable) category.

The Secondary Survey

The secondary survey comprises the subjective interview and the objective examination: taking vital signs and conducting the head-to-toe survey to look for specific signs and symptoms

The three examination rules are (1) Explain to the patient what you are going to do. (2) Obtain consent. (3) At all times take care not to aggravate possible spinal injuries.

Throughout the process of assessment and emergency care, make four kinds of observations. Observe the patient (1) for anything that looks wrong, (2) for level of consciousness, (the Glasgow Coma Scale may be used), (3) for changes in his condition, and (4) for skin condition.

In the interview, look over the scene, look over the patient, and look for medical identification devices. Gather information by asking specific questions and listening to the patient's and bystanders' responses. If the patient is suffering pain or distress, ask PQRST questions (regarding the Provocation, Quality, Region, Referral, Recurrence, Relief, Severity, and Time of the pain or distress). To get patient history, ask AMPLE questions (regarding Allergies, Medications, Previous medical history, Last meal, and Events leading up to this incident).

The two parts of the examination phase of the secondary survey are (1) taking vital signs and (2) the head-to-toe survey.

For vital signs, determine radial pulse rate and character. Measure respiratory rate and note the character of respirations. Measure blood pressure by auscultation or palpation. Determine relative skin temperature. At this time also note skin color and the general condition of the skin. You must repeat vital sign readings, constantly monitoring and re-assessing the patient.

Head-to-Toe Survey:

NECK—Gently examine for cervical point tenderness, midline deformity, and muscle spasms. Check to see if the patient is a neck breather: Examine for neck injury. Look for a medical identification necklace.

HEAD—Check scalp for cuts, bruises, swellings, and other signs of injury. Examine the skull for deformities, depressions, and other signs of injury. Include the facial bones. Inspect the eyelids for injury and do the same for the eyes. Determine pupil size, equality, and reactivity. Check for abnormal eye tracking. Note any discoloration on the inner eyelid. Look for blood, clear fluids, or bloody fluids in the ears and nose. Examine the mouth for obstructions, bleeding, and any odd odors.

CHEST—Examine for injury (cuts, bruises, penetrations, impaled objects, and fractures). Use compression as a test for fractures. Check for equal expansion and watch for unusual chest movements. Listen for equal air entry (and assess breathing sounds).

ABDOMEN—Examine for injuries (cuts, bruises, penetrations, and impaled objects). Check for local and general pain as you examine the abdomen for tenderness, distention, masses, and rigid areas.

LOWER BACK—Feel for deformity and point tenderness.

PELVIS—Use compression to check for fractures and look for signs of injury.

GENITAL REGION—Note any obvious injury. Look for priapism when assessing male patients suspected of having spinal injuries.

LOWER EXTREMITIES—Examine for injury (deformities, swellings, discolorations, bone protrusions, and fractures). Run point tenderness tests on suspect fracture sites. Confirm a distal pulse in each limb, and check each lower limb for nerve function. Capillary refill may be checked at this time. Check sensation and movement in all extremities.

UPPER EXTREMITIES—Examine for injury (deformities, swellings, discolorations, bone protrusions, and fractures). Run point tenderness tests on suspected fracture sites. Confirm a radial pulse for each wrist and check for nerve function. Check for a medical identification bracelet. Capillary refill may be checked at this time.

BACK AND BUTTOCKS—Examine for bleeding and obvious injury, if indicated.

As an EMT your overriding concern is your own safety. For the patient your major concerns, in order, are (1) to identify and treat life-threatening conditions, (2) to make a status decision on the patient's stability and possible need for immediate transport, (3) to identify any other injuries and medical conditions and provide emergency care, and (4) to keep the patient stable.

Special Assessment Concerns

As an EMT you will have to assess medical patients and trauma patients, conscious patients and unconscious patients. You must learn to deal with unfavorable scenes, environments and locations, special or uncooperative patients and bystanders, severe or grotesque injuries patients with multiple injuries, and more than one patient.

You must tailor assessment and care procedures to the situation and according to local protocols. You must fill out the required forms completely and accurately.

4

On the Scene

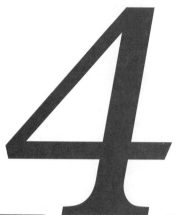

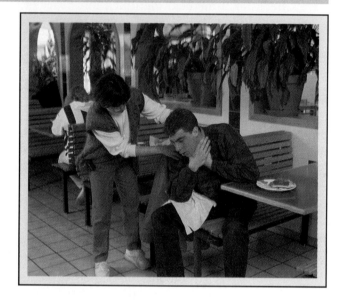

You are having dinner with your family in your favorite restaurant. After you order, you observe a man two tables away. It isn't difficult to notice him, because he is very loud and abusive to the waitress and seems drunk. You hope he isn't driving.

Suddenly, the man clutches his throat with both hands. His face is turning red, and he appears overcome with panic. You recognize the signs of choking and go to his aid.

You: CAN YOU SPEAK?

Man: (Shakes his head frantically.)

You: I'm an Emergency Medical Technician. I can help you. (As you begin to act, you explain . . .) This is called the Heimlich maneuver. It'll get that food out of your throat.

The restaurant has become quiet. The manager approaches and you instruct him to call 911 for EMS. Your first few attempts to relieve the obstruction do not work, but you are not discouraged. You reposition your hands and try again. Suddenly a large piece of meat flies out of the man's mouth. He begins to gasp, then cough.

You remain with the man and encourage him to keep coughing to bring up any remaining pieces of food. You carefully monitor him until the ambulance arrives. When the ambulance crew comes in, you provide a full report on what happened. They transport the man to the hospital. You return to your table but are a little too excited to eat!

The skills you learn as an EMT will be with you even when you are not on the ambulance. Obtaining and maintaining a good airway is perhaps the most important of these skills. The knowledge is never wasted. You never know when you may need it to help a stranger, a friend—or even a member of your own family.

The Airway and Rescue Breathing

There are several conditions that can rapidly cause death: breathing stops, or breathing and heartbeat stop, or there is severe bleeding, or the patient goes into severe shock. When a patient has one or more of these life-threatening conditions, you must be prepared to administer basic life support, techniques to keep a patient alive until definitive care can be undertaken by others. As an EMT you must know how to do this using a minimum of equipment—in some cases with no more than your hands and your breath.

The procedures of basic life support will be discussed in this and the next few chapters: Chapter 4, resuscitation when breathing stops (rescue breathing requiring no special equipment); Chapter 5, resuscitation when breathing and heartbeat both stop (CPR and defibrillation); Chapter 6, equipment-assisted breathing aids and oxygen therapy; Chapter 7, control of bleeding; and Chapter 8, control of shock.

Expected Outcome, Chapter 4: *You will be able to evaluate a patient's airway and breathing and undertake basic procedures to clear the airway and provide rescue breathing.*

Note: Procedures discussed in the following chapters are those usually done by the EMT. If you run into problems on the scene or during transport, follow local protocols for calling for paramedic assistance.

WARNING: Protect yourself from infectious diseases by using appropriate barrier devices such as a pocket face mask with one-way valve, face shield, or bag-valve mask; goggles or eye shield; and disposable gloves. Always conform to your local EMS system's infection exposure control plan.

THE RESPIRATORY SYSTEM
  The Importance of Breathing
  Clinical Death and Biological Death
  Respiratory System Anatomy
  Respiration

RESPIRATORY FAILURE
  Opening the Airway
  Rescue Breathing

AIRWAY OBSTRUCTION
  Causes of Airway Obstruction
  Techniques for Clearing the Airway
  Procedures for Clearing the Airway
  Procedures for an Adult
  Procedures for a Child
  Procedures for an Infant

Knowledge *After reading this chapter you should be able to*

1. State three reasons why breathing is essential to life. (pp. 102-104)

2. Define and compare clinical death and biological death. (p. 104)

3. Name and label the major structures of the respiratory system. (pp. 104-105)

4. Name the major muscles used in breathing. (p. 105)

5. Relate changes in volume and pressure to the process of breathing. (pp. 105-106)

6. List the signs of adequate and of inadequate breathing. (p. 106)

7. Describe, step by step, the head-tilt, the head-tilt, chin-lift, and the jaw-thrust maneuvers. (pp. 109-110)

8. Explain why mouth-to-mask ventilation is preferred over ventilations involving direct contact. (p. 111)

9. List, step by step, the actions taken when providing mouth-to-mouth ventilation. (pp. 111, 113-114)

10. Compare and contrast mouth-to-nose ventilation and mouth-to-stoma ventilation with the mouth-to-mouth techniques. (pp. 114-117)

11. List, step by step, the actions taken when providing rescue breathing to an infant or a child. (p. 117)

12. State what the EMT can do to correct problems of gastric distention caused by artificial ventilation. (pp. 117-118)

13. Describe the recovery position and explain the circumstances in which a patient should be placed in this position. (p. 118)

14. List FIVE factors that may cause partial or complete airway obstruction. (p. 119)

15. List THREE major signs of partial airway obstruction. (pp. 119-120)

16. State when you must treat a partial airway obstruction as if it were a complete airway obstruction. (p. 120)

17. Describe the signs displayed by a conscious and an unconscious patient with a complete airway obstruction. (p. 120)

18. Describe, step by step, the procedures used in correcting airway obstructions, including

---

Before studying this chapter, you may want to review Chapter 2, in which the anatomy and physiology of the human body were introduced; particularly, review the information on body cavities (especially the thoracic cavity, or chest cavity). Also review the Anatomy and Physiology Plate on the Respiratory System at the end of this book.

THE RESPIRATORY SYSTEM

The Importance of Breathing

Ensuring breathing, or **respiration,** takes precedence over all other emergency care measures. The reason is stated simply: If a person cannot breathe, he cannot survive.

The body's cells must be provided with *oxygen* and have *carbon dioxide* removed. Both oxygen and carbon dioxide are gases. During the first half of the process of respiration, breathing in brings oxygen from the atmosphere to the gas exchange levels of the lungs. There the oxygen moves into the bloodstream, which carries it to the cells. Conversely, carbon dioxide moves from the cells into the bloodstream, which carries it into the lungs. There, the other half of the process of respiration, breathing out, takes the carbon dioxide out of the body into the atmosphere.

Chemical processes within the body's cells continually convert food into the energy that is needed for life. These processes are collectively called *metabolism.* An adequate and continuous supply of oxygen is required for many of these metabolic processes. Oxygen is needed to make energy-rich compounds, and is also needed to help break these compounds down. The energy

- The Heimlich maneuver (pp. 121-122)
- Chest thrusts (pp. 122-123)
- Back blows and chest thrusts for infants (pp. 123-124)
- Finger sweeps (pp. 124-125)

19. State the criteria for success in clearing an airway obstruction. (p. 125)

20. State the sequence of procedures for correcting an airway obstruction in a conscious adult, an adult who loses consciousness, and an adult who is unconscious when you find him. (pp. 126-128)

21. State the sequence of procedures for correcting an airway obstruction in a conscious child, a child who loses consciousness, and child who is unconscious when you find him. (pp. 128-129)

22. State the sequence of procedures for correcting an airway obstruction in a conscious infant, an infant who loses consciousness, and an infant who is unconscious when you find him. (pp. 129-131)

Skills *As an EMT you should be able to*

1. Determine if a patient has adequate or inadequate breathing or if the patient is in respiratory arrest.

2. Open a patient's airway using the head-tilt, chin-lift, or the jaw-thrust maneuver.

3. Correctly perform rescue breathing with mouth-to-mask, mouth-to-mouth, mouth-to-nose, and mouth-to-stoma ventilations.

4. Correctly perform rescue breathing on infants and small children.

5. Identify and prevent gastric distention while performing rescue breathing.

6. Place a patient in the recovery position.

7. Determine if a patient has a partial or a complete airway obstruction.

8. Perform the Heimlich maneuver and chest thrusts to clear airway obstructions in adults and children.

9. Perform back blows and chest thrusts to clear airway obstructions in infants.

released is used to contract muscles, send nerve impulses, build new tissues, digest foods, and carry out all other life processes.

Carbon dioxide is a waste product of certain metabolic processes. If allowed to accumulate in the body, carbon dioxide can become a deadly poison. As the concentration of carbon dioxide increases, a person will start panting (increase the respiratory rate), trying to rid the body of the carbon dioxide. Heart rate and blood pressure increase. Soon, brain cells start to malfunction. The person may appear sleepy and difficult to arouse. If the patient's brain is also receiving inadequate oxygen, the patient may become restless or combative. As more carbon dioxide builds up in the body, the person may start to hallucinate, owing to the toxic effects of the excess carbon dioxide. The person is soon likely to lose consciousness. Unless corrected, many body functions, including respiration, will fail, causing death.

The process of respiration does more than supply oxygen and remove carbon dioxide. It also helps the body to maintain its chemical balance. Many reactions in our bodies tend to throw the body out of chemical balance. Some of these reactions make the blood too acidic, while others make it too basic (alkaline). The respiratory system plays a key role in preventing this by regulating the amount of carbon dioxide that is in circulation. The carbon dioxide helps to regulate acid-base balance by producing compounds known as buffers. When breathing becomes inadequate, the acid-base balance of the blood becomes upset, causing cells to die. Some of the cells most sensitive to this imbalance are those in the brain.

The brain and the other structures of the nervous system are very sensitive to a lack of oxygen, an increase in carbon dioxide, or an acid-base imbalance. The brain uses approximately 20% of the oxygen that is in the circulatory system. Even a slight decrease in available oxygen can affect brain function. A marked decrease can lead to drastic changes and, eventually, to death.

REMEMBER: Breathing provides needed oxygen for the cells, removes potentially dangerous carbon dioxide, and helps to maintain the acid-base balance of the blood.

Clinical Death and Biological Death

The process of respiration cannot be separated from the process of circulation. It is not enough to receive oxygen at the exchange level of the lungs. The oxygen must be transported by the blood to the cells. Likewise, carbon dioxide must be carried by the blood to the lungs for removal from the body. You must always relate breathing to circulation, making sure that both processes are taking place. (Heart action and circulation will be considered in Chapter 5.)

Understanding the relationship between respiration and circulation is basic to understanding *clinical death* and *biological death*. As an EMT, you must know the difference between these two definitions of death (Figure 4-1).

- **Clinical Death**—*A patient is clinically dead the moment breathing and heartbeat stop.*
- **Biological Death**—*A patient is biologically dead when the brain cells die.* If a patient is not breathing and the heart is not circulating oxygenated blood, potentially lethal changes begin to take place in the brain within 4 to 6 minutes; brain cells usually begin to die within 10 minutes (this can be delayed by cold temperatures, see Chapter 20).

You may be able to reverse clinical death, but biological death is irreversible.

Respiratory System Anatomy

The major structures of the **airway** include

- **Nose**—the primary pathway for air to enter and leave the system
- **Mouth**—the secondary pathway for air
- **Pharynx** (FAR-inks)—the throat; the passageway for both air and food
- **Larynx** (LAR-inks)—the neck structure that connects the pharynx and the trachea. The voicebox is contained in the larynx. When viewed externally, the most prominent fea-

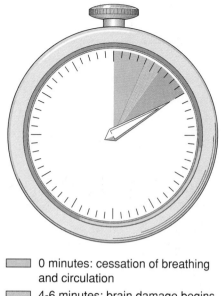

	0 minutes: cessation of breathing and circulation
	4-6 minutes: brain damage begins
	10 minutes: brain cells begin to die

Figure 4-1 The death of brain cells.

ture is the **thyroid** (THY-roid) **cartilage**, or Adam's apple. A trap-door-like structure in the larynx, the **epiglottis** (EP-i-GLOT-is), normally prevents food, liquids, and foreign objects from entering the trachea and lungs as they pass through the larynx en route to the stomach.

- **Trachea** (TRAY-ke-ah)—the windpipe
- **Bronchial Tree**—branching from the trachea to the microscopic air sacs of the lungs. The first branches are the right and left main stem (primary) **bronchi** (BRONG-ke). These branch into secondary bronchi. The smaller branches coming off the secondary bronchi are called the **bronchioles** (BRONG-ke-olz).
- **Lungs**—the spongy, elastic organs containing **alveoli** (al-VE-o-li), the microscopic air sacs where oxygen and carbon dioxide exchange takes place.

Those structures found superior to the larynx are called the **upper airway**. The **lower airway** comprises all the structures from the larynx to the alveoli.

The structures of the airway do more than provide a passageway for air to and from the lungs. As air passes through the upper airway, it is filtered, adjusted to body temperature, and humidified. Hairs in the nose start the filtration process, trapping large particles. The mucus on

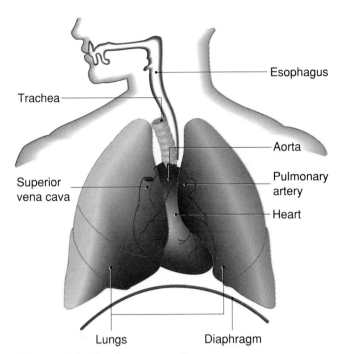

Trachea — Esophagus

Aorta

Superior vena cava — Pulmonary artery

Heart

Lungs   Diaphragm

Figure 4-2 The thoracic cavity.

the surface of the airway lining picks up most of the smaller particles. The blood vessels in the airway lining can either provide heat to air that is below body temperature or absorb heat from air that is too warm. The tissues of the lining add water to the air so that it is nearly saturated with moisture. These processes combine to condition the air to help prevent lung damage.

Most of the trachea and all of the lungs are situated in the thoracic, or chest, cavity (Figure 4-2).

Respiration

The physical process of respiration is so constant in a healthy person that he is seldom aware of his own breathing. Breathing is an automatic function. We can, for short periods, control the rate and depth of our breathing. However, most of the time breathing is involuntary, controlled by respiratory centers in the brain. These respiratory centers are sensitive to the levels of carbon dioxide and oxygen in our blood. If the carbon dioxide level becomes too high or the oxygen level too low, our respiratory centers automatically direct us to breathe faster and deeper.

If you try to hold your breath, the respiratory centers in your brain urge you to breathe. You can't run while taking slow, shallow breaths, because your respiratory centers automatically adjust the rate, depth, and rhythm of

breathing to suit the needs of your cells. When you go to sleep, the respiratory centers are still at work, instructing your body to breathe.

Inspiration and Expiration The work of breathing changes pressures inside the thoracic cavity and the lungs. These changes in pressure result from the combined actions of the **intercostal** (in-ter-KOS-tal) **muscles**, which are the muscles attached to the rib cage, and of the **diaphragm** (DI-ah-fram), the dome-shaped muscle that separates the chest from the abdomen. An **inspiration** (the process of breathing in, or inhaling) takes place when these muscles contract. An **expiration** (the process of breathing out, or exhaling), takes place when the intercostal muscles and diaphragm relax.

A basic law of physics governs breathing: AS VOLUME INCREASES, PRESSURE DECREASES. Just prior to inspiration, the thoracic cavity has a certain volume and pressure, and so do the lungs, which are located within the thoracic cavity. Inspiration begins when the diaphragm contracts and flattens downward while the intercostal muscles contract and pull the ribs outward. These movements increase the volume of (amount of space inside) the thoracic cavity and the lungs. As the volume increases, the pressure decreases. When the pressure inside the lungs drops below the pressure of the atmosphere outside the body, air will enter the lungs to equalize the pressure. The air at the higher pressure of the atmosphere will move to the area of lower pressure inside the lungs.

The opposite happens during expiration. The intercostal muscles and diaphragm relax. This decreases the volume of (amount of space inside) the thoracic cavity and lungs. When the volume decreases, the pressure inside the lungs increases. The air will move from the higher pressure in the lungs to the lower pressure of the atmosphere.

These pressure changes are not large (Figure 4-3). The changes in pressure are just enough to cause air to flow in and out of the lungs. Injuries that penetrate the chest and disturb this delicate pressure balance are life threatening. Such injuries will be discussed in Chapter 14.

The process of breathing is repeated 12 to 20 times per minute in the average adult at rest. Each breath will move about 500 mL (milliliters) of air. This approximate amount can also be expressed as ½ liter, 500 cc (cubic centimeters), or 1 pint. In times of stress or physical exertion, our respiratory rate and volume usually increase.

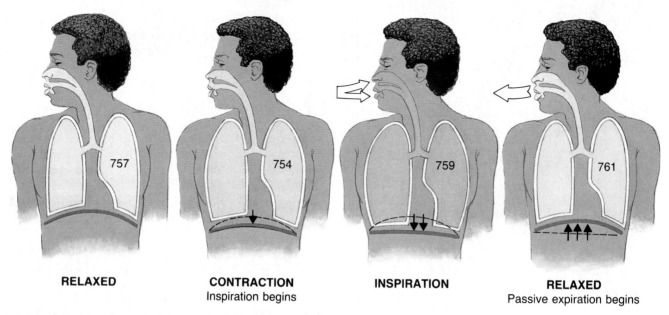

ATMOSPHERIC PRESSURE 760 mmHg

RELAXED	CONTRACTION	INSPIRATION	RELAXED
	Inspiration begins		Passive expiration begins

Figure 4-3 Changes in volume and pressure produce inspirations and expirations (mmHg = millimeters of mercury pressure).

RESPIRATORY FAILURE

Simply stated, **respiratory failure** is either the cessation of normal breathing or the reduction of breathing to the point where oxygen intake is not sufficient to support life. When breathing stops completely, the patient is in **respiratory arrest**. Respiratory arrest can develop during heart attack, stroke, airway obstruction, drowning, electrocution, drug overdose, poisoning, brain injury, severe chest injury, suffocation, and prolonged respiratory failure.

Patient Assessment—Respiratory Failure

Signs

To determine the signs of ADEQUATE BREATHING, you should

- [ ] LOOK for the even (bilateral) rise and fall of the chest associated with breathing.
- [ ] LISTEN for air entering and leaving the nose or mouth. The sounds should be typical, free of gurgling, gasping, crowing, and wheezing.
- [ ] FEEL for air moving out of the nose or mouth.
- [ ] Check for typical skin coloration. There should be no blue or gray colorations.

- [ ] Note a rate and depth of breathing typical for a person at rest (see Chapter 3).

The following are signs of INADEQUATE BREATHING.

- [ ] Chest movements are absent, minimal, or uneven.
- [ ] Movements associated with breathing are limited to the abdomen (abdominal breathing).
- [ ] No air can be felt or heard at the nose or mouth, or exchange is evaluated as below normal.
- [ ] Noises such as wheezing, snoring, gurgling, or gasping are heard during breathing.
- [ ] The rate of breathing is too rapid or too slow (see Chapter 3).
- [ ] Breathing is very shallow, very deep, or appears labored.
- [ ] The patient's skin, lips, tongue, ear lobes, or nailbeds are blue or gray. This is called **cyanosis** (sigh-ah-NO-sis). The patient is said to be cyanotic (sigh-ah-NOT-ik).
- [ ] Inspirations are prolonged (indicating a possible upper airway obstruction) or expirations are prolonged (indicating a possible lower airway obstruction).
- [ ] The patient is unable to speak, or the patient cannot speak full sentences because of shortness of breath.

106   Basic Life Support

Emergency Care Steps

When the patient's signs indicate inadequate or no breathing, prompt action must be taken. The result of uncorrected respiratory failure, and certainly of respiratory arrest, is often death. The procedures by which life threatening respiratory problems are treated are

1. Opening the airway
2. Rescue breathing

These procedures are discussed in detail below.

The procedures for airway evaluation, opening the airway, and rescue breathing are best carried out with the patient lying supine, or flat on his back. Patients who are found in positions other than supine should be moved to the floor or stretcher for evaluation and treatment (Figure 4-4). If spinal injury is suspected, stabilize the head and neck as you move the patient to the floor.

Any movement of a trauma patient before patient assessment and any necessary immobilization of spinal injuries and fractures can produce serious injury to the patient. Breathing, however, is one of our first priorities and must be assured as quickly as possible. If the trauma patient must be moved, every effort must be made to protect the patient's neck and spine during repositioning. In Chapter 3, a method for repositioning the patient was discussed. Scan 4-1 reviews this procedure.

Use the following as indications that head, neck, or spinal injury may have occurred—especially when the patient is unconscious and cannot tell you what happened.

- The mechanism of injury is one that can cause head, neck, or spinal injury. A patient who is found on the ground near a ladder or stairs, for example, may have such injuries. Motor vehicle accidents are another common cause of head, neck, and spinal injuries.
- Any injury at or above the level of the shoulders indicates that head, neck, or spinal injuries may also be present.
- Family or bystanders may tell you that an injury to the head, neck, or spine has occurred or may give you information that leads you to suspect it.
- The patient is unconscious.

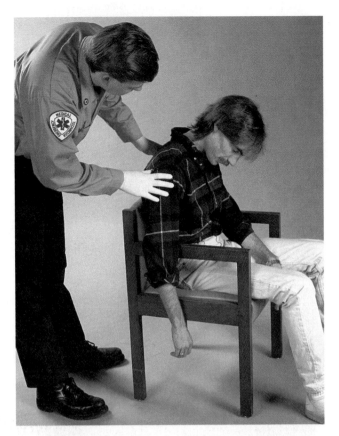

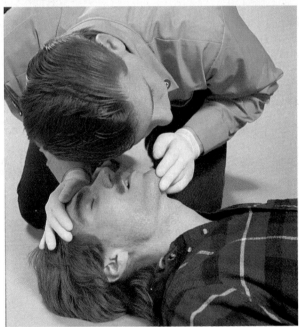

Figure 4-4 Positioning the patient for airway evaluation and care.

Opening the Airway

As an EMT you must ensure an open airway during the primary survey. You must open and maintain the airway in any patient who cannot

Repositioning the Patient for Basic Life Support

Warning: This maneuver is used to initiate airway evaluation, rescue breathing, or CPR when you must act alone. For all other repositionings, use the four-rescuer log roll (Chapter 12).

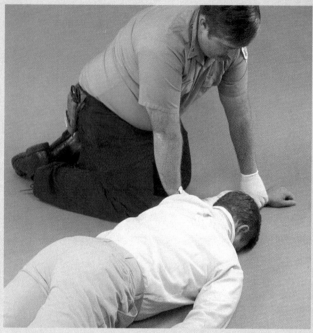

1. Straighten the legs and position the closest arm above the head.

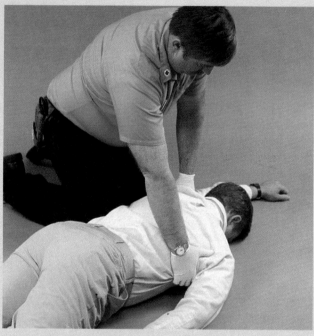

2. Cradle the head and neck. Grasp under the distant armpit.

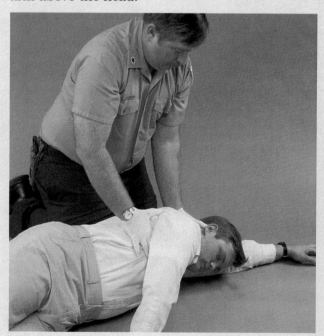

3. Move the patient as a unit onto his side.

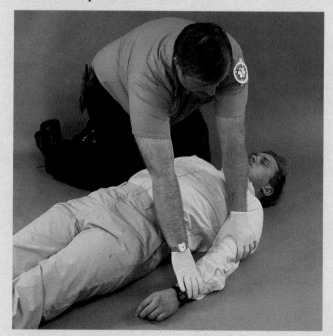

4. Move the patient onto his back and reposition the extended arm.

do so for himself. This includes patients who are semiconscious, unconscious, or in respiratory or cardiac arrest.

Most airway problems are caused by the tongue. As the head flexes forward, the tongue may slide into the airway, causing an obstruction. If the patient is unconscious, the tongue loses muscle tone and muscles of the lower jaw relax. Since the tongue is attached to the lower jaw, the risk of airway obstruction by the tongue is even greater during unconsciousness. The basic procedures for opening the airway help to correct the position of the tongue (Figure 4-5).

There are three procedures commonly recommended for opening the airway: the head-tilt maneuver; the head-tilt, chin-lift maneuver; and the jaw-thrust maneuver. The first two are *not* recommended when head, neck, or spinal injury is suspected.

Head-Tilt Maneuver This procedure (Figure 4-6) can be used on a conscious or non-trauma patient who is in need of airway maintenance. It may be used for a patient who is semiconscious and needs some assistance to keep the airway open. Airway assistance and positioning such as this may help prevent unconsciousness or respiratory arrest.

Warning: If any indication of head, neck, or spine injury is present, DO NOT USE THE HEAD-TILT MANEUVER. Remember that any unconscious patient, or any trauma patient whether unconscious or conscious, may be suspected of having an injury to the head, neck, or spine.

Follow these steps to perform the head-tilt maneuver.

1. If you find the patient with a compromised airway in a sitting position, move him to a supine position on the floor or stretcher for best airway care.
2. If you find the patient lying down with his head resting on some object or on pillows, move the patient from the object or remove the pillows to prevent the head from flexing forward and closing the airway.
3. To perform the head-tilt procedure, simply reposition the head by placing your palm on the forehead and applying gentle, firm, backward pressure to tilt the patient's head back.

Head-Tilt, Chin-Lift Maneuver This technique (Figure 4-7) provides for the maximum opening of the airway. It is useful on all patients

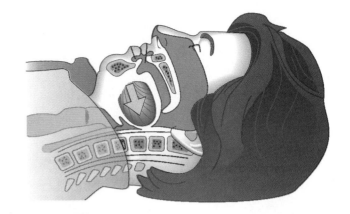
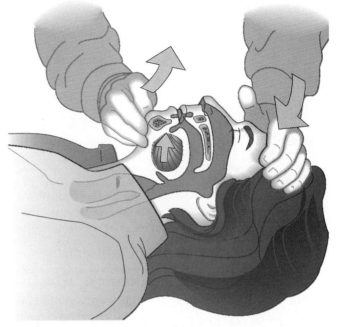

Figure 4-5 Procedures for opening the airway help reposition the tongue.

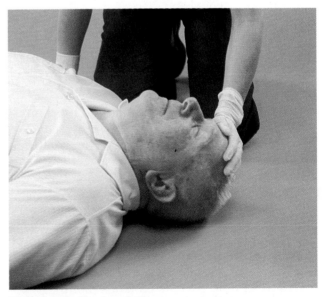

Figure 4-6 The head-tilt maneuver.

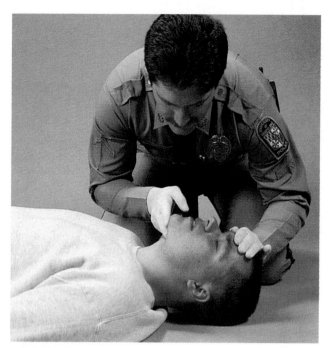

Figure 4-7 The head-tilt, chin-lift maneuver.

who are in need of assistance in maintaining an airway or breathing. It is one of the best methods for correcting obstructions caused by the tongue.

Warning: If any indication of head, neck, or spine injury is present, DO NOT USE THE HEAD-TILT, CHIN-LIFT MANEUVER. Remember that any unconscious and many conscious trauma patients may be suspected of having an injury to the head, neck, or spine.

Follow these steps to perform the head-tilt, chin-lift maneuver.

1. Once the patient is supine, place one hand on the forehead and place the fingertips of the other hand under the bony area at the center of the patient's lower jaw.
2. Tilt the head by applying gentle pressure to the patient's forehead.
3. Use your fingertips to lift the chin and to support the lower jaw. Move the jaw forward to a point where the lower teeth are almost touching the upper teeth. *Do not* compress the soft tissues under the lower jaw, which can obstruct the airway.
4. *Do not* allow the patient's mouth to be closed. To provide an adequate opening at the mouth, you may need to use the thumb of the hand supporting the chin to pull back the patient's lower lip. *Do not* insert your thumb into the patient's mouth.

Jaw-Thrust Maneuver This procedure (Figure 4-8) is most commonly used to open the airway of an unconscious patient or one with suspected head, neck, or spinal injuries.

Note: THE JAW-THRUST MANEUVER IS THE *ONLY* WIDELY RECOMMENDED PROCEDURE FOR USE ON UNCONSCIOUS PATIENTS OR PATIENTS WITH POSSIBLE HEAD, NECK, OR SPINAL INJURIES.

Follow these steps to perform the jaw-thrust maneuver.

1. Carefully keep the patient's head, neck, and spine aligned, moving him as a unit, as you place him in the supine position.
2. Kneel at the top of the patient's head, resting your elbows on the same surface on which the patient is lying.
3. Carefully reach forward and gently place one hand on each side of the patient's lower jaw, at the angles of the jaw below the ears.
4. Stabilize the patient's head with your forearms.
5. Using your index fingers, push the angles of the patient's lower jaw forward.
6. You may need to retract the patient's lower lip with your thumb to keep the mouth open.
7. *Do not* tilt or rotate the patient's head. REMEMBER, THE PURPOSE OF THE JAW-THRUST MANEUVER IS TO OPEN THE AIRWAY WITHOUT MOVING THE HEAD OR NECK.

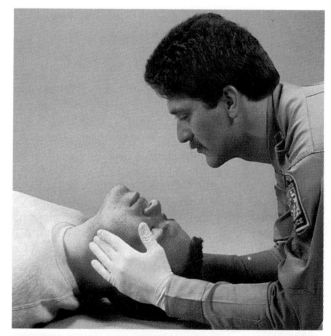

Figure 4-8 The jaw-thrust maneuver.

Rescue Breathing

Rescue breathing is also called *pulmonary resuscitation* (PUL-mo-ner-e re-SUS-si-TAT-shun) or *artificial ventilation*. Although there are many names and several variations, the purpose of this technique is to provide oxygen to, and allow carbon dioxide to be removed from, a patient who has stopped breathing or whose breathing is inadequate to sustain life. The procedure may not cause normal breathing to resume, but it will keep the patient alive until more advanced techniques can be applied.

Many students wonder how artificial ventilations provide enough oxygen to the patient, since the air has already been in the rescuer's lungs. Atmospheric air contains 21% oxygen. The air you exhale contains 16% oxygen. This means that the air you provide for the non-breathing patient still contains about three times the amount of oxygen (5%) that is normally removed from atmospheric air by the lungs. In other words, the air you provide contains enough oxygen to supply the patient's needs.

To make artificial ventilations more effective, supplemental oxygen should be provided. The use of supplemental oxygen increases the patient's chance of survival. (Supplemental oxygen devices will be discussed in Chapter 6.) The start of respirations should not be delayed, however, if oxygen is not available; rather oxygen should be administered as soon as possible after the start of ventilations. As an EMT you should be able to provide ventilations both with and without supplemental oxygen.

Mouth-to-Mask Ventilation You will be instructed in the basic procedures of mouth-to-mouth, mouth-to-nose, and mouth-to-stoma ventilations according to American Heart Association guidelines. It is recommended, however, that you provide breaths to patients using a barrier device such as a pocket face mask (Scan 4-2) or a bag-valve mask which offers protection from infectious diseases (Figure 4-9). The use of these and other protective barrier devices will be covered in Chapter 6. Follow your local protocols in regard to how rescue breathing is to be done in your EMS system.

Mouth-to-Mouth Ventilation This technique (Figure 4-10) can be performed by one person with no special equipment.

Warning: When possible, use a barrier device (pocket face mask) for infection control.

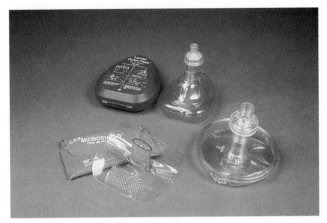

Figure 4-9A Barrier devices.

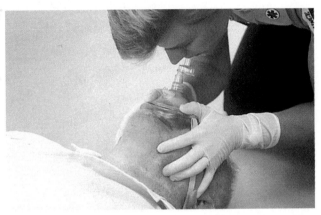

Figure 4-9B Providing breaths with a pocket face mask.

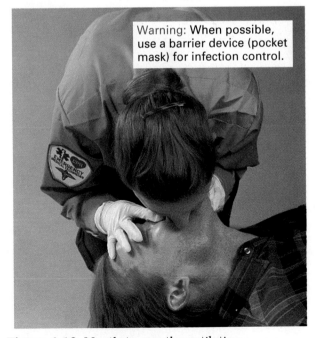

Warning: When possible, use a barrier device (pocket mask) for infection control.

Figure 4-10 Mouth-to-mouth ventilation.

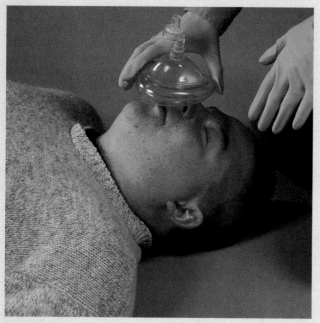

1. Position the patient and prepare to place the mask.

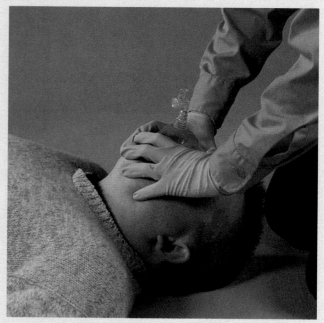

2. Seat the mask firmly on the patient's face.

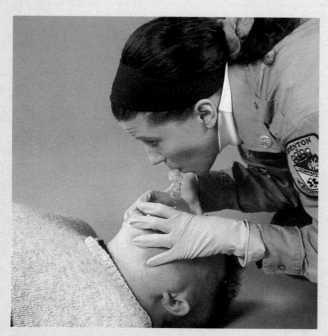

3. Open the patient's airway and watch the chest rise as you ventilate through the one-way valve.

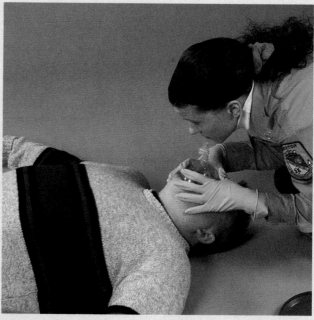

4. Watch the patient's chest fall during exhalation.

Mouth-to-mouth ventilation is used when the patient is in respiratory arrest, that is, when he is no longer breathing. The procedure is also used when a patient's respiratory rate or depth is not sufficient to sustain life. When performing mouth-to-mouth ventilations, remember that you will need to open and maintain the airway using the head-tilt, chin-lift method, or, on patients with suspected head, neck or spine injuries, the jaw-thrust maneuver.

When providing mouth-to-mouth ventilations for an adult patient (See Table 4-1 and see also "Ventilating Infants and Children" later in this chapter), you should follow the steps below. Remember that you will be safer if you employ a pocket face mask with one-way valve (see Chapter 6).

1. Establish if the patient is unresponsive (tap the shoulder and ask, "Are you OK?").
2. If the adult patient is unresponsive and you are working alone, immediately telephone 911 or your designated emergency number, or radio your EMS dispatch center for help, BEFORE BEGINNING ARTIFICIAL VENTILATIONS.
3. Properly position the patient and open the airway.
4. Determine if the patient is breathing and if the breathing is adequate (see "Patient Assessment—Respiratory Failure," earlier in this chapter). Take 3 TO 5 SECONDS to determine if the patient is breathing.
5. Maintain the patient in the optimum head-tilt position and pinch the nose closed with the thumb and forefinger of the hand you are using to hold the patient's forehead. If using a pocket face mask, place it over the

patient's mouth and nose. Hold the apex (point) in place with the edge of your hand that does the head tilt. Hold the base in place with the thumb of the hand that does the chin lift.

6. Deliver two slow breaths (1½ to 2 seconds each) as follows:
   - Open your mouth wide and take a deep breath. Place your mouth on the mask's chimney or around the patient's mouth, making a tight seal with your lips against the patient's face. Exhale into the mask or the patient's mouth until you see his chest rise and feel the resistance offered by his expanding lungs. Stop when you see the chest rise so that you do not overventilate the patient. Break contact with the face mask or the patient's mouth (allowing the nostrils to open) to allow him to exhale passively.
   - Take in another deep breath and exhale this air into the patient's airway. Allow the patient to exhale. (**Note:** If these initial attempts to ventilate fail, reposition the patient's head and try again. If necessary, remove any vomitus, bloody fluids, or foreign objects obstructing the airway—see "Techniques for Clearing the Airway" later in this chapter.)
7. If the patient does not begin spontaneous breathing after these initial breaths, check for a carotid pulse. If the patient has no pulse, begin cardiopulmonary resuscitation (CPR—see Chapter 5). If there is a pulse, but no breathing, continue with the following cycle
   - Take a deep breath and pinch the patient's nostrils closed; form a seal with

TABLE 4-1   Rescue Breathing and Clearing the Airway

	Adult	Child	Infant
Age	8 yrs and older	1–8 yrs	birth–1 yr
Initial ventilation	1 ½ to 2 sec.	1 to 1 ½ sec.	1 to 1 ½ sec.
Ventilation rate	10–12 breaths/min.	20 breaths/min.	20 breaths/min.
Heimlich maneuver	Series of 5 abdominal thrusts	Series of 5 abdominal thrusts	NOT USED FOR INFANTS
Chest thrusts (if obese or pregnant); back blows and chest thrusts (for infants)	Series of 5 thrusts to chest—arms locked, hands in CPR position	NOT USED FOR CHILDREN	Series of: 5 back blows 5 chest thrusts, using 2-3 fingers
Working alone: Call 911 or emergency dispatcher	After establishing unresponsiveness— before beginning resuscitation	After establishing unresponsiveness and 1 minute of resuscitation	After establishing unresponsiveness and 1 minute of resuscitation

the patient's mouth and exhale air into the patient's airway. (Or use a pocket face mask with one-way valve.)

- Break contact with the mask or patient's mouth (allowing the nostrils to open).
- Air should be passively released from his lungs while you . . .
- Turn your head to watch the patient's chest fall and listen and feel for the return of air.
- Take another deep breath and begin the cycle again.

Important: For artificial respirations provided to the adult patient, after the initial two slow breaths, you must deliver breaths to the patient at ONE EVERY 5 OR 6 SECONDS to give a rate of 10 TO 12 BREATHS PER MINUTE. A respiratory cycle—inhalation/exhalation—takes 5 to 6 seconds. Watch the chest rise as you ventilate, then watch the chest fall as the patient exhales and ventilate again.

Once you are breathing for the patient, you must continue to do so until he starts to breathe on his own (spontaneous breathing) or until you transfer the responsibility to another trained person. If you detect cardiac arrest, you must begin cardiopulmonary resuscitation (CPR), continuing to breathe for the patient as part of this procedure.

You will know that you are adequately ventilating the patient if you

- SEE the chest rise and fall
- HEAR and FEEL air leaving the patient's lungs
- FEEL resistance to your ventilations as the patient's lungs expand

You also may note that the patient's color improves or remains normal. In some cases, another rescuer may note that the pupils of the patient's eyes react to light.

The most common problems with the mouth-to-mouth technique include

- Failure to form a tight seal over the patient's mouth (with your mouth or pocket face mask)
- Failure to pinch the nose completely closed in mouth-to-mouth procedures
- Failure to establish an open airway because of inadequate head tilt or head positioning

- Failure to have the patient's mouth open wide enough to receive ventilations
- Failure to clear the upper airway of obstructions.

Many students wonder how big the rescue breath should be. The clearest guideline is that it must be big enough to make the patient's chest rise, but not bigger. That is why it is so important to watch the patient's chest rise and feel for resistance to your breaths. As stated earlier, the average breath of an adult at rest moves 500 mL of air. More air is needed for an effective artificial ventilation. The size should be somewhere between a normal breath and a double-sized breath. You are trying to deliver at least 800 to 1,200 mL of air to the adult patient. Often, each breath turns out to be around 500 mL if you try to deliver the breaths too quickly. If the volume of air is too great or delivered too quickly, it can also overwhelm the ability of the patient's trachea to accept the breath and cause gastric distention (discussed later in this chapter).

Remember: If there is a possibility of spinal injury, employ the jaw-thrust maneuver to open the airway. If you are using your hands to maintain the jaw thrust, then you must use your cheek to seal the nose if you are doing mouth-to-mouth rescue breathing. This technique is difficult, even when practiced on a regular basis, and is very tiring for the rescuer. If the jaw thrust is used, the mouth-to-nose technique or use of a pocket face mask or bag-valve-mask is preferred.

Mouth-To-Nose-Ventilation Occasionally, you will not be able to ventilate a nonbreathing patient by the mouth-to-mouth technique. An accident victim may have severe injuries to the mouth and lower jaw. A patient lacking teeth or dentures may make it difficult to get a good seal. For this patient, you may have to use the mouth-to-nose technique (Figure 4-11). Most of the procedure is very similar to the mouth-to-mouth technique. The airway must be opened and two slow breaths delivered. As with the mouth-to-mouth procedure, breaths are then delivered ONE EVERY 5 OR 6 SECONDS to give a rate of 10 TO 12 BREATHS PER MINUTE. The following are ways in which the mouth-to-nose procedure differs from the mouth-to-mouth procedure.

- You must keep one hand on the patient's forehead to maintain an open airway and

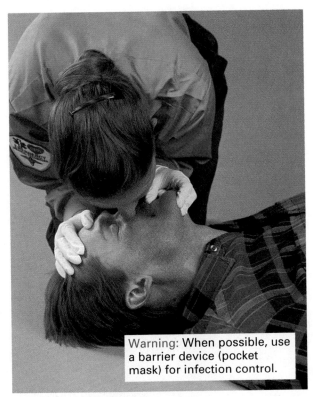

Figure 4-11 Mouth-to-nose ventilation.

Warning: When possible, use a barrier device (pocket mask) for infection control.

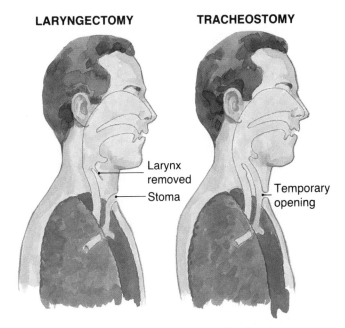

LARYNGECTOMY   TRACHEOSTOMY

Larynx
removed

Stoma

Temporary
opening

Figure 4-12 Differences between the laryngectomy and the tracheostomy.

use your other hand to close the patient's mouth.

- The patient's nose is left open.
- To provide breaths, you must seal your mouth around and deliver ventilations through the patient's nose. The patient's mouth must be kept shut during delivery of the ventilation.
- When allowing the patient to exhale passively, you must break contact with his nose and slightly open his mouth. Keep your hand on the patient's forehead to help keep his airway open as he exhales.

Remember: The jaw thrust should be used if there is a possibility of spinal injury. For the mouth-to-nose technique, do not allow the lower lip to retract as you push with your thumbs. Use your cheek to seal the patient's mouth.

Ventilating Neck Breathers Although such occasions are rare, you may have to ventilate a neck breather, or laryngectomy patient. A **laryngectomy** (LAR-in-JEK-to-me) is a surgical procedure in which part or all of the larynx has been removed. The trachea is shortened and is usually brought to the front of the neck as a permanent opening called a **stoma** (STO-mah—Fig-

ure 4-12). The patient is called a laryngectomee (LAR-in-JEK-to-me). At present, there are approximately 30,000 laryngectomees in the United States.

A laryngectomy requires the construction of a permanent stoma. A **tracheostomy** (TRAY-ke-OS-to-me), the creation of an artificial opening into the trachea through the neck, may be temporary or permanent, depending on the reason for the surgery (Figure 4-12).

The opening of a tracheostomy is round and usually no more than several millimeters in diameter. This opening often contains two concentric metal tubes, although some patients may have only one tube made of metal or plastic. When two tubes are used, there is an outer tube and an inner one passing from outside the skin to the trachea. In the laryngectomy, the opening is large and round and the edge of the tracheal lining can be seen attached to the skin. There is no metal tube. The method of ventilation is the same for both types of patients.

When you examine a patient's stoma, you may find that there is a breathing tube (or tubes) in the opening. This tube may become clogged and need cleaning. Do not remove the tube. The tube should be cleaned while in place. Quickly clean the neck opening of encrusted mucus and foreign matter using a gauze pad or handkerchief (*do not* use tissue). Pass a sterile suction catheter tube through the stoma and into the

INSERT 3 TO 5 INCHES

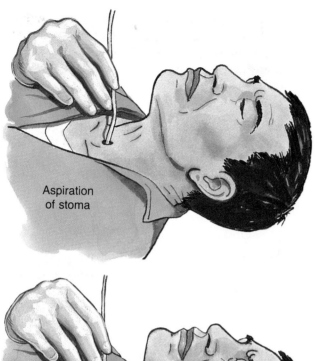

Aspiration
of stoma

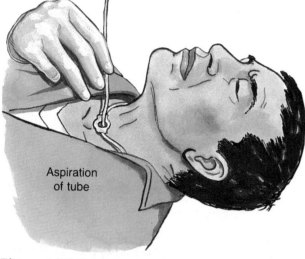

Aspiration
of tube

Figure 4-13 Suctioning techniques for the laryngectomy and tracheostomy patient.

trachea (Figure 4-13). *Do not* insert the catheter more than 3 to 5 inches into the trachea. Allow suctioning to take place for a few seconds while withdrawing the catheter (see Chapter 6). *Do not* waste time by attempting to do a complete suctioning. Once the airway is partially open, start mouth-to-stoma ventilations. If approved in your EMS system, protect yourself by using a pediatric pocket face mask over the top of the stoma.

Since the patient's airway from throat to trachea has been interrupted, you will have to use the mouth-to-stoma technique on neck breathers (Figure 4-14). Use the same basic technique as for mouth-to-mouth ventilation, but

- Do not tilt the head. Best results come from keeping the patient's head straight and his shoulders slightly elevated.

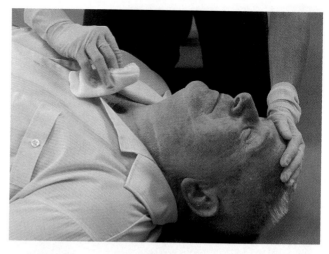

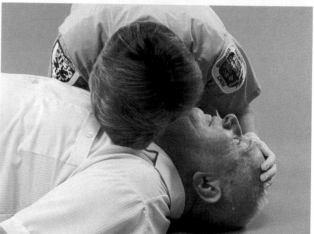

Figure 4-14 Mouth-to-stoma ventilations. Use a pediatric-sized pocket face mask.

- Place your mouth directly over the patient's stoma rather than his mouth.
- Use the same size breaths you normally would during mouth-to-mouth resuscitation, and provide VENTILATIONS AT THE RATE OF ONE EVERY 5 OR 6 SECONDS OR 10 TO 12 BREATHS PER MINUTE.
- Make certain that you watch for the patient's chest to rise and fall as you provide ventilations. If the patient's chest does not rise, it may mean that the patient is a partial neck breather. This type of patient does take in and expel some air through the mouth and nose. In such cases, you will have to pinch closed the nose and seal the mouth with the palm of your hand.

Note: Other special patients, including the elderly, near-drowning victims, and accident victims, will be covered later in this text. The special problems of airway obstruction and artificial ventilation will be discussed when these cases are presented.

Warning: You may be exposed to infectious diseases when using the mouth-to-stoma technique. Follow local protocols in regard to the use of a pediatric-sized pocket face mask or other suitable barrier.

Ventilating Infants and Children In basic life support, an **infant** is any patient from birth to 1 year of age, a **child** is any patient from 1 to 8 years of age, and an **adult** is any patient older than 8 years of age.

To provide ventilations to the infant or child (Figure 4-15 and Table 4-1), you should

1. Establish whether the patient is responsive. (Tap the patient. Ask a child, "Are you OK?" An infant should move or cry when tapped or spoken to loudly.)
2. Lay an infant or child on a hard surface. A small infant may be held in your arms.
3. Open the airway and determine if the patient is breathing. Take 3 TO 5 SECONDS to determine breathlessness.

Warning: A slight head tilt is all that is required to open the airway of an infant or child. Some rescuers provide too great a tilt, which may actually obstruct the airway of a young infant. On the other hand, some rescuers are too cautious with the head tilt. If the patient's chest does not rise when you provide a breath, it may be due to an improper head tilt. Make certain that you do not underventilate the patient because of failure to maintain an open airway.

4. Take a breath and cover both the mouth and nose of the infant or small child patient (mouth-to-mouth-and-nose technique). If a

pocket face mask is used, it must be the correct size for the patient.

5. Deliver TWO SLOW BREATHS (1 to 1 ½ seconds per breath). Pause to take a breath between the two ventilations. Only small breaths are required to ventilate infants.

Warning: You must stay alert for resistance to your ventilations and for chest movements. If you are too forceful with your ventilations, air will be forced into the patient's stomach. Provide a breath that is just large enough to make the patient's chest rise. If your efforts are met with resistance, there may be an upper airway obstruction (discussed later in this chapter). Do not use excessive pressure to force air into the lungs.

6. When allowing the patient to exhale, uncover both mouth and nose. Allow for deflation between breaths.
7. If the infant or child patient is unresponsive and you are working alone, PROVIDE ARTIFICIAL VENTILATIONS FOR 1 MINUTE BEFORE BREAKING to telephone 911 or your local emergency number, or to radio for help.
8. If the patient is not breathing after two initial ventilations, determine pulselessness. If there is no pulse, start cardiopulmonary resuscitation (CPR—see Chapters 5 and 17). If the patient has a pulse, start rescue breathing and . . .
9. Provide ventilations to infants and children at the rate of ONE BREATH EVERY 3 SECONDS in order to deliver 20 BREATHS PER MINUTE. The volume should be that which makes the patient's chest rise without overinflating. Watch as the patient exhales, then re-inflate enough to make the chest rise.

Gastric Distention Rescue breathing can force some air into the patient's stomach, and the stomach becomes distended (bulges). This may indicate that the airway is blocked, that there is improper head position, or that the ventilations being provided are too great or too quick to be accommodated by the lungs or the esophagus. This problem is seen most frequently in infants and children but can occur with any patient.

A slight bulge is of little worry, but a major distention can cause two serious problems. First, the air-filled stomach reduces lung volume by forcing up the diaphragm. Second, regurgita-

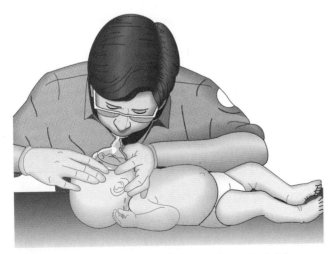

Figure 4-15 Ventilating infants and small children.

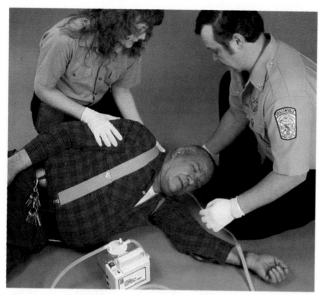

Figure 4-16 Be prepared for vomiting when attempting to relieve gastric distention.

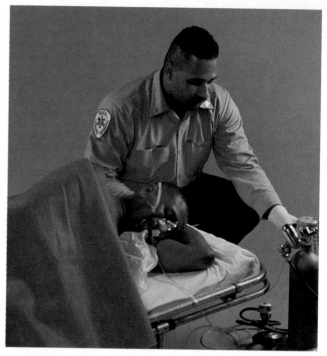

Figure 4-17 Place the breathing but unresponsive patient who has no head, neck, or spine injury in the recovery position to protect the airway.

tion (the slow expulsion of fluids and partially digested foods from the stomach into the throat) or vomiting (the forceful expulsion of the stomach's contents) are strong possibilities. This could lead to additional airway obstruction or the **aspiration** (AS-pir-AY-shun), or breathing in, of vomitus into the patient's lungs. When this happens, lung damage can occur and a lethal form of pneumonia may develop.

The best way to avoid gastric distention, or to avoid making it worse once it develops, is to position the patient's head properly, avoid too forceful and too quickly delivered ventilations, and limit the volume of ventilations delivered. The volume delivered should be limited to the size breath that causes the chest to rise. This is why it is so important to watch the patient's chest rise as each ventilation is delivered and to feel for resistance to your breaths.

When gastric distention is present, be prepared for vomiting (Figure 4-16). If the patient does vomit, roll the entire patient onto his side. (Turning just the head may allow for aspiration of vomitus as well as aggravating any possible neck injury.) Protect the head and neck of the patient as you roll him. Be prepared to use suction to clear the patient's mouth and throat of vomitus.

Manually pressing on the abdomen to relieve distention in the prehospital setting is *not* recommended.

The Recovery Position Patients who resume adequate breathing and pulse after resuscitation are placed in the recovery position

(Figure 4-17). This position is also suitable for patients who are unconscious with adequate pulse and respirations. The recovery position allows for drainage from the mouth and prevents the tongue from falling backward and causing an airway obstruction.

The patient should be rolled onto his side. This should be done moving the patient as a unit, that is, *not* twisting the head, shoulders, or torso. The patient may be rolled onto either side; however it is preferable to have the patient facing the EMT so that monitoring and suctioning may be more easily performed.

If the patient does not have respirations that are sufficient to support life, the recovery position must not be used. The patient should be placed supine and his ventilations assisted.

Warning: *Do not* use the recovery position for patients who have possible spinal injuries.

AIRWAY OBSTRUCTION

Causes of Airway Obstruction

Every year in the United States, as many as 3,000 people die of airway obstruction. In basic life support, establishing an open airway may be

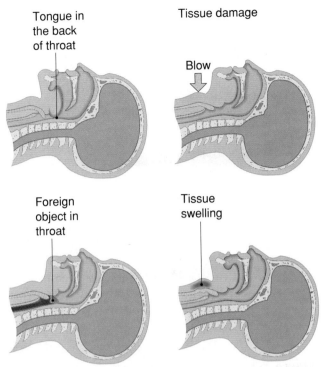

Tongue in the back of throat

Tissue damage

Blow

Foreign object in throat

Tissue swelling

Figure 4-18 Four possible causes of airway obstruction.

the face, breathing hot air (as in fires), poisons, and severe injury due to blows to the neck or chest. **Edema** (e-DE-mah), or swelling, of the pharynx and tracheal tissues presents a major problem in providing emergency care.

- Diseases—Respiratory infection, allergic reactions, and certain chronic illnesses such as asthma can cause edema or bronchial spasms that will obstruct the airway.

There is little that the EMT can do to clear obstructions from the lower airway. Most of the time, such obstructions are due to respiratory disease. Upper airway obstruction caused by the tongue or by foreign objects may be cleared using a few simple techniques.

Airway obstructions are one of two types: partial or complete. Each type of obstruction has different characteristics that may be noted during assessment, and each type has a different procedure of care. It is important to know the differences between partial and complete obstruction and the correct care for each.

critical. As an EMT you must be able to quickly detect and, when possible, correct airway obstructions.

Many factors can cause the patient's airway to become partially or completely obstructed, including (Figure 4-18):

- Obstruction by the Tongue—As noted earlier, the tongue can fall back and block off the pharynx. This often occurs when a patient's head flexes forward and is allowed to remain in that position. This problem is most commonly seen with unconscious patients and patients who have abused alcohol or some other drug.
- Obstruction by the Epiglottis—Attempts by the patient to force inspirations may create a negative pressure that forces the epiglottis (and tongue) to block the airway.
- Foreign Objects or Materials—These can include pieces of food, ice, toys, dentures, broken teeth, vomitus, and liquids pooling in the back of the throat. This problem is most commonly seen with children and with patients who have abused alcohol or drugs.
- Tissue Damage—Accident-related tissue problems can be caused by puncture wounds to the neck, crushing wounds to

---

**Patient Assessment—
Partial Airway Obstruction**

Keep in mind the mechanisms of injury. Look over the scene for clues that tell you to be alert for airway problems. Something as simple as noticing a half-eaten sandwich may make a difference.

Signs

Be on the alert for partial airway obstruction if you note

☐ Unusual Breathing Sounds—Listen for
Snoring—probably caused by the tongue obstructing the pharynx.
Gurgling—often due to a foreign object or blood and other fluids in the trachea.
Crowing—probably caused by spasms in the larynx.
Wheezing—This may not indicate any major problems but should not be treated lightly since it may be due to serious edema or spasms along the airway.

☐ Skin Discoloration—The patient is breathing, but there is a noticeable blue or gray color to the skin, lips, tongue, ear lobes, or nailbeds. This is recorded as cyanosis.

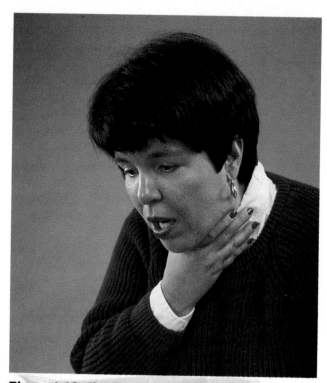

Figure 4-19 The distress signal for choking.

poor air exchange, begin to treat the patient AS IF THERE IS A COMPLETE AIRWAY OBSTRUCTION (see below).

Patient Assessment—Complete Airway Obstruction

Signs

☐ The Conscious Patient—The conscious patient with a complete airway obstruction will try to speak, but he will not be able to do so. He will also not be able to breathe or cough. Usually, he will display the distress signal for choking by clutching the neck between thumb and fingers.

☐ The Unconscious Patient—The unconscious patient with a complete airway obstruction is more difficult to identify. The patient is found in respiratory arrest. Only when ventilation attempts are unsuccessful (the rescue breather discovers resistance to ventilations that changing the head position does not correct; the chest will not rise; there is no observable exchange of air) does it become apparent that there is an obstruction. Clues to an airway obstruction may also be found at the scene (bystanders report that the patient collapsed while eating dinner, for example).

☐ Changes in Breathing—The patient's breathing may keep changing from near normal to very labored and back again.

A conscious patient trying to indicate an airway problem will usually point to his mouth or hold his neck (Figure 4-19). Many do this even when a partial obstruction does not prevent speech. Ask the patient if he is choking, or ask if he can speak or cough. If he can, then the obstruction is partial.

Patient Care—Complete Airway Obstruction

Follow the procedures described under "Techniques for Clearing the Airway" and "Procedures for Clearing the Airway," below.

Patient Care—Partial Airway Obstruction

For the conscious patient with an apparent partial airway obstruction, have him cough. A strong and forceful cough indicates he is exchanging enough air. Continue to encourage the patient to cough in the hope that such action will dislodge and expel the foreign object. *Do not* interfere with the patient's efforts to clear the partial obstruction by means of forceful coughing.

Warning: In cases where the patient has an apparent partial airway obstruction but he cannot cough or has a very weak cough, or the patient is cyanotic or shows other signs of

Techniques for Clearing the Airway

When you have determined that the airway is obstructed, you must take appropriate measures to clear it.

1. *Open the airway.* Since so many obstructions are caused by the tongue, you must first make certain that the airway is open (by using a head-tilt, head-tilt, chin-lift, or jaw-thrust maneuver, as described earlier in this chapter).

2. *Provide artificial ventilations for the unconscious, nonbreathing patient.* When the patient is unconscious, once the airway is open but the patient is not breathing, do

not waste time looking for or trying to remove a foreign object; attempt to provide the two initial ventilations that are part of rescue breathing (don't forget that adjusting the head position will sometimes solve the problem if the first attempts are unsuccessful). If the initial ventilations are unsuccessful, assume that there is foreign matter in the airway. (Make this assumption without attempting artificial ventilations for the conscious patient who is able to indicate that he is choking on a foreign object.)

3. *Remove any foreign object.* If you have assured that the airway is open (and have unsuccessfully attempted artificial ventilation if the patient is unconscious and not breathing), two techniques are recommended for removal of a foreign object:
   - Manual thrusts (including the Heimlich maneuver)
   - Finger sweeps

On any given patient you may have to use both techniques. These techniques are discussed in detail below.

The methods for clearing the airway vary depending on whether the patient is conscious, loses consciousness while being treated, or is already unconscious, and whether the patient is an adult, child, or infant. The techniques for correcting airway obstructions (manual thrusts and finger sweeps) are described below under "Techniques for Clearing the Airway." The procedures for applying these techniques to each type of patient are then described under "Procedures for Clearing the Airway."

Note: If the cause of airway obstruction is blood, liquids, or vomitus pooling in the throat, you should consider suctioning to clear the airway (see Chapter 6). However, do not delay efforts to clear the airway in order to locate and set up suctioning equipment.

The Heimlich Maneuver—Abdominal Thrusts In the **Heimlich maneuver**, developed by Dr. Henry Heimlich, manual thrusts to the abdomen are used to force bursts of air from the lungs that will be sufficient to dislodge an obstructing object (Figure 4-20 and Table 4-1).

Warning: Do not use the Heimlich maneuver on patients in late stages of pregnancy (when the uterus is so large that it intrudes into the area of the abdomen where you would apply the thrusts). Also do not use the Heimlich maneuver on infants (from birth to 1 year of age).

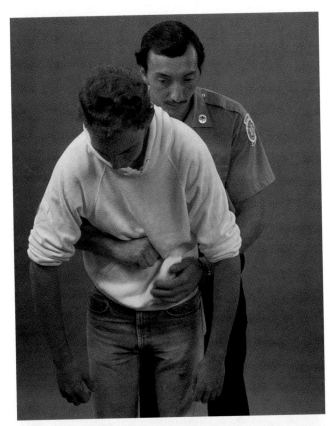

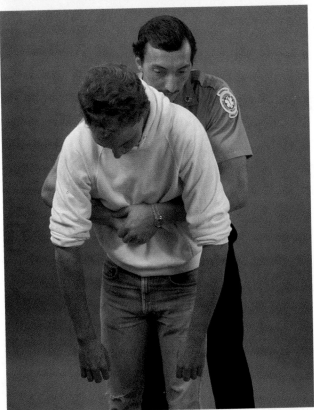

Figure 4-20 The Heimlich maneuver. Place your fist on the patient's midline, between the waist and rib cage. Grasp this fist and rapidly deliver five inward and upward thrusts.

For the conscious adult or child (not infant) patient who is standing or sitting

1. While standing behind the patient, reach underneath the patient's arms to his front. Wrap your arms around his waist.
2. Make a fist and place the thumb side of this fist against the midline of the patient's abdomen, between the waist and rib cage. Avoid touching the patient's chest, especially the area immediately below the sternum (the region of the xiphoid process).
3. Grasp your properly positioned fist with your other hand and apply pressure inward and up toward the patient's diaphragm in one smooth, quick movement. This will cause your fist to press into the patient's abdomen. Deliver a series of FIVE RAPID INWARD THRUSTS up toward the diaphragm. Each new thrust should be separate and distinct, delivered with the intent of relieving the obstruction.

For the unconscious adult or child (not infant) patient or for a conscious patient who cannot sit up or be seated with your assistance, or if you are too short to reach around the patient and deliver upward thrusts

1. Move the patient into a supine position (Figure 4-21).
2. Kneel and straddle the patient at the level of the thighs, facing his chest.
3. Place the heel of your hand on the midline of his abdomen, slightly above the navel and well below the xiphoid process.

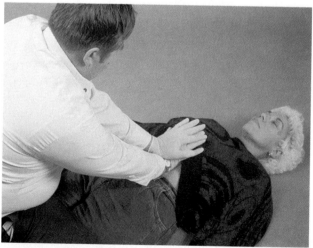

Figure 4-21 The Heimlich maneuver used on a patient who is supine.

4. Now place your free hand over the positioned hand. Your shoulders should be directly over the patient's abdomen. Be sure that you are positioned over the midline of the abdomen so that thrusts will be delivered straight up, not off to one side.
5. Deliver the thrusts by pressing your hands inward and upward toward the patient's diaphragm. Deliver FIVE RAPID THRUSTS. Each new thrust should be separate and distinct, delivered with the intent of relieving the obstruction.

If you complete a series of five thrusts and the obstruction is still present, if the patient is conscious quickly reassess your hand position and the victim's airway. Repeat the thrusts in series of five until the object is expelled or there is a change in the patient's airway and breathing status. If the patient is unconscious, open the airway, use finger sweeps to attempt to remove the obstruction, and attempt to ventilate before doing another series of thrusts.

If the patient is very large or if you are a small individual, you can deliver more effective thrusts if you straddle one leg of the patient.

Chest Thrusts Chest thrusts (Table 4-1) are used in place of abdominal thrusts when the patient is in the late stages of pregnancy (Figure 4-22), or when the patient is too obese for abdominal thrusts to be effective.

For the conscious adult patient who is standing or sitting

1. Position yourself behind the patient and slide your arms under his armpits, so that you encircle his chest.
2. Form a fist with one hand and place the thumb side of this fist on the patient's sternum. You should make contact with the midline of the sternum, about two to three finger widths above the xiphoid process. This results in the fist being placed over the lower half of the sternum, but not in contact with the edge of the rib cage.
3. Grasp the fist with your other hand and deliver FIVE CHEST THRUSTS directly backward toward the spine until the obstruction is relieved. Do not exert this force in an upward or downward direction or off to one side.

If the obstruction is not relieved, quickly

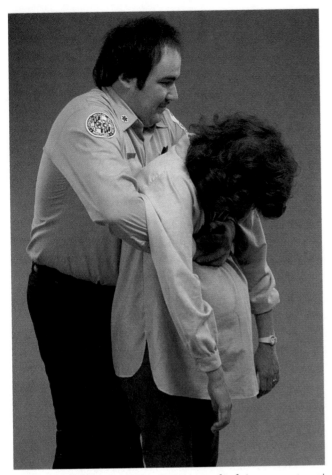

Figure 4-22 The chest thrust applied to a pregnant patient.

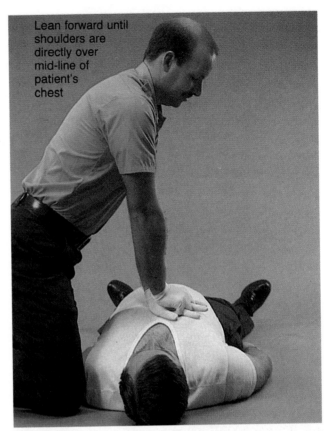

Lean forward until shoulders are directly over mid-line of patient's chest

Figure 4-23 The chest thrust method can be used when the patient is lying on his back.

reassess your position and the patient's airway and continue delivering series of five thrusts.

For the unconscious adult patient chest thrusts are best carried out when the patient is supine (Figure 4-23). In this position, chest thrusts are delivered as you would for CPR. Once the patient is properly positioned, you should

1. Kneel alongside the patient at the level of his chest. Have both of your knees facing the patient's chest.
2. Position the heel of one hand on the midline of the sternum, two to three finger widths above the xiphoid process (your fingers should be perpendicular to the sternum). Lift and spread your fingers to avoid applying too much pressure to the ribs.
3. Place your other hand on top of the first, interlocking your fingers. Lock your elbows and lean forward until your shoulders are

directly over the midline of the patient's chest.
4. Deliver FIVE SLOW, DISTINCT THRUSTS in a downward direction, applying enough force to compress the chest cavity. Continue until the object is expelled.

For an infant, back blows are alternated with chest thrusts (Figure 4-24).

1. Lay the infant face down along your forearm with the head lower than the trunk. Support the head by placing your hand around the jaw. You may need to add support by resting your forearm on your thigh. Rapidly deliver FIVE BACK BLOWS (in 3 to 5 seconds) using the heel of your hand. Strike forcefully directly between the shoulder blades.
2. Place your free arm on the infant's back. Support the head with your hand and sandwich him between your two arms. Turn the infant over so his back is along your forearm. Place your forearm against your

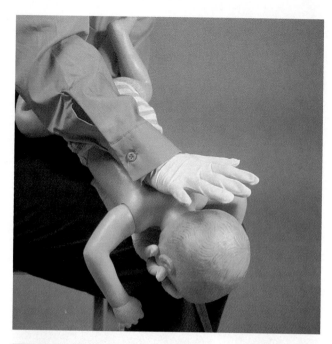

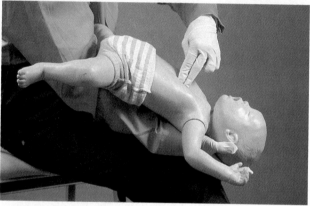

Figure 4-24 To clear an airway obstruction in an infant, alternate back blows with chest thrusts.

thigh again. The head should be lower than the trunk.

3. Rapidly deliver FIVE CHEST THRUSTS, using the tips of two or three fingers. Apply pressure along the midline of the sternum. The fingers should be placed one finger width below an imaginary line drawn directly between the nipples.

4. If the airway remains obstructed, continue back blows and chest thrusts.

Note: *Do not* place infants or small children into the head-down position if they have a partial obstruction and can breathe adequately in an upright position. Keep in mind that forceful coughing is a good sign in cases of partial airway obstruction.

Airway maintenance, rescue breathing, CPR, and other basic life support procedures for infants and children will be summarized in Chapter 17.

Finger Sweeps A finger sweep is an attempt to manually remove an airway obstruction that has become dislodged or partially dislodged. Using a gloved hand to protect from infectious agents, sweep the mouth from one side to the other. Take care not to force the object farther down the patient's throat. The finger sweep technique should not be used for infants and children unless the object can actually be seen. "Blind" finger sweeps are especially dangerous in these smaller patients; if the obstruction is in sight, use your little finger to remove it.

You can open an *unconscious* patient's mouth and airway by using the *tongue-jaw-lift* procedure (Figure 4-25). This requires you to grasp both tongue and lower jaw between your gloved thumb and fingers and lift to move the tongue away from the back of the pharynx. This movement will also move the tongue away from any foreign object that might be lodged in the back of the throat. The procedure may partially solve the problem of obstruction. However, it will be necessary to keep the patient's face up and insert the index finger of your free gloved hand into the patient's mouth and move this finger along the inside of the cheek to the base of the tongue. Using your finger as a hook, attempt to dislodge the object and sweep it into the mouth so it can be removed.

In some cases, it may be necessary to use your index finger to push the foreign object against the opposite side of the patient's throat in order to dislodge and lift the object. During such a procedure, you must take extra care not to push the object farther down the patient's throat.

You can also use the *crossed-fingers technique* to open the mouth of an unconscious patient (Figure 4-25). Use one gloved hand to steady the patient's forehead. Place your thumb against the patient's lower lip and your index finger against his upper teeth. Crossing the thumb and finger will force open the patient's mouth. Once the mouth is open, hold the lower jaw so that it cannot close.

Once you have opened the patient's mouth, release the patient's forehead and use the index finger of this hand to dislodge the foreign object as you would in the tongue-jaw-lift procedure.

Warning: A *conscious* patient has a gag reflex that can induce vomiting. This vomitus can be

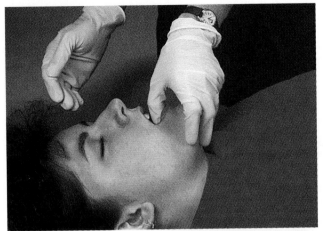

A.

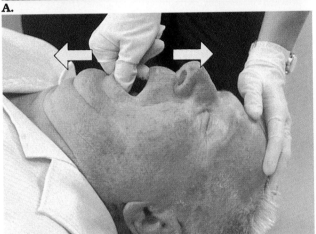

B.

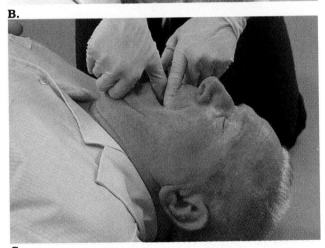

C.

Figure 4-25 Open the patient's mouth using **(A)** the tongue-jaw lift or **(B)** the crossed-fingers technique. Use **(C)** finger sweeps to remove foreign objects from the airway and mouth.

aspirated into the lungs. This is why most EMS Systems do not sanction the use of finger sweeps on conscious patients. Some localities believe that there are situations in which aggressive actions must be taken during basic life sup-

port. If an obstructing object becomes visible, the EMT can use a finger sweep to dislodge and remove the object. If you are using a finger sweep method on a conscious patient, or you are trying to grasp a dislodged object, take great care not to induce vomiting or force the object farther down the patient's airway. Stay alert to avoid being bitten by the patient.

Remember: When using the finger sweep technique, if the object comes within reach grasp the object and remove it. Be careful not to push it down the patient's airway. Be aware of a possible gag reflex and be prepared for the patient to vomit.

Procedures for Clearing the Airway

The following pages contain procedures and sequences to use in the event of a complete airway obstruction or a partial airway obstruction with poor air exchange (Table 4-2). These procedures or combinations of procedures are considered to have been effective if any of the following happens.

- The patient re-establishes good air exchange or spontaneous breathing.
- The foreign object is expelled from the mouth.
- The foreign object is expelled into the mouth where it can be removed by the rescuer.
- The unconscious patient regains consciousness.
- The patient's skin color improves.

When an obstruction is not easily corrected, you will have to combine procedures in an attempt to open the airway.

The use of the Heimlich maneuver or of chest thrusts requires a little common sense. Even though five thrusts are called for, if the first one works, the remaining thrusts are not needed. You must stay aware of what is happening to the patient when applying the procedure. Remember that each manual thrust should be performed with the intent of relieving the obstruction.

The thrusts are to be delivered rapidly, but some restraint is needed. Too forceful and too rapid a blow may injure the patient. An improperly delivered thrust may cause damage in the thoracic or abdominal cavity. Trying to do the thrusts as quickly as you can move will probably cause you to lose your balance and deliver an improper and possibly harmful thrust. You must

TABLE 4-2 Airway Clearance Sequences

	Adult	Child	Infant
Age	8 yrs and older	1–8 yrs	birth–1 yr
Conscious	Ask, "Are you choking?" or "Can you speak?" Series of 5 Heimlich maneuvers.	Ask, "Are you choking?" or "Can you speak?" Series of 5 Heimlich maneuvers.	Observe signs of choking (small objects or food, wheezing, agitation, cyanosis, absence of respirations). Series of: 5 back blows 5 chest thrusts.
Loses consciousness during procedure	Assist patient to floor. Establish unresponsiveness (ask "Are you OK?"). If alone, call for help, then . . . Open airway. Attempt to ventilate. Heimlich maneuver or chest thrusts (as appropriate). Finger sweeps. (Repeat as needed.)	Assist patient to floor. Establish unresponsiveness (ask "Are you OK?"). Open airway. Heimlich maneuver. Remove visible objects (NO blind sweeps). (Repeat as needed.) After 1 minute, call for help if alone.	Establish unresponsiveness (tap or speak loudly). Attempt to ventilate. Back blows and chest thrusts. Remove visible objects (NO blind sweeps). (Repeat as needed.) After 1 minute, call for help if alone.
Unconscious when found	Establish unresponsiveness. If alone, call for help, then . . . Open airway Attempt to ventilate. Heimlich maneuver or chest thrusts (as appropriate). Finger sweeps. (Repeat as needed.)	Establish unresponsiveness. Open airway. Attempt to ventilate. Heimlich maneuver. Remove visible objects (NO blind sweeps). (Repeat as needed.) After 1 minute, call for help if alone.	Establish unresponsiveness. Open airway. Attempt to ventilate. Back blows and chest thrusts. Remove visible objects (NO blind sweeps). (Repeat as needed.) After 1 minute, call for help if alone.

practice these techniques on the manikins provided in your course and keep your skills up to date.

If a person has only a partial airway obstruction and is still able to speak and cough forcefully, do not interfere with his attempts to expel the foreign body. Carefully watch him, however, so that you can immediately provide help if this partial obstruction becomes a complete one.

An unconscious patient or a conscious patient with total airway obstruction will present the greatest problems (Scans 4-3 and 4-4).

Warning: If the patient has no pulse or at any point becomes pulseless, CPR must be initiated (see Chapter 5).

Remember: Although the Heimlich maneuver is specified in the procedures described below, chest thrusts must be used for very obese patients, and for patients in late stages of pregnancy, alternating back blows and chest thrusts for infants.

Procedures for an Adult

The following are procedures for clearing an obstructed airway in an adult (Scan 4-3).

Conscious Adult If the adult patient is conscious, you should

1. Determine if there is a COMPLETE OBSTRUCTION or a PARTIAL OBSTRUCTION WITH POOR AIR EXCHANGE. Look, listen, and feel for the signs of obstruction. Be certain to ask, "Are you choking?" or "Can you speak?" If the patient can speak, see if he can produce a forceful cough. If the patient has a complete obstruction or poor air exchange . . .
2. Provide FIVE THRUSTS OF THE HEIMLICH MANEUVER in rapid succession. If the manual thrusts have not expelled the obstruction . . .
3. Re-evaluate your hand position and repeat the thrusts until you are successful or the patient loses consciousness.

Clearing the Airway—Adult

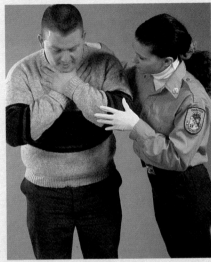

1. Recognize and assess that patient is choking. Ask, "Can you speak?" or "Are you choking?"

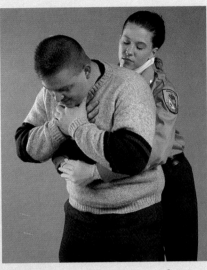

2. Position yourself to perform the Heimlich maneuver.

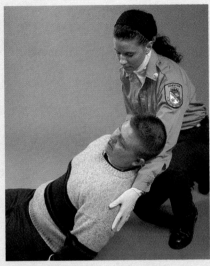

3. If the patient becomes weak or unconscious, assist him to the floor.

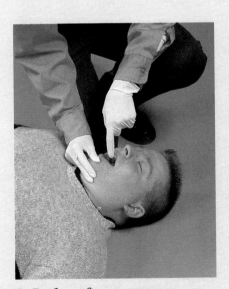

4. Perform finger sweeps.

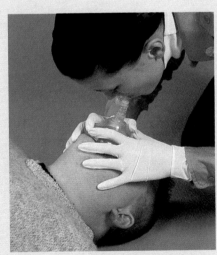

5. Attempt to ventilate. If you are not successful . . .

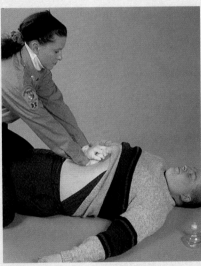

6. Perform the Heimlich maneuver.

Adult Loses Consciousness If the patient loses consciousness, you should

1. Protect the patient who suffers a loss of consciousness from possible injury due to falling.
2. Establish unresponsiveness. If you are working alone, call 911, or telephone your local emergency number, or radio the EMS dispatch center *immediately*, before attempting patient care.
3. Use the tongue-jaw lift to open the mouth. Perform finger sweeps.
4. Open the airway and attempt to ventilate. If this fails . . .
5. Deliver FIVE THRUSTS OF THE HEIMLICH MANEUVER.
6. Repeat the tongue-jaw lift and finger sweeps.
7. Open the airway and repeat your attempt to ventilate the patient. If this fails . . .
8. Continue with the following cycle until you are successful.
   - Heimlich maneuver
   - Finger sweeps
   - Attempt to ventilate

Unconscious Adult If the patient is unconscious when you arrive

1. Establish unresponsiveness. If you are working alone, call 911, or telephone your local emergency number, or radio the EMS dispatch center *immediately*, before attempting patient care.
2. Position the patient on his back with arms at his sides.
3. Attempt to open the patient's airway by the head-tilt, chin-lift (if there is no possible head, neck, or spinal injury) or jaw-thrust maneuver (if there is a possibility of trauma). Remember to look, listen, and feel for breathing.
4. Provide mouth-to-mask ventilations. (If you use mouth-to-mouth ventilations, remember to pinch the patient's nostrils closed. Typically, this is done with the hand used to hold the patient's forehead.) Try to give TWO SLOW VENTILATIONS (1 ½ to 2 seconds each) as described in the section on mouth-to-mouth ventilation earlier in this chapter. If your attempts to ventilate the patient fail, you should . . .
5. Reposition the patient's head, attempt to create an open airway, and try again to ventilate. If this fails . . .

6. Deliver FIVE THRUSTS OF THE HEIMLICH MANEUVER. If this fails . . .
7. Use the tongue-jaw lift and attempt finger sweeps. After removing the object, or if you cannot find and remove the obstruction, you should . . .
8. Open the airway and attempt to ventilate. If attempts to ventilate fail . . .
9. Continue with the cycle of Heimlich maneuver, finger sweeps, and attempts to ventilate until successful.

If you are unable to dislodge the obstruction, you have a critical emergency, requiring transport to a medical facility without delay. You must continue efforts to clear the obstruction, even if you can do no more than partially dislodge the object. The chances of at least partially dislodging the object will improve with time as the muscles of the patient's jaw and upper airway relax. Once the object is partially dislodged, you should be able to keep the patient alive by artificial ventilations. Keep in mind that CPR may be necessary.

Remember: You must persist in your efforts until the airway is clear or until you have dislodged the object enough to allow for you to provide artificial ventilations. If the patient's brain cells do not receive oxygen, they will begin to die within 10 minutes. Keep in mind that procedures used to clear the airway may at first fail, only to be successful later as muscles in the patient's body relax.

Procedures for a Child

The following are procedures for clearing an obstructed airway in a child.

Conscious Child Start by determining if there is an airway obstruction. Ask the child, "Are you choking?" "Can you speak?" "Can you cough?" If the child cannot cough or has an ineffective cough, or if the child's breathing problems continue to worsen, perform FIVE THRUSTS OF THE HEIMLICH MANEUVER. Continue with the thrusts until the object is expelled or the child loses consciousness.

Child Loses Consciousness If the child who has an airway obstruction loses consciousness while you are providing care, provide the same care as you would for an adult, but DO NOT ATTEMPT BLIND FINGER SWEEPS. (Look for and remove any *visible* foreign objects.) The

Heimlich maneuver is best delivered if you kneel at the child's feet. You may place the child on a table and stand at his feet.

If your attempts to clear the airway fail, continue the cycle of Heimlich maneuver, attempts to remove *visible* foreign objects, and attempts to ventilate until you are successful.

If you are working alone when the child loses consciousness, break to telephone or radio for assistance after 1 minute of attempts to clear the airway and ventilate.

Unconscious Child If the child is unconscious when you arrive, carry out the same procedures as you would for an adult patient. The Heimlich maneuver is best delivered if you kneel at the child's feet. You may place the child on a table and stand at his feet.

DO NOT ATTEMPT BLIND FINGER SWEEPS. (Look for and remove any *visible* foreign objects.)

If you fail at your attempts to clear the airway, repeat the cycle of Heimlich maneuver, attempts to remove *visible* foreign objects, and attempts to ventilate until you are successful.

If you are working alone, break to telephone or radio for assistance after 1 minute of attempts to clear the airway and ventilate.

Procedures for an Infant

The following are procedures for clearing an obstructed airway in an infant (Scan 4-4).

Conscious Infant If the patient is a conscious infant who requires your assistance to clear an airway obstruction, you should

1. Determine that there is an airway obstruction. An infant is not yet old enough to display the universal choking sign. Indications that an infant is choking are
   - Evidence of small objects or food around the infant
   - Wheezing or other unusual airway noises
   - Agitation or a look of panic
   - Blue or gray skin discoloration (cyanosis)
   - Absence of respirations
   - Inability to ventilate
2. Lay the infant face down along your forearm with the head lower than the trunk. Support the head by placing your hand around the jaw. Add support by resting your forearm on your thigh.
3. Deliver FIVE BACK BLOWS in 3 to 5 seconds. Deliver the blows forcefully with the

heel of your hand between the infant's shoulder blades. If this fails . . .
4. Support the infant's head and sandwich him between your two hands. Turn the infant over onto his back, keeping the head lower than the trunk.
5. Deliver FIVE CHEST THRUSTS, using the tips of two or three fingers. Apply pressure along the midline of the sternum. The fingers should be placed one finger width below an imaginary line drawn directly between the nipples.
6. Continue with the sequence of back blows and chest thrusts until the object is expelled or the infant loses consciousness.

Note: The above procedures are recommended only in cases where the infant's problem is a known or strongly suspected obstruction due to a foreign object, vomitus, or blood. If the problem is caused by tissue swelling related to an allergy or infection, transport the infant and follow the care protocol for epiglottitis as explained in Chapter 17.

Infant Loses Consciousness If the infant suffers a loss of consciousness while you are attempting to clear the airway, you should

1. Establish unresponsiveness (the infant does not move or cry when tapped or spoken to loudly. Do not shake the infant).
2. Position the patient and use the tongue-jaw lift. Look for and remove any visible foreign objects. DO NOT ATTEMPT BLIND FINGER SWEEPS.
3. Attempt to ventilate. If this fails . . .
4. If working alone, call 911, telephone your local emergency number, or radio the EMS dispatch center after 1 minute of attempts to clear the airway and ventilate.
5. Deliver FIVE BACK BLOWS. If this fails . . .
6. Deliver FIVE CHEST THRUSTS.
7. Employ the tongue-jaw lift and look for and remove any foreign objects. DO NOT ATTEMPT BLIND FINGER SWEEPS.
8. Re-attempt to ventilate. If this fails . . .
9. Continue with the sequence of back blows, chest thrusts, foreign object removal (not "blind"), and attempts to ventilate until you are successful.

Unconscious Infant If the infant is unconscious when you arrive

1. Establish unresponsiveness.

Clearing the Airway— Unconscious Infant

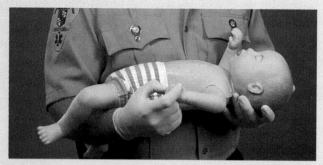

1. Establish unresponsiveness. Position the infant.

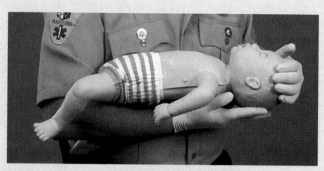

2. Open airway. Establish breathlessness.

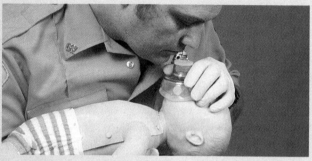

3. Attempt to ventilate. If this fails, reposition head and try again.

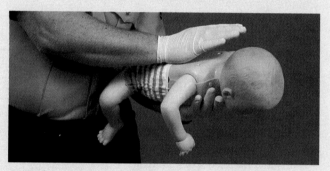

4. Deliver 5 back blows.

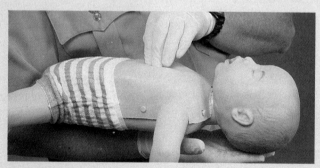

5. Deliver 5 chest thrusts.

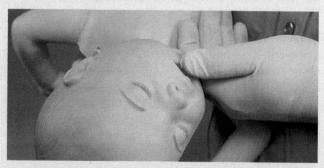

6. Remove visible objects.

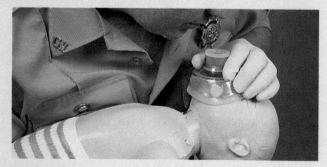

7. Re-attempt to ventilate.

8. Repeat the sequence of
- Back blows
- Chest thrusts
- Removing visible objects
- Re-attempting ventilations.

2. Place the infant on its back, supporting the head and neck.
3. Open the airway and establish breathlessness.
4. Attempt to ventilate, using the mouth-to-mouth-and-nose or mouth-to-mask technique. Should this fail . . .
5. Reposition the infant's head and attempt to ventilate. If this fails . . .
6. If working alone, call 911, telephone your local emergency number, or radio the EMS dispatch center after 1 minute of attempts to clear the airway and ventilate.
7. Lay the infant face down along your forearm with the head lower than the trunk. Support the head by placing your hand around the jaw. Support your forearm on your thigh. Deliver FIVE BACK BLOWS in 3 to 5 seconds. If this fails . . .
8. Sandwich the infant between your arms and turn him over onto his back, keeping the head lower than the trunk. Deliver FIVE CHEST THRUSTS. If this fails . . .
9. Insert your gloved thumb into the mouth, over the tongue. Wrap your fingers around the lower jaw and lift the tongue and jaw forward, opening the patient's mouth. Look for any objects causing the obstruction. If you can see the object, remove it using your little finger, but do not attempt "blind" finger sweeps. If you cannot see and remove an object . . .
10. Open the airway and attempt to ventilate using the mouth-to-mouth-and-nose or mouth-to-mask technique.
11. Repeat the following sequence until you are successful.
    • Five back blows
    • Five chest thrusts
    • Looking for and removing visible objects (no "blind" finger sweeps)
    • Attempts to ventilate

Should the infant develop respiratory arrest, and you have cleared enough of the obstruction to provide adequate ventilation, provide two breaths and check for heart action to see if CPR must be initiated (see Chapters 5 and 17).

CHAPTER REVIEW

KEY TERMS

You may find it helpful to review the following terms.

adult—in basic life support, anyone over 8 years of age.

airway—the passageway for air entering or leaving the body. The structures of the airway are the nose, mouth, pharynx, larynx, trachea, bronchial tree, and lungs.

alveoli (al-VE-o-li)—the microscopic air sacs of the lungs where gas exchange with the bloodstream takes place.

aspiration (AS-pir-AY-shun)—the breathing in of vomitus or other foreign matter into the lungs.

biological death—when the brain cells die.

bronchial (BRONG-ke-ul) **tree**—the branching of the airway from the trachea to the air sacs of the lungs.

bronchioles (BRONG-ke-olz)—the smaller branches of the airway that connect the bronchi to the air sacs of the lungs.

bronchi (BRONG-ke)—the two large sets of branches that come off the trachea and enter the lungs. There are right and left bronchi.

child—in basic life support, anyone from 1 to 8 years of age.

clinical death—when breathing and heart action stop.

cyanosis (sigh-ah-NO-sis)—when the skin, lips, tongue, ear lobes, or nailbeds turn blue or gray from lack of oxygen in circulation. The patient is said to be cyanotic (sigh-ah-NOT-ik).

diaphragm (DI-ah-fram)—the dome-shaped muscle of respiration that separates the chest from the abdomen.

edema (e-DE-mah)—swelling due to the accumulation of fluid in the tissues.

epiglottis (EP-i-GLOT-is)—the trapdoor-like structure at the entrance to the trachea.

expiration (ex-pir-AY-shun)—breathing out, or exhaling.

Heimlich maneuver—manual thrusts to the abdomen to force bursts of air from the lungs to dislodge an airway obstruction.

infant—in basic life support, anyone from birth to 1 year of age.

inspiration (in-spir-AY-shun)—breathing in, or inhaling.

intercostal (in-ter-KOS-tal) **muscles**—the muscles between the ribs.

laryngectomy (LAR-in-JEK-to-me)—a surgical procedure in which all or part of the larynx is removed. An opening is usually made in the neck, through which the patient breathes.

larynx (LAR-inks)—the portion of the airway connecting the pharynx and the trachea. It contains the voicebox and vocal cords.

lower airway—the structures of the airway from the larynx to the air sacs of the lungs.

lungs—the organs where exchange of oxygen and carbon dioxide take place.

pharynx (FAR-inks)—the throat.

rescue breathing—providing artificial ventilations (or pulmonary resuscitation to a person who has stopped breathing on his own or whose breathing is inadequate).

respiration (RES-pir-AY-shun)—breathing.

respiratory (RES-pir-uh-tor-e) **arrest**—when a person stops breathing completely.

respiratory (RES-pir-uh-tor-e) **failure**—either the cessation of normal breathing or the reduction of breathing to the point where oxygen intake is insufficient to support life.

resuscitation (re-SUS-i-TAY-shun)—any efforts used to artificially restore breathing or breathing and heart function.

stoma (STO-mah)—the permanent neck opening created in a laryngectomy or tracheostomy.

thyroid (THY-roid) **cartilage**—the Adam's apple.

trachea (TRAY-ke-ah)—the windpipe.

tracheostomy (TRAY-ke-OS-to-me)—a surgical procedure in which an artificial opening into the trachea is made through the neck.

upper airway—the structures of the airway superior to the larynx.

SUMMARY

The Respiratory System

We breathe to bring in oxygen, to remove carbon dioxide, and to help regulate the acid-base balance of our blood. Air flows in and out of the lungs as the diaphragm and intercostal muscles contract and relax, producing changes of volume and pressure in the thoracic cavity and lungs.

Clinical death occurs when an individual stops breathing and the heart stops beating. Biological death occurs when the brain cells die; this takes place when the brain cells are without oxygen.

The airway is the passageway through which air moves in and out of the body. The upper airway includes the nose, mouth, and pharynx (throat). The lower airway includes the larynx (including the voicebox and the epiglottis), trachea (windpipe), bronchial tree (from bronchi through the bronchioles), and lungs with their microscopic alveoli.

Respiratory Failure

When evaluating a patient for adequate or inadequate breathing, look for the chest movements associated with breathing, listen and feel for air exchange, and note anything that may indicate problems with breathing (unusual rate or depth; skin color changes; inability to speak in full sentences).

The most common cause of airway obstruction is the tongue. Opening the airway will move the tongue away from the back of the throat. Sometimes this alone will allow respirations to resume. If the patient does not have spinal injuries, the airway may be opened by the head-tilt or the head-tilt, chin-lift maneuver. If there is a possibility of neck or spinal injury, the jaw thrust must be used. Do not hyperextend the neck of an infant or small child, but make certain that the airway is open to allow for adequate ventilation.

It is strongly recommended that EMTs use a pocket face mask, bag-valve mask, or other approved barrier device to avoid contact with the patient's body fluids.

Mouth-to-mouth ventilation is used on adults and children. In some situations, mouth-to-nose or mouth-to-stoma ventilation must be used. Infants are ventilated using a mouth-to-mouth-and-nose technique. (All of these can be replaced with a mouth-to-mask technique.)

Review Scans 4-1 and 4-2 and Table 4-1 for rescue breathing techniques and rates for adults, children, and infants.

Be on the alert for gastric distention which results when artificial ventilations are too rapid or too great in volume, forcing air into the patient's stomach. If gastric distention develops, reposition the patient's head, deliver slow ventilations, and do not overinflate the patient. Gastric distention may cause vomiting, so have suction equipment ready for use. Do not press on the abdomen to relieve distention.

If a patient's respirations resume and are adequate to support life, place him in the recovery position. Do not use this position if the patient has possible spinal injuries.

Airway Obstruction

Five possible causes of partial or complete airway obstruction are the tongue, the epiglottis, foreign objects, tissue damage, and disease. Conscious patients with complete airway obstruction will often display the universal sign of choking (hands clutched at the throat) and display a panicked look on their faces. They will be unable to speak or to cough.

Patients with a partial airway obstruction may have a good or poor air exchange. Patients with a good air exchange will cough forcefully. Patients with a poor air exchange may have snoring, gurgling, crowing, or wheezing respirations and a weak cough. This poor air exchange is not enough to sustain life and must be dealt with in the same way as a complete obstruction.

Conscious patients with a complete obstruction or a partial obstruction and poor air

exchange are treated with the Heimlich maneuver or chest thrusts. Unconscious patients are often discovered to have airway obstructions when rescuers are unable to ventilate them. If the airway has been repositioned and is still obstructed, the Heimlich maneuver or chest thrusts are used, followed by finger sweeps and re-attempting to ventilate.

The Heimlich maneuver should not be used on patients in late stages of pregnancy or on infants. For pregnant patients, the chest thrust is used. Alternating series of back blows and chest thrusts are used for infants. All procedures are used in series of five until the obstruction is relieved. Procedures for clearing an airway obstruction are considered successful when the patient establishes good air exchange, the foreign object is expelled from or into the mouth, the unconscious patient regains consciousness, and the patient's skin color improves.

The exact procedures for specific patients (adult, child, and infant who are conscious, lose consciousness, or are unconscious when you arrive) are described at the end of the chapter. Make sure you can perform each sequence correctly.

Review Scans 4-3 and 4-4 and Tables 4-1 and 4-2 for techniques for clearing the airway for adults, children, and infants.

5

On the Scene

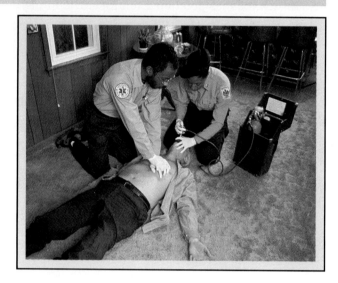

After a large holiday meal, 61-year-old George Stewart begins to look ill. He is sweating and clutching at his chest. He won't admit that he feels bad, but realizing that something is wrong, the family immediately calls 911.

At the ambulance station, you get the call as "man, possible heart attack, 114 State Street." En route, the dispatcher, who has kept the family on the line, reports that the patient has lost consciousness and pulse and that his son, who took an American Red Cross course in cardiopulmonary resuscita-

tion, is now doing CPR. In addition, an advanced life support unit is responding from the other side of town.

On arrival, you hurry in with your oxygen kit and assessment kit while your partner brings in the suction unit. You find Mr. Stewart on his back, chest bared, somewhat blue around the lips, and CPR in progress.

You (to George's son who is doing CPR): I'm an Emergency Medical Technician from the ambulance. When I give the signal, I want you to stop so I can check for a pulse. . . STOP COMPRESSIONS. (The son stops, and you palpate the carotid artery, noting that there is no pulse.) My partner and I will take over now. You did a great job, son.

You quickly take over chest compressions while your partner delivers oxygen-assisted ventilations. Moments later, the paramedics arrive and set up defibrillation equipment to deliver electric shocks to Mr. Stewart's chest.

This patient was lucky: His family wasted no time calling 911; his son knew how to perform CPR; the dispatcher acted swiftly; and EMTs and paramedics were able to provide essential care within minutes. A few weeks later, you and your partner are thrilled to hear that George Stewart is home from the hospital and on his way to recovery.

CPR—Cardiopulmonary Resuscitation

One of the leading causes of death in the United States continues to be heart disease. Often there are warning signs, but heart attacks also often happen with no advance warning. So it is no surprise that most sudden cardiac deaths occur outside a hospital, usually at home. Many factors influence whether a person will survive a heart attack, but the most significant factor is how quickly the person gets help. Heart attack death rates go down when the public is educated to call 911 immediately and when many people in a community are trained in CPR. Ever-improving response times by EMTs and paramedics with CPR and advanced skills also improve survival rates dramatically.

Expected Outcome, Chapter 5: *You will understand the basic structure and function of the heart and the circulatory system and you will be able to perform CPR. (With additional training and equipment, if approved or mandated by your local system, you may also learn to perform automated defibrillation as part of your EMT course or as part of a separate course.)*

> **WARNING:** Protect yourself from infectious diseases by using appropriate barrier devices such as a pocket face mask with one-way valve, face shield, or bag-valve mask; goggles or eye shield; and disposable gloves. Always conform to your local EMS system's infection exposure control plan.

Knowledge *After reading this chapter you should be able to*

1. List and define the FIVE main components of the circulatory system. (p. 137)

2. Locate the anatomical position of the heart, describe the circulation of blood through the four chambers of the heart and the pulmonary and systemic circulations, and describe the heart's conduction system. (pp. 137-138)

3. Describe the relationship of heart, lung, and brain activity. (pp. 138-139)

4. Define and describe major causes of cardiac arrest. (pp. 139-140)

5. Define CPR and explain how CPR works. (pp. 140-142)

6. List the assessment steps that lead to a decision on whether to start CPR. (pp. 142-143)

7. List, step by step, the procedures for performing CPR on adults. (pp. 143-147)

8. Compare one-rescuer CPR and two-rescuer CPR, for adults. (pp. 147-152)

9. Explain how to join CPR in progress. (pp. 152-153)

10. List, step by step, the sequence of procedures for changing positions during two-rescuer CPR. (pp. 153-154)

11. List, step by step, the procedures for performing CPR on infants and children. (pp. 153, 156-157)

12. Compare rates and ratios of compressions and ventilations of one- and two-rescuer CPR for adults, children, and infants. (Table 5-1, pp. 147, 149, 151-152, 157)

13. State how the EMT can determine that CPR is effective. (p. 157)

14. State ways to counter deficiency in CPR. (p. 157)

15. List factors that may make CPR ventilations and compressions ineffective. (pp. 157-158)

16. List reasons why CPR may be interrupted. (p. 158)

17. Describe how to move a patient, while performing CPR, down stairs, through narrow hallways and doorways, and while loading on and off the ambulance. (pp. 158, 159)

18. List possible complications of CPR. (pp. 158, 160)

19. Explain circumstances in which, even though a patient has no pulse, CPR should not be started and explain circumstances in which CPR may be terminated. (pp. 160-161)

Optional Objectives, Defibrillation

20. Explain the importance of early defibrillation. (p. 162)

21. List two shockable and two non-shockable heart rhythms. (p. 163)

22. Explain how defibrillation works. (pp. 163-164)

23. List four phases of the time period from collapse to defibrillation and explain ways in which each can be shortened. (pp. 164-165)

24. Explain the safety guidelines for operating automated defibrillators. (p. 165)

25. Explain how to attach a defibrillator and how to operate fully automatic and semi-automatic defibrillators. (pp. 165-168)

Skills *As an EMT you should be able to*

1. Correctly evaluate a patient to detect cardiac arrest.

2. Perform one-rescuer CPR on adults, children, and infants.

3. Perform two-rescuer CPR, including the proper change of positions.

4. Perform CPR on a patient while he is being moved.

Optional Objective, Defibrillation

5. Safely operate a defibrillator if you have been trained in its use.

Before studying this chapter, you may want to review Chapter 2 in which the anatomy and physiology of the human body were introduced; particularly, review the information on body cavities (especially the thoracic cavity, or chest cavity) and position of the heart. Also look over the Anatomy and Physiology Plate on the Circulatory (Cardiovascular) System at the back of this book.

THE HEART

This chapter introduces you to the **circulatory system**. This system is composed of the

- **Heart**—acting as a pump to circulate the blood
- **Arteries**—the vessels that carry blood away from the heart
- **Veins**—the vessels that return blood to the heart
- **Capillaries**—the microscopic vessels where exchange between the blood and the body's tissues takes place
- **Blood**—the fluids and cells that are circulated to carry oxygen and nutrients to and wastes away from the body's tissues

From the above description, you can see why the circulatory system is also called the *cardiovascular system,* from *cardio,* meaning "heart," and *vascular,* meaning "(blood) vessels." It is the system made up of the heart and the vessels that circulate blood throughout the body.

The Anatomy of the Heart

The human heart is a muscular organ about the size of your fist, located in the center of the thoracic cavity (Figure 5-1). The heart has four chambers: two upper chambers called **atria** (AY-tre-ah—the singular is *atrium*) and two lower chambers called **ventricles** (VEN-tri-kulz).

The atria both contract at the same time. When they contract, the blood is forced into the heart's lower chambers, the ventricles. Both ventricles receive blood from their respective atria and then contract simultaneously to pump blood out of the heart. The path the blood takes on its journey through the body is as follows: *right atrium to right ventricle to lungs to left atrium to left ventricle to body*—then back to the right atrium to start its journey all over again. Below, this path of the circulatory system is described in a little more detail.

- Right Atrium—The **venae cavae** (the *superior vena cava* and the *inferior vena cava*) are the two large veins that return blood to the heart. The right atrium receives this blood and, upon contraction, sends it to the right ventricle.
- Right Ventricle—The right ventricle receives blood from the chamber above it, the right atrium. When the right ventricle contracts, it pumps this blood out to the lungs via the **pulmonary arteries**. Remember, this blood is very low in oxygen and is carrying waste carbon dioxide that was picked up as the blood circulated through the body. While this blood is in the lungs, the carbon dioxide is excreted (taken out of the blood to be carried out of the body when the person breathes out), and oxygen is obtained (taken into the blood from air the person has breathed in). The oxygen-rich blood is now returned to the left atrium via the **pulmonary veins**.
- Left Atrium—The left atrium receives the oxygen-rich blood from the lungs. When it contracts, it sends this blood to the left ventricle.
- Left Ventricle—The left ventricle receives oxygen-rich blood from the chamber above it, the left atrium. When it contracts, it pumps this blood into the **aorta**, the body's largest artery, for distribution to the entire body. Since the blood must reach all parts of the body, the left ventricle is the most muscular and strongest part of the heart.

Two more terms help to describe the path of circulation (Figure 5-2). These are **pulmonary circulation**, the term for the transport of blood from the heart to the lungs and back again (*pulmonary* refers to the lungs), and **systemic circulation**, the term for the transport of blood from the heart to all parts of the body and back to the heart (*systemic* refers to the entire body system).

Between each atrium and ventricle is a one-way valve to prevent blood in the ventricle from being forced back up into the atrium when the ventricle contracts. The pulmonary artery also has a one-way valve so that blood does not return to the right ventricle. The aorta also has a one-way valve to prevent backflow to the left ventricle. This system of one-way valves keeps the blood moving in the correct direction along the path of circulation.

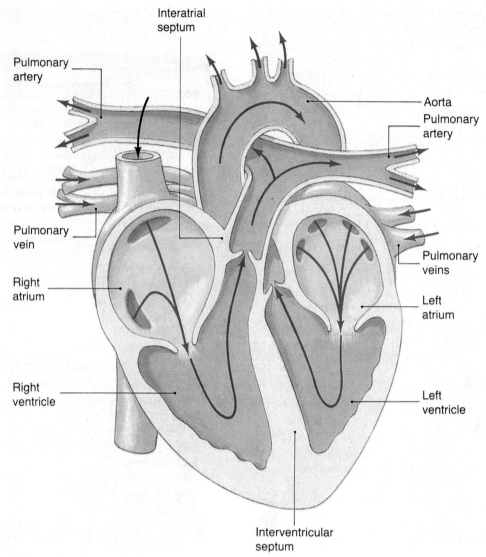

Interatrial septum

Pulmonary artery

Aorta
Pulmonary artery

Pulmonary vein

Pulmonary veins

Right atrium

Left atrium

Right ventricle

Left ventricle

Interventricular septum

Figure 5-1 Structures of the heart.

The contractions, or beating, of the heart is an automatic, involuntary process. The heart has its own natural "pacemaker" and a system of specialized muscle tissues that conduct electrical impulses that stimulate the heart to beat. This network is called the **conduction system**. Regulation of rate, rhythm, and force of heartbeat comes, in part, from the cardiac control centers of the brain. Nerve impulses from these centers are sent to the pacemaker and conduction system of the heart. These nerve impulses and chemicals released into the blood (e.g., epinephrine) control the heart's rate and strength of contractions.

The Heart-Lung-Brain Relationship

There is a close relationship between the functions of the heart, lungs, and brain. This relationship may be seen in the following scenarios.

- A person develops a complete airway obstruction. With this obstruction, the patient is unable to breathe. The heart continues to beat for a short time, but there is no fresh oxygen being picked up by the blood as it passes through the lungs, therefore no fresh oxygen being carried to the brain and other tissues of the body. In response to the lack of oxygen, the brain

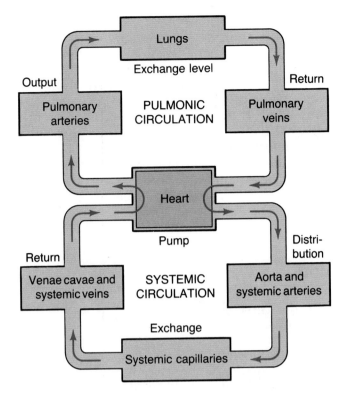

Figure 5-2 The heart pumps blood through pulmonary and systemic circulation.

begins functioning improperly and the patient loses consciousness. The heart itself begins to feel the lack of oxygen. It begins to beat improperly, then not at all. Blood, even poorly-oxygenated blood, is no longer being circulated to the brain. Without respiration and heartbeat—and thus without oxygen—the brain dies.

- A person has a massive heart attack which causes his heartbeat abruptly to stop. When the heartbeat stops, blood is not being carried to the brain and the brain centers that control breathing cease to function. Without heartbeat and respiration, the brain dies.

In the first scenario, breathing stopped first and this caused the heart to stop. In the second scenario, the heart stopped first and this caused breathing to cease. As you know, the brain requires a constant supply of oxygen that must be breathed in and carried to the brain by the blood. As soon as the brain's oxygen supply is lessened or interrupted by cessation of—or inadequate—breathing and/or heartbeat, the brain in its turn stops supporting breathing and

heartbeat. In a short time the lack of oxygen causes the brain itself to die.

In other words, the functions of breathing, heartbeat, and brain are so interdependent that each depends on the other two and the failure of any of them will cause the failure of the others.

Heart Function and Cardiac Arrest

The heart may be compared to a pump—a very efficient pump. When the average adult is at rest, the heart will pump 10 pints (about 5 liters) of blood each minute, more when the body is active. On the average, the heart pumps more than 16,000 pints of blood each day. In an average lifetime, this human pump is required to beat over 2.5 billion times in order to move over 450 million pints of blood. Unlike a mechanical pump, the heart accomplishes this remarkable feat without interruption.

The heart and blood vessels are not totally maintenance free. There are a number of risk factors that are associated with heart disease, heart attack, and stroke. They are

- High blood pressure
- Elevated cholesterol and triglyceride levels
- Cigarette smoking (and passive inhalation of others' smoke)
- Lack of exercise
- Obesity
- Stress

It is never too late to eliminate these risk factors, stop the ongoing damage, and even improve the health of the circulatory system. Lifestyle changes such as adopting a more healthful diet, exercising, and quitting smoking are invaluable. Regular physical exams can help monitor blood cholesterol and triglyceride levels and blood pressure, which can be treated through medication and/or diet. There are many ways to avoid and lower stress.

Cardiac arrest means that the heart has stopped beating. There can be a number of causes of cardiac arrest, including the risk factors listed above. Almost all victims of cardiac arrest that has not resulted from an external cause such as drowning, electrocution, suffocation, drug intoxication, or trauma, however, have some degree of **atheroschlerosis** (ATH-er-o-skle-RO-sis). That is, like most Americans, they have cholesterol plaques lining and narrowing the inside of their arteries. The coronary arteries, too, develop this plaque, a condition known as

coronary artery disease (CAD). These plaques reduce the amount of oxygen-carrying blood that can flow through the artery in a given period of time.

Atherosclerosis usually does not produce advance symptoms but rather, if the narrowing reaches an advanced stage, may result in a sudden cardiac event—usually a coronary artery spasm or a myocardial infarction (heart attack)—which may end in cardiac arrest.

- **Coronary Artery Spasm**—A common cause of cardiac arrest, a coronary artery spasm is a brief contraction of the muscular wall of a coronary artery. If the artery is already significantly narrowed due to the presence of cholesterol plaque, this spasm may result in a temporary interruption of blood flow to the part of the heart distal to the spasm. Even a brief interruption of blood supply in some people is enough to cause the heart to begin beating erratically and, ultimately, to fibrillate (quiver ineffectively). These individuals may collapse suddenly with no warning symptoms.

- **Myocardial Infarction (Heart Attack)**—A somewhat less common cause of cardiac arrest is actual blockage of a coronary artery, usually by a blood clot at a point where the artery is already narrowed by cholesterol plaque. When this happens, the interruption of the blood supply to the part of the heart distal to the blockage deprives the heart muscle of oxygen. This can lead to ventricular fibrillation (discussed later in this chapter). If prolonged, parts of the heart muscle begin to die, a condition known as myocardial infarction or, more commonly, as heart attack.

While most people do not suffer cardiac arrest with their first heart attack, up to 45% of all cardiac arrests occur as the result of heart attacks. This means simply that there are many more heart attacks than there are cardiac arrests. A person experiencing a heart attack will generally complain of pain in the chest, jaw, left arm, or indigestion-like pains in the upper abdomen, shortness of breath, sweating, and so on, although the duration of symptoms prior to suffering a cardiac arrest is highly variable and may be short. (Myocardial infarction and other heart problems will be discussed in detail in Chapter 15.)

Note: EMTs are not immune to diseases of the heart and blood vessels. An EMT's lifestyle is too often one of long hours, stress, and poor diet. EMTs constantly see the ravages of cardiovascular disease, but many do nothing to prevent its happening to themselves or those they love! Your agency may offer blood pressure screenings to your community as a public service as well as counseling to reduce stress and other health services. EMTs need to take advantage of such programs and to spread the word about them. In this way, you can not only treat the victims of cardiovascular disease, but you can also help prevent it by being a good role model.

CPR

As you learned in Chapter 4, when a patient's breathing and heartbeat cease, *clinical death* occurs. This condition may be reversible. When the brain cells die, *biological death* occurs. This usually happens within 10 minutes of clinical death and is not reversible. This is not to say that a person who has been in a state of clinical death for 8 to 10 minutes cannot survive. There are some factors that may delay biological death. These factors will be discussed later in this chapter.

The American Heart Association has developed the concept of the *Chain of Survival*. Since we know that clinical death quickly progresses to biological death, emergency medical assistance must get to the patient rapidly, and this depends on the smooth functioning of an unbroken chain of help for the patient.

The first link in the chain is usually a friend or member of the patient's family or of the public who recognizes the warning signs or witnesses the heart attack and calls 911. Obviously, if the bystander fails to access EMS, the Chain of Survival is broken at its start. The bystander can further strengthen the chain if he or she has taken advantage of an American Heart Association or American Red Cross course and can provide **cardiopulmonary resuscitation** (KAR-de-o PUL-mo-ner-e re-SUS-i-TA-shun), or **CPR**—artificial support of breathing and circulation—to delay biological death until help arrives.

The next link in the chain is the Emergency Medical Dispatcher (EMD) or other dispatcher who receives the call for help and activates the EMS system, deciding which services are needed and sending them to the scene, possibly also providing instructions by telephone to the person who called for help.

You, as an EMT, provide the next link in the chain by continuing or initiating CPR and, if they are not already on the way, calling for advanced life support (ALS) units that can deliver **defibrillation** (de-FIB-ri-LAY-shun), an electrical current applied to the outside of the patient's chest that can "shock" the heart out of certain lethal rhythms. In some EMS systems, EMTs are trained and equipped to deliver automated defibrillation (which will be discussed later in this chapter).

The final link in the Chain of Survival is early advanced care. Advanced care consists of administering specialized medications, fluids, and advanced airway procedures. These procedures are usually carried out by paramedics or, in some localities, by advanced EMTs.

When any link in the chain is weak, the patient's chance of survival is much reduced. The key role of the EMT in the Chain of Survival is CPR.

How CPR Works

Cardiopulmonary resuscitation is the basic life support measure applied when a patient's heart and lung actions have stopped. During CPR, you will have to

- Maintain an open airway.
- Breathe for the patient.
- Perform chest compressions to force the patient's blood to circulate.

These steps are related to and follow the sequence of the ABCs of the primary survey in which A = Airway, B = Breathing, and C = Circulation (Figure 5-3).

CPR is a method of artificial breathing and circulation. When natural heart action and breathing have stopped, we must provide an artificial means to oxygenate the blood and keep it in circulation. This is accomplished by providing **chest compressions** and **ventilations.**

- *To provide chest compressions,* you place the patient supine on a hard surface and compress the chest by applying downward pressure with your hands. This action causes an increase of pressure inside the chest and possible actual compression of the heart itself, one or both of which force the blood out of the heart and into circulation. When pressure is released, the heart refills with blood. The next compression

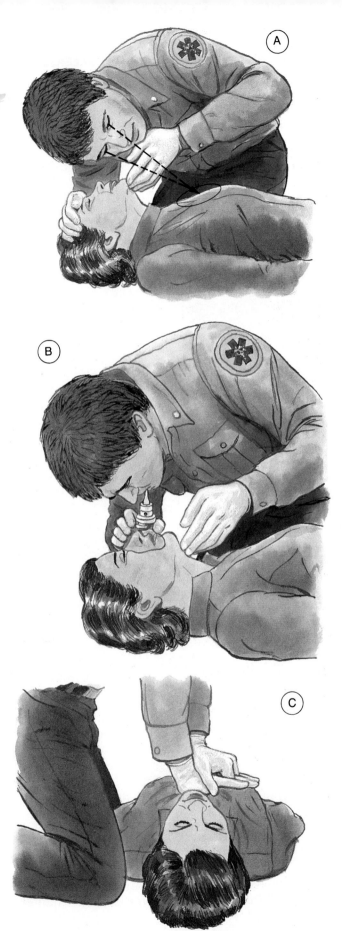

Figure 5-3 The ABC technique of CPR.

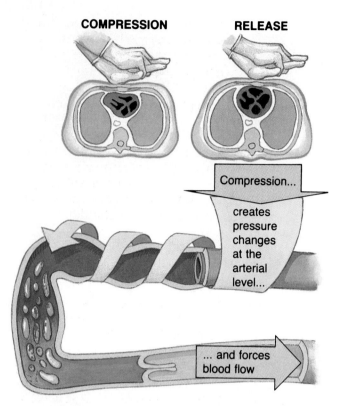

COMPRESSION   RELEASE

Compression...

creates pressure changes at the arterial level...

... and forces blood flow

Figure 5-4 During CPR, compressions cause pressure changes that cause the blood to circulate.

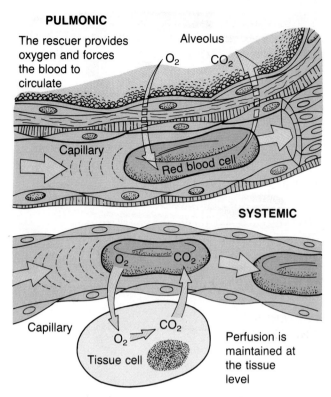

PULMONIC

The rescuer provides oxygen and forces the blood to circulate

Alveolus

O_2 CO_2

Capillary

Red blood cell

SYSTEMIC

O_2 CO_2

Capillary CO_2

O_2 CO_2

Tissue cell

Perfusion is maintained at the tissue level

Figure 5-5 CPR provides the patient with oxygen.

sends this fresh blood into circulation and the cycle continues (Figure 5-4).

- *To provide ventilations,* you use mouth-to-mask, mouth-to-mouth, mouth-to-nose, or mouth-to-stoma methods as described in Chapter 4. IT IS HIGHLY RECOMMENDED THAT CPR BE PERFORMED USING A POCKET FACE MASK OR OTHER BARRIER DEVICE AS PROTECTION AGAINST INFECTIOUS DISEASES.

Remember: Both compressions and ventilations are necessary in CPR. One does little good without the other. Compressions without ventilations would circulate blood without enough oxygen in it to sustain brain or heart function. Ventilations without compressions would force oxygen into the lungs without circulating the blood to pick up the oxygen and deliver it to the body (Figure 5-5).

Assessment: Knowing When to Do CPR

The decision to begin CPR must come from the results of the primary survey. Review Chapter 4 if necessary for more detail on all the steps through rescue breathing.

Warning: Performing CPR on a patient who has a pulse may result in serious medical complications. Therefore, YOU MUST PERFORM THE ABCs OF THE PRIMARY SURVEY to establish whether the patient has an open airway, is or is not breathing, and has or does not have a pulse *before* deciding whether to initiate CPR.

In addition to the danger of performing CPR on a patient who has a pulse, keep in mind these other reasons always to perform the entire sequence of ABC assessment and care.

- Open Airway—Artificial ventilations are not effective unless there is an open airway.
- Breathing—Circulating blood will not be effective unless the blood is oxygenated.
- Circulation—Artificial ventilation is not effective unless the blood is circulating.

The steps leading to the beginning of CPR should be

1. ESTABLISH UNRESPONSIVENESS—Is the patient responsive? Gently shake the patient's shoulder and shout, "ARE YOU OKAY?" If the patient is conscious and able

to speak, you know that his ABCs are all right for the present; he would not be conscious or able to speak if he did not have an open airway, breathing, and heartbeat.

Note: If mechanism of injury suggests possible spinal injury, protect the head and spine while establishing unresponsiveness.

2. CALL FOR HELP—*If the patient is unresponsive,* you know that he may have an obstructed airway, may be without respirations, and/or may be without circulation. If you are working alone, however, DO NOT BEGIN RESUSCITATION BEFORE YOU HAVE CALLED FOR HELP. Call 911 or your local emergency number or radio to your dispatch center, *then* immediately continue your rapid assessment and care for the ABCs.

3. REPOSITION THE PATIENT, if necessary, placing the patient supine on a hard surface. Be sure to turn the patient as a unit, protecting the alignment of head and spine.

4. ESTABLISH AN OPEN AIRWAY—This should be done by the head-tilt, chin-lift, or jaw-thrust maneuvers (use the jaw thrust if spinal injury is suspected). Usually at this time, you can easily check to see if the patient is a neck breather.

5. CHECK FOR BREATHING—Use the LOOK, LISTEN, and FEEL method, taking no more than 3 to 5 seconds to determine if the patient is breathing. A patient who is breathing does not immediately need either rescue breathing or CPR. If the patient is not breathing, you should . . .

6. DELIVER TWO BREATHS—Use rescue breathing techniques. Each of the two initial breaths should take 1½ to 2 seconds. Allow time for deflation and to take your own replenishing breath between the rescue breaths. If the breaths are unsuccessful, reposition the patient's head to try to correct the airway opening, then deliver two more breaths. If these breaths are unsuccessful and you believe there may be an upper airway obstruction, begin techniques to clear the airway (e.g., Heimlich maneuver or chest thrusts and finger sweeps). If the patient's airway is clear and he is still in respiratory arrest . . .

7. CHECK FOR A CAROTID PULSE—Maintain the head tilt with one hand on the patient's forehead and use your other hand to feel for a carotid pulse in the patient's neck (see Chapter 3 on how to find the carotid pulse). It is important to check the carotid pulse rather than the radial (wrist) pulse because a weak heartbeat may not be felt at the more distal sites of the body but may be felt in the large arteries such as the carotid artery (the easiest to find and feel). *If there is a pulse but the patient is not breathing,* continue rescue breathing. *If there is no pulse* after 5 to 10 seconds of palpation (longer if the patient has been submerged in cold water—see Chapter 21), the patient is in cardiac arrest and you should . . .

8. BEGIN CPR.

Remember: DO NOT INITIATE CPR ON ANY PATIENT WHO HAS A CAROTID PULSE.

Note: Bleeding can prevent proper and adequate circulation. If a patient has lost too much blood, then CPR will not be effective. When bleeding is very profuse, as in the case of a severed major artery, CPR might speed up the patient's blood loss; oxygenated blood would be circulated, but the patient would bleed to death. If CPR accelerates blood loss, the bleeding may have to be quickly controlled (see Chapter 7). This situation is rare, but it is critical when it occurs.

How to Do CPR

CPR can be done by one or by two rescuers. All of the information below under "Positioning the Patient," "Finding the CPR Compression Site," "Providing Chest Compressions," and "Providing Ventilations" applies to both one-rescuer and two-rescuer CPR. Specific information about each type of CPR then follows under "One-Rescuer CPR" and "Two-Rescuer CPR." Scans 5-1, 5-2, 5-3, 5-4, and 5-5 can help you follow and review these procedures as they are described below.

Positioning the Patient The cardiac arrest patient must be placed supine on a hard surface, such as the floor or ground or a spine board (Figure 5-6). If the patient is in bed or on an ambulance stretcher, a backboard or similar rigid object should be placed under the patient. *Do not* delay CPR to find a rigid object if one is not at hand. Instead, move the patient to the floor. CPR cannot be delayed because of patient injury. If you are alone, *do not* try to immobilize the spine or splint fractures before initiating CPR. It is critical that CPR be started as soon as possible without regard to injuries or aggrava-

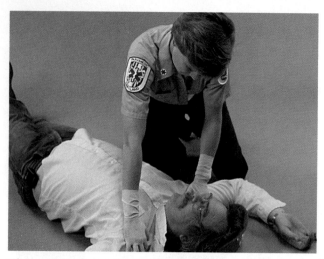

Figure 5-6 Properly position the patient for CPR.

tion of injuries that may result—except for taking due care to attempt to keep the head and neck aligned while moving the patient and using the jaw-thrust maneuver to open the airway if spinal injury is suspected. Saving the patient's life is the first consideration.

Finding the CPR Compression Site First visualize the location of the heart, which lies at about the midline of the body between the **sternum**, or breastbone, and the spinal column. The upper seven pairs of the ribs attach to the sternum. These, along with the **clavicles** (KLAV-i-kuls), or collarbones, support the sternum over the heart.

To be effective and prevent serious injury to the patient, chest compressions must be delivered to the **CPR compression site** on the sternum (Scan 5-1). Locate the CPR compression site by using the following technique.

1. Kneel alongside the patient. Face the patient with your knees at the level of the patient's shoulders. This will allow you to perform rescue breathing and chest compressions without having to move your knees. Have your knees shoulder-width apart for balance and stability.

2. Use the index and middle fingers of your hand closest to the patient's feet to locate the lower margin (border) of the rib cage. Do this on the side of the chest closest to your knees.

3. Move your fingers along the rib cage toward the center of the patient's body. Stop when you find the location where the ribs meet the sternum. This area is called the **substernal notch**. Keep your middle finger at this notch and your index finger resting on the lower tip of the sternum.

4. Now move your other hand and place it so the heel of that hand is resting against your index finger and is centered on the sternum. This is the CPR compression site. Your hand is placed over the lower half of the sternum, centered from side to side.

5. The hand that was used to locate the substernal notch is now placed over the hand on the CPR compression site (Figure 5-7). The fingers of both hands are pointing away from your body. You may interlace or extend your fingers, but you must KEEP YOUR FINGERS OFF THE PATIENT'S CHEST.

This position provides a centered compression and avoids injury to the patient's ribs or internal organs. You are now ready to provide compressions.

Providing Chest Compressions To summarize what has been done so far: The patient has been positioned supine on a hard surface. You are on your knees, which are shoulder-

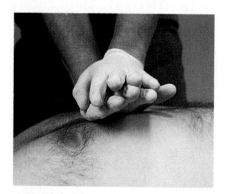 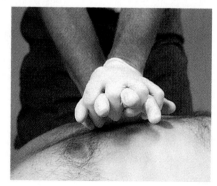 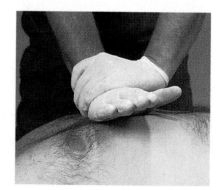

Figure 5-7 Hand placement for compressions.

Locating the CPR Compression Site

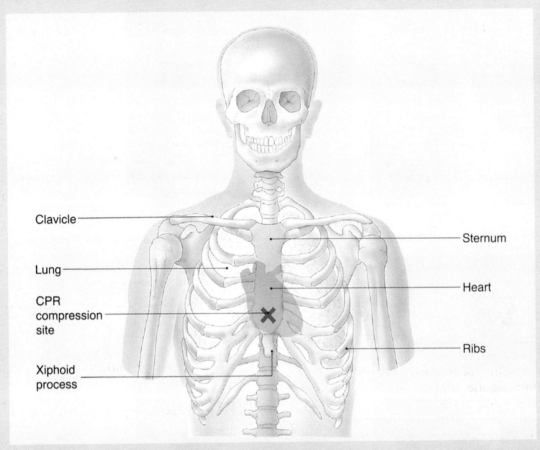

Clavicle

Lung

CPR compression site

Xiphoid process

Sternum

Heart

Ribs

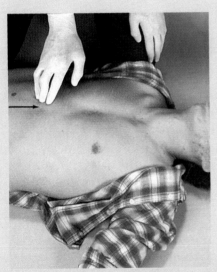

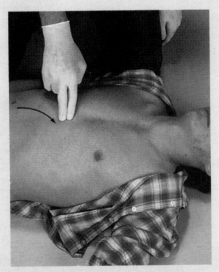

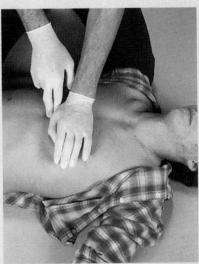

1. Use the index and middle fingers of the hand that is closest to the patient's feet to locate the lower border of the rib cage.

2. Move your fingers along the rib cage until you find the point where the ribs meet the sternum, the substernal notch. Keep your middle finger at the notch and your index finger resting on the lower tip of the sternum.

3. Move your other hand to the midline. Place its thumb side against the index finger of the lower hand.

145

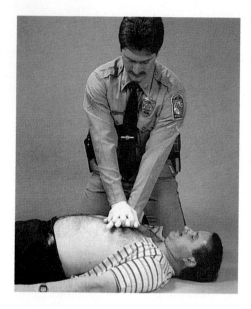

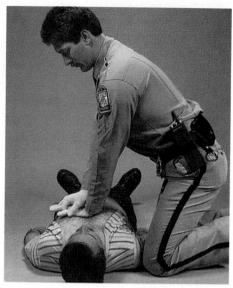

Figure 5-8 The shoulders are placed directly over the compression site.

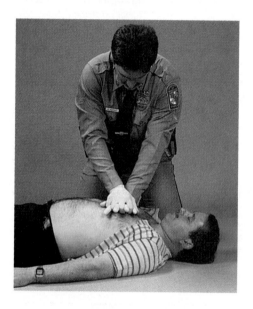

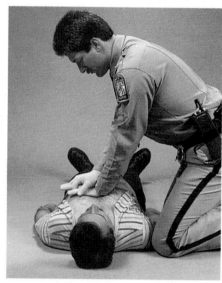

Figure 5-9 Compressions are delivered straight down.

width apart. Your hands are properly positioned on the CPR compression site, which is midline and on the lower half of the sternum. Now . . .

1. Straighten your arms and lock your elbows (Figure 5-8). You must not bend the elbows when delivering or releasing compressions.
2. Make certain that your shoulders are directly over your hands (directly over the patient's sternum). This will allow you to deliver compressions straight down onto the site. Keep both of your knees on the ground or floor.
3. Deliver compressions STRAIGHT DOWN, with enough force to depress the sternum of a typical adult 1½ to 2 inches (Figure 5-9).

Note: Monitoring the depth of your compressions is one way to determine if they are adequate—the *only* way, if you are working alone. Another method for determining whether your compressions are adequate is to have someone else feel for a carotid pulse while you perform compressions. When CPR compressions are being performed properly, they should produce a carotid pulse. Never try to feel for a carotid pulse during compressions if you are by yourself; rather, perform compressions at 1½ to 2 inches until help arrives.

4. Fully release pressure on the patient's sternum, but *do not* bend your elbows and *do*

not lift your hands from the sternum, which can cause you to lose correct positioning of your hands. Your movement should be from your hips, the hips acting as a fulcrum. Compressions should be delivered in a rhythmic, not a "jabbing," fashion. THE AMOUNT OF TIME YOU SPEND COMPRESSING SHOULD BE THE SAME AS THE TIME FOR THE RELEASE. This is known as the **50:50 rule**: 50% compression, 50% release.

Providing Ventilations Ventilations are given between sets of compressions. You are to use the same techniques that you learned for rescue breathing (see Chapter 4). Mouth-to-mask, mouth-to-mouth, mouth-to-nose, or mouth-to-stoma methods can be used as needed (Figure 5-10). REMEMBER THAT USE OF A POCKET FACE MASK OR OTHER BARRIER DEVICE IS RECOMMENDED AS PROTECTION AGAINST INFECTIOUS DISEASES. Provide each ventilation with enough force so that you observe the patient's chest rise. Breaths provided slowly (at 1½ to 2 seconds for each breath) and with adequate but not too great force will help prevent gastric distention, which is caused when air is forced into the stomach.

One-Rescuer CPR

Refer to Scan 5-2, which shows all the techniques of one-rescuer CPR for the adult patient.

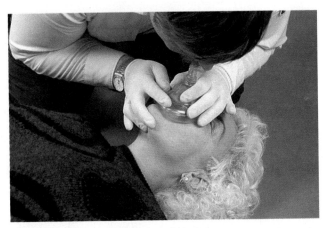

Figure 5-10 Providing ventilations.

Follow this page step by step as you practice on the adult manikins provided for your training.

Compressions and Ventilations: Rates and Ratios One-rescuer CPR is delivered as follows (see also Table 5-1).

- COMPRESSIONS—80 to 100 per minute (15 compressions every 10 seconds will put you in the middle of this range)
- VENTILATIONS—2 breaths after every 15 compressions, each breath 1½ to 2 seconds in duration (exhalation takes place naturally; do not delay return to compressions to watch for exhalation)
- RATIO—15 compressions to 2 ventilations (15:2)

TABLE 5-1 CPR for Adults, Children, and Infants

	Adult	*Child*	*Infant*
Age	8 yrs and older	1-8 yrs	birth-1 yr
Compression depth	1½ to 2 inches	1 to 1½ inches	½ to 1 inch
Compression rate	80-100/min	100/min	at least 100/min
Each ventilation	1½ to 2 seconds	1 to 1½ seconds	1 to 1½ seconds
Ventilation rate	10-12 breaths/min	20 breaths/min	20 breaths/min
Pulse check location (throat)	carotid artery (throat)	carotid artery (upper arm)	brachial artery
One-rescuer CPR compressions-to-ventilations ratio	15:2	5:1	5:1
Two-rescuer CPR compressions-to-ventilations ratio	5:1	5:1	5:1
Working alone: Call 911 or emergency dispatcher	After establishing unresponsiveness— before beginning resuscitation	After establishing unresponsiveness and 1 minute of resuscitation	After establishing unresponsiveness and 1 minute of resuscitation

One-Rescuer CPR

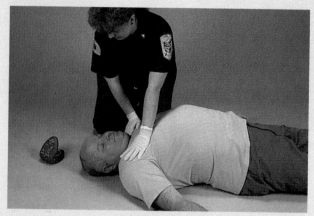

1. Establish unresponsiveness and reposition. (Call for help if you are working alone.)

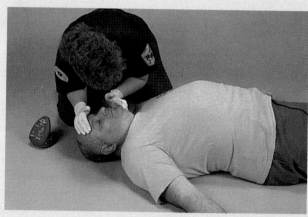

2. Open airway.

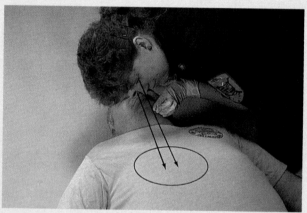

3. Look, listen, and feel for breath (3-5 seconds).

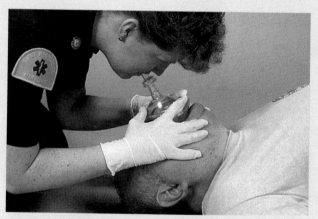

4. Ventilate twice (1½ to 2 sec/ventilation). When possible, use a pocket face mask.

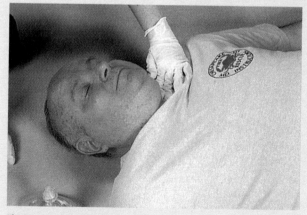

5. No pulse (5-10 seconds).

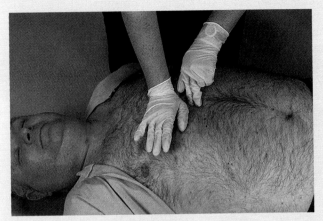

6. Locate compression site.

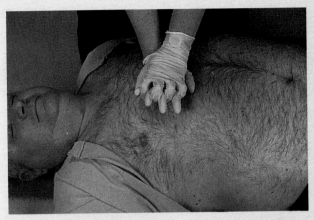

7. Position hands.

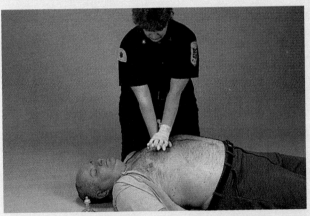

8. Begin compressions (Compressions at depth of 1½ to 2 inches, delivered at a rate of 80-100/minute).

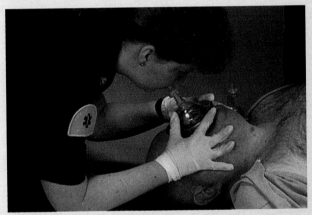

9. Ventilate twice. (Provide 2 ventilations every 15 compressions.)

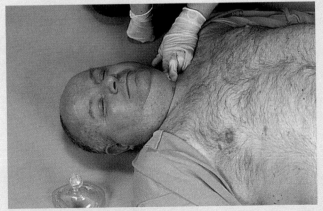

10. Recheck pulse and breathing after 4 cycles, then every few minutes.

Remember: When alone, call for help as soon as unresponsiveness is established.

During one-rescuer CPR, time is taken away from compressions in order to provide ventilations. Even though you are delivering compressions at the rate of 80 to 100 per minute, usually only 60 compressions are delivered in 1 minute because of the breaks for ventilation. To be certain that you are delivering compressions at the correct rate, you should say "One-and, two-and, three-and, four-and, five-and, . . ." until you reach 15 compressions. Don't take time to say "and" after "fifteen," but pause immediately to deliver two ventilations, relocate the CPR compression site, and begin the next set of 15 compressions.

Once CPR is begun it should not be interrupted unless absolutely necessary. Interruptions in CPR are discussed later in the chapter.

Checking for Pulse and Breathing CPR should be carried out for approximately ONE MINUTE, or FOUR CYCLES of 15 compressions and 2 ventilations. At this point you should check for a carotid pulse (3 to 5 seconds). At the same time look, listen, and feel for breathing. If there is no pulse, return to CPR. If there is a pulse but no breathing, perform rescue breathing. If there are both pulse and breathing, continue to monitor both carefully, taking care to check every few minutes for a carotid pulse.

CPR should not be delayed for more than a few seconds for a pulse-and-breathing check. If CPR is continued after the first check, break to check for a carotid pulse and the return of spontaneous breathing every few minutes thereafter.

Considerations for the Single Rescuer Remember, you may be called upon to perform CPR while off duty or even on duty, but by yourself. Begin the sequence for CPR by checking for responsiveness. ONCE YOU FIND THE PATIENT UNRESPONSIVE, ACTIVATE THE EMS SYSTEM BEFORE ANY FURTHER ASSESSMENT OR CPR. Call 911 or your local emergency number. If you have a radio, contact the EMS dispatcher for assistance. Provide the dispatcher

1. The location of the emergency (with cross streets or roads, if possible)
2. The telephone number you are calling from
3. What you believe has happened (e.g., heart attack, fall, vehicle collision)
4. How many persons need help
5. The condition of the patient or patients
6. What aid you are giving or plan to give the patient or patients
7. What additional help is needed (e.g., advanced cardiac life support, fire department)

8. Any other information the dispatcher requests

Relay the information accurately but swiftly and return to the patient.

Remember that it is recommended that CPR be conducted using a pocket face mask or other barrier device as protection against infectious diseases. Any of these devices that have a strap that holds the mask on the patient's face is best for one-rescuer CPR. It will hold the mask in place while you are doing compressions. Devices that do not have this strap will need to be placed on the patient's face after each set of compressions.

Two-Rescuer CPR

Refer to Scan 5-3, which shows all the techniques of two-rescuer CPR for the adult patient. Follow this page step by step as you practice on the adult manikins provided for your training. In the Scan, both rescuers are shown on the same side of the patient to allow you to see what each person is doing. The procedure goes more smoothly if the rescuers are on opposite sides of the patient, as in Figure 5-11. This is particularly true when position changes are taking place. Once in the ambulance, the procedure will have

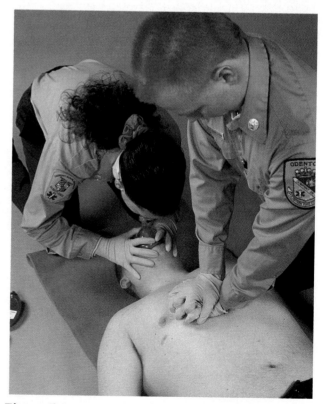

Figure 5-11 Opposite-side positioning in two-rescuer CPR.

Two-Rescuer CPR

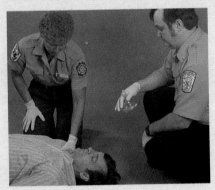

1. Determine unresponsive-ness. Reposition patient.

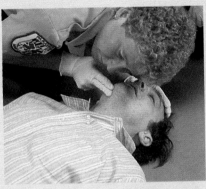

2. Open the airway and look, listen, and feel for breath (3-5 seconds).

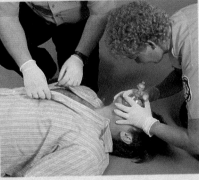

3. Ventilate twice (1½ to 2 sec/ventilation).

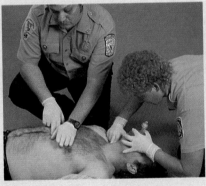

4. Determine pulselessness. Locate CPR compression site.

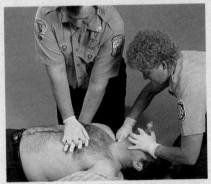

5. Say "no pulse." Begin compressions.

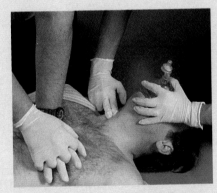

6. Check compression effective-ness. Deliver 5 compressions in 3-4 seconds (rate = 80-100/minute).

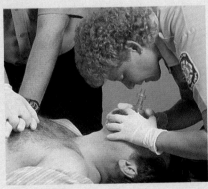

7. Ventilate once (1½ to 2 sec/ventilation). Stop for venti-lation.

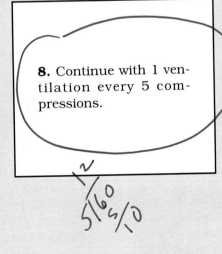

8. Continue with 1 ven-tilation every 5 com-pressions.

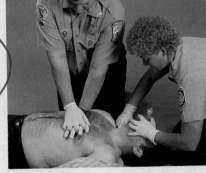

9. After a few minutes, reassess breathing and pulse. No pulse—ventilate and say "Continue CPR." Pulse—say, "Stop CPR."

Note: Assess for spontaneous breathing and pulse at the end of the first minute, and then every few minutes thereafter.

to be done with one rescuer providing ventilations with supplemental oxygen while positioned at the patient's head.

There are several advantages to two-rescuer CPR. The patient receives more oxygen (since ventilations are given more frequently and by a rescuer whose main responsibility is ventilation rather than chest compressions), circulation and blood pressure improve (since chest compressions, though interrupted more frequently, are not interrupted for as long), and the problem of rescuer fatigue is lessened. CPR with two rescuers also makes it easier to use barrier devices such as pocket face masks and bag-valve devices since there is not the difficulty posed by a single rescuer having to move from ventilations to chest compressions and back again.

Compressions and Ventilations: Rates and Ratios Two-rescuer CPR is delivered as follows (see also Table 5-1).

- COMPRESSIONS—80 to 100 per minute (about 15 compressions every 10 seconds)
- VENTILATIONS—1 breath after every 5 compressions, each breath 1½ to 2 seconds in duration (exhalation takes place naturally during the next compression)
- RATIO—5 compressions to 1 ventilation (5:1)

The compressor counts out loud saying, "One and two and three and four and five, breathe." The compressor pauses for 1½ to 2 seconds to allow the ventilator to deliver a breath. After the breath has been delivered, the compressor resumes. Between ventilations, the ventilator may check the carotid pulse to determine the effectiveness of compressions.

Note: If the ventilator misses a breath, he should not wait for the next fifth stroke to provide the ventilation. Instead, he should deliver this missed ventilation on the upstroke of the next compression.

Checking for Pulse and Breathing After the first minute of CPR and every few (three to four) minutes thereafter, the ventilator should check to see if the patient has a carotid pulse and also to look for spontaneous breathing. Since compressions will cause a pulse, to get a true check of the patient's status (whether spontaneous heartbeats have resumed) compressions must be stopped for pulse checks. A pulse check during CPR should take only 3 to 5 seconds. If a pulse is detected, the ventilator should say, "Stop compressions." Rescue breathing should

be provided if needed. If there is no pulse, the ventilator should say, "No pulse. Continue CPR."

How to Join CPR in Progress If you wish to join another member of the EMS System who has initiated CPR, you should

1. Ask to help.
2. Allow the first rescuer to complete a cycle of 15 compressions and 2 ventilations.
3. Assume the responsibility for compressions and allow the first rescuer to become the ventilator.

If CPR has been started by someone who is certified but not part of the EMS System and you join this person to start CPR

1. Identify yourself and state that you are an EMT and you are ready to perform two-rescuer CPR.
2. While the first rescuer is providing compressions, spend five seconds checking for a carotid pulse produced by each compression. This is to determine if the compressions being delivered are effective. Inform the first rescuer if there is or is not a pulse being produced.*
3. You should say, "Stop compressions" and check for spontaneous pulse and breathing. This should take only a few seconds.
4. If there is no pulse, you should ventilate once and state, "No pulse. Continue CPR."
5. The switch from one-rescuer to two-rescuer CPR should take place after the first rescuer has completed a cycle of 15 compressions and 2 ventilations.
6. The first rescuer resumes compressions, and the second rescuer provides a ventilation during a brief pause after every fifth compression. If desired, the second rescuer can start compressions and allow the first rescuer to provide the ventilations.

Note: If you are off duty and arrive after CPR has been started, let the first rescuer know that you know CPR and that you are an EMT. If you find that the first rescuer does not know CPR, stop him and take over, providing one-rescuer techniques. Always verify that someone has activated the EMS system.

Should you find yourself providing CPR while off duty, you may be able to have a bystander assist you in the two-rescuer method. However, be certain that the bystander has been

*If the first rescuer cannot deliver effective compressions, you will have to take over for him once CPR is resumed.

trained by the American Heart Association or the American Red Cross in CPR. Too often people wish to help thinking they know the procedure based on what they have seen on television, without the benefit of formal CPR training. If you begin two-rescuer CPR with the aid of a bystander and find that he is unable to perform properly and you cannot quickly correct the problem, stop the two-rescuer procedure and begin one-rescuer CPR. The volunteer may be sent to confirm that EMS is en route or to direct the incoming ambulance crew to the patient.

How to Change Positions When two rescuers are performing CPR, one of the rescuers may wish to change positions (Scan 5-4). Often the compressor is the one who becomes fatigued, but the ventilator also may request a change. The most important factor in the change is that it be done in as little time as possible. The compressor controls the change and will signal the pending change at the beginning of a series of compressions as follows: "CHANGE. One and two and three and four and five, BREATHE." The ventilator will provide one full breath, and the two rescuers will quickly change positions.

The rescuer who was previously providing compressions is now the ventilator. This rescuer opens the airway immediately upon reaching the patient's head and checks for a carotid pulse and respirations. These checks should take no more than 3 to 5 seconds. If a change takes place every 2 minutes or less, a check of pulse and breathing does not need to be done on every change.

CPR Techniques for Infants and Children

The techniques of CPR for infants and small children are essentially the same as those used for adults (See Scan 5-5; see also Chapter 17). You will have to

1. Establish unresponsiveness.
2. Correctly position the patient.
3. Open the airway (head-tilt, chin-lift, or jaw-thrust).
4. Establish respiratory arrest (3 to 5 seconds).
5. Provide artificial ventilations and clear the airway, if necessary.
6. Establish the lack of pulse in 5 to 10 seconds.
7. Provide chest compressions and ventilations.
8. Do frequent assessments of pulse and breathing. This is to be done every few minutes.

Some procedures and rates differ when the patient is an infant or a child. If younger than 1 year of age, the patient is considered to be an infant. Between 1 and 8 years of age, the patient is considered to be a child. Over the age of 8 years, adult procedures apply to the patient. Keep in mind that the size of the patient can also be an important factor. A very small 9-year old may have to be treated as a child.

Positioning the Patient When CPR must be performed, adults, children, and infants are placed on their backs on a hard surface. For an infant, the hard surface can be the rescuer's hand or forearm.

Opening the Airway For an infant or a child, use the head-tilt, chin-lift or the jaw-thrust technique, but apply only a slight tilt for an infant. Too great a tilt may close off the infant's airway; however, make certain that the opening is adequate (note chest rise during ventilation). Always be sure to support an infant's head.

Establishing a Pulse Take these steps to establish a pulse in an infant or a child.

- INFANT—For infants, you should use the **brachial** (BRAY-key-al) **pulse**. This is the pulse that can be felt when compressing the major artery of the upper arm, the brachial artery (Figure 5-12). Do not use the carotid or radial pulse. To find the brachial pulse

  1. Locate the point halfway between the infant's elbow and shoulder.
  2. Place your thumb on the lateral side of the upper arm at this midway point.

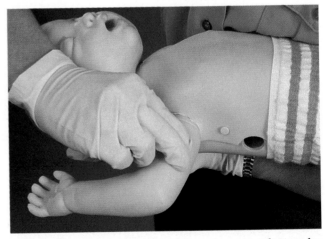

Figure 5-12 For infants, determine circulation by feeling for a brachial pulse.

Changing Positions

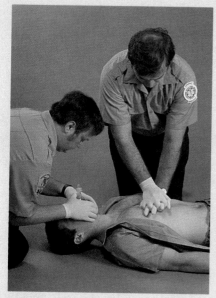

1. When fatigued, the compressor calls for the switch. Give a clear signal to change.

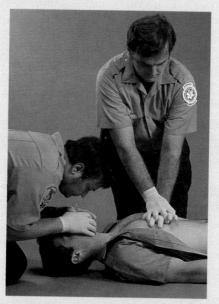

2. Compressor completes fifth compression. Ventilator provides one ventilation.

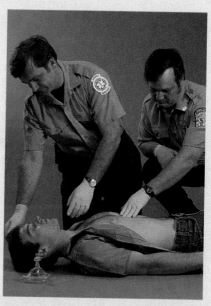

3. Ventilator moves to chest and begins to locate compression site. Compressor begins to move to head.

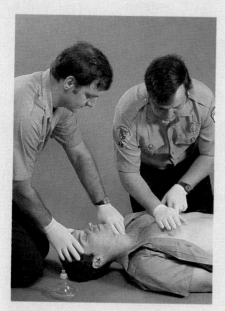

4. New compressor finds site. New ventilator checks carotid pulse.

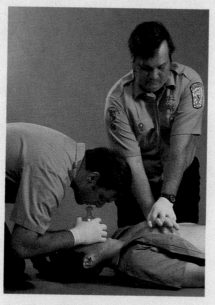

5. New ventilator says, "No pulse," and ventilates once (1½ to 2 seconds), using his own pocket face mask.

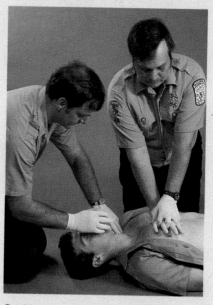

6. New compressor delivers 5 compressions (3-4 seconds) at a rate of 80-100 per minute. New ventilator assesses compressions.

Note: Both rescuers are shown on same side of patient for purpose of clarity. See Figure 5-11 for proper positioning on opposite sides of patient.

CPR Summary

ONE RESCUER	FUNCTIONS		TWO RESCUERS
	• Establish unresponsiveness • If there's no response, call 911 • Position patient • Open airway • Look, listen, and feel (for 3-5 seconds)		
	• Deliver 2 breaths (11/2 - 2 sec/ventilation)		
	• Check carotid pulse. . . (5-10 seconds) If no pulse. . . • Begin chest compressions		
	DELIVER COMPRESSIONS		
	80-100/min (15/9-11 sec)	80-100/min (5/3-4 sec)	
	DELIVER VENTILATIONS **10-12 breaths/min**		
	2/15	1/5 (Pause to allow ventilations)	
	• Do 4 cycles • Check pulse	• Ventilator checks effective-ness	
	CONTINUE PERIODIC ASSESSMENT		

Changing Postions

• Compressor-signal to change; provide 5 compressions • Ventilator-one ventilation	New ventilator checks pulse provides 1 ventilation (uses new mask)	Continue CPR sequence

NOTE: Wear gloves and use either a pocket mask with one-way valve or bag valve mask

3. Place the tips of your index and middle fingers at the midway point on the medial surface of the infant's upper arm. You will feel a groove in the muscle at this location.

4. Press your index and middle fingers in toward the bone, taking care not to exert too much pressure. To do so may collapse the artery, stopping circulation to the lower arm and perhaps causing you to miss feeling the pulse.

5. Take 5 to 10 seconds to determine pulselessness.

- CHILD—Determine circulation in the same manner as for an adult. Check 5 to 10 seconds at the carotid artery for a pulse.

If you are acting alone and you find an unresponsive infant or child, continue the ABCs of the primary survey and start CPR. DO CPR FOR 1 MINUTE BEFORE ACTIVATING THE EMS SYSTEM.

Chest Compressions Follow these procedures to provide chest compressions to an infant or a child (Figure 5-13).

- INFANT—Compressions are delivered to an infant on the midline of the sternum, one finger-width below an imaginary line drawn between the infant's nipples. This position is easily located by placing the index finger on the imaginary line between the nipples. This places the middle and ring fingers in the proper area for compressions. The infant's sternum should be depressed ½ to 1 inch.

- CHILD—Compressions are applied using the heel of one hand. The compression site is the lower third of the sternum one finger-width above the substernal notch, located using the same procedure that is applied to the adult patient. The child's sternum should be depressed 1 to 1½ inches.

Ventilations Follow the procedures below to provide ventilations to an infant or a child. AS WITH ADULTS, USE A POCKET FACE MASK OR OTHER BARRIER DEVICE.

- INFANT—The rescuer should provide a slow, gentle breath of air using the mouth-to-mouth-and-nose with barrier protection or approved mouth-to-mask. It is essential to watch the rise and fall of the infant's chest. The rescuer should deliver just

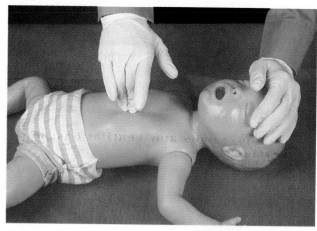

A.

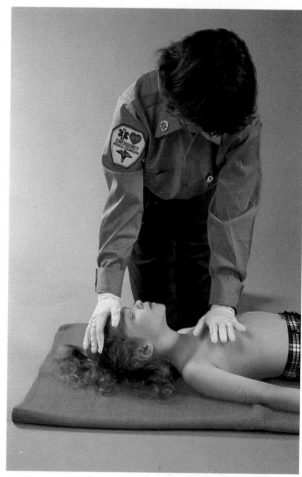

B.

Figure 5-13 Chest compressions for infants and children. (A) Infants: Use tips of fingers and light pressure. (B) Children: Use heel of one hand only.

enough air to cause the infant's chest to rise, taking 1 to 1½ seconds per ventilation.

- CHILD—A slow, gentle breath is provided to the child patient, taking 1 to 1½ seconds per ventilation. Again, only enough air is

156 Basic Life Support

delivered to cause the patient's chest to rise. Mouth-to-mouth or mouth-to-nose with barrier protection or approved mouth-to-mask techniques are usually employed. If the patient is a small child, you may have to use the mouth-to-mouth-and-nose method with barrier protection.

Compressions and Ventilations: Rates and Ratios For infants and children, deliver compressions and ventilations as follows (See also Table 5-1).

- INFANT—Deliver compressions at the rate of at least 100 per minute (5 compressions in no more than 3 seconds). Pause to give a slow (1 to 1½ seconds) gentle breath every 5 compressions to give a ratio of 5:1.
- CHILD—Deliver compressions at the rate of 100 per minute (5 compressions every 3 seconds). Pause to give a slow (1 to 1½ seconds) gentle breath every 5 compressions to give a ratio of 5:1.

Note: To establish the correct rate for infants, count: "One, two, three, four, five, breathe." Provide the ventilation during a pause immediately after "five." For children, count: "One and two and three and four and five, breathe." Pause and provide the ventilation immediately after "five."

Special Considerations in CPR

How to Know if CPR Is Effective To determine if CPR is effective

- *If possible have someone else feel for a carotid pulse* during compressions and watch to see the patient's chest rise during ventilations.
- *Listen for exhalation of air*, either naturally or during compressions, as additional verification that air has entered the lungs.

In addition to these events, any of the following indications of effective CPR may be noticed.

- Pupils constrict.
- Skin color improves.
- Heartbeat returns spontaneously.
- Spontaneous, gasping respirations are made.
- Arms and legs move.
- Swallowing is attempted.

- Consciousness returns.

Even at best, the CPR you provide will be only 25% to 33% as effective as normal heart action. To counter this deficiency, you may take several actions.

- Perform CPR as closely as possible to the recommended guidelines.
- Consider using a mechanical-compressor to assist chest compressions if your EMS system provides them and you are trained in their use.
- Avoid stopping CPR or keep interruption of CPR to a minimum.
- Deliver supplemental oxygen. Use an oxygen delivery system that provides 90% to 100% oxygen with each ventilation. (Even though supplemental oxygen is significant in basic life support, do not delay or stop CPR in order to set up an oxygen delivery system.)
- Provide defibrillation if you are trained to do so (as discussed later in this chapter), or call for assistance from those who can provide it as quickly as possible.
- Call for advanced cardiac life support assistance as quickly as possible.

If you speak with experienced EMTs, you will learn that CPR rarely causes the return of spontaneous heartbeat and breathing. The main objective of CPR is to keep a patient who is clinically dead from reaching the irreversible point of biological death. Often defibrillation and advanced life support measures such as medications and advanced airway techniques are required to fully reverse the patient's condition. REMEMBER, WITHOUT YOUR EFFORTS AT CPR, THERE WOULD BE NO HOPE AT ALL!

If you perform CPR and the patient does not survive, it is most likely because the patient had experienced a severe heart attack with death of heart muscle, had already reached irreversible biological death before CPR could begin, or had injuries too severe to survive. Whether it is your first or your hundredth time, the death of a patient is a traumatic event. Share your feelings with others; everyone has had similar feelings. (See "EMT Stress Syndrome," Chapter 21.)

Factors That May Make CPR Ineffective Ineffective CPR refers to the application of *improper* resuscitative techniques. The patient's chances for survival greatly improve if CPR is done efficiently. Problems that may decrease the efficiency of CPR include

For ventilations (see Chapter 4)
- The patient's head is not placed in the proper head-tilt, chin-lift or jaw-thrust position for ventilations.
- The patient's mouth is not opened wide enough for air exchange.
- There is not an effective seal made against the patient's face, mouth, or nose.
- The patient's nose is not pinched shut during mouth-to-mouth ventilations.
- The patient's mouth is not closed completely during mouth-to-nose ventilations.
- The ventilations are delivered too rapidly or at too great a volume, and gastric distention develops as air intended for the lungs goes into the stomach.

For chest compressions
- The patient is not lying on a hard surface.
- The rescuer's hands are incorrectly placed.
- There are prolonged interruptions.
- The chest is not sufficiently compressed.
- The compression rate is too rapid or too slow.
- Compressions are jerky, not smooth with 50% of the cycle being compression and 50% being the release of compression.

Interrupting CPR Once you begin CPR, you may interrupt the process for no more than a few seconds to check for pulse and breathing or to reposition yourself and the patient. The first recommended pulse and breathing check is after the first minute of CPR. You should continue to check for these vital signs every few minutes.

In addition to these built-in interruptions, you may interrupt CPR to

- Move a patient onto a stretcher
- Move a patient down a flight of stairs or through a narrow doorway or hallway, or on and off the ambulance (see "Moving Patients During CPR" below)
- Suction to clear vomitus or airway obstructions
- Allow for defibrillation or advanced cardiac life support measures to be initiated

Moving Patients During CPR CPR must be continued while the patient is on the stretcher and being transferred to the ambulance, as shown in Scan 5-6. Ideally, CPR should not be interrupted for more than a few seconds during transfer. When moving the stretcher down stairs or through narrow spaces or in loading it on and off the ambulance, however, interruptions to CPR may take longer than a few seconds. These interruptions can be minimized as follows.

- Stairs—It is difficult to perform CPR on stairs. Perform CPR at the top of the stairs then, on a signal, move the patient down the stairs where CPR is quickly resumed. If there are multiple flights of stairs, stop on each landing to perform CPR before moving to the next level.
- Narrow Hallways and Doors—It is also difficult to position an EMT beside the stretcher while moving through doorways or proceeding down narrow hallways. In these situations, perform CPR until it is time to move through the narrow spot. On signal, discontinue CPR and resume it as quickly as possible when you reach an open area.
- Loading into the Ambulance—Other brief interruptions may be encountered while loading the patient into the ambulance. Delays may be shortened by having an EMT in the ambulance, ready to start CPR when the stretcher is loaded. The reverse should be done on arrival at the hospital with an EMT or hospital personnel prepared to begin CPR when the stretcher reaches the ground.

CPR *must be continued once the patient is loaded into the ambulance.* The procedures should continue uninterrupted except for suctioning or other essential procedures until the emergency department staff takes over CPR or the physician on duty tells you to stop your CPR efforts.

Complications of CPR

Injury to the rib cage is the most common complication of CPR. When the hands are placed too high on the sternum, fractures to the upper sternum and the clavicles may occur. If the hands are too low on the sternum, the xiphoid may be fractured or driven down into the liver, producing severe lacerations (cuts) and profuse internal bleeding. When the hands are placed too far off center, or when they are allowed to slip from their position over the CPR compression site, the ribs or their cartilage attachments may be fractured (Figure 5-14).

Even when CPR is correctly performed, cartilage attached to the ribs may separate or ribs may be fractured. In such cases, *do not stop CPR.* Simply reassess your hand position and

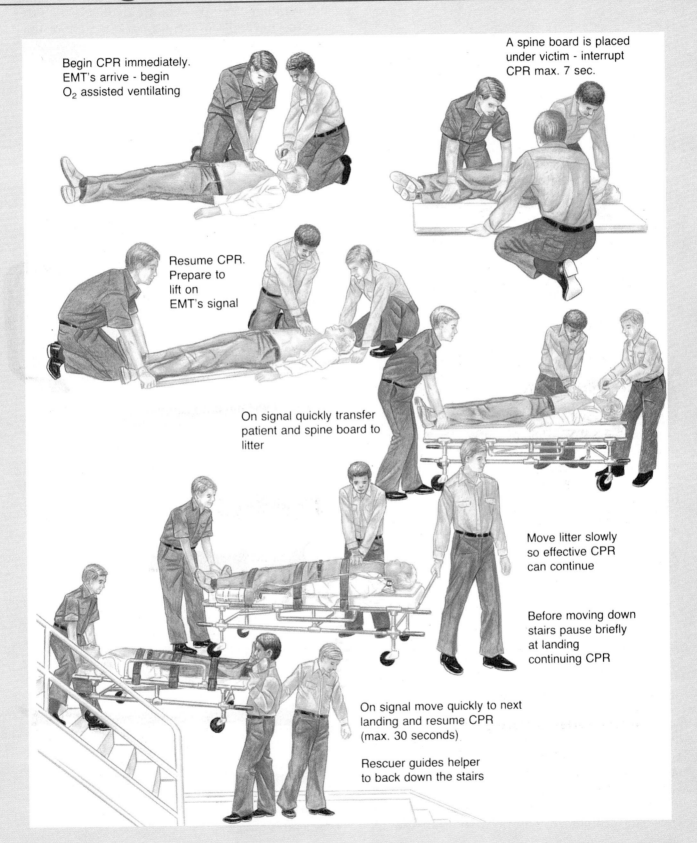

Begin CPR immediately. EMT's arrive - begin O₂ assisted ventilating

A spine board is placed under victim - interrupt CPR max. 7 sec.

Resume CPR. Prepare to lift on EMT's signal

On signal quickly transfer patient and spine board to litter

Move litter slowly so effective CPR can continue

Before moving down stairs pause briefly at landing continuing CPR

On signal move quickly to next landing and resume CPR (max. 30 seconds)

Rescuer guides helper to back down the stairs

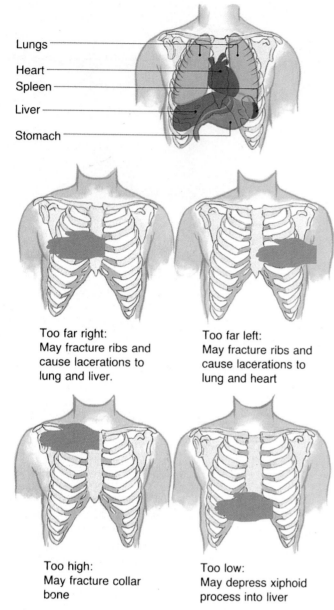

Lungs
Heart
Spleen
Liver
Stomach

Too far right:
May fracture ribs and cause lacerations to lung and liver.

Too far left:
May fracture ribs and cause lacerations to lung and heart

Too high:
May fracture collar bone

Too low:
May depress xiphoid process into liver

Figure 5-14 Improper positioning of the hands during CPR can damage the rib cage and underlying organs.

compression depth and continue CPR. It is far better that the patient suffer a few broken ribs and live than die because you did not continue to perform CPR for fear of inflicting additional injury.

Often when CPR is performed on elderly patients, the first few compressions will separate rib cartilage. When this happens, you may hear a "crunch" as you apply a compression. *Do not stop CPR.* Again, reassess your hand position and the depths of your compressions and continue CPR.

The problem of gastric distention that is

associated with pulmonary resuscitation (see Chapter 4) also may occur when performing CPR. When performing one-rescuer CPR, the rescuer often rushes to get to the patient's head and ventilate. Ventilations are delivered too fast and too hard. To prevent gastric distention (or ineffective respirations), adequately position the head to open the airway for every ventilation and provide slow (1½ to 2 seconds for adults; 1 to 1½ seconds for infants and children) ventilations that are just adequate to make the chest rise. When gastric distention is present, be alert for vomiting.

Other complications may result from improper CPR efforts, but most are easy to avoid by following American Heart Association guidelines for CPR.

When Not to Begin or to Terminate CPR

As discussed earlier in this chapter, CPR should *not* be initiated when you find that the patient—even though unresponsive and perhaps not breathing—*does have a pulse.* In addition, there are special circumstances in which CPR should not be initiated *even though the patient has no pulse.*

- Obvious mortal wounds—These include decapitation, incineration, a severed body, and injuries that are so extensive that CPR cannot be effectively performed (e.g., severe crush injuries to the head, neck, and chest).
- Rigor mortis—This is the stiffening of the body and its limbs that occurs after death, usually within 4 to 10 hours.
- Obvious decomposition.
- A line of lividity—Lividity is a red or purple skin discoloration that occurs when gravity causes the blood to sink to the lowest parts of the body and collect there. Lividity usually indicates that the patient has been dead for more than 15 minutes unless hypothermia is present (see Chapter 21). Using this sign requires special training that is usually not part of the basic EMT program.
- Stillbirth—CPR should not be initiated for a stillborn infant who has died hours prior to birth. This patient may be recognized by blisters on the skin, a very soft head, and a strong disagreeable odor (see Chapter 18).

In all cases, if you are in doubt, radio for a physician's advice.

Except in the above instances, when dealing with a patient in cardiac arrest, your duty as an EMT is to begin CPR immediately. Even though the patient may have a terminal illness or he may be very old, you cannot decide to withhold CPR. Bystanders may ask you not to begin CPR. Family members may say that the patient would not want your help, but you have no proof of this. Even though many states are now recognizing that resuscitation may violate certain persons' rights to die with dignity, you cannot make such a decision. It would be rare, but it is possible that the people at the scene want the patient to die for less noble reasons.

To refrain from performing resuscitation, you must have written documentation that is accepted by your EMS System. This documentation must be immediately available. You cannot delay starting CPR while someone searches for the document. Once CPR is started, it should be stopped only if the following criteria have been met: At the hospital, the physician's written order sheet can be used to authorize cessation of resuscitation by the professional medical staff. Such an order sheet is often called a "Do Not Resuscitate" or "DNR" order. Your instructor can tell you if DNR orders may be honored in the field in your region or state. Become familiar with the form or forms required. In the absence of these regulations, the only person who can tell you not to resuscitate a clinically dead patient is a physician, either on the scene or via radio or telephone. Remember, YOU MUST FOLLOW LOCAL PROTOCOLS.

CPR is most effective if started immediately after cardiac arrest occurs. If a patient has been in arrest for more than ten minutes, resuscitation efforts usually are not effective. However, there are documented cases of adults who were in arrest for more than ten minutes being resuscitated with no major brain damage. Some have survived after being in arrest for well over 30 minutes. Cold air temperatures appear to prolong the time someone can be in arrest before biological death occurs; cold water is even more effective in delaying biological death (see Chapter 21). Also keep in mind that children and infants may tolerate longer periods of cardiac arrest than can adults.

Do not refuse to begin CPR because someone is thought to have been in cardiac arrest for more than 10 minutes. The moment the patient was seen to collapse and the moment of cardiac arrest are not usually the same. A patient can be unconscious with minimum effective lung and heart action for quite some time before actual cardiac arrest occurs. Once you have started CPR, you must continue to provide CPR until

- Spontaneous circulation occurs . . . then provide artificial respiration as needed.
- Spontaneous circulation and breathing occur.
- Another trained rescuer can take over for you.
- You turn care of the patient over to ALS medical personnel or a physician.
- You are too exhausted to continue.
- You receive a "no CPR" order from a physician or other authority per local protocols.

If you turn the patient over to another rescuer, this person must be trained to your level or higher. This does not mean that the person has to be an EMT. The new rescuer must have certification (American Heart Association or American Red Cross) in basic cardiac life support. First Responders can take over CPR for you if they are certified in CPR. If you do turn over resuscitation to a person who is certified, but not an EMT, it should be because you are exhausted, you need to set up oxygen delivery or defibrillation equipment, or are other patients who have life-threatening emergencies. You must supervise the person who has taken over CPR, since you are still responsible for the patient.

Many students have fears of having to stop CPR because of exhaustion. As a member of the EMS System, you have to be realistic about patient care and know when you have done all you can for a patient. If you are isolated and have provided CPR for 30 minutes to an hour and are too exhausted to go on, remember that there are physical limitations to the care you can provide. Few patients having received CPR for such a long period of time will survive. You will have done all you could for the patient and should not feel guilty at having to stop CPR.

You lessen the chances of physical exhaustion if you learn to control rescuer hyperventilation. When providing CPR, you establish an irregular pattern of breathing for yourself. This may cause you to begin to breathe very quickly and deeply, unable to regain control. You can help prevent this by keeping in good physical condition and learning not to try to take a breath with each compression. You have to learn to establish a normal breathing rate when delivering chest compressions.

Special Situations There are special situations that require CPR and other basic life support measures. These include near-drownings, electric shocks, accidents producing crushing chest injuries, drug overdoses, and toxic gas inhalations. The problems of resuscitation as they relate to these special problems will be covered in later chapters.

Keeping CPR Skills Current CPR skills can be quickly lost when not regularly practiced. As an EMT be certain to practice CPR on infant, child, and adult manikins. Ideally you should complete a CPR course once every year. One way to stay current in the technique is to become a CPR instructor for the American Heart Association or American Red Cross and teach CPR to the citizens in your community.

DEFIBRILLATION

In many EMS systems, defibrillation is performed by paramedics who are part of advanced life support units. In some EMS systems, EMTs are being trained in automated defibrillation, either as part of their basic EMT course or in a separate course. The information that follows is intended to introduce basic facts about defibrillation and how it can be coordinated with CPR to EMTs who will not be trained to perform defibrillation as well as to those who will undertake this special training. It is not intended to replace or to be the text for a course in defibrillation.

Reading the following information is optional, to be assigned at the discretion of your instructor.

The Importance of Early Defibrillation

Although many factors influence whether a person will survive an out-of-hospital cardiac arrest (the person's age and prior medical history, for example), the most significant factor is the total time elapsed from collapse to defibrillation—the delivery of an electrical shock through the chest.

Until recently, defibrillation was a skill performed only by EMS personnel with hundreds of hours of training. It has been demonstrated, however, that basic EMTs with only a few hours of additional training can safely and effectively perform the skills of defibrillation with an **automated external defibrillator (AED)**. In one study, the survival rate of persons experiencing out-of-hospital cardiac arrest was more than five times higher in small communities where the EMTs had been trained to defibrillate than in communities where they could not.

The reason for this has become increasingly clear: long-term survival is unusual in cases where more than 8 minutes have elapsed between collapse and defibrillation. Defibrillating a person this quickly (and even more quickly is ideal) will be possible only if emergency responders are trained and equipped to defibrillate in the field.

In some states, with the additional training in defibrillation that is required, you can achieve the designation EMT-D (for Emergency Medical Technician-Defibrillation). You will either receive this training as part of your basic EMT course or will receive it in a separate course.

Automated Defibrillation

The user of a standard, manually operated defibrillator must be able to make rapid and correct interpretation of electrocardiogram (ECG) rhythm sounds and decisions as to whether a shock is indicated. One drawback of using this type of defibrillator is the difficulty of maintaining crisp skills, especially in communities where the skills are rarely used in actual patient care activities. Frequent periodic recertification sessions that include thorough and strict evaluation of rhythm recognition and defibrillation skills are an absolute requirement when manual defibrillators are used.

Technological advances have now made it possible for a defibrillator itself to recognize ECG rhythms that should be shocked and to either automatically charge up and deliver a shock or advise the rescuer to deliver a shock. These new defibrillators, called automated external defibrillators (AEDs), are so simple to operate that defibrillation can now be considered a skill well within the reach of every EMT and First Responder. The development of the AED has made effective emergency cardiac care outside a hospital a realistic goal for communities of all sizes.

Cardiac rhythm recognition and the operation of a standard manual defibrillator will not be discussed in this chapter because EMTs are more likely to use one of the automated external defibrillators than a manually operated defibrillator.

What Everyone Should Know About Cardiac Arrest and Defibrillation

Usually, but not always, a cardiac event such as a coronary artery spasm or myocardial infarction (heart attack) are associated with a disturbance of the heart's electrical, or conduction, system, which must function normally if the heart is to continue to beat with a regular rhythm. The most common conditions that result in cardiac arrest are

Shockable Rhythms
- Ventricular Fibrillation—The primary electrical disturbance resulting in cardiac arrest is called **ventricular fibrillation** (ven-TRIK-u-ler fib-ri-LAY-shun) **(VF)**. Between 50% and 60% of all cardiac arrest victims will be in VF if EMS personnel arrive in the first 8 minutes or so. The heart in VF may have plenty of electrical energy, but it is totally disorganized. Chaotic electrical activity originating from many sites in the heart prevents the heart muscle from contracting normally and thus pumping blood. If you could see a heart in VF, it would appear to be quivering like a bag of worms. VF is considered a shockable rhythm, one for which defibrillation is effective.
- Ventricular Tachycardia—Automated external defibrillators are also designed to shock a rhythm known as **ventricular tachycardia** (ven-TRIK-u-ler tak-i-KAR-de-uh) **(V-Tach)** if it is very fast. In ventricular tachycardia (a very unusual cardiac arrest rhythm observed in less than 10% of all out-of-hospital cases), the heartbeat is organized, but it is usually quite rapid. The faster the heart rate, the more likely it is that ventricular tachycardia will not allow the heart's chambers to fill with enough blood between beats to produce blood flow sufficient to meet the body's needs, especially that of the brain. Pulseless V-Tach is considered a shockable rhythm.

Nonshockable Rhythms
- Electromechanical Dissociation—In 15% to 20% of cardiac arrest victims, the heart muscle itself fails even though the electrical rhythm remains relatively normal. This condition of relatively normal electrical activity but no pumping action—called **electromechanical dissociation** (el-EK-tro-mek-AN-i-kul dis-so-see-AY-shun) **(EMD)** because the electrical activity is dissociated, or separated, from the mechanical, or pumping activity—means that the heart muscle is severely and almost always terminally sick. Defibrillation cannot help these people because their heart's electrical

rhythm is already organized and slow (unlike ventricular tachycardia, wherein the rhythm is organized but very fast). EMD is not considered a shockable rhythm.
- Asystole—In the remaining 20% to 25% of cardiac arrest victims, the heart has ceased generating electrical impulses altogether. When this happens, a condition called **asystole** (ah-SIS-to-le), there is no repetitive electrical stimulus to cause the heart muscle to contract, and so it does not. As a result, there is no blood flow, and the patient has no pulse or regular respirations and is unconscious. (This condition is commonly called "flatline," because the wavy line displayed on an ECG when there is electrical activity goes flat with asystole.) Asystole is not considered a shockable rhythm.

If you have been adding up the numbers, you know by now that automated defibrillators will shock only about six or seven of every ten cardiac arrest patients to whom they are attached: those suffering from the disturbed rhythms of ventricular fibrillation or ventricular tachycardia. For patients suffering from electromechanical dissociation (heart muscle failure) or asystole (complete lack of electrical activity), defibrillation will not be effective.

Note: As an EMT you cannot diagnose heart ailments or causes of cardiac arrest. You must initiate CPR and defibrillation as rapidly as possible and, if defibrillation is not successful in restoring heart function, continue CPR to prevent biological death until the patient's care can be taken over at the medical facility or by those with advanced skills.

How Defibrillation Works

Contrary to popular opinion, defibrillation is not "jump-starting" a dead heart. In fact, it is just the opposite. The therapeutic action of a defibrillatory shock is the sudden termination of a heart's electrical activity, often enabling the heart to restart in a coordinated fashion.

For defibrillation to be of benefit to a person, the heart must have enough life left in it that it will be capable of beating on its own once the chaotic pattern has been disrupted. The amount of life left in a heart is evidenced by the coarseness (amplitude) of the ventricular fibrillation. The coarser the fibrillation the more likely it is that defibrillation will be successful. Since the coarseness of VF is determined in part by the total time in cardiac arrest, and since the extent of damage to the brain is certainly influenced by the total time in cardiac arrest, it should be clear that the sooner a person is defibrillated, the more likely he is to survive.

It should also be clear that delivering shocks to a person in asystole or even in very fine ventricular fibrillation will rarely result in the development of a spontaneous organized rhythm because there is simply not enough energy remaining in the heart to allow it to function on its own.

The Importance of Speed

Recall that a major factor in the survival of a person who is in cardiac arrest is the amount of time that elapses from the moment of collapse until the start of defibrillation. This time period has four phases.

1. EMS access time
2. Dispatch time
3. Ambulance response time
4. Assessment and shock time

For an EMS system to be effective, each of these time segments must be as short as possible (Table 5-2).

EMS Access Time This is the time that passes from the time a person collapses in cardiac arrest until someone notifies the EMS system. A person who collapses in front of another person (witnessed arrest) should have a far greater chance of survival than a person who collapses in an isolated place away from other people; the person seeing the collapse can call for an ambulance.

That someone sees a person collapse in cardiac arrest is no guarantee that an ambulance will be called immediately, however. In fact, most witnesses to a collapse delay calling for an ambulance for 2 minutes or more, and many delay calling for 4 to 6 minutes and longer. The typical witness of a cardiac arrest is a woman 65 years old, alone with her husband at the time of his collapse, and not trained in CPR. Even though CPR training programs are available for members of the public, few senior citizens attend.

Obviously, members of the public should be trained in CPR. But the public should also be trained to call for an ambulance immediately upon seeing someone collapse, even though they know CPR. Any delay in activating the community EMS system results in delayed defibrillation.

Dispatch Time The second phase of a defibrillation effort begins with receipt of the call for help by a dispatcher and ends with the alerting of an ambulance crew. This time segment should be kept as short as possible. The dispatcher rapidly determines whether the call is for a cardiac problem (by asking the caller about difficult breathing, unconsciousness, unresponsiveness, and the like). Then the dispatcher immediately sends out an emergency medical service unit with a defibrillator. Once this is done, the dispatcher acquires additional information from the caller while the ambulance is on the way.

Ambulance Response Time The third phase of the collapse-to-defibrillation period is

TABLE 5-2 Minimizing the Time from Collapse to Defibrillation

Time Component	Objective	Goal	Method
EMS access time	To minimize the time from collapse until someone places a call for help	1.0 min	An increased community awareness of the need for quickly calling for an ambulance; more public CPR programs
Dispatch time	To minimize the time it takes for an EMS dispatcher to elicit information from a caller and get a defibrillator-equipped unit on the road	0.5 min	Better dispatcher training, improved call handling procedures
Response time	To minimize the time it takes to get a trained defibrillator team to the patient	3.0 min	Strategic placement of automated defibrillators with first-response personnel
Shock time	To minimize the time it takes to deliver the first shock	1.5 min	Use automated defibrillators; continually practice to maintain peak efficiency

the time from dispatch until the ambulance arrives at the location of the stricken person. Ambulance response time varies considerably from community to community, as well as from one area to another within large communities. Response times are often long in large cities where congested roads are a problem and in small communities where volunteers must respond to the ambulance garage from homes and places of business. The fastest ambulance response times are generally in towns and small cities that are large enough to have an ambulance service that is staffed around the clock by in-station crews, but small enough that traffic and response distances are not problems.

One way to shorten the time from dispatch to the arrival of a defibrillator in communities that do not have in-station crews is to station an AED with a trained EMT 24 hours a day. Thus, when a call for a potential cardiac problem is received, that trained individual can respond directly to the scene with the defibrillator while other EMTs respond to the station to get the ambulance. This approach works. In one group of small communities, the time it took to get a defibrillator on the road was reduced from 7.5 minutes to 2.5 minutes. Placing automated defibrillators with first responders in large cities has proved equally effective in reducing the response time of a trained individual with a defibrillator.

Assessment and Shock Time The final phase of a defibrillation period is the time that elapses from the time that a rescuer arrives at the side of the stricken person to the time the first shock is delivered. As with each of the other phases of the collapse to defibrillation period, this time segment must be kept as short as possible if life-saving efforts are to be effective—ideally 1 minute or less.

The shorter the collapse-to-defibrillation time, the greater the chance for survival. A person who can be shocked in 4 to 6 minutes or less after collapse has a good chance of surviving. A person who cannot be shocked within 8 minutes of the moment of collapse has only a slim chance of surviving.

Because the ambulance response time alone approaches 8 minutes in many communities, the importance of implementing creative approaches to shortening the various components of the time from collapse to shock cannot be overemphasized. The goals listed in Table 5-2, if achieved, should result in a witnessed VF survival rate of 25% or higher.

Operating Automated Defibrillators Safely

Ambulance and rescue services can choose between fully automatic and semi-automatic (shock advisory) defibrillators, depending on personal preference and the medical director's judgment. The general operation of both types of defibrillator will be discussed here. The following "don'ts" apply to both types.

- Never activate an automated defibrillator unless the patient is in full cardiac arrest as evidenced by unconsciousness, the absence of a pulse, and the absence of other than agonal respirations.
- Never activate an automated defibrillator unless the patient is lying still and not in contact with rescuers or bystanders.
- Never activate an automated defibrillator in a moving ambulance. If defibrillation must be attempted again during transport, have the ambulance operator pull over and stop during defibrillation.
- Do not operate in the rain, in a puddle, or on a steel or other metal boat deck.
- Do not position the pads closer than 5 inches from a pacemaker battery.
- Do not neglect to wipe off nitro paste or pads from the chest prior to applying the defibrillator pads.

Attaching the Defibrillator to the Patient
The basic steps for attaching an automated defibrillator to a patient are the same regardless of whether the unit is automatic or semi-automatic.

All automated external defibrillators use self-adhesive monitor/defibrillation pads rather than the standard monitoring electrodes and hand-held defibrillation paddles used with manual defibrillators (Figure 5-15). The self-adhesive

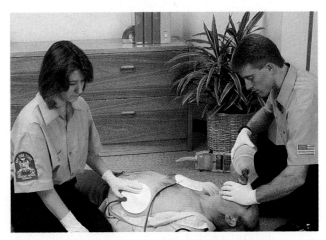

Figure 5-15 Using an automated defibrillator.

pads allow for both monitoring of the patient's heart rhythm and for delivery of the shock. Correct placement of the pads is accomplished in the following manner.

While your partner initiates CPR
- Expose the patient's chest and quickly wipe it dry, if necessary. Do not take the time to shave any chest hair from the pad sites. Every second counts.
- Remove two pads from their protective packages immediately upon arrival at the patient's side.
- Connect the cables that lead from the automated defibrillator according to the manufacturer's instructions and be sure that the connections are tight.
- Taking care not to tear the pad, remove the plastic backing from one pad and place it on the right upper chest with one edge of the pad next to, but not on, the sternum, and the top edge just touching the clavicle. Use a rolling motion when applying the pads to ensure that air is not trapped underneath.
- Press on the adhesive portion of the pad to ensure good contact with the skin. Do not press on the center of a pad that has a gel-sponge center; to do so will squeeze gel into the adhesion area and prevent the pad from sticking to the skin.
- Remove the backing from the second pad and place it over the apex of the heart (below and to the left of the nipple) in the same manner.

Although either pad may be attached to either cable, it is recommended for consistency that units employing color-coded cables or pads be placed as follows.

- The red color (cable or pad, depending on the manufacturer) should be applied over the apex area.
- The white color (cable or pad, depending on the manufacturer) should be applied over the right border of the sternum.

This placement ensures correct positioning of the patient's ECG signal into the monitor circuitry. If the pad/cable connections are not secure or if the pads are not firmly adhered to the patient's chest, all automated defibrillators will announce a warning to check the electrodes. An automated defibrillator will not function until the pads and cables are securely attached and properly connected.

Operating a Fully Automatic Defibrillator
A fully automatic defibrillator will assess the patient's rhythm and determine whether a shock is needed. If it senses that a shock is needed, a fully automatic defibrillator will automatically charge to a preset energy level and deliver the shock, all without any further action by the rescuer. The newest models of fully automatic defibrillators have only two controls: an ON button and an OFF button. Fully automatic defibrillators also make use of voice synthesizers to verbally announce instructions and warnings such as "STOP CPR" and "STAND BACK" and "CHECK BREATHING AND PULSE."

Before operating a fully automatic defibrillator
- Assess your patient's breathing and pulse.

If the person is not breathing and does not have a pulse, and you are working with a partner
- Direct your partner to begin CPR while you prepare the defibrillator and attach the pads to the patient.

If you are working alone
- Prepare the defibrillator, attach the pads to the patient, and then begin CPR to get some oxygenated blood moving.

When the defibrillator is attached to the patient
- Clear everyone—including yourself—from contact with the patient.
- Press the ON button. The defibrillator will announce "STOP CPR" and begin analyzing the patient's rhythm. If a shock is indicated, the fully automatic defibrillator will repeatedly announce "STAND BACK," charge to 200 joules of energy, and deliver the shock. Do not touch or move the patient when you hear the warning "STAND BACK."
- Remain clear of the patient. Immediately following delivery of the first shock, the fully automatic defibrillator will again analyze the rhythm. If the patient still has a rhythm for which a shock is indicated, the defibrillator will once again warn "STAND BACK" and charge to 200-300 joules of energy. The second shock will be delivered as soon as the charging process is complete.*
- Remain clear of the patient. The process continues automatically until the third

---

* The most common energy levels are noted in the text (200/200-300/360 joules). Local medical control always has the option of changing these levels.

shock of 360 joules has been delivered or until the patient has a rhythm for which shocking is not indicated. With the newer fully automatic defibrillators, energy selection is not under the control of the rescuer.

After three shocks have been delivered or if the patient has a rhythm that should not be shocked, the defibrillator will announce "CHECK BREATHING AND PULSE" and then enter an inactive monitoring mode.

At this point
- Check carefully for spontaneous pulses and respirations.

If a pulse is present
- Immediately prepare the patient for transportation to a hospital. Leave the defibrillator connected to the patient. Continue life-support measures as necessary, including the administration of oxygen and assisting ventilations.

If there is no pulse
- Leave the defibrillator connected and resume CPR.

In either case, after 60 seconds the fully automatic defibrillator will prompt you to "STOP CPR," following which it will again analyze the patient's rhythm. If a shock is indicated, the defibrillator will warn you to "STAND BACK" and then deliver up to three more shocks.

If a shock is not indicated or after the three additional shocks have been delivered, the fully automatic defibrillator will prompt you to "CHECK BREATHING AND PULSE," following which it will enter a perpetual monitoring mode. If CPR is indicated, perform it. If the patient has a pulse, continue preparations for transportation.

During the perpetual monitoring mode, the fully automatic defibrillator will continually assess the patient's heart rhythm, although it will not be able to deliver additional shocks without further action on your part, even if a rhythm develops for which a shock is indicated. If this should happen, you will hear a beep followed by the prompt "CHECK BREATHING AND PULSE." Stop immediately if you are performing CPR and carefully check for a spontaneous pulse and regular respirations. If there is no pulse, clear the area, press the ON button, and repeat the steps outlined above.

Remember: Not all models of fully automatic defibrillators function in exactly the same manner as described here. Consult the user's manual for the defibrillator you will be using for accurate and detailed instructions.

Operating a Semi-automatic Defibrillator
A semi-automatic, or shock advisory, defibrillator requires more rescuer interaction than does a fully automatic model. Once attached and activated, a semi-automatic defibrillator will assess the patient's rhythm and, if a shock is indicated, begin charging to 200 joules. Once fully charged, however, a semi-automatic defibrillator will not automatically deliver the shock, but instead will prompt you to press a button and thus shock the patient. The safety precautions for fully automatic defibrillators also apply to semi-automatic models: before pressing the shock delivery button, ensure that everyone, including yourself, is clear from contact with the patient.

Before operating a semi-automatic defibrillator

If the person is not breathing and does not have a pulse, and you are working with a partner
- Direct your partner to begin CPR while you prepare the defibrillator and attach the pads to the patient.

If you are working alone
- Prepare the defibrillator, attach the pads to the patient, and then begin CPR to get some oxygenated blood moving.

When the defibrillator is connected to the patient:
- Turn on the unit by lifting open the display module.

The message screen will display a variety of information, including the command "PRESS TO ANALYZE" with an arrow pointing to the appropriate button. Pressing the button will cause the defibrillator to analyze the patient's rhythm.

If a shock is indicated, the semi-automatic defibrillator will begin charging to 200 joules of energy. The charging process may or may not be accompanied by a voice prompt to "STAND BACK," depending on the model of defibrillator being used. Once fully charged, a prompt will appear on the LCD screen to press the indicated button in order to deliver the shock.

When the prompt appears
- Make sure that everyone is clear of the patient, including yourself; then press the indicated button.

Following delivery of the shock
- Press the analyze button and repeat the procedure to deliver the second shock at 200-300 joules.

If a third shock is indicated, the energy level can be increased to 360 joules by pressing the indicated button during the charging process.

If no shock is indicated, a semi-automatic defibrillator will display a message to that effect.

When this occurs
- Carefully check for spontaneous pulses and respirations.

If pulses and respirations are absent
- Resume CPR.

If pulses and respirations are present
- Prepare the patient for immediate transportation to a hospital.

The maximum number of shocks allowed and the energy levels to be used should be dictated by local physician-determined standing orders.

As with fully automatic defibrillators, differences exist in the operation of various models of semi-automatic defibrillators. Consult the user's manual for accurate and detailed operating instructions.

Medical Control and Quality Assurance
Although automated defibrillators are easy to operate and their use is encouraged in most EMS systems, no defibrillator should be used by EMS and rescue personnel unless authorized and monitored by a physician medical director. The physician must develop and/or approve a patient care protocol that defines exactly how the defibrillator is to be used in the field. Defibrillation is a potentially hazardous medical procedure that can be performed only under the direction of a licensed physician.

Because the necessity for speed requires that defibrillation-trained rescuers operate without direct medical control, there must be a mechanism for monitoring the performance of the rescuers and the AED. Accordingly, automated defibrillators are equipped with either a dual-channel cassette tape recorder (or similar device) or a medical control module for recording the events of the resuscitation attempt. It is beyond the scope of this chapter to discuss the features or operation of the various recording devices currently available. You should be aware, however, that it is only through careful review of these recordings that the correct operation of the defibrillator can be ensured. Every effort must be made to ensure that complete recordings are made of each resuscitation effort and that these recordings are promptly reviewed by the physician medical director or his or her designee.

Remember: Defibrillation equipment must be checked at the beginning of every shift and maintained in working order at all times.

CHAPTER REVIEW

KEY TERMS

You may find it helpful to review the following terms.

aorta (a-OR-tah)—the largest artery in the body. It transports blood from the left ventricle to begin systemic circulation.

arteries—the vessels that carry blood away from the heart.

asystole (ah-SIS-to-le)—a condition in which the heart has ceased generating electrical impulses.

atheroschlerosis (ATH-er-o-skle-RO-sis)—a narrowing of the coronary arteries caused by deposits of cholesterol plaques.

atria (AY-tree-ah)—the two upper chambers of the heart. There is a right atrium (which receives unoxygenated blood returning from the body) and a left atrium (which receives oxygenated blood returning from the lungs).

automated external defibrillator (AED)—a machine that automatically recognizes shockable chaotic heart rhythms and delivers a shock to the outside of the patient's chest. See also *defibrillation.*

blood—the fluids and cells that are circulated to carry oxygen and nutrients to and wastes away from the body's tissues.

brachial (BRAY-key-al) **pulse**—the pulse measured by palpating the major artery (brachial artery) of the arm. This pulse is used to detect heart action and circulation in infants.

capillaries—the microscopic vessels where exchange between the blood and the body's tissues takes place.

cardiac arrest—when the heart stops circulating blood or stops beating entirely.

cardiopulmonary resuscitation (KAR-de-o PUL-mo-ner-e re-SUS-i-TA-shun), **CPR**—heart-lung resuscitation. A combined effort is made to restore or maintain respiration and circulation, artificially.

chest compressions—during cardiopulmonary resuscitation, pushing motions that depress the sternum (breastbone) to artificially circulate the blood when the heart has stopped beating.

circulatory system—the system composed of the heart, arteries, veins, and capillaries that circulates blood through the body; also called the *cardiovascular system.*

clavicles (KLAV-i-kulz)—the two collarbones, one attached to the right side of the superior sternum and one attached to the left side.

conduction system—specialized heart muscle that acts as nervous tissue to initiate heart contraction.

coronary artery disease (CAD)—narrowing of the coronary arteries by deposits of cholesterol plaque.

coronary artery spasm—a brief contraction of the muscular wall of a coronary artery which may result in cardiac arrest.

CPR compression site—for the adult and child, this is the placement of the hands approximately one finger-width above the substernal notch. For infants it is the point on the midline of the sternum that is one finger-width lower than an imaginary line drawn between the nipples.

defibrillation (de-FIB-ri-LAY-shun)—an electrical current applied to the outside of a patient's chest to stop all electrical activity, often enabling the heart to restart in a coordinated fashion.

electromechanical dissociation (el-EK-tro-mek-AN-i-kul dis-so-see-AY-shun) **(EMD)**—a condition in which the heart's electrical rhythm remains relatively normal, yet the mechanical pumping activity fails to follow the electrical activity, causing cardiac arrest.

50:50 rule—the rule that CPR compressions and releases should be equal: 50% compression, 50% release.

heart—the muscular organ that acts as a pump to circulate the blood.

myocardial infarction (heart attack)—the death of heart muscle caused by blockage of a coronary artery and prolonged interruption of blood flow to the heart muscle.

pulmonary (PUL-mo-nar-e) **arteries**—the blood vessels that carry blood from the right ventricle of the heart to the lungs.

pulmonary circulation—the transport of blood from the right ventricle of the heart to the lungs, where the blood excretes carbon dioxide and picks up oxygen, then back to the left atrium of the heart.

pulmonary veins—the vessels that carry oxygenated blood from the lungs to the left atrium of the heart.

sternum (STER-num)—the breastbone.

substernal notch—a general term for the lowest region on the sternum to which the ribs attach.

systemic (sis-TEM-ik) **circulation**—the transport of blood from the left ventricle of the heart to the body, where the blood provides oxygen to the tissues and picks up waste carbon dioxide, then back to the right atrium of the heart.

veins—the vessels that return blood to the heart.

venae cavae (VE-ne KA-ve)—the *superior vena cava* and the *inferior vena cava.* These two major veins return blood from the body to the right atrium.

ventilations—breaths provided artificially, called *CPR ventilations* when provided between series of chest compressions during cardiopulmonary resuscitation.

ventricles (VEN-tri-kulz)—the two lower chambers of the heart. There is a right ventricle (which sends blood to the lungs) and a left ventricle (which sends oxygenated blood to the body).

ventricular fibrillation (ven-TRIK-u-ler fib-ri-LAY-shun) **(VF)**—a condition in which the heart's electrical impulses are disorganized, preventing the heart muscle from contracting normally.

ventricular tachycardia (ven-TRIK-u-ler tak-i-KAR-de-uh) **(V-Tach)**—a condition in which the heartbeat is quite rapid; if rapid enough, ventricular tachycardia will not allow the heart's chambers to fill with enough blood between beats to produce blood flow sufficient to meet the body's needs.

The Heart

The circulatory system consists of the heart, arteries, veins, capillaries, and blood. The heart is located in the center of the thoracic cavity and pumps blood through the pulmonary circulation (to and from the lungs) and systemic circulation (to and from the body).

The functions of heart, lungs, and brain are interdependent. Without intervention, the failure of one will cause the failure of the others.

Cardiac arrest is the stopping of the heartbeat. It can result from an external cause such as drowning, electrocution, suffocation, drug intoxication, or injury, or it can result from internal disease, principally atheroschlerosis, the narrowing of the arteries by deposits of cholesterol plaques. Events that may result in cardiac arrest include coronary artery spasm or myocardial infarction, both caused by interruption of blood flow to the heart.

CPR

When someone stops breathing and the heart stops beating, clinical death occurs. Within approximately 10 minutes, biological death can result. CPR can prevent the patient from reaching biological death until definitive care can be provided.

During CPR you will have to maintain an open airway, provide ventilations to the patient, and perform chest compressions to circulate the patient's blood.

To assess the patient in order to decide if CPR must be done: (1) establish unresponsiveness, (2) call for help if you are working alone, (3) reposition the patient, (4) establish an open airway, (5) check for breathing using the look, listen, feel method, (6) deliver two breaths, (7) check for a carotid pulse, and (8) begin CPR. *Remember that it is dangerous to initiate CPR on any patient who has a pulse.*

To do CPR: (1) position the patient, (2) find the CPR compression site on the midline of the lower half of the sternum, (3) provide chest compressions, and (4) provide ventilations. CPR can be done by one or by two rescuers. Review Table 5-1 to compare elements of one- and two-rescuer CPR for adults, children, and infants.

Signs that CPR is effective include a carotid pulse felt during compressions and exhalation of air observed after ventilations. Other signs of effective CPR: pupils constrict, skin color improves, heartbeat returns spontaneously, spontaneous respirations are made, arms and legs move, swallowing is attempted, or consciousness returns.

CPR is only about 25% to 33% as effective as normal heart action. To counter this deficiency, follow CPR guidelines, avoid interrupting CPR, consider using a mechanical compressor, deliver supplemental oxygen, provide or call for defibrillation, call for advanced life support assistance.

Factors that can make CPR ventilations ineffective include improper head position, mouth not open enough, ineffective seal, nose not pinched shut during mouth-to-mouth ventilations, mouth not closed during mouth-to-nose ventilations, ventilations too rapid or too great in volume. Factors that can make CPR compressions ineffective include patient not on a hard surface, hands incorrectly placed, prolonged interruptions, chest insufficiently compressed, compression rate too rapid or too slow, jerky compressions (not 50% compressions, 50% release).

CPR may be interrupted for these reasons: to check for return of spontaneous breathing and pulse, to move the patient onto a stretcher, down stairs, through a narrow hall or door, or on and off the ambulance, to suction the airway, or to allow for defibrillation or advanced cardiac life support measures.

Fractures of the rib cage and sternum and internal injuries are complications that may result from CPR but are not reasons to stop CPR. CPR should not be initiated when there are obvious mortal wounds, rigor mortis, decomposition, lividity, or stillbirth of an infant that has obviously died hours prior to birth. You must follow local protocols about honoring "Do Not Resuscitate" orders.

Once you have started CPR, you must continue it until the heartbeat starts spontaneously (continue rescue breathing as needed), heart beat and breathing start spontaneously, another trained rescuer takes over, you turn over care of the patient to a physician or medical facility, or you are too exhausted to continue.

Defibrillation

Defibrillation is the application of an electrical shock to the external chest. It stops certain potentially lethal rhythms and allows the heart to start beating again in a coordinated manner. Early defibrillation (optimally within 4 to 6 minutes of collapse) is extremely important in improving the chances of surviving cardiac arrest. Manual defibrillation is usually provided by paramedics. In some EMS systems, EMTs are trained to operate automated external defibrillators (AEDs).

The section of this chapter on defibrillation and the AED was written by Kenneth R. Stults, M.S., Director of The University of Iowa Hospitals and Clinics, Emergency Medical Services Learning Resources Center, and modified for style by the authors of this text.

On the Scene

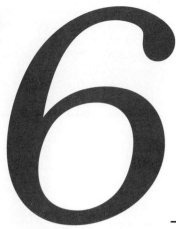

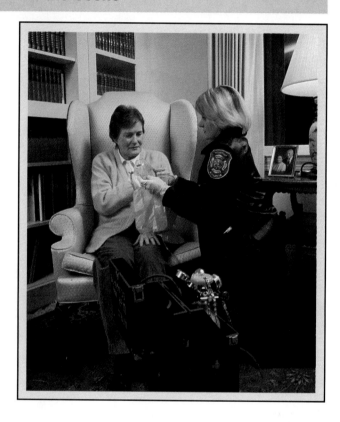

Fifty-six-year-old Martha Quick is having an argument with her husband, Ralph. In mid-argument, Martha begins to develop chest pain. Ralph rushes to call 911 for EMS. When you and your partner arrive, he leads you to his wife, explaining about the argument and subsequent chest pain. After being introduced, you begin your exam.

You: *Mrs. Quick, could you tell me about the pain?*

Mrs. Quick: *It's right here. (She motions to the center of her chest.) It feels like something is squeezing my chest.*

You: *On a scale of 1 to 10, how bad is the pain?*

Mrs. Quick: *It's bad. I guess 7 or 8.*

You: *I'm going to put an oxygen mask on your face. When you get chest pain, it may be your body's way of telling you that you need oxygen. This mask may be a little uncomfortable, but it's important. (Then, after administering the oxygen . . .) How bad is the pain now—scale of 1 to 10?*

Mrs. Quick *(gratefully): About 2. It's a lot better.*

Oxygen is a drug. Since it is not in a pill or a bad-tasting liquid, we often forget this fact. Oxygen is one of the best treatments we can provide as EMTs. In fact, we administer oxygen on most emergency calls, since there are few patients who cannot benefit from oxygen—usually the sooner the better. Oxygen is used for many problems including trauma, bleeding, shock, and—as the hospital confirmed in Mrs. Quick's case—heart problems.

Weeks later, you learn that Mrs. Quick is doing well under a doctor's guidance. The Quicks are both grateful for your prompt response and care. Neither can remember what they were arguing about.

Breathing Aids and Oxygen Therapy

Chapter Overview

In Chapters 4 and 5 you learned about the most essential basic life support procedures you will carry out as an EMT: establishing and maintaining an open airway and performing rescue breathing and CPR. As noted in those chapters, these are procedures that you can carry out with nothing more than your breath and your hands (although you must use barrier devices to protect against infection if at all possible).

Basic life support can be substantially improved, however, through the use of breathing aids and oxygen-delivery systems, which you will learn about in this chapter. Think about the benefits of oxygen as you read all of the other chapters in this text.

Expected Outcome, Chapter 6: *You will be able to use airway adjuncts, ventilation devices, and suction equipment to assist in airway maintenance and artificial ventilations, and you will be able to use special equipment to administer oxygen to breathing and nonbreathing patients.*

> **Warning:** Protect yourself from infectious diseases by using appropriate barrier devices such as a pocket face mask with one-way valve, face shield, or bag-valve mask; goggles or eye shield; and disposable gloves. Always conform to your local EMS system's infection exposure control plan.

BREATHING AIDS
    Airway Adjuncts
    Suctioning and Suction Devices
    Artificial Ventilation Adjuncts (Barrier Devices)

OXYGEN THERAPY
    The Importance of Supplemental Oxygen
    Hypoxia
    Hazards of Oxygen Therapy
    Oxygen Therapy Equipment
    Administering Oxygen
    Delivering Oxygen to the Breathing Patient
    Administering Oxygen to the Nonbreathing Patient
    Automatic Resuscitators

Knowledge *After reading this chapter, you should be able to*

1. State THREE major benefits of using breathing aids. (p. 174)

2. Define and explain the purpose of *oropharyngeal airways* and *nasopharyngeal airways*. (p. 176)

3. Describe how to insert an oropharyngeal airway and a nasopharyngeal airway. (pp. 176-178)

4. State the purpose of suctioning and the components of a suction unit. (pp. 179-181)

5. Describe, step by step, the techniques of suctioning. (pp. 181, 183; Scan 6-1)

6. Explain how to perform artificial ventilations using a pocket face mask. (pp. 183-184)

7. Explain how to perform artificial ventilations using a face shield. (p. 184)

8. Explain how to perform artificial ventilations using a bag-valve mask system. (pp. 184-186)

9. State the advantages and the disadvantages of oxygen therapy. (pp. 186-188)

10. Define *hypoxia* and list several causes of this condition. (pp. 186-187)

11. Describe D, E, M, G, and H oxygen cylinders and state how to determine the expected duration of flow for any given cylinder. (pp. 188-189; Table 6-1)

12. List rules for the safe handling and operation of oxygen cylinders. (pp. 189-190)

13. Define *pressure regulator* and describe how to connect this device to an oxygen supply cylinder. (p. 190)

14. Compare and contrast the Bourdon gauge flowmeter, the pressure-compensated flowmeter, and the constant flow selector valve. Describe how to connect a flowmeter to an oxygen delivery system. (pp. 190-191)

15. Describe the correct procedures for the field use of a humidifier, stating when this device is to be used. (pp. 191-192)

I t is vitally important that the EMT know how to provide basic life support—establishing and maintaining an open airway, rescue breathing, and CPR—without using any special equipment. However, there are a number of breathing aids, devices that can assist the EMT in these essential tasks. In addition, the administration of oxygen substantially improves the quality of artificial ventilations as well as being effective therapy for a number of medical problems.

BREATHING AIDS

There are many special devices available to assist in the support of airway and breathing. These devices provide three major benefits.

- Improved Airway Maintenance—Devices that are commonly referred to as **airway adjuncts** help maintain an open airway by preventing the tongue from falling against the back of the throat.

- Increased Oxygen Delivery—While mouth-to-mouth and similar procedures provide oxygen to the patient at about 16%, there are many oxygen delivery devices that can increase delivered oxygen to almost 100%.

- Infection Control—There are several types of **barrier device** currently available that prevent the EMT from coming in contact with a patient's body fluids while delivering ventilations.

These devices, when used properly, benefit both the patient and the EMT. It is important to remember that YOU SHOULD NEVER DELAY RESUSCITATION MEASURES IN ORDER TO LOCATE, RETRIEVE, OR SET UP SPECIAL EQUIPMENT OR OXYGEN DELIVERY DEVICES. In order to prevent a delay in beginning resuscitation while still protecting yourself and benefiting the patient

16. Identify a nasal cannula, a simple face mask, a partial rebreather mask, a nonrebreather mask, and a Venturi mask. (pp. 192-193, 197-198)

17. For each of the above oxygen delivery devices state the range of percentage of oxygen delivered, the approximate range of liter per minute flow needed, and the typical patients for whom each device can be used. (pp. 192-193, 197-198; Table 6-2)

18. State how the pocket face mask and a bag-valve mask unit can be used to deliver oxygen to a nonbreathing patient. (p. 198)

19. Define *demand-valve resuscitator*, *positive-pressure resuscitator*, *multiple-function resuscitator*, and *automatic transport resuscitator* and describe whether and how each device can be used to ventilate the breathing or nonbreathing patient. (pp. 198-199)

20. Describe, step by step, how to set up oxygen equipment, administer oxygen to a patient, and perform the procedures for discontinuing the administration of oxygen. (Scans 6-2 and 6-3)

Skills *As an EMT you should be able to*

1. Determine if an airway adjunct is needed, insert the proper-sized device, and provide ventilation.
2. Correctly use both fixed (installed) and portable suction equipment.
3. Provide ventilation with a bag-valve mask unit.
4. Use a pocket mask or face shield to provide ventilation.
5. Select the correct oxygen delivery device for a patient.
6. Properly set up oxygen equipment, deliver oxygen to a patient, and discontinue the administration of oxygen.
7. Assemble, test, disassemble (when appropriate), and clean all equipment used to ensure an airway, suction, provide ventilation, and deliver oxygen to a patient.

- *Know how to use your equipment before you have to use it in an emergency.* Become familiar and drill frequently with resuscitation equipment. When the time comes to use it, you will perform quickly and accurately.

- *Keep equipment in stock and available.* Have airway adjuncts and equipment for supplemental oxygen where it can be easily obtained. It should take a prominent position in the equipment that is brought to the patient. The ABCs are our first priority in patient care. The equipment for the maintenance and support of the ABCs should be easily retrieved, both in our "kits" and in the ambulance. There should be a size available to fit every patient.

- *Make sure that all airway equipment is in working order.* Having to repair equipment on the scene causes unnecessary and embarrassing delays. Check this equipment on each shift. Clean and maintain it properly after each use.

Remember: The airway equipment that will be discussed in this chapter will only *assist* you in the care of your patient. Often the use of adjunct devices requires you to monitor the patient *more closely* once you begin using the device. No equipment will replace the care that can be given by an EMT!

Aids to breathing can be divided into several categories: airway adjuncts, suctioning devices, and ventilation adjuncts (now frequently called barrier devices). Oxygen-delivery devices, which aid breathing and also serve other medical purposes, will be discussed later in this chapter.

Airway Adjuncts

Once you gain access to a patient and begin the primary survey, your first course of action is to establish an open airway. This airway must be maintained throughout all care procedures.

The most common impediment to an open airway is the tongue. When a patient becomes unconscious, the muscles relax. The tongue will slide back into the pharynx and obstruct the airway. Even though a jaw-thrust, head-tilt, or chin lift maneuver will help open the airway of a patient, the tongue may return to its obstructive position once the maneuver is released. Sometimes, even when the jaw-thrust or head-tilt is maintained, the tongue will "fall back" into the pharynx.

Airway adjuncts, devices that aid in maintaining an open airway, may be used early in the treatment of the unresponsive patient and continue throughout your care. There are several types of airway adjuncts. In this chapter, only the devices that are a part of the standard EMT-Basic course—those whose main function is to keep the tongue from blocking the airway—will be discussed.

The two most common airway adjuncts for the EMT are the **oropharyngeal airway** and the **nasopharyngeal airway**. The structure and use of these airways can be understood by analyzing their names. *Oro* refers to the mouth, *naso* the nose, and *pharyngeal* the throat. Oropharyngeal airways are inserted into the mouth and help keep the tongue from falling back into the throat. Nasopharyngeal airways are inserted through the nose and rest in the throat, also helping keep the tongue from becoming an airway obstruction.

Rules for Using Airway Adjuncts Some general rules apply to the use of both the oropharyngeal and the nasopharyngeal airway.

- Use an airway on all unconscious patients who do not exhibit a gag reflex. The gag reflex causes vomiting or retching when something is placed in the throat.
- Open the patient's airway manually before using an adjunct device.
- When inserting the airway, take great care not to push the patient's tongue back into the throat.
- Do not continue inserting the airway if the patient begins to gag. Continue to maintain the airway manually and *do not* use an adjunct device. If the patient remains unconscious for a prolonged time, you may later attempt to insert an airway to determine if the gag reflex is still present.
- When an airway is in place, YOU MUST STILL MAINTAIN A HEAD-TILT AND MONITOR THE AIRWAY.

- If the patient regains consciousness or develops a gag reflex, remove the airway immediately.
- Use infection control practices while maintaining the airway. Wear disposable gloves. In airway maintenance there is a chance of a patient's body fluids coming in contact with your face and eyes. Wear goggles or other appropriate devices to prevent this contact.

Oropharyngeal Airways Once a patient's airway is opened, an oropharyngeal airway can be inserted to help keep it open. An oropharyngeal airway is a curved device, usually made of plastic, that can be inserted through the patient's mouth. The oropharyngeal airway has a flange that will rest against the patient's lips. The rest of the device holds down the tongue as it curves back to the throat. The proper use of an oropharyngeal airway greatly reduces the chances of the patient's airway becoming obstructed.

There are standard sizes of oropharyngeal airways (Figure 6-1). Many manufacturers make a complete line, ranging from airways for infants to large adult sizes. An entire set should be carried in one case to allow for quick, proper selection.

The device *cannot* be used effectively unless you select the correct airway size for the patient. An airway of proper size will extend from the corner of the patient's mouth to the tip of the earlobe on the same side of the patient's face. An alternative method is to measure from the center of the patient's mouth to the angle of the lower jaw bone (mandible). *Do not* use an airway unless you have measured it against the patient and it is verified as being the proper size. If the

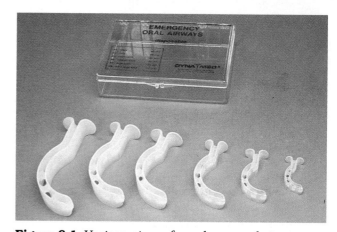

Figure 6-1 Various sizes of oropharyngeal airways.

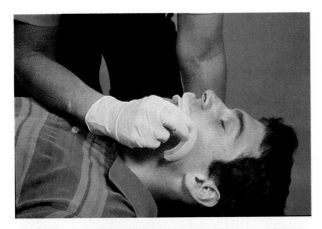

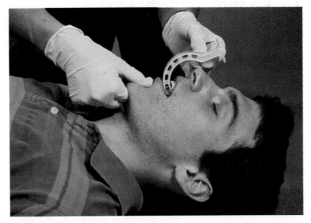

Figure 6-3 The airway is inserted with the tip pointing to the roof of the patient's mouth.

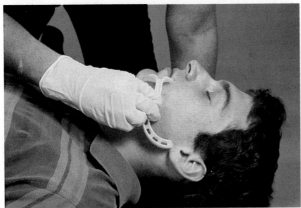

Figure 6-2 The airway is chosen and is checked for correct size.

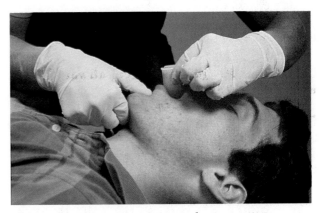

Figure 6-4 The airway is rotated into position.

airway is not the correct size, do not use it on the patient (Figure 6-2).

To insert an oropharyngeal airway

1. Place the patient on his back. When caring for a medical patient with no indications of spinal injury, the neck may be hyperextended. If there are possible spinal injuries, use the jaw-thrust maneuver, moving the patient no more than necessary to ensure an open airway (the airway takes priority over the spine). Extreme care must be taken.

2. Cross the thumb and forefinger of one hand and place them on the upper and lower teeth at the corner of the patient's mouth. Spread your fingers apart to open the patient's jaws (the crossed-fingers technique, see Chapter 4). Hold the mouth open using these same fingers.

3. Position the correct size airway so that its tip is pointing toward the roof of the patient's mouth (Figure 6-3).

4. Insert the airway and slide it along the roof

of the patient's mouth, past the soft tissue hanging down from the back (the uvula), or until you meet resistance against the soft palate. Be certain not to push the patient's tongue back into the throat. Any airway insertion is made easier by using a tongue blade (tongue depressor). In a few cases, you may *have* to use a tongue blade to hold the tongue in place. *Watch* what you are doing when inserting the airway. This procedure should not be performed by "feel" only.

5. GENTLY rotate the airway 180 degrees so that the tip is pointing down into the patient's throat (Figure 6-4). This method prevents pushing the tongue back.

6. Place the nontrauma patient in a maximum head-tilt position. Minimize all movements of the head if there are possible spinal injuries.

7. Check to see that the flange of the airway is against the patient's lips (Figure 6-5). If the

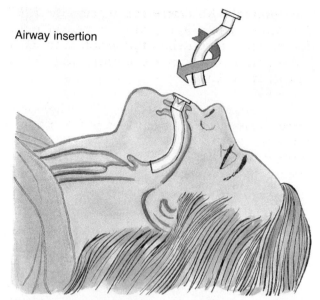

Airway insertion

Figure 6-5 Note that when the airway is properly positioned, the flange rests against the patient's lips.

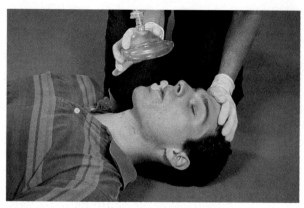

Figure 6-6 The patient is ready for ventilation.

airway is too long or too short, remove the airway and replace it with the correct size.

8. Provide mouth-to-adjunct ventilation as you would provide mouth-to-mouth ventilation, or place the mask you will use for ventilation over the in-place airway adjunct (Figure 6-6).

9. Monitor the patient closely. If there is a gag reflex, remove the airway at once. Remove the adjunct by following the anatomical curvature. You do not need to rotate the device when removing it.

Note: Some EMS systems allow an oropharyngeal airway to be inserted with the tip pointing to the side of the patient's mouth. The device is then rotated 90 degrees so that its tip is pointing

down the patient's throat. Do not use this approach unless it is part of the protocol of your EMS system.

Nasopharyngeal Airways Many EMS systems now allow use of the nasopharyngeal airway. This device has gained in popularity because it often does not stimulate the gag reflex. This allows the nasopharyngeal airway to be used in patients who have a reduced level of consciousness but still have an intact gag reflex. Other benefits include the fact that it can be used when the teeth are clenched and when there are oral injuries.

Use the soft flexible latex nasal airway and not the rigid clear plastic airways in the field. The soft ones are less likely to cause soft tissue damage or bleeding. The typical sizes for adults are 34, 32, 30, and 28 French.

To insert a nasopharyngeal airway (Figure 6-7)

1. Select the largest nasopharyngeal airway that will fit into the patient's nostril without using any force. This is approximately the diameter of the patient's little finger.

2. Lubricate the outside of the tube with a water-based lubricant before insertion. *Do not* use a petroleum jelly or any other type of non-water-based lubricant. Such substances can damage the tissue lining the nasal cavity and the pharynx, or cause an aspiration pneumonia if they get into the lungs.

3. Gently push the tip of the nose upward. Keep the patient's head in a neutral position. Most nasopharyngeal airways are designed to be placed in the right nostril. The bevel (angled portion at the tip of the airway) should face toward the nasal septum.

4. Insert the airway into the nostril. The airway is advanced until the flange rests firmly against the patient's nostril. Never force a nasopharyngeal airway. If you experience difficulty advancing the airway, pull the tube out, rotate it 180°, and try the other nostril.

Caution: Do not attempt the use of a nasopharyngeal airway if there is evidence of clear (cerebrospinal) fluid coming from the nose or ears. This may indicate a skull fracture in the area where the airway would pass.

Oropharyngeal and nasopharyngeal airways can be a tremendous asset to the EMT when

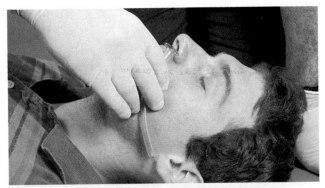

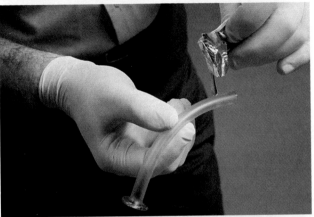

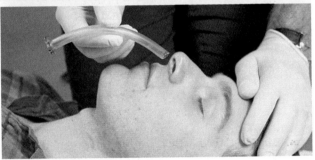

Ⓓ Airway insertion

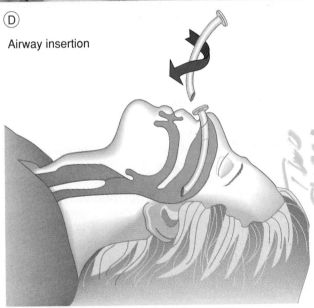

Figure 6-7 Inserting a lubricated nasopharyngeal airway.

used properly. No device can replace the EMT. The proper use of these airways or any other device depends on the appropriate use, good judgment and adequate monitoring of the patient by the EMT.

Advanced Airway Devices There are many airway adjuncts that traditionally fall into the advanced life support category. Endotracheal intubation has been primarily an advanced procedure; however many EMS systems are training EMTs in endotracheal intubation or esophageal intubation devices that prevent regurgitation during an arrest.

Even if you will not be allowed to perform this technique, you may work with advanced EMTs or provide transfers between hospitals with intubated patients. A basic understanding of this procedure will help in those circumstances. Appendices 1 and 2 explain intubation devices in detail.

Suctioning and Suction Devices

The patient's airway must be kept clear of foreign materials, blood, vomitus, and other secretions. Materials that are allowed to remain in the airway may be forced into the trachea and eventually into the lungs. This will cause complications ranging from severe pneumonia to complete airway obstruction. Suctioning is the method of removing such materials. Before learning the techniques of suctioning we will discuss the types of suction equipment available and how each works.

Each **suction unit** consists of a suction source, a collection container for materials you suction, tubing, and suction tips or catheters. Systems are either installed in the ambulance or are portable and may be brought to the scene.

Fixed (Installed) Systems Many ambulances have a suction unit installed in the patient compartment (Figure 6-8). These units are usually installed near the head of the stretcher so they are easily used. Installed systems, often called "on-board" units, create a suctioning vacuum produced by the engine's manifold or an electrical power source. To be effective, suction devices must furnish an air intake of at least 30 LPM (liters per minute) at the open end of a collection tube. This will occur if the system can generate a vacuum of no less than 300 mmHg (millimeters of mercury) when the collecting tube is clamped.

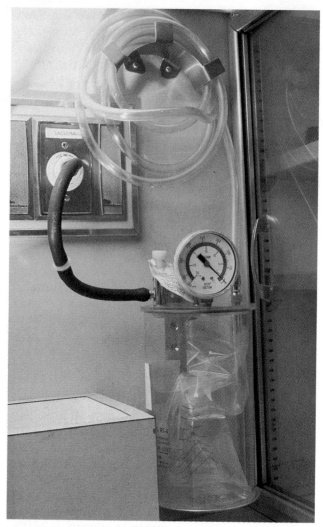

Figure 6-8 Fixed (installed) suction unit for ambulance patient compartments.

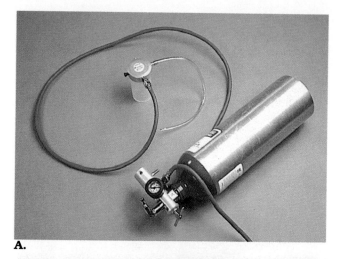

A.

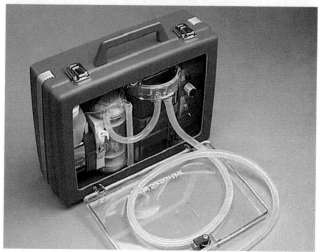

B.

Figure 6-9 A. An oxygen-powered portable suction unit. B. A portable suction unit that is powered by electricity.

Portable Suction Units There are many different types of portable suction units (Figure 6-9). They may be electrically powered (by batteries or household current), oxygen- or air-powered, or manually operated. The requirement for the amount of suction a portable unit must provide is identical to the fixed unit (30 LPM, 300 mmHg). It is important to have the ability to suction anywhere. Portable suction gives us that ability.

Tubing, Tips, and Catheters For suctioning to be effective, the proper equipment must be used. While a suction unit might be the most powerful available, it will do no good unless used with the proper attachments.

- Tubing—The tubing attached to a suction unit must be thick walled, non-kinking, wide bore tubing. This is because the tub-

ing must not collapse due to the suction, must allow "chunks" of suctioned material to pass, and must not kink, which would reduce the suction. The tubing must be long enough to comfortably reach from the suction unit to the patient.
- Suction Tips—Currently the most popular type of suction tip is the rigid pharyngeal tip, also called a "Yankauer" or tonsil-tip suction. This rigid device allows the EMT to suction the mouth and throat with excellent control over the distal end of the device. It also has a larger bore than flexible catheters. Caution must be used with rigid tip suction. When the tip is placed into the pharynx, the gag reflex may be activated, producing additional vomiting. It is also possible to stimulate the vagus nerve in the

back of the throat, which can slow the heart rate. So be careful not to suction more than a few seconds with a rigid tip and never lose sight of the tip.

- Suction Catheters—Suction catheters are plastic tubes that are used for suctioning. They come in various sizes identified by a number "French." The larger the number, the larger the catheter. A "14 French" catheter is larger than an "8 French" catheter. These catheters are usually not large enough to suction vomitus or thick secretions and may kink. Flexible catheters are designed to be passed through a tube such as a nasopharyngeal or endotracheal tube.

Another important part of a suction device is the collection container. All units should have a non-breakable container to collect the suctioned materials. These containers must be easily removed and decontaminated. Remember to wear gloves, goggles, and mask not only while suctioning, but while cleaning the equipment as well. Most newer suction devices have disposable containers to eliminate the time and risks involved in decontamination.

Suction units must also have a container of sterile water nearby. This water is used to clear matter that is partially blocking the tubing. When this partial blockage of the tube occurs, place the suction tip or catheter in the container of water. This will cause a stream of water to flow through the tip and tubing, usually forcing the clog to dislodge. When the tip or tubing becomes clogged with an item that will not dislodge, replace it with a new tip or catheter.

In the event of copious, thick secretions or vomiting, consider removing the rigid tip or catheter and using the large bore, rigid suction tubing. After you are finished, place the standard tip back on for further suctioning.

Techniques of Suctioning Although there may be some variations in suction technique (a suggested technique is shown in Scan 6-1), there are a few rules that always apply.

- *Always use appropriate infection control practices while suctioning.* These practices include the use of goggles, mask, and disposable gloves. Proper suctioning requires you to have your fingers around and sometimes inside the patient's mouth. Disposable gloves prevent contact between the EMT and the patient's bodily fluids. Goggles and mask are also recommended since

these fluids might splatter, or the patient may gag or cough, sending droplets to the EMT's face, eyes, and mouth.

- *Never suction for longer than a few seconds,* since supplemental oxygen or ventilations cease while suctioning, keeping oxygen from the patient.

Patients who need airway control and suctioning are often unconscious and may be in cardiac or respiratory arrest. Oxygen delivery to this patient is very important. During suctioning, the ventilations or other method of oxygen delivery is discontinued to allow for the passage of the suction catheter. To prevent critical delays in oxygen delivery, limit suctioning to a few seconds, then resume ventilations or oxygen delivery.

You may **hyperventilate** (HI-per-VENT-i-late) a patient before and after suctioning. That is, you may ventilate a patient who is receiving artificial ventilations at a slightly faster rate before and after suctioning to compensate for the oxygen not delivered during suctioning.

- *Place the tip or catheter where you want to begin the suctioning and suction on the way out.* Most suction tips and catheters do not produce suction at all times; the suctioning must be started by the EMT. The tip or catheter will have an open distal end where the suction is delivered. It will also have an opening, or port, in the proximal portion. When the EMT's finger is placed over the proximal port, suctioning begins from the distal end.

Measure the suction catheter in a manner similar to an oropharyngeal airway. The length of catheter that should be inserted into the patient's mouth is equal to the distance between the corner of the patient's mouth and earlobe.

Carefully bring the tip of the catheter to the area where suctioning is needed. Never "jab" or force the suction tip into the mouth or throat. Then place your finger over the proximal opening to begin the suctioning, and suction as you slowly withdraw the tip from the patient's mouth. It is not necessary to measure when using a rigid tip. Rather, you should be sure not to lose sight of the tip when inserting it.

Suctioning is usually delivered with the patient turned on his side. This allows free secretions to flow from the mouth while suctioning is being delivered. Caution must be used in

Techniques of Suctioning

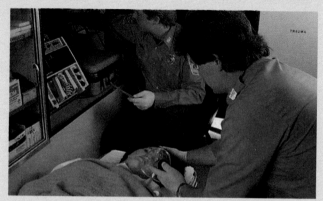

1. Position yourself at the patient's head and turn the patient to the side.

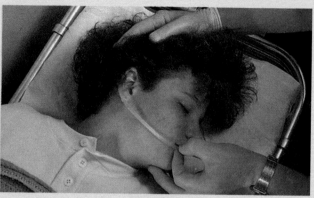

2. Measure flexible suction catheter: the distance between the patient's earlobe and the corner of the mouth, or center of the mouth to the angle of the jaw. A rigid tip does not need to be measured; simply do not lose sight of the tip.

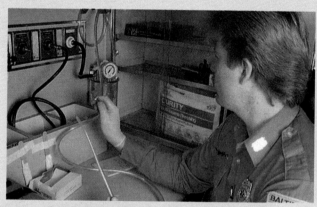

3. Turn unit on and test for suction.

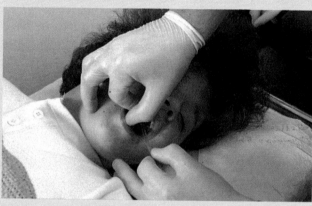

4. Open the patient's mouth by the crossed-finger technique and clear mouth.

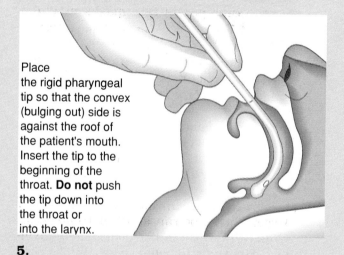

Place the rigid pharyngeal tip so that the convex (bulging out) side is against the roof of the patient's mouth. Insert the tip to the beginning of the throat. **Do not** push the tip down into the throat or into the larynx.

5.

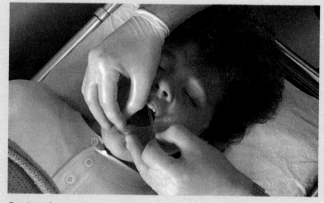

6. Apply suction **only** after the tip of the catheter or the rigid tip is in place. Suction on the way out.

Note: Suction is controlled by placing your finger over the port in the flexible catheter or rigid suction tip.

patients with suspected neck or spinal injuries. If the patient is fully and securely immobilized, the entire backboard may be tilted to place the patient on his side. For the patient for whom such injuries are suspected but who is not immobilized, suction as best you can without turning the patient. If all other methods have failed, as a last resort you may turn the patient's body as a unit, attempting to keep the neck and spine in line. Suctioning should not be delayed to immobilize a patient.

The suction tip or catheter should be moved into place carefully and not forced. Rigid suction devices may cause tissue damage and bleeding. Never probe into wounds or attempt to suction away attached tissue with a suction device. Certain skull fractures may actually cause brain tissue to be visible in the throat. If this occurs, do not suction near this tissue; limit suctioning to the mouth.

Suction devices may also cause activation of the gag reflex and stimulate vomiting. In a patient who already has secretions that need to be suctioned, vomiting only makes things worse. If you advance a suction catheter or rigid suction tip and the patient begins to gag, withdraw the tip to a position that does not cause gagging and begin suctioning.

Artificial Ventilation Adjuncts (Barrier Devices)

There are several devices available to assist in artificial ventilation. The three major categories of these devices are pocket face masks, face shields, and bag-valve masks. The benefits of these adjuncts are

- *To provide supplemental oxygen.* As stated in Chapter 4, the breaths a rescuer provides contain only about 16% oxygen. Many ventilation adjuncts provide a mechanism to administer supplemental oxygen, which helps increase the efficiency of rescue breathing or CPR.
- *To act as a barrier device.* A ventilation adjunct acts as a barrier, preventing the EMT from coming in contact with the patient's body fluids and breath, which are possible sources of infection.

The Pocket Face Mask The **pocket face mask** is a modification of a resuscitator facepiece. It is made of soft, collapsible material and can be carried in the rescuer's pocket, jacket, or purse (Figure 6-10). Many EMTs purchase their

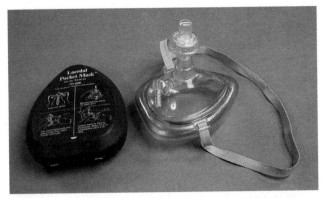

Figure 6-10 Pocket face masks. Note the chimney with one-way valve for mouth-to-mask ventilations.

own pocket face masks for their workplace or automobile first aid kits.

Face masks have important infection control features. Most masks have a one-way valve. This valve allows the EMT's ventilations to enter but prevents the patient's exhaled air from coming back through the valve and into contact with the EMT. Since ventilations are delivered through the one-way valve, the EMT does not have direct contact with the patient's mouth.

Some pocket masks have oxygen inlets. When oxygen is attached to the inlet and supplied at 10 liters per minute, an oxygen concentration of approximately 50% is delivered. This is significantly better than the 16% delivered by mouth-to-mask without oxygen.

Most pocket face masks are made of a clear plastic. This is important because the EMT must be able to observe the patient's mouth and nose for vomiting or secretions that need to be suctioned. The EMT also needs to observe color of the lips, an indicator of the respiratory status of the patient. Some pocket face masks may also have a strap that goes around the patient's head. This is helpful during one-rescuer CPR since it holds the mask on the patient's face while the rescuer is performing compressions.

To provide mouth-to-mask ventilation, you should

1. Position yourself at the patient's head and open the airway. It may be necessary to clear the airway. Insert an oropharyngeal airway to help keep the patient's airway open.
2. Connect oxygen to the inlet on the face mask. Oxygen should be run at 10 to 15 liters per minute. *If oxygen is not immediately available, do not delay mouth-to-mask ventilations.*
3. Position the mask on the patient's face so that the apex (top of the triangle) is over the

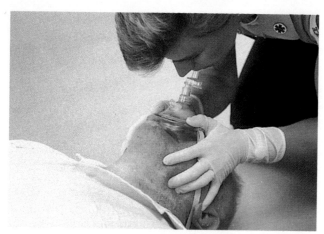

Figure 6-11 Providing mouth-to-mask ventilations. Note the placement of the EMT's hands.

bridge of the nose and the base is between the lower lip and prominence of the chin.

4. Hold the mask firmly in place while maintaining the proper head tilt (Figure 6-11) by placing
   • Both thumbs on the sides of the mask
   • Index, third and fourth fingers of each hand grasping the lower jaw on each side between the angle of the jaw and the ear lobe to lift the jaw forward
5. Take a deep breath and exhale into the port or one-way valve at the top of the mask port. Each ventilation should be delivered over 1½ to 2 seconds in adults, 1 to 1½ seconds in infants and children. Watch for the patient's chest to rise.
6. Remove your mouth from the port and allow for passive exhalation. Continue as you would for mouth-to-mouth ventilations or CPR.

The Face Shield A **face shield** is a thin, see-through barrier that is placed over the face of the patient. It helps prevent contact between the mouths of the patient and the EMT, reducing the risk of infectious disease transmission.

The face shield is applied over the patient's face and ventilations are delivered through small holes or permeable material in the same manner as in mouth-to-mouth ventilation. The EMT is positioned at the side of the patient. A seal will be made against the patient's mouth through the shield. The nose should be pinched during ventilations. Oropharyngeal airways may be used if available.

Since shields are thin and small, they are even easier and less expensive to carry than a pocket face mask. For the same reason, face shields are also popular for personal and workplace first aid kits. A drawback for the on-duty EMT is that most face shields do not have the ability to accept supplemental oxygen, which should be used whenever possible.

The Bag-Valve Mask Ventilator The **bag-valve mask** is a hand-held ventilation device. It may also be referred to as a bag-valve mask unit, system, device, resuscitator, or simply BVM. The bag-valve mask unit is the preferred method of ventilating a nonbreathing patient and is also helpful to assist ventilations in the patient whose own respiratory attempts are not enough to support life, such as a patient in respiratory failure or drug overdose. The BVM also provides an infection-control barrier between the patient and the EMT. The use of the bag-valve mask in the field is often referred to as "bagging" the patient.

Bag-valve mask units come in neonatal (newborn), pediatric, and adult sizes. (Figure 6-12). Many different types of bag-valve mask systems are available; however, all have the same basic parts as shown in Figure 6-13. The bag must be a self-refilling shell. The system must have an oxygen inlet port and a reservoir system to allow for maximum oxygen delivery. The valve should be nonrebreathing (preventing the patient from rebreathing his own exhalations) and not subject to freezing in cold temperatures. Most systems have a standard 15/22 mm respiratory fitting to ensure a proper fit with other respiratory equipment, face masks, and endotracheal tubes.

Warning: Many older bag-valve masks have "pop-off" valves. These valves were designed to open after certain pressures were obtained. Studies have shown that these pop-off valves may prevent adequate ventilations. BVM systems with pop-off valves should be replaced. BVM systems should also have a clear face mask so that the EMT can observe the lips for cyanosis and monitor the airway in case suctioning is needed.

The mechanical workings of a bag-valve mask device are simple. Oxygen, flowing at 10 to 15 LPM, is attached to the BVM and enters the reservoir. When the bag is squeezed, the air inlet to the bag is closed, and the oxygen is delivered to the patient. BVM systems without a reservoir supply approximately 50% oxygen. Systems with an oxygen reservoir provide nearly 100% oxygen.

When the squeeze of the bag is released, a passive expiration by the patient will occur. While the patient exhales, oxygen enters the reservoir to be delivered to the patient the next time the EMT squeezes the bag. The bag itself

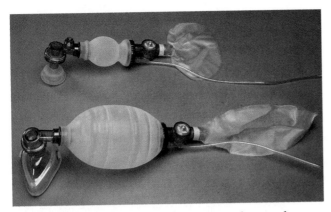

Figure 6-12 Pediatric and adult bag-valve mask units.

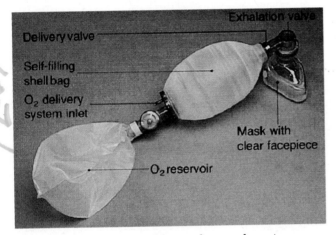

Delivery valve

Self-filling shell bag

O₂ delivery system inlet

Exhalation valve

Mask with clear facepiece

O₂ reservoir

Figure 6-13 The typical bag-valve mask system.

will hold anywhere from 1,000 to 1,600 milliliters of air, depending on the age of the BVM system. Newer models are designed to hold more air. According to American Heart Association guidelines, at least 800 milliliters of air must be delivered to the patient. This means that the bag-valve mask system must be used properly and efficiently.

Warning: When working alone, it may be very difficult to use the bag-valve mask system properly. To do so requires extensive practice. Since one hand must be available to squeeze the bag, this leaves only one hand to maintain a seal between the mask and the patient's face *and* maintain the required head tilt. Many EMS systems require the bag-valve mask unit to be used by two rescuers. One rescuer uses both hands to maintain the mask seal and head tilt. The second rescuer squeezes the bag. If a second rescuer is not available to assist in the BVM procedure, some EMS systems mandate the use

of a pocket mask with supplemental oxygen instead of the BVM.

When using the bag-valve mask device you should

1. Position yourself at the patient's head and establish an open airway. If necessary, clear the patient's airway.
2. Insert an oropharyngeal airway.
3. Be certain to use the correct size mask for the patient. The apex or top of the triangular mask should be over the bridge of the nose. The base of the mask should rest between the patient's lower lip and the prominence of the chin.
4. Be certain to hold the mask firmly in position, with
   • The thumb holding the upper part of the mask
   • The index finger between the valve and the lower cushion
   • The third, fourth, and fifth fingers on the lower jaw, between the chin and ear. This may vary slightly depending on the size of the rescuer's hands. With some units, you will have to hold your palm over the facepiece and hook your fingers under the patient's jaw (Figure 6-14).
5. With your other hand, squeeze the bag ONCE EVERY 5 SECONDS. The squeeze should be a full one, causing the patient's chest to rise. For infants and children, squeeze the bag ONCE EVERY 3 SECONDS. Make certain you use the correct size mask for infants and children.
6. Release pressure on the bag and let the patient exhale passively. While this occurs the bag is refilling from the oxygen source or atmosphere.

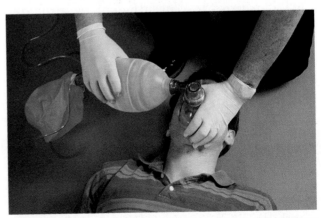

Figure 6-14 Hand positioning for using the bag-valve mask.

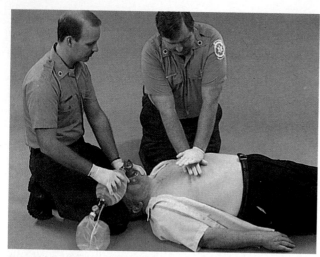

Figure 6-15 Two-rescuer CPR using a bag-valve mask system.

The BVM may also be used during CPR (Figure 6-15). The bag is squeezed once each time a ventilation is to be delivered. In one-rescuer CPR, it is preferable to use a pocket mask with supplemental oxygen rather than a BVM system. A single rescuer would take too much time picking up the BVM and obtaining a face seal each time a ventilation is to be delivered.

The EMT must know the workings of the bag-valve mask so it may be disassembled after calls and disinfected. Several disposable BVM systems are also available.

OXYGEN THERAPY

The Importance of Supplemental Oxygen

Administration of oxygen is perhaps one of the most important and beneficial treatments an EMT can provide. The atmosphere provides approximately 21% oxygen. If a person is without illness or injury, that 21% is enough to support normal functioning. The fact is, however, people that EMTs come in contact with *are* sick or injured and often require supplemental oxygen. Conditions that may require oxygen include

- Respiratory or Cardiac Arrest—In Chapter 5 you learned that CPR is only 25 to 33% as effective as normal circulation. High-concentration oxygen administration provides a better chance of survival for the patient in respiratory or cardiac arrest.
- Heart Attacks and Strokes—These emer-

gencies result from an interruption of blood to the heart or brain. When this occurs, tissues are deprived of oxygen. Providing extra oxygen is extremely important.

- Shock—Since shock is the failure of the cardiovascular system to provide sufficient blood to all the vital tissues, all cases of shock reduce the amount of oxygenated blood reaching the tissues. Administration of oxygen helps the blood that does reach the tissues deliver the maximum amount of oxygen.
- Blood Loss—Whether bleeding is internal or external, there is a reduced amount of circulating blood and red blood cells, so the blood that is circulating needs to be saturated with oxygen.
- Lung Diseases—The lungs are responsible for turning oxygen over to our blood cells to be delivered to the tissues. When the lungs are not functioning properly, supplemental oxygen helps assure that the body's tissues receive adequate oxygen.
- Broken Bones, Head Injuries, and More—There are very few emergencies where oxygen administration would not be appropriate. All our body's systems work together. An injury in one part may cause shock that affects the rest of the body.

Hypoxia

Hypoxia is an insufficiency in the supply of oxygen to the body's tissues. Sometimes the term *anoxia* is used to mean the same thing; however, this term means a complete lack of oxygen. There are several major causes of hypoxia. Consider the following scenarios where patients develop hypoxia.

- A victim is trapped in a fire. The air that the victim breathes contains smoke and reduced amounts of oxygen. Since the victim cannot breathe in enough oxygen, hypoxia develops.
- A patient has emphysema. This lung disease decreases the efficiency of the transfer of oxygen between the atmosphere and the body. Since the lungs cannot do their function properly, hypoxia develops.
- A patient overdoses on a drug that has a depressing effect on the respiratory system. The patient's respirations are only 5 per minute. In this case, the victim is not breathing frequently enough to support the oxygen needs of the body.

- A patient has a heart attack. The lungs function properly by taking atmospheric air and turning it over to the blood for distribution. The damaged heart, however, cannot pump the blood throughout the body, and hypoxia develops.

There are many causes of hypoxia, including the examples above, stroke, shock, and others. The most important thing to know is how to recognize signs of hypoxia so that it may be treated. Hypoxia may be characterized by a blue or grey color to the skin (cyanosis). When the brain suffers hypoxia, the patient's level of consciousness may deteriorate. Restlessness or confusion may result. As you read Chapter 8, you will notice that this is closely related to the condition called shock.

As an EMT your concern will be to prevent hypoxia from developing or becoming worse and, when possible, to reduce the level of hypoxia. The way that this is done is with the administration of oxygen.

Hazards of Oxygen Therapy

Although the benefits of oxygen are great, oxygen must be used carefully. The hazards of oxygen therapy may be grouped into two categories: nonmedical and medical.

The *nonmedical hazards of oxygen* include

- The oxygen used in emergency care is stored under pressure, usually 2,000 to 2,200 pounds per square inch (psi) or greater in a full cylinder. If the tank is punctured, or a valve breaks off, the supply tank can become a missile (damaged tanks have been able to penetrate concrete walls). Imagine what would happen in the passenger compartment of an ambulance if such an accident occurred.
- Oxygen supports combustion, causing fire to burn more rapidly. It can saturate towels, sheets, and clothing, greatly increasing the risk of fire.
- Under pressure, oxygen and oil do not mix. When they come into contact, a severe reaction occurs which, for our purposes, can be termed an explosion. This is seldom a problem, but it can easily occur if you try to lubricate a delivery system or gauge with petroleum products, or allow contact with a petroleum-based adhesive (e.g., adhesive tape).

These nonmedical hazards are extremely rare and can be avoided totally if oxygen and oxygen equipment are treated properly.

The *medical hazards of oxygen* rarely affect the patients treated by the Emergency Medical Technician. There are certain patients who, when exposed to high concentrations of oxygen for a prolonged time, may develop negative side effects. These situations are rarely seen in the field, but in order to have a full understanding of oxygen delivery, they are presented here.

- Oxygen Toxicity or Air Sac Collapse—These problems are caused in some patients whose lungs react unfavorably to the presence of oxygen and also may result from too high a concentration of oxygen for too long a period of time. The body reacts to a sensed "overload" of oxygen by reduced lung activity and air sac collapse (atelectasis). Like the other conditions listed here, these are extremely rare in the field.
- Infant Eye Damage—This may occur when newborns are given too much oxygen. These infants may develop scar tissue behind the lens of the eye (retrolental fibroplasia) as a result of elevated blood oxygen concentrations. This does *not* occur from infant's eyes being exposed to oxygen. This should never be a problem in field situations.
- Respiratory Depression or Respiratory Arrest—This problem may result when patients having **chronic obstructive pulmonary disease (COPD)**, including emphysema, chronic bronchitis, and black lung, are given high concentrations of oxygen for a prolonged time.

As an EMT you probably will not see oxygen toxicity or air sac (alveolar) collapse or most of the other adverse conditions that can result from oxygen administration. The time required for such conditions is too long to cause any problems during emergency care in the field.

Oxygen should not be withheld from any infant or premature infant for fear of eye damage. Again, the amount of time oxygen is in contact with infants in the field will not cause harm.

COPD patients are a special case. They are usually on a **hypoxic drive**. They have developed a tolerance to carbon dioxide levels that usually govern breathing. In hypoxic drive, the body determines the need to breathe based on oxygen rather than carbon dioxide and may interpret the higher oxygen levels that result from oxygen administration as a signal to reduce or stop breathing.

If the COPD patient appears to have mild respiratory distress or other minor problems, oxygen may be administered by a low concentration device. Appropriate oxygen concentrations for this patient are 24 to 28%.

Even the COPD patient, however, must receive a high concentration of oxygen if he needs it. This patient's risk of respiratory depression or arrest should prompt the EMT to monitor closely and be prepared to resuscitate. It should *not* prompt the EMT to withhold needed oxygen. (See more about COPD and oxygen therapy in Chapter 15.)

Rule: The benefits of oxygen far exceed the medical or nonmedical hazards. Never withhold oxygen from the patient who really needs it!

Always follow your local protocols for oxygen administration guidelines. If you are uncertain of what concentration or method of oxygenation to use, radio medical control or the medical facility for instructions.

Oxygen Therapy Equipment

In the hospital setting, oxygen is delivered to the patient from conveniently located oxygen tanks or regulators. In the field, oxygen must be safe, lightweight, portable, and dependable.

Some field oxygen systems are very portable so they may be brought almost anywhere. Other systems are installed inside the ambulance so that oxygen can be delivered during transportation to the hospital. Most oxygen delivery systems contain several items (Figure 6-16): oxygen cylinders, pressure regulators, and a delivery device (face mask or cannula). When the patient is not breathing, additional devices (such as a bag-valve mask) can be used to force oxygen into the patient's lungs.

Oxygen Cylinders Outside a medical facility, the standard source of oxygen is the **oxygen cylinder**, a seamless steel or lightweight alloy cylinder filled with oxygen under pressure, equal to 2,000 to 2,200 psi (pounds per square inch) when the cylinders are full. Cylinders come in various sizes, identified by letters (Figure 6-17). Those in common use in emergency care include

- D cylinder—contains about 350 liters of oxygen
- E cylinder—contains about 625 liters of oxygen
- M cylinder—contains about 3,000 liters of oxygen

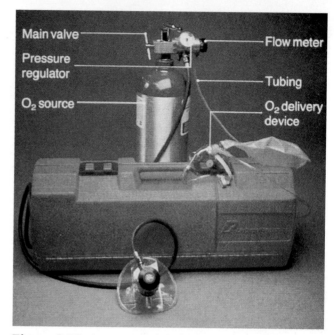

Figure 6-16 An oxygen delivery system.

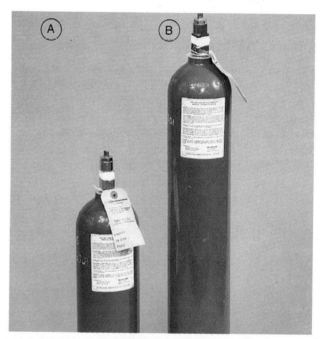

Figure 6-17 A. D cylinder. B. E cylinder. These cylinders still have the suppliers' plastic wrappers over the outlets. Do not use adhesive tape.

Fixed systems on ambulances include the M cylinder and larger cylinders (Figure 6-18):

- G cylinder—contains about 5,300 liters of oxygen
- H cylinder—contains about 6,900 liters of oxygen.

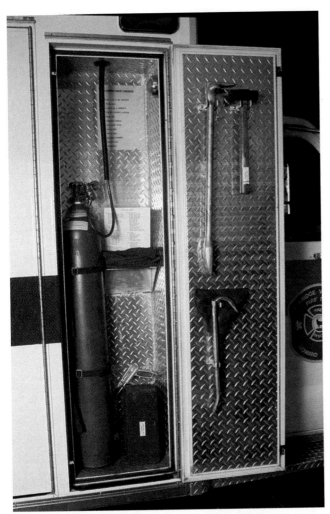

Figure 6-18 Larger cylinders are used for fixed systems on ambulances.

TABLE 6-1 Oxygen Cylinders: Duration of Flow

SIMPLE FORMULA		
$\dfrac{\text{Gauge pressure in psi} - \text{the safe residual pressure} \times \text{constant}}{\text{Flow rate in liters/minute}}$	=	duration of flow in minutes

RESIDUAL PRESSURE = 200 psi

CYLINDER CONSTANT (based on size)

D = 0.16	G = 2.41
E = 0.28	H = 3.14
M = 1.56	K = 3.14

Determine the life of an M cylinder that has a pressure of 2000 psi and a flow rate of 10 liters/minute.

$$\frac{(2000-200) \times 1.56}{10} = \frac{2808}{10} = \begin{array}{l}281 \text{ minutes}\\ \text{or 4 hours and}\\ 41 \text{ minutes}\end{array}$$

The United States Pharmacopoeia has assigned a color code to distinguish compressed gases. Light green and white cylinders have been assigned to all grades of oxygen. Unpainted stainless steel and aluminum cylinders are also used for oxygen. Regardless of the color, always check the label to be certain you are using medical grade oxygen.

Part of your duty as an EMT is to make certain that the oxygen cylinders you will use are full and ready before they are needed to provide care. The length of time you can use an oxygen cylinder depends on the pressure in the cylinder and the flow rate. You cannot tell if an oxygen cylinder is full, partially full, or empty by lifting or moving the cylinder. The method of calculating cylinder duration is shown in Table 6-1. Oxygen cylinders should never be allowed to empty below the safe residual. The safe residual for an oxygen cylinder is when the pressure

gauge reads 200 psi or above. Below this point there is not enough oxygen in the cylinder to allow for proper delivery to the patient. Before the cylinder reaches the 200 psi reading, you must switch to a fresh cylinder.

SAFETY is of prime importance when working with oxygen cylinders. You should

- NEVER drop a cylinder or let it fall against any object. When transporting a patient with an oxygen cylinder, make sure the oxygen cylinder is strapped to the stretcher or otherwise secured.
- NEVER leave an oxygen cylinder standing in an upright position without being secured.
- NEVER allow smoking around oxygen equipment in use. Clearly mark the area of use with signs that read "OXYGEN—NO SMOKING."
- NEVER use oxygen equipment around an open flame.
- NEVER use grease, oil, or fat-based soaps on devices that will be attached to an oxygen supply cylinder. Take care not to handle these devices when your hands are greasy. Use greaseless tools when making connections.
- NEVER use adhesive tape to protect an oxygen tank outlet or to mark or label any oxygen cylinders or oxygen delivery apparatus. The oxygen can react with the adhesive and debris and cause a fire.
- NEVER try to move an oxygen cylinder by dragging it or rolling it on its side or bottom.
- ALWAYS use the pressure gauges, regulators, and tubing that are intended for use with oxygen.

- ALWAYS use nonferrous metal oxygen wrenches for changing gauges and regulators or for adjusting flow rates. Other types of metal tools may produce a spark should they strike against metal objects.
- ALWAYS ensure that valve seat inserts and gaskets are in good condition. This prevents dangerous leaks. Gaskets on D and E oxygen cylinders should be replaced each time a cylinder change is made.
- ALWAYS use medical grade oxygen. Industrial oxygen contains impurities. The cylinder should be labeled "OXYGEN U.S.P." The oxygen must not be more than 5 years old.
- ALWAYS open the valve of an oxygen cylinder fully, then close it half a turn to prevent someone else from thinking the valve is closed and trying to force it open. The valve does not have to be turned fully to be open for delivery.
- ALWAYS store reserve oxygen cylinders in a cool, ventilated room, properly secured in place.
- ALWAYS have oxygen cylinders hydrostatically tested EVERY 5 YEARS. The date a cylinder was last tested is stamped on the cylinder. Some cylinders can be tested every 10 years. These will have a star after the date (e.g., 4M86★).

Pressure Regulators The pressure in an oxygen cylinder is too high to be delivered to a patient. A **pressure regulator** must be connected to the cylinder to provide a safe working pressure of 30 to 70 psi.

On cylinders of the E size or smaller, the pressure regulator is secured to the cylinder valve assembly by a yoke assembly. The yoke is provided with pins that must mate with corresponding holes in the valve assembly. This is called a pin-index safety system. Since the pin position varies for different gases, this system prevents an oxygen delivery system from being connected to a cylinder designed to contain another gas.

Cylinders larger than the E size have a valve assembly with a threaded outlet. The inside and outside diameters of the threaded outlets vary according to the gas in the cylinder. This prevents an oxygen regulator from being connected to a cylinder containing another gas. In other words, a nitrogen regulator cannot be connected to an oxygen cylinder, and vice versa.

Cylinder pressure can be reduced in one or two steps (Figure 6-19). For a one-step reduction, a single-stage pressure regulator is used. A two-step reduction requires a two-stage regulator.

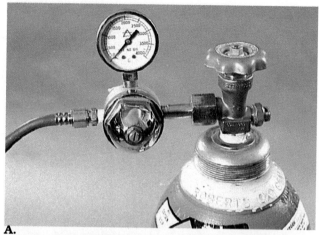

A.

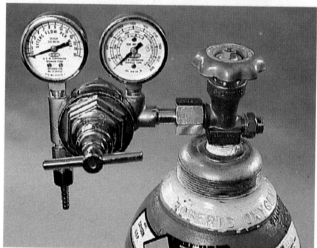

B.

Figure 6-19 A. Single-stage regulator. B. Two-stage regulator for D and E size cylinders.

Most regulators used in emergency care are the single-stage variety. This type will allow for the use of a demand valve (discussed later in this chapter).

Before connecting the pressure regulator to an oxygen supply cylinder, stand to the side of the main valve opening and open (crack) the cylinder valve slightly for just a second to clear dirt and dust out of the delivery port or threaded outlet.

Note: You must maintain the regulator inlet filter. It has to be free of damage and clean to prevent contamination of and damage to the regulator.

Flowmeters A **flowmeter** allows control of the flow of oxygen in liters per minute. It is connected to the pressure regulator. Most jurisdictions keep the flowmeter permanently attached to the pressure regulator.

Three major types of flowmeters are available. For use in the field, the pressure-compen-

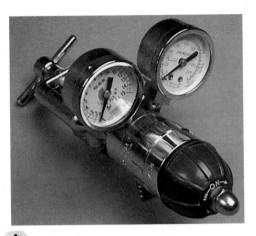
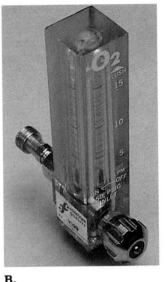
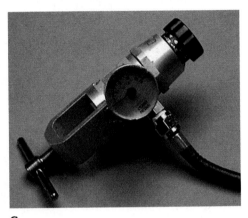

A.   **B.**   **C.**

Figure 6-20 A. Bourdon gauge flowmeter (pressure gauge). B. Pressure-compensated flowmeter. C. Constant flow selector valve.

sated flowmeter is considered to be superior to the Bourdon gauge flowmeter; however, it is more delicate than the Bourdon gauge and must be operated in an upright position. For these reasons, many EMS systems use the pressure-compensated flowmeter for fixed oxygen systems only.

- Bourdon Gauge Flowmeter (Figure 6-20A)— This unit is a pressure gauge calibrated to indicate flow in liters per minute. The meter is fairly inaccurate at low flow rates and has often been criticized as being unstable. However, it is rugged and will operate at any angle. It is a useful gauge for most portable units.

  The major fault with this type of flowmeter is its inability to compensate for back pressure. A partial obstruction (as from kinked tubing) will be reflected in a reading that is higher than the actual flow. The gauge may read 6 liters per minute and only be delivering 1 liter per minute. This type of gauge contains a filter that can become clogged, causing the gauge to read higher than the actual flow. Inspect and change the filter as recommended by the manufacturer.

- Pressure-Compensated Flowmeter (Thorpe tube-type flowmeter, Figure 6-20B)—This meter is gravity dependent and must be in an upright position to deliver an accurate reading. The unit has an upright, calibrated glass tube in which there is a ball float. The float rises and falls according to the amount

of gas passing through the tube. This type of flowmeter indicates the actual flow at all times, even though there may be a partial obstruction to gas flow (as from a kinked delivery tube). If the tubing collapses, the ball will drop to show the lower delivery rate. This unit is not practical for many portable delivery systems.

- Constant Flow Selector Valve (Figure 6-20C)—This type of flowmeter is gaining in popularity. It has no gauge. It allows for the adjustment of flow in liters per minute in stepped increments (2, 4, 6, 8 . . . 15 liters per minute). When using this type of flowmeter, make certain that it is properly adjusted for the desired flow and monitor the meter to make certain that it stays properly adjusted. This type of meter should be tested for accuracy as recommended by the manufacturer.

Humidifiers A **humidifier** can be connected to the flowmeter to provide moisture to the dry oxygen coming from the supply cylinder (Figure 6-21). Dry oxygen can dehydrate the mucus membranes of the patient's airway and lungs. In most short-term use, the dryness of the oxygen is not a problem; however, the patient is usually more comfortable when given humidified oxygen. This is particularly true if the patient has COPD.

A humidifier is usually no more than a nonbreakable jar of water attached to the flowmeter. Oxygen passes (bubbles) through the water to become humidified. As with all oxygen delivery

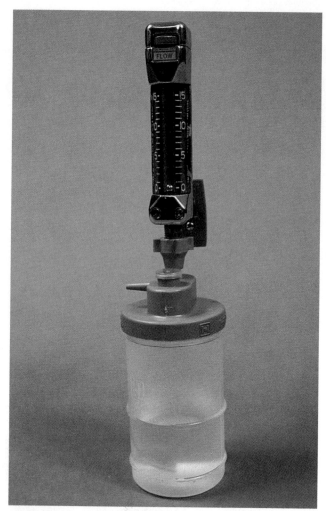

Figure 6-21 A simple oxygen humidifier.

equipment, the humidifier must be kept clean. The water reservoir can become a breeding ground for algae, harmful bacteria, and dangerous fungal organisms. Always use fresh water in a clean reservoir for each shift. Sterile single-patient-use humidifiers are available and preferable.

Note: Humidifiers are no longer used in many EMS systems. These devices are generally not used in short-term emergency calls. The humidifier may be beneficial for long-distance-transfer patients and for those with epiglottitis or croup (see Chapter 17).

Administering Oxygen

Scans 6-2 and 6-3 will take you step by step through the process of administering oxygen and discontinuing the administration of oxygen. *Do not* attempt to learn on your own how to use oxygen delivery systems. You should work with your instructor and follow his or her directions for the specific equipment you will be using.

Oxygen is administered to *breathing patients* for a variety of conditions. Oxygen is also administered to assist in the delivery of artificial ventilations to *nonbreathing patients*. A number of oxygen-delivery devices and systems are used. Each has benefits and drawbacks. A device that is good for one patient may not be ideal for another. The goal is to use the oxygen delivery device that is *best* for each patient.

Delivering Oxygen to the Breathing Patient

For the patient who is breathing and requires supplemental oxygen due to hypoxia the following devices (Table 6-2) are available to assist the patient's ventilations.

- Nasal Cannula—A **nasal cannula** provides low concentrations of oxygen (between 24% and 44%). Oxygen is delivered to the patient by two prongs that rest in the patient's nostrils. The device is usually held to the patient's face by placing the tubing over the patient's ears and securing the slip-loop under the patient's chin (Figure 6-22).

  Cannulas are often used on patients with medical emergencies who are not in distress, but where oxygen may still be helpful. *Patients who have chest pain, signs of shock, hypoxia, or other more serious problems need a higher concentration than can be provided by a cannula.* Some patients will not tolerate a mask-type delivery device because they feel "suffocated" by the mask. For the patient who refuses to wear an oxygen face mask, the cannula is better than no oxygen at all.

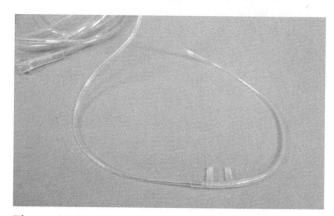

Figure 6-22 A loop type nasal cannula.

TABLE 6-2 Oxygen Delivery Devices

Oxygen Delivery Device	Flow Rate	% Oxygen Delivered	Special Use
Nasal cannula	1-6 LPM	24-44%	Patients who cannot tolerate a mask; some COPD patients
Simple face mask Partial rebreather mask	6-10 LPM	35-60%	May be used on some medical patients or those with minor trauma; most EMS systems recommend the *nonrebreather* mask for patients who require oxygen
Nonrebreather mask	8-15 LPM	80-95%	Delivery device of choice for patients with hypoxia, shock, or the potential for shock; use with caution in COPD patients
Venturi mask	4-8 LPM	24-40%	COPD patients in minor to moderate distress; long term use

When a cannula is used, the liters per minute delivered should be no more than 4 to 6. At higher flow rates the cannula begins to feel more uncomfortable and dries out the nasal mucus membranes.

Many COPD patients use a nasal cannula to receive oxygen at home. In the event you respond to the residence of a COPD patient, you may find oxygen already in use. If your EMS system allows, and the patient has minor distress, oxygen may be continued through the patient's cannula. Usually patients are on 1 to 2 liters at home. This may be increased to 2 to 3 liters en route to the hospital.

- Simple Face Mask—The **simple face mask** is a soft, clear plastic mask that will conform to the contours of the patient's face (Figure 6-23). There are small perforations on the side of the mask to allow atmospheric air to enter and exhaled air to escape. The mask is used to deliver moderate concentrations of oxygen (35% to 60%) with a flow rate of 6 to 8 liters per minute. An infant-sized face mask can be placed over the stoma of a neck-breather.

Caution: Always start with 6 liters per minute of flow when using the simple face mask. If you start with less, carbon dioxide can build up in the mask. At a flow rate of 1 liter per minute, the patient gets less oxygen than from atmospheric air.

- Partial Rebreather Mask—A **partial rebreather mask** combines a face mask and a reservoir bag (Figure 6-24). The mask will only function properly if it is well fitted to the patient's face. Oxygen should be in the reservoir before you place the mask on the patient's face. The reservoir bag must be

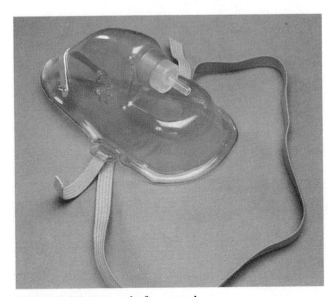

Figure 6-23 A simple face mask.

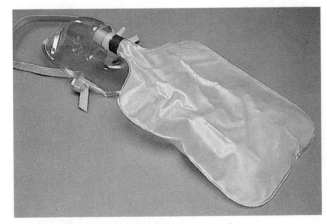

Figure 6-24 A partial rebreather mask.

Preparing the Oxygen Delivery System

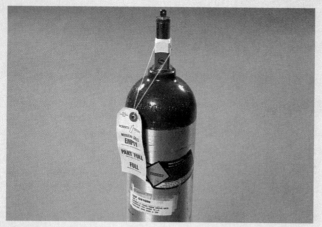

1. Select desired cylinder. Check label, "Oxygen U.S.P."

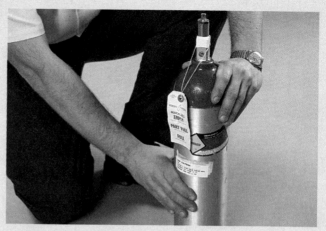

2. Place the cylinder in an upright position and stand to one side.

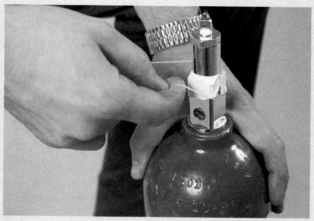

3. Remove the plastic wrapper or cap protecting the cylinder outlet.

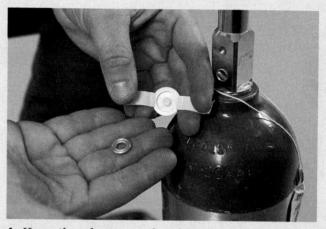

4. Keep the plastic washer (some set-ups).

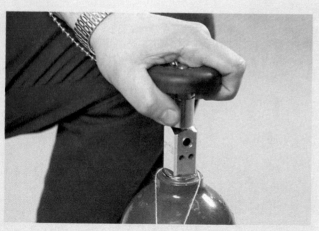

5. "Crack" the main valve for one second.

PIN   DISS

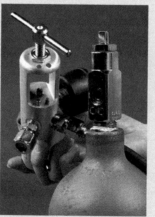

6. Select the correct pressure regulator and flowmeter.

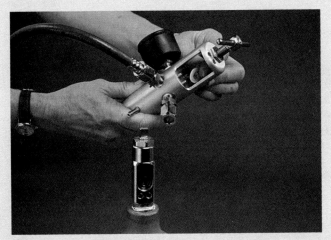

7. Place cylinder valve gasket on regulator oxygen port.

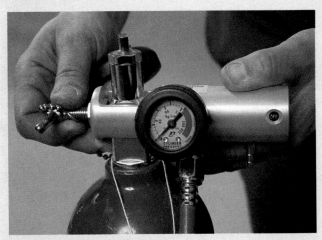

8. Make certain that the pressure regulator is closed.

PIN   DISS

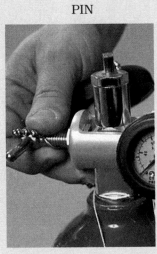

9. Align pins, for DISS, thread by hand.

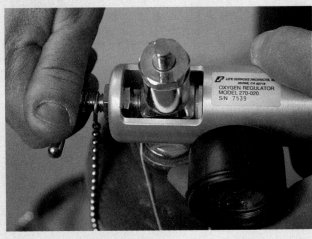

10. Tighten T-screw for pin-index.

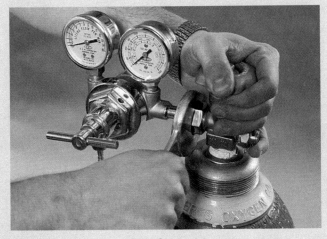

Tighten with a wrench for DISS.

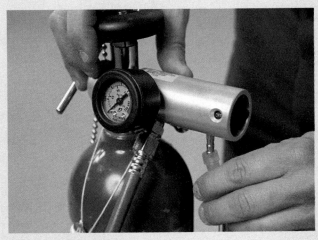

11. Attach tubing and delivery device.

Administering Oxygen

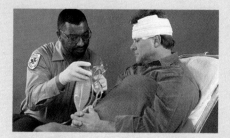

1. Explain to patient the need for oxygen.

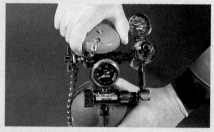

2. Open main valve—adjust flowmeter.

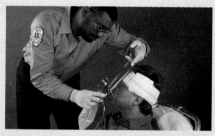

3. Place oxygen delivery service.

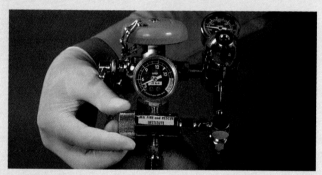

4. Adjust flowmeter.

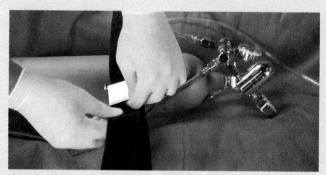

5. Secure during transfer.

Discontinuing Oxygen

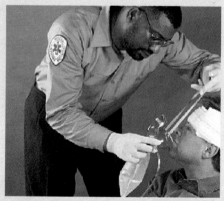

1. Remove delivery device.

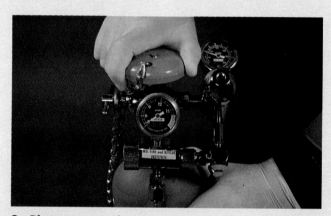

2. Close main valve.

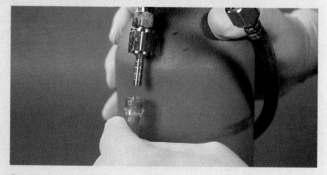

3. Remove delivery tubing.

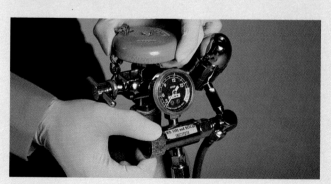

4. Bleed flowmeter.

filled with enough oxygen so that it does not collapse by more than one third when the patient inhales. Part of the patient's oxygen-enriched exhaled air will enter the reservoir bag to be mixed with oxygen (the reason for the name "partial rebreather" is that the patient will rebreathe some of his own exhaled air), the rest will escape through perforations in the mask. Concentrations of 35% to 60% can be delivered when flow rates are between 6 and 10 liters per minute.

- Nonrebreather Mask—Excluding the bag-valve mask system used with oxygen and the demand-valve resuscitator, the **nonrebreather mask** is the EMT's best way to deliver high concentrations of oxygen (Figure 6-25). This device must be placed properly on the patient's face to provide the necessary seal to ensure high concentration delivery. The reservoir bag must be inflated before the mask is placed on the patient's face. To inflate the reservoir bag, use your finger to cover the exhaust portal or the connection between the mask and the reservoir. The reservoir must always contain enough oxygen so that it does not deflate by more than one third when the patient takes his deepest inspiration. This can be maintained by the proper flow of oxygen. Air exhaled by the patient does not return to the reservoir (is not rebreathed). Instead, it escapes through a flutter valve in the facepiece.

This mask will provide concentrations of oxygen ranging from 80% to 95%. The minimum flow rate is 8 liters per minute. Depending on the manufacturer and the fit of the mask, the maximum flow can range from 12 to 15 liters per minute. New design features allow for one emergency port in the mask so that the patient can still receive atmospheric air should the oxygen supply fail. This feature keeps the mask from being able to deliver 100% oxygen but is a neces-

sary safety feature. The mask is excellent for use in shock and for severely hypoxic patients who do not suffer from COPD.

Note: Some devices are made so that they can be rebreather or nonrebreather masks, depending on a valve adjustment.

- Venturi Mask—A **Venturi mask** (Figure 6-26) is specifically designed for use when low concentrations of oxygen (24% to 40%) are required. The oxygen is delivered into the mask by way of a jet that pulls in atmospheric air to mix it with the oxygen. The flow is rapid enough to flush out the carbon dioxide that tends to accumulate in a face mask. Various-sized color-coded adaptors can be attached to the device to control the oxygen flow to the patient. Standard sizes include 3, 4, and 6 LPM adaptors. If a 4-liter adaptor is in place and you attempt to deliver 8 liters of oxygen per minute, the jet will draw in more atmospheric air to mix with the oxygen. This "Venturi effect" draws in enough air so that only 4 liters of oxygen per minute reaches the patient. Since Venturi masks often come in several parts, become familiar with this mask and how to use it before using it in the field.

Note: The Venturi is the only face mask recommended for COPD patients in minor respiratory distress. COPD patients with signs of more serious distress or hypoxia require a higher concentration of oxygen, administered with caution.

In practice, the simple face mask and the partial rebreather mask are rarely used. In most cases, if a patient needs only a low concentration of oxygen, a nasal cannula or Venturi mask is used. If the patient fears a mask, a nasal can-

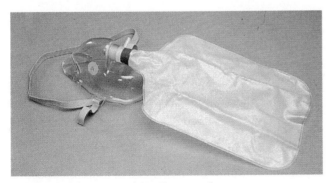

Figure 6-25 A nonrebreather mask.

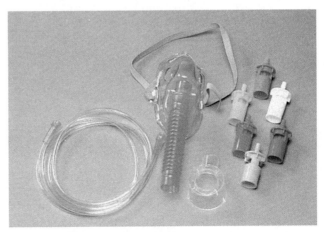

Figure 6-26 A Venturi mask.

nula may be used at 6 LPM. For other patients who need oxygen, most EMS systems recommend using a nonrebreather mask. The in-between oxygen concentrations offered by the simple face mask and the partial rebreather mask are seldom indicated or recommended.

Administering Oxygen to the Nonbreathing Patient

When a patient is found to be apneic (without respirations), artificial ventilation begins. The pocket face mask and the bag-valve mask are two devices used to assist the EMT in delivering artificial ventilations.

- **Pocket Face Mask**—The pocket face mask is placed over the patient's mouth and nose. The EMT ventilates into a one-way valve on top of the mask to ventilate the patient. Supplemental oxygen may be attached to many pocket face masks. At a flow rate of 10 liters per minute, 50% oxygen may be delivered to the patient during artificial ventilations.

  The pocket face mask is popular because of its ease of use. Since both hands are on the mask, a seal between the mask and the patient's face is easily obtained. Many EMS systems prefer the pocket face mask over the bag-valve mask for this reason.

- **Bag-Valve Mask**—The bag-valve mask is another method of forced ventilations for the nonbreathing patient. A mask is placed on the victim's face and the bag is squeezed, forcing air into the patient's lungs. The BVM should also have an oxygen inlet and reservoir bag that, when used with oxygen at 15 LPM, delivers over 90% oxygen to the nonbreathing patient. The BVM can also be used to provide ventilations to assist the patient whose respiratory attempts are not enough to support life.

Caution: Bag-valve masks are difficult to use. To become proficient with a BVM system you will need considerable practice. The mask-to-face seal can only be done with one hand since the other hand is needed to squeeze the bag. Without a proper face seal and a full compression of the bag, ventilations will be ineffective. BVM systems are best used when there are two rescuers available for ventilations. If one rescuer cannot use the BVM effectively, a pocket face mask with supplemental oxygen should be used.

Automatic Resuscitators

Since oxygen is kept under pressure in cylinders, some oxygen-delivery devices use that pressure to force air into the patient's lungs. Some are suitable for breathing patients, some for nonbreathing patients, some for both.

- **Demand-Valve Resuscitator**—The demand-valve resuscitator is a device that delivers oxygen "on demand." A mask connected to the demand-valve system is sealed on the patient's face. When the patient inhales, the valve opens and 100% oxygen is delivered to the patient. The flow of oxygen continues until the patient exhales. THE PATIENT MUST BE BREATHING to open up the valve and receive the oxygen.
- **Positive-Pressure Resuscitator**—A positive-pressure resuscitator is controlled by the rescuer. Oxygen flows into the patient's lungs when the rescuer pushes a button. The ventilation continues until a preset pressure is reached in the lungs (usually about 40 mmHg) or until the button is released.

  The positive-pressure device is popular because a two-hand mask seal can be

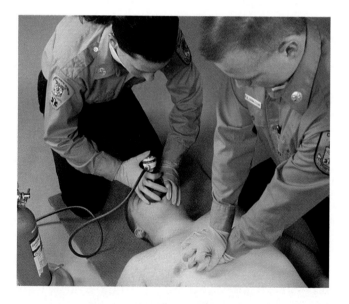

- BREATHING PATIENT
  Demand-valve model delivers as patient starts an inspiration
- NONBREATHING PATIENT
  Manually triggered positive-pressure mode delivers when rescuer depresses control button

Figure 6-27 Multiple-function (demand-valve, positive-pressure) resuscitator.

used. Only one finger is required to push the button to initiate the ventilation, in contrast to the BVM which requires the whole hand.

Caution must be used with positive-pressure devices. Although easier to use than the BVM, the positive-pressure resuscitator does not allow the EMT to "feel" the lung compliance during ventilation. Positive-pressure units *must* be used with a reducing valve to prevent excessive pressure resulting in gastric distention or injury to the lungs.

- **Multiple-Function Resuscitators**—Many oxygen-powered resuscitators combine the demand-valve system with the positive-pressure resuscitator (Figure 6-27). This resuscitator can be used as a demand valve for the breathing patient. If the patient should cease breathing, or his respirations are not sufficient to support life, they may be assisted with positive-pressure ventilations controlled by the rescuer.
- **Automatic Transport Ventilator (ATV)**—Transport ventilators are relatively new to EMS. These devices may be the next generation of positive-pressure resuscitator. The automatic transport ventilator delivers ventilations at a set volume, pressure, and interval. These ventilators are designed to attach to an endotracheal tube and automatically provide ventilations.

An additional benefit is that a mask seal can be held with both hands since the automatic ventilator provides the ventilation. There is no bag to squeeze or button to push. Gastric distention is minimized since the ventilation is delivered at a lower pressure over a period of 1 ½ to 2 seconds.

ATVs may play an increasing role in the future of prehospital resuscitation.

Warning: Do not use demand-valve or positive-pressure resuscitators on infants and children. Severe lung damage may occur. While these devices may be used on the COPD patient, caution should be used.

Note: Always follow your local protocols for artificial ventilation with adjunct breathing devices. PATIENTS BEING VENTILATED FOR ANY REASON SHOULD HAVE AN OROPHARYNGEAL OR NASOPHARYNGEAL AIRWAY IN PLACE.

CHAPTER REVIEW

KEY TERMS

You may find it helpful to review the following terms.

airway adjunct—a device placed in a patient's mouth or nose in order to help maintain an open airway. See *oropharyngeal airway* and *nasopharyngeal airway*.

automatic transport ventilator (ATV)—a device that automatically delivers ventilations at a set volume, pressure, and interval.

bag-valve mask—a hand-held unit with a self-refilling bag, directional valve system, and face mask. The bag is squeezed to deliver atmospheric air to the patient. This unit can be set up to deliver nearly 100% oxygen when connected to a supplemental oxygen supply system.

barrier device—a device such as a pocket face mask, face shield, bag-valve mask, disposable gloves, or goggles that prevent direct contact with a patient or the patient's breath or body fluids.

chronic obstructive pulmonary disease (COPD)—a group of diseases and conditions including emphysema, chronic bronchitis, and black lung.

demand-valve resuscitator—an oxygen-powered breathing device that will deliver oxygen when the patient attempts an inspiration.

face shield—a thin, transparent barrier device that protects against direct contact with the patient during artificial ventilations.

flowmeter—a valve that indicates the flow of oxygen in liters per minute.

humidifier—a device connected to the flowmeter to add moisture to the dry oxygen coming from the cylinder.

hypoxia (hi-POK-se-ah)—an inadequate supply of oxygen reaching the body's tissues.

hypoxic (hi-POK-sik) **drive**—a condition common to COPD patients in which the body determines the need to breathe based on oxygen rather than carbon dioxide and may interpret the higher oxygen levels that result from oxygen administration as a signal to reduce or stop breathing.

hyperventilate (HI-per-VENT-i-late)—in suctioning, to provide ventilations at a higher rate to compensate for oxygen not delivered during suctioning.

multiple-function resuscitator—an oxygen-powered breathing device that combines demand-valve and positive-pressure functions. See *demand-valve resuscitator* and *positive-pressure resuscitator*.

nasal cannula (NAY-zl KAN-yuh-luh)—a device that delivers low concentrations of oxygen through two prongs that rest in the patient's nostrils.

nasopharyngeal (na-zo-fah-RIN-je-al) **airway**—a flexible breathing tube inserted through the patient's nose into the pharynx.

nonrebreather mask—a face mask and reservoir bag device that delivers high concentrations of oxygen. All of the patient's exhaled air escapes through a valve and is not rebreathed.

oropharyngeal (or-o-fah-RIN-je-al) **airway**—a curved airway adjunct inserted through the patient's mouth into the pharynx.

oxygen cylinder—a cylinder filled with oxygen under pressure.

partial rebreather mask—a face mask and reservoir bag device that delivers moderate concentrations of oxygen. Part of the patient's exhaled air enters the reservoir to mix with the oxygen and be rebreathed.

pocket face mask—a device with a one-way valve to aid in mouth-to-mouth resuscitation. It can be used with supplemental oxygen when fitted with an oxygen inlet.

positive-pressure resuscitator—a manually triggered, oxygen-powered breathing device.

pressure regulator—a device connected to an oxygen cylinder to reduce cylinder pressure to a safe pressure for delivery of oxygen to a patient.

simple face mask—a soft mask through which moderate concentrations of oxygen can be delivered.

suction unit—a device that is used to remove blood, secretions, or other fluids from a patient's mouth, throat, or stomach.

Venturi (ven-TUR-e) **mask**—a mask that delivers consistently regulated low concentrations of oxygen.

SUMMARY

The EMT must be able to provide basic life support—airway, breathing, and circulation—without any special equipment. However breathing aids and oxygen administration improve the quality of artificial ventilation, and oxygen is effective therapy for a number of medical problems.

Breathing Aids

Breathing aids provide three major benefits: improved airway maintenance, increased oxygen delivery, and infection control. However, *never delay resuscitation to locate special equipment.*

Airway adjuncts can be used to maintain an open airway. There are two major types, oropharyngeal and nasopharyngeal airways.

Oropharyngeal airways will help keep the patient's tongue from slipping back into the throat. These airways should be used for unconscious patients who have no gag reflex. Before insertion, airways must be measured to insure that they are the proper size. The oropharyngeal airway is inserted with the tip toward the roof of the mouth and then rotated into position. Once inserted the flange must rest against the patient's lips.

Nasopharyngeal airways must be lubricated with a water-based lubricant. These devices may be used in a semi-conscious patient since they are less likely to activate a gag reflex.

Fluids can be removed from a patient's mouth and throat through the use of suction. A suction unit consists of a suction source, a collection container, tubing, and suction tips or catheters. Suction units may be fixed units, such as the ones mounted in the ambulance, or portable units that may be brought to the patient. Suction should always be performed while withdrawing the tip or catheter from the mouth. Suction should never be continued for more than a few seconds.

There are a number of artificial ventilation adjuncts (barrier devices). Pocket face masks and face shields serve as barrier devices for infection control. Pocket face masks often accept supplemental oxygen, but face shields ordinarily do not. Both are small and inexpensive enough to carry when off duty or in personal first aid kits.

Bag-valve mask systems with oxygen inlets and reservoirs are another type of artificial ventilation adjunct. While this system provides high-concentration oxygen and a barrier against infection, they are difficult to use. BVM systems should be used by two EMTs when possible or by single EMTs who are proficient in their use.

Oxygen Therapy

Hypoxia is an insufficiency of oxygen at the tissue level. This can result from trauma, smoke inhalation, lung disease, drug overdose, heart attack, stroke, shock, and other causes. Administration of oxygen is the chief therapy to prevent or reduce hypoxia.

There are several nonmedical hazards to guard against when dealing with oxygen. Oxygen is under high pressure and can become a powerful missile if the tank is punctured or a valve breaks off. Oxygen supports combustion and so is a fire hazard. Oxygen and petroleum products, including adhesives, can cause a violent reaction when they come in contact with each other. The medical hazards of oxygen—including oxygen toxicity or collapse of air sacs in the lungs, infant eye damage, and respiratory depression or arrest—result from high concentrations delivered for a prolonged time and are thus rarely caused by or seen in prehospital care.

COPD patients are on a hypoxic drive. This means that the body determines the need to breathe based on oxygen rather than carbon dioxide. Oxygen at a high percentage for a prolonged period of time may cause respiratory depression or arrest. The EMT must monitor and be prepared to resuscitate but must not withhold needed oxygen.

Despite any potential hazards, *never withhold oxygen from a patient who needs it.*

Oxygen cylinders come in various sizes, identified by the letters D, E, M, G, and H. Oxygen cylinders should never be allowed to empty below the safe residual of 200 psi (pounds per square inch) as indicated on the cylinder's pressure gauge.

Oxygen is supplied in pressurized cylinders. These cylinders may become projectiles if they are dropped and the valve ruptures. Oxygen also supports combustion and can detonate if mixed with oil. Regulators should never be oiled or taped. Safety rules for working with oxygen cylinders must be followed at all times.

The oxygen in a cylinder is under high pressure of 2,000 to 2,200 psi. A pressure regulator must be connected to the cylinder to provide a safe working pressure of 30 to 70 psi. A flowmeter attached to the pressure regulator allows control of the flow of oxygen in liters per minute. A humidifier can be connected to the flowmeter to counteract the dryness of the oxygen that can dehydrate the patient's mucus membranes. This is seldom done in EMS systems except, in some cases, for long-distance transfer and for patients with epiglottitis or croup.

There are several methods of delivering oxygen to patients who are breathing. The nasal cannula provides 24% to 44% oxygen. It may be helpful to patients who have COPD or who cannot tolerate a face mask. The simple face mask or the partial rebreather mask provides an intermediate level of oxygen, 35% to 60% (many EMS systems do not recommend the use of these intermediate-level masks). The nonrebreather mask is for patients who are hypoxic but without COPD involvement. It can provide over 90% oxygen. The Venturi Mask is designed to provide oxygen to the COPD patient. Most Venturi masks have settings to deliver between 24% and 40% oxygen.

Oxygen can be delivered to nonbreathing patients in conjunction with a pocket face mask or a bag-valve mask. There are also several oxygen-powered breathing devices available. Demand-valve devices provide 100% oxygen "on demand." When the patient breathes, a valve opens and allows the patient to breathe oxygen. Upon expiration, the valve closes. Positive-pressure devices use the pressurized oxygen to force a ventilation to the patient who isn't breathing. This is often done at high pressures and may cause gastric distention. A positive-pressure resuscitator is easier to use than a bag-valve mask since two hands can be used to hold the mask in place. Demand-valve and positive-pressure resuscitators are sometimes available in the same unit, called a multiple-function resuscitator. The automatic transport ventilator is designed to attach to an endotracheal tube and provide ventilations automatically.

Positive-pressure and demand-valve resuscitators should never be used on infants and children.

Patients being ventilated for any reason should have an oropharyngeal or nasopharyngeal airway in place at all times.

Infection control procedures must always be followed. Disposable gloves should always be worn. Mask and goggles should be worn during suctioning or at any other time there is a chance of body fluids splashing to the face.

CHAPTER 7

On the Scene

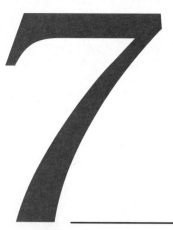

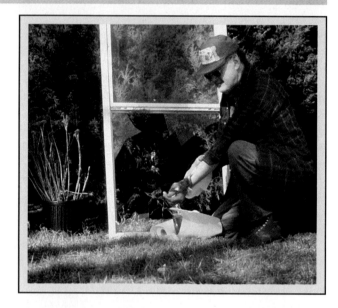

Bill Hopkins is cleaning windows when he slips and puts his arm through a pane of glass. Bill does not initially feel the pain. The first thing he observes is the blood flowing freely from the laceration on his forearm. Bill's wife Nancy hears the glass breaking and comes out to see what the problem is. She gives Bill a cloth to help stop the bleeding and goes to phone 911. Your EMS unit is dispatched for a "severe laceration with profuse bleeding."

As you arrive on the scene, you see Bill sitting on the ground with the cloth wrapped around his arm. As you exit the ambulance, you remind your partner to put on gloves, goggles, and gown for infection control.

You: Sir, we're Emergency Medical Technicians. Let me take over the pressure on the cloth. Can you tell me what happened?

Bill Hopkins: I was trying to put this storm window back in, and I slipped. Put my arm right through it.

You: Did you fall or pass out?

Bill Hopkins: No. I just sat down here afterwards. Good thing my wife was home.

You: Yes it was. I'm going to replace this cloth with a sterile dressing and keep pressure on your arm. My partner is going to put an oxygen mask on you, because it looks like you've lost some blood.

As you replace the cloth with your dressing, you are able to briefly examine the wound. The flow of dark red blood has almost stopped, but there is still some oozing of blood from around the wound. You place a sterile 5 x 9 gauze over the wound and wrap it with a wide bandage to create a pressure dressing, then ask Bill to hold his forearm above the level of his heart. You have additional bulky dressings at hand in case the bleeding resumes. As you prepare for transportation, you check vital signs, including capillary refill, and assess the injured arm to be sure the injury or tight dressing has not interfered with distal circulation, sensation, and movement.

Nancy Hopkins follows in her car as you transport her husband to the hospital.

Bleeding

Profuse external bleeding is one of the conditions that you will look for as part of your check of circulation—the "C" step during the ABCDEs of the primary survey. You will also look for signs of severe internal bleeding during both the primary and the secondary survey. Profuse bleeding, whether external or internal, is life threatening. For the EMT, the ability to control bleeding is an essential skill.

Expected Outcome, Chapter 7: *You will be able to detect, evaluate, and control external and internal bleeding.*

Warning: Protect yourself from infectious diseases by using appropriate barrier devices such as a pocket face mask with one-way valve, face shield, or bag-valve mask; goggles or eye shield; and disposable gloves. Always conform to your local EMS system's infection exposure control plan.

THE BLOOD AND BLOOD VESSELS

EXTERNAL BLEEDING
    Evaluating External Bleeding
    Controlling External Bleeding

INTERNAL BLEEDING
    Causes and Significance
    Detecting Internal Bleeding
    Evaluating Internal Bleeding
    Controlling Internal Bleeding

Knowledge *After reading this chapter, you should be able to*

1. List the FIVE major functions of blood. (p. 205)
2. List the THREE major types of blood vessels and describe their functions. (pp. 205-206)
3. Relate the types of blood vessels to the THREE kinds of external bleeding. (p. 206)
4. List observations at the scene and signs of shock that indicate possible severe blood loss. (p. 207)
5. List the FOUR major methods of controlling external bleeding. (p. 207)
6. Describe direct pressure methods of controlling mild and profuse bleeding. (pp. 208-209)
7. Describe the application of a pressure dressing. (p. 209)
8. Describe the use of elevation in the control of external bleeding and note when it should not be used. (pp. 209-210)
9. Define *pressure point* and list and locate the major pressure point sites used in EMT-level emergency care. (p. 210)
10. Describe, step by step, the use of pressure points to control bleeding from the upper and lower limbs. (pp. 210-211)
11. Explain why tourniquets are used only after other methods of controlling profuse bleeding have failed. (pp. 211-212)
12. Describe, step by step, the procedures for applying a tourniquet, including all precautions for the procedure. (p. 212)
13. Describe how a blood pressure cuff, splinting, cold applications, and pneumatic anti-shock garments can be used to control bleeding. (p. 213)
14. List causes of internal bleeding. (pp. 213-214)
15. List FOUR indications that internal bleeding may have occurred, the signs of internal bleeding, the signs and symptoms of shock associated with internal bleeding, and SIX indications that internal bleeding is severe. (pp. 214-215)
16. Describe the procedures for controlling internal bleeding. (pp. 215-216)

Skills *As an EMT you should be able to*

1. Evaluate the seriousness of bleeding and the approximate blood loss.
2. Control external bleeding by
   - Direct pressure
   - Direct pressure and elevation
   - Arterial pressure point
   - Tourniquet
3. Use the following devices to assist with the control of bleeding.
   - Pressure bandage
   - Blood pressure cuff
   - Splinting
   - Cold applications
   - Anti-shock garments (if recommended by local protocols)

Profuse bleeding is a life-threatening condition that requires immediate emergency care. In fact, any significant bleeding must be controlled before the patient is delivered to the staff of a medical facility. An understanding of the blood and blood vessels is basic to understanding both internal and external bleeding and the methods of controlling it.

THE BLOOD AND BLOOD VESSELS

Blood is a living tissue made up of plasma (PLAZ-mah) and formed elements (Figure 7-1).

- **Plasma**—Plasma is a watery, salty fluid that makes up over half the volume of the blood.
- **Formed Elements**—The formed elements include

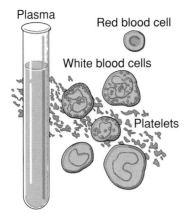

Figure 7-1 The major components of blood.

TABLE 7-1 Blood Volumes

Patient	Total Blood Volume	Lethal Blood Loss if Not Replaced (rapid)
Adult male (154 pounds)	5.0 to 6.6 liters	2.0 liters
Adolescent (105 pounds)	3.3 to 4.5 liters	1.3 liters
Child (early to late childhood . . . depends on size)	1.5 to 2.0 liters	0.5 to 0.7 liter
Infant (newborn, normal weight range)	300+ milliliters	30 to 50 milliliters

Note: One liter equals about two pints. One milliliter is about the same as 20 drops from a medicine dropper.

Red Blood Cells—also called RBCs, erythrocytes, or red corpuscles. Their primary function is to carry oxygen to the tissues and carbon dioxide away from the tissues.

White Blood Cells—also called WBCs, leukocytes, or white corpuscles. They are involved in destroying microorganisms (germs) and producing substances called antibodies that help the body resist infection.

Platelets (PLATE-lets)—membrane-enclosed fragments of specialized cells. When these fragments are activated, they release chemical factors needed to form blood clots.

The functions of blood are

- Transportation of Gases—to carry oxygen from the lungs to the tissues and to carry carbon dioxide from the tissues to the lungs
- Nutrition—to carry food substances from the intestine or storage tissues (fatty tissue, the liver, and muscle cells) to the rest of the body tissues
- Excretion—to carry wastes away from the tissues to the organs of excretion (kidneys, large intestine, skin, and lungs)
- Protection—to defend against disease-causing organisms by engulfing and digesting (eating) them, or by producing antibodies against them (immunity)
- Regulation—to carry hormones, water, salt, and other chemicals that control the functions of organs and glands. The regulation of body temperature is aided by the blood, which carries excessive body heat to the lungs and skin surface.

The volume of blood differs from person to person, based on body size (Table 7-1). The typical adult male has about 5 liters of blood, or slightly over 10 pints, or 7% of the body weight. The loss of blood volume is very significant, not only in terms of the loss of formed elements but also in loss of plasma. Keep in mind that each person has a minimum volume of blood that is needed in circulation to keep the cardiovascular system working efficiently enough to maintain life.

A general classification of blood volume can be based on the age of the patient. An infant may have only 300 milliliters (ml) of blood (1 ml equals about 20 drops from a medicine dropper, 15 ml equals 1 tablespoon). Depending on size, children have from 1.5 to 2 liters of blood. Adolescents usually have from 3.3 to 5.0 liters of blood depending on their size.

Blood vessels are the means by which blood is transported throughout the body. There are three major types of blood vessels (Figure 7-2). They are

- **Artery**—a blood vessel with thick, muscular walls that carries blood away from the heart

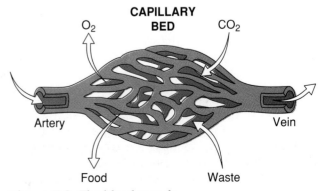

Figure 7-2 The blood vessels.

- **Capillary**—a microscopic blood vessel where oxygen/carbon dioxide and nutrient/waste exchange takes place
- **Vein**—a blood vessel that carries blood back to the heart. A vein contains one-way valves that keep the blood flowing in the proper direction.

As the heart beats, it circulates blood. Blood travels through the arteries into the capillaries where oxygen and nutrients are exchanged for carbon dioxide and waste products. After the blood exits the capillaries it enters the veins to return to the heart and lungs, where the circulation began.

Although they are very small, the capillaries are an important part of the circulatory system. Because the capillaries are where the transfer of oxygen, nutrients, and waste products to and from the cells takes place, it is vital that blood reach each capillary throughout the body. When blood reaches and fills the capillaries, it is called **perfusion**. Without perfusion of the capillaries, oxygen does not reach vital tissues and organs, and dangerous waste products build up in the cells and tissues.

Bleeding has a devastating effect on perfusion. There is only so much blood to circulate. Once a certain amount of the body's blood volume is lost, perfusion of all capillaries will not occur. The parts of the body that are not perfused will eventually experience tissue death. The brain, nerve cells, and kidneys are especially sensitive to decreased perfusion.

The term **hemorrhage** (HEM-o-rej) means bleeding. Bleeding can be classified as external or internal.

EXTERNAL BLEEDING

In addition to being classified as external or internal, bleeding can be classified as to the type of vessel losing the blood. At the EMT level of care, this is done only for external bleeding. External bleeding (Figure 7-3) is classified into three types.

- Arterial Bleeding—the blood loss from an artery. Remember that the artery is the first vessel the blood is pumped into as it leaves the heart. Arteries have strong walls that hold blood under high pressure. Therefore, the bleeding from an artery is often rapid, spurting with each heartbeat, and profuse.

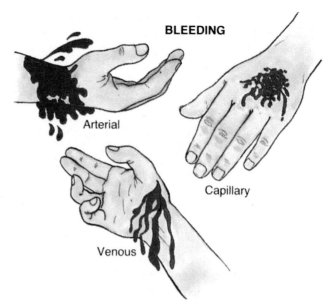

Figure 7-3 The three types of external bleeding.

The blood that comes from an artery is usually bright red.
- Venous Bleeding—the loss of blood from a vein. Veins carry blood under lower pressures and return it to the heart. Venous bleeding is usually a steady flow and can be quite heavy. Venous blood is usually dark red or maroon in color.
- Capillary Bleeding—the loss of blood from a capillary. Since capillaries are very small, bleeding from a capillary area, or capillary "bed," is usually slow, often described as "oozing." The color of the blood is red, usually less bright than arterial blood.

Although the treatments for all types of external bleeding are the same, the type of bleeding (arterial, venous, or capillary) may alert the EMT to some additional information. Arterial bleeding is often profuse. Since it is under high pressure, clot formation (which stops bleeding naturally) is difficult. Bleeding control measures may be required during the entire trip to the hospital. Veins sometimes pose special problems. Large veins may suck in debris and air bubbles. This is a serious problem with large veins, such as those in the neck. A bubble of air in the bloodstream, known as an air **embolism,** may be carried directly to the heart and interfere with or actually stop the heartbeat. The lungs and brain are also sensitive to air emboli.

Capillary bleeding is usually the result of a minor wound or scrape. This type of injury is often associated with contamination of the skin and the chance of infection. Large wounds often have capillary bleeding from the edges in addition to another type of bleeding from a vessel deeper in the wound.

Evaluating External Bleeding

Serious blood loss is a life-threatening condition. The amount of blood that can be lost before death occurs will vary from individual to individual (see Table 7-1). Usually a loss of 25% to 40% of a person's blood volume will create a life-threatening condition.

Certain guidelines can be used that do not require calculating an individual patient's total blood volume. A rapid loss of 1 liter of blood by an adult must be considered to be life threatening. Depending on body size and weight, a loss of one-fourth to one-half liter of blood by a child will be life threatening. For an infant, 24 ml. of blood loss *must* be viewed as life threatening.

Detecting and stopping life-threatening external bleeding are part of the primary survey. Priority is given to heavy blood flow, usually from arteries and large veins.

Patient Assessment—External Bleeding

An estimate of the amount of external blood loss is important in terms of predicting possible shock, sorting patients for triage, and identifying bleeding that must be treated during the primary survey. (Slow bleeding that normally could wait until the secondary survey may be a primary survey concern if it has been steady for a long period of time and the blood loss has become significant.)

Estimating external blood loss may be difficult. Blood may flow to the floor or may be absorbed by furniture, carpeting, or clothing. In any event, it is difficult to make an objective determination of the amount of blood loss. To help form a concept of blood loss, pour a pint of water on the floor next to a fellow student or a manikin. Try soaking an article of clothing with a pint of water and note how much of the article is wet and how wet it feels to your touch. (See also Figure 7-4).

Since it is difficult to determine the quantity of blood loss, it is important also to observe the patient for other signs of hemorrhage.

Signs

A patient who has experienced significant blood loss will display signs of shock (shock

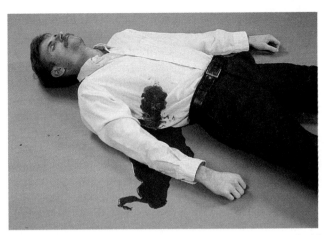

Figure 7-4 Estimating external blood loss: one-half liter (approximately 1 pint).

will be discussed in Chapter 8). These signs may include

- ☐ Rapid pulse rate
- ☐ Rapid, shallow respirations
- ☐ Cool, clammy skin
- ☐ Combative, confused or restless behavior, or a change in the level of consciousness.

Remember: Regardless of the apparent volume of blood loss, if the patient has any of the indications of shock, then the bleeding must be classified as serious. However, the EMT should not wait for signs of shock to be present before beginning treatment. In fact, *when shock is evident it may be too late!* Any patient with a significant amount (more than a small cut or scrape) of blood loss should cause the EMT to be alert for, and prevent, the development of shock.

Controlling External Bleeding

The control of external bleeding is an important skill. If left uncontrolled, bleeding may lead to shock and death.

Patient Care—External Bleeding

Emergency Care Steps

The major methods used to control external bleeding are

- ☐ Direct pressure
- ☐ Elevation
- ☐ Pressure Points
- ☐ Applying a Tourniquet

Other methods used to assist in bleeding control are splinting, cold application, and the use of an anti-shock garment. These methods will be discussed in detail below.

In addition to these manual methods of bleeding control, an important treatment for any bleeding patient is

☐ Oxygen—Since blood loss prevents the perfusion of oxygen to the tissues, the use of supplemental oxygen is vital. Oxygen should be administered after the bleeding has been controlled. Never delay the manual methods of bleeding control to set up or deliver oxygen to the patient.

Remember: Infection control is another important consideration for the EMT when attempting to control bleeding. Always wear disposable gloves while performing bleeding control, applying dressings, or cleaning up after a bleeding patient, and follow your local infection exposure control plan with regard to disposing of blood-stained sheets and other materials. When there is spurting or possible splashing of blood, wear a mask, goggles or eyeshield, and a protective gown.

Direct Pressure The most acceptable method of controlling external bleeding is by applying pressure directly to the wound (Figure 7-5). Direct pressure can be applied by your gloved hand, by a dressing and your hand, or by a pressure dressing. Always wear protective gloves.

When bleeding is MILD, you should

1. Apply pressure to the wound, preferably with a sterile dressing held against its surface. (A clean handkerchief or cloth can be used if a sterile dressing is not immediately available.)
2. Hold pressure firmly on the wound for 10 to 30 minutes. This will usually stop the bleeding. Your aim is to control the bleeding and limit additional significant blood loss.
3. Once bleeding is controlled, secure the dressing in place with bandaging.
4. *Never* remove a dressing once it is in place. To do so may restart bleeding or cause additional injury to the site. Apply another dressing on top of the blood-soaked one and hold them both in place. Continue this

DIRECT PRESSURE

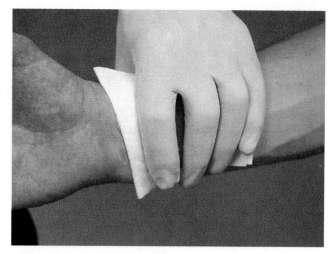

Apply pressure with dressing.

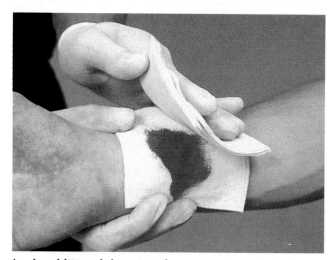

Apply additional dressing if necessary.

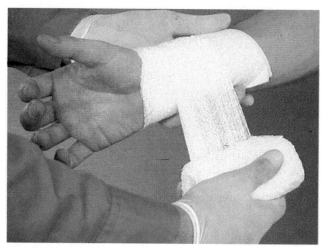

Bandage wound.

Figure 7-5 Direct pressure is applied until bleeding is controlled.

procedure until bleeding is controlled, or until you deliver the patient to the staff of a medical facility.

If bleeding is PROFUSE, you should

1. *Not* waste time trying to find a dressing (Figure 7-6).
2. Place your gloved hand directly on the wound and exert firm pressure.
3. Keep applying steady, firm pressure until the bleeding is controlled.
4. Once bleeding is controlled, bandage a dressing firmly in place to form a pressure dressing.

A **pressure dressing** can be applied to establish enough direct pressure to control most bleeding. Several sterile gauze pad dressings are placed on the wound. A bulky dressing is placed over the gauze pads. An efficient bulky dressing for a severely bleeding wound is the combined, or multitrauma, dressing. Sanitary napkins also can be used. The dressings should be held in place with a self-adhering roller bandage wrapped tightly over the dressing and above and below the wound site. Enough pressure must be created to control the bleeding.

Note: After controlling the bleeding from an extremity using a pressure dressing, check for a distal pulse to be certain that the dressing has not restricted blood flow in the treated limb. If you do not feel a pulse, you may have to adjust the pressure to reestablish circulation. Frequent checks of the distal pulse should continue throughout your care for the patient. In some cases, the severing of a major artery will stop the circulation needed to produce a pulse.

The dressings should not be removed once they are applied. If bleeding continues, more pressure can be added using the palm of your gloved hand, or a tighter bandage can be applied. In some cases, you may have to create more bulk by adding dressings. In rare cases, you may have to remove a blood-soaked bulky bandage leaving the initial dressing in place so that bleeding can be controlled by direct pressure.

A variety of dressings can be used in emergency situations. Some of these are shown in Figure 7-7.

Be aware that, in certain areas of the body, you may be unable to apply an effective pressure dressing, for example, when bleeding is from the armpit. You may have to maintain pressure by

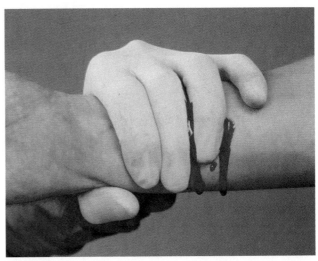

Figure 7-6 In cases of profuse bleeding, *do not* waste time hunting for a dressing.

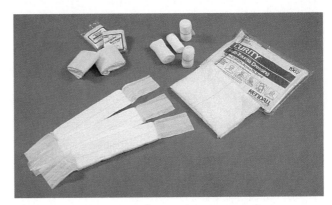

Figure 7-7 Dressings for use in emergencies.

holding your gloved hand directly over the wound. Even though you may be contaminating the wound, the risk of uncontrolled bleeding far outweighs that of possible infection.

Remember: Direct pressure is usually the quickest and most efficient means of controlling external bleeding.

Elevation This method is used along with direct pressure. When an injured extremity is elevated so that the wound is above the level of the heart, gravity helps to reduce blood pressure, thus bleeding is slowed (Figure 7-8). This method should not be used if there are possible fractures or dislocations to the extremity, objects impaled in the extremity, or possible spinal injury. To use elevation, you should

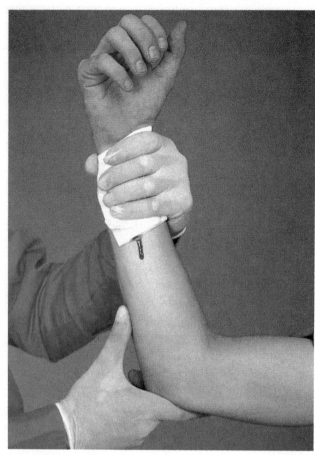

Figure 7-8 Combine direct pressure and elevation.

1. Apply direct pressure to the site of bleeding.
2. Elevate the injured extremity. If the forearm is bleeding, simply elevate the forearm. You do not have to elevate the entire limb.

Pressure Points If direct pressure or direct pressure and elevation fail, your next approach may be the use of pressure points (Figure 7-9). A **pressure point** is a site where a main artery lies near the surface of the body and directly over a bone (these correspond well to pulse sites). Six sites (three on each side) are used to control profuse bleeding in field emergency care. These sites are the

- **Brachial** (BRAY-ke-al) **Artery**—for bleeding from the upper limb (Figure 7-10).
- **Femoral** (FEM-o-ral) **Artery**—for bleeding from the lower limb (Figure 7-11).
- **Temporal** (TEMP-o-ral) **Artery**—for bleeding from the scalp.

The use of pressure points requires skill on the part of the rescuer. Unless you know the exact location of the point and how much pressure to apply, the pressure point technique is of no use.

Remember: Pressure point techniques are to be used only after direct pressure or direct pressure and elevation have failed to control the bleeding.

Following are guidelines for controlling bleeding from the extremities using pressure points.

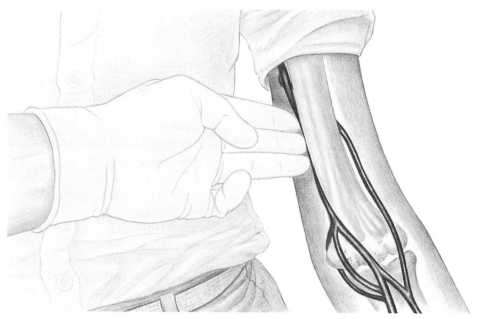

Figure 7-9 Using pressure points can stop profuse bleeding from an arm or leg.

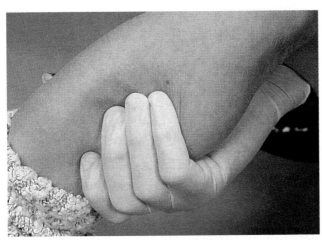

Figure 7-10 Apply pressure to the brachial artery pressure point to control bleeding from the arm.

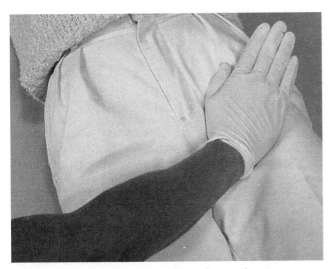

Figure 7-11 Apply pressure to femoral artery pressure point to control bleeding from the leg.

- Bleeding from the Upper Extremity—Apply pressure to a point over the brachial artery. To find the artery, hold the patient's arm out at a right angle to his body, with the palm facing up. (If it is not possible to raise the arm this far, do the best you can without forcing the arm or aggravating an injury.) Find the groove between the biceps muscle and the arm bone (humerus), about midway between the elbow and the armpit. Cradle the upper arm in the palm of your hand and position your fingers into this medial groove. You can now compress the brachial artery against the underlying bone by pressing your finger into this groove. If pressure is properly

applied, you will not be able to feel a radial pulse. If the wound is to the distal end of the limb, bleeding may not be effectively controlled by this method. This is because blood is being sent to this region from many smaller arteries that have branched off of the major arteries in the limb.

- Bleeding from the Lower Extremity—Apply pressure to a point over the femoral artery. Locate this artery on the medial side of the thigh where it joins the lower trunk. You should be able to feel pulsations at a point just below the groin. Place the heel of your hand over the site and exert pressure downward toward the bone until it is obvious that the bleeding has been controlled. You will need more pressure than that applied for the brachial artery pressure point. Considerable force must be exerted if the patient is very muscular or obese. If pressure is properly applied, a distal pulse cannot be felt. As discussed above for the upper extremity, this method may not control bleeding for distal wounds.

Tourniquet A **tourniquet** (TURN-i-ket) is a device that constricts *all* blood flow to and from an extremity. THIS PROCEDURE IS A LAST RESORT, used only when other methods to control life-threatening bleeding have failed. Experienced EMTs realize that the use of a tourniquet is a "life or limb" situation. The use of the tourniquet will stop the life-threatening bleeding, but it often results in the loss of the limb the tourniquet is applied to.

Fortunately, when direct pressure and pressure dressings, elevation, and pressure points are used effectively, tourniquets are rarely needed.

Clean-edged amputations often do not require the application of a tourniquet. This is because many of the injured blood vessels seal shut as a result of spasms produced in their muscular walls (vasospasms). Bulky pressure dressings are very effective in controlling the bleeding associated with this type of injury. Rough-edged amputations, usually produced by crushing or tearing injuries, often bleed freely since the nature of the injury does not allow for effective vasospasms. This type of amputation may cause more persistent bleeding that may require a tourniquet to control. However, never apply a tourniquet before trying direct pressure, elevation, and pressure points first.

Tourniquets are used only for wounds of the extremities. *Do not* apply a tourniquet directly over the knee or elbow.

The tourniquet should be made of a wide material, preferably 2 to 3 inches in width. There are commercially made tourniquets, or a makeshift device may be made from a cravat, a wide belt, or other wide, soft material. Among the items that should *never* be used as a tourniquet are ropes, wires, and other narrow items that may cut into the patient's skin.

Once a tourniquet is in place, it should not be removed or loosened. Loosening of the tourniquet may dislodge clots and cause bleeding to resume. This additional bleeding will add to the patient's blood loss that occurred prior to tourniquet application and almost certainly cause severe shock. Another complication of tourniquet removal or loosening is **tourniquet shock**. Severely injured tissues release harmful substances that gather below the level of the tourniquet. If the tourniquet is loosened or released, these substances are released in high concentrations to the rest of the body. If you keep the tourniquet in place, the patient has a better chance of survival, even if it means the loss of a limb.

Remember: The tourniquet is only to be used as a last resort. The device itself should be made of a wide material that will not cut into a patient's skin. The devices are only to be used on extremities but not directly over a joint. Once a tourniquet has been applied, it should not be loosened or removed in the field.

While you are applying a tourniquet, you may have another rescuer apply direct pressure and pressure point techniques. This may slow the bleeding and reduce blood loss until the tourniquet is in place. To apply a tourniquet, you should (Figure 7-12)

1. Select a place between the heart and the wound, as close as possible to, but not even with, the edge of the wound. This should be within 2 inches of the wound. If the wound is on a joint, apply the tourniquet above the joint (toward the heart).
2. Place a pad made from a dressing (a roll of gauze bandage) or a folded handkerchief over the main supplying artery before applying the constricting band. This will help protect the site and will apply additional pressure over the artery.
3. If a commercial tourniquet is used, carefully place it around the limb at the site and pull the free end of the band through the buckle or friction catch and draw this end tightly over the pad. You should tighten the tourniquet to the point where bleeding is

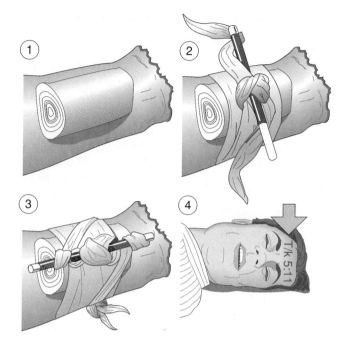

Figure 7-12 Application of a tourniquet.

controlled. Do not tighten the tourniquet beyond this point.

If you are using a cravat or other piece of material, carefully slip the material around the injured limb and tie a knot with the ends of the tourniquet. The knot should be over the pad. A stick, rod, or similar device should be inserted into the knot and used to tighten the tourniquet. Turn the device until bleeding is controlled. Do not tighten beyond this point. Tape or tie the tightening device in place. KEEP THE TOURNIQUET IN PLACE. DO NOT LOOSEN.

4. Attach a notation to the patient to indicate that a tourniquet has been applied and the time of application. If a tag is not available, mark the patient's forehead in ink. Write "TK" and the time of application so that the tourniquet does not go unnoticed by the emergency department staff. Make certain that you do not cover the extremity to which the tourniquet has been applied. This is done for the visual monitoring of the effectiveness of the tourniquet and to ensure that the tourniquet does not go unnoticed.

It is the EMT's responsibility to advise the emergency department staff of the application of a tourniquet. Even if this is done via radio, it must also be done in person at the hospital.

There may be instances in which you arrive at a scene and find that bystanders have applied a tourniquet. Most EMS systems have standard operating procedures that must be followed in such cases. Sometimes bystanders apply tourniquets thinking that this is a proper procedure for all bleeding. If the EMT can determine that the bleeding was not severe and may be controllable by means other than a tourniquet and that the tourniquet has not been in place for long, and if your local EMS guidelines permit, the tourniquet may be released *slowly* while someone applies direct pressure to the wound site. Follow your local EMS guidelines. If in doubt, radio for medical control advice.

Blood Pressure Cuff This device can be applied as a tourniquet to control apparently life-threatening arterial bleeding from an extremity. The cuff is placed above the wound (between the wound and the heart) and inflated to the pressure required to control the bleeding. This is usually in the 150-mmHg range for persons with normal blood pressure. A dressing and bandage is secured after the bleeding is controlled. The cuff can safely be left inflated for 30 minutes or more; however, it must be closely monitored to make certain that cuff pressure is not lost. The use of the blood pressure cuff may prove to be the only way to control bleeding for patients who are trapped in wreckage.

A blood pressure cuff can also be used after a dressing has been applied to make a pressure dressing.

Splinting The splinting of fractures will be covered in Chapters 10 and 11. Often when a fractured extremity is splinted, bleeding associated with the fracture may be controlled (Figure 7-13). This occurs when the sharp ends of broken bones are stabilized, preventing additional damage to blood vessels at the injury site.

Inflatable splints, also called air splints, are sometimes used to help control internal and external bleeding from an extremity, even when there is no fracture. They may be useful when a severe laceration (cut) extends over the length of the extremity. The pressure produced by the splint is a form of direct pressure.

Since these splints are inflated by mouth, there is a limit to the amount of pressure produced. The pressure may not be sufficient to control *arterial* bleeding and may even make it worse. However, these devices can be helpful in maintaining pressure after other manual methods have already controlled bleeding.

Cold Application The application of ice or coldpacks to an injury has been done for centuries. Cold minimizes swelling and reduces bleeding by constricting blood vessels. It does not, by itself, control bleeding, but it may be useful in combination with other techniques. Cold application can also help reduce the pain of the injury that caused the bleeding.

Ice or cold packs should never be applied directly to the skin. Prolonged contact may actually cause frostbite. Wrap the ice pack in a cloth or towel before placing it against the skin, and do not leave it there for more than 20 minutes at a time.

Anti-Shock Garments Although the use of anti-shock garments is controversial, most experts agree that they are useful for controlling bleeding from areas the garment covers. This device will be discussed at length in Chapter 8. Refer to your local protocols for information on how your EMS system uses anti-shock garments.

INTERNAL BLEEDING

Internal bleeding is bleeding that occurs within the body and cannot be seen. It can be minor or severe and life threatening. There are many spaces inside the body that can hold enough blood to allow a patient to bleed to death without any external, observable bleeding.

Causes and Significance

Internal bleeding can be minor. For instance, a small contusion (bruise) is an example of internal bleeding. By itself, a small bruise is of minor importance.

Other cases of internal bleeding, however, are major. There can be enough internal blood loss to bring about shock, heart and lung failure, and eventual death. Blood vessel ruptures in the chest or abdomen can cause death in minutes or seconds.

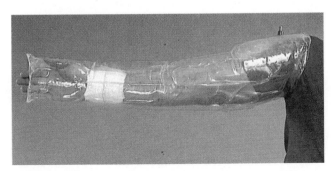

Figure 7-13 Immobilizing a fractured extremity can help control bleeding.

Crushing injuries, ruptured or lacerated organs and blood vessels, bleeding ulcers, and severely bruised tissues can all produce serious internal blood loss. Internal bleeding can occur with wounds that are deep enough to sever major arteries and veins. A deep chest or abdominal wound can cut through many blood vessels, causing blood to flow freely into the body cavity. Any cut into muscle or the fracturing of bone will also cause internal blood loss.

Be alert to the fact that many cases of internal bleeding occur when there are no cuts in the skin or cavity walls. Blunt trauma, an injury produced by an object that was not sharp enough to penetrate the skin, may cause major internal bleeding. The force is carried into the body, rupturing vessels and organs. Patients who are thrown against dashboards, steering wheels, armrests, and other objects in vehicle collisions can suffer from internal injuries that produce serious internal bleeding.

A blow delivered to one side of the body may cause internal bleeding on the opposite side. For example, although such an injury would be unusual, a blow to the right side of the abdomen may rupture the spleen (on the left side of the body) and release a liter or more of blood.

Detecting Internal Bleeding

Internal bleeding may be indicated by a serious external wound or injury. Often, however, the external signs of internal bleeding are minor or nonexistent. There may be only minor external bleeding. In blunt trauma situations, a minor externally visible bruise may be the only indication that an internal organ has been ruptured.

Patient Assessment—Internal Bleeding

You may detect internal bleeding by looking for

- Mechanisms of Injury—sources of blunt trauma that may have produced internal injuries and that may have few or no external signs
- External Wounds and Injuries—that may produce or be associated with internal injuries, detected during the primary survey
- Signs of Internal Injury—as detected in the head-to-toe physical exam during the secondary survey (see below)
- Signs and Symptoms of Shock—(see below)

Signs of Internal Bleeding

The signs listed below follow the order you may encounter them during the head-to-toe examination of the secondary survey. Assume internal bleeding whenever you detect

- Bruises or penetrating trauma on the neck
- Wounds that have penetrated the skull
- Blood or bloody fluids in the ears or nose
- Vomiting or coughing up blood (coffee-ground or frothy red in appearance)
- Bruises on the chest or the signs of possible rib fracture
- Wounds that have penetrated the chest or abdomen
- Areas of bruised or swollen abdomen
- Abdominal tenderness, rigidity, or spasms (the patient may guard the abdomen)
- Blood in the urine
- Rectal or vaginal bleeding
- Bone fractures, especially the pelvis and the long bones of the arm and thigh.

Signs and Symptoms of Shock

Shock will be discussed in more detail in Chapter 8. For now, consider some of the following signs of shock closely associated with internal bleeding.

- Restlessness (a reliable early sign) or combativeness
- Altered level of consciousness
- Breathing—rapid, possibly becoming shallow
- Pulse—rapid and weak
- Blood pressure—a marked drop, usually to 90/60 mmHg or lower (usually a late sign)
- Skin—pale, cool, and clammy, often with profuse sweating (usually found first at the extremities)
- Eyes—pupils may be dilated
- Body—shaking and trembling (rare)

The following symptoms of shock are closely related to internal bleeding.

- Anxiety or restlessness
- Weakness
- Thirst
- Complaints of feeling cold

Remember: You may detect internal bleeding by looking for mechanisms of injury, wounds and injuries that often produce internal bleeding, and certain signs and symptoms of shock.

Evaluating Internal Bleeding

Special tests and procedures are done at the hospital to determine the approximate amount of internal blood loss. At the scene, it is difficult for the EMT to know how serious internal bleeding may be.

Patient Assessment—Internal Bleeding

Signs

Consider internal bleeding to be *severe* if *any* of these signs is present.

☐ The patient is vomiting or coughing up blood. This blood may look like coffee grounds. Pink, frothy blood in the mouth or nose often indicates bleeding in the lungs.
☐ There is rigidity or spasms of the abdominal wall muscles.
☐ There is penetration of the chest cavity or the abdomen.
☐ There is a fracture to the femur or pelvis (assume a blood loss of 1 liter or more).
☐ There are deep bruises. Since it is difficult to estimate internal blood loss, assume a 10% blood loss for every deep bruise the size of a man's fist that is found on the chest or abdomen (Figure 7-14). Even though this may not be true for a particular patient, it is better to overestimate the significance of possible internal bleeding.
☐ Any of the signs or symptoms of shock is present.

Remember: There may be severe internal bleeding with no external bleeding or bruising, so be alert for *any* of the above signs as an indication of possible internal bleeding.

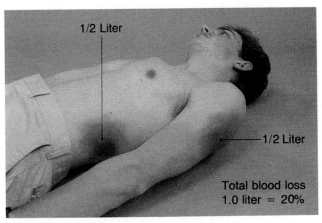

Figure 7-14 Estimating internal blood loss.

Carefully evaluating the patient's signs and symptoms and quickly estimating internal blood loss will help you determine the possibilities of your patient developing severe shock or cardiac arrest. Remember, when there is more than one patient, the order of care and transport may be affected by internal blood loss.

Controlling Internal Bleeding

Control of internal bleeding depends on the location of the injury and the cause of the bleeding.

Patient Care—Internal Bleeding

Minor internal bleeding related to a blunt injury to an extremity may be controlled by a pressure dressing and bandage. The pressure applied will tend to close off the ends of bleeding vessels. Extreme care must be taken, however, since a fracture may have been produced by the accident. The careless application of a pressure bandage to a closed fracture site may injure soft tissues or aggravate the fracture. Special care must be taken to avoid additional injury to the spine, chest, and pelvis.

The application of a splint to an injured extremity often will help control internal bleeding related to fractures. Inflatable splints are useful for such cases.

Injury-related or illness-induced bleeding into the thoracic or the abdominopelvic cavity may not be controllable at the accident scene, even when using pneumatic anti-shock garments.

You must continue to ensure an open airway and monitor vital signs. Patients with possible neck or spinal injuries must be given special care to avoid aggravation of these injuries. Profuse external bleeding must be cared for immediately.

Emergency Care Steps

When providing care for a patient with possible internal bleeding, you should

1 Maintain an open airway.
2 Reassure the patient and provide emotional support throughout all aspects of care. A calm patient has a better chance for survival. The stress and anxiety produced by the emergency will increase the patient's pulse rate, thus increasing bleeding.
3 Keep the patient lying down and at rest.

4. Control all serious bleeding. If the bleeding is in an extremity, use a snug bandage over a bulky pad applied directly over the injury site, taking care not to aggravate fractures. Remember that applying a splint serves both to immobilize an injured limb and to control bleeding.
5. Apply PASG if indicated in your local protocols.
6. Position and treat for shock, as described in Chapter 8. You may have to first immobilize fractures before positioning for shock.
7. ADMINISTER A HIGH CONCENTRATION OF OXYGEN AS SOON AS POSSIBLE.

8. Loosen restrictive clothing at the neck and waist.
9. Provide appropriate care for fractures.
10. Give nothing to the patient by mouth. ANTICIPATE VOMITING, having suction available for immediate use.
11. Monitor vital signs every 5 minutes.
12. Keep the patient warm.
13. Transport as soon as possible to a medical facility. Avoid rough and excessive handling. Remember, patients with bleeding into the chest and abdominal cavities are HIGH-PRIORITY PATIENTS.

CHAPTER REVIEW

KEY TERMS

You may find it helpful to review the following terms.

artery—any major blood vessel carrying blood away from the heart.
brachial (BRAY-ke-al) **artery**—the major artery of the upper arm. Some types of external bleeding from the upper extremity can be controlled by applying pressure to the brachial artery pressure point.
capillary—the thin-walled, microscopic blood vessels where oxygen/carbon dioxide and nutrient/waste exchange with the tissues takes place.
embolism (EM-bo-liz-m)—a moving blood clot or foreign body, such as fat or an air bubble inside a blood vessel. (The plural is *emboli*.)
femoral (FEM-o-ral) **artery**—the major artery supplying the thigh. Some types of external bleeding from the lower extremity can be controlled by applying pressure to the femoral artery pressure point.
formed elements—red blood cells, white blood cells, and platelets.
hemorrhage (HEM-o-rej)—internal or external bleeding.

liter (LE-ter)—metric measurement of liquid volume that is equal to 1.057 quarts. One pint is almost equal to one-half liter.
perfusion—the constant flow of blood through capillaries.
plasma (PLAZ-mah)—the fluid portion of the blood. It is the blood minus the formed elements.
pressure dressing—a bulky dressing held in position with a tightly wrapped bandage to apply pressure to help control bleeding.
pressure point—a site where a main artery lies near the surface of the body and directly over a bone. Pressure on such a point can stop distal bleeding.
temporal (TEMP-o-ral) **artery**—the major artery in the region of the temple. Some types of external scalp bleeding can be controlled by applying pressure to the temporal pressure point.
tourniquet (TURN-i-ket)—a device that constricts all blood flow to and from an extremity.
tourniquet shock—a dangerous condition caused when a tourniquet is loosened or released, and toxic substances that have gathered distal to the tourniquet are released in high concentrations to the rest of the body.
vein—any major blood vessel returning blood to the heart.

SUMMARY

The Blood and Blood Vessels

The blood is living tissue which is made up of plasma (the fluid portion of the blood) and formed elements (the red and white blood cells and the platelets). Blood has many functions within the body, including transportation of gasses, nutrition, excretion, protection, and regulation.

All humans have a certain blood volume. This volume is dependent on the size and weight of the person. When a person loses 25 to 40 % of blood volume, a life-threatening condition exists. A very small amount of blood loss is critical to a child.

The blood is carried through the body by three types of blood vessels: arteries, capillaries, and veins.

Arteries are muscular and carry blood away from the heart at high pressures.

Capillaries are microscopic vessels between the veins and arteries.

Veins return blood to the heart. They contain blood at a lower pressure than arteries. Veins contain valves that keep blood flowing in the proper direction.

Bleeding may be internal or external.

External Bleeding

External bleeding is visible outside the body. Bleeding from an artery is called arterial bleeding. This type of bleeding is difficult to control and is characterized by bright red, spurting blood. Bleeding from a vein is called venous bleeding and is usually flowing rather than spurting and dark red or maroon in color. Bleeding from capillaries is usually slow or oozing, and not as bright as arterial blood.

In addition to observed bleeding, a trail or pool of blood and signs of shock including a rapid pulse, rapid and shallow breathing, and restless or combative behavior indicate possible severe blood loss.

Infection control practices should always be used when there is external bleeding. The four major methods of external bleeding control are direct pressure, elevation, use of pressure points, and—as a last resort—application of a tourniquet.

Use a gloved hand to apply direct pressure over a bleeding wound. If possible, use a sterile dressing. Once a dressing is placed directly over a wound, never remove it. On extremities, a pressure bandage may be applied to help stop bleeding.

Use elevation, usually in combination with direct pressure, to control bleeding from an extremity, when there is no fracture or spinal injury.

Use external hand pressure to compress pressure points along an artery proximal to the bleeding. This is most often performed on the brachial (arm), or femoral (leg) arteries.

Using a tourniquet to control bleeding is a *last resort*, as it may cause loss of the limb. Place the tourniquet over a pad that has been set close to the wound, over the main supplying artery between the site of the wound and the patient's heart. Tighten the tourniquet to the point at which the bleeding stops and fix the tourniquet in place at this point. A plainly visible notation must be made that a tourniquet is in use. ONCE THE TOURNIQUET IS IN PLACE, DO NOT LOOSEN IT. A blood pressure cuff may also be used as a tourniquet.

Additional means of controlling or helping to control external bleeding include splinting, cold applications, and application of anti-shock garments. Anti-shock garments are used only if local protocols permit.

Internal Bleeding

Internal bleeding can be very serious. Look for mechanisms of injury that may cause internal bleeding, and look for wounds associated with this type of bleeding, look for signs of internal bleeding, and signs and symptoms of shock.

Signs of internal bleeding include (in the order you may discover them during a head-to-toe survey): bruises on the neck, wounds to the skull, blood or blood fluids in the ears or nose, vomiting or coughing up blood, bruises on the chest or signs of rib fracture, wounds that have penetrated the chest or abdomen, bruises or swellings of the abdomen, abdominal tenderness, rigidity or spasms, blood in the urine, rectal or vaginal bleeding, and bone fractures especially to the pelvis and the long bones of the arm and thigh.

Any time that a patient is suspected of having internal bleeding, check for shock. Signs and symptoms of shock associated with internal bleeding include anxiety or restlessness, weakness, thirst, and feeling cold. If the patient has signs of shock with no outward injuries, always consider internal bleeding.

Management of the patient with internal injuries is centered around treatment for shock. This is discussed in the next chapter. In addition, pressure dressings and splints can be applied for external bleeding that is found in an extremity.

Remember: Administration of a high concentration of oxygen is an important treatment for a patient with any kind of bleeding or potential for shock.

CHAPTER

8

On the Scene

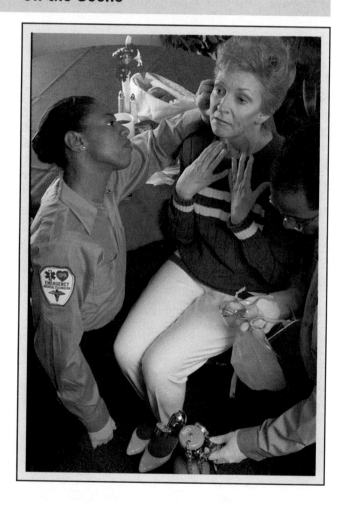

A coworker notices the look of concern on Allyson's face. Hives, too, are now visible on her face and neck. The coworker asks Allyson if she wants an ambulance, and Allyson gasps "yes." When you arrive, you can see from across the room that Allyson is having considerable difficulty breathing. As a coworker leads you to her, he tells you, "I think she's having a heart attack."

You: Ms. Wells, I'm Felicia Richardson, an EMT from the ambulance. Can you tell me what's wrong?

Allyson Wells: I just can't catch my breath. My chest is tight, too. It all came on so suddenly.

You: My partner is setting up some oxygen to put on. That should help your breathing. Has this ever happened before?

Allyson Wells: Well, yes, I have some allergies. I'm careful not to eat shellfish.

While you continue your assessment, your partner applies a nonrebreather oxygen mask. The restaurant manager approaches and asks if she can help. You ask if there were any shellfish in Allyson's dinner. The manager checks with the chef and reports that shrimp and lobster shells were used in making the sauce.

Allyson Wells has just had a promotion. To celebrate, she is having dinner with friends from work. Just into the main course, Allyson suddenly develops chest tightness and difficulty breathing. Initially, Allyson thinks it may be from the excitement of the promotion and the dinner. As the chest tightness worsens, she knows it is more serious.

It appears that Allyson is having anaphylactic shock, an allergic reaction, and not a heart attack. But this does not mean that her condition is not serious. Anaphylactic shock is a life-threatening condition. You arrange for immediate transport with paramedic intercept en route.

Shock

Shock is a life-threatening condition that can be the result of any serious injury and many medical conditions. As an EMT you must be familiar with the variety of causes of shock (profuse bleeding is the most common but not the only cause) and have a general knowledge of the physiology of shock (what goes on inside the body when shock occurs). More important, you must be able to recognize shock or the potential for shock in your patient and provide treatment to prevent the condition from developing or worsening and to keep the patient stable until advanced or definitive care can begin at the hospital.

Expected Outcome, Chapter 8: *You will understand how shock occurs and you will be able to help prevent and treat for shock.*

> **Warning:** Protect yourself from infectious diseases by using appropriate barrier devices such as a pocket face mask with one-way valve, face shield, or bag-valve mask; goggles or eye shield; and disposable gloves. Always conform to your local EMS system's infection exposure control plan.

ABOUT SHOCK
  Causes of Shock
  Types of Shock

TREATING FOR SHOCK
  Detecting Shock
  Preventing and Managing Shock
  Anaphylactic Shock
  Fainting

ANTI-SHOCK GARMENTS
  How Anti-Shock Garments Work
  Controversy About Anti-Shock Garments
  Indications
  Contraindications
  Applying an Anti-Shock Garment
  Removing an Anti-Shock Garment

Knowledge *After reading this chapter, you should be able to*

1. Define shock and match the causes of shock to the types of shock. (pp. 220-222)

2. List the signs and symptoms of shock. (pp. 222-224)

3. Define *compensated shock* and *decompensated shock* and list the signs of compensated shock. (pp. 224-225)

4. Describe, step by step, the procedures used in the prevention and the care for shock. (pp. 225-227)

5. Describe anaphylactic shock in terms of what it is, how serious it is, and what causes it. (p. 227)

6. List the signs and symptoms of anaphylactic shock. (p. 228)

7. Describe the care that should be provided for anaphylactic shock. (pp. 228-229)

8. Describe how to reduce a patient's chances of fainting. (p. 230)

Anti-Shock Garments

9. Define *anti-shock garment* and explain two mechanisms by which anti-shock garments work. (pp. 230-231)

10. List the indications for the use of anti-shock garments. (p. 231)

11. State the absolute contraindication and the relative contraindications for the use of the anti-shock garment. (pp. 231-232)

12. Describe how to apply an anti-shock garment. (p. 232; Scan 8-1)

13. Describe how to remove an anti-shock garment. (pp. 232; 235)

Skills *As an EMT you should be able to*

1. Survey for shock and anaphylactic shock.

2. Apply the measures needed to prevent shock and to care for shock.

3. Apply the measures needed to care for anaphylactic shock.

4. Carry out appropriate procedures to help prevent fainting.

Optional Objectives, Anti-Shock Garments

5. Correctly apply an anti-shock garment.

6. Correctly remove an anti-shock garment.

The first hour after injury is known as the golden hour. If advanced life support is started and the required surgery can begin during this hour, many trauma patients have an improved chance of survival. The major problem to be cared for during this hour is shock. Once shock reaches a certain level of severity, the patient cannot be saved.

ABOUT SHOCK

Shock is the body's response to a failure of adequate perfusion, or blood flow through the capillaries, to all tissues and organs. There are a number of possible causes of shock, resulting from severe illness or injury.

Causes of Shock

The heart and the blood vessels make up the **vascular container**, the system that contains the body's blood. To function properly, this container must be filled with blood and must be efficiently pumped by the heart. The failure of perfusion that causes shock happens when the vascular container is not filled.

Three elements of the vascular system—the heart, the blood, and the blood vessels—can be related to the failure to keep the vascular container full and the consequent development of shock.

- The Heart—If the heart fails to pump blood efficiently enough to keep the vascular container filled, shock will develop.
- The Blood—There cannot be too little blood

to fill the vascular container. A serious loss of blood or plasma will lead to shock.

- The Blood Vessels—The vascular container cannot be too large for the volume of blood. Dilation (expansion) of blood vessels, without sufficient constriction (shrinking or contraction) of other blood vessels to compensate (make up for the expanded vessels) can cause shock.

If there is a failure of any of these three factors—the pumping of the heart, the supply of blood, or the dilation and compensatory constriction of the blood vessels—perfusion in the brain, lungs, and other body organs will not be adequate.

Understanding the role of the blood vessels in the development of shock is important. Blood vessels can change their diameter. If an area of the body requires more blood because it is doing more work, the vessels in that area dilate as needed to allow greater flow. At the same time, another area of the body that does not require the extra blood flow may constrict its vessels to reduce the blood flow in that area and help keep the overall system filled with blood. If you are running, blood flow to the muscles increases through dilated arteries. At the same time, blood flow to the stomach and intestines lessens because vessels supplying these organs have constricted. If all the vessels in the body dilated at once, there would not be nearly enough blood to fill the entire system, causing circulation to fail. Whenever too many vessels dilate to allow for adequate perfusion (filling the capillaries), shock develops.

As shock develops, the failure of any one part of the vascular system can create problems in the other parts. For example, if blood is being lost through bleeding, the heart rate will increase in an effort to circulate blood to all the vital tissues. This action causes more blood to be lost. Immediately, the body will react to this additional blood loss by again increasing the heart rate. This process will continue, leading to the death of the patient.

At the onset of shock, the body tries to adjust to the loss of blood, improper heart activity, or the dilation of too many blood vessels. However, at a certain point in some types of shock, enough blood has been lost so that the system is no longer filled, no matter how hard the heart pumps or how much the blood vessels constrict. In other cases of shock, the heart becomes too inefficient in circulating blood and perfusion fails. There are also cases in which there is no loss of blood volume and the heart is performing properly, but too many vessels are dilated. For these cases, there is too much volume (capacity) in the system to be filled by the available blood.

Regardless of the mechanism, shock is the failure of the cardiovascular system to provide sufficient blood to all the vital tissues of the body.

Remember: Shock may develop (1) if the heart fails as a pump, or (2) blood volume is lost, or (3) blood vessels dilate to create a vascular container capacity too great to be filled by the available blood.

Types of Shock

Shock may accompany many emergency situations; thus treatment for it is included in emergency care procedures for virtually every serious injury and medical problem.

There is more than one type of shock. A patient may develop

- *Hypovolemic* (HI-po-vo-LE-mik) *Shock*—caused by the loss of blood or other body fluids. When shock develops due to blood loss or loss of plasma, this form of hypovolemic shock is called *hemorrhagic* (HEM-or-RAJ-ik) *shock*. Dehydration due to diarrhea, vomiting, or heavy perspiration can also lead to the development of hypovolemic shock.
- *Cardiogenic* (KAR-di-o-JEN-ic) *Shock*—caused by the heart failing to pump blood adequately to all vital parts of the body
- *Neurogenic* (NU-ro-JEN-ic) *Shock*—caused by the failure of the nervous system to control the diameter of blood vessels (seen with spinal injury). Once the blood vessels are dilated, there is not enough blood in circulation to fill this new volume, causing shock.
- *Anaphylactic* (AN-ah-fi-LAK-tik) *Shock*—a life-threatening reaction of the body to a substance to which the patient is extremely allergic.
- *Psychogenic* (SI-ko-JEN-ic) *Shock*—is fainting, a nervous system reaction. It is often brought about by fear, bad news, the sight of blood, or a minor injury. A sudden dilation of the blood vessels takes place and the proper blood flow to the brain is momentarily interrupted, causing the patient to faint.

This is a temporary condition and is considered a self-correcting form of shock.

- *Metabolic* (MET-ah-BOL-ik) *Shock*—associated with changes in body chemistry, including salt balance and acid-base balance. Failure of the adrenal, thyroid, or pituitary glands may lead to metabolic shock.
- *Septic Shock*—caused by severe infection. Toxins (poisons) are released into the bloodstream and cause blood vessels to dilate, increasing the volume of the circulatory system beyond functional limits. In addition, plasma is lost through vessel walls, causing a loss in blood volume. This type of shock is seldom seen by the EMT in the field since the patient is usually hospitalized before it occurs.

The most common form of serious shock associated with injury is the form of hypovolemic shock known as hemorrhagic shock (think of the word *hemorrhage*, meaning "bleeding"), due to the loss of blood. Bleeding can be external or internal. In addition to the loss of whole blood, enough plasma may also be lost to result in a severe drop in blood volume. This may be the case with burns and crushing injuries. A pre-existing condition of dehydration will hasten the reaction. Be alert to this in areas of high temperatures, such as warehouses and factories. This also can be a problem if the patient was sweating profusely prior to injury, as in sports and hunting accidents. Certain strenuous work situations, such as those of dockworkers and steelworkers, may cause enough body fluid loss prior to the accident to quicken the effects of blood loss.

Cardiogenic shock is usually brought about by injuries to the heart, heart attacks, or electrical shock. Many diseases, if allowed to go untreated, may eventually do enough heart damage to cause cardiogenic shock. Be on the alert for low blood pressure, edema (swelling) of the ankles, and the signs of heart failure (see Chapter 15).

In neurogenic shock due to nerve paralysis caused by spinal cord or brain injuries, there is no actual loss of blood but rather a dilation of blood vessels that increases the volume of the circulatory system beyond the point where it can be filled. Blood can no longer adequately fill the entire system and pools in the blood vessels in certain areas of the body. Severe blows to the abdomen also can disrupt nerves, possibly bringing about neurogenic shock.

TREATING FOR SHOCK

Detecting Shock

Shock sometimes occurs very rapidly, placing the patient in a critical condition long before you arrive at the scene. In other cases, the patient may develop shock slowly as you provide care. There is a saying used by EMS personnel: "Patients can go into shock a little at a time." For such patients, you will have warning signs, but never assume that an apparently stable patient will not go into shock. *Monitor your patients!*

Patient Assessment—Shock

The signs and symptoms of shock usually develop in a specific order, which will be discussed later in this chapter. However, as an EMT, you are likely to encounter the patient after he has begun to develop shock, so you may not be able to observe the full sequence of development.

Imagine that you have just arrived at an accident scene. Look over the signs and symptoms listed below and consider how you might obtain them during a patient assessment (Figure 8-1 and Figure 8-2).

Signs

☐ ENTIRE BODY: Look for evidence of
- Restlessness or signs of fear
- Profuse external bleeding
- Mechanism of injury suggesting internal bleeding
- Nausea and/or vomiting
- Shaking and trembling (rare)

☐ LEVEL OF CONSCIOUSNESS: Sudden unresponsiveness, faintness, loss of consciousness, or changes in behavior (confusion, agitation)

☐ PULSE: Rapid and weak (an early sign)

☐ BREATHING: Shallow and rapid

☐ BLOOD PRESSURE: Low. The blood pressure may be 90/60 or lower (a late sign).

☐ SKIN: Pale, moist, and cool. There is often profuse sweating and a clammy feel to the touch.

☐ EYES: Lackluster, dilated pupils

☐ FACE: Pale, often with cyanosis (bluish color) at the lips and earlobes.

☐ CAPILLARY REFILL: Slow. When you apply pressure to the tip of a nail bed, it will turn

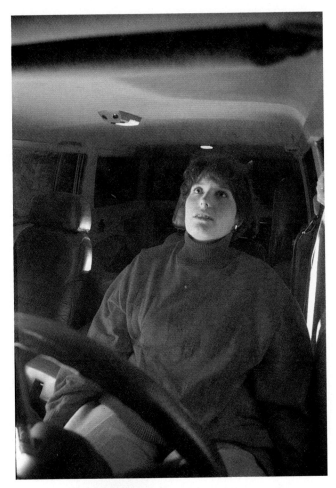

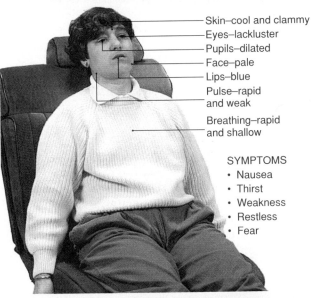

Skin–cool and clammy
Eyes–lackluster
Pupils–dilated
Face–pale
Lips–blue
Pulse–rapid and weak
Breathing–rapid and shallow

SYMPTOMS
• Nausea
• Thirst
• Weakness
• Restless
• Fear

SIGNS
• Restlessness   • Becomes unresponsive

Figure 8-1 and **Figure 8-2** Signs and symptoms of shock.

white. (In infants and children, compress the entire back of the hand or foot.) When pressure is released, it should regain nor-

mal color in 2 seconds or less. When capillary refill time takes longer than 2 seconds, it may be an indication of shock. A simple rule to follow is that the refill should take place in less time than it takes to say "capillary refill."

Symptoms

☐ Nausea
☐ Thirst
☐ Weakness
☐ Dizziness
☐ Feeling cool or cold
☐ A feeling of impending doom.

Note: Blood pressure is a late sign in the development of shock. A good EMT will expect shock and have started treatment before the blood pressure begins to drop. Because a patient has a blood pressure of 90/60 or even below may not in itself indicate shock. Some patients have normally low blood pressure. A reading of 88/56 may be normal for them. Low blood pressure must also be correlated with other signs of shock. *When a patient has low blood pressure, a rapid pulse, and cool, clammy skin, this WHOLE PICTURE indicates shock.*

Caution: Children and young adults may not show signs of shock until an extremely large volume of blood has been lost. Some children will not experience a decreased blood pressure until *40% of the circulating blood volume is lost.* This means that they will not display a lowered blood pressure until they are near death! Do not be fooled by this phenomenon in the field.

All the symptoms and signs of shock are usually not present at once, nor do they occur in the order in which they may be detected during the patient assessment. It is important that the EMT constantly re-evaluate any patient with the potential for shock. In most cases, as shock develops, the sequence of events is as follows (Figure 8-3).

Early development: The body compensates for shock.

1. *Increased pulse rate* indicates that the body is adjusting to the loss of blood, plasma, or other body fluids, or that it is trying to adjust for some other cause of inefficient circulation. Unlike the rapid pulse rate associated with the stress and fear of the emergency, this increased rate will not slow down. The rate may rise significantly when the patient assumes an erect or sitting position.

Early Development	Loss of Compensation	Late Development
Increased pulse rate	Skin color changes	Changes in levels of consciousness
Increased respirations	Rapid, weak pulse	Marked drop in blood pressure
Restlessness	Labored breathing	Weak pulse
Fearfulness	Weakness	Weakened respirations
Increased capillary refill time	Thirstiness	
	Nausea	

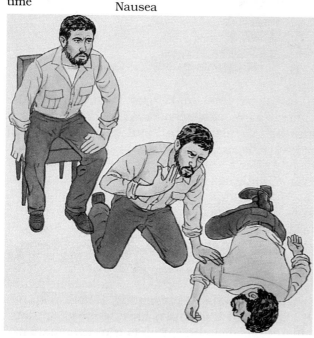

Figure 8-3 The development of shock.

2. *Increased breathing rate* occurs next, but not in all cases. The patient developing shock has inefficient circulation. This means that his tissues may not be receiving enough oxygen and that carbon dioxide is increasing at the tissue level. His body attempts to compensate by increasing the rate of breathing. This rate will not slow down as it does in cases of stress.

3. *Restlessness or combativeness* is the patient's reaction to his body's attempt to compensate for the developing shock. This may be the first detectable sign in some cases. He often "feels" that something is wrong. In many cases, the patient looks afraid.

Full-blown shock: The body stops compensating.

4. *Skin changes and increase of capillary refill time to greater than 2 seconds* will be detected. Skin changes start early in the development of shock, but they may not be noticed until the latter stages. The patient's skin will turn pale and his lips, nailbeds, and the membranes in his mouth will show cyanosis. Diaphoresis (profuse sweating) is usually present.

5. *Thirst, weakness, and nausea* may be noticed.

6. *Rapid, weak pulse and labored, weakened respirations* indicate that the body is failing in its attempts to compensate for the circulatory system failure.

Late developments

7. *Changes in level of consciousness* may occur. This may precede detection of weakened respiratory efforts. The effects of inadequate circulation to the brain will cause the patient to become confused, disoriented, sleepy, or unconscious.

8. *A marked drop in blood pressure* will occur, indicating the failure of the patient's body to compensate for the developing shock. This may be delayed in children and young adults.

Preventing and Managing Shock

The same basic care should be used to keep a patient from *developing* shock and to manage a patient who is *in* shock. *The best management for shock is prevention.*

Note: Whenever there is even the possibility of shock developing, treat for shock by administering a high concentration of oxygen.

Patient Assessment—Compensated Shock

Keep in mind that a patient's body may be able to compensate for the early effects of shock, especially if the patient is young and in good physical condition. This is known as **compensated shock**, and its signs may appear in this order.

1. A slight increase in pulse rate
2. Increased capillary refill time
3. A slight drop in systolic blood pressure and an increase in diastolic pressure

This type of patient will appear to be stable, but he is actually at his limit in being able to compensate. Unless he receives immediate effective care for shock, his body will no longer be able to compensate adequately and he will rapidly decline, quickly showing the symptoms and signs of life-threatening shock, or **decompensated shock**, that were listed under "Detecting Shock," above.

When the nature of the injury or illness or the mechanism of injury indicates that shock is a possibility, care for shock, regardless of the patient's symptoms or signs. The following is an example of this kind of patient.

A 29-year-old female is driving home from work when she is involved in a motor vehicle collision. The damage to her car is extensive, but she claims to be "OK" except for some minor pain in her abdomen. An exam by an EMT reveals a bruise on the left side of the patient's abdomen. Her pulse is 112 and capillary refill time is 3 seconds.

This patient has the signs and symptoms of compensated shock. Her pulse is elevated, capillary refill time is greater than 2 seconds, and the damage to her vehicle and subsequent abdominal bruising provide a mechanism of injury that points to internal bleeding.

An EMT who did not understand shock might take a blood pressure, get a "normal" reading, and not treat the patient for her likely injuries.

Remember: When the nature of the illness or injury or the mechanism of injury indicates that shock is a possibility, care for shock, regardless of the patient's signs or symptoms.

Shock can be the result of many types of medical and trauma (injury) emergencies. The EMT's main treatments for trauma-related shock are controlling external bleeding, administering oxygen, and reassuring the patient. The next phase of care, which is beyond the EMT level and usually provided at the hospital, is definitive treatment, which includes advanced life support measures and, most important in cases of trauma, surgery.

The "golden hour of trauma," within which definitive care must be given, was mentioned at the beginning of this chapter. When treating the critical trauma patient on the scene, the "platinum ten minutes" must be kept in mind, the ten minutes during which emergency care for life-threatening conditions, including bleeding and shock, must be initiated if at all possible (obviously this may not be possible if, for example, the patient is pinned inside a vehicle). Patients in any type of shock, or with the potential for shock, must be transported to the hospital without delay.

Remember: Prompt transportation should be considered a treatment for all patients in shock.

Patient Care—Shock

As you read the following list of care measures for patients with shock or the potential for shock, consider that steps 1-4 may be done on the scene. These include the ABCs, oxygen, spinal precautions, and backboarding. Steps 5-11 may be done en route to the hospital.

Emergency Care Steps

1. *Ensure an open airway and breathing* (see Chapters 4, 5, and 6). As in all cases, if the patient is breathing, maintain an adequate airway. If the patient is not breathing, establish an airway and provide rescue breathing. Have suction equipment ready and stay alert for vomiting. If both respiration and circulation have stopped, initiate CPR measures. If this is a trauma patient, use the jaw thrust maneuver for airway control.

2. *Control bleeding* (see Chapter 7). Use direct pressure, elevation, pressure points, or other methods as required. The loss of blood volume is life threatening for the shock patient. Apply an anti-shock garment when local protocols recommend (see later in this chapter).

3. *Administer oxygen as soon as possible* (see Chapter 6). An oxygen deficiency will result from the reduced circulation taking place in shock. Provide a high concentration of oxygen. STAY ALERT FOR VOMITING.

4. Immobilize for possible spinal injuries.

5. *Splint fractures* (see Chapters 10 and 11). Splinting slows bleeding and reduces pain, both of which aggravate shock. AVOID ROUGH HANDLING since body motion has a tendency to aggravate shock.

6. *Position the patient* (Figure 8-4). You have three choices of patient position, depending on the patient's problem and local policies.

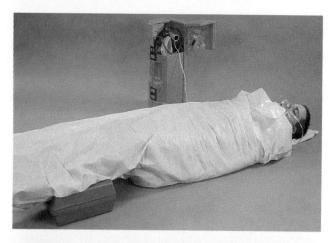

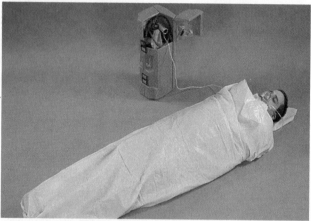

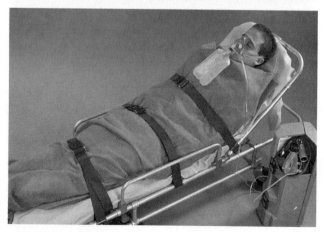

Figure 8-4 Positioning the shock patient.

- LOWER EXTREMITY ELEVATION: This is the most recommended position. Raise the patient's legs slightly, about 12 inches. If there are fractures of the lower extremities, they cannot be major and they must be splinted before being elevated. Do not use this procedure if there are indications of neck or spinal injuries, head injuries, chest injuries,

abdominal injuries, hip dislocations or fractures, or pelvic fractures. Do not tilt the patient's entire body into a head-down position. To do so will press the abdominal organs against the diaphragm.

- SUPINE: The patient is placed flat on his back, with adequate padding to provide comfort. This position is often used if there are serious injuries to the extremities.
- SEMISEATED (semi-Fowler's): This position is used for conscious medical patients with indications of respiratory or heart problems. It is not recommended for patients with the signs and symptoms of internal or external bleeding. If blood pressure is low, the patient should remain flat to help raise blood pressure.

The idea is to keep the patient as comfortable as possible and to allow him to find the position that provides for the easiest breathing. Regardless of the position used, monitor the patient's vital signs and be alert for vomiting.

7 REASSURE THE PATIENT.

8 *Keep the patient lying still.* The more at rest a shock patient remains, the better are his chances for survival.

9 *Prevent loss of body heat.* Your goal is to keep the patient's body temperature as near to normal as possible. Place a blanket under and over the patient (ground placement of the blanket is best done when positioning the patient so as not to increase body movement). Prevent heat loss, but DO NOT ALLOW THE PATIENT TO OVERHEAT. When possible, remove any wet clothing. *Do not* move patients with head, neck, or spinal injury for the purpose of placing a blanket under them.

10 *Give nothing by mouth.* The patient in shock or developing shock may develop a dry mouth and thirst. Also, the oxygen being administered may dry the patient's oral and nasal pathways. If oxygen is to be used for long periods, the humidification of the oxygen should be considered. *Do not* give the patient anything to drink, including ice. *Do not* give any food or medications orally. To do so will probably induce vomiting.

11 *Monitor the patient.* You must take vital signs and record the results when you do the patient assessment. Check and record

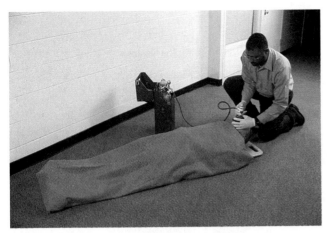

Figure 8-5 Managing the shock patient.

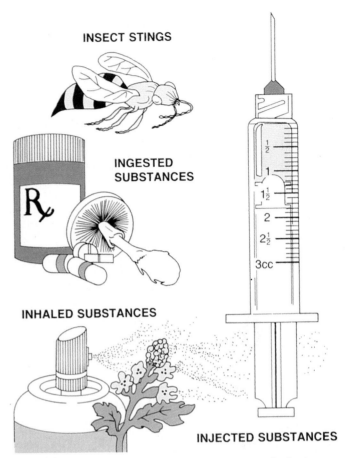

Figure 8-6 Substances that can cause anaphylactic shock.

these signs EVERY 5 MINUTES until you deliver both patient and information to a medical facility staff (Figure 8-5).

The use of anti-shock garments may be part of your EMS System's protocol for certain shock patients. See the end of this chapter for details.

Anaphylactic Shock

Anaphylactic shock results from a severe allergic reaction. It must always be considered to be life threatening.

Almost any of a wide variety of substances can be an **allergen**, something that causes an adverse physical reaction in some persons who come in contact with it. For example, cat dander can be an allergen. A person who is allergic to cat dander will sneeze and itch whenever a cat is nearby. This is a minor allergic reaction. Other allergic reactions are more severe. Consider bee stings. Some people have no reaction other than pain and some swelling at the sting site. A few people have more serious reactions to bee stings, developing anaphylactic shock.

In anaphylactic shock, exposure to the allergen will cause blood vessels to dilate rapidly and cause a drop in blood pressure (hypotension). The tissues that line the respiratory system may swell and obstruct the airway, leading to respiratory failure.

Causes of anaphylactic reactions include (Figure 8-6)

- INSECT STINGS—The stings of bees, yellow jackets, wasps, and hornets can cause rapid and severe reactions.

- INGESTED SUBSTANCES—Foods such as nuts, spices, berries, fish, and shellfish, as well as certain drugs can cause reactions. In most cases, the effect is slower than that seen with insect stings.
- INHALED SUBSTANCES—Dust, pollens, and chemical powders can often cause very rapid and severe reactions.
- INJECTED SUBSTANCES—Antitoxins and drugs such as penicillin may cause severe reactions.
- ABSORBED SUBSTANCES—Certain chemicals, when in contact with the skin, produce severe reactions.

Patient Assessment—Anaphylactic Shock

There is no way to predict the exact course of anaphylactic shock. Severe reactions may take place immediately or be delayed 30 minutes or more. A very mild allergic reaction may turn into more serious anaphylactic shock in a matter of minutes.

SIGNS OF ALLERGY SHOCK

- Restlessness

- Fainting, coma

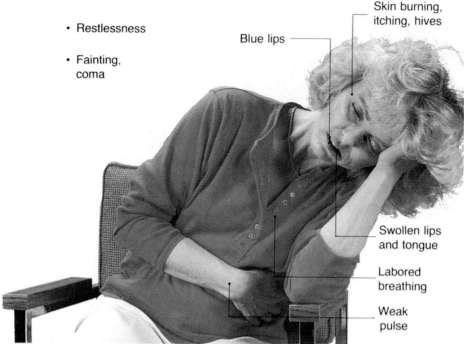

Skin burning, itching, hives

Blue lips

Swollen lips and tongue

Labored breathing

Weak pulse

Figure 8-7 Signs of anaphylactic shock.

Signs

The signs of anaphylactic shock can include (Figure 8-7)

- ☐ LEVEL OF CONSCIOUSNESS: Restlessness, often followed by fainting or unconsciousness
- ☐ BREATHING: Difficult, sometimes with wheezing or rales
- ☐ PULSE: Rapid and very weak or imperceptible
- ☐ BLOOD PRESSURE: Above normal at first and then it may drop to shock level
- ☐ SKIN: Obvious irritation or blotches (such as hives)
- ☐ FACE: Marked swelling of the face and tongue, often with cyanosis of lips and paleness around the mouth and tongue
- ☐ VOMITING
- ☐ EXTREMITIES: Often there is swelling of the ankles and/or wrists

Symptoms

The symptoms of anaphylactic shock can include

- ☐ Itching and burning skin, especially about the face, chest, and back

- ☐ Painful constriction of the chest with difficult breathing
- ☐ Dizziness
- ☐ Feelings of restlessness and anxiety
- ☐ Nausea, abdominal pain, or diarrhea
- ☐ Headache
- ☐ Temporary loss of consciousness (rare)

Again, relate the signs and symptoms listed above to the patient assessment process.

Patient Care—Anaphylactic Shock

Anaphylactic shock is a serious emergency requiring the injection of medications to combat the allergic reaction.

Emergency Care Steps

Initial emergency care efforts should be directed toward basic life support. As an EMT, you should

1. *Provide basic life support measures.* Maintain an open airway and perform rescue breathing or CPR as required.
2. *Provide a high concentration of oxygen and care for shock.*

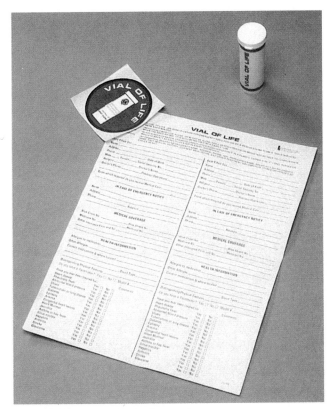

Figure 8-8 A "Vial of Life" sticker.

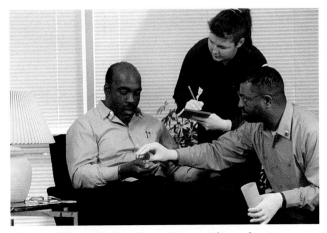

Figure 8-9 Assisting the patient with medications.

3 *Transport to a medical facility immediately.* Notify the facility by radio on the way. Place the alert patient in a supine or semi-Fowlers position. If the information is available, tell the staff the substance causing the reaction and the means of patient contact (e.g., sting, inhalation). Continue basic life support measures during transport.

Note: In some jurisdictions, protocols call for the EMT to provide basic life support and wait for an advanced life support response.

When interviewing a patient, it is always helpful to ask if they have any allergies. This includes allergies to food, environmental items, medications, and so on. Unexplained symptoms may be explained by an allergic reaction.

Patients who have known severe allergic reactions may have medication to take immediately after coming in contact with an allergen. If you are in the patient's residence, you may find a "Vial of Life" (Figure 8-8) or similar type of sticker on the main outside door, the closest window to the main door, or the refrigerator door. The sticker indicates that patient informa-

tion and medications can be found in the refrigerator. Often the EMT is asked to assist in administering this medication (Figure 8-9). Many of these medications are in an injectable form and beyond the level of training of the EMT. In this situation the EMT should rely on local protocols to guide their actions. If there are questions, medical control may be contacted for advice.

Fainting

As noted in our classification of shock, fainting (**syncope**, SIN-ko-PE) is a self-correcting form of shock resulting from a temporary lack of adequate blood flow to the brain. Usually, the serious problems related to fainting are injuries that occur during falls that result from the temporary loss of consciousness. Fainting may be caused by stressful situations. However, it may be an indication that the patient has blood pressure problems (a sudden drop or elevation) or some other serious medical problem. Brain tumors, heart disease, undetected diabetes, and inner ear disorders are just a few medical problems that may first present themselves through fainting. Fainting in an older person is a serious sign more often than with younger patients. Often, it may indicate a serious cardiovascular problem that may prove to be lethal.

Patient Assessment—Fainting

Take the pulse and blood pressure of anyone who faints. The pulse may be rapid or, in some cases, very slow.

Emergency Care Steps

FOR A PATIENT WHO HAS FAINTED

1. *Recommend seeing a physician if additional care is refused.* If you are called to the scene of a fainting and the patient refuses to be transported for additional care, recommend that he see a physician as soon as possible.

2. *Advise against driving or operating machinery.* In a polite but firm manner, tell the patient not to drive or operate any machinery until he has been examined by a physician.

3. *Document refusal of care.* Make certain that you have the patient's witnessed refusal in writing, relay information to the medical facility, and write an extensive documentation about refusal.

4. *Provide emotional support.*

FOR A PATIENT WHO FEELS FAINT

1. *Most patients*—Seat the patient with head between knees if there is no injury or heart condition. You can often prevent a patient from fainting by placing him in a seated position and lowering his head to a level between the knees (Figure 8-10). Do not do this for patients with fractures, possible neck or spinal injuries, or severe head injuries. This procedure is not recommended for anyone having difficulty breathing or who has a known heart problem.

2. *Patients with breathing or heart problems*—Have a patient with difficulty breathing or a heart problem lie down with the feet slightly elevated and give emotional support. This will provide protection and may prevent fainting.

3. *Patients with congestive heart failure or COPD*—Place the patient who is suffering from congestive heart failure or COPD (chronic obstructive pulmonary disease, see Chapter 15) in a semiseated position. This will provide comfort and allow you to protect him in case he faints.

ANTI-SHOCK GARMENTS

In some EMS systems, the use of anti-shock garments is not recommended because of potential problems that will be discussed in the next segment. In systems where they are used, protocols and guidelines for their use vary from locality to locality. Follow the recommendations of your instructor and local protocols with regard to the use of anti-shock garments.

An **anti-shock garment** is a garment that covers the abdomen and lower extremities and is inflated to apply pneumatic counterpressure. *Pneumatic counterpressure* refers to the use of air to create pressure against something. In the case of anti-shock garments, the pressure is applied against the flow of blood. These devices are referred to as *pneumatic anti-shock garments (PASG), military anti-shock trousers (MAST),* and *pneumatic counter pressure devices.* The term *anti-shock garment* will be used in this section.

The anti-shock garment has many uses, some of which are controversial. These uses include treatment of severe hypovolemic shock, control of bleeding, splinting, and more. This text may describe uses for the anti-shock garment that are not recommended in your area. Always follow the protocols of your local EMS system regarding use of anti-shock garments.

How Anti-Shock Garments Work

The anti-shock garment is designed to counteract hypovolemia (low circulating blood volume) and occasionally is effective against certain internal bleeding. The garment does this by developing an encircling pressure around both lower extremities, the pelvis, and the abdomen. This pressure slows or stops bleeding in the

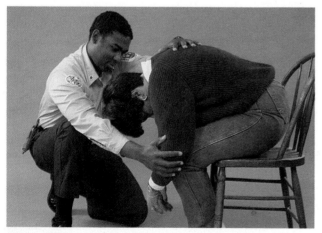

Figure 8-10 Protect the patient and try to prevent fainting.

areas of the body that are enclosed by the pressurized garment. Bleeding is controlled by direct pressure the garment places on the damaged vessel or vessels.

The anti-shock garment causes an elevation of blood pressure. The rise in blood pressure may be caused by one or more of the following mechanisms.

- The anti-shock garment may cause blood from the lower extremities to be pushed up into the central circulation. This has been called an "autotransfusion" of blood.
- The second possible mechanism is an increase in systemic vascular resistance. This means that the anti-shock garment creates a constriction of the blood vessels which, in turn, causes an increase in blood pressure.

There are a number of advantages associated with the use of an anti-shock garment other than the effect on blood pressure. Among these are

- The garment can be applied quickly and not inflated until it is needed.
- An anti-shock garment could serve as an air splint for a fractured pelvis and lower extremity fractures.
- Electrocardiograms and x-rays can be taken and a Foley catheter (used to drain the urinary bladder) can be inserted while the patient is in an inflated garment.
- Intravenous lines can be started more easily in some cases due to the increase in the volume of blood in the vascular beds in the upper extremities.

Some of the disadvantages of using anti-shock garments include

- There may be an increase of fluids in the lungs of some elderly patients.
- There may be increased difficulty in breathing or discomfort during breathing for some patients.
- Bleeding may increase in areas not enclosed by the device.
- There may be a worsening of injury at the diaphragm (traumatic diaphragmatic herniation).
- Nausea and vomiting will increase for some patients.
- Problems can occur with defecation and urination.

- There may be an increased mortality of patients with certain types of chest trauma.

Controversy About Anti-Shock Garments

There is a certain amount of controversy regarding the use of the anti-shock garment. Some experts believe that the garment may actually make some patients worse. Injuries such as penetrating thoracic injuries, fluid on the heart (cardiac tamponade), and internal bleeding from the major vessels within the chest may be complicated by use of the anti-shock garment. More will be known about anti-shock garments as information is compiled through further research and use.

Keep in mind the controversial nature of the anti-shock garment as you read the following information about how anti-shock garments may be used. Remember that the final decision about field use, indications, and contraindications are governed by your local EMS system.

Indications

Use of an anti-shock garment should be considered for a patient with

- A systolic blood pressure of less than 80 mmHg
- A systolic blood pressure of less than 100 mmHg and evidence of the classic signs of shock
- Profuse bleeding from an injury or injuries to the lower extremities
- A fracture or fractures of the lower extremities
- A fracture or fractures of the pelvis or femur, with shock
- Closed abdominal injury, with shock
- Multiple trauma, with shock
- A pregnant patient with shock. Only the leg compartments of the garment will be inflated. This approach may also be taken for some obese patients.

Contraindications

A contraindication is the opposite of an indication: It is when the anti-shock garment should *not* be used. Decisions should be based on regulations set forth by your local medical control.

The primary contraindication to application and inflation of the anti-shock garment is

- **Pulmonary Edema**—fluid in the lungs. The pulmonary blood vessels and the alveoli (air sacs) contain excess fluids, a serious condition. Pulmonary edema causes decreased oxygen delivery to the cells. This may be identified by using a stethoscope to listen to the lungs. Pulmonary edema is characterized by rales, an abnormal lung sound produced when air is moved through fluids in the bronchial tree.* The patient with pulmonary edema may also have distended (bulging) neck veins. (See Chapter 15.)

Pulmonary edema is an *absolute* contraindication to the use of the anti-shock garment. (An absolute contraindication is one that will always prevent application of the garment.) Other conditions may not be ideal for the garment, but the prevention of serious shock is more important than the problems it may cause. These are called *relative* contraindications. (The contraindication must be weighed relative to the need to control shock in deciding whether to use the garment.) Some of these relative contraindications are

- *Massive bleeding into the thoracic cavity.* (Many physicians feel that this is an absolute contraindication.)
- *Uncontrolled bleeding above the level of the suit* that cannot be controlled by direct pressure or pressure dressing. (Many physicians feel that this is an absolute contraindication.)
- *Pregnancy.* If the pregnant patient has signs of shock, the leg sections may be inflated and the abdominal section left uninflated. A physician may order you to inflate the abdominal compartment of the garment.
- *Abdominal injury with evisceration or abdominal impaled object.* Many systems recommend inflation of only the leg compartments of the garment when there is an open abdominal injury.
- *Chest pain, heart attack, and stroke.* Use of the garment with these conditions depends on the blood pressure, presence of pulmonary edema, and other factors.

Note: Some EMS systems have a protocol that does not allow for the application of anti-shock garments in cases involving injury to the head. The reason is to help

prevent an increase in intracranial pressure. However, some protocols now allow for the application of the garment when there is a head injury *and* signs and symptoms of shock. Often when there is a head injury and low blood pressure, the reduction in blood pressure is from internal bleeding in the chest or abdomen. In this situation, the garment can be used to treat hypovolemic shock with little chance of increasing intracranial pressure. Remember, follow your local guidelines.

Applying an Anti-Shock Garment

An anti-shock garment is to be applied in accordance with local protocols. In many localities, application requires the order from a physician. The procedure for application of the garment is shown in Scan 8-1.

There are three major types of anti-shock garments in use. The plain garment does not have any pressure gauges. The one-gauge garment measures individual pressures, one compartment at a time. The three-gauge garment has a pressure gauge for each compartment.

When internal abdominal bleeding is suspected, inflate all the compartments at the same time. The patient's clothing should not be left on under the garment. The removal of the patient's lower outer garments improves the application of the garment and allows for the easier insertion of a Foley catheter at a later time. If this is not possible, then remove the patient's belt and any sharp objects found in the pockets before applying the garment. Since transport will be required, the anti-shock garment should be placed on the patient-carrying device before the patient.

Note: Vital signs are to be taken before applying an anti-shock garment and should be monitored EVERY 5 MINUTES thereafter.

Removing an Anti-Shock Garment

The garment should be removed only when a physician is present and

- The physician orders the removal of the garment.
- Intravenous correction of volume loss has begun.
- Vital signs have just been monitored and recorded, noting that the patient is stable.
- An operating room is available.

---

* Studies show that few EMTs can adequately assess breath sounds. If you suspect but cannot confirm pulmonary edema, seek advice from medical control.

Application of an Anti-Shock Garment

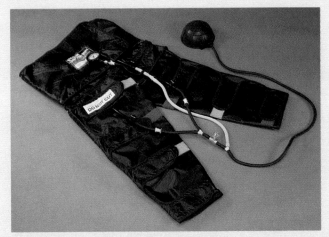

Adult garment and inflation pedal.

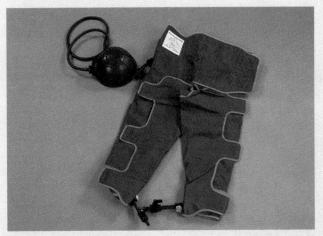

Pediatric garment.

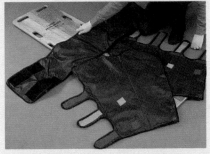

1. Unfold the garment and lay it flat. It should be smoothed of wrinkles.

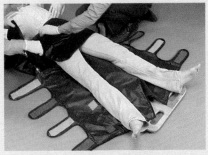

2. Log roll the patient onto the garment, or slip it under him. The upper edge of the garment must be just below the rib cage.

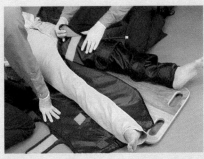

3. Check for a distal pulse and enclose the left leg, securing the Velcro straps.

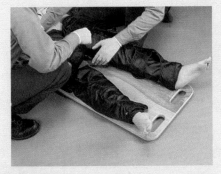

4. Check for a distal pulse and enclose the right leg, securing the Velcro straps.

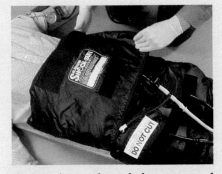

5. Enclose the abdomen and pelvis, securing the Velcro straps.

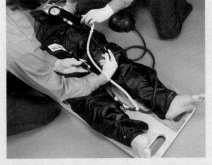

6. Check the tubes leading to the compartments and the pump.

Note: Patient's clothing remains on for demonstration purposes. In actual use, clothing should be removed. Anti-shock garment can be placed over traction splint.

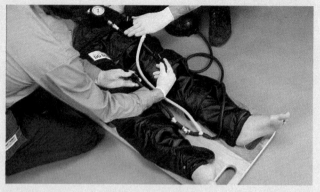

7. Open the stopcocks to the legs and close the abdominal compartment stopcock.

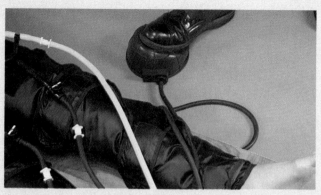

8. Use the foot pedal to inflate the lower compartments simultaneously, or the required lower extremity compartment. Inflate until air exhausts through the relief valves, the Velcro makes a crackling noise, or the patient's systolic blood pressure is stable at 100 to 110 mmHg or higher.

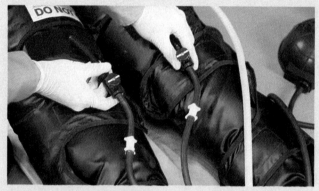

9. Close the stopcocks.

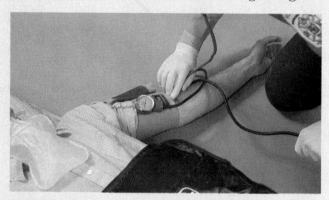

10. Check the patient's blood pressure.

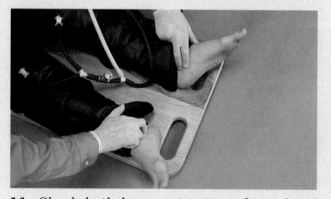

11. Check both lower extremities for a distal pulse.

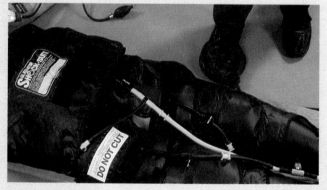

12. If BP is below 100 mmHg, open the abdominal stopcock and inflate abdominal compartment. Close stopcock.

Note: Monitor and record vital signs every 5 minutes. If the garment loses pressure, add air as needed. Some protocols call for the inflation of all three compartments of the garment simultaneously.

In some cases the garment may have to remain inflated until the patient is taken into surgery. The garment should only be deflated and removed by someone trained in its use and familiar with the type of garment being used. To remove an anti-shock garment, have someone continually monitor vital signs and

1. Slowly deflate the abdominal compartment, checking the patient's systolic blood pressure after each small increment of deflation. If the patient's blood pressure drops 6 mmHg or more, stop the deflation and wait for fluids or blood to be infused to stabilize the patient. If at any time the patient shows a sudden drop in blood pressure (a drop of 10 mmHg or more), the garment will have to be reinflated. Once the abdominal compartment has been deflated . . .

2. Slowly deflate one leg compartment following the same procedures as above. (The time this should take varies with different protocols. Some methods have the rescuer continue immediately with the deflation if the patient's blood pressure is stable. Other methods require 20 minutes between deflating each compartment. Follow your local protocol.) Then . . .

3. Slowly deflate the other leg compartment, following the same procedure as above.

Remember: Discontinue deflation if the systolic blood pressure drops more than 6 mmHg from its previous level or if the systolic blood pressure is 100 mmHg or less. Additional intravenous infusion is needed before deflation can continue.

Warning: Currently, many EMS systems have no indications for the prehospital removal of anti-shock garments once they are inflated. Where removal is allowed, it is done for patients who develop shortness of breath, pulmonary edema, or hypertension.

CHAPTER REVIEW

KEY TERMS

You may find it helpful to review the following terms.

allergen—something to which a person is allergic; something that causes an adverse physical response.

anaphylactic (an-ah-fi-LAK-tik) **shock**—the most severe type of allergic reaction in which a person develops shock when he encounters a substance to which he is allergic. This is a true, life-threatening emergency.

anti-shock garment—a garment that covers the lower body and lower extremities and inflates to exert air pressure and increase blood flow to the central body, heart, and brain.

compensated shock—a condition in early shock in which the body is compensating for, and to a degree masking, the presence of shock. Its signs may include a heart rate above 100, a slight drop in blood pressure, an increase in capillary refill time, and a slight drop in systolic with an increase in diastolic blood pressure.

decompensated shock—when the body can no longer compensate for the conditions that cause shock and the patient begins to show the symptoms of full-blown, life-threatening shock.

pulmonary edema (PUL-mo-nar-e ed-EE-mah)—fluid in the lungs. Pulmonary edema is an absolute contraindication to the use of anti-shock garments.

shock—a life-threatening condition with a variety of possible causes; most commonly the reaction of the body to the failure of the cardiovascular system to provide an adequate supply of blood to all vital parts of the body.

syncope (SIN-ko-pe)—fainting; a self-correcting, temporary form of shock.

vascular container—the system that contains the body's blood; the heart and the blood vessels.

SUMMARY

About Shock

There are various types of shock. The most common results from the inability of the cardiovascular system to fill the vascular container, that is, failure to provide sufficient oxygenated blood to all the vital tissues of the body through perfusion of all the capillaries.

The types of shock include hypovolemic (caused by loss of blood or other body fluids), cardiogenic (caused by failure of the heart to pump blood adequately), neurogenic (caused by failure of the nervous system to control blood vessel diameter), anaphylactic (caused by a severe allergic reaction), psychogenic (a nervous system reaction caused by fear or other psychological stress), metabolic (caused by changes in body chemistry), and septic (caused by toxins, or poisons, in the bloodstream).

Treating for Shock

The signs of shock can include restlessness, profuse external bleeding, mechanism of injury suggesting internal bleeding, nausea or vomiting, shaking and trembling, altered levels of consciousness, rapid and weak pulse, shallow and rapid breathing, a drop in blood pressure, moist and cool skin, lackluster eyes, dilated pupils, pale face and cyanosis at the lips or ear lobes. Increased capillary refill time may be observed. The symptoms of shock can include nausea, thirst, weakness, dizziness, coolness, and the feeling of impending doom.

During compensated shock, the body works to make up for the early effects of shock. Signs of compensated shock are an increase in pulse rate, increased capillary refill time, and a slight drop in systolic blood pressure with an increase in diastolic pressure. Do not wait for signs of shock to develop, however, but act to prevent shock whenever the mechanism of injury or other circumstances signal the potential for shock.

Prevention and management of shock are basically the same. Maintain an adequate airway and control major bleeding. *Administer oxygen as soon as possible.* Immobilize the patient if spinal injury is suspected. Splint fractures, keep the patient at rest, lying down and covered to stay warm but not overheated. In most cases, the patient will benefit if the lower extremities are elevated. A supine or semiseated position may be more useful, depending on the nature of the patient's illness or injury. Give nothing by mouth. Provide emotional support. *Monitor vital signs* and *be on the alert for vomiting.*

Anaphylactic shock is a *life-threatening emergency.* This type of shock is brought about when the patient comes into contact with a substance to which he is allergic (bee stings, insect bites, chemicals, dusts, pollens, drugs, foods). The signs of anaphylactic shock can include restlessness, becoming unresponsive, difficult breathing, a rapid and very weak pulse, high blood pressure later dropping to shock level, hives or blotchy skin, swelling of the face and tongue, cyanosis, and vomiting, and possible swelling of the ankles or wrists. The symptoms of anaphylactic shock include complaints of itching and burning skin, chest pains with difficult breathing, dizziness, restlessness, nausea, headache, and, rarely, temporary loss of consciousness. The care for anaphylactic shock includes basic life support measures, oxygen, and the same care as for all shock patients. Transport the patient to a medical facility immediately. Some local protocols call for paramedic intercept. Remember to ask the patient about allergies during the interview. Be certain to look for medical identification devices or a "Vial of Life" or similar sticker. Follow local protocols with regard to assisting a patient with medications.

Fainting is a mild form of self-correcting shock; however, it may be a sign of serious problems. Always look for injuries caused by falls due to fainting. Take the patient's pulse and blood pressure and provide emotional support. If the patient refuses transport, encourage him to see a physician. Discourage the patient from driving or operating machinery until he is examined by a physician. Fainting can often be prevented by placing the patient in a seated position and lowering his head to a level between the knees. Do not follow this procedure for patients having fractures, spinal injuries, heart problems, or difficult breathing. Have patients with breathing or heart problems or low blood pressure lie supine or with legs elevated.

Anti-Shock Garments

An anti-shock garment is a garment that covers the abdomen and lower extremities and is inflated to apply pneumatic counterpressure against the flow of blood. The garment causes an increase in blood pressure and can help to control internal bleeding. The rise in blood pressure may be caused by pushing blood from the lower extremities up into the central circulation or by increasing constriction of the blood vessels.

Indications for use of an anti-shock garment include systolic blood pressure of less than 80 mmHg or of less than 100 mmHg with evidence of shock, profuse bleeding from the lower extremities, fracture of the lower extremities, pelvis, or femur, closed abdominal injury, or multiple trauma in conjunction with evidence of shock. The one absolute contraindication (when the garment must *not* be used) is pulmonary edema. Relative contraindications (which *may* be outweighed by the need to use the garment to control shock) include massive bleeding into the thoracic cavity, uncontrolled bleeding above the level of the garment, pregnancy, abdominal evis-ceration or impalement, chest pain, heart attack, or stroke. Current research indicates that massive bleeding into the thoracic cavity and uncontrolled bleeding above the level of the garment may be considered as absolute contraindications.

Review Scan 8-1 regarding how to apply an anti-shock garment. An anti-shock garment should be removed only in the presence of a physician or under orders from medical control with slow deflation, intravenous correction of volume loss in progress, operating room available, and constant monitoring of vital signs. Some EMS systems have *no* indications for pre-hospital removal of an anti-shock garment, or, if it is allowed, only for patients who develop shortness of breath, pulmonary edema, or hypertension.

Always follow your local protocols with regard to the use of anti-shock garments.

On the Scene

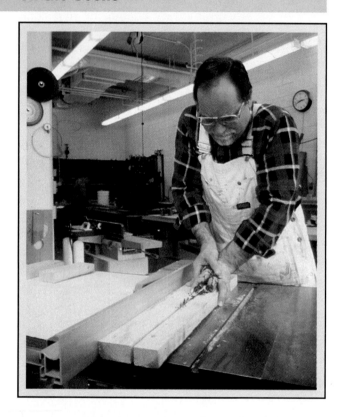

Martin Clark works at a furniture manufacturing company. While he is pushing a piece of hard wood through his table saw, his hand slips, and he is horrified to see that the saw blade has severed the first two joints of his index finger.

Mr. Clark feels faint but is able to yell to a coworker who calls 911. When you arrive,

Mr. Clark is sitting on a bench. He is pale and holding a bloody towel over his right hand. You introduce yourself and ask if you can help. Mr. Clark eagerly agrees.

You: *Can you tell me what happened, Mr. Clark?*

Mr. Clark: *My hand slipped over the saw. My finger . . . well . . . it's gone.*

Coworker *(stepping forward, triumphantly): I found the finger! I took it to the lunchroom and packed it in ice so they can sew it back on!*

Your Partner *(to the coworker): Thank you very much, sir. May I have it? (He retrieves the amputated finger.)*

You: *Is your hand the only place you're hurt, Mr. Clark?*

Mr. Clark: *Yes, it really hurts. Can they put my finger back on?*

You: *That's for the doctors to decide. But we'll bring along the finger and take care of you so you'll have the best chance.*

While your partner removes the amputated finger from the ice and packages it properly, you examine Mr. Clark. He appears pale and weak although there is minimal bleeding. You move him to the ambulance, dress the wounded stump and finger, administer oxygen, and notify the hospital.

Soft Tissues and Internal Organs

Chapter Overview

As an EMT you will deal with two kinds of emergencies: injuries and medical conditions. This is the first of six chapters on injuries. The next five chapters will take up musculoskeletal injuries (to the upper extremities and lower extremities), skull and spine injuries, injuries to the soft tissues of the head and neck, and injuries to the chest, abdomen, and genitalia.

In this chapter you will begin your study of injuries by considering general kinds of soft tissue and internal organ injuries and basic care, including dressing and bandaging skills.

Expected Outcome, Chapter 9: *You will be able to identify, assess, and care for closed and open wounds to the soft tissues.*

Warning: Protect yourself from infectious diseases by using appropriate barrier devices such as a pocket face mask with one-way valve, face shield, or bag-valve mask; goggles or eye shield; and disposable gloves. Always conform to your local EMS system's infection exposure control plan.

THE SOFT TISSUES

TYPES OF SOFT TISSUE INJURIES
Closed Wounds
Open Wounds

TREATMENT OF SOFT TISSUE INJURIES
Treatment of Closed Wounds
Treatment of Open Wounds

Knowledge *After reading this chapter, you should be able to*

1. Define soft tissues. (pp. 240-241)
2. Label and define the THREE major layers of the skin. (pp. 241-242)
3. Define *closed wound* and *open wound*. (pp. 242, 243)
4. Classify closed wounds as contusions, internal lacerations, internal punctures, crush injuries, or ruptures. (pp. 242-243)
5. Classify open wounds as abrasions, incisions, lacerations, punctures, avulsions, amputations, or crush injuries. (pp. 243-245)
6. Cite possible underlying injuries indicated by bruises in various locations and the basic procedures used in caring for a closed wound. (p. 246; Table 9-1)
7. Define *dressing, multitrauma dressing, occlusive dressing*, and *bandage*. (pp. 247-250)
8. State the FOUR basic rules that apply to the dressing of wounds. (p. 250)
9. State the FIVE basic rules that apply to bandaging. (p. 251)
10. Cite the basic procedures used in caring for most open wounds. (p. 252)
11. Cite the basic procedures used in caring for abrasions, incisions, lacerations, and puncture wounds. (pp. 252-253)
12. List NINE steps used in caring for wounds involving impaled objects. (pp. 253-254)
13. Cite the basic procedures used in caring for avulsions, amputations, crush injuries, and protruding organs. (pp. 254-255)

Skills *As an EMT you should be able to*

1. Determine types of soft tissue injuries.
2. Control bleeding and provide emergency care for open wounds.
3. Provide basic emergency care for closed wounds.

There are several kinds of soft tissue injuries. As an EMT you must learn what the soft tissues are, what the kinds of soft-tissue injuries are, what these injuries are called in medical terminology, and basic methods of treating them.

THE SOFT TISSUES

The soft tissues of the body include the skin, fatty tissues, muscles, blood vessels, fibrous tissues, membranes (tissues that line or cover organs), glands, and nerves (Figure 9-1). The teeth, bones, and cartilage are considered hard tissues.

The most obvious soft tissue injuries involve the skin (Figure 9-2). Most people do not think of the skin as a body organ, but it is. In fact, it is the largest organ of the human body. The major functions of the skin include

- Protection—The skin serves as a barrier to keep out microorganisms (germs), debris, and unwanted chemicals. Underlying tissues and organs are protected from environmental contact. This helps preserve the chemical balance of body fluids and tissues.
- Water Balance—The skin helps prevent water loss and stops environmental water from entering the body.
- Temperature Regulation—Blood vessels in the skin can dilate (increase in diameter) to carry more blood to the skin, allowing heat to radiate from the body. When the body needs to conserve heat, these vessels constrict (decrease in diameter) to prevent heat loss. The sweat glands found in the skin produce perspiration, which will evaporate

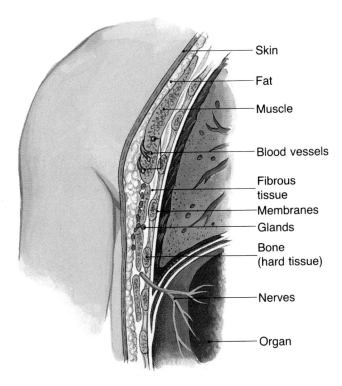

Figure 9-1 Soft tissues.

Skin
Fat
Muscle
Blood vessels
Fibrous tissue
Membranes
Glands
Bone (hard tissue)
Nerves
Organ

and help cool the body. The fat that is part of the skin serves as a thermal insulator.

- Excretion—Salts, carbon dioxide, and excess water can be released through the skin.
- Shock (impact) Absorption—The skin and its layers of fat help protect the underlying organs from minor impacts and pressures.

The skin has three major layers: the epidermis, the dermis, and the subcutaneous layer.

The outer layer of the skin is called the **epidermis** (ep-i-DER-mis). It is composed of four layers (strata) except for the skin of the palms of the hands and soles of the feet. These two regions have five layers. The outermost layers are composed of dead cells, which are rubbed off or sloughed off and are replaced. The pigment granules of the skin and living cells are found in the deeper layers. The cells of the innermost layer are actively dividing, replacing the dead cells of the outer layers.

The epidermis contains no blood vessels or nerves. Except for certain types of burns and

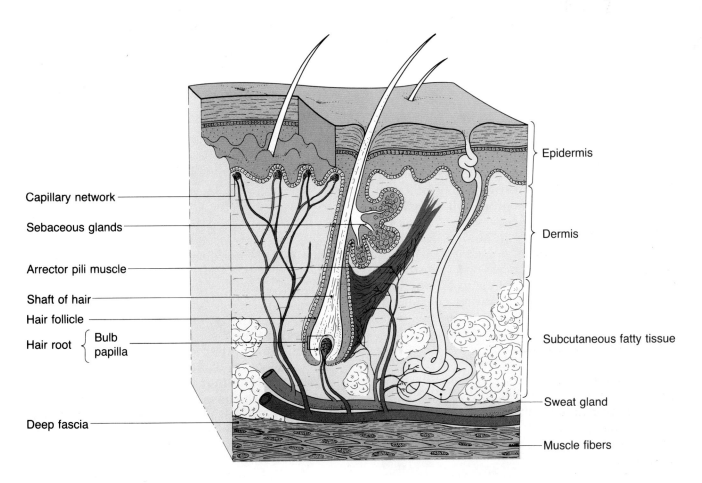

Capillary network
Sebaceous glands
Arrector pili muscle
Shaft of hair
Hair follicle
Hair root { Bulb / papilla
Deep fascia

Epidermis
Dermis
Subcutaneous fatty tissue
Sweat gland
Muscle fibers

Figure 9-2 The skin.

injuries due to cold, injuries of the epidermis present few problems in EMT-level care.

The layer of skin below the epidermis is the **dermis** (DER-mis). This layer is rich with blood vessels, nerves, and specialized structures such as sweat glands, sebaceous (oil) glands, and hair follicles. Specialized nerve endings are found in the dermis. They are involved with the senses of touch, cold, heat, and pain.

Once the dermis is opened to the outside world, contamination and infection become major problems. The wounds can be serious, accompanied by profuse bleeding and intense pain.

The layers of fat and soft tissue below the dermis are called the **subcutaneous** (SUB-ku-TA-ne-us) **layers**. Shock absorption and insulation are major functions of this layer. Again, there are the problems of tissue and blood-stream contamination, bleeding, and pain when these layers are injured.

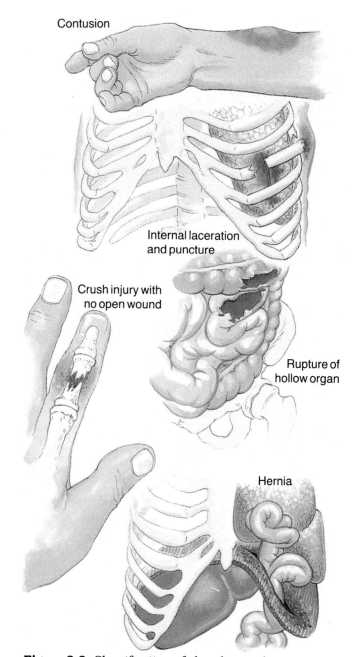

Figure 9-3 Classification of closed wounds.

TYPES OF SOFT TISSUE INJURIES

Soft tissue injuries are generally classified as closed wounds or open wounds.

Closed Wounds

A **closed wound** is an internal injury, that is, there is no open pathway from the outside to the injured site. These wounds usually result from the impact of a blunt object. Although the skin itself may not be broken, there may be extensively crushed tissues beneath it. Closed wounds can be simple bruises, internal lacerations (cuts), and internal punctures caused by fractured bones, crushing forces, or the rupture (bursting open) of internal organs (Figure 9-3). Bleeding can range from minor to life threatening. As an EMT, you should always consider the possibility of closed soft tissue injuries when there are fractures and blunt trauma..

Contusions A **contusion** (kun-TU-zhun) is a bruise (Figure 9-4). A variable amount of bleeding occurs at the time of injury and may continue for a few hours after the trauma. Swelling at the wound site may occur immediately, or it may be delayed as much as 24 to 48 hours. This swelling is caused by a collection of blood under the skin or in the damaged tissues. Blood almost always collects at the injury site and the resulting "blood tumor" is called a **hematoma** (hem-ah-TO-mah). Blood seeping into the surrounding tissues forms the characteristic "black and blue" mark (**ecchymosis—EK-i-MO-sis**). When you perform the patient assessment, the color of the bruise will probably be blue to reddish purple. With time, the blood at the site undergoes changes, causing the color of the bruise to turn to a brownish yellow.

Internal Lacerations and Punctures When bones are fractured, sharp ends or fragments

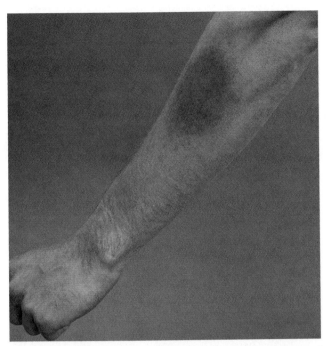

Figure 9-4 Contusions are the most common form of closed wounds.

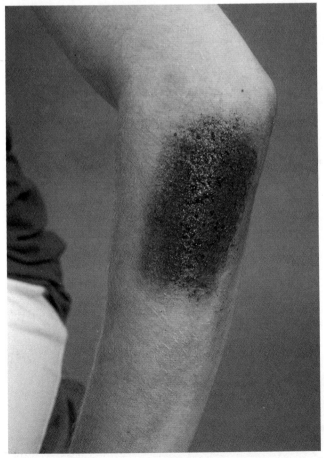

Figure 9-5 Abrasions are the least serious form of open wound.

can cut or puncture internal body structures. The lungs, heart, liver, kidneys, and spleen can be lacerated by fractured ribs. Ends of fractured ribs may also puncture a lung, allowing inspired air to flow into the pleural cavity. On rare occasions, the urinary bladder can be lacerated or punctured as a result of pelvic fractures. A fractured bone can damage muscles, blood vessels, nerves, organs and glands, and other structures composed of soft tissues.

Crush Injuries and Ruptures Force can be transmitted from the body's exterior to its internal structures, even when the skin remains intact and even in cases in which the only indication of injury is a simple bruise. This force can cause the internal organs to be crushed or to rupture and bleed internally. Solid organs such as the liver and spleen normally contain considerable amounts of blood. When crushed, they bleed severely. Contents of hollow organs, such as digested food or urine, can leak into the body cavities, causing severe inflammation and tissue damage.

Organ coverings and cavity linings also can rupture during injury. Parts of organs or muscles may be forced through these openings; yet all the damage is internal and is not usually directly visible on the outside of the body. This type of injury is often called a rupture but is actually classified as a **hernia** (HER-ne-ah).

Open Wounds

An **open wound** is an injury in which the skin is interrupted, exposing the tissues underneath. The cause of the interruption can come from the outside, as a laceration, or from the inside when a fractured bone end tears outward, through the skin.

Abrasions The classification of **abrasion** (ab-RAY-zhun) includes simple scrapes and scratches in which the outer layer of the skin is damaged but all the layers are not penetrated (Figure 9-5). Skinned elbows and knees, "road rash," "mat burns," "rug burns," and "brush burns" are examples of abrasions. There may be no detectable bleeding or only the minor ooze of blood from capillary beds. The patient may be experiencing great pain, even though the injury is minor. Because of dirt ground into the skin, the opportunity for infection is great with this type of injury.

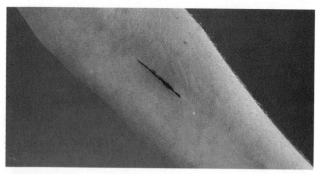

Figure 9-6 The edges of an incision wound are smooth.

Incisions An **incision** is a smooth cut, usually made by a sharp object, such as a knife or razor blade. The edges of the cut skin and the underlying tissues are smooth due to the sharpness of the object inflicting the injury (Figure 9-6). If the wound is deep, large blood vessels and nerves may be severed.

Lacerations A **laceration** is a jagged cut. The tissues are snagged and torn, forming a rough edge around the wound (Figure 9-7).

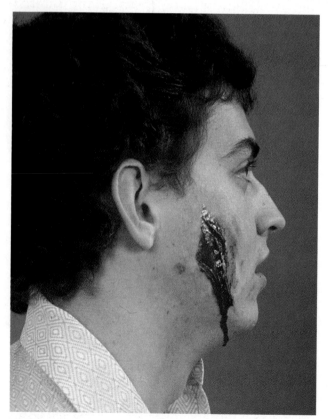

Figure 9-7 The edges of a laceration are jagged and rough.

Often, this type of wound is caused by objects having sharp, irregular edges, such as broken glass or a jagged piece of metal. However, a laceration can also result from a severe blow or impact with a blunt object. The rough edges of a laceration tend to fall together and obstruct the view as you try to determine the wound depth. It is usually impossible to look at the outside of a laceration and determine the extent of the damage to underlying tissues. If significant blood vessels have been torn, bleeding will be considerable, but usually less than that seen with incisions. Sometimes the bleeding is partially controlled when blood vessels are stretched and torn. This is due to the natural curling and folding of the cut ends that aid in rapid clot formation.

Punctures When a sharp, pointed object passes through the skin or other tissue, a **puncture wound** has occurred. Typically, puncture wounds are caused by sharp, pointed objects: nails, ice picks, splinters, or knives. Often, there is no severe external bleeding problem, but internal bleeding may be profuse. Contamination must always be viewed as serious. There are two types of puncture wounds. A **penetrating puncture wound** can be shallow or deep (Figure 9-8). In either case, tissues and blood vessels are injured. A **perforating puncture wound** has both an *entrance wound* and an *exit wound* (Figure 9-9). The object causing the injury passes through the body and out to create an exit wound. In many cases, the exit wound is more serious than the entrance wound. A "through-and-through" gunshot wound is an example of a perforating puncture wound.

Avulsions In an **avulsion** (a-VUL-shun), flaps of skin and tissues are torn loose or pulled off completely (Figure 9-10). When the tip of the nose is cut or torn off, this is an avulsion. The same applies to the external ear. A glove avulsion occurs when the hand is caught in a roller. In this type of accident, the skin is stripped off like a glove. An eye pulled from its socket (extruded) is a form of avulsion. The term *avulsed* is used in reporting the wound, as in "an avulsed eye," or "an avulsed ear."

Amputations The extremities are sometimes subject to **amputation**. The fingers (Figure 9-11), toes, hands, feet, or limbs are completely cut through or torn off. Jagged skin and bone edges can be observed. There may be massive bleeding; however, the force that amputates a

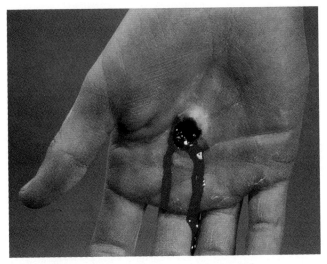

Figure 9-8 A penetrating puncture wound.

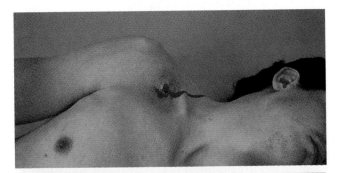

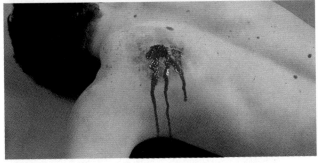

Figure 9-9 A perforating puncture wound has an entrance and exit.

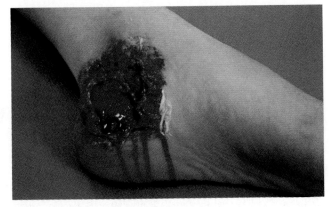

Figure 9-10 Avulsed skin.

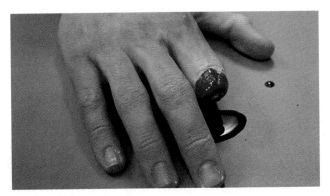

Figure 9-11 An amputation.

limb may close off torn blood vessels, limiting the amount of bleeding. Often, blood vessels collapse or retract and curl closed to limit the bleeding from the wound site.

Crush Injuries A **crush injury** can result when an extremity is caught between heavy items, such as pieces of machinery. Blood vessels, nerves and muscles are involved and swelling may be a major problem with resulting loss of blood supply distally. Bones are fractured and may protrude through the wound site. Soft tissues and internal organs can be crushed to produce both profuse external and internal bleeding (Figure 9-12). Patients who are pinned under heavy objects may suffer "tourniquet shock" (see Chapter 7) when the object is removed and toxins that have built up behind the blockage are suddenly released into the bloodstream. Sometimes, external bleeding may be mild or totally absent.

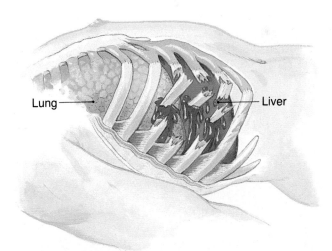

Figure 9-12 Both soft tissues and internal organs are damaged in crush injuries.

TREATMENT OF SOFT TISSUE INJURIES

The EMT cannot repair *blood vessel* and *nerve* damage, although additional injury can be prevented through prompt and efficient care. Controlling bleeding, protecting from additional wound contamination, and initiating certain procedures to reduce pain and prevent shock are some of the important prehospital measures taken by the EMT. There is no direct EMT-level care for *muscle* injury other than treating wounds and perhaps immobilizing the injured limb. However, the control of bleeding and proper wound care are critical and may be the determining factors in patient survival (Figure 9-13).

The body's *organs* and *glands* are composed of soft tissues. Injuries to these structures can range from minor to immediate life-threatening problems. At the EMT-level of care, little can be done directly to organ and gland injuries, but what can be done may be a major factor in patient survival.

The detection of organ and gland injury and how this knowledge affects care, priority of care, and order of transport are of great importance in emergency medicine. As an EMT you must know the organs and major glands and where they are located. You must know which are solid organs and which are hollow so you can consider the possible types of injuries based on the mechanism of injury, extent of internal bleeding, and complications due to a ruptured organ. As you learn more about the body organs, remember to relate the organs of the abdominopelvic cavity to the abdominal quadrants (see Chapter 2).

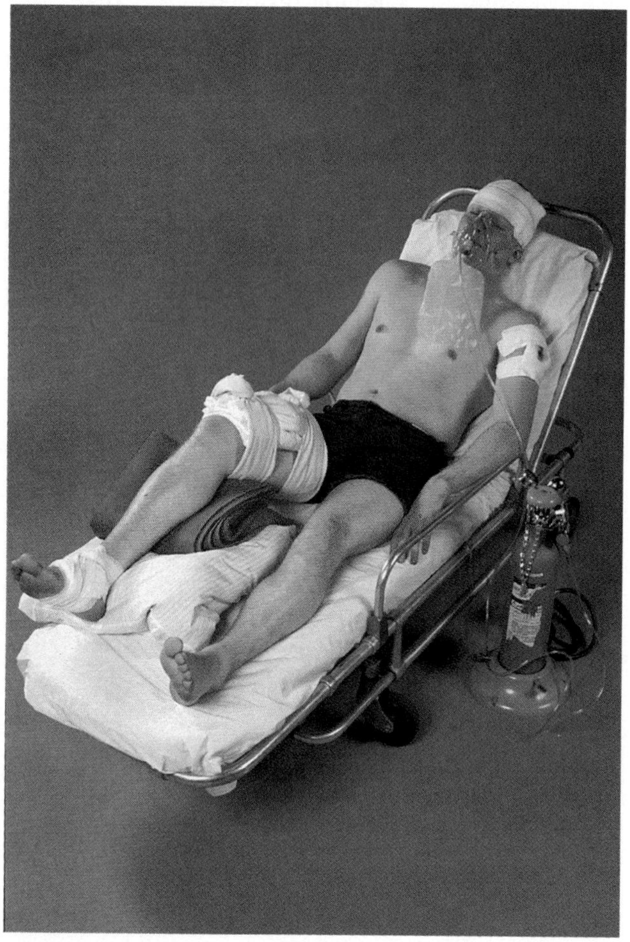

Treatment of Closed Wounds

Contusions are the most frequently encountered closed wounds. Most simple bruises will not require emergency care in the field.

Figure 9-13 Control of bleeding and wound care are critical.

Patient Assessment—Closed Wounds

Signs

A bruise *may* be an indication of internal injuries and related internal bleeding. Each of the signs listed in Table 9-1 indicates possible serious internal injuries requiring special care.

Patient Care—Closed Wounds

Emergency Care Steps

1. *Position the patient so that a minimum of weight is placed on a bruised area* when the patient's injuries allow you to do so.
2. *MANAGE AS IF THERE IS INTERNAL BLEEDING, AND CARE FOR SHOCK* if you believe that there is a possibility of internal injuries.
3. *Stay alert for the patient to vomit.*
4. *Continue to monitor the patient* for the development of shock and transport as soon as possible.
5. *Administer oxygen at the highest possible concentration (Figure 9-14).*
6. *Apply anti-shock garment* when appropriate and local protocols permit.

Later, we will cover the care you need to render in specific cases of internal injuries to the soft tissues and body organs.

TABLE 9-1 Contusions (Bruises) as Signs of Soft Tissue Injury

Sign	Indicates
Large bruise or bruised areas directly over body organs such as the spleen, liver, or kidneys	Possible injury to underlying organs
Swelling or deformity at site of bruise	Possible underlying fracture
Contusion on the head or neck	Possible injury to the cervical spine. Search for blood in the mouth, nose, and ears.
Bruise on the trunk or signs of damage to the ribs or sternum	Possible chest injury. Determine if the patient is coughing up frothy red blood, which may indicate a punctured lung, and assess him for difficult breathing. Use your stethoscope to listen for equal air entry and any unusual breathing sounds.
Bruise on the abdomen	Possible injury to the abdominal organs. Look to see if the patient has vomited. If so, is there any substance in the vomitus that looks like coffee grounds (partially digested blood)? Use the methods described in Chapter 3 to detect if the patient's abdomen is rigid or tender.

Note: Treatment for internal bleeding was discussed in Chapter 7. Treatment of head, chest, and abdominal injuries will be discussed in Chapters 12, 13, and 14.

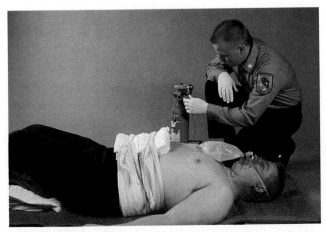

Figure 9-14 Administer a high concentration of oxygen and care for shock.

Treatment of Open Wounds

There are few cases of open wound care that do not require the application of dressings and bandages (Scan 9-1). At one time it was necessary to learn many complicated dressing and bandaging techniques for a variety of wounds. (Later in the text you will learn some special techniques for specific injuries.) However modern dressing materials and self-adhering roller bandages make it possible to apply a set of basic dressing and bandaging skills, described below, to most soft tissue injuries.

Dressings and Bandages To start with, you should know the following definitions (Figure 9-15).

- **Dressing**—Any material applied to a wound in an effort to control bleeding and prevent further contamination. Dressings should be sterile.
- **Bandage**—Any material used to hold a dressing in place. Bandages need not be sterile.

Warning: Be certain to wear disposable gloves and other barrier devices to avoid contact with the patient's blood and body fluids and follow infection control procedures.

Various dressings are carried in emergency care kits. These dressings should be sterile, meaning that all microorganisms and spores that can grow into active organisms have been

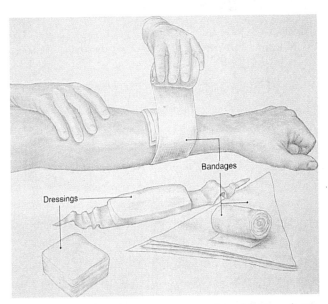

Figure 9-15 Dressings cover wounds, while bandages hold dressings in place.

Examples of General Dressing and Bandaging

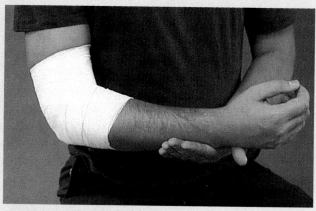

FOREHEAD (NO SKULL INJURY) OR EAR Place dressing and secure with self-adhering roller bandage.

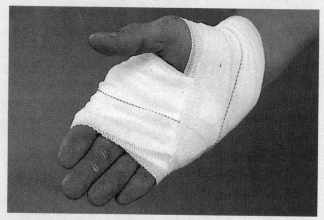

ELBOW OR KNEE Place dressing and secure with cravat or roller bandage. Apply roller bandage in Figure 8 pattern.

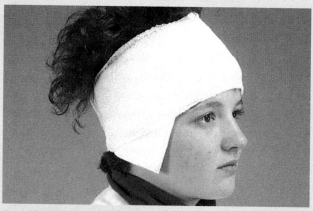

FOREARM OR LEG Place dressing and secure with roller bandage, distal to proximal. Better protection is offered if palm or sole is wrapped.

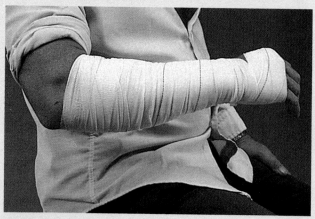

HAND Place dressing, wrap with cravat, and secure at wrist. Use same pattern for roller bandage. Bandage in position of function.

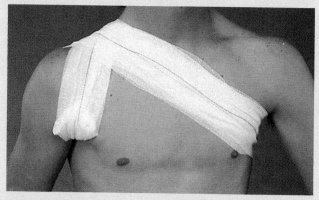

SHOULDER Place dressing and secure with Figure 8 of cravat or roller dressing. Pad under knot if cravat is used.

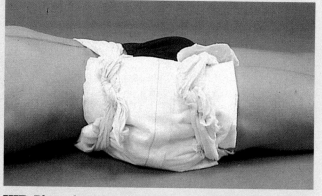

HIP Place bandage and large dressing to cover hip. Secure with first cravat around waist and second cravat around thigh on injured side.

Note: Always leave fingertips or toes showing to assess circulation.

248

killed. Dressings also should be aseptic, meaning that all dirt and foreign debris have been removed. In emergency situations, when commercially prepared dressings are not available, clean cloth, towels, sheets, handkerchiefs, and other similar materials may be suitable alternatives.

The most popular dressings are individually wrapped sterile gauze pads, typically 4 inches square. A variety of sizes are available, referred to according to size, such as 2 by 2s, 4 by 4s, 5 by 9s, and 8 by 10s.

Large bulky dressings, such as the universal or **multitrauma dressings**, are available when bulk is required for profuse bleeding or when a large wound must be covered. These dressings are especially useful for stabilizing impaled objects. Sanitary napkins can sometimes be used in place of the standard bulky dressings. Although not sterile, they are separately wrapped and have very clean surfaces (do not apply any adhesive surface of the napkin directly to the wound). Of course, bulky dressings can be made by building up layers of gauze pads.

Note: Large bulky dressings are not meant to be used to cover multiple wound sites. With the exception of closely spaced shotgun pellet wounds and other similar puncture wounds, each wound should be dressed independently to ensure proper bleeding control and dressing techniques.

The **occlusive dressing** is used when it is necessary to form an airtight seal. This is done when caring for open wounds to the abdomen,* for external bleeding from large neck veins, and for open wounds to the thorax. Sterile, commercially prepared occlusive dressings are available in two different forms. There are plastic wrap and petroleum gel-impregnated gauze occlusive dressings. Local protocols vary as to which form to use. Nonsterile wrap and foil also can be used in emergency situations. In emergencies, EMTs have been known to fashion occlusive dressings from plastic credit cards, plastic bags, aluminum foil wrappers, and ECG electrodes.

Warning: Some EMS Systems report that aluminum foil has caused lacerations of exposed abdominal organs.

Large dressings are sometimes needed in emergency care. Sterile, disposable burn sheets are commercially available. Bed sheets can be sterilized and kept in plastic wrappers to be later used as dressings. These sheets can make effec-

*Occlusive dressings are used for open abdominal wounds to help prevent the loss of moisture.

tive burn dressings or may be used in some cases to cover exposed abdominal organs.

Bandages are provided in a wide variety of types. The preferred bandage is the self-adhering, form-fitting roller bandage (Figure 9-16). It

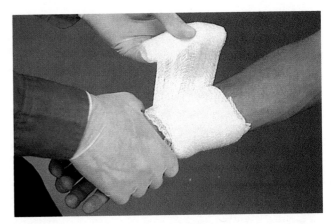

A.

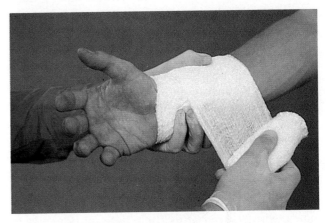

B.

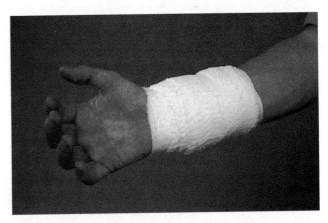

C.

Figure 9-16 Applying a self-adhering roller bandage: (A) Secure with several overlying wraps. (B) Overlap the bandage, keeping it snug. (C) Cut and tape or tie into place.

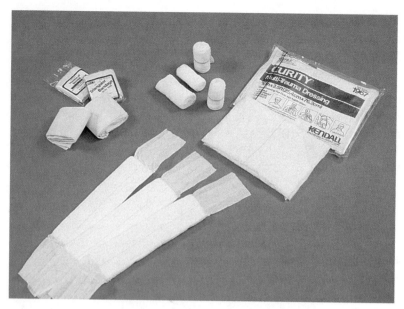

Figure 9-17 Materials used for dressings and bandages.

eliminates the need to know many specialized bandaging techniques developed for use with ordinary gauze roller bandages.

Dressings can be secured using adhering or nonadhering gauze roller bandage, triangular bandages, or strips of adhesive tape (Figure 9-17). In a situation where one of these is not available, you can use strips of cloth, handkerchiefs, and other such materials. Elastic bandages that are used in the general care of strains and sprains should not be used to hold dressings in place. They can become constriction bands, interfering with circulation. This is very likely to occur as the tissues around the wound site begin to swell after the elastic bandage is in place.

Patient Care—Dressing Open Wounds

Emergency Care Steps

The following rules apply to the general dressing of wounds.

1 USE STERILE OR VERY CLEAN MATERIALS—Avoid touching the dressing in the area that will come into contact with the wound. Grasp the dressing by the corner, taking it directly from its protective pack, and place it on the wound.
2 COVER THE ENTIRE WOUND—The entire surface of the wound and the immediate surrounding areas should be covered.
3 CONTROL BLEEDING—With the exception of the pressure dressing, a dressing should

not be bandaged into place if it has not controlled the bleeding. You should continue to apply dressings and pressure as needed for the proper control of bleeding.
4 DO NOT REMOVE DRESSINGS—Once a dressing has been applied to a wound, it must remain in place. Bleeding may restart and tissues at the wound site may be injured if the dressing is removed. If the bleeding continues, put new dressings over the blood-soaked ones.

There is an exception to the rule prohibiting the removal of dressings. If a bulky bandage has become blood-soaked, it may be necessary to remove the bandage so that direct pressure can be reestablished or a new bulky bandage can be added and a pressure dressing created. Protection for the wound site is better maintained if one or more simple gauze dressing pads are placed over the top of the injured tissues prior to the placement of the bulky bandage. This will allow for the removal of a bulky bandage without disturbing the wound.

Remember: Do not remove the dressings that lie in contact with the wound, as you may disturb the clots that have formed. Doing so may cause the bleeding to start again.

Patient Care—Bandaging Open Wounds

Emergency Care Steps

The following rules apply to general bandaging.

1 DO NOT BANDAGE TOO TIGHTLY—All dressings should be held snugly in place, but they must not restrict the blood supply to the affected part.

2 DO NOT BANDAGE TOO LOOSELY—Hold the dressing by bandaging snugly, so the dressing does not move around or slip from the wound. Loose bandaging is a common error in emergency care.

3 DO NOT LEAVE LOOSE ENDS—Any loose ends of gauze, tape, or cloth may get caught on objects when the patient is moved.

4 DO NOT COVER THE TIPS OF FINGERS AND TOES—When bandaging the extremities, leave the fingers and toes exposed whenever possible to observe skin color changes that indicate a change in circulation and to allow for easier neurologic reassessment. Pain, pale or blue-colored skin, cold skin, numbness, and tingling are all indications that a bandage may be too tight. If the fingers or toes are burned, they will have to be covered.

5 COVER ALL EDGES OF THE DRESSING—This will help to reduce additional contamination. The exception is found in the procedures for open chest wounds (see Chapter 14).

There are two special problems that occur when bandaging an extremity. First, point pressure can occur if you apply the bandage around a very small area. It is best to wrap a large area of the extremity, ensuring a steady, uniform pressure. Apply the bandage from the smaller diameter of the limb to the larger diameter (distal to proximal) to help ensure proper pressure and contact. Second, the joints of the extremity have to be considered. You can bandage across a joint, but do not bend the limb once the bandage is in place. To do so may restrict circulation, loosen the dressing and bandage, or cause both to happen. In some cases, it may be necessary to apply an inflatable or rigid splint, or to use a sling and swathe to prevent movement of the joint after bandaging.

Principles of Open Wound Care There are some general principles of emergency care for most open wounds (Figure 9-18).

Warning: Be certain to wear disposable gloves and other barrier devices to avoid contact with the patient's blood and body fluids and follow infection control procedures.

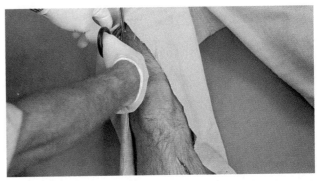
A.

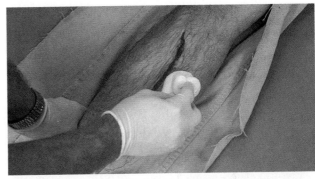
B.

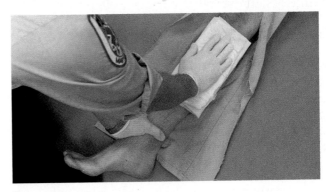
C.

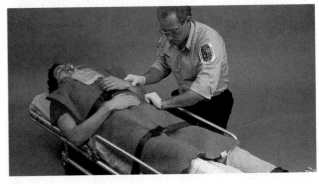
D.

Figure 9-18 Care for open wounds. A. Expose wound. B. Clean wound surface. C. Apply direct pressure. D. Keep patient at rest.

Emergency Care Steps

For most open wounds follow these steps.

1. *Expose the wound.* Clothing that covers a soft tissue injury must be lifted, cut, or split away. For some articles of clothing, this is best done with scissors or a seam cutter. Do not attempt to remove clothing in the usual manner. To do so may aggravate existing injuries and cause additional damage and pain.

2. *Clean the wound surface.* Do not waste time trying to pick out embedded particles and debris from the wound. Simply remove large pieces of foreign matter from its surface. Proper wound cleaning must be done by a physician. When possible, use a piece of sterile dressing to brush away large debris from the surface while protecting and reducing contamination from contact with your soiled gloves.

3. *Control bleeding.* Start with direct pressure or direct pressure and elevation. When necessary, employ pressure point procedures or use a blood pressure cuff. Remember, a tourniquet is used only as a last resort (see Chapter 7).

4. *Prevent further contamination.* Use a sterile dressing, if possible. When none is available, use the cleanest cloth material at the scene.

5. *Bandage the dressing in place after bleeding has been controlled.* If an extremity is involved, check for a distal pulse to make certain that circulation has not been interrupted by the application of a tight bandage. With the exception of a pressure dressing, bleeding must be controlled before bandaging is started. Periodically recheck the bandage to make certain that bleeding has not restarted.

6. *Keep the patient lying still.* Any patient movement will increase circulation and could restart bleeding.

7. *Reassure the patient.* This will help ease the patient's emotional response and perhaps lower his pulse rate and blood pressure. In some cases this may help to reduce the bleeding rate. Also, a patient who feels reassured will usually be more willing to lie still, reducing the chances of restarting controlled bleeding.

8. *Care for shock.* For all serious wounds, care for shock, including the administration of a high concentration of oxygen.

Emergency care steps specific to the various kinds of open wounds are detailed below.

Abrasions, Incisions, and Lacerations In treating *abrasions*, care should be provided to reduce wound contamination. Bleeding from a long, deep *incision* may be difficult to control, but direct pressure over a dressing usually works well. The air-inflated splint can be useful in the management of this type of wound when it is applied over top of a dressing. *Do not* pull apart the edges of a *laceration* in an effort to see into the wound.

Most incisions and lacerations can be cared for by bandaging a dressing in place. Some EMS systems recommend using a butterfly bandage for minor incisions and lacerations. A gauze dressing should be bandaged over the butterfly strip.

Note: Do not underestimate the effects of an incision or laceration. When evaluating a distal pulse, also check for sensory and motor function distal to the injury. The patient may need stitches, plastic surgery, or a tetanus shot at the hospital. So do not put on butterfly bandages and leave the patient at the scene. A serious infection or scarring can result.

Puncture Wounds Use caution when caring for puncture wounds. An object that appears to be embedded *only* in the skin may actually go all the way to the bone. In such cases, it is possible that the patient may not have any serious pain. Even an apparently moderate puncture wound may cause extensive internal injury with serious internal bleeding. What appears at first to be a simple, shallow puncture wound may be only part of the problem. There also could be a severe exit wound that requires immediate care, so be sure to search for one.

Gunshot wounds are puncture wounds that can fracture bones and cause extensive soft tissue and organ injury. The seriousness of the wound cannot be determined by the caliber of the bullet or the point of entry and exit. The bullet may have tumbled through tissues, been deflected off a bone, fragmented, or exploded inside the body. All bullet wounds are to be considered to be serious. If the bullet has penetrated the body, you *must* assume that there is considerable internal injury. Close-range shootings often have burns around the entry wound. Air guns fired at close range can cause serious damage by injecting air into the tissues.

When caring for a patient with a moderate or serious puncture wound

1. *Reassure the alert patient.* Such wounds are frightening to the patient.
2. *Search for an exit wound* when there is a gunshot wound. Control of bleeding and adequate wound treatment require care of both the *entry* and the *exit* wounds.
3. *Assess the need for basic life support measures* whenever there is a gunshot wound. Care for shock, administering oxygen at a high concentration.
4. *Immobilize the patient's spine* when the head, neck, or torso is involved.

Impaled Objects As an EMT you may have to care for patients with puncture wounds containing impaled objects (Figure 9-19). The object may be a knife, a fence post or guard rail, a shard of glass, or even a wooden stick, piercing any part of the body. Even though it is rare, you may be confronted with a long impaled object that must be shortened before care can begin or transport is possible. In such cases, contact the emergency department physician for specific directions. Usually, someone must hold the object, keeping it very stable, while you gently saw it through at the desired length. A fine-toothed saw with rigid blade support (e.g., a hack saw or reciprocating saw) should be used.

In general, when caring for a patient with a puncture wound involving an impaled object

1. *DO NOT REMOVE THE IMPALED OBJECT.* The object may be plugging bleeding from a major artery while it is in place, so to remove it may cause severe bleeding when the pressure is released. Removal of the object may cause further injury to nerves, muscles, and other soft tissues.

2. *Expose the wound area.* Cut away clothing to make the wound site accessible. Take great care not to disturb the object. Do not attempt to lift clothing over the object; you may accidentally move it. Long impaled objects may have to be stabilized by hand during the exposure, bleeding control, and dressing steps.
3. *Control profuse bleeding by direct pressure if possible.* **Caution:** Position your gloved hands on either side of the object and exert pressure downward. Do not put pressure on the object. This pressure must be applied with great care if the object has a cutting edge, such as a knife or a shard of glass; otherwise, you may cause additional injury to the patient. Be careful not to injure your hands.
4. *Stabilize the impaled object with a bulky dressing.* While you continue to stabilize the object and control bleeding, have another trained rescuer place several layers of bulky dressing around the injury site so that the dressings surround the object on all sides. Manual stabilization must continue until the stabilizing dressings are secured in place.

The second EMT will begin by placing folded multitrauma pads, sanitary napkins, or some other bulky dressing material on opposite sides of the object, along the vertical line of the body or affected limb. For long or large objects, folded towels, blankets, or pillows may have to be used in place of dressing pads. Remove your hands from under the pads. Place them on top and apply pressure as each layer is placed in position. The next layer of pads should be placed on opposite sides of the object, perpendicular to the first layer. Continue

A.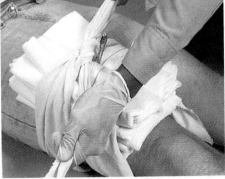

B.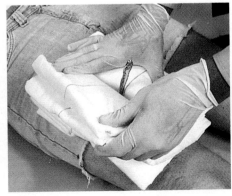

Figure 9-19 Impaled objects. A. Expose the wound and control bleeding. B. Stabilize the impaled object.

this process until as much of the object as possible has been stabilized.

Once bandaged into place, the dressings will stabilize the object and exert downward pressure on bleeding vessels. Keep in mind that there is a limited amount of time that can be given to impaled object stabilization. Stay in contact with the emergency department for directions and recommendations.

5. *Hold the dressings in place.* Adhesive strips may hold the dressings in place; however, blood around the wound site, sweat, and body movements may not allow you to use tape. Triangular bandages folded into strips (*cravats*) can be applied, tying one above and one below the impaled object. The cravats should be wide (no less than four inches in width once folded). A thin rigid splint can be used to push the cravats under the patient's back when they are needed to care for objects impaled in the trunk of the body (Figure 9-20).

6. *Care for shock and provide oxygen at the highest possible concentration.* When appropriate, the administration of oxygen and the covering of the patient to conserve body heat should be done as soon as possible. When working by yourself, these may have to be delayed while you attempt to control bleeding.

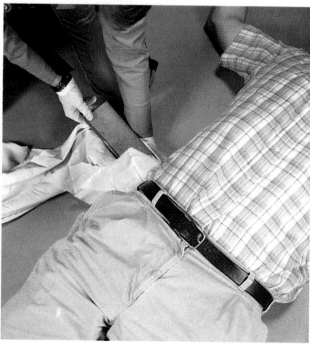

Figure 9-20 A flat splint or coat hanger can be used to position the cravat.

7. *Keep the patient at rest and provide emotional support.* Position the patient for minimum stress. If possible, immobilize the affected area the same as you would for a possible fracture.

8. *Carefully transport the patient as soon as possible.* Avoid any movement that may jar, loosen, or dislodge the object. If the object was removed by bystanders before you arrived, bring it to the hospital for examination by a physician.

9. *Reassure the patient throughout all aspects of care.* An alert patient with an impaled object is usually very frightened.

NOTE: Special procedures are used when caring for objects impaled in the eye and in the cheek. These procedures will be covered in Chapter 13.

Avulsions Emergency care for avulsions requires the application of large, bulky pressure dressings. In addition, you should make every effort to preserve any avulsed parts and transport them to the medical facility along with the patient. It may be possible to surgically restore the part or use it for skin grafts.

In cases in which flaps of skin have been torn loose but not off

1. *Clean the wound surface.*
2. *Fold the skin back to its normal position* as gently as possible.
3. *Control bleeding and dress the wound* using bulky pressure dressings.

Should skin or another body part be torn from the body

1. *Control bleeding and dress the wound* using a bulky pressure dressing.
2. *Save the avulsed part* by wrapping it in a *dry sterile* gauze dressing secured in place by self-adherent roller bandage and placing the wrapped part in a plastic bag, plastic wrap, or aluminum foil, in accordance with local protocol. If none of these items is available at the scene, wrap the avulsed part in a lint-free, sterile dressing. Your EMS system may require that the sterile wrap be soaked with sterile saline. Make certain that you label the part, noting what it is and the patient's name, date, and time the part was wrapped and bagged. Your records should show the approximate time of the avulsion.
3. *Keep the avulsed part as cool as possible,*

without freezing. Place the wrapped and bagged part in a cooler or any other available container so that it is on top of a cold pack or a SEALED bag of ice (do not use dry ice). *Do not* immerse the avulsed part in ice, cooled water, or saline. Label the container the same as the label used for the saved part.

Remember: Serious avulsions can be frightening. You must reassure the patient.

Note: The care of avulsed tissues is directed by local protocols, often written to match the reimplantation procedures of the hospitals in your EMS system. Some EMS systems prefer that the dressing used to wrap the avulsed part be moistened with normal sterile saline (sterile distilled water is not recommended). This saline must be from a fresh sterile source. Keep in mind that once a sterile source of saline has been opened it is no longer considered sterile. Take great care if you use this method since the saline may carry microorganisms from your gloved hand through the dressing to the avulsed part.

Amputations As in other external bleeding situations, the most effective method to control bleeding is a snug pressure dressing.

1. *Place the pressure dressing over the stump.*
2. *Use pressure point techniques or a blood pressure cuff* if required to control bleeding.
3. *A tourniquet should not be applied* unless other methods used to control bleeding have failed.
4. *When possible, wrap the amputated part in sterile dressing* and secure the dressing material in place with self-adhesive gauze bandage. Wrap or bag the amputated part in plastic, label it, and transport the part with the patient. The amputated part should be kept cool in the same manner as an avulsed part.
5. *Do not immerse the amputated part directly in water or saline.* It can be sealed in a plastic bag and the bag placed in a bedpan with water kept cool by cold packs.

Crush Injuries If a crush injury to an extremity has resulted in severe arterial bleeding, a blood pressure cuff can be applied as a

tourniquet above the wound. Inflate the cuff to the pressure necessary to control the bleeding (see Chapter 7). Dress and bandage the wound after the bleeding has been controlled.

Protruding Organs Open wounds of the abdomen may be so large and deep that organs protrude through the wound opening. This is known as an **evisceration** (e-vis-er-A-shun). In such cases

1. *Administer oxygen in a high concentration* as soon as possible.
2. *Care for shock,* positioning the patient to provide for a clear airway and minimum stress to the wound site.
3. *Do not touch or try to replace the organ.*
4. *Expose the wound site,* cutting away clothing. Do not attempt to pull away any article or piece of clothing that does not lift off easily.
5. *Flex the patient's uninjured legs at the hips and knees,* if possible, to reduce tension on the abdominal muscles.
6. *Cover the exposed organ and wound opening* with sterile plastic wrap (or aluminum foil—remembering that foil can lacerate an organ—in accordance to local protocol. Some EMS systems apply a sterile, lint-free dressing that is soaked with sterile saline before the occlusive dressing). The dressing should extend at least two inches beyond the wound edges or the edges of the exposed organ.
7. *Create an occlusive dressing* by taping the dressing in place, sealing the edges. This will help prevent the loss of moisture from the internal organs, membranes, and tissues.
8. *Apply a thick dressing pad* or clean towel over the top of the first dressing. This will help to prevent heat loss. Hold this in place with cravats.
9. *Apply an anti-shock garment and inflate the leg sections* if appropriate and local protocols permit. (Do not inflate the garment on the eviscerated organs).
10. *Reassure the patient* through all steps of care.

More specifics for this type of wound care will be presented in Chapter 14.

KEY TERMS

You may find it helpful to review the following terms.

abrasion (ab-RAY-zhun)—a scratch or scrape.

amputation—the surgical removal or traumatic severing of a body part. The most common usage in emergency care refers to the traumatic amputation of an extremity or part of an extremity.

avulsion (ah-VUL-shun)—the tearing away or tearing off of a piece or flap of skin or other soft tissue. This term also may be used for an eye pulled from its socket or a tooth dislodged from its socket.

bandage—any material used to hold a dressing in place.

closed wound—an internal injury with no open pathway from the outside.

contusion (kun-TU-zhun)—a bruise.

crush injury—an injury that results when an extremity is caught between heavy items or is subjected to great pressure. Blood vessels, nerves, and muscles are damaged. Bones may be fractured.

dermis (DER-mis)—the inner (second) layer of skin found beneath the epidermis. It is rich in blood vessels and nerves.

dressing—any material (preferably sterile) used to cover a wound that will help control bleeding and help prevent additional contamination.

ecchymosis (EK-i-MO-sis)—the discoloration of the skin due to internal bleeding.

epidermis (ep-i-DER-mis)—the outer layer of skin.

evisceration (e-vis-er-A-shun)—when an organ or part of an organ protrudes through a wound opening.

hematoma (hem-ah-TO-mah)—a swelling caused by the collection of blood under the skin or in damaged tissues as a result of an injured or broken blood vessel.

hernia (HER-ne-ah)—part of a muscle or organ forced through an opening in the lining of the organ or body cavity; also called a *rupture*.

incision—a smooth cut.

laceration—a jagged cut.

multitrauma dressing—a bulky dressing.

occlusive dressing—any dressing that forms an airtight seal.

open wound—an injury in which the skin is interrupted, exposing the tissue beneath.

puncture wound—an open wound that tears through the skin and destroys underlying tissues. A **penetrating puncture wound** can be shallow or deep. A **perforating puncture wound** has both an entrance and an exit wound.

rupture—see *hernia*.

subcutaneous (SUB-ku-TA-ne-us) **layers**—the layers of fat and soft tissues found below the dermis.

SUMMARY

Warning: Be certain to wear disposable gloves and other barrier devices to avoid contact with the patient's blood and body fluids and follow infection control procedures.

The Soft Tissues

The soft tissues of the body include the skin, fatty tissues, muscles, blood vessels, fibrous tissues, membranes (tissues that line or cover organs), glands, and nerves. The major layers of the skin are the dermis, the epidermis, and the subcutaneous layer.

Types of Soft Tissue Injuries

Soft tissue damage may be classified as *closed wounds* and *open wounds*. Closed wounds are internal, with no pathway from the outside. Open wounds are those in which the skin has been interrupted.

Contusions (bruises) are the most common type of closed wound and may indicate significant injury to underlying organs, tissues, and structures. Other closed wounds include internal lacerations, internal punctures, crush injuries, and ruptures or hernias.

Abrasions, incisions, and lacerations are the most common types of open wounds. Puncture wounds are open wounds classified as penetrating or perforating. Perforating wounds have both an entrance wound and an exit wound. Avulsions occur when skin or certain body parts are torn loose or from the body. Amputation is the cutting or tearing off of a finger, hand, arm, toe, foot, or leg. Crush injuries can create external and internal injury with severe tissue damage. Both internal and external bleeding are seen with such injuries.

Treatment of Soft Tissue Injuries

Always care for closed wounds as if there is internal bleeding. Be alert for vomiting. Administer oxygen. Monitor and treat for shock.

When caring for open wounds, wear disposable gloves and take all necessary protective measures. Most open wounds require the application of dressings and bandages. Commonly used dressings include gauze pads, bulky or multitrauma dressings to control profuse bleeding, and occlusive dressings when an airtight seal is necessary. Common bandages include self-adhering roller bandages, nonadhering gauze roller bandages, triangular bandages, cloth strips or cravats, and adhesive tape.

The rules for dressing an open wound are as follows: (1) Use sterile or very clean materials. (2) Cover the entire wound. (3) Control bleeding, with pressure if necessary. (4) Leave dressings in place. Do not remove or you may restart the bleeding. Add more dressings if necessary.

The rules for bandaging an open wound are as follows: (1) Do not bandage too tightly or blood supply may be restricted. (2) Do not bandage too loosely or dressings may move or slip. (3) Do not leave loose ends that can get caught.

(4) Leave fingers and toes exposed so circulation and nerve function in the extremity can be monitored. (5) Cover all edges of the dressing.

The procedure of care for most open wounds is as follows: (1) Expose the wound. (2) Clean the wound surface. (3) Control bleeding. (4) Prevent further contamination. (5) Bandage dressing in place. (6) Keep patient lying still. (7) Reassure the patient. (8) Care for shock. Use this procedure for abrasions, incisions, and lacerations.

If the patient has a puncture wound, assume there are serious internal injuries with bleeding. Look for an exit wound and care for both entrance and exit wounds. Keep in mind that patients suffering from blood loss do better when you administer oxygen and treat for shock.

Do not remove impaled objects. Control bleeding and stabilize the impaled object.

Partially avulsed skin can be folded gently back to its normal position after the wound surface is cleaned. If skin is torn off, preserve the part in a secured wrap of sterile gauze dressing and place it in a plastic bag. Be certain to properly label the saved part. Transport the avulsed part with the patient, keeping it cool but out of direct contact with ice or cooled water.

For an amputation, attempt to control bleeding by direct pressure applied to a bulky dressing held directly over the stump, or use a pressure dressing. Care for the amputated part the same as for an avulsed part. If necessary, use pressure point techniques to help control bleeding from the stump.

When there is a crush injury to an extremity, the application of a blood pressure cuff may be the best way to control severe external bleeding. The last resort is a tourniquet.

Do not try to replace protruding organs. Control bleeding and cover with an occlusive dressing. Keep the organs warm and moist. Care for shock.

10

On the Scene

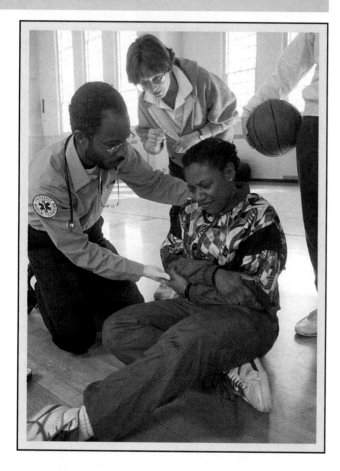

Seventeen-year-old Nancy Addison was attempting to retrieve a rebound when she collided with another player. Knocked off balance, she fell to the floor on her outstretched arm. When Nancy hit the floor, she could feel the pain in her lower arm.

The coach and the other players soon realized Nancy was hurt. After looking at her arm, the coach suspected it was broken. A teacher was sent to call 911. You receive the call for a "broken arm" at a high school basketball game. When you arrive, Nancy is sitting on the gym floor surrounded by concerned teammates and her coach. She has an icepack on her arm.

You: *"Hi. We're from the ambulance. Can you tell me what happened?"*

Nancy: *"I was jumping for the ball and I fell down. I landed pretty hard on my arm. I think I felt a snap."*

You: *"Did you pass out when you fell?"*

Nancy: *"No."*

You: *"OK. I'm going to check for other injuries. Do you hurt anywhere else?"*

Nancy may very well have a broken radius and ulna. Her arm appears discolored and swollen. The fact that Nancy heard a "snap" is significant. Often patients will hear a snap or feel bone ends "grinding together." But a broken arm may not be Nancy's only injury. Since she admits that she "fell pretty hard," there may be other injuries along the path of the force. You know that since she fell on an outstretched arm, the energy may have been transmitted to her elbow, humerus, shoulder, or neck. You can tell from the swelling and discoloration that there has also been damage to the soft tissues of her forearm.

This is not a life-or-death emergency— Nancy's injuries are unlikely to be life threatening. But the care you provide reduces her pain and prevents further damage and possible disability.

The Upper Extremities

Splinting a broken arm is the kind of activity most people think of when they think of emergency care. However, an injured bone or joint is not, by itself, life threatening. So assessing and caring for such injuries is an important concern, but never the first concern at the emergency scene.

In this chapter you will learn about the musculoskeletal system, where the care of bone and joint injuries fits among the priorities of emergency care, and specifically about injuries to the upper extremities. In the next chapter you will learn about injuries to the lower extremities.

Expected Outcome, Chapter 10: *You will be able to assess and care for musculoskeletal injuries to the upper extremities.*

WARNING: Protect yourself from infectious diseases by using appropriate barrier devices such as a pocket face mask with one-way valve, face shield, or bag-valve mask; goggles or eye shield; and disposable gloves. Always conform to your local EMS system's infection exposure control plan.

THE MUSCULOSKELETAL SYSTEM
    The Muscles
    The Skeletal System
    The Human Skeleton
    The Axial Skeleton
    The Appendicular Skeleton

TYPES OF BONE AND JOINT INJURIES
    Fractures
    Other Injuries

TREATMENT OF INJURIES TO THE EXTREMITIES
    Total Patient Care
    General Care for Skeletal Injuries

COMPLICATIONS OF MUSCULOSKELETAL INJURIES
    Complications
    Special Considerations

Knowledge *After reading this chapter you should be able to*

1. List the FOUR major functions of the skeletal system. (p. 262)

2. Define *bone*, *joint*, *ligament*, and *tendon*. (pp. 262, 270)

3. Label the major anatomical structures of a long bone. (pp. 262-263)

4. Describe the special healing properties of bone. (p. 263)

5. Define *axial skeleton* and *appendicular skeleton*. (pp. 263-267)

6. Distinguish between *skull*, *cranium*, and *face*. (p. 264)

7. Name and label the FIVE major divisions of the spinal column. (pp. 264-265)

8. Define *thoracic cage* in terms of its skeletal components. (p. 265)

9. Locate and name the major bones of the extremities. (p. 266)

10. Define *open fracture* and *closed fracture*, listing signs and symptoms associated with both. (pp. 267-269)

11. Define *angulated fracture*, noting when special care should be provided for this type of fracture. (pp. 267, 272, 274, 275)

12. Define *dislocation*, *sprain*, and *strain*. (pp. 269-271)

13. Explain where the care of bone and joint injuries fits among the priorities of emergency care. (p. 271; Table 10-1)

14. State the basic care provided for injuries of the upper extremities, including soft and rigid splinting procedures. (pp. 272-285)

15. Describe the procedures used to determine muscle damage, impaired circulation, and nerve damage of the extremities. (pp. 286-287)

Skills *As an EMT you should be able to*

1. Assess injuries to the upper extremities based on signs and symptoms.

2. Provide soft tissue care for injuries to the upper extremities.

3. Provide care for injuries to the bones and joints of the upper extremities, including
   • Fractures and dislocations of the pectoral girdle
   • Fractures of the humerus
   • Fractures and dislocations of the elbow
   • Fractures of the forearm and wrist
   • Fractures of the hand, including fingers

4. Use basic splints, including rigid splints and various kinds of soft splints.

5. Straighten closed angulated fractures, when appropriate.

6. Evaluate muscle, nerve, and vascular function of the upper extremities.

7. Make and use noncommercial splints for emergency situations.

8. Provide total patient care for patients with fractures.

Many students have an interest in extremity injuries and eagerly await the part of their training in which they will study injuries to the bones and joints. A few hours of disciplined study enable them to learn the names and locations of the bones, how to classify and detect probable fractures, and how to apply splints to these injuries. However, while they are learning this new information, some students may neglect what they have been taught about soft tissues. The muscles, nerves, connective tissues, and blood vessels are no longer considered as they should be in care procedures. This can carry over into the field: Some EMTs become so concerned about detecting and caring for fractures that they fail to notice other injuries or give fractures too high a priority.

Remember: When a bone is fractured, the damage to blood vessels, nerves, and other soft tissues may be of greater significance than the fracture. Proper care of bone and joint injuries must include efficient soft tissue care.

THE MUSCULOSKELETAL SYSTEM

Figure 10-1 shows the major blood vessels and muscles, along with a few of the major nerves found in the upper extremities. As an EMT you do not need to know every structure found in an extremity. However, you will need to remember how complex these structures are and consider the damage that may be done to soft tissues in cases of possible fracture or dislocation.

Bones are a part of a more complex system called the musculoskeletal system. This system is composed of all the bones, joints, and muscles, as well as tendons, ligaments, and cartilages in the body.

The Muscles

Muscles are involved with *body movement*, with *moving food*, *fluids*, or *blood* through structures in the body, with *body posture*, and with helping to make up certain *body structures* (e.g., the wall of the intestine). When people refer to the musculoskeletal system, they are usually referring to the muscles involved with body movement.

There are three types of muscles in the body (Figure 10-2).

- Skeletal Muscle—This is *voluntary muscle*, meaning that its actions are controlled by conscious thought. It is fast to contract and fast to relax and be ready for its next contraction. Skeletal muscle connects to bones directly or by way of tendons.

- Smooth Muscle—This is *involuntary muscle*, meaning that its actions cannot be controlled by conscious thought. It is slow to contract and slow to relax and be ready for its next contraction. Smooth muscle helps to make up the walls of internal organs, with the exception of the heart.

- Cardiac Muscle—This is a highly specialized form of *involuntary muscle* that makes up the walls of the heart. When the body is

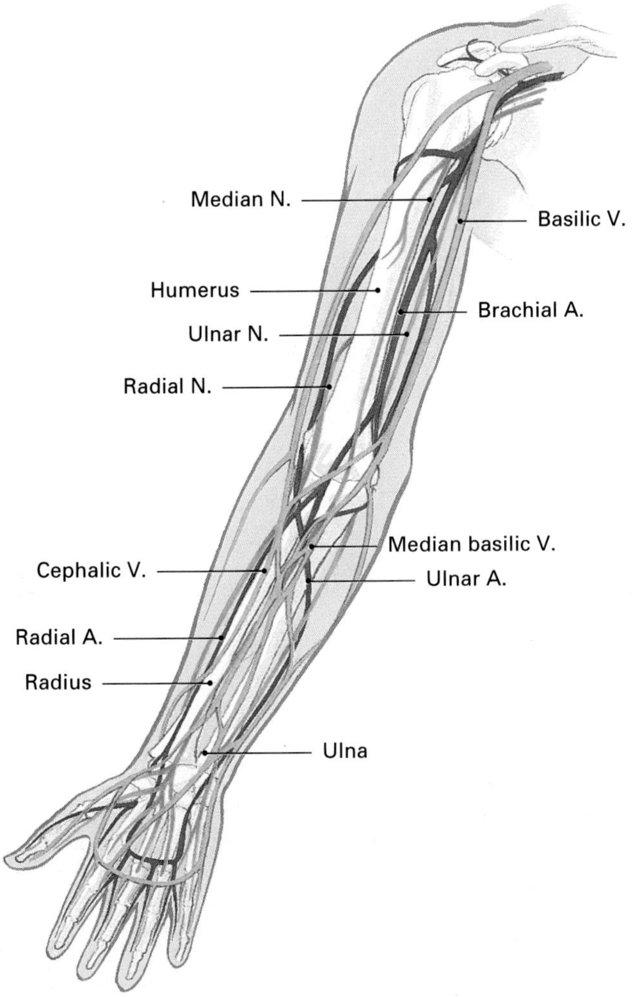

Median N.

Basilic V.

Humerus

Brachial A.

Ulnar N.

Radial N.

Median basilic V.

Cephalic V.

Ulnar A.

Radial A.

Radius

Ulna

Figure 10-1 The complex anatomy of the arm. (A, artery; N, nerve; V, vein)

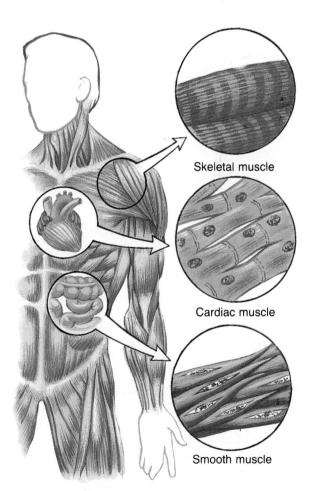

Skeletal muscle

Cardiac muscle

Smooth muscle

Figure 10-2 The three types of muscles.

at rest, cardiac muscle can contract and relax and be ready for its next contraction in approximately 0.8 second.

The *diaphragm* is a special type of voluntary muscle. Even though you can have conscious control of its contractions, you cannot hold your breath for too long a time before the involuntary nervous system takes over.

Most of the emergency care of muscle injury is associated with care of soft tissue injury and possible fractures. Dressing open wounds, immobilizing the injured part, and treating for shock are the basic care procedures for serious muscle injuries.

The Skeletal System

The skeletal system is made up of all the bones and joints in the body.

Bones are not simply mineral deposits that require less care than other living tissues of the body. If you do not realize that bones are hard yet somewhat flexible living structures, you may find yourself providing improper care.

Functions of the Skeletal System The skeletal system serves four major functions: support, movement, protection, and blood cell production.

The bones *support*, creating a framework to give the body form and to provide a rigid structure for the attachment of muscles and other body parts. Bones **articulate** (ar-TIK-u-late), or connect to other bones to form **joints**, most of which are movable. Acting with muscles, bones and their joints allow for *body movement*.

Bones also provide *protection* for the vital organs. The skull protects the brain; the spinal column encloses and protects the spinal cord; the ribs protect the heart, lungs, liver, stomach, and spleen; and the bones of the pelvis protect the urinary bladder and the internal reproductive organs. Bones also protect a soft tissue called marrow that is found within them. Some bones have red bone marrow that contains cells involved in *blood cell production*.

The Anatomy of Bone Bones are classified according to their appearance (Figure 10-3). There are long, short, flat, and irregular bones. The bones found in the arm and thigh are examples of **long bones**. The major **short bones** of the body are in the hands and feet. Among the **flat bones** are the sternum, shoulder blades,

and ribs. The vertebrae of the spinal column are examples of **irregular bones**.

The outward appearance of a typical long bone creates the impression that it is a simple, rigid structure, made of the same material throughout. As you will see, it is actually quite complex.

Most people are aware that bone contains calcium, making it very hard. Bone also contains protein fibers that give it a degree of flexibility. The strength of our bones is a combination of this hardness and flexibility. As we age, there is less protein being formed in the bones and less calcium being stored. As a result, bones become brittle and fracture more easily than when we are young.

Bones are covered by a strong, white, fibrous material called the **periosteum** (per-e-OS-te-um). Blood vessels and nerves pass through this membrane as they enter and leave the bone. When bone is exposed as a result of injury, the periosteum becomes visible. You may see fragments of bones and foreign objects on this covering, but do not remove them. If they have pierced this tissue,

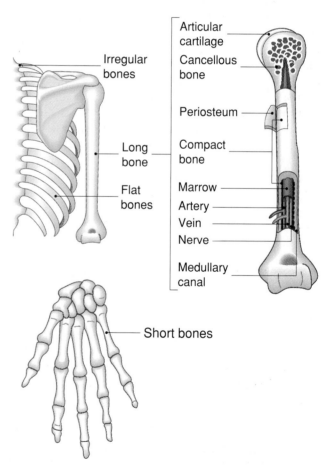

Figure 10-3 The anatomy of bone and classification by shape.

262　Trauma

the objects may be held firmly in place and offer a great deal of resistance to any pulling or sweeping efforts. In addition, you will not be able to tell if the object has entered the bone or is impaled in an underlying blood vessel or nerve.

The typical long bone has a **shaft** that is cylindrical in shape. The shafts of bones appear to be straight, but each bone has its own unique curvature. When the end of a bone is involved in forming a ball-and-socket joint, it will be rounded to allow for rotational movement. This rounded end is called the **head** of the bone. It is connected to the shaft by the **neck**. The ends of bones forming joints are covered with cartilage called **articular cartilage**. Bone marrow is contained in the center of bones. In long bones, this is found in a marrow cavity known as the **medullary** (MED-u-lar-e) **canal**.

The Self-Healing Nature of Bone Before discussing fractures and emergency care procedures, let us examine how a broken bone repairs itself. Understanding this process will give you an appreciation of why a broken bone must be immobilized quickly and must remain immobilized to heal properly.

The first effect of an injury to a bone is the swelling of soft tissues and the formation of a blood clot in the area of the fracture. Both are due to the destruction of blood vessels in the periosteum and the bone and to the loss of blood from adjacent damaged vessels. Interruption of the blood supply causes death to the cells at the injury site.

Cells a little farther from the fracture site remain intact, and within a few hours of the trauma, they begin to divide rapidly to form a mass of new tissue that eventually grows together to form a collar of tissue that completely surrounds the fracture site. New bone is generated from this mass to eventually heal the damaged bone. The whole process can take weeks or months, depending on the bone that has been fractured, the type of fracture, and the health and age of the patient.

Should the fractured bone be mishandled early in care, more soft tissues may be damaged requiring a longer period for the formation of a tissue mass and replacement of the bone. If the bone ends are disturbed during regeneration, proper healing will not take place and a permanent disability may result. In children the majority of the growth of a long bone occurs in the area known as the growth plate, which is near the ends of the shaft. If a fracture in this area is not properly handled, the child may grow up with one leg shorter than the other.

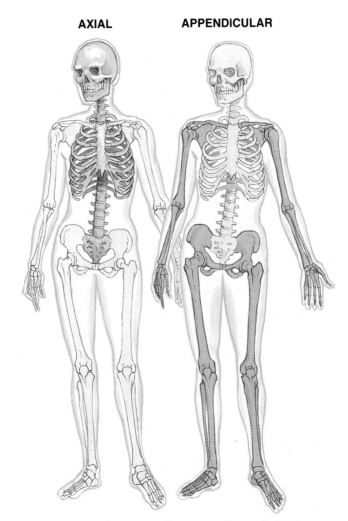

Figure 10-4 The major divisions of the skeletal system.

The Human Skeleton

There are 206 bones in the human body. Each bone is a part of one of the two major divisions of the skeletal system (Figure 10-4).

- **Axial** (AK-si-al) **Skeleton**—all the bones forming the upright axis of the body, including the skull, spinal column, sternum, and ribs.
- **Appendicular** (AP-en-DIK-u-ler) **Skeleton**—all the bones forming the upper and lower **extremities**, including clavicles, scapulae, arms, forearms, wrists, hands, pelvis, thighs, legs, ankles, and feet.

The Axial Skeleton

The axial skeleton is composed of the *skull*, the vertebral (VER-te-bral) column or *spinal column*, the *ribs*, and the *sternum* (Figure 10-5). It makes up the longitudinal axis of the human body.

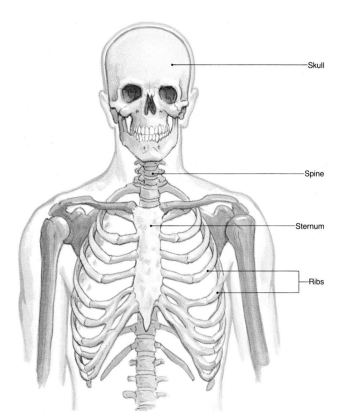

Figure 10-5 The axial skeleton.

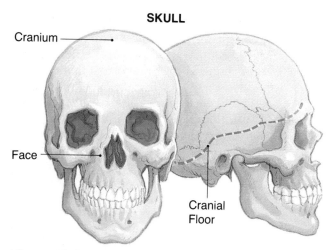

Figure 10-6 Divisions of the skull.

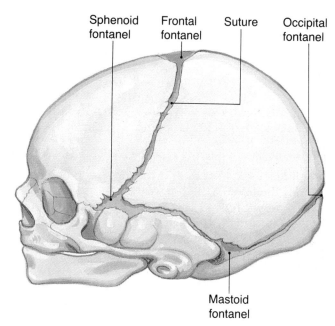

Figure 10-7 The infant skull.

The Skull The **skull** is made up of 22 bones that form the **cranium** (KRAY-ni-um) and the **face** (Figure 10-6).

The 8 bones of the cranium are classified as flat bones and are irregular in shape. These bones begin to fuse together strongly at approximately 12 to 18 months of age to produce immovable joints, forming the rigid brain case surrounding the cranial cavity (see Chapter 2). The point at which two bones of the cranium articulate (join together) is known as a **suture**. The fusion is not complete in infants, causing "soft spots" (fontanelles) in a baby's cranium (Figure 10-7). This is why one must be careful in applying any pressure to the skull of an infant. Whenever care procedures call for you to support the head of an infant, spread your fingers to reduce pressure, avoiding these "soft spots."

The cranium forms the forehead and upper orbits of the eyes, the top and back of the skull, and the sides of the upper skull. In addition, its bones fuse to form an internal structure called the **cranial floor**. This is the inferior wall of the brain case, containing numerous small openings to provide passageways for nerves and blood vessels that lead to and from the brain.

Note: Many people use the term *skull* to mean cranium. In most cases, when you hear that a patient has a skull fracture, you can be certain that the cranium is the injury site.

The remaining 14 bones of the skull form the face. These bones are highly irregular in shape, but when fused together, they give the face its characteristic shape. As in the case of the cranium, the facial bones are fused into immovable joints, except for the lower jaw or **mandible** (MAN-di-bl). The anatomy of the face will be discussed in Chapter 12.

The Spinal Column The **spinal column** is made up of 33 irregularly shaped bones known as **vertebrae** (VER-te-bre). This column of bones gives support to the head and upper body, provides a point of attachment for the pelvis, and

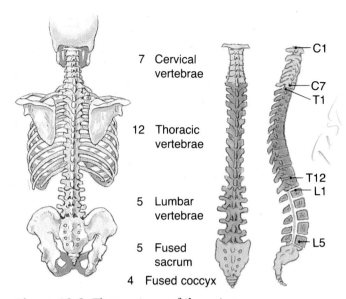

7 Cervical vertebrae

12 Thoracic vertebrae

5 Lumbar vertebrae

5 Fused sacrum

4 Fused coccyx

C1

C7
T1

T12
L1

L5

Figure 10-8 The anatomy of the spine.

protectively houses the spinal cord within the spinal cavity (see Chapter 2). Each bone has a posterior spinous process, many of which can be felt along the midline of a person's back.

The vertebrae are connected by *ligaments*. Located between each two vertebrae is a *disk* of cartilage, hard enough in composition to prevent collapse, yet soft enough to serve as a cushion. Since the spinal cord must be protected and an upright posture is to be maintained, spinal column movement is limited. The spinal column has five divisions: **cervical vertebrae**, **thoracic vertebrae**, **lumbar vertebrae**, **sacrum**, and **coccyx** (Figure 10-8) .

The Thoracic Cage The **thoracic cage** is composed of 12 pairs of ribs, 12 thoracic vertebrae, and the sternum.

There are 12 pairs of ribs in the human body, the same for both male and female. All of the ribs connect posteriorly to the thoracic vertebrae. The upper 7 pairs of ribs attach directly to the **sternum**, or breastbone, by way of cartilage. The next 3 pairs of ribs connect to the cartilage of the seventh pair of ribs. The term *floating ribs* is given to the last two pairs of ribs. These ribs are connected to the spine, but they do not attach to the sternum or the cartilages of the ribs located above them. Anteriorly, all the ribs are palpable, except for the first pair, which lie behind the clavicles.

The points of attachment for rib pairs 6 through 10 can be easily felt on each side of the sternum. The cartilage attachment points on each side are referred to as the **costal** (KOS-tal) **margin**. The costal margins combine to form the **costal arch**.

The sternum is part of the axial skeleton. In addition to the attachment of the ribs, the sternum also articulates with the **clavicles**, or collarbones. A visible depression occurs at this point known as the **jugular notch** (suprasternal notch). The lower extension of the sternum is the **xiphoid process**.

The chest surrounds and protects the lungs and the pleura, the heart and the pericardial sac, part of the trachea, part of the esophagus, and the great blood vessels (aorta and superior and inferior venae cavae). The rib cage extends downward to offer protection to portions of the liver, gallbladder, stomach, and spleen (Figure 10-9).

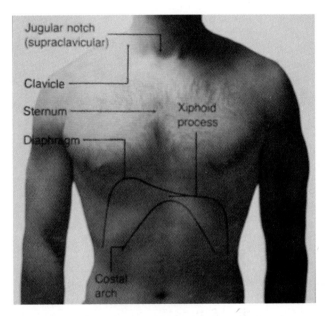

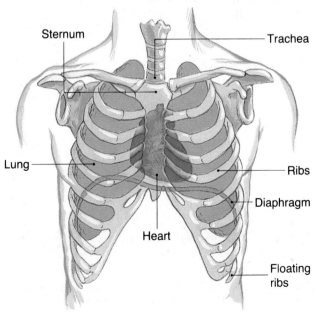

Figure 10-9 The anatomy of the chest.

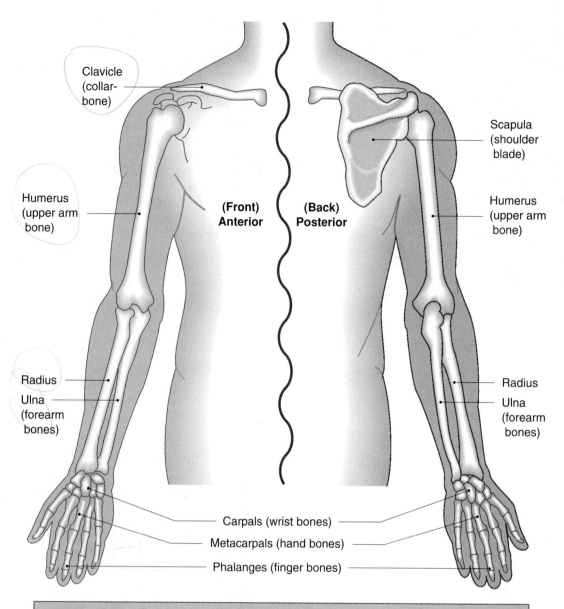

Clavicle (collar-bone)

Humerus (upper arm bone)

Radius

Ulna (forearm bones)

(Front) Anterior

(Back) Posterior

Scapula (shoulder blade)

Humerus (upper arm bone)

Radius

Ulna (forearm bones)

Carpals (wrist bones)

Metacarpals (hand bones)

Phalanges (finger bones)

THE UPPER EXTREMITIES

COMMON NAME	ANATOMICAL NAME
Shoulder girdle	Pectoral girdle (pek-TOR-al): clavicle, scapula, and head of humerus
Collarbone (1/side)	Clavicle (KLAV-i-kul)
Shoulder blade (1/side)	Scapula (SKAP-u-lah)
Arm bone (1/limb, from shoulder to elbow)	Humerus (HU-mer-us)
Forearm bones (2/limb, from elbow to wrist: 1/medial, 1/lateral)	Ulna (UL-nah)– medial Radius (RAY-de-us)– lateral
Wrist bones (8/wrist)	Carpals (KAR-pals)
Hand bones (5/palm, palm bones)	Metacarpals (meta-KAR-pals)
Finger bones (14/hand)	Phalanges (fah-LAN-jez)

Figure 10-10 Bones of the upper extremity.

The Appendicular Skeleton

The appendicular skeleton is composed of the upper and lower extremities. In this chapter, we will consider, in detail, the structures making up the upper extremities. The lower extremities will be covered in Chapter 11.

The Upper Extremities As an EMT you will be expected to know the medical names for the major bones in the body. This will allow you to communicate better with the other members of the patient care team and to use materials available for your continuing education. Should you ever forget the medical name of a bone when presenting information to the emergency department staff, use the common name of the bone. This is better than losing your credibility by using the incorrect term.

The bones of the upper extremities are shown in Figure 10-10.

Note: When a physician uses the term *arm*, it is to make reference to the upper arm or humerus. The lower arm is the *forearm*. The entire structure, from shoulder to fingertips, is the *upper extremity*.

TYPES OF BONE AND JOINT INJURIES

Structures of the musculoskeletal system are subject to injury in the form of fractures, dislocations, sprains, and strains.

Fractures

By definition, a **fracture** is any break in a bone, including chips, cracks, splintering, and complete breaks. There are two basic types of fractures: closed fractures and open fractures (Figure 10-11).

A **closed fracture** occurs when a bone is broken but there is no penetration extending from the fracture through the skin. In other words, pieces of bone have not been forced outward to rip through the skin. In many cases of closed fracture, soft tissue damage is minor. In some cases, because of bone end displacement or bone splintering, soft tissue damage may be great, with the damage being difficult to detect. Internal bleeding may be profuse.

An **open fracture** can occur in one of two ways. First, a bone can be fractured with soft tissues damaged from the fracture outward through the skin. Pieces of bone may actually pierce through the skin. Second, a penetrating wound can produce fractures. The wound is open from the skin to the injured bone. If there is a cut at the fracture site, you should assume an open fracture, even if the bone is not sticking out.

An **angulated fracture** involves a broken bone with the limb or joint taking on an abnormal shape (the humerus may be bent or twisted between the shoulder and the elbow). Angulated fractures can be mild or very severe, occurring with both open and closed fractures (Figure 10-11).

Causes of Fractures The force necessary to fracture a bone can be applied in a variety of ways (Figure 10-12). Direct force can fracture a

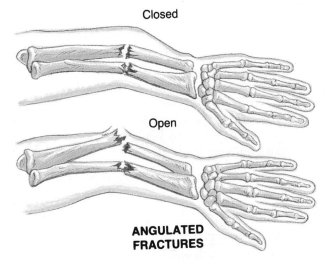

Closed

Open

ANGULATED FRACTURES

Figure 10-11 Basic types of fractures.

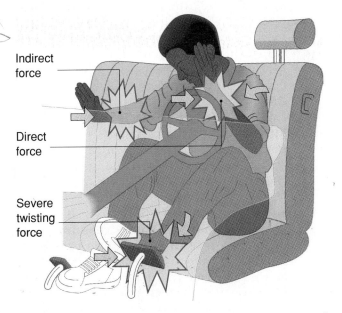

Indirect force

Direct force

Severe twisting force

Figure 10-12 Bones may be fractured in a variety of ways.

CHAPTER 10 The Upper Extremities **267**

bone at the point of contact. A person may be struck by the bumper of an automobile and suffer a fracture at the point where the leg was hit. Indirect force also can fracture bones. This happens when forces are carried from the point of impact to the bone, as when a person falls on his hand and receives a broken arm or clavicle. Twisting forces, as in sports injuries, can cause bones to break. Such injuries often occur in football and skiing accidents when a person's foot is caught and twisted with enough force to fracture a leg bone. Aging and bone disease can increase the risk of fractures (pathologic fractures), with bones being broken even during minor accidents, such as a hip fracture from tripping on a rug.

Patient Assessment—Fractures

Fractures may be hard to detect. When assessing a patient, you should always consider if the mechanism of injury is the type that might cause broken bones. Also consider the age and general health of the patient.

Signs and Symptoms

The signs and symptoms of a fracture (Figure 10-13) can include

- Feeling or Sound—The patient says that he felt a bone break or heard the bone snap.
- Tenderness and Pain—Pain is often severe and constant. The patient may hold the injured part, attempting to prevent additional pain from being produced by movement (guarding). The tissues directly over the fracture will be very tender. You should gently touch the area along the line of a bone in order to determine whether or not there is a possible fracture and the exact location of the injury site. *Do not* probe into or near the edges of open fractures. *Point tenderness* at the injury site is a strong indicator of a possible fracture.
- Deformity—If a part of a limb appears different in size, shape, or length than the same part on the opposite side of the patient's body, you must assume that there is a fracture. If a bone or a joint appears to have an unusual angle, consider this deformity to be a reliable sign of fracture. Gently feel along the patient's limbs noting any lumps, fragments, or ends of fractured bones.

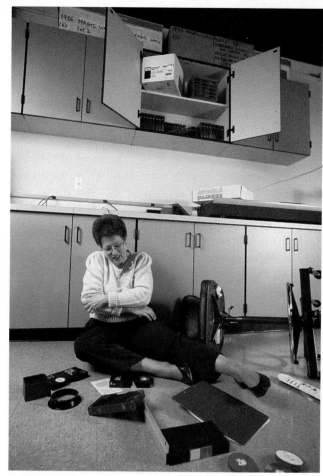

Figure 10-13 Typical signs of a fracture.

- Swelling and Discoloration—These begin shortly after injury. Discoloration may start as a reddening of the skin. Black and blue bruises will usually not occur for several hours.
- Crepitus—**Crepitus** (KREP-i-tus) is a *symptom* when the patient tells you that he heard noises or felt a grating sensation when he moved a limb. This sound or sensation is caused when the broken bone ends rub together. *Do not* ask the patient to move the limb so that you may hear the noise. Crepitus also can be a *sign*. When the patient moves, you may hear a grating sound or feel unusual vibrations through the patient's skin. If you detect crepitus, *do not* ask the patient to move again so that you can confirm the sign.
- Loss of Function—The patient may not be able to move a limb or part of a limb. Sometimes he will be able to move a limb, but the movement will produce intense

pain. If the patient reports that he can move the arm but not the fingers, or if he can move the leg but not the toes, there may be a fracture that has caused damage to adjoining nerves and blood vessels.

- ☐ Loss of Distal Pulse—This is very serious, indicating the interruption of circulation.
- ☐ Loss of Sensation—Bones or bone fragments may have injured nerves.
- ☐ Numbness or Tingling Sensations—Displaced bones or bone fragments may have injured blood vessels or nerves.
- ☐ Exposed Bone—Fragments or the ends of fractured bone may be visible where they break through the skin in some cases of open fractures.
- ☐ False Motion—When the patient moves, the injured bone will display abnormal motion along the shaft, indicating that the bone has been fractured into separate segments. *Do not* ask the patient to move in order to check for this sign.
- ☐ Muscle Spasms—Involuntary contractions in the injured extremity.

Note: Any of the above signs or symptoms gives enough evidence to assume a fracture.

Other Injuries

The most severe injuries to *bones* are fractures. Severe injuries to *joints* can be the result of fractures, dislocations, or a combination of both.

Joints occur wherever two or more bones articulate. The resulting joint can be immovable, as seen when two bones join together to form part of the cranium. Most joints are movable joints, such as the hinge joint of the elbow and the ball-and-socket joint of the hip.

A movable joint consists of the ends of the two joining bones, with these ends usually covered by articular cartilage. The highly movable joints in the body are **synovial** (si-NO-ve-al) **joints** (Figure 10-14). They are surrounded by a fibrous **joint capsule** and contain membranes that produce a slippery fluid (synovial fluid) to lubricate joint movements. Injury to synovial joints can include damage to the capsule, the bone ends, and the ligaments that hold the bone ends in place.

Dislocations When one end of a bone making up a joint is pulled or pushed out of place, a **dislocation** occurs. Usually, the dislocated bone is pulled from its socket. Soft tissue

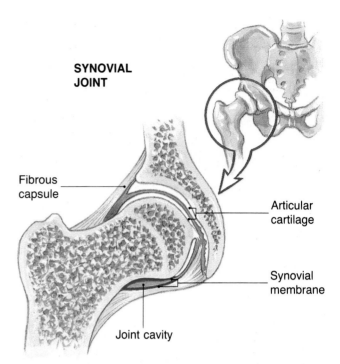

SYNOVIAL JOINT

Fibrous capsule

Articular cartilage

Synovial membrane

Joint cavity

Figure 10-14 The anatomy of a synovial joint.

injury can be very serious, including damage to blood vessels, nerves, and the joint capsule. Major blood vessels and nerves tend to be well protected in most parts of the body. However, in a movable joint these structures lie close to the bones forming the joint and are quite vulnerable to injury when there is a dislocation.

Patient Assessment—Dislocations

The signs and symptoms of a dislocation are usually obvious.

Signs and Symptoms

- ☐ An obvious deformity of the joint
- ☐ Swelling at the joint
- ☐ Pain, which increases with movement
- ☐ The patient may lose use of the joint or may complain of a "locked" or "frozen" joint.

If the patient's only sign is deformity of a joint, a dislocation is more likely than a fracture. However, you *must* still consider a fracture to be a possibility. Even when you believe that a dislocation has occurred, you cannot rule out a *combined injury* of dislocation and fracture.

Sprains Bone is connected to bone by **ligaments**, which hold the bone ends in place to help form and strengthen joints (Figure 10-15). When a ligament is torn, a **sprain** occurs.

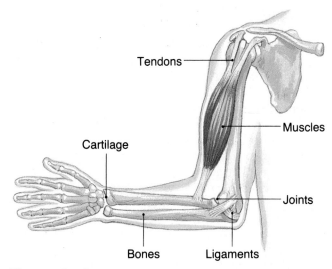

Figure 10-15 Ligaments, tendons, and joints.

Patient Assessment—Sprains

Sprains can sometimes be difficult to tell from fractures and dislocations.

Signs and Symptoms

Signs and symptoms of a sprain typically include

- ☐ Swelling
- ☐ Discoloration
- ☐ Pain on movement

While both swelling and deformity are associated with fractures and dislocations, a typical sprain should have the swelling, because of soft tissue injury, but *without* the deformity. As an EMT, however, you should assume that what appears to be a sprain may be fracture.

Strains A **strain** is different from a sprain. Sprains involve torn ligaments; a strain is a stretching of the muscles or of the **tendons** that connect muscle to bone, or a mild tearing of the muscle.

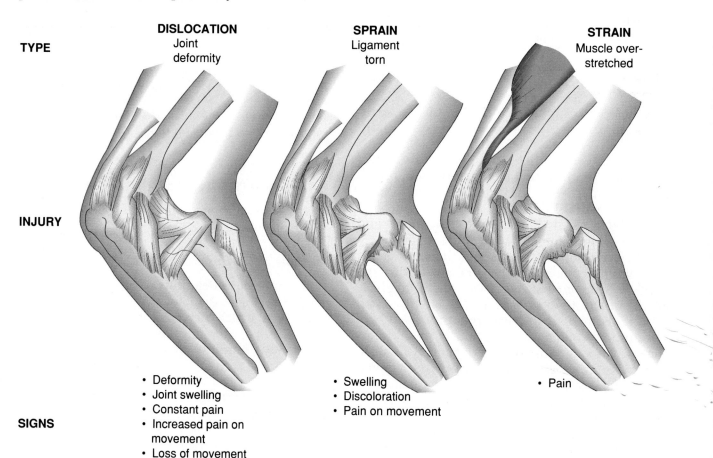

TYPE	DISLOCATION Joint deformity	SPRAIN Ligament torn	STRAIN Muscle over-stretched

INJURY

SIGNS:
- Deformity
- Joint swelling
- Constant pain
- Increased pain on movement
- Loss of movement
- "Frozen joint"

- Swelling
- Discoloration
- Pain on movement

- Pain

Figure 10-16 Injuries other than fractures.

A strain does not usually provide the severe signs or symptoms of a sprain, dislocation, or fracture.

Symptoms

The only symptom of a strain may be

☐ Pain

Even if the patient's only symptom is pain and you suspect a strain, you cannot rule out the possibility of a fracture.

Remember: It is difficult to distinguish dislocations, sprains, and some strains from fractures (Figure 10-16). Therefore, whenever there is evidence of a musculoskeletal injury to an extremity—given the conditions at the accident scene, the diagnostic equipment you carry, and your level of training as an EMT—you must assume that the injury is or involves a fracture.

Patient Care—Fractures, Dislocations, Sprains, and Strains

You will usually have to treat all musculoskeletal injuries to the extremities as if they were fractures, as detailed in "Treatment of Injuries to the Extremities" on the following pages.

TREATMENT OF INJURIES TO THE EXTREMITIES

While some fractures, especially open fractures, appear gruesome and very serious, few present a real threat to life. Your unhurried but efficient action, however, may mean the difference between a rapid and complete recovery and a long, painful hospitalization and rehabilitation. When dealing with fractures, one of your main duties is to immobilize the injured limb. No matter how near you are to the medical facility, you should immobilize fractures and dislocations to prevent aggravation of the injury. Of course, basic cardiac life support situations and certain critical multiple injuries may necessitate transport before such care can be rendered. In these cases the patient should be carefully placed on a long backboard, which acts as a temporary splint.

Total Patient Care

Many untrained people arrive at the scene of an accident and try to start caring for fractures. When caring for a person with an injury to the bone or joint of an extremity, it is first necessary to resolve other more serious problems. Remember to conduct a primary survey and a secondary survey, including physical exam, vital signs, and an interview. You must detect life-threatening problems and correct these problems as quickly as possible. Table 10-1 shows where injuries to the bones and joints fit into the priorities of emergency care.

Provide emotional support to patients with possible fractures. You may need to remind the patient that fractured bones will heal. Tell the concerned patient that new techniques in the care of fractures often reduce the time a patient spends wearing a cast and receiving rehabilita-

TABLE 10-1   Bone and Joint Injuries and the Priorities of Emergency Care

Problems That Demand Care before Bone and Joint Injuries
Airway
Breathing
Circulation
Disability
Shock
Neck and spinal injuries
Open chest wounds
Open abdominal wounds
Serious burns
Priority of Care for Fractures

First priority:
    Fractures of the spine
 	
 Second priority:
    Fractures to the head, rib cage, pelvis
 	
 Lowest priority:
    Fractures of the extremities

Priority of Care for Extremity Fractures
Lower extremities before upper extremities
Pelvis
Femurs
Joints
Long bones

tive therapy. Your emotional support may help keep the patient at rest and help to control blood pressure, pulse, and breathing rate.

General Care for Skeletal Injuries

The proper time to care for a specific bone or joint injury is when the patient is reasonably stable. Be certain that serious bleeding is controlled and that all open wounds have been dressed with sterile dressings. The general care procedures for suspected fractures and dislocations are shown in Scan 10-1. The exceptions to this approach will be covered under specific care procedures in the rest of this chapter.

Repositioning Limbs A realistic approach must be taken when splinting a patient's possible fractures. In some cases, especially those involving motor vehicle accidents, it will be necessary to slightly reposition a limb or perhaps the entire patient to allow for splinting to take place, or to allow for the patient to be removed from the debris or wreckage after splinting is completed. Variations in splinting procedures occur when the questions of straightening a limb or straightening an angulated fracture are considered.

Each EMS system has its own protocols for the repositioning of limbs and straightening of angulated fractures. These protocols are formulated after considering typical response and transport times, the specialized training of the EMTs, methods of splinting and the types of splints used, the type of medical facility that will receive the patient, and the care procedures that will be used at the medical facility. All EMS systems recognize that some movement of a limb may be necessary to allow for a splint to be applied. Usually, a combination of two or more of the following protocols will be used. Your instructor will explain which of these protocols are followed in your EMS System. Check off these protocols as you are provided with the information concerning your EMS System. YOU MUST FOLLOW LOCAL PROTOCOLS.

- Place angulated long bone fractures (no joint involvement) in anatomical position before splinting or traction (tension) is applied unless there is an associated dislocation or resistance is met. (Seek recommendation of emergency department physician.)

- Splint all dislocations in the position in which they are found.
- If pulse is absent distal to long bone injury, splint as above and expedite transport.

When in doubt as to the correct protocol, contact the emergency department physician. Such contact is recommended for any case that involves a patient who does not have a distal pulse or has evidence of nerve damage.

Straightening Angulated Fractures Straightening angulations of closed long bone fractures is within the scope of EMT-level care. If appropriate, slightly angulated closed fractures of the extremities can usually be straightened and immobilized with few problems. However, severely angulated fractures can pose serious problems. Angulations make splinting and transport more difficult. They can pinch or cut through nerves and blood vessels and usually are painful for the patient. They must, however, be repositioned so they can be splinted. *Not* to splint would be more dangerous.

Warning: DO NOT ATTEMPT TO STRAIGHTEN ANGULATED FRACTURES OF THE SHOULDER OR WRIST. Major nerves and blood vessels pass through these joints, close to the major bones. Attempts to straighten dislocations may cause serious, even permanent, damage. DO NOT ATTEMPT TO STRAIGHTEN ANY DISLOCATED JOINT.

Gently attempt to straighten the limb (Figure 10-17). If the joint shows evidence of a crush injury, do not attempt to straighten it. Whenever there is no distal pulse, transport the patient as soon as possible.

The patient's pain may increase during the process of straightening an angulation. This will be temporary, with the pain lessening and muscle spasms being reduced as splinting is completed. **Manual traction (tension)**—the procedure for straightening closed angulated fractures other than those to the shoulders, elbows, wrists, or knees—is done as follows.

1. CAREFULLY cut away clothing that lies over the fracture site.
2. Grasp the upper extremity above and below the fracture site and apply smooth, steady tension along the long axis of the limb. Gently attempt to align the limb to its anatomical position. Hold the limb so that you maintain alignment and tension until your partner can apply a splint.

General Care for Skeletal Injuries

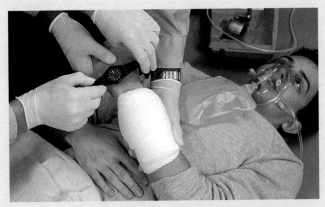

1. Determine signs and symptoms of skeletal injury through patient assessment. Expose site and control bleeding with appropriate dressing. One EMT stabilizes injury site throughout the procedure.

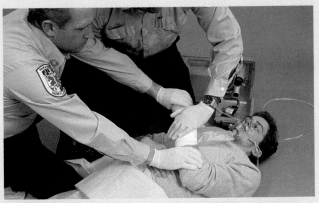

2. Begin treating for shock as soon as possible by providing oxygen and maintaining body temperature.

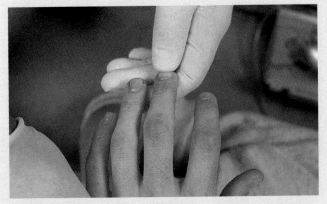

3. Check for impairment of circulation by palpating distal pulse and checking capillary refill time.

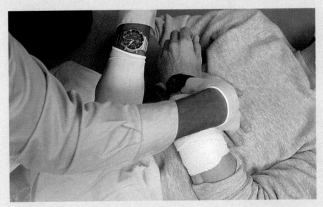

4. Check neurological function. Is patient able to sense your touch or make slight movement of extremity?

273

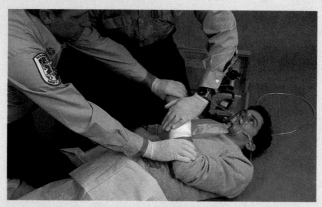

5. Straighten angulated closed fractures by gently attempting to return limb to anatomical or splinting position. Splint in position found if resistance is met or patient feels severe pain. Do not attempt to straighten any dislocation.

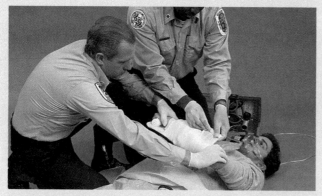

6. One EMT applies manual traction (tension) while another EMT immobilizes the injury site.

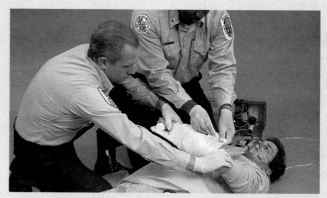

7. Secure the splint snugly, distal to proximal, but do not impair circulation. Package the limb so that the joints immediately above and below the fracture site are immobilized.

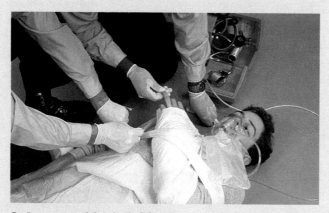

8. Leave nail beds (of fingers or toes) exposed. Monitor circulation and nerve function. Continue treatment for shock and monitor vital signs.

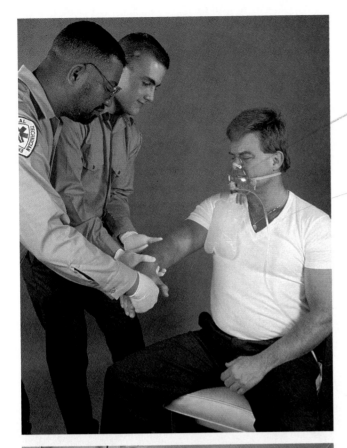

stitute support must be provided to immobilize the bone to prevent further injury. Splinting is the process used to achieve these goals.

Any item that will immobilize a fracture or a dislocation is called a **splint**. The splint must immobilize the fractured bone ends and the joints immediately proximal (above) and distal (below) to the broken bone. If a joint is injured, the splint should immobilize the joint and the bones proximal and distal to the joint.

There are a number of reasons for splinting. In addition to immobilizing the injured extremity, splinting helps to prevent or reduce the severity of the complications that accompany fractures and dislocations. These complications include

* Pain—Much of the pain experienced by the patient is associated with the unrestricted movement of bone ends and fragments. In cases of dislocation, splinting may prevent bone ends from placing additional pressure on nerves, blood vessels, and sensitive tissues.
* Damage to Soft Tissues—The processes of fracturing and dislocation cause soft tissue injuries that will be aggravated if the extremity is not immobilized. Nerves can be damaged beyond repair if the extremity is not immobilized.
* Bleeding—Dislocated bones, the ends of fractured bones, and bone fragments can damage blood vessels.
* Restricted Blood Flow—Dislocated bones, the ends of fractured bones, and bone fragments can press against blood vessels, reducing or shutting off the flow of blood.
* Closed Fractures Becoming Open Fractures—The sharp edges of fractured bones may tear through the patient's skin to produce an open fracture.

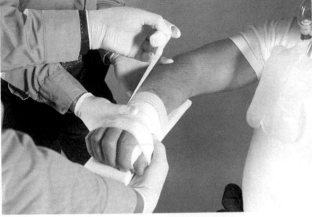

Figure 10-17 Procedure for straightening and immobilizing an angulated closed fracture.

Note: If a firm resistance is felt while you are applying tension, crepitus occurs, or the patient experiences a significant increase in pain, do not try to correct the angulation. Attempt to correct the angulation only once. Be certain that your actions do not displace a joint. Any additional attempts require a physician's approval.

Splinting A bone is a supporting structure. When it is broken or dislocated, some sub-

Types of Splints There are two types of splints for upper extremities: rigid and soft (Scan 10-2).

The process of splinting is easier to understand if you consider **rigid splints**. As the name implies, these splints are stiff, with very little flexibility. When applied along an injured bone, they serve to immobilize the bone and the joints immediately above and below the injury site, preventing the movement of the injured bone. A rigid splint also will allow for repositioning and transfer of the patient with a minimum of movement of the injured extremity.

There are many types of commercial rigid splints, including those made of wood, alu-

Splints and Accessories

Splints and accessories for extremity fractures. Rigid or soft splints—including board, inflatable, blanket, and pillow—are used for the upper extremities.

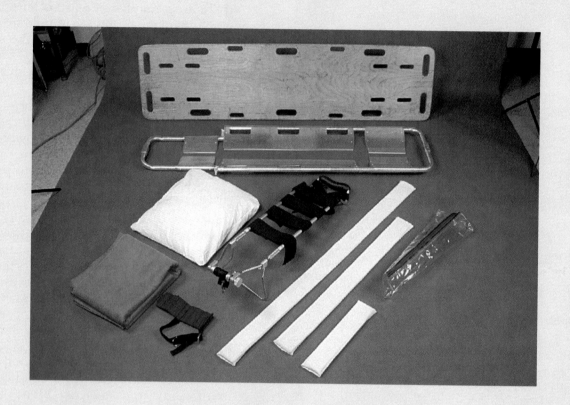

minum, compressed wood fibers, cardboard, wire, and plastic. Some come with their own washable pads; others require padding to be applied before being secured to the patient. Most ambulances carry short padded board splints (18 inches long), medium padded board splints (3 feet long), and long padded board splints (at least 4½ feet long).

Soft splints can be of two types. One type is the **air-inflatable splint**. This splint is classified as a soft splint even though it is rigid when finally applied to the site of injury (see Scan 10-7 on air-inflated splints). There may be problems experienced when using this type of splint. Air may leak from the splint, the air pressure may change as temperature and altitude change, and the size of the splint may not be adequate for many patients. It is not practical to attempt a distal pulse evaluation once the splint is inflated. Usually, an evaluation of circulation will have to be done. All of these problems faced in the field and the fact that many emergency departments have reported significant pain to the patient when the splint is removed have led some EMS systems to drop air-inflated splints from their approved equipment lists.

The second type of soft splint is the **vacuum splint**. Other soft splints are pillows, blankets, towels, and dressings. One of the most useful soft-splinting techniques is the application of a sling and swathe (see Scan 10-3). Be sure always to immobilize the two adjacent joints.

There will be times when you do not have enough splints at the scene of an accident or you are responding while you are off duty and do not have any commercial splints. You will have to make your own splints from materials at the scene. Your emergency splints may be soft splints such as pillows or rolled blankets, or they may be rigid splints made from a variety of materials. You can use pieces of lumber, plywood, compressed wood products, cardboard, rolled newspapers or magazines, umbrellas, canes, broom handles, shovel handles, sporting equipment (a catcher's or hockey goalie's shin guards have been used), or tongue depressors (for fractured fingers).

Some of these items can be found at the scene of a typical accident. Ask bystanders to help you find something that can be used as a splint. Give them suggestions and ask if they have any ideas. Having bystanders check the trunks of their cars usually produces results. Tell them you are looking for something rigid and long enough to hold the fractured bone and the joints immediately above and below this bone.

In some cases, it will be necessary to splint the injured limb to an unaffected limb, thus using the patient's own body as a splint. For example, an injured finger may be taped to an adjoining uninjured finger, or it may be necessary to tie a patient's lower limbs together or to secure the arm to the chest.

Splinting the Upper Extremities There are eight basic rules to keep in mind as you apply splints for injuries to the extremities.

- WHEN IN DOUBT, SPLINT.
- Patients with possible fractures or dislocations should be treated for shock and, when appropriate, administered a high concentration of oxygen.
- Always be sure that a rigid splint is padded before it is applied to a patient.
- When securing a splint to an extremity, wrap it from distal to proximal.
- Be certain that you have not disrupted vascular or nerve function during the splinting process. Check the distal pulse, capillary refill, and nerve function before and after splinting. Remember to record your findings on your prehospital care report. Monitor these factors and distal skin color and temperature during transport.
- When possible, splint fractures of the forearm or hand with the hand in its position of function. This is the position the hand would be in if the patient were to reach out and pick up a palm-sized round object. A roll of bandage placed in the patient's hand will help maintain the position of function.
- When possible, elevate an injured extremity after it is immobilized to reduce swelling.
- Continue to check air-inflated splints to be certain that they have not lost or gained pressure. Altitude or temperature changes will affect splint pressure. Leaks may occur from punctures or the deterioration of valves or zippers.

Musculoskeletal (orthopedic) injuries can be frightening to the patient. Always reassure the conscious patient, explaining what you must do. Many patients assume that a splint means that they definitely have a fracture. Unless the fracture is obvious, let patients know that you are suspicious of a fracture and the splinting process is a precaution.

The Shoulder Girdle Injuries to the shoulder girdle involve some special assessment and care considerations.

Patient Assessment— Shoulder Girdle Injuries

Be aware of the signs and symptoms that point to shoulder girdle injury.

Signs and Symptoms

- [ ] Pain in the shoulder may indicate several types of injury. Look for specific signs.
- [ ] A dropped shoulder, with the patient holding the arm of his injured side against the chest, often indicates a fracture of the clavicle or scapula (Figure 10-18).
- [ ] Indications of a severe blow to the back over the scapula. (All the bones of the shoulder girdle can be felt except the scapula. Only the superior ridge of the scapula, called the spine, can be easily palpated. Injury to the scapula is rare but must be considered if there are indications of a severe blow at the site of this bone.)
- [ ] Check the entire shoulder girdle.
  1. Check for deformity where the clavicle attaches to the sternum—possible fracture or dislocation.
  2. Feel for deformity where the clavicle joins the scapula (acromioclavicular joint, ak-KRO-me-o-klav-IK-u-lar)—possible dislocation.
  3. Feel and look along the entire clavicle for deformity—possible fracture.
  4. Note if the head of the humerus can be felt or moves in front of the shoulder—possible anterior dislocation. This displacement also may be due to a fracture.

Patient Care—Shoulder Girdle Injuries

Learn the emergency care steps to follow when you suspect a shoulder girdle injury.

Emergency Care Steps

1. Check for a radial pulse on the injured side. If there is no pulse, immobilize and transport as soon as possible, notifying the receiving facility.
2. Determine nerve function by checking for feeling and movement of the fingers on the injured side. If there is possible nerve damage, immobilize and transport as soon as possible.
3. It is not practical to use a rigid splint for injuries to the clavicle, scapula, or the head of the humerus. Use a sling and swathe (see Scan 10-3). If there is possible cervical spine injury, do not tie a sling around the neck.
4. If there is evidence of a possible anterior dislocation of the head of the humerus, place a thin pillow between the patient's arm and chest before applying the sling and swathe.
5. *Do not* attempt to straighten or reset any dislocations.

Note: Sometimes a dislocated shoulder will reduce itself ("pop back into place"). When this happens, you should check for a distal pulse and nerve function. Apply a sling and swathe and transport the patient. The patient must be seen by a physician. Be certain to note the self-reduction on the patient form and to report the event to the emergency department staff.

The following section—Scans 10-3 through 10-7—contains additional information on emergency care for injuries to the upper extremities. As an EMT you are responsible for knowing how to care for injuries to the entire upper extremity.

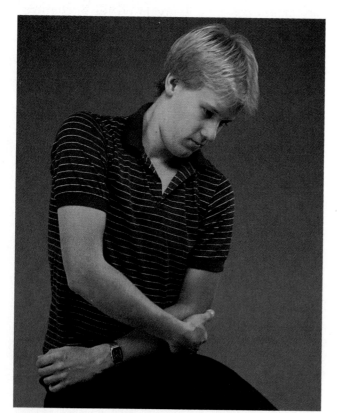

Figure 10-18 Fractured clavicle, noted by "dropped" shoulder.

Sling and Swathe

Dough Logan
Scott Champion

A sling is a triangular bandage used to support the shoulder and arm. Once the patient's arm is placed in a sling, a swathe can be used to hold the arm against the side of the chest. Commercial slings are available. Roller bandage can be used to form a sling and swathe. Velcro straps can be used to form a swathe. Use whatever materials you have on hand, provided they will not cut into the patient.

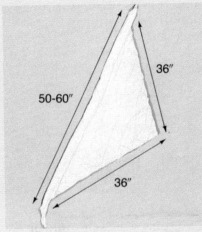

1. The sling should be in the shape of a triangle.

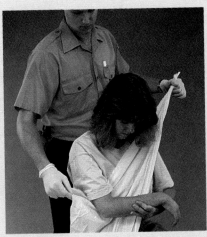

2. Position the sling over the top of the patient's chest as shown. Fold the patient's injured arm across the chest.

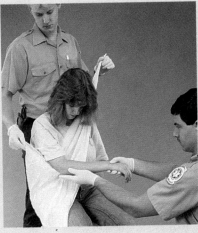

3. If the patient cannot hold his arm, have someone assist until you tie the sling.

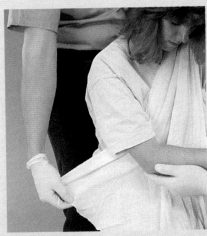

4. One point of the triangle should extend behind the elbow on the injured side.

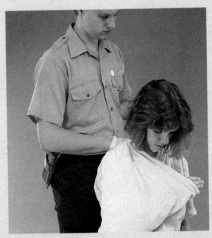

5. Take the bottom point of the triangle and bring this end up over the patient's arm. When you are finished, this point should be taken over the top of the patient's injured shoulder.

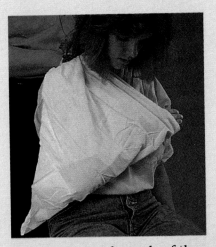

6. Draw up on the ends of the sling so that the patient's hand is about four inches above the elbow (exceptions are discussed later).

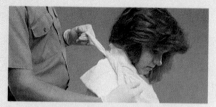

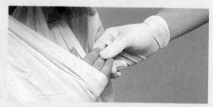

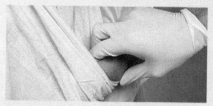

7. Tie the two ends of the sling together, making sure that the knot does not press against the back of the patient's neck. The area can be padded with bulky dressings or sanitary napkins.

8. Leave the patient's fingertips exposed to detect any color or skin temperature changes that indicate the lack of circulation.

9. Check for a radial pulse. If the pulse has been lost, take off the sling and repeat the procedure. Check neurologic function. Repeat sling procedure if necessary.

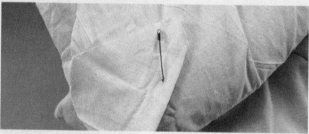

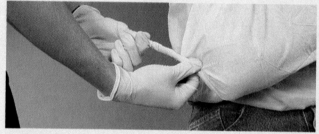

10A. Take hold of the point of material at the patient's elbow and fold it forward, pinning it to the front of the sling. This forms a pocket for the patient's elbow.

10B. If you do not have a pin, twist the excess material and tie a knot in the point.

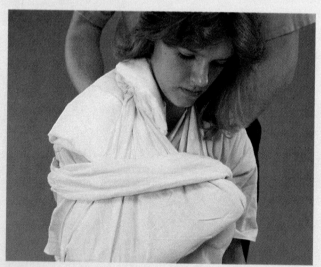

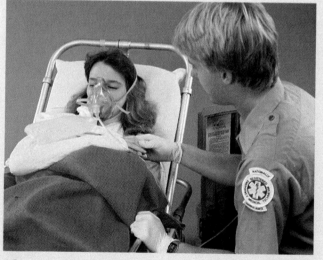

11. A swathe can be formed from a second piece of triangular material. This swathe is tied around the chest and the injured arm, over the sling. Do not place this swathe over the patient's arm on the uninjured side.

12. • Assess distal pulse and neurologic function. • Treat for shock. • Provide a high concentration of oxygen. • Continue to reassure the patient. • Take vital signs.

Note: If the patient has a cervical spine injury, do not tie sling around neck.

Injuries to the Humerus—
Soft Splinting

SIGNS: Injury to the humerus can take place at the proximal end (shoulder), along the shaft of the bone, or at the distal end (elbow). Deformity is the key sign used to detect fractures to this bone in any of these locations; however, assess for all signs of skeletal injury. Follow the rules and procedures for care of an injured extremity.

Note: **RIGID SPLINTING IS PREFERRED.**

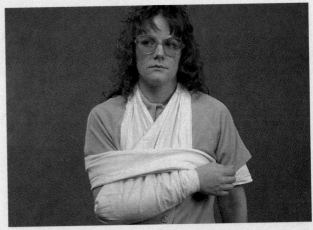

1. Fracture at proximal end. Gently apply a sling and swathe. If you have only enough material for a swathe, bind the patient's upper arm to his body, taking great care not to cut off circulation to the forearm.

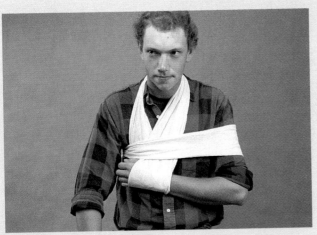

2. Fracture of the shaft. Use rigid splints whenever possible; otherwise, gently apply a sling and swathe. The sling should be modified so that it supports the wrist only.

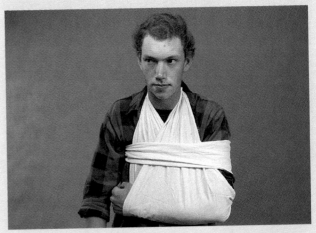

3. Fracture at distal end. Gently apply a full sling and swathe. Do not draw the hand upward to a position above the elbow. Instead, keep elbow flexion as close to a 90° angle as possible.

Warning: Before applying a sling and swathe to care for injuries to the humerus, check for nerve function and circulation. If you do not feel a pulse, attempt to straighten any slight angulation if the patient has a closed fracture (follow local protocol). Otherwise, prepare for immediate immobilization and transport. Should straightening of the angulation fail to restore the pulse or function, splint with a medium board splint (36 inches), keeping the forearm extended. If there is no sign of circulation or nerve function, you will have to attempt a second splinting. If this fails to restore circulation and nerve function, transport immediately. Do not try to straighten angulation of the humerus if there are any signs of fracture or dislocation of the shoulder or elbow.

Arm and Elbow Fractures and Dislocations

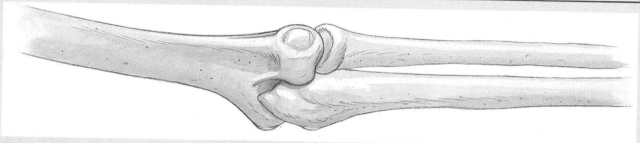

The elbow is a joint and not a bone. It is composed of the distal humerus and the proximal ulna and radius, forming a hinge joint. You will have to decide if the injury is truly to the elbow. Deformity and sensitivity will direct you to the injury site.

Care: If there is a distal pulse, the dislocated elbow should be immobilized in the position in which it is found. The joint has too many nerves and blood vessels to risk movement. Be certain to check for circulation and nerve impairment before and after splinting. When a distal pulse is absent, make one attempt to slightly reposition the limb after contacting the emergency department physician. Do not force the limb into its normal anatomical position.

Elbow in or Returned to Bent Position

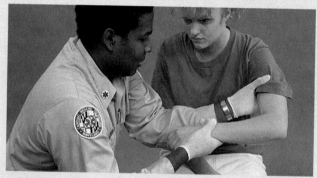

1. Slight repositioning of the limb may be necessary to allow for proper splinting. **Do not** continue if you meet resistance or significantly increase the pain.

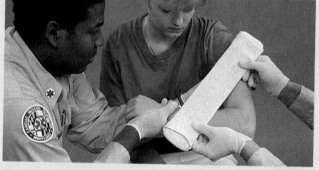

2. Use a padded board splint that will extend 2 to 6 inches beyond the arm and wrist when placed diagonally.

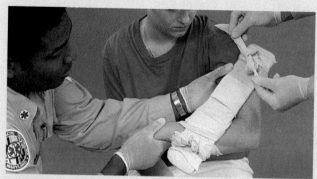

3. Place the splint so it is just proximal to the shoulder and to the wrist. Use cravats to secure to the forearm, then the arm.

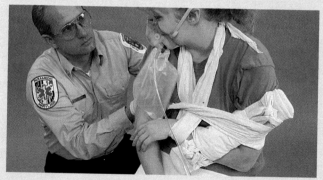

4. A wrist sling can be applied to support the limb; keep the elbow exposed. Apply a swathe if possible.

Elbow in Straight Position

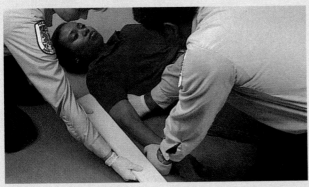

1. Use a padded board splint that extends from under the armpit to a point past the fingertips.

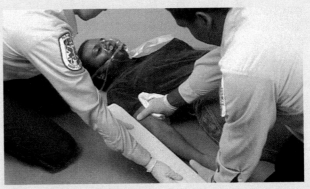

2. Pad the armpit and place a roll of bandages in the patient's hand to help maintain position of function.

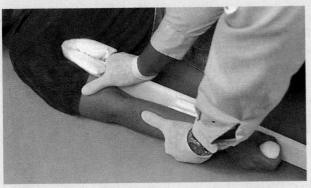

3. Place padded side of board against medial side of limb. Pad all voids.

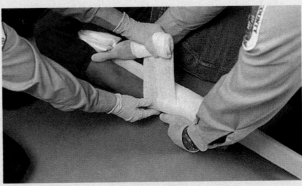

4. Secure splint, bandaging from distal to proximal. Leave fingertips exposed. Reassess distal pulse and neurologic signs.

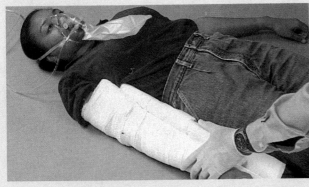

5. Place pads between patient's side and splint.

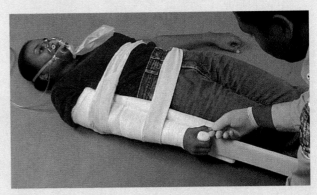

6. Secure splinted limb to body with two cravats. Avoid placing over suspected injury site.

Injuries to the Forearm, Wrist, and Hand

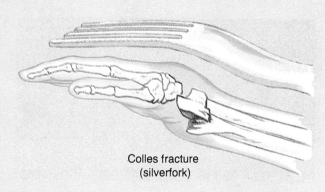

Colles fracture
(silverfork)

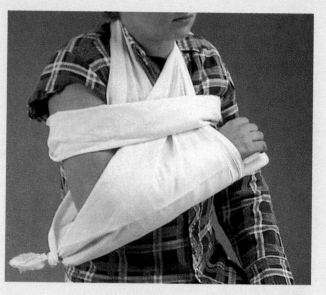

SIGNS:

- Forearm—deformity and tenderness. If only one bone is broken, deformity may be minor or absent.
- Wrist—deformity and tenderness, with the possibility of a Colles (KOL-ez) fracture that gives a "silverfork" appearance to the wrist.
- Hand—deformity and pain. Dislocated fingers are obvious.

CARE: Check for circulation and nerve impairment before and after splinting. Fractures occurring to the forearm, wrist, or hand can be splinted using a padded rigid splint that extends from the elbow past the fingertips. The patient's elbow, forearm, wrist, and hand all need the support of the splint. Tension must be provided throughout splinting. Roller bandage should be placed in the hand to ensure the position of function. After rigid splinting, apply a sling and swathe.

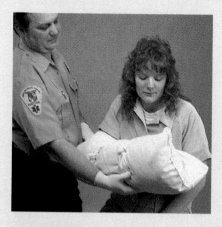

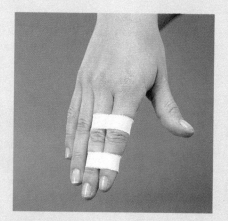

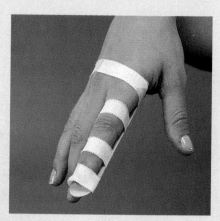

ALTERNATIVE CARE: Fractures of the hand and dislocations of the wrist can be cared for with soft splinting by placing the hand in the position of function and tying the forearm, wrist, and hand into the fold of one pillow or between two pillows. An injured finger can be taped to an adjacent uninjured finger or splinted with a tongue depressor. Some emergency department physicians prefer that care be limited to a wrap of soft bandages. **DO NOT** try to "pop" dislocated fingers back into place.

Scan 10-7
Air-Inflated Splints

WARNING! Air-inflated splints may leak. Make certain that the desired pressure is maintained. When applied in cold weather, an inflatable splint will expand when the patient is moved to a warmer place. Variations in pressure also occur if the patient is moved to a different altitude. Occasionally monitor the pressure in the splint with your fingertip. Air-inflated splints may stick to the patient's skin in hot weather.

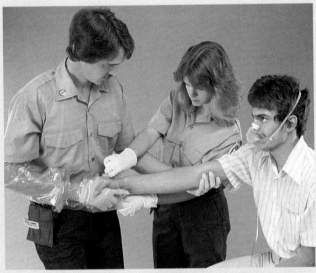

1. Slide the uninflated splint up your forearm, well above the wrist. Use this same hand to grasp the hand of the patient's injured limb as though you were going to shake hands and apply steady tension.

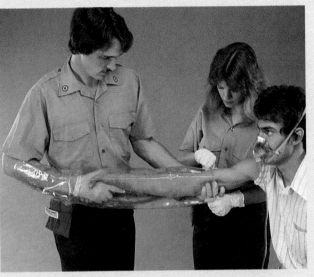

2. While you support his arm in this fashion, your partner gently slides the splint over your hand and onto the patient's injured limb. The lower edge of the splint should be just above his knuckles. Make sure the splint is properly placed and free of wrinkles.

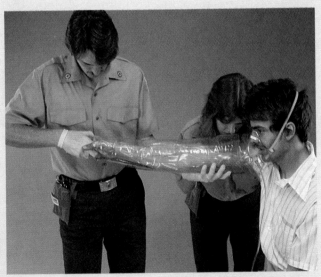

3. Continue to support the patient's arm while you have your partner inflate the splint by mouth to a point where you can make a slight dent in the plastic when you press your thumb against the splint surface.

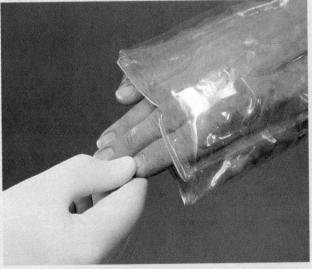

4. Monitor the patient's fingernail beds and fingertips for indications of circulation impairment. Continue to assess neurologic function.

285

COMPLICATIONS OF MUSCULOSKELETAL INJURIES

A number of complications and special considerations may be associated with musculoskeletal injuries to the extremities.

Complications

Injuries to bones and joints may also result in muscle damage, impaired circulation, nerve damage, or wound contamination (Figure 10-19).

Muscle Damage Muscle is often damaged when there are injuries to the joints and bones. In addition to this damage, injuries such as lacerations, punctures, damage from impaled objects, and serious contusions can occur to muscle. The principles of soft tissue injury care must be applied to open wounds involving muscles. Splinting is often desirable even when there are no indications of fractures. Immobilizing the limb will help prevent additional injury to muscle tissue and help control internal bleeding.

Impaired Circulation Fractures and dislocations can cause blood vessels to be lacerated or pinched shut. The major arteries of the extremities lie close to the bones, especially at the joints. As part of the care provided, you must take a distal pulse when evaluating the extent of injury and after you splint an extremity. No pulse indicates a lack of circulation below the injury site. When the extremity is deficient in circulation distal to the injury site, the limb is said to be **ischemic** (is-KE-mik). After about 90 to 120 min-

utes, ischemic tissue will begin to die, or become **necrotic**. Therefore, circulation must be restored as quickly as possible to a pulseless extremity.

Other signs can indicate impaired circulation. **Capillary refill** should be evaluated as a standard procedure before and after splinting. Carefully examine the skin at the distal end of the injured limb and compare what you find with the same area on the opposite side of the body. If the skin color has turned blue (cyanosis) or pale (pallor), or the skin is cold by comparison to the uninjured limb, circulation is probably inadequate. Next, exert pressure over a nailbed on the injured limb, then release the pressure. The nail bed should appear white (blanched) for a brief moment, then regain color as the capillaries refill. If capillary refilling does not take place within 2 seconds, there may be impaired circulation. This is not a very reliable sign if the patient has been exposed to a cold environment.

Nerve Damage Just as blood vessels can be cut or have too much pressure placed on them, so can the nerves running through the extremities. Even when there is no spinal damage, the patient with nerve damage due to a fracture may be unable to move his fingers or toes, depending on the site of the injury. A fracture of the humeral shaft can interrupt the radial nerve, limiting the patient's ability to extend the hand at the wrist. Elbow injuries can damage the ulnar nerve, limiting muscular action or sensation in the hand, particularly in the fourth (ring) and fifth (little) fingers. Lack of movement at the ankles with no response to stimulus along the superior surface of the foot is seen in some cases of fibula fractures in which nerves are damaged.

Wound Contamination In the case of open fractures, a common complication is contamination. *Do not* reach into the wound or try to clean the surface of the exposed bone. In the case of long bone open fractures, contamination is a major problem in the long-term care of the patient. Improper initial care can lead to serious infection. Detached bone fragments outside the body should be cared for and transported the same as an avulsed tissue.

Special Considerations

There are some special considerations to be noted when providing care for a patient having suspected fractures or dislocations.

1. If there is no distal pulse, evidence of defi-

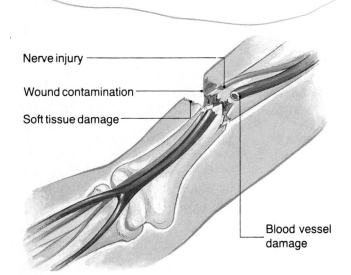

Nerve injury

Wound contamination

Soft tissue damage

Blood vessel damage

Figure 10-19 Complications with fractures.

cient circulation (very weak pulse, the limb feels cold, poor capillary refilling), or poor neurologic function, *the suspected fracture or dislocation takes on a higher priority.*

2. An injured extremity is usually elevated after completion of splinting to help reduce swelling. However, *this should not be done if*

there are any signs of inadequate circulation in the limb.

3. The exposed bone ends and fragments of an open fracture may re-enter the wound as the injured extremity is splinted. *The medical facility staff must be informed if this has happened.*

CHAPTER REVIEW

KEY TERMS

You may find it helpful to review the following terms.

air-inflatable splint—a splint that is classified as a soft splint but becomes rigid when inflated.

angulated fracture—a break to a bone causing the limb or joint to take on an unnatural shape or bend.

appendicular (AP-en-DIK-u-ler) **skeleton**—that part of the skeleton in the upper and lower extremities.

articular cartilage (ar-TIK-u-lar KAR-te-lij)—an elastic tissue that covers the ends of bones forming joints.

articulate (ar-TIK-u-late)—to meet, as in the formation of a joint where two or more bones come together.

axial (AK-si-al) **skeleton**—the skull, spine, ribs, and sternum.

bones—hard but flexible living structures that provide support for the body and protection to vital organs. Types of bones are **long**, **short**, **flat**, and **irregular**. The typical long bone has a cylindrical **shaft**, and a rounded end, or **head**, which is connected to the shaft by the **neck**.

capillary (KAP-i-lar-e) **refill**—the return of blood to the microscopic blood vessels known as capillaries after blood has been forced out by pressure that is then released. Normal refill time is 2 seconds.

cervical (SER-vi-kal) **vertebrae**—the seven vertebrae in the neck.

clavicles (KLAV-i-kuls)—the collarbones.

closed fracture—a broken bone with no associated opening in the skin.

coccyx (KOK-siks)—the four fused vertebrae that form the terminal bone of the spine; the "tailbone."

costal (KOS-tal) **arch**—the arch of cartilage formed by the costal margin.

costal margin—the cartilage attachment points for ribs 6 through 10. It forms the costal arch.

cranium (KRAY-ne-um)—the bones forming the brain case of the skull.

cranial (KRAY-ne-ul) **floor**—the fused bones of the cranium that form the internal, inferior wall of the brain case.

crepitus (KREP-i-tus)—a grating sensation or sound made when fractured bone ends rub together.

dislocation—injury causing the end of a bone to be pulled or pushed from its joint.

extremities (ex-TREM-i-teez)—the portions of the appendicular skeleton that include the clavicles, scapulae, arms forearms, wrists, and hands (upper extremities); the pelvis, thighs, legs, ankles, and feet (lower extremities).

face—the anterior portion of the head.

fracture (FRAK-cher)—any break in a bone.

ischemic (is-KE-mik)—deficient in oxygen because of reduced circulation or blood supply.

joint capsule—a fibrous structure that surrounds a synovial joint and contains the membranes that produce synovial fluid.

joints—places where bones articulate, or meet. Most joints are movable.

jugular notch—the visible depression where the clavicles and sternum meet.

ligaments—tissues that connect bone to bone.

lumbar (LUM-bar) **vertebrae**—the five vertebrae of the midback.

mandible (MAN-di-bul)—the lower jaw.

manual traction—the process of applying tension to straighten and realign a fractured limb before splinting. Also known as *tension.*

medullary (MED-u-lar-e) **canal**—the cavity in long bones containing bone marrow.

necrotic (nek-ROT-ik)—having suffered necrosis (nek-ROS-is) or tissue death.

open fracture—either a broken bone with the ends or fragments tearing outward through the skin or a penetrating wound with an associated fracture.

periosteum (per-e-OS-te-um)—the white fibrous membrane covering a bone.

rigid splint—a stiff device used to immobilize a fracture or dislocation.

sacrum (SAY-krum)—the five fused vertebrae of the lower back.

skull—the bony structure of the head made up of 22 bones that form the cranium and the face.

soft splints—air-inflatable splints, vacuum splints, or cushioning items such as pillows, towels, blankets, or dressings that help immobilize a fracture or dislocation.

spinal column—the column of bones known as vertebrae that houses the spinal cord and supports the head and upper body.

splint—a device used to immobilize fractures and dislocations so that there is a minimum of movement to the bone and to the joints above and below the bone.

sprain—a partially torn ligament.

sternum—the breastbone.

strain—the overstretching or mild tearing of a muscle.

suture (SU-cher)—the point or seam where two bones, especially cranial bones, articulate, or join together.

synovial (si-NO-ve-al) **joints**—the highly movable joints in the body, such as the elbow, consisting of the ends of two joining bones surrounded by a joint capsule and lubricated by synovial fluid.

tendons—tissues that connect muscle to bone.

tension—see *manual traction*.

thoracic (tho-RAS-ik) **cage**—the bony structure that protects the heart, lungs, and other organs in the chest. It is made up of 12 pairs of ribs, the 12 thoracic vertebrae, and the sternum, or breastbone.

thoracic vertebrae—the 12 vertebrae to which the ribs attach.

vacuum splint—a type of soft splint.

vertebrae (VER-te-bre)—the 33 irregularly shaped bones of the spinal column.

xiphoid (ZIF-oid) **process**—the lower extension of the sternum.

Note: The study of medicine that deals with musculoskeletal injury and disease is orthopedics. The term comes from *ortho* (to straighten or correct) and *pedio* (pertaining to the child). The term literally means to straighten the child. The first orthopedists provided care for the deformities of children.

SUMMARY

The Musculoskeletal System

The bones, joints, and muscles make up the musculoskeletal system. There are three types of muscle: skeletal, smooth, and cardiac. Skeletal muscle is considered when studying musculoskeletal injuries.

The four major functions of the skeletal system are body support, body movement, organ protection, and certain aspects of blood cell production. Bones have self-healing properties. A fractured bone must be immobilized quickly and remain immobilized so that proper healing is not prevented.

There are two major divisions to the skeletal system: the axial skeleton and the appendicular skeleton. The axial skeleton is composed of the skull (cranium and face), the spinal column (five divisions: cervical, thoracic, and lumbar vertebrae, sacrum, and coccyx), ribs, and sternum.

The upper and lower extremities are part of the appendicular skeleton. Each upper extremity consists of the scapula (shoulder blade), clavicle (collarbone), humerus (arm), ulna and radius (forearm), carpals (wrist), metacarpals (hand), and phalanges (fingers).

Types of Bone and Joint Injuries

If a part of a fractured bone tears through the patient's skin, the injury is an open fracture. This also is the case when a penetrating wound accompanies a fracture. If the fractured bones do not tear through the patient's skin to open the fracture to the outside, the injury is a closed fracture. When a bone is broken, it will often bend or twist to form an angulated fracture.

Any break of a bone is a fracture. A dislocation occurs when a bone is pulled out from a joint. Partially torn ligaments produce sprains.

Stretching or minor tearing of muscles produces strains.

The signs and symptoms of fracture may include the feeling or sound of breaking bone, tenderness or pain, deformity, swelling, discoloration, crepitus, loss of function, loss of distal pulse, loss of sensation, numbness or tingling, exposed bone, false motion, or muscle spasms. Dislocation usually has deformity, swelling, pain, and loss of function. Sprains normally have swelling, discoloration, and pain on movement but no deformity. Pain is usually the only sign of strain.

Treatment of Injuries to the Extremities

As an EMT you should never become so preoccupied with fractures that you forget to conduct a primary survey and a secondary survey with an interview. Remember that the airway, breathing, circulation, and disability are your first priorities. Shock, neck, spinal, chest, abdominal, and head injuries, and serious burns are all to be treated before fractures.

The order of care for fractures is: first priority, spine fractures; second priority, fractures of the head, rib cage, and pelvis; third priority, fractures of the extremities, lower extremities first.

You should apply sterile dressings, when possible, to all open fractures of the extremities.

Angulations can be straightened by manual traction (tension): grasping the limb above and below the site of the fracture and gently pulling with the hand you have placed below the site. Basically, fractures should be realigned unless they involve a joint. *Do not* attempt to straighten dislocations. Splint dislocations in the position they are found.

Splinting is used to immobilize fractures. The application of a splint can also help to prevent or reduce the severity of complications such as pain, soft tissue damage, bleeding, restricted blood flow, and closed fractures becoming open fractures. The process can be carried out using rigid or soft splints. In some cases, it may be necessary to splint one body part to another.

As an EMT you must be able to use noncommercial splints. Consider such items as lumber and sporting equipment when you need to make an emergency splint.

WHEN IN DOUBT, SPLINT.

Remember first to control bleeding, dress open wounds, and care for shock, administering a high concentration of oxygen. Assess the injury, Check for a distal pulse and assess nerve function before and after splinting. Cut away, remove, or lift away the patient's clothing over the injury site and remove all jewelry from the affected limb before splinting. When possible, straighten closed angulated fractures. Apply manual traction. Splint, wrapping from distal to proximal.

A rigid splint should immobilize the bone and the joints directly above and below the injured bone. All rigid splints should be padded before they are secured to the patient. When possible, an injured limb should be elevated once it is splinted to reduce swelling. However, *do not* elevate if there is evidence of impaired circulation. Check air-inflated splints to be sure they have not gained or lost pressure.

Be aware of the special signs of injury to the shoulder girdle, especially a dropped shoulder indicating clavicular fracture. Immobilize with sling and swathe.

Patients with possible fractures and dislocations need to be reassured throughout the care process.

Whenever possible, immobilize all fractures and dislocations before moving the patient.

Complications of Musculoskeletal Injuries

Injuries to bones and joints may also result in muscle damage, impaired circulation, nerve damage, and wound contamination. Soft tissue care and splinting are beneficial for muscle injuries. Give a higher priority to any fracture or dislocation when circulation appears impaired. Avoid excessive movement of joints that may aggravate blood vessel and nerve damage. Minimize contamination by not reaching into or touching the bone in an open wound. Report to the medical facility staff any instance in which the bone ends re-enter an open fracture wound.

11

On the Scene

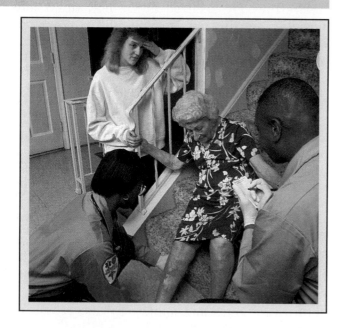

Eighty-eight-year-old Margaret Berlowitz is upstairs when she hears the doorbell ring. In her haste to answer the door, she misses the last step and falls to the entryway floor. Mrs. Berlowitz feels an immediate intense pain in her lower leg. The neighbor at the door, who has heard her fall, enters and calls 911 for EMS. She also calls Mrs. Berlowitz's daughter at her nearby job.

Your EMS unit is dispatched for "a fall." When you arrive, Mrs. Berlowitz's daughter is pulling into the driveway just ahead of you. The neighbor meets you and your partner and the daughter at the door and fills

you in on the details of the accident. Your patient is in considerable pain.

You: Hello, Mrs. Berlowitz. We're from the ambulance, and we'd like to help you. Can you tell me what happened?

Mrs. Berlowitz: I was coming downstairs to answer the door, and I slipped. I'm not as young as I used to be. (She tries to laugh through the pain.)

You: Did you feel dizzy or pass out before you fell?

Mrs. Berlowitz: Oh, no. I just plain slipped.

You: I can see you're in a lot of pain. We're going to check you over. We'll take care of your leg and see if there's anything else that needs looking after.

As you proceed through your primary and secondary surveys, you do not find any other significant injuries. Mrs. Berlowitz appears to have a fracture of the tibia, and you and your partner apply a rigid board splint. Although Mrs. Berlowitz appears to be fine except for her leg, you realize the potential for blood loss and shock and make sure to administer a high flow of oxygen.

En route to the hospital, you listen sympathetically as your patient's daughter "vents" her frustration about her mother's not being as steady on her feet as she once was. Now, she says, she will carry out the plan she and her mother have talked about, to hire someone to look in on Mrs. Berlowitz regularly on the days when her daughter is at work.

The Lower Extremities

In the last chapter you learned about the musculoskeletal system and about injuries to to the bones and joints, especially of the upper extremities. In this chapter you will learn about the lower extremities.

Expected Outcome, Chapter 11: *You will be able to assess and care for musculoskeletal injuries to the lower extremities.*

WARNING: Protect yourself from infectious diseases by using appropriate barrier devices such as a pocket face mask with one-way valve, face shield, or bag-valve mask; goggles or eye shield; and disposable gloves. Always conform to your local EMS system's infection exposure control plan.

THE LOWER EXTREMITIES

INJURIES TO THE BONES AND JOINTS
     Fractures
     The Pelvis
     The Femur

GENERAL TREATMENT OF INJURIES TO THE
LOWER EXTREMITIES
     Pulse Assessment
     Nerve Function Assessment
     Manual Traction (Tension)
     Spinal Protection

TREATMENT OF SPECIFIC INJURIES TO THE
LOWER EXTREMITIES
     Fractures of the Pelvis
     Hip Dislocations
     Hip Fractures
     Femoral Shaft Fractures
     Knee Injuries
     Fractures of the Leg
     Injuries to the Ankle and Foot

Knowledge *After reading this chapter, you should be able to*

1. Locate and name the major bones of the lower extremities. (pp. 292-294)

2. Explain, in terms of its anatomy, why special consideration is given to injury to the bones of the pelvis. (pp. 295-297)

3. Relate the significance of the muscle mass of the thigh to the care procedures for a fractured femur. (pp. 297-298, 300)

4. Describe the basic care provided for given injuries of the lower extremities, including pulse and nerve function assessment, manual traction (tension), and spinal protection. (pp. 298-300)

5. Describe how an EMT can determine if a patient has a possible fracture of the pelvis, an anterior dislocation of the hip, or a posterior dislocation of the hip. (pp. 300-301, 301-302)

6. Describe emergency care for pelvic fractures, hip dislocations, hip fractures, femoral shaft fractures, knee injuries, leg fractures, and ankle and foot injuries. (pp. 301-303, 311-313, 321; Scans 11-3 through 11-8)

7. Describe, step by step, traction splinting procedures. (Scans 11-1A, B, and C; Scan 11-2)

Skills *As an EMT you should be able to*

1. Identify injuries to the lower extremities based on signs and symptoms.

2. Provide soft tissue care for injuries to the lower extremities.

3. Provide care for injuries to the bones and joints of the lower extremities, including
   - Pelvic fractures
   - Hip fractures
   - Anterior and posterior hip dislocations
   - Fractures of the femur
   - Fractures and dislocations of the knee
   - Fractures of the leg
   - Fractures and dislocations of the ankle
   - Fractures of the foot

4. Use the basic splints that are a part of EMT-level care at the accident scene, including rigid, soft, and traction splints.

5. Properly straighten closed angulated fractures, when appropriate.

6. Evaluate vascular and nerve function for the lower extremities.

7. Make and use noncommercial splints for emergency situations.

8. Provide total patient care for patients with injury to the lower extremities.

Injuries to the bones and joints of the lower extremities often require emergency care at the scene of an accident. Although not life-threatening by themselves, such injuries cause great pain to the patient and, if not quickly immobilized, may not heal correctly. In addition, bone and joint injuries often involve other kinds of damage as well.

Remember: When a bone is fractured, the damage to blood vessels, nerves, and other soft tissues may be of greater significance than the fracture. Proper care of bone and joint injuries *must* include efficient soft tissue care.

THE LOWER EXTREMITIES

As you learned in Chapter 10, the appendicular skeleton is composed of the upper and lower extremities. In this chapter we will consider the structures making up the lower extremities. The lower extremities are composed of the pelvis and the two lower limbs. The bones of the lower extremities are shown in Figure 11-1.

Each limb consists of the femur, patella, tibia, fibula, tarsals, metatarsals, and phalanges. The joint between the pelvis and the head of the femur is called the hip. The knee

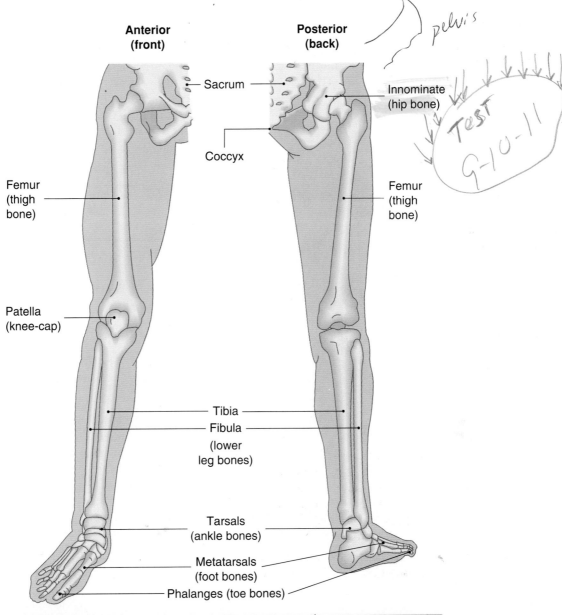

Anterior (front)

Posterior (back)

Sacrum

Innominate (hip bone)

Coccyx

Femur (thigh bone)

Femur (thigh bone)

Patella (knee-cap)

Tibia

Fibula (lower leg bones)

Tarsals (ankle bones)

Metatarsals (foot bones)

Phalanges (toe bones)

pelvis

Test 9-10-11

THE LOWER EXTREMITIES

COMMON NAMES

Pelvic girdle (pelvis or hips)

Thigh bone (1/limb)
Kneecap (1/limb)
Leg bones (shin bones, 2/leg, 1 medial, 1 lateral)
Ankle bones (7/foot)

Foot bones (5/foot)
Toe bones (14/foot. some people have two bones in their little toe, others may have three)

ANATOMICAL NAMES

Innominate on each side made up of the fused ilium, ischium, and pubis bones, as well as sacrum and coccyx posteriorly

Femur (FE-mer)
Patella (pah-TEL-lah)
Tibia (TIB-e-ah) – medial
Fibula (FIB-yo-lah) – lateral
Tarsals (TAR-sals)

Metatarsals (meta-TAR-sals)
Phalanges (Fah-LAN-jez)

Figure 11-1 Bones of the lower extremity.

joint is composed of the distal femur, the proximal tibia, and the patella. The distal tibia and fibula join with the tarsals to form the ankle.

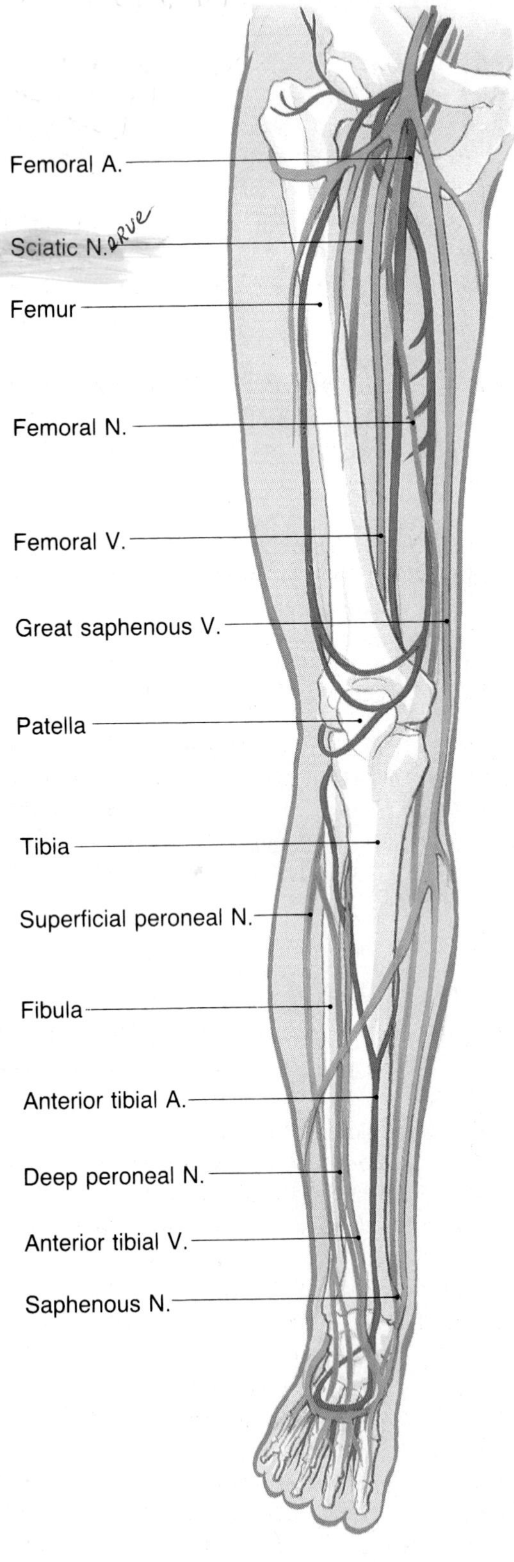

Note: To a physician, the *hip* is the joint formed by the pelvis and the head of the femur. Many patients commonly refer to the lateral pelvis as their hip. The medical staff will call the upper leg the *thigh* and the lower leg the *leg*. From pelvis to the tips of the toes is the lower extremity.

Figure 11-2 shows the major blood vessels and muscles, along with a few of the major nerves found in the lower limb.

INJURIES TO THE BONES AND JOINTS

Structures of the musculoskeletal system are subject to injury in the form of fractures, dislocations, sprains, and strains.

Fractures

As discussed in Chapter 10, a fracture is any break in a bone. Fractures can be open or closed, depending on whether or not the bone end protrudes or has protruded through the skin (Figure 11-3).

There are other classifications of fractures that are based on x-ray appearance (Figure 11-4). Obviously, this is not part of the knowledge, skills, and equipment of the EMT. However, you will hear these terms at the medical facility when

Femoral A.

Sciatic N.

Femur

Femoral N.

Femoral V.

Great saphenous V.

Patella

Tibia

Superficial peroneal N.

Fibula

Anterior tibial A.

Deep peroneal N.

Anterior tibial V.

Saphenous N.

Figure 11-2 The complex anatomy of the lower extremity (A, artery; N, nerve; V, vein).

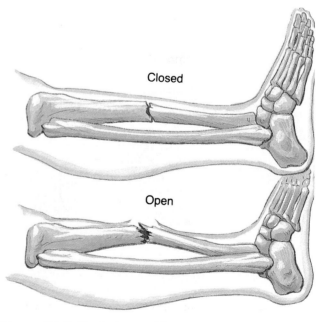

Closed

Open

Figure 11-3 Basic types of fractures

discussing fractures. The x-ray classifications are

State test

- Transverse—The break is straight across the shaft of a bone.
- Oblique—The break forms an angle to the shaft.
- Spiral—The fracture has the appearance of a spring. The break twists around the shaft of the bone.
- Greenstick—The fracture is incomplete and is so called because it looks like a green stick that is bent but not broken. Some fibers are separated, while others remain intact. This type of fracture is common in infants and children whose bones are still soft and pliable.
- Impacted—The ends of broken bones are jammed into each other.
- Comminuted—The bone is fragmented. A severe crush injury may cause a bone to break into many pieces.

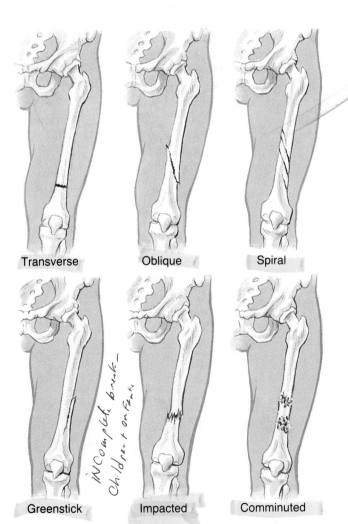

Transverse   Oblique   Spiral

Greenstick   Impacted   Comminuted

Incomplete break—Children often

Figure 11-4 Classification of fractures

The Pelvis

The pelvis is sometimes called the pelvic girdle. It is composed of two large hip bones, one on each side. Each large hip bone is made up of three bones fused together tightly (Figure 11-5).

- **Ilium** (IL-e-um)—Each ilium forms an upper "wing" of the pelvis. If you ask someone to place his hands on his hips, he will usually place them over the ilia (plural of ilium) of the pelvis.
- **Ischium** (IS-ke-um)—Each ischium forms the lower, posterior portion of the pelvis. Part of the ischium can be felt as a ridge of bone underneath the muscles of the buttock.
- **Pubis** (PYOO-bis) or **Pubic** (PYOO-bik) **Bone**—The right and left pubic bones join to form the medial, anterior section of the pelvis.

The pelvic bones join with the sacrum and coccyx of the spine to encircle the pelvic cavity.

Patient Assessment—Pelvic Injuries

All injuries involving the bones of the pelvis must be considered to be serious. Patients with possible pelvic bone injury must be seen by a physician as soon as possible. Four anatomical factors make this special caution necessary.

☐ The pelvis surrounds and protects the urinary bladder, part of the large intestine, and the internal reproductive organs. Injury to the pelvic bones also may mean injury to the internal organs and, frequently, severe internal bleeding.

☐ Many major nerves are associated with the pelvis. The spinal cord does not pass through the entire spinal column. It stops at the level of the lower border of the first lumbar vertebra. A large number of nerves originate from this level, sweeping downward (Figure 11-6). Injury to the ilia also may mean injury to many of these nerves.

☐ The pelvis joins with the sacrum. If there is injury to the pelvis, there may be injury to the spine. There is a rule to follow in EMT-level care: if the mechanism of injury produced enough force to damage the strong bones of the pelvis, then assume that there is also spinal injury.

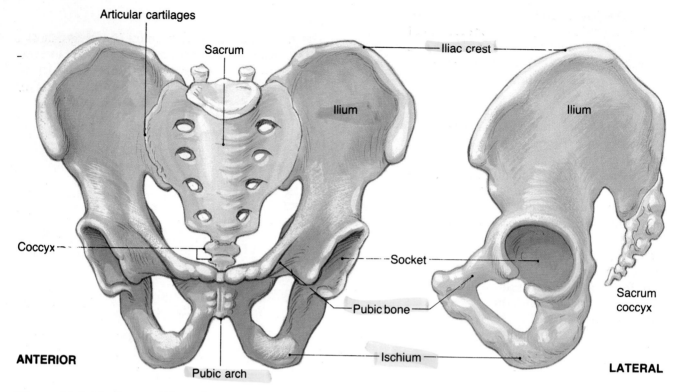

Figure 11-5 The bones of the pelvis.

ANTERIOR

LATERAL

Articular cartilages

Sacrum

Iliac crest

Ilium

Ilium

Coccyx

Socket

Sacrum coccyx

Pubic bone

Ischium

Pubic arch

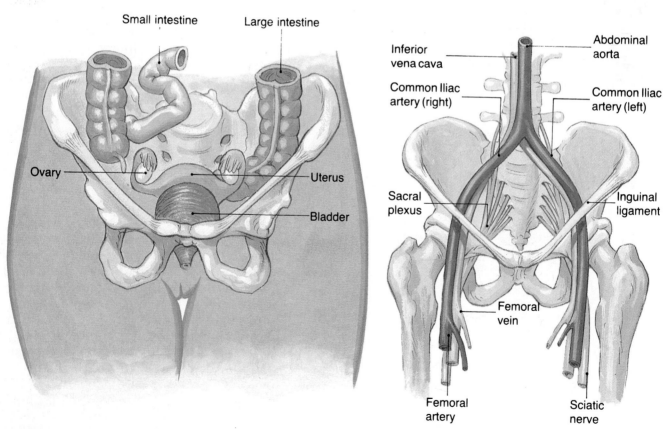

Figure 11-6 Injury to the pelvis may damage internal organs and major blood vessels and nerves.

Small intestine

Large intestine

Ovary

Uterus

Bladder

Inferior vena cava

Abdominal aorta

Common Iliac artery (right)

Common Iliac artery (left)

Sacral plexus

Inguinal ligament

Femoral vein

Femoral artery

Sciatic nerve

The lower limbs join with the pelvis. This means that major arteries, veins, and nerves must be associated with the pelvis and the hip joints. Damage to the pelvic bones or the joints with the femurs may mean significant blood vessel damage and blood loss or serious nerve injury.

As noted, the pelvic bones are very strong bones; however, the force applied to these bones during motor vehicle collisions and falls may produce serious injury. About 3% of all fractures involve the pelvis, with the percentage increasing for elderly patients. Fractures to the pelvis are second to skull fractures in terms of complications and death. Depending on the location of the fracture site and its severity, the mortality rate for pelvic fractures is from 5% to 20%. The most serious complication is usually severe internal bleeding that rapidly leads to hypovolemic shock.

The Femur

The femur is the long bone of the thigh. It is a large, strong bone, surrounded by a large muscle mass. Major blood vessels and nerves pass close to the hip joint and are associated with the femur and the muscles of the thigh and leg.

Patient Assessment—Femoral Injuries

The large muscle mass of the thigh can complicate fractures to the femur (Figure 11-7). There may be internal or external bleeding from arteries deep in the thigh that is difficult to detect or control. Contractions of the thigh muscle may cause the ends of a completely fractured femur to ride over one another and, if it is an open fracture, cause the bone ends to recede, making detection of the open fracture difficult.

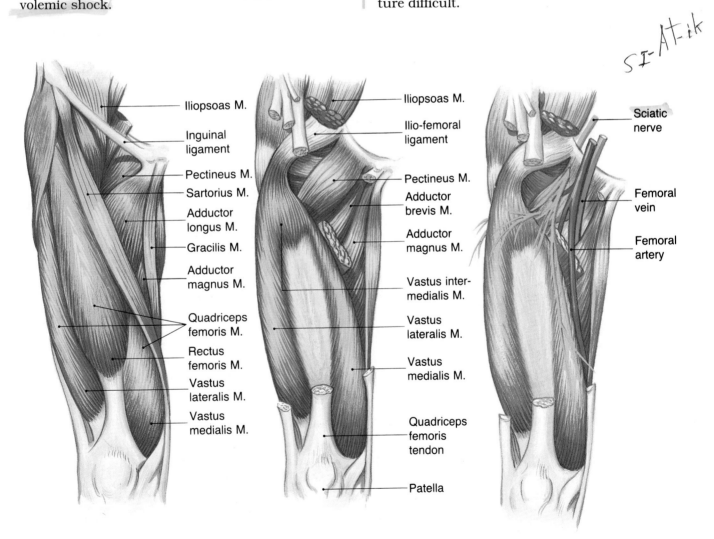

Figure 11-7 Injury to the femur is complicated by the muscle mass of the thigh and its major vessels and nerves.

In addition, if the mechanism of injury produced enough force to fracture the femur, it is reasonable to assume that there may be

☐ Associated injury to the hip joint, pelvis, or spine
☐ Impairment of circulation in the lower extremity
☐ Impairment of nerve function in the lower extremity
☐ Severe internal or external bleeding with a blood loss of 1 pint or more occurring rapidly

Patient Care—Injuries to the Lower Extremities

Emergency care for injuries to the lower extremities is discussed throughout the rest of this chapter: first, general guidelines on treating injuries to the lower extremities, then specific assessment and care procedures for injuries to the pelvis, hip, femur, knee, leg, ankle, and foot.

GENERAL TREATMENT OF INJURIES TO THE LOWER EXTREMITIES

The basic rules for patient care and the splinting of the upper extremities (see Chapter 10) also apply to the lower extremities (Figure 11-8). Special consideration must be given to assessment of a distal pulse and nerve function, providing manual traction (tension), use and application of a traction splint, and procedures to protect possible spinal injuries.

Pulse Assessment

Circulation must be assessed distal to (beyond) the injury site. One of two pulse sites (Figure 11-9) can be used.

- Posterior Tibial Pulse—This site is recommended if the patient's shoe cannot be removed and there is no serious injury to the posterior ankle. The pulse site can be found on the medial side of the limb, posterior to the "ankle bone." To feel the pulse, apply pressure using the tips of two fingers placed in the groove found between the ankle bone and the **Achilles** (ah-KIL-ez) **tendon**.

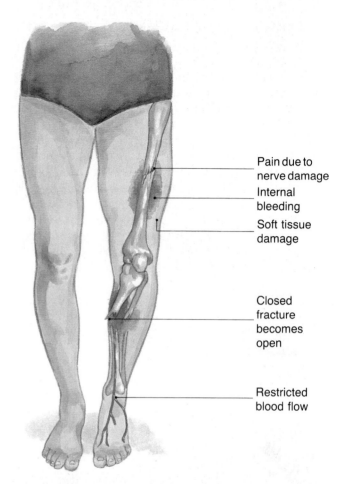

Pain due to nerve damage

Internal bleeding

Soft tissue damage

Closed fracture becomes open

Restricted blood flow

Figure 11-8 Splinting can prevent or lessen the complications associated with bone and joint injury.

- Dorsalis Pedis Pulse—This site is on the anterior surface of the foot, lateral to the tendon of the great toe. The pulse may be felt by applying pressure with the tips of two fingers. The patient's shoe must be removed for proper pulse assessment. As noted in Chapter 3, this pulse site is more reliable than the posterior tibial but may be difficult to feel. If the pulse is hard to find and you will need to check it again, make a small x on the skin with your pen.

Nerve Function Assessment

Nerve function distal to the injury site must be assessed. Different approaches are used for the conscious and unconscious patient.

- **Conscious Patient**—Touch a toe and ask the patient to tell which one you touched.
- **Unconscious Patient**—Assume spinal injury and nerve damage. Avoid pinching a distal

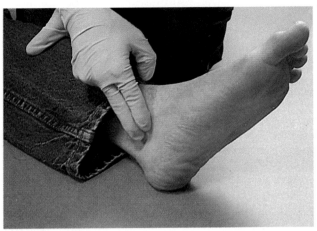

A.

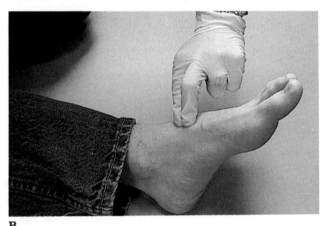

B.

Figure 11-9 Establishing distal pulse. A. Posterior tibial. B. Dorsalis pedis.

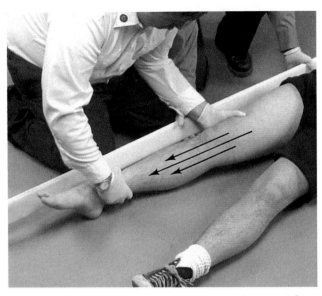

Figure 11-10 Applying manual traction (tension) for leg fractures.

area to check for a possible reflex which may cause movement that will aggravate the injury.

Manual Traction (Tension)

Depending on the injury site, manual traction (tension) is applied in one of two ways and is maintained until the completion of splinting.

Manual Traction (Tension) for Leg Injuries Manual traction (tension) is applied in the same fashion that was used for the upper extremities. The EMT uses one arm to stabilize the patient's limb at the fracture site and the other arm to provide the manual traction (tension) and gently attempt to align the limb to its anatomical position.

The manual traction (tension) should not be applied until you and your partner are ready to apply the splint. This is because the procedure of manual traction (tension) *must* be a continuous one until the splint takes over for the rescuer. Since providing manual traction (tension) to a lower limb is a tiring procedure, splinting must be done immediately to avoid the loss of traction (tension).

Two EMTs are needed so that one can lift and support the limb, the second can apply manual traction (tension), and the first then moves so he can apply the splint.

If the fracture is to the tibia or fibula (Figure 11-10)

1. Kneel alongside the injured limb, with your knee that is closest to the patient's head kept at the level of his knee.
2. Using the hand closest to the patient's head, grasp the back of the patient's thigh above the knee. This would be just above the rounded distal ends of the femur known as the femoral **condyles** (KON-diles). These rounded ends form what most persons call the "sides" of their knees.
3. Grasp the injured leg at the calf with your other hand, below the fracture site and as close to the ankle as possible while still providing support for the injury site.
4. Warn the conscious patient that there may be a temporary increase in pain. While supporting the knee and thigh, use the hand at the distal end of the limb to apply manual traction (tension). Sometimes the patient will tell you that the limb feels better after you have applied manual traction (tension).

5. At the same time that you are applying manual traction (tension), gently lift the limb so that the heel is about 10 inches off the ground. This lift will allow the splint to be secured to the leg without having to reposition the limb.

Manual Traction (Tension) for Thigh Injuries The weight of the thigh and its strong muscle mass requires that manual traction (tension) be applied with the pulling action of two hands (Figure 11-11). When possible, another person should support the thigh while manual traction (tension) is applied.

1. Kneel alongside the injured limb, with your knee closest to the patient's head at the level of his knee. This should be a comfortable position since care procedures and splinting of the injured limb may take a few minutes.
2. Using the hand closest to the patient's head, grasp the back of the thigh above the femoral condyles.
3. Using your free hand, grasp the injured limb above the ankle, leaving room for the ankle strap that is used for traction splinting.
4. Use both hands to apply traction (tension).
5. At the same time, gently lift the patient's limb so that the heel is about 10 inches off the ground. (The fracture site will have to be supported by another EMT as you lift.)
6. Brace yourself to hold manual traction (tension) throughout the traction splinting process. Some rescuers have found that they can place the knee that is closest to the patient's ankle against the elbow of the arm used to grasp the ankle.

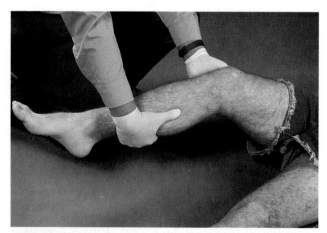

Figure 11-11 Applying manual traction (tension) to the thigh.

Note: The traction splint should not be applied if there are lower leg fractures on the same limb. Some EMS systems use the traction splint only for fractures of the femur.

Spinal Protection

After splinting, the patient should be placed on a rigid surface to help protect and support the spine. The long spine board or orthopedic (scoop-style) stretcher can be used, in accordance with local protocols (see Chapters 12 and 25). This procedure should be done for all injuries to the pelvis, hip, and femur. The orthopedic stretcher is useful for injuries to the pelvis and hip. The long spine board is recommended for patients with injuries to the femur, after splinting has been completed.

TREATMENT OF SPECIFIC INJURIES TO THE LOWER EXTREMITIES

There are specific characteristics, as well as assessment and care procedures, for injuries to the pelvis, hip, femur, knee, leg, ankle, and foot. These are discussed on the following pages.

Fractures of the Pelvis

Fractures of the pelvis may occur with falls, in motor vehicle collisions, or when a person is crushed by being squeezed between two objects. Pelvic fractures may be the result of direct or indirect force.

Patient Assessment—Pelvic Fractures

WARNING: Indications of pelvic fractures mean that there may be serious damage to internal organs, blood vessels, and nerves. Internal bleeding may be profuse, leading to shock. Any force strong enough to fracture the pelvis also can cause injury to the spine.

Signs and Symptoms

☐ Complaint of pain in pelvis, hips, groin, or back. This may be the only indication, but it is significant if the mechanism of injury indicates possible fracture. Usually, obvious deformity will be associated with the pain.

- Painful reaction when pressure is applied to the **iliac crest** (wings of the pelvis) or to the pubic bones.
- Patient complains that he cannot lift his legs when lying on his back. (*Do not* test for this, but do check for sensation.)
- The foot on the injured side may turn outward (lateral rotation). This also may indicate a hip fracture.
- The patient has an unexplained pressure on the urinary bladder and the feeling of having to void the bladder.

Patient Care—Pelvic Fractures

Note: It may be very difficult to tell a fractured pelvis from a fractured hip. When there is doubt, care for the patient as if there is a pelvic fracture in order to protect blood vessels and nerves associated with the joint. Remember, there may be spinal injuries.

Emergency Care Steps

1. MOVE THE PATIENT AS LITTLE AS POSSIBLE. Any moves should be done so that the patient moves as a unit. Never lift the patient with the pelvis unsupported.
2. Determine the status of circulation and nerve function distal to the injury site.
3. Straighten the patient's lower limbs into the anatomical position if there are no injuries to the hip joints and lower limbs and if it is possible to do without meeting resistance or causing excessive pain. **Warning:** DO NOT USE A LOG ROLL TO MOVE A PATIENT WITH A SUSPECTED PELVIC FRACTURE.
4. Prevent additional injury to the pelvis by stabilizing the lower limbs. Place a folded blanket between the patient's legs, from the groin to the feet, and bind them together with wide cravats. Thin rigid splints can be used to push the cravats under the patient. The cravats can then be adjusted for proper placement at
   - Upper thigh
   - Above knee
   - Below knee
   - Above ankle
5. Assume that there are spinal injuries and immobilize the patient on a long spine board or use an orthopedic stretcher (see Chapters 12 and 25). When securing the

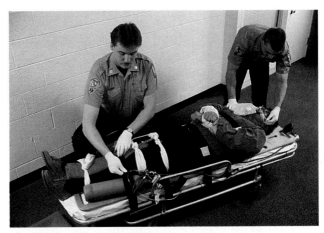

Figure 11-12 Immobilizing a patient with hip or pelvic injuries on a long spine board.

patient, avoid placing the straps or ties over the pelvic area (Figure 11-12).
6. Reassess distal circulation and nerve function.
7. Care for shock, providing a high concentration of oxygen.
8. Transport the patient as soon as possible.*
9. Monitor vital signs.

Note: Some EMS systems use the anti-shock garment for a patient with a possible pelvic fracture. The garment should be placed on the spine board prior to moving the patient onto the board. When pelvic fracture is a possibility, always be alert for shock and possible injuries to internal organs.

Hip Dislocations

A hip dislocation occurs when the head of the femur is pulled or pushed from its pelvic socket.

Patient Assessment—Hip Dislocation

It is difficult to tell a hip dislocation from a fracture to the proximal femur. Conscious patients will complain of intense pain with both types of injury.

*Some EMS Systems allow for adjustments to be made prior to transport. Once the patient is in the ambulance and prepared for transport, the EMT is allowed to make adjustments to improve patient comfort and reduce muscle spasms of the abdomen and lower limb. This can be done by gently flexing the patient's legs and placing a pillow under the knees. If you are allowed to follow this protocol, a warning must be issued since the patient may have associated spinal injuries.

Signs

☐ Anterior hip dislocation—The patient's entire lower limb is rotated *outward* and the hip is usually *flexed*.

☐ Posterior hip dislocation (most common)—The patient's leg is rotated *inward*, the hip is flexed, and the knee is bent. The foot may hang loose (footdrop), and the patient is unable to flex the foot or lift the toes. Often, there is a lack of sensation in the limb. These signs indicate possible damage caused by the dislocated femoral head, to the **sciatic** (si-AT-ik) **nerve**, the major nerve that extends from the lower spine to the posterior thigh. This injury often occurs when a person's knees strike the dashboard during a motor vehicle collision (Figure 11-13).

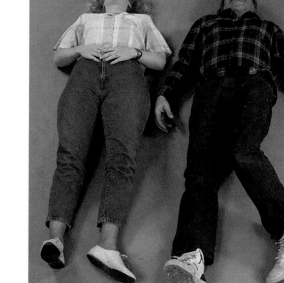

Patient Care—Hip Dislocation

Checking for circulation and nerve impairment, and treating for shock are important in caring for hip dislocation.

Emergency Care Steps

1. Check for circulation and nerve impairment.
2. Move patient onto a long spine board. Some systems use a scoop-style stretcher. When this device is used, the limb should be immobilized (see Step 3) prior to placing the patient on the stretcher.
3. Immobilize the limb with pillows or rolled blankets.
4. Secure the patient to the board with straps or cravats.
5. Reassess circulation and nerve function. IF THERE IS A PULSE OR SENSORY PROBLEM, NOTIFY THE MEDICAL FACILITY and transport immediately.
6. Care for shock, providing a high concentration of oxygen.
7. Transport carefully, monitor vital signs, and continue to check for nerve and circulation impairment.

Note: If the head of the femur slides or pops back into place, note this on the patient form and report the event to the emergency department staff so that the previous dislocation does not go unnoticed. If you have what you believe is a fractured femur and the leg is flexed and will not straighten, you may also

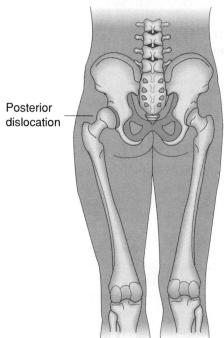

Posterior view

Posterior dislocation

Figure 11-13 Signs of anterior and posterior hip dislocation.

have a dislocated hip. In this case the traction splint will not help, and the long spine board and board splints are more appropriate.

Hip Fractures

A hip fracture is a fracture to the uppermost portion of the femur, not to the pelvis. The fracture can occur to the femoral head, the femoral neck, or at the proximal end of the femur just below the neck of the bone. Direct force (motor vehicle collision) and twisting forces (falls) can cause a hip fracture. Elderly people are more susceptible to this type of injury because of brittle bones or bones weakened by disease.

Patient Assessment—Hip Fractures

Consider the mechanism of injury that may have caused a hip fracture. Consider the pathophysiology that may have caused an elderly patient to fall.

Signs and Symptoms

☐ Pain is localized, but some patients complain of pain in the knee.
☐ Sometimes the patient is sensitive to pressure exerted on the lateral prominence of the hip (greater trochanter).
☐ Surrounding tissues are discolored. This may be delayed.
☐ Swelling is evident.
☐ Patient is unable to move limb while on his back.
☐ Patient complains about being unable to stand.
☐ Foot on injured side usually turns outward; however, it may rotate inward (rarely).
☐ Injured limb may appear shorter.

Patient Care—Hip Fractures

Be certain to check for nerve and circulatory impairment. This must be continued during transport. The patient should be managed for shock and receive oxygen at a high concentration. It is recommended that the patient be placed on a spine board or orthopedic stretcher after splinting.

Emergency Care Steps

One of the following methods can be used to stabilize a hip fracture.

☐ Bind the legs together—Place a folded blanket between the patient's legs and bind the legs together with wide straps, Velcro-equipped straps, or wide cravats.

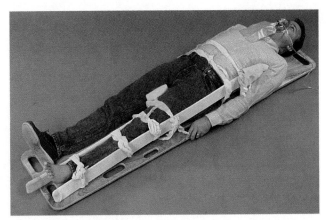

Figure 11-14 Long board splinting for a fractured hip (padded splint).

Carefully place the patient on a long spine board and use pillows to support the lower limbs. Secure the patient to the board. An orthopedic stretcher can be used in place of the long spine board.

☐ Padded boards—Push cravats or straps under the patient at the natural voids (e.g., small of the back and back of the knees) and readjust them so that they will pass across the chest, the abdomen, just below the belt, below the crotch, above and below the knee, and at the ankle. Use thin splints to push the cravats or straps under the patient to avoid the unnecessary moving of the patient. Splint with two long padded boards. Ideally, one padded board should be long enough to extend from the patient's armpit to beyond the foot. Splint with another padded board that is long enough to extend from the crotch to beyond the foot. Cushion with padding in the armpit and crotch and pad all voids created at the ankle and knee. Secure the boards with the cravats or straps (Figure 11-14).

☐ Traction splinting (see Scans 11-1A, B, and C and 11-2)*—This procedure is acceptable for most patients. Many systems recommend this method for the elderly patient only if transport is to take more than 30 minutes or will be very rough. Traction splinting usually reduces patient pain and will help reduce muscle spasms in the lower limb.

☐ Apply an anti-shock garment if indicated as per local protocols (see Chapter 8).

*Most EMS Systems restrict the use of the traction splint to the care of patients who have possible fractures to the *shaft* of the femur.

The Fernotrac Traction Splint — Preparing the Splint

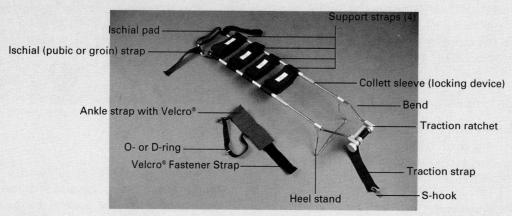

Support straps (4)
Ischial pad
Ischial (pubic or groin) strap
Collett sleeve (locking device)
Bend
Ankle strap with Velcro®
Traction ratchet
O- or D-ring
Velcro® Fastener Strap
Traction strap
Heel stand
S-hook

1. The Fernotrac Traction Splint

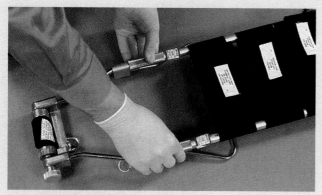

2. Loosen sleeve locking device.

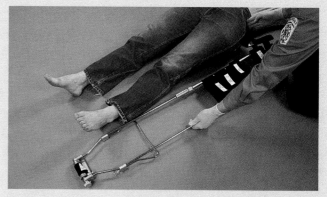

3. Place next to uninjured leg—ischial pad next to iliac crest.

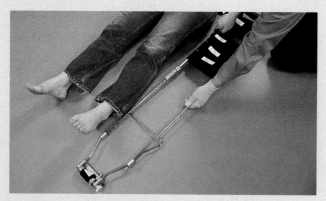

4. Hold top and move bottom until bend is at heel.

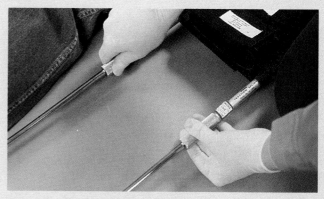

5. Lock sleeve.

Note: Some splints in use are measured by placing the ring at the level of the bony prominence that can be felt in the middle of each buttock (ischial [IS-ke-al] tuberosity) and the distal end of the splint placed 8 to 10 inches beyond the foot.

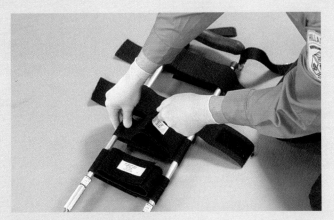

6. Open support straps.

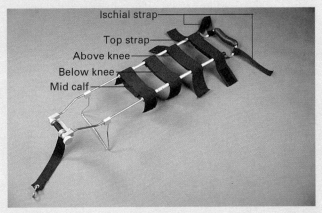

7. Place straps under splint.

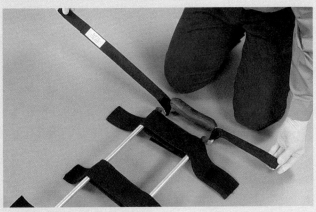

8. Release ischial strap. Attached ends should be next to ischial pad.

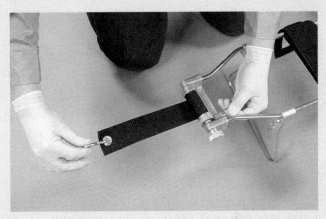

9. Pull release ring on ratchet and . . .

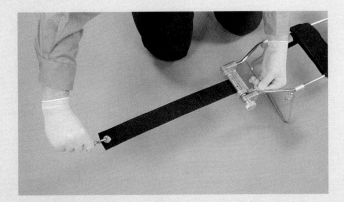

10. Release the traction strap.

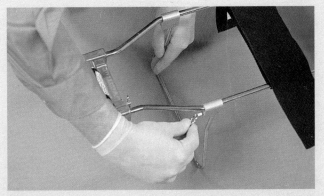

11. Extend and position heel stand after splint is in position under patient.

Note: Traction splints vary depending on the manufacturer. Learn to use the equipment supplied in your area and keep up to date with new equipment as it is approved for use.

Traction Splinting — Applying the Splint

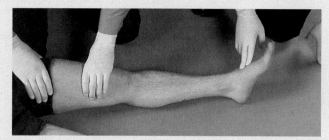

1. EMT 1 stabilizes injury with hands positioned above and below fracture site on thigh; EMT 2 has exposed injury site, dresses any open wounds, and assesses neurological function, distal pulse, and capillary refill.

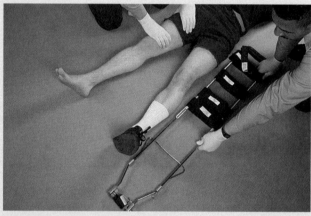

2. EMT 1 continues stabilization as EMT 2 measures and prepares the traction splint.

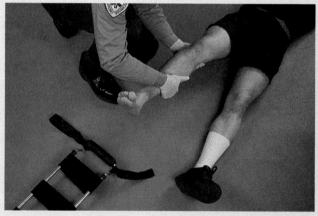

3. EMT 1 positions self to take manual traction and maintain throughout splinting. One hand slides to mid-calf to lift and support lower leg; one hand slides behind knee to support and maintain traction. The knee is gripped and raised and the lower leg is lifted and remains level with floor.

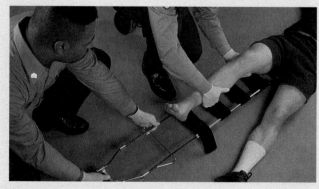

4. EMT 2 places splint under leg so that the ischial pad is against the bony prominence of the buttocks (ischial tuberosity). When the splint is in position, extend the kickstand.

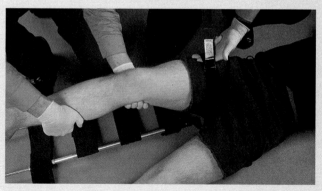

5. EMT 2 attaches ischial strap over groin and thigh. Pull the strap up over the thigh muscle. (Be careful of genitalia.) Some protocols may require padding under the strap.

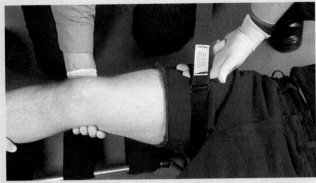

6. Secure strap with Velcro fastener and test tightness. Two fingers should fit under the buckle.

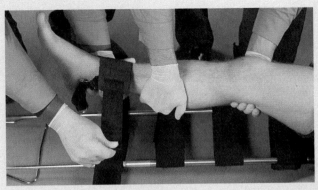

7. EMT 2 places ankle hitch snugly around ankle and secures Velcro Fasteners. Patient's foot should be in upright position.

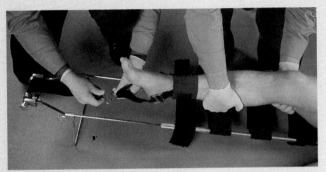

8. EMT 2 attaches S-hook to D-ring.

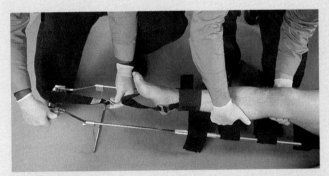

9. EMT 2 begins to apply mechanical traction by turning windlass. EMT 1 gently lowers limb onto splint as traction is applied and pulling leg straight.

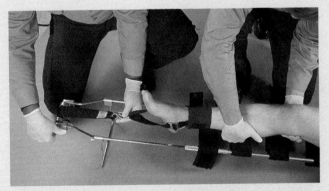

10. *Conscious Patient*: Full traction is applied when manual traction is taken over by mechanical traction and patient pain and muscle spasms are reduced. *Unconscious Patient*: Full traction is applied when manual traction is taken over by mechanical traction and the injured limb is extended to about the same length as the uninjured one.

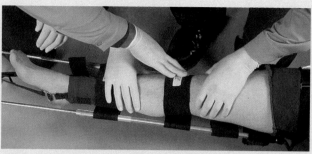

11. EMT 1 now positions hands on top of lower leg to stabilize. EMT 2 fastens support straps: one just above the ankle hitch, one just below the knee, one just above the knee, and one at the top of the thigh, just below the pubic strap. (DO NOT fasten a strap over the fracture site. Secure that strap underneath the splint to provide added support.)

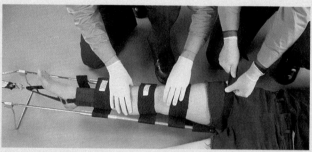

12. EMT 1 continues to stabilize as EMT 2 rechecks and tightens pubic strap.

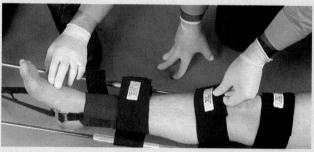

13. EMTs will recheck distal pulse, neurological response, capillary refill, and tightness of support straps.

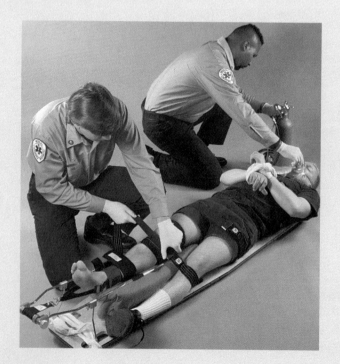

14. Package the patient and place on a long board or lift with scoop onto stretcher. Treat for shock by providing a high concentration of oxygen, monitoring vital signs, maintaining body warmth, and monitoring vital signs. Periodically monitor splint and distal functions of injured leg.

Traction Splinting—Variation

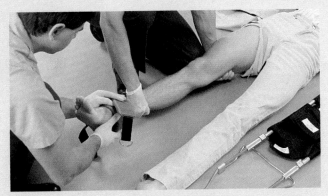

1. Some systems attach the ankle hitch prior to applying manual traction (tension). EMT 1 should apply the hitch while EMT 2 stabilizes the limb.

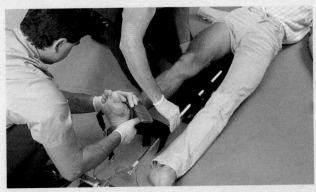

2a. While EMT 1 applies manual traction (tension), EMT 2 can support the injured thigh and position the splint.

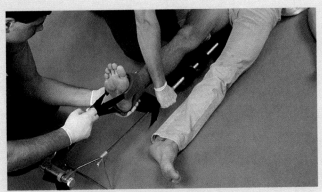

2b. Some systems allow manual traction to be applied by grasping the D-ring and ankle.

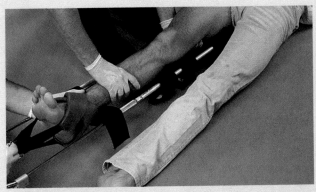

3. EMT 1 maintains manual traction (tension) and lowers the limb onto the cradles of the splint.

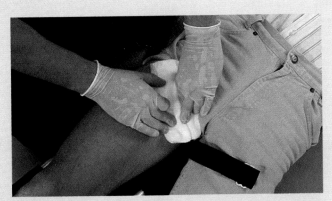

4. While EMT 1 maintains manual traction, EMT 2 applies padding to the groin area before securing the ischial strap. **Note:** Some EMS systems do not apply padding in order to reduce slippage.

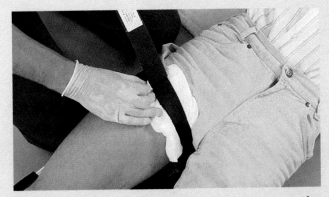

5. EMT 2 secures the ischial strap, connects the ankle hitch to the windlass, tightens the ratchet to equal manual traction (tension), and secures the cradle straps.

The Sager Traction Splint

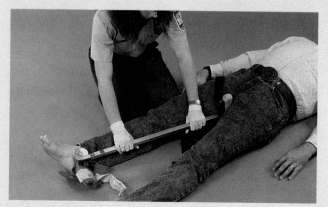

1. Splint will be placed medially.

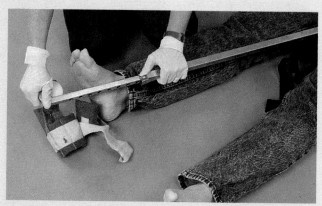

2. Length should be from groin to 4 inches past heel. Unlock to slide.

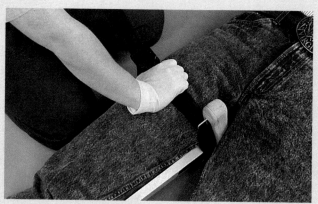

3. Secure thigh strap.

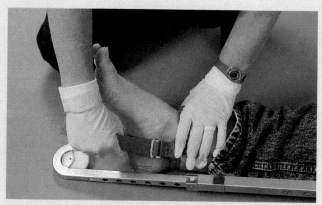

4. Wrap ankle harness above ankle (malleoi) and secure under heel.

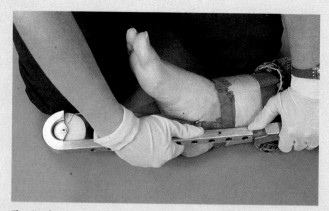

5. Release lock and extend splint to achieve desired traction (in pounds on pulley wheel).

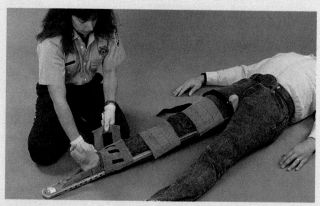

6. Secure straps at thigh, lower thigh and knee, and lower leg. Strap ankles and feet together. Secure to spine board.

Femoral Shaft Fractures

Because the femur is a large, strong bone, considerable force is necessary to cause a fracture of the femoral shaft.

Patient Assessment— Femoral Shaft Fractures

As noted earlier, the thigh's large muscle mass can complicate femoral fractures. Muscle contractions can cause bone ends to ride over each other or to recede from an open fracture wound. You must check for the signs of an open fracture and never assume that a wound on the thigh is of external origin.

Signs and Symptoms

☐ Pain, often intense
☐ Often there will be an open fracture with deformity and sometimes with the end of the bone protruding through the wound. When the injury is a closed fracture, there will be deformity with possible severe angulation.
☐ The injured limb may appear to be shortened because the contraction of the thigh muscles has caused the bone ends to override each other.

Warning: Studies of mechanisms of injury indicate that pediatric patients with fractured femurs often have injury to internal organs.

Patient Care—Femoral Shaft Fractures

In addition to splinting the fractured bone, you must attempt to control serious bleeding from deep thigh arteries. This can be difficult because of the barrier of the thigh's muscle mass.

Emergency Care Steps

1. Control bleeding by applying direct pressure (avoiding a possible fracture site) forcefully enough to overcome the barrier of muscle mass. The femoral artery pressure point may be used. (See Chapter 7 on bleeding and pressure points.)
2. As soon as possible, manage the patient for shock and provide a high concentration of oxygen.
3. Check circulatory and nerve impairment.
4. Apply a traction splint.

Warning: The traction splint should not be applied if you suspect that there may be additional injuries or fractures to the area of the knee or tibia/fibula of the same limb. An anti-shock garment can be used if there are multiple leg fractures. Its use for shock is the priority, but it can also serve as a splint. It is not, however, a good splint for the lower leg since it does not immobilize the ankle.

Traction splints are used to immobilize broken bone ends of a fractured femur so that further damage is avoided. Traction is the application of just enough force to stabilize the broken bone. It is *not* the stretching or moving of the fractured bone until the ends are aligned.

When a bone breaks completely, the normal tendency of the muscles to contract often causes bone ends to slip past one another, or "override." When muscles are large and powerful, as in the thigh, the tendency is more pronounced. Patient movement and the movement necessary during transport can increase the override and cause serious soft tissue damage, including a closed fracture becoming an open fracture. Scans 11-1A, B, and C and 11-2 show the procedures and variations in procedures for applying a traction splint. Whenever possible, three rescuers should be used to apply the splint. This allows one rescuer to support the injury site when the limb is lifted to place the splint.

If a traction splint is not available, bind the legs together after placing them in the anatomical position and checking for pulse and sensation.

Note: Most of the splints in use today require that the patient's shoe be removed for proper traction splinting. With some older splints, the patient's shoe may remain in place if neurologic and pulse assessment is possible, if the shoe will not prevent the ankle hitch from being properly placed, and if the shoe will not slip off after mechanical traction (tension) is applied.

Knee Injuries

The knee is a *joint* and not a single bone. Fractures can occur to the distal femur, to the proximal tibia and fibula, and to the patella (kneecap).

Patient Assessment—Knee Injuries

What may appear to be a dislocation may prove to be a fracture or a combined fracture and dislocation. Even if you believe that the patient has suffered a dislocated patella and the kneecap has repositioned itself, realize that other damage may be hidden. Whether the patient has a fracture, dislocation, sprain, or strain (Figure 11-15), always manage as if there is a fracture and transport.

Signs and Symptoms

☐ Pain and tenderness
☐ Deformity with obvious swelling

Patient Care—Knee Injuries

Do not confuse a knee dislocation with a patella dislocation. The patella can become displaced by ligament damage when the lower leg and knee are twisted, as in a skiing or racketball accident. A knee dislocation happens when the tibia is forced posteriorly by blunt force to the anterior proximal tibia, as when the knee strikes the dash in a motor vehicle collision. Always check for a distal pulse, since the dislocated knee joint can compress the posterior tibial artery and stop the major blood supply to the lower leg. If there is no pulse, this is a TRUE EMERGENCY. Contact the emergency physician for permission to gently move the lower leg anteriorly to allow for a pulse, and transport immediately.

DO NOT ATTEMPT TO STRAIGHTEN ANGULATIONS if there is evidence of dislocation of the knee. Remember to check for circulatory and nerve impairment. If there is no indication of dislocation, an attempt may be made to place the leg in anatomical position if this is required to move or otherwise manage the patient. DO NOT FORCE THE LEG. Stop if there is any resistance or increase in pain for the patient. Make only one attempt to straighten the leg. If this attempt fails, call the emergency department physician.

Once splinting is done, monitor the patient. If there is a loss of distal pulse, a loss of sensation, or if the foot becomes discolored (white, mottled or blue, or a loss of tone) and turns cold, transport the patient without delay. Notify the emergency department while en route.

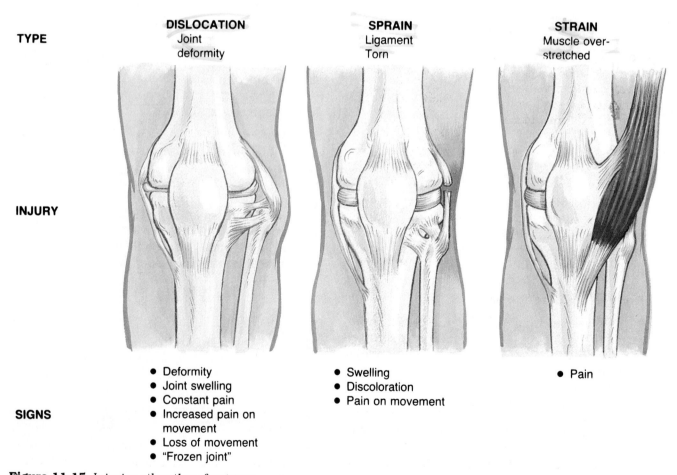

| TYPE | DISLOCATION
Joint deformity | SPRAIN
Ligament Torn | STRAIN
Muscle over-stretched |

INJURY

| SIGNS | • Deformity
• Joint swelling
• Constant pain
• Increased pain on movement
• Loss of movement
• "Frozen joint" | • Swelling
• Discoloration
• Pain on movement | • Pain |

Figure 11-15 Injuries other than fractures.

Emergency Care Steps

There are two general methods of immobilizing the knee, one if the knee is bent, the other if it is straight.

- Knee Bent—Immobilize in the position in which the leg is found if resistance and pain prevent straightening. Tie two padded board splints to the thigh and above the ankle so that the knee is held in position (Scan 11-3). A pillow can be used to support the leg.
- Knee Straight or Returned to Anatomical Position—Immobilize with two padded board splints or a single padded splint and an ankle hitch (Scans 11-4 through 11-6). When using two padded boards, one medial and one lateral offer the best support. Remember to pad the voids created at the knee and ankle.

Fractures of the Leg

Either or both of the long bones of the lower leg—the tibia or the fibula—may be fractured.

Patient Assessment—Leg Fractures

You might expect to see a deformity of the lower leg when the tibia or fibula is fractured. However, such deformity is often absent.

Signs and Symptoms

- Pain and tenderness
- Swelling

Patient Care—Leg Fractures

Immobilizing the legs by application of a splint may also help to relieve pain and control bleeding.

Emergency Care Steps

1. Care for shock, administering a high concentration of oxygen.
2. Check for circulatory and nerve impairment.
3. Splint.
   - Air-inflated splint—Apply an air-inflated splint (Figure 11-16). Slide the uninflated splint over your hand and gather it in place until the lower edge clears your wrist. Grasp the patient's foot with one hand and his leg just above the injury

site using your free hand. While maintaining manual traction (tension), have your partner slide the splint over your hand and onto the injured leg. Your partner must make sure that the splint is relatively wrinkle free and that it covers the injury site. Continue to maintain traction (tension) while your partner inflates the splint. Test to see if you can cause a slight dent in the plastic with fingertip pressure. Remember to check periodically to see that the pressure in the splint has remained adequate and has not decreased or increased. Note that there are problems associated with the use and removal of this type of splint. See the warnings in Chapter 10 concerning the use of air-inflated splints.
   - Two-splint method—You can immobilize the fracture using two rigid board splints (Scan 11-7).
   - Single splint with ankle hitch—A single splint with an ankle hitch can be applied (Scan 11-8).
4. Monitor distal pulse, neurological functions, and vital signs.

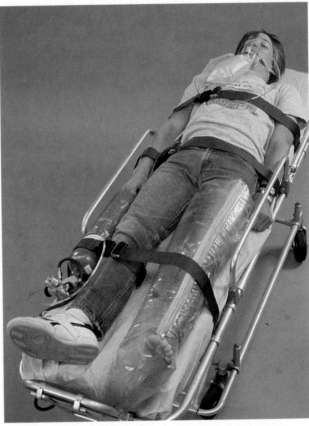

Figure 11-16 Using an air-inflated splint for lower leg fractures.

Knee Injuries—Knee Bent— Two Splint Method

If there is a distal pulse and nerve function, or the limb cannot be straightened without meeting resistance or causing severe pain, knee injuries should be splinted with the knee in the position in which it is found.

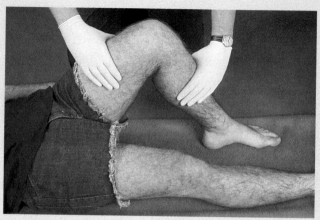

1. Without applying traction, attempt to place the knee in anatomical position if allowed to do so in your EMS system. If this fails . . .

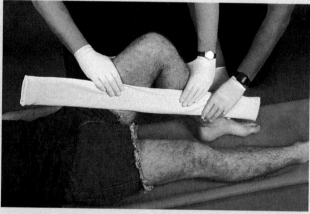

2. The splints should be equal and extend 6-12 inches beyond the mid thigh and mid calf.

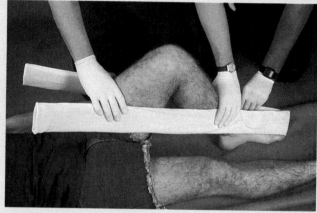

3. Place padded side of splints medially and laterally.

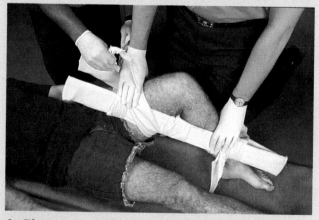

4. Place a cravat through the knee void and tie the boards together.

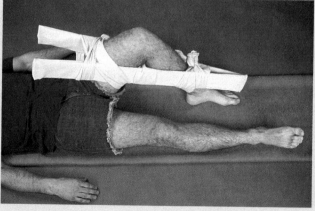

5. Using a figure eight, secure one cravat to the ankle and the boards, secure the second cravat to the thigh and the boards.

Scan 11-4
The Ankle Hitch

The ankle hitch can be used with a single padded board splint to immobilize injured knees and legs. It is made with a 3-inch-wide cravat.

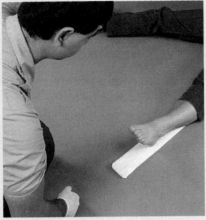

1. Kneel at distal end of injured limb.

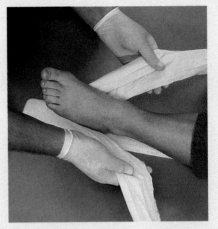

2. Center cravat in arch.

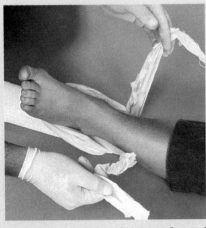

3. Place cravat along sides of foot and cross cravat behind ankle.

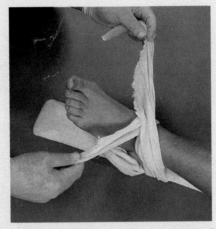

4. Cross cravat ends over top of ankle.

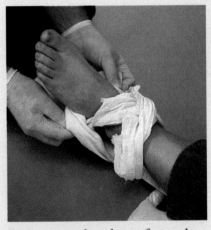

5. A stirrup has been formed.

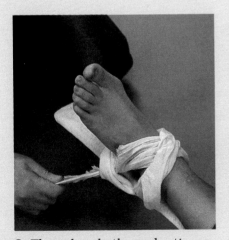

6. Thread ends through stirrup.

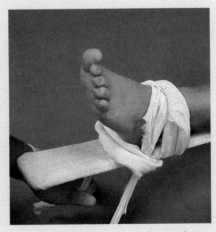

7. Pull ends downward to tighten.

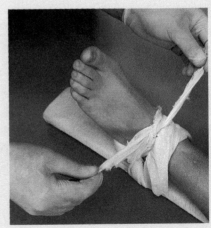

8. Pull upward and tie over ankle wrap.

Knee Injuries—Knee Straight—Single Splint Method

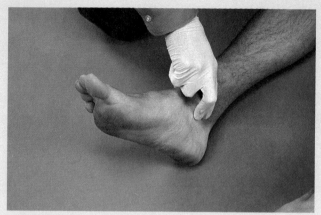

1. Assess distal pulse and nerve function.

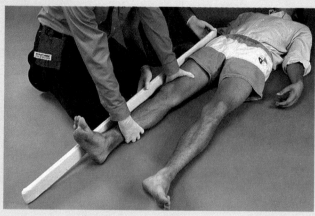

2. Use a padded board splint that extends from buttocks to 4 inches beyond heel.

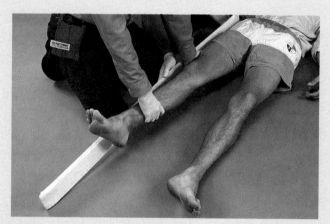

3. Stabilize and lift the limb.

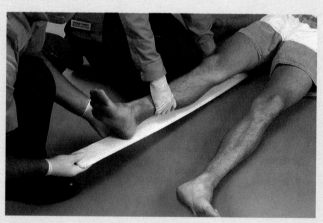

4. Place splint along posterior of limb.

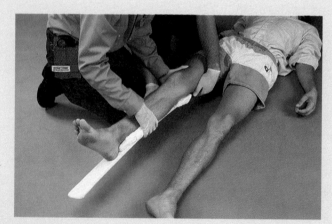

5. Pad voids.

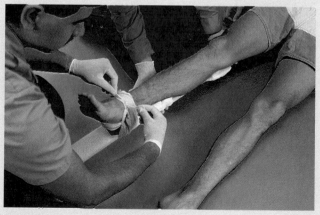

6. Apply an ankle hitch (see Scan 11-4)

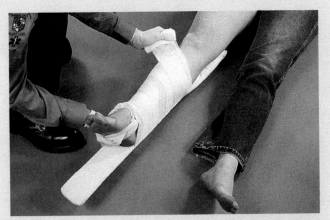

7. Use 6-inch self-adhering roller bandage. Apply distal to proximal, or use cravats.

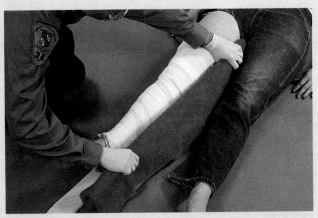

8. Place folded blanket between legs, groin to feet.

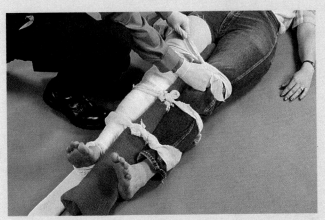

9. Tie thighs, calves, and ankles together; knot over uninjured limb.

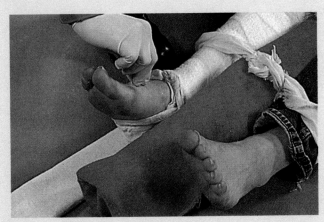

10. Reassess distal pulse and nerve function.

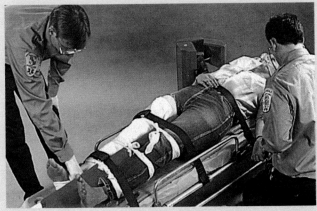

11. Care for shock and continue to provide a high concentration of oxygen.

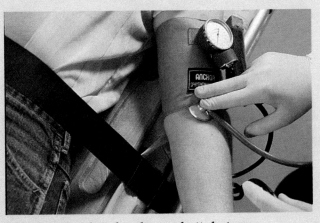

12. Monitor distal pulse and vital signs.

Knee Injuries—Knee Straight or Returned to Anatomical Position— Two Splint Method

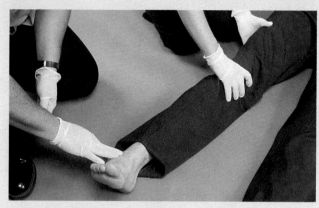

1. Assess distal pulse and nerve function.

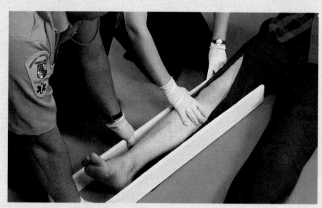

2. Select two padded board splints. Medial = groin to 4 inches beyond foot. Lateral = iliac crest to 4 inches beyond foot.

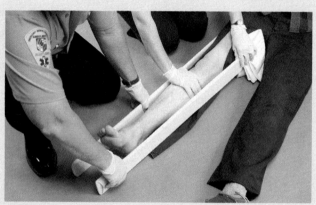

3. Stabilize the limb and pad groin.

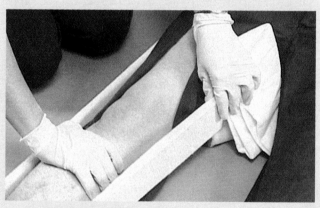

4. Position splints.

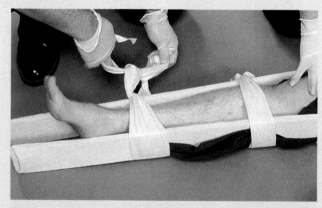

5. Secure splints at thigh, above and below knee, and at mid calf. Pad voids.

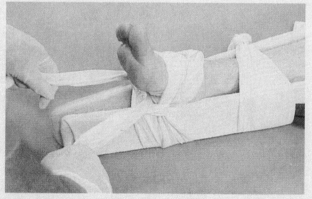

6. Cross and tie two cravats at the ankle or hitch the ankle.

Remember to reassess distal pulse and nerve function. Care for shock and continue to provide a high concentration of oxygen.

Leg Injuries—
Two Splint Method

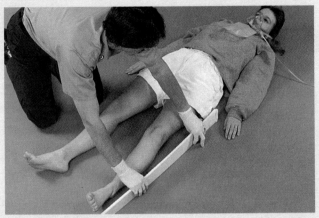

1. Measure splint. It should extend above the knee and below the ankle.

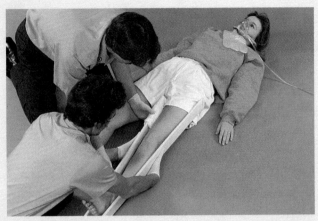

2. Apply manual traction (tension) and place one splint medially and one laterally. Padding is toward the leg.

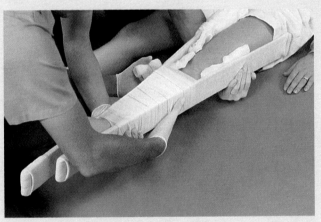

3. Secure splints distal to proximal, padding voids.

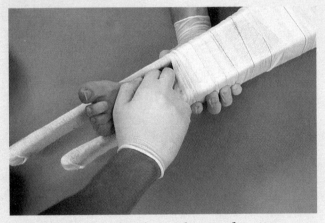

4. Reassess distal pulse and nerve function.

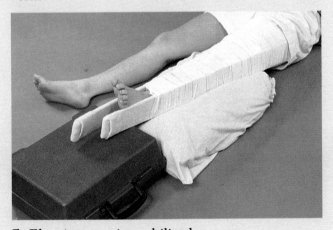

5. Elevate, once immobilized.

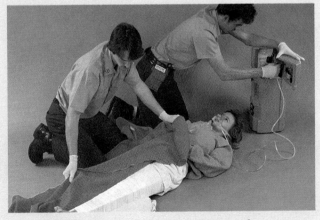

6. Treat for shock and continue to administer a high concentration of oxygen. Transport on a long spine board for additional support.

319

Leg Injuries—
Single Splint Method

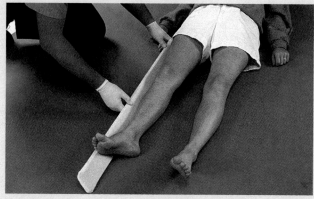

1. Measure splint. It should extend from mid thigh to 4 inches below ankle.

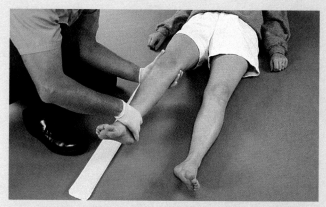

2. Apply manual traction (tension) and lift limb 10 inches off ground.

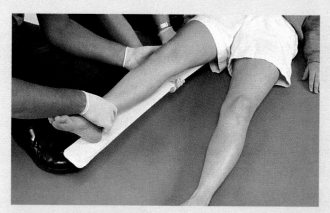

3. Place splint along the posterior of the limb, at mid thigh.

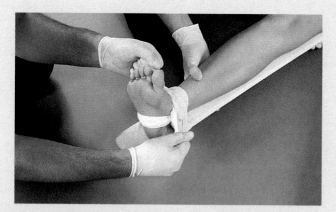

4. Apply ankle hitch (see Scan 11-4).

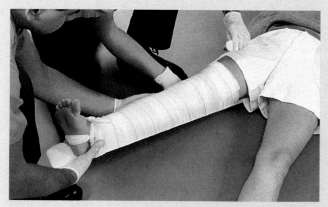

5. Secure, distal to proximal.

Note: Reassess distal pulse and nerve function. Elevate the injured limb, care for shock, and continue to administer a high concentration of oxygen.

Injuries to the Ankle and Foot

Sprains (torn ligaments) and fractures are the most common musculoskeletal injuries to the ankle and foot.

It is often difficult to distinguish between fractures and sprains to the foot or ankle.

Signs and Symptoms

Both fractures and sprains are characterized by

- ☐ Pain
- ☐ Swelling

Do not attempt to distinguish between or care differently for a sprain or a fracture to the ankle or foot. Treat either as if it is a fracture.

Emergency Care Steps

Long splints, extending from above the knee to beyond the foot, can be used. However, soft splinting is an effective, rapid method and is recommended for most patients (Figure 11-17). To soft splint, you should

1. Assess distal pulse and nerve function.
2. Stabilize the limb.
3. Remove the patient's shoe if possible, but only if it removes easily and can be done with no movement to the ankle.
4. Lift the limb, but *do not* apply traction (tension).
5. Place three cravats under the ankle.
6. Place a pillow, lengthwise under the ankle, on top of the cravats. The pillow should extend 6 inches beyond the foot.

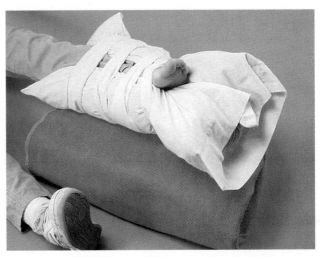

Figure 11-17 Pillow splinting an injured ankle.

7. Gently lower the limb onto the pillow, taking care not to change the position of the ankle. Stabilize by tying the cravats.
8. Adjust the cravats so that they are at the top of the pillow, midway, and at the heel.
9. Tie the pillow to the ankle and foot, distal to proximal.
10. Tie a fourth cravat loosely at the arch of the foot.
11. Elevate with a second pillow or blanket.
12. Reassess distal pulse and nerve function.
13. Care for shock if needed. If there are no other injuries, and no symptoms or signs of shock, oxygen is usually not administered. Some EMS Systems now recommend that oxygen be provided at a high concentration for all patients who may have any possible fractures.
14. An ice pack can be applied to the injury site to reduce bleeding and swelling. *Do not* apply the ice pack directly to the skin.

Note: A commercial splint with a foot and leg that extends above the knee may be better than a pillow since it will immobilize the joints adjacent to the ankle.

KEY TERMS

You may find it helpful to review the following terms.

Achilles (ah-KIL-ez) **tendon**—the common term for the tendon that connects the posterior lower leg muscles to the heel. The anatomical term is calcaneal (kal-KA-ne-al) tendon.

condyles (KON-diles)—the large, rounded projections at the distal end of the femur and the proximal end of the tibia. Some persons refer to these as the sides of their knees.

iliac (IL-e-ak) **crest**—the upper, curved boundary of the ilium.

ilium (IL-e-um)—the upper portions of the pelvis, forming the wings of the pelvis.

ischium (IS-ke-em)—the lower, posterior portions of the pelvis.

pubic (PYOO-bik) **bone**, **pubis** (PYOO-bis)—the middle (medial), anterior portion of the pelvis.

sciatic (si-AT-ik) **nerve**—the major nerve that extends from the lower spine to the posterior thigh.

traction splints—special splints that apply a constant pull along the length of a lower extremity. This helps to stabilize the fractured bone and reduce muscle spasms in the limb. Traction splints are used primarily to treat femoral shaft fractures.

SUMMARY

The Lower Extremities

The lower extremities are composed of the pelvis and two lower limbs. Each limb consists of the femur (thigh), patella (kneecap), tibia and fibula (leg), tarsals (ankle), metatarsals (foot), and phalanges (toes).

Injuries to the Bones and Joints

Many different types of injuries can occur to structures of the musculoskeletal system (such as fractures, dislocations, sprains, and strains).

Injuries to the pelvis and femur are especially serious. Pelvic fractures have a high mortality rate. Because the pelvis protects many organs, because major nerves and blood vessels pass near the pelvis, and because the pelvis joins the sacrum (lower spine), injury to the pelvis is often associated with other serious injuries. The femur is a very strong bone surrounded by a large muscle mass. Consequently, a force great enough to break the femur can also be assumed to have caused other serious injuries.

There are some SPECIAL SIGNS you need to know.

- Pelvic pain when you compress the patient's hips = pelvic fracture.
- Pelvic injury with patient's foot turning outward = pelvic fracture.
- Lower limb rotates outward = possible anterior hip dislocation, hip fracture, or pelvic fracture.
- Lower limb rotates inward and knee and hip are bent = possible posterior hip dislocation or hip fracture.

322 Trauma

General Treatment of Injuries to the Lower Extremities

Frequent assessment of pulse (for circulation) and nerve function is important before, during, and after emergency care for injuries to the extremities. Manual traction (tension) and spine protection are important in caring for lower extremity injuries.

Treatment of Specific Injuries to the Lower Extremities

It is important to learn specific soft and rigid splinting procedures for injuries to the pelvis, hip, femoral shaft, knee, leg, ankle, and foot. Application of traction splints for femoral shaft fractures and, in some EMS systems, for hip fractures, must also be mastered.

12

On the Scene

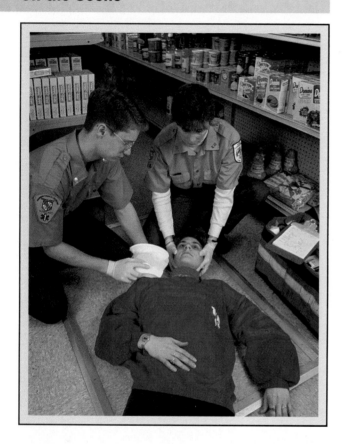

Nineteen-year-old Sandy McGill works at the local convenience store. Her parents were worried about her taking a job where she would be working alone, but Sandy argued that it was a way to earn money for college. It turns out Sandy's parents were right. Early one morning, someone strikes Sandy on the back of the head with an object she never saw coming.

The robber scoops out the cash drawer and escapes just minutes before a patron stops in and finds Sandy lying unconscious on the

floor between shelves. Fighting panic, the patron phones 911. Your ambulance service receives the call as "unknown injuries from an assault." You arrive at the scene to find the police already there. A sergeant explains what has happened. As you approach you discover Sandy is conscious, but a police officer has told her not to move or try to get up.

You: Hi. We're from the ambulance. Can you tell me what happened?

Sandy: I must have gotten hit over the head with something. Real hard.

You: Did you pass out?

Sandy: I don't even remember getting hit. This man asked me to find something for him on the shelf. I had my back to him hunting for what he wanted, and the next thing I know I'm on the floor with a police officer standing over me.

You: I'm going to check you over to see where you're hurt. My partner is going to hold your head still just so we don't injure your spine. Do you hurt any place other than your head?...

You and your partner perform a thorough patient assessment. Since Sandy told you that she was struck on the head with considerable force, you take precautions for neck and back injuries. The remainder of the assessment is negative, and you place Sandy in a cervical collar, move her onto a backboard, and transport her to the hospital.

A week later you learn that Sandy suffered no permanent injuries, but her parents have talked her out of returning to work at the store.

The Skull and Spine

Chapter Overview

Almost everyone realizes that injuries to the skull, brain, and spine are potentially extremely serious, possibly producing paralysis or even death. Incorrect treatment for such injuries can aggravate them, or even produce new injuries. In this chapter you will learn step-by-step procedures for assessing and caring for such injuries.

Expected Outcome, Chapter 12: You will understand the anatomy of the axial skeleton and nervous system and be able to assess and provide emergency care for injuries to the skull, brain, and spine.

WARNING: Protect yourself from infectious diseases by using appropriate barrier devices such as a pocket face mask with one-way valve, face shield, or bag-valve mask; goggles or eye shield; and disposable gloves. Always conform to your local EMS system's infection exposure control plan.

THE AXIAL SKELETON
> The Skull
> The Spine

THE NERVOUS SYSTEM

INJURIES TO THE SKULL AND BRAIN
> Types of Skull and Brain Injuries
> Cranial Fractures and Brain Injuries
> Facial Fractures
> Injuries to the Mandible
> Care for Patients Wearing Helmets

INJURIES TO THE SPINE
> Types of Spinal Injuries
> Mechanisms of Injury
> Total Body Immobilization Devices
> Application of a Short Spine Board or
>   Extrication Device
> Immobilization for Removal From a Vehicle

Knowledge *After reading this chapter you should be able to*

1. Define *axial skeleton*. (pp. 326-327)

2. Distinguish between cranium and face. (p. 327)

3. Define *suture, cranial floor, temporal bone, mandible, maxillae,* and *temporomandibular joint.* (p. 327)

4. Name and label the FIVE major divisions of the spinal column. (pp. 327-328)

5. Define *central nervous system, peripheral nervous system, somatic nervous system,* and *autonomic nervous system.* (pp. 328-329)

6. Define *open head injury, closed head injury, direct brain injury,* and *indirect brain injury.* (p. 329)

7. List the signs and symptoms of possible cranial fracture and brain injury. (pp. 331-334)

8. List, step by step, the care for injury to the cranium or brain. (pp. 334-336)

9. Describe THREE types of LeForte fracture. (p. 336)

10. List the signs of a facial fracture. (pp. 336-337)

11. List, step by step, the care for injury to the face. (pp. 337)

12. List the signs and symptoms of injury to the mandible. (p. 337)

13. List the steps for caring for a fracture or dislocation of the mandible. (pp. 337-338)

14. Describe how to remove a helmet from an injured patient. (p. 338; Scan 12-1)

15. List the types of injuries to the spine and relate these injuries to mechanisms of injury. (pp. 338, 340)

16. State how to determine possible spinal injury, including assessment strategies and signs and symptoms. (pp. 340-344; Scan 12-2)

17. Describe how to apply a rigid cervical or extrication collar. (pp. 344-345; Scan 12-3)

18. Describe basic strategies for transferring and securing a patient to a long spine board. (p. 345; Scan 12-4)

19. Describe how and in what circumstances to transfer a patient to a long spine board using a rope sling. (p. 345)

20. Describe, step by step, how to secure a patient to a short spine board or flexible extrication device. (pp. 352-353; Scan 12-6)

21. Explain how to extricate a patient from a vehicle onto a long spine board. (pp. 353, 357)

Skills *As an EMT you should be able to*

1. Assess a patient for possible cranial, brain, facial, mandible, or spinal injuries.

2. Provide emergency care for patients with possible cranial, brain, facial, mandible, or spinal injuries.

3. Apply an extrication collar and transfer and secure a patient to a long spine board.

4. Apply an extrication collar and a short spine board or extrication device.

5. Carry out extrication of a patient from a vehicle onto a long spine board.

When you study injuries to the skull and the spine, it is first necessary to review and expand your knowledge of the anatomy and physiology of the axial skeleton and nervous system. Then you will study the mechanisms and kinds of injuries that can occur to the skull and spine, the signs and symptoms of such injuries, and emergency care.

THE AXIAL SKELETON

In Chapter 10, we divided the skeleton into two subdivisions: the axial skeleton and the appendicular skeleton. The axial skeleton (Figure 12-1) is composed of the skull, the spinal column or vertebral (VER-te-bral) column, the ribs, and the sternum. It makes up the longitudinal axis of the human body.

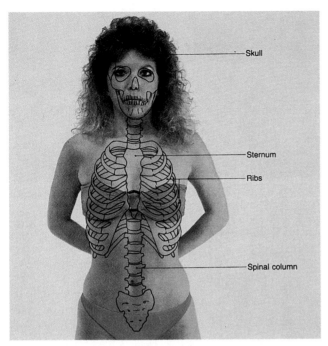

Figure 12-1 The axial skeleton.

In this chapter, we will consider the skull, the vertebral column, and the close relationship of the axial skeleton to the nervous system. The soft tissues of the head and neck will be covered in Chapter 13. The ribs, sternum, and the remaining structures of the chest will be discussed in Chapter 14.

The Skull

The skull is made up of the **cranium** (KRAY-ni-um) and the facial bones (Figure 12-2). The cranium forms the forehead (frontal), top (parietal), back (occipital), and upper sides (temporal) of the skull. The **cranial floor** is the inferior wall of the brain case—the bony floor beneath the brain. The cranial bones are fused together to form immovable joints. The point at which two bones of the cranium articulate (join together) is known as a **suture**.

There are fourteen irregularly shaped bones forming the face. The facial bones are fused into immovable joints, except for the **mandible** (MAN-di-bl). It joins on each side of the cranium with a **temporal** (TEM-por-al) **bone** to form the **temporo-mandibular** (TEM-po-ro-man-DIB-u -lar) **joint**. This joint is sometimes referred to as the TM joint.

The upper jaw is made up of two fused bones called the **maxillae** (mak-SIL-e). Each is known as a *maxilla* (mak-SIL-ah). The upper third, or bridge, of the nose contains two **nasal bones**. There is a cheek bone on each side of the skull. The cheek bone can be called the **malar** (MA-lar) or the *zygomatic* (zi-go-MAT-ik) *bone*. The malars and the maxillae form a portion of the **orbits** (sockets) of the eyes.

The Spine

The divisions of the spinal column were presented in Chapter 10. Figure 12-3 serves to review these divisions.

SKULL

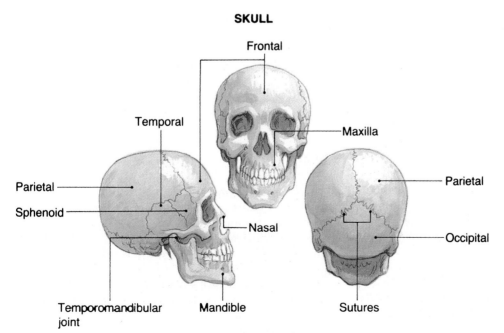

Figure 12-2 The bones of the skull.

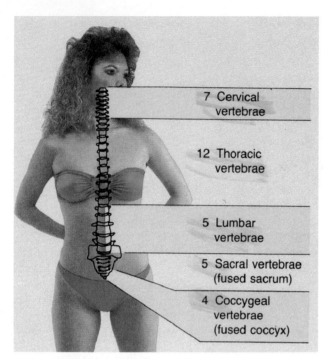

Figure 12-3 The divisions of the spinal column.

7 Cervical vertebrae

12 Thoracic vertebrae

5 Lumbar vertebrae

5 Sacral vertebrae (fused sacrum)

4 Coccygeal vertebrae (fused coccyx)

THE NERVOUS SYSTEM

When evaluating a patient for injuries to the head and spine, always consider the possibility of nervous system damage. The same holds true for many types of chest injuries, since the thoracic spine as well as the chest nerves may have been injured.

Anatomically, the nervous system (Figure 12-4) is divided into three systems: (1) the **central nervous system (CNS)**, (2) the **peripheral nervous system (PNS)**, and (3) the autonomic nervous system. The central nervous system consists of the brain and the spinal cord. The peripheral nervous system includes the nerves that enter and leave the spinal cord and those nerves that travel between the brain and organs without passing through the spinal cord (e.g., the optic nerve between the eye and brain). Messages sent from the body to the brain are carried by sensory nerves. The nerves sending messages from the brain to the muscles are called motor nerves. These nerves are responsible for voluntary motion. They control voluntary movements, those we consciously control, such as walking or grasping.

The final component of the nervous system is the **autonomic** (aw-toh-NOM-ik) **nervous system**. The motor nerves of this system connect

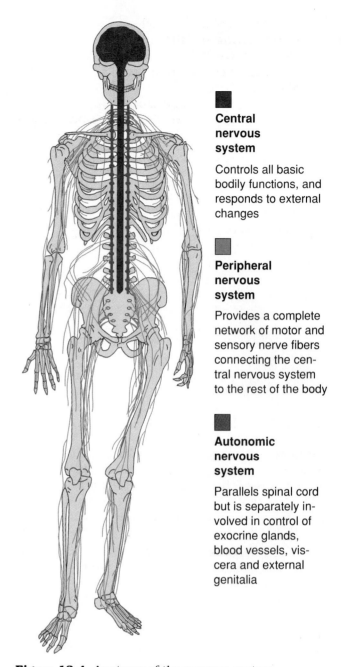

Central nervous system

Controls all basic bodily functions, and responds to external changes

Peripheral nervous system

Provides a complete network of motor and sensory nerve fibers connecting the central nervous system to the rest of the body

Autonomic nervous system

Parallels spinal cord but is separately involved in control of exocrine glands, blood vessels, viscera and external genitalia

Figure 12-4 Anatomy of the nervous system.

the brain and spinal cord to the heart muscle (myocardium), glands, smooth muscles in the walls of hollow organs, and the smooth muscles in the walls of the blood vessels in the skin, skeletal muscles, and organs. The autonomic system controls involuntary functions, those we do not consciously control, including

- Slowing or increasing heart rate
- Increasing or decreasing the strength of heart contractions

- Constricting blood vessels in the skin
- Constricting or dilating blood vessels in skeletal muscles
- Dilating or constricting blood vessels in the abdominal organs
- Changing bronchial diameter
- Contracting and relaxing the urinary bladder
- Dilating or constricting the pupils of the eye
- Increasing or decreasing the secretion of saliva and digestive juices

Any injury that interferes with or stops an autonomic function can be life threatening.

The brain is the master organ of life, the center of consciousness, self-awareness, and thought. It controls basic functions, including breathing and, to some degree, heart activity. Messages from all over the body are received by the brain, which decides how to respond to changing conditions both inside and outside the body. The brain sends messages to the muscles so that we can move, or to a particular organ so that it will carry out a desired function. Any major skull injury can damage the brain, causing vital body functions to fail.

The spinal cord is a relay between most of the body and the brain. A large number of the messages to and from the brain are sent through the spinal cord. Damage to the cord can isolate a part of the body from the brain. Function of this part can be lost, possibly forever.

Reflexes allow us to react quickly to such things as pain and excessive heat, without the brain having to send orders. The spinal cord is the center of reflex activity. Damage to the cord can destroy reflex function in certain areas of the body.

The healing power of the brain and nerve tissue is limited. Once this tissue is damaged to a certain extent, function is lost and cannot be restored. As an EMT your initial care will often prevent additional damage to the brain, spinal cord, and major nerves of the body.

INJURIES TO THE SKULL AND BRAIN

Types of Skull and Brain Injuries

Skull Injuries Skull injuries include fractures to the cranium and fractures to the face. If severe enough, these injuries can include direct and indirect injuries to the brain. In addition, there can be cuts to the scalp and other soft tissue injuries, as covered in Chapters 9 and 13.

A practical classification of injuries to the skull corresponds to the classification of fractures and wounds, namely, either open or closed. However, the words "open" and "closed" refer to the skull bones. When the bones of the cranium are fractured, if the dura is broken, even though the scalp is not lacerated, the patient has an *open head injury*. In a closed head injury, there may be a laceration of the scalp; however, if the cranium is intact, or free of fractures, the term *closed head injury* is used. In practice, it may not be possible for the EMT to determine if a head injury is open or closed. It is safest for the EMT to assume that there may be an open head injury beneath any contusion or laceration of the scalp.

There are four major types of skull fractures. A *linear skull fracture* is a thin line crack in the cranium. A *comminuted* (KOM-i-nu-ted) *skull fracture* has cracks radiating out from the center of the point of impact. A *depressed skull fracture* is one in which bone fragments are separated from the skull and driven inward by the object that struck the head. Fractures to the cranial floor are called *basal skull fractures*. Analysis by a physician is needed to detect these fractures; however, clear or bloody fluids in the nose and ears suggests a basal skull fracture.

Sometimes the term *penetrated skull* will be used as a fifth type of skull fracture. This is actually a type of injury, not a type of fracture. It can be caused by bullets, knife blades, or some other object penetrating the cranial bones. A penetrated skull injury may produce any or all of the four types of skull fracture.

Brain injuries Brain injuries can be classified as *direct* or *indirect*. Direct injuries can occur in open head injuries, with the brain being lacerated, punctured, or bruised by the broken bones of the skull, by bone fragments, or by foreign objects.

In cases of closed head injuries and certain types of open head injuries, damage to the brain can be indirect. The shock of impact is transferred to the brain. Like any other mass of tissue, the brain swells when it is injured. This swelling is serious since there is little room for expansion within the cranium. It becomes more difficult for blood to get into the head. The tissues become low in oxygen and high in carbon

CONCUSSION

- Mild injury usually with no detectable brain damage
- Usually no loss of consciousness
- Headache, grogginess, and short term memory loss common

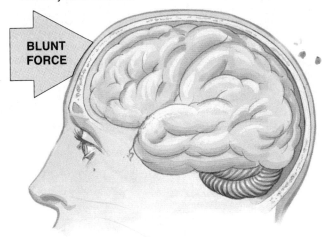

BLUNT FORCE

CONTUSION

- Unconsciousness or decreased level of consciousness
- Bruising or rupturing of brain tissue and vessels at any of these levels:

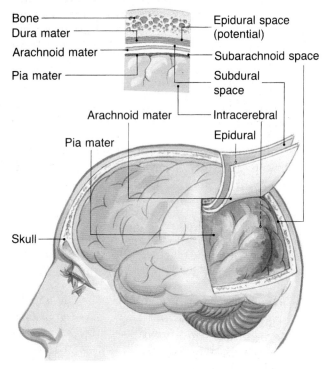

Bone
Dura mater
Arachnoid mater
Pia mater

Epidural space (potential)
Subarachnoid space
Subdural space

Arachnoid mater
Pia mater
Skull

Intracerebral
Epidural

Figure 12-5 Closed head injuries.

dioxide, which increases the swelling further. Indirect injuries to the brain include (Figure 12-5)

- **Concussion**—A concussion may be so mild that the patient is unaware of the injury. When a person strikes his head in a fall, or is struck by a blunt object, a certain amount of the force is transferred through the skull to the brain. Usually there is no detectable damage to the brain and the patient may or may not become unconscious. Most patients with a concussion will feel a little "groggy" after receiving a blow to the head. Headache is common. If there is a loss of consciousness, it usually lasts only a short time and does not tend to recur. Some loss of memory (amnesia) of the events surrounding the accident is fairly common. Long-term memory loss associated with concussion is rare.

- **Contusion**—A bruised brain can occur with closed head injuries, sometimes as the result of a concussion, when the force of the blow is great enough to rupture blood vessels found on the surface of, or deep within, the brain. Since there is little space for the brain to move before striking the walls of the cranial cavity, this bruise or contusion often takes place on the side of the brain *opposite* the point of impact. A contusion is usually caused by acceleration/deceleration injuries in which the brain hits the inside of the skull on acceleration, bounces off the opposite side on deceleration, and rebounds to strike the first side of the skull again. When the bruising of the brain occurs on the side of the injury, it is called a *coup*; when it occurs on the side opposite the injury it is called a *contracoup*. The inside of the skull has many sharp, bony ridges that can lacerate a moving brain.

With time, as you practice emergency care, you will hear of or care for a patient with a **subdural hematoma** (sub-DU-ral he-mah-TO-mah) (Figure 12-6). When the brain is bruised, lacerated, or punctured, blood from ruptured vessels can flow between the brain and its protective covering, the **meninges** (me-NIN-jez). The thick outer layer of the meninges is known as the *dura mater*. A subdural hematoma is situated between the dura mater and the brain.

Often, this bleeding is a slow venous flow. Even when the bleeding stops, the hematoma will continue to grow in size as it absorbs tissue fluids. Since there is no room for expansion in the cranium, severe pressure can be placed on the brain. Death can occur if vital brain centers

CRANIAL HEMATOMAS

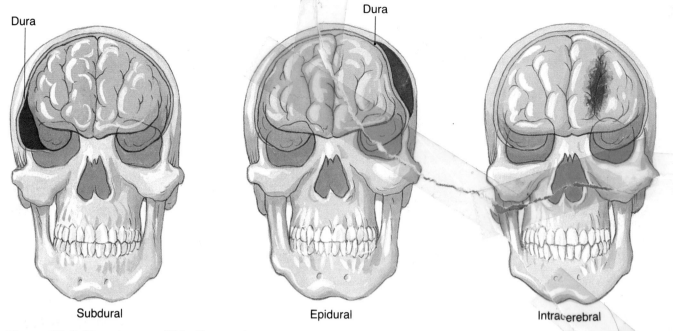

Figure 12-6 Hematomas within the cranium.

are damaged. This type of hematoma may occur rapidly or over a prolonged period of time.

Two other types of hematomas are related to head injuries (see Figure 12-6). The **epidural** (ep-i-DU-ral) **hematoma** occurs when blood flows between the meninges and the cranial bones (above the dura). Most of this flow is profuse arterial bleeding, causing a TRUE EMERGENCY. This type of hematoma is often associated with severe blows to the temples, in front of and just above the ears and is the reason for batters' helmets in baseball. Often the patient will at first be unconscious, followed by a fully conscious period (the lucid interval), only to suffer a second loss of consciousness.

An **intracerebral** (in-trah-SER-e-bral) **hematoma** occurs when blood pools within the brain itself, pushing tissues against the bones of the cranium. Depending on the severity of injury, the time from injury to TRUE EMERGENCY can vary greatly. Death can occur before transport.

A **laceration** can occur to the brain as a result of a penetrating or perforating wound of the cranium. Not only is there the problem of direct injury, but there may also be severe indirect injury due to hematoma formation.

NOTE: Signs and symptoms of possible injury to the skull or brain should alert you to the strong additional possibility of cervical spine injury.

Cranial Fractures and Brain Injuries

The signs and symptoms of cranial fractures and of brain injuries overlap but also differ in some respects. However, as described below, emergency treatment for a patient with either or both is the same.

Patient Assessment—Cranial Fractures

Visible bone fragments and perhaps even bits of brain tissue are the most obvious signs of cranial fracture, but the majority of cranial fractures do not produce these signs.

Signs and Symptoms

You should consider the possibility of a cranial fracture whenever you note (Figure 12-7)

- Decreased Consciousness—The patient is unconscious after injury or displays a decreased level of consciousness or confusion. Use the AVPU scale. This is the most important sign.
- Deep Laceration or Severe Bruise—an injury that has produced a deep laceration or severe bruise to the scalp or forehead. *Do not probe into the wound or separate the wound opening to determine wound depth.*

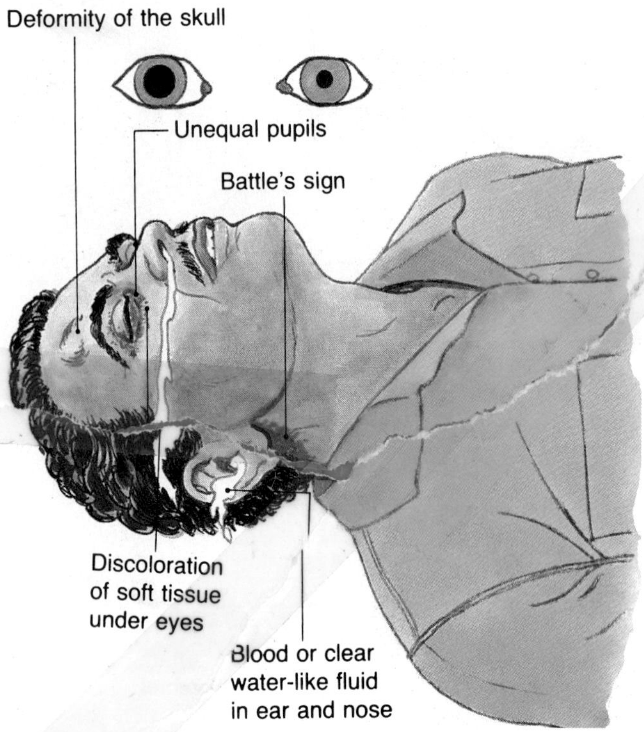

Figure 12-7 Signs of cranial fracture.

tain cerebrospinal fluid unless you gently absorb some fluid onto a gauze dressing and watch the clear fluid separate out from the spot of blood ("targeting" or "halo test"). This test is not always reliable.

Remember that damage to the brain can be *indirect*, not signaled by an open skull wound or not adjacent to the wound site. The shock of impact transferred to the brain can cause concussion, contusion, or subdural, epidural, or intracranial hematoma.

Signs and Symptoms

In cases of head injury, you should consider the possibility of a brain injury if you note

- ☐ Pain—ranging from a headache to severe discomfort
- ☐ Decreased Level of Consciousness—loss of consciousness, altered states of consciousness, amnesia, or confusion, usually increasing as time passes (the most important sign or symptom)
- ☐ Personality Changes—ranging from irritable to irrational behavior (a major sign)
- ☐ Blood Pressure and Pulse Rate—Blood pressure may be elevated while the pulse rate decreases (this is called Cushing's syndrome).
- ☐ Respirations—may change pattern, becoming labored, then rapid, and then stopping for a few seconds
- ☐ Temperature—may increase (late sign due to inflammation, infection, or damage to temperature-regulating centers)
- ☐ Pupils—unequal and/or unresponsive
- ☐ "Doll's Eye Response"—Ordinarily, when the head turns the eyes remain fixed in the original direction, moving left when the head turns right, for example. When there is a brain injury, the eyes may move with the head, staying in midline position like a doll's eyes. DO NOT ASK THE PATIENT TO MOVE HIS HEAD. THIS WOULD RISK FURTHER CERVICAL INJURY.
- ☐ Vision—disturbed in one or both eyes
- ☐ Hearing—may be impaired, or ringing in the ears
- ☐ Equilibrium—Patient may be unable to stand still with eyes closed or stumbles

opposite of shock

- ☐ Pain or Swelling—any severe pain or swelling at the site of a head injury. Pain may be a symptom of skull injury. *Do not* palpate the injury site.
- ☐ Deformity of the Skull—depressions in the cranium, large swellings ("goose eggs"), or anything that looks unusual about the shape of the cranium
- ☐ "Battle's Sign"—any bruise or swelling behind the ear. This is a late sign.
- ☐ Unequal pupils—The pupils are not the same size. This is a late sign caused by compression of the optic nerve that controls pupil constriction.
- ☐ "Raccoon's Eyes"—black eyes or discoloration of the soft tissues under both eyes. This is usually a delayed finding.
- ☐ Sunken Eye—One eye appears to be sunken.
- ☐ Bleeding—from the ears and/or the nose
- ☐ Clear Fluid—flowing from the ears and/or the nose. This could be **cerebrospinal** (ser-e-bro-SPI-nal) **fluid**, also called **CSF**. This fluid surrounds the brain and spinal cord. It cannot come out through the ears or nose unless the cranium has been fractured and the meninges are torn.

If fluids coming from the ears or nose are bloody, you will not be able to tell if they con-

when attempting to walk. (Do not test for this.)

- ☐ Vomiting—often forceful or projectile
- ☐ Posturing—When painful stimulus is applied, the patient flexes the arms and wrists and extends the legs and feet in response (called *decorticate posture*) or extends the arms with the shoulders rotated inward and the wrists flexed, legs extended (*decerebrate posture*). These postures may also be assumed spontaneously, without painful stimulus. These are significant signs of deep cerebral or upper brainstem injury.
- ☐ Paralysis—often to one side of the body
- ☐ Signs of a Skull Fracture—any head injury in which signs of skull fracture are present
- ☐ Deteriorated Vital Signs—any head injury when the patient displays a deterioration of vital signs

Note: Shock is not a sign of head injury but may be present if there is severe bleeding. If there is head injury with shock, look for indications of blood loss.

With so many factors to consider, the mechanism of injury and the location of the injury site become very important when trying to determine if there is possible brain damage. *Some of the signs and symptoms of brain injury can cause untrained personnel to assume that a patient with a brain injury is merely intoxicated or abusing other drugs. Never assume intoxication or drug abuse.*

Warning: If an unconscious patient regains consciousness, only to lose consciousness again, you must report this to the emergency department staff. This is a strong indication of possible life-threatening brain injury.

Level of Consciousness and Neurological Assessment ALL patients having head injury or suspected brain damage must be carefully monitored during transport. Have suction available at all times. Be prepared in case the patient has a seizure (see Chapter 16). Keep a constant watch over the patient. What you observe and report can have a great bearing on the initial actions taken by the emergency department staff.

Part of the Champion Sacco trauma score discussed in Chapter 3 was the Glasgow Coma Scale. Many EMS systems use this scale to record data on patients with possible head and brain injury. The scale is shown in Table 12-1. When using this scale, remember

TABLE 12-1   The Glasgow Coma Scale

Eye opening	Spontaneous	4
	To voice	3
	To pain	2
	None	1
Verbal response	Oriented	5
	Confused	4
	Inappropriate words	3
	Incomprehensible words	2
	None	1
Motor response	Obeys command	6
	Localizes pain	5
	Withdraws from pain	4
	Flexion from pain	3
	Extension from pain	2
	None	1
Glasgow Coma Scale Points: TOTAL =		

Reduction of Glasgow Coma Scale points for use in a trauma score:

14-15 = 5	5-7 = 2
11-13 = 4	3-4 =1
8-10 = 3	

NOTE: There are updated variations of this scale. Use the scale provided by your EMS system. See Chapter 3 for more information.

1. Note if there are eye injuries or injuries to the face that prevent the patient from opening the eyes. If the injuries are more than minor ones, do not ask the patient to open his eyes.
2. Spontaneous eye opening means that the patient has the eyes open without your having to do anything. If his eyes are closed, then you should say, "Open your eyes" to see if the patient will obey this command. Try a normal level of voice. If this fails, shout the command. Should the patient's eyes remain closed, apply an accepted painful stimulus (e.g., pinch a toe, scratch the palm or sole, rub the sternum).
3. When evaluating the patient's verbal responses, use the following criteria.
   - Oriented—The patient, once aroused, can tell you who he is, where he is, and the year and month or day of the week. A person who can answer these questions appropriately is said to be alert on the AVPU scale.
   - Confused—The patient cannot answer the above questions, but he can speak in phrases and sentences.
   - Inappropriate words—The patient says or shouts a word or several words at a time.

Usually this requires physical stimulation. The words do not fit the situation or a particular question. Often, the patient curses.

- Incomprehensible sounds—The patient responds with mumbling, moans, or groans.
- No verbal response—Repeated stimulation, verbal and physical, does not cause the patient to speak or make any sounds.

4. The following are the criteria used to evaluate motor response.

- Obeys command—The patient must be able to understand your instruction and carry out the request. For example, you can ask (when appropriate) for the patient to hold up two fingers.
- Localizes pain—Should the patient fail to respond to your commands, apply pressure to one of the nail beds for 5 seconds or firm pressure to the sternum. Note if the patient attempts to remove your hand. Do not apply pressure over an injury site. Do not apply pressure to the sternum if the patient is experiencing difficult breathing.
- Withdraws—after painful stimulation. Note if the elbow flexes, he moves slowly, there is the appearance of stiffness, he holds his forearm and hand against the body, or the limbs on one side of the body appear to be paralyzed (hemiplegic position).
- Posturing—after painful stimulation. Note if the legs and arms extend, there is apparent stiffness with these moves, and if there is an internal rotation of the shoulder and forearm.

Since a number of observations concerning neurologic condition have to be made at relatively close intervals, many ambulances are provided with locally designed neurologic observation forms. An example of the information contained on many local forms is shown in Figure 12-8. Proper use of these forms will allow you to provide emergency department personnel with an accurate record of your observations. If your EMS System does not use a specialized form, you should use the AVPU approach described in Chapter 3.

Patient Care— Cranial Fractures and Brain Injuries

The following procedures apply to patients with cranial injuries, with or without possible damage to the brain.

NEUROLOGICAL ASSESSMENT FORM			
TIME	INITIAL ASSESS- MENT ____		
CONSCIOUS	YES/NO	YES/NO	YES/NO
ORIENTED	YES/NO	YES/NO	YES/NO
RESPONSIVE TO VOICE	YES/NO	YES/NO	YES/NO
RESPONSIVE TO COMMAND	YES/NO	YES/NO	YES/NO
TALKS	YES/NO	YES/NO	YES/NO
REACTS TO PAIN	YES/NO/NA	YES/NO/NA	YES/NO/NA
ABILITY TO MOVE ● LEFT LEG ● RIGHT LEG ● LEFT ARM ● RIGHT ARM			
PUPILS ● REACTIVITY ● SIZE	L | R	L | R	L | R

Figure 12-8 Neurologic observations form.

Emergency Care Steps

When caring for patients with injuries to the cranium, you should assume that neck or spinal injuries also exist and

1. *Ensure an open airway.* Careful handling is essential since there may be associated spinal injury. For such cases, American Heart Association guidelines call for the use of the jaw-thrust. If there are open injuries to the skull, or if skull fracture is obvious, always use the jaw-thrust technique.
2. *Maintain an open airway.* Monitor the conscious patient for changes in breathing. For the unconscious patient, an oropharyngeal airway should be inserted. This must be done without hyperextending the neck. Have suctioning equipment ready for immediate use.*
3. *Provide resuscitative measures if needed.*

* Nasal airways should not be used if basal skull fractures are suspected or nasal and orbital fractures are present.

④ *Immobilize the neck and spine.* Apply a rigid collar and place the patient on a spine board.

⑤ *Administer oxygen.* This is critical should there be brain damage. Deliver as high a concentration of oxygen as possible.

Note: Most EMS systems have adopted a special protocol for hyperventilating patients with a head injury. This protocol requires the EMT to deliver oxygen-assisted ventilations (bag-valve mask or positive pressure) at the rate of 25+ per minute rather than the usual 12 ventilations per minute. This procedure is called "hyperventilating the patient." The hyperventilation will help reduce brain tissue swelling by lowering carbon dioxide levels and raising oxygen levels.

⑥ *Control bleeding.* Do not apply pressure if the injury site shows bone fragments or depression of the bone or if the brain is exposed. Do not attempt to stop the flow of blood or cerebrospinal fluid from the ears or the nose. If the skull is fractured, you may increase intracranial pressure and may also increase the risk of infection. Use a loose gauze dressing.

⑦ *Keep the patient at rest.* This can be a critical factor.

⑧ *Monitor vital signs.*

⑨ *Talk to the conscious patient.* Ask the patient questions so that he will have to concentrate. This procedure will help you to detect changes in the patient's level of consciousness.

⑩ *Dress and bandage open wounds.* Stabilize any penetrating objects. (Do not remove any objects or fragments of bone.)

⑪ *Manage the patient for shock* even if shock is not present, to prevent shock from developing. Avoid overheating.

⑫ *Elevate the head of the spine board slightly* if there is no evidence of shock.

⑬ *Provide emotional support.*

⑭ *Position the patient properly and be prepared for vomiting* (as discussed below under "Positioning the Patient With Cranial Injury").

Positioning the Patient With Cranial Injury Proper patient positioning is important in caring for patients with head injuries. Conscious patients with apparently minor closed head injuries and *absolutely no signs of neck or spinal injuries* can be positioned in one of two ways.

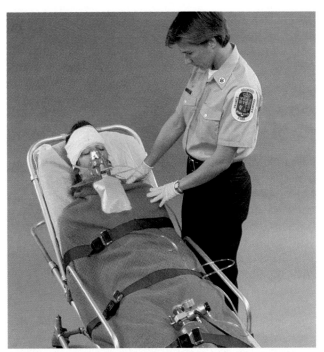

Figure 12-9 Head-elevated position for conscious patients with minor closed head injury and no signs of spinal injury.

1. Head elevated—To reduce the risk of intracranial pressure buildup, elevate the entire upper body or slant the entire body to a head-elevated position (Figure 12-9). Do not simply elevate the patient's head at the neck. To do so may partially obstruct the airway. Placing the patient's upper body at an angle gives better control should the patient vomit.

2. Supine—Some systems have adopted a positioning that places the patient flat on his back. They believe that there is little risk of intracranial pressure buildup in this position and that it helps prevent shock. If you use this positioning, you *must* have suction equipment ready and monitor continuously for vomiting.

If you are not certain as to the severity of the patient's injuries, if there is evidence of cervical spine injury, or if the patient with a head injury is unconscious, then a rigid cervical or extrication collar must be applied and the patient positioned on a long spine board. With the entire head, neck, and body rigidly immobilized, the patient may be rotated into a lateral recumbent position so that blood and mucus can drain freely, and if the patient vomits, as brain-injured patients are likely to do, the vomitus is less likely to cause an airway obstruction or be aspirated (breathed into the lungs). Some patients with a head injury will vomit without warning. Many vomit without first experiencing nausea. If injuries prevent such positioning, constant monitoring and frequent suctioning are required.

Cranial Injuries With Impaled Objects If there is an object impaled in the patient's cranium, do not remove it. Instead, stabilize the object in place with bulky dressings. This, plus care in handling, minimizes accidental movement of the object during the remainder of care and transport.

In some situations you may be confronted with a patient whose skull has been impaled by a long object. This can make transporting of the patient impossible until the object is cut or shortened. Pad around the object with bulky dressings, then carefully (and rigidly) stabilize the object on both sides of where the cut will be made. Cutting should be done with a tool that will not cause the object to move or vibrate when it is finally severed. Often, a hand hacksaw with a fine tooth blade is the best tool to use because it can be carefully controlled and produces only a small amount of heat. In any case in which you may have to cut a long impaled object, call and seek advice from the emergency department physician.

Facial Fractures

Facial fractures are usually produced by an impact, as when a child is struck in the face by a baseball bat or when someone is thrown against the windshield during a motor vehicle crash.

Depending upon the mechanism of injury, the face can be fractured at any site. Some commonly occurring facial fractures are classified into three types called **LeForte fractures**. A LeForte I fracture transverses the upper jaw or maxilla. It falls between the nose and the upper gum line, separating the hard palate or roof of the mouth from the rest of the maxilla. A LeForte II fracture is pyramidal in shape. It extends from the corner or extreme lateral edges of the maxilla (where the last teeth are found in the gum) upward under the eye orbits and across the nasal bone. This fracture separates the entire upper jaw and nose from the rest of the face. A LeForte III fracture is higher on the face, extending from the temporomandibular joint slightly

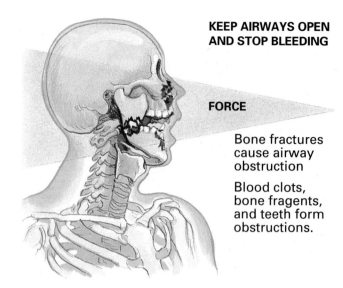

KEEP AIRWAYS OPEN AND STOP BLEEDING

FORCE

Bone fractures cause airway obstruction

Blood clots, bone fragents, and teeth form obstructions.

Figure 12-10 Potential complications from facial fractures.

A B C

upward and laterally through the orbits and above the nose. This fracture separates the entire face from the remainder of the skull. The Type III fracture can be extensive enough to produce a basal skill fracture and leakage of cerebrospinal fluid.

Patient Assessment—Facial Fractures

Facial fractures can be so simple that they go undetected, or they may produce serious, grotesque injuries. Of primary concern is the state of the patient's airway (Figure 12-10). Bone fragments may lodge in the back of the throat, causing airway obstruction. Blood, blood clots, and dislodged teeth, or a separated palate also may cause partial or total airway obstruction.

Signs

Consider the possibility of facial fractures when you note (Figure 12-11)

☐ Blood in the airway
☐ Facial deformities
☐ False face bone movements (e.g., the movement of the upper jaw bones)
☐ Black eyes or discoloration below the eyes
☐ A swollen lower jaw, poor jaw function, or poor alignment of teeth
☐ Teeth that are loose or have been knocked out, or broken dentures

336 Trauma

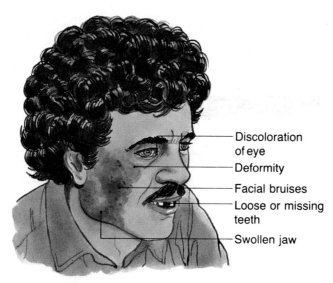

Figure 12-11 Signs of facial fracture.

- Discoloration of eye
- Deformity
- Facial bruises
- Loose or missing teeth
- Swollen jaw

☐ Large facial bruises
☐ Any other indications of a severe blow to the face

Patient Care—Facial Fractures

When confronted with a patient having possible facial fractures, your principal concerns are to support the spine, to keep the airway open, and to stop profuse bleeding.

Emergency Care Steps

1 Spinal Support—If the patient is unconscious, or if there are indications of possible facial fractures, apply a rigid or extrication collar. Such patients must be transported with support provided for the entire spine. Immobilize the spine by securing the patient to a long spine board.

2 Airway Maintenance—Clear the mouth of debris and establish an airway. If there has been a Type I LeForte fracture, the hard palate may have fallen back over the nasopharynx and you may have to lift the maxilla outward and hold it in place with a gloved hand to assure an open airway. Other types of facial fracture also cause facial bones to move freely and may require manual management.

3 Drainage—You must maintain drainage during care at the scene and in transport to keep the airway clear. Positioning the patient for drainage is essential. The patient and the long spine board to which he is secured may need to be rotated to allow for drainage. If both sides of the face are injured, a supine position with suction may be used. Aggressive suctioning may be required whatever the patient's position.

4 Control of Bleeding—Direct pressure is the usual method used to control bleeding, but care must be exercised not to apply pressure over a probable fracture site.

5 Treatment of Impaled Objects—If there is an object impaled in the patient's face, do not remove it. Instead, as described above for cranial impalements, stabilize the object with bulky dressings. The exception to this stabilization procedure occurs when the object is impaled in the soft tissues of the cheek and has entered the oral cavity. Care for such cases is presented in Chapter 13.

Injuries to the Mandible

The mandible is subject to dislocation as well as to fracture.

Patient Assessment—Mandible Injury

Signs and Symptoms

The signs and symptoms for these injuries include

☐ Pain
☐ Discoloration
☐ Swelling
☐ Facial distortion
☐ Loss of use of the lower jaw or difficulty with speech
☐ Malocclusion—the improper alignment of the upper and lower teeth when the jaw is closed. (Do not test for this.)
☐ Bleeding around teeth

Patient Care—Mandible Injury

Care is the same for both fractures and dislocations of the mandible.

Emergency Care Steps

1 Maintain an open airway.
2 Dress any open wounds.

3 Apply a cervical or extrication collar if indicated.
4 Properly position the patient.
5 Care for shock.
6 Provide a high concentration of oxygen.
7 Transport, monitoring vital signs.

Care for Patients Wearing Helmets

Helmets are worn in many sporting events and by many motorcycle riders. Facial, neck, and spinal injury care may call for the removal of the helmet. The helmet should not prevent you from reaching the patient's mouth or nose if resuscitation efforts are needed. Protection shields can be lifted and face guards can be cut away. If the face guard is to be cut, one EMT must steady the patient's head and neck with manual stabilization. The other EMT should snap off the guard or unscrew it.

Do not attempt to remove a helmet if doing so causes increased pain, or if the helmet proves difficult to remove, unless there is a possible airway obstruction or pulmonary resuscitation must be provided.*

When a helmet must be removed, it is a two-rescuer procedure (Scan 12-1). After fully explaining to the patient what you are going to do, follow this procedure.

1. EMT 1 is positioned at the top of the patient's head and maintains manual stabilization with a hand on the lower jaw. The construction of the helmet may require stabilization to be applied with the fingers while the rest of the hand is placed on the side of the helmet.
2. EMT 2 opens, cuts, or removes the chin strap, then places one hand on the patient's chin and, using the other hand, applies stabilization at the occipital region.
3. EMT 1 can now release manual stabilization and slowly remove the helmet. The lower sides of the helmet will have to be gently pulled out to clear the ears. Eyeglasses will have to be removed.
4. EMT 1, after removing the helmet, re-establishes manual stabilization and maintains an open airway by using the jaw-thrust.
5. EMT 2 can release manual stabilization and apply an extrication collar. The patient should then be secured to a long spine board.

*Follow your local protocols. Some EMS systems call for helmet removal in all cases to allow for proper securing of the patient to a long spine board.

Note: This method has not been adopted by all EMS Systems. Your instructor will inform you of local policies.

INJURIES TO THE SPINE

Types of Spinal Injuries

Injuries to the spine must always be considered when you find serious injury to the body. Remember that spinal injury can be associated with head, neck, and back injuries. Do not overlook the possibility of spinal injury when dealing with chest, abdominal, and pelvic injuries. Even injuries to the upper and lower extremities can be associated with forces intense enough to also produce spinal injury. Remember, you must always do a complete secondary survey, except when a patient is categorized as C (critical) or U (unstable) and given immediate transport. Failure to complete the patient survey will reduce your chances of detecting possible spinal injury.

Injuries to the spinal column include

- Fractures, with and without bone displacement
- Dislocations
- Ligament sprains
- Disk injury, including compression

The vertebral column may be injured without damage to the spinal cord or spinal nerves. For example, a fractured coccyx is below the level of the spinal cord. Ligament sprains are relatively simple injuries. However, when displaced fractures and dislocations occur, the cord, disk, and spinal nerves may be severely injured. Serious contusions and lacerations, accompanied by pressure-producing swelling, can take place. The entire column can become unstable, leading to cord compression that may produce paralysis or death.

Mechanisms of Injury

Note: There is a simple rule you can follow. If the mechanism of injury exerts great force on the upper body (Figure 12-12) or if there is any soft tissue damage to the head, face, or neck due to trauma (e.g., from being thrown against a dashboard), you may then assume that there is a possible cervical spine injury. Any blunt trauma above the clavicles may damage the cervical spine.

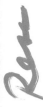

Helmet Removal From Injured Patient

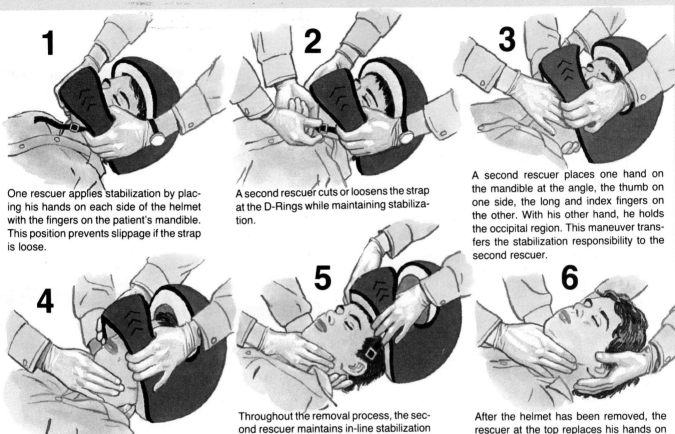

1

One rescuer applies stabilization by placing his hands on each side of the helmet with the fingers on the patient's mandible. This position prevents slippage if the strap is loose.

2

A second rescuer cuts or loosens the strap at the D-Rings while maintaining stabilization.

3

A second rescuer places one hand on the mandible at the angle, the thumb on one side, the long and index fingers on the other. With his other hand, he holds the occipital region. This maneuver transfers the stabilization responsibility to the second rescuer.

4

The rescuer at the top removes the helmet.
Three factors should be kept in mind.
(a) The helmet is egg-shaped and therefore must be expanded laterally to clear the ears.
(b) If the helmet provides full facial coverage, glasses must be removed first.
(c) If the helmet provides full facial coverage, the nose will impede removal. To clear the nose, the helmet must be tilted backward and raised over it.

5

Throughout the removal process, the second rescuer maintains in-line stabilization from below in order to prevent head tilt.

6

After the helmet has been removed, the rescuer at the top replaces his hands on either side of the patient's head with his palms over the ears, taking over stabilization.

Summary:
The helmet must be maneuvered over the nose and ears while the head and neck are held rigid.
(a) Stabilization is applied from above.
(b) Stabilization is transferred below with pressure on the jaw and occiput.
(c) The helmet is removed.
(d) Stabilization is re-established from above.

7

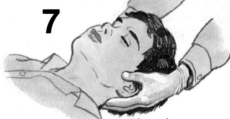

Stabilization is maintained from above until a cervical collar and a spine board are in place.

Note: If the patient has shoulder pads and you are removing a football helmet, remember to pad behind the head to keep it aligned with the padded shoulders.

From John E. Campbell, M.D., and Alabama Chapter, American College of Emergency Physicians, *BTLS Basic Prehospital Trauma Care*, The Brady Company, 1988.

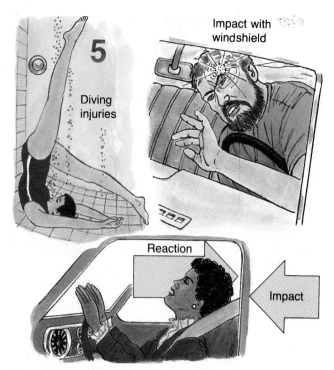

Figure 12-12 Mechanisms of neck injury.

Some parts of the spine are more susceptible to injury than others. Because they are somewhat splinted by the attached ribs, the segments of the thoracic spine are not usually damaged except in the most violent accidents or in gunshot wounds. The pelvic-sacral spine attachment helps to protect the sacrum in the same way. On the other hand, the cervical and lumbar vertebrae are susceptible to injury because they are not supported by other bony structures.

Remember that the adult skull weighs more than 17 pounds, and it rests on a very small area of the cervical spine (sometimes described as like a pumpkin on a broom handle). Motor vehicle collisions produce violent whiplash injuries because of the speed and sudden deceleration of the vehicle. When a vehicle strikes another vehicle or a fixed object head on, the neck can whip quickly back and forth. The vehicle decelerates abruptly, but the head continues to travel forward at the same rate of speed that the vehicle was traveling, even though the body is held by seat restraints. This neck movement may exceed the normal range of motion. Virtually the same thing occurs when the vehicle is struck from behind.

A fall can produce spinal injury when the victim strikes an object, the ground, or the floor. The force generated during a fall may be enough to fracture, crush, or dislocate vertebrae. Cases

of needless disability have been reported when head injuries or other injuries were noted and cared for but spinal injuries were overlooked.

Today more and more people are participating in sports of all kinds: roller-blading, bicycling, surfing, rock climbing, and others too numerous to mention. Many sports accidents can cause spinal injury. A sledding or skiing accident may hurl a person into a tree or other fixed object, twisting or compressing the spinal column. There may be no open wound or fracture of an extremity, or signs of injury may be hidden by bulky clothing. As a result, improper care may be rendered as the victim with a possible spinal injury is placed on a stretcher without adequate examination and immobilization.

Diving accidents often produce injury to the cervical spine. When the diver strikes the diving board, the side or bottom of the pool, or an underwater object, the head can be severely forced beyond its normal limits of motion (flexion, extension, or compression). Cervical vertebrae may be fractured or dislocated, ligaments may be severely sprained, and the spinal cord may be compressed or otherwise traumatized in the cervical region and at other spots along the cord.

Football and other contact sports can cause accidents severe enough to produce spinal injury. Whenever the game involves player contact or falling to the ground, be on the alert for spinal injury.

Remember: Any violent or falling accident can produce spinal injury. The most common causes of spinal cord injury are motor vehicle collisions, fractured spines in the elderly (often caused by falls, or spontaneous fractures of brittle bones that, in turn, cause falls), diving accidents, and gunshot wounds. You must do a complete survey of the patient. You should assume that all unconscious trauma patients have spinal injury. Whenever you are in doubt, assume that there are spinal injuries and immobilize the torso and the head and neck.

Patient Assessment—Spinal Injury

Remember: Any unconscious patient who is the victim of an accident *must* be assumed to have spinal injury.

Spinal injuries can be difficult to detect. Your chances of finding possible spinal injury will increase if you

1. *Consider the mechanism of injury.* Is the accident the type that can produce spinal injury? Serious falls, motor vehicle collisions, diving accidents, and cave-ins often cause spinal damage.

2. *Observe breathing patterns.* During normal respiration, the rib cage rises during inspiration and falls during expiration. Damage to the nerves that control the movement of the rib cage can prevent this. The nerve that controls the diaphragm is located high in the cervical area and is often unharmed, but the intercostal nerves that control the chest muscles are often damaged in cervical and thoracic injuries. As a result, when the diaphragm moves downward to pull in air, the ribs, instead of expanding, collapse; when the diaphragm relaxes and air is expelled, the rib cage rises—the opposite of the normal pattern. This is called *neurogenic paradoxical respiration,* a characteristic only of spinal cord injury. Check abdominal movement from the side by placing your hand on the patient's abdomen and looking for reversed movements during respiration.

3. *Observe the position (posturing) of the patient.* The patient in a supine position may have the arms stretched out above the head, flexed across the chest, or extended along the sides with wrists flexed.

4. *Question the patient and bystanders about the accident.* They may be able to report a mechanism of injury that is not obvious or movement prior to being pulled from the car or swimming pool.

5. *Conduct a head-to-toe examination.*
   - Are there injuries that you can associate with spinal injuries? Facial injury, head wounds and fractures, neck wounds, blunt trauma to the head, neck, back, or chest, pelvic fractures, hip dislocations, and severing or penetrating wounds of the neck or trunk indicate a mechanism of injury that may have produced damage to the spine.
   - Are there signs and symptoms indicating possible spinal injury?
   - Does a neurologic survey indicate any problem with nerve function?

6. *Monitor the patient to note any changes associated with spinal injury.* Numbness and tingling in the extremities may begin, or paralysis may occur. Document sensory and motor response in all four extremities before and after immobilization.

Signs and Symptoms

The following signs and symptoms of spinal injury (Scan 12-2) are discussed more fully below.

- Pain without movement
- Pain with movement
- Tenderness
- Deformity (rare)
- Impaired breathing
- Priapism
- Posturing
- Loss of bowel or bladder control
- Paralysis or nerve impairment of the extremities
- Severe shock

Note: Paralysis, pain without movement, pain with movement, and tenderness anywhere along the spine are reliable indicators of possible spinal injury in the conscious patient. If these are present, you have sufficient reason to immobilize the patient before proceeding with the survey. If immediate immobilization is not possible, use extreme care in handling the patient. In the field, it is not possible to rule out spinal injury even in cases in which the patient has no pain and is able to move his limbs. The mechanism of injury alone may be the deciding factor.

Pain Without Movement The pain is not always constant and may occur anywhere from the top of the head to the buttocks. Pain in the leg is common for certain types of injury to the lower spinal cord and vertebral column. Other painful injuries can mask out this symptom of spinal injury.

Pain With Movement The patient normally tries to lie perfectly still to prevent pain on movement. You should not request the patient to move just to determine if pain is present. However, if the patient complains of pain in the neck or back experienced with voluntary movements, you must consider this to be a symptom of possible spinal injury. Pain with movement in apparently uninjured shoulders and legs is a good indicator of possible spinal injury.

Tenderness Gentle palpation of the injury site, when accessible, may reveal point tenderness.

Deformity The removal of clothing to check the back for deformity of the spine is not

Assessing Patients for Spinal Injuries

Signs and Symptoms

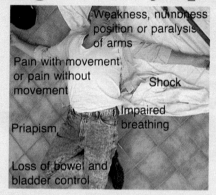

Weakness, numbness position or paralysis of arms

Pain with movement or pain without movement

Shock

Priapism

Impaired breathing

Loss of bowel and bladder control

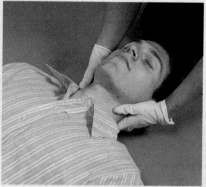

Point cervical tenderness and deformity

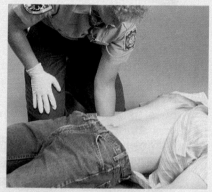

Point spinal column tenderness and deformity

Conscious—Lower Extremities Assessment

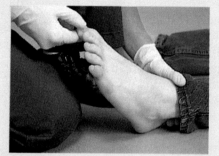

Touch toe

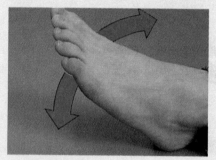

Foot wave

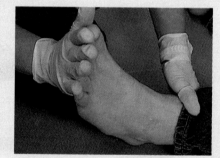

Foot push

RESULTS: If the patient can perform these tasks, there is little chance of severe injury to the cord anywhere along its length. However, immobilizing the spine is called for since this test does not rule out all types of injuries, including vertebral fractures. If the tests can only be performed to a limited degree and with pain, there may be pressure somewhere along the cord. When a patient is not able to perform any of the tests, you must assume that there is spinal injury damage.

Conscious—Upper Extremities Assessment

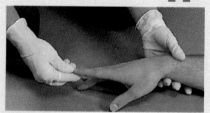

Touch finger

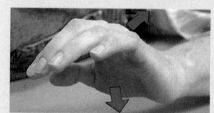

Hand wave

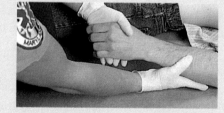

Hand squeeze

RESULTS: Performance of all tests indicates little chance of damage in the cervical area but does not rule out all possibilities. Limited performance and pain—pressure on cord in cervical area. Failure to perform any test and negative lower extremity results—assume severe cord injury in neck.

UNCONSCIOUS PATIENTS: Test the responses to painful stimuli (pinching) applied to the distal limb. If removal of shoes may aggravate existing injuries, apply the stimuli to the skin around the ankles.

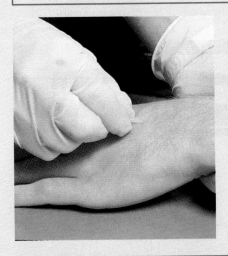
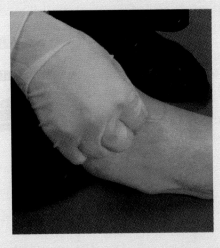

REMEMBER
It is difficult to survey the unconscious patient with accuracy. A deeply unconscious patient will not pull back from a painful stimulus. Should the mechanism of injury indicate possible spinal damage, or if the trauma patient is unconscious, assume that spinal injury is present.

RESULTS: Slight pulling back of foot—cord usually intact. NO foot reaction—possible damage anywhere along the cord. Hand or finger reaction—usually no damage to cervical cord. No hand or finger reaction—possible damage to the cervical cord.

Summary of Observations and Conclusions

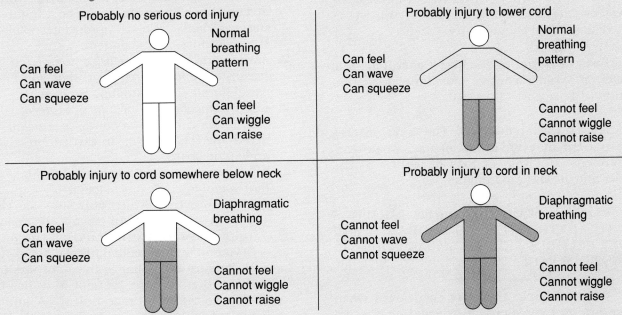

Probably no serious cord injury

Can feel
Can wave
Can squeeze

Normal breathing pattern

Can feel
Can wiggle
Can raise

Probably injury to lower cord

Can feel
Can wave
Can squeeze

Normal breathing pattern

Cannot feel
Cannot wiggle
Cannot raise

Probably injury to cord somewhere below neck

Can feel
Can wave
Can squeeze

Diaphragmatic breathing

Cannot feel
Cannot wiggle
Cannot raise

Probably injury to cord in neck

Cannot feel
Cannot wave
Cannot squeeze

Diaphragmatic breathing

Cannot feel
Cannot wiggle
Cannot raise

WARNING: If the patient is unconscious or the mechanism of injury indicates possible spinal injury, assume that spinal injury is present.

recommended. OBVIOUS SPINAL DEFORMITIES ARE RARE. However, if you note a gap between the **spinous processes** (bony extensions) of the vertebrae or if you can feel a broken spinous process, you must consider the patient to have serious spinal injuries. It is also possible to feel tight muscles in spasm.

Impaired Breathing Neck injury can impair nerve function to the chest muscles. Watch the patient breathe. If there is only a slight movement of the abdomen, with little or no movement of the chest, it is safe to assume that the patient is breathing with the diaphragm alone (diaphragmatic breathing). This is also true if there is a reversal of normal breathing patterns with the rib cage collapsing on inspiration, rising on expiration. Panting due to respiratory insufficiency may develop.

Priapism Persistent erection of the penis is a reliable sign of spinal injury affecting nerves to the external genitalia.

Posturing In some cases of spinal injury, motor nerve pathways to the muscles that extend the arm can be interrupted, but those that lead to the muscles that bend the elbow and lift the arm remain functional. The patient may be found on his back, with the arms extended above the head, which may indicate a cervical spine injury. Arms flexed across the chest or extended along the sides with wrists flexed also signal spinal injury.

Loss of Bowel or Bladder Control Loss of bowel or bladder control may indicate spinal injury.

Nerve Impairment to the Extremities The patient may have loss of use, weakness, numbness, tingling, or loss of feeling in the upper and/or lower extremities.

Paralysis of the Extremities PARALYSIS OF THE EXTREMITIES IS PROBABLY THE MOST RELIABLE SIGN OF SPINAL INJURY IN CONSCIOUS PATIENTS.

Severe Shock This may occur even when there are no indications of external or internal bleeding. It can be caused by the failure of the nervous system to control the diameter of blood vessels (neurogenic shock).

Patient Care—Spinal Injury

Regardless of where the apparent spinal injury is located on the cord, care is the same.

Emergency Care Steps

For all patients with possible spinal injury, and for all accident victims when there is doubt as to the extent of injury, you should

1. Provide manual stabilization for the head and neck.
2. Apply an extrication or rigid collar and continue to maintain manual stabilization.
3. Secure the patient on a long spine board.
4. Administer oxygen in high concentration. Edema to the cord may impair oxygen delivery to the cord. When this occurs, cellular death can take place.

Total Body Immobilization Devices

The techniques for applying an extrication collar and placing and securing a patient onto a long spine board are presented in Scans 12-3 and 12-4. Before you study the Scans, consider the following.

1. *Always reassure the patient.* Having an extrication collar applied and being strapped to a spine board can be a frightening experience. When appropriate, explain the procedures to the patient.
2. *Make certain that you have completed an accurate primary survey* and that you have cared for all life-threatening problems.
3. *Use the mechanism of injury, state of consciousness, and a secondary survey* to determine the need for an extrication collar and spine board.
4. *Always apply a rigid collar when you believe that spinal injury is a possibility.*
   - Make certain that you assess the patient's neck prior to placing the collar. Take special care to look for tracheal deviation and distended jugular veins.
   - Make sure the collar is the right size for the patient. A large patient may not be able to wear a large collar. A small patient with a long neck may need your largest collar. The front width of the collar should fit between the point of the chin and the chest at the suprasternal

(jugular) notch. Once in place, the collar should rest on the clavicles and support the lower jaw.

- Remove necklaces and large earrings before applying the collar.
- Keep the head in the anatomical position when applying manual stabilization and the collar. Be certain to keep the patient's hair out of the way.
- Maintain manual stabilization while the collar is secured, and continue to manually immobilize the head and neck until the patient is secured to a long spine board.

5. *When a patient is secured to a long spine board, the order of straps goes from chest to foot and the head is to be secured last,* using 3-inch tape. The tape offers support, especially if the patient and board are to be tilted to allow for drainage. However, blood on the patient's skin and hair may make using tape impractical. You should learn to use cravats as a backup method. Do not tape or tie the cravats across the patient's eyes.

6. *Additional immobilization for the head and neck can be provided* with light foam filled sandbags, a commercial head immobilization device, blanket rolls, or similar objects or devices. If used, these would be applied after securing the patient's body to the long spine board but before securing the head with tape or cravats.

7. *Always manage the patient for shock and administer a high concentration of oxygen.*

Remember: You may doubt that there is injury to a patient's spine because of a lack of obvious symptoms and signs. Nevertheless, when there is *any* possibility of spinal injury, APPLY RIGID IMMOBILIZATION and transport as though you know for sure that damage to the spinal cord has occurred.

Note: Some authorities recommend securing the patient's head first when placing him on a long spine board. However, since the patient may shift or need to be turned to his side due to vomiting as straps are applied, possibly aggravating existing injuries, the "head last" protocol is shown in this text.

A variety of full body immobilization devices, including various types of long spine boards, are available (Scan 12-5).

Transferring a Patient with a Rope Sling

In some accident situations, it may not be possible for rescuers to position themselves around a patient during the transfer effort. He may be under a vehicle or a piece of machinery or in a pocket of debris. A 1-inch-diameter rope sling or loop can be used to great advantage in situations like these. Rope slings are especially efficient when there are only two EMTs (Figure 12-13).

1. Manually stabilize the head and neck, and apply an extrication or rigid collar. The head and neck are manually stabilized until the patient is secured to the long spine board.

2. Slip the rope sling over the person's chest and under his arms.

3. If the sling is adjustable, slide the steel rings down the rope. Position them as close to the person's head as possible. This will assure that a straight pull is made, and the doubled rope will help to support the person's head.

4. Slightly raise the person's head and shoulders just enough to permit your partner to slide the end of the board under them.

5. Exert a smooth, steady pull on the rope to move the person onto the board. Keep your hands as low to the board as you can to assure that the person's spine is kept straight.

6. Continue to pull on the rope until the person is completely on the board.

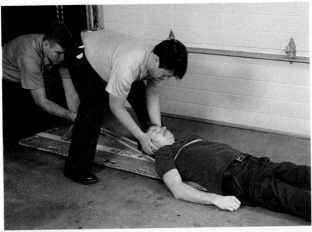

Figure 12-13 Moving a patient onto a long spine board using a rope sling.

Spinal Injuries—Rigid Collars

Extrication and Rigid Collars

Rigid cervical and extrication collars are applied to protect the cervical spine. **Do not** apply a soft collar.

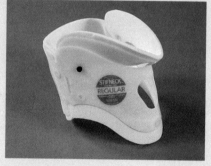

STIFNECK™—Rigid extrication

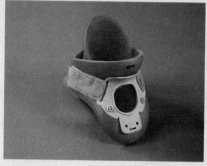

PHILADELPHIA CERVICAL COLLAR™

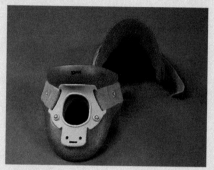

PHILADELPHIA CERVICAL COLLAR™—Opened

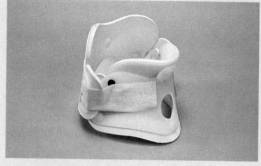

NEC-LOC™—Rigid extrication

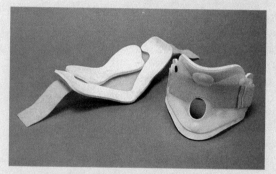

NEC-LOC™—Opened

Applying Manual Stabilization

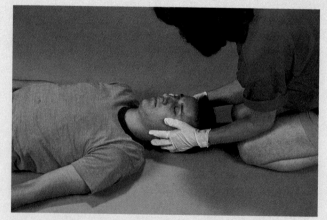

Properly position both hands. Maintain stabilization, keeping head in neutral alignment.

Do not apply traction to the head and neck, or pull and twist the head. You are trying to stabilize the head and neck.

Stifneck™ Collar—Seated Patient

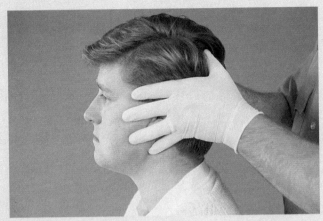

1. Stabilize the head and neck from the rear.

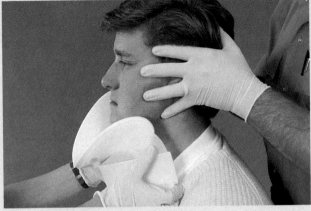

2. Properly angle the collar for placement.

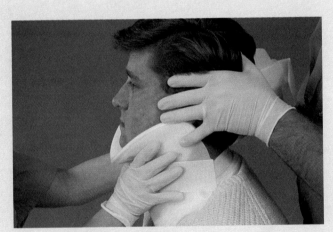

3. Position the collar bottom.

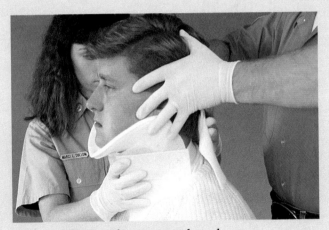

4. Set collar in place around neck.

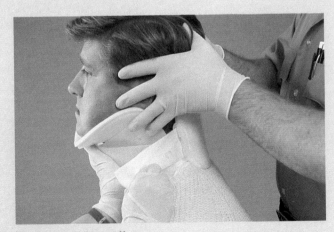

5. Secure the collar.

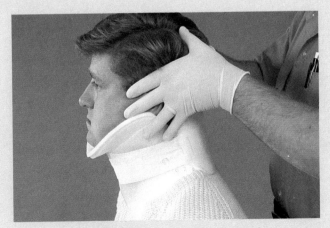

6. Spread fingers and maintain support.

347

Stifneck™ Collar—Supine Position

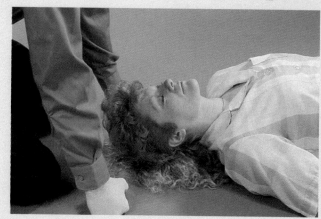

1. Kneel at patient's head.

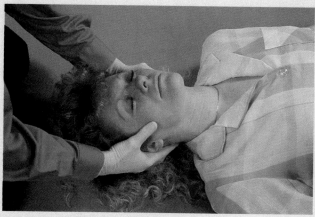

2. Stabilize the head and neck.

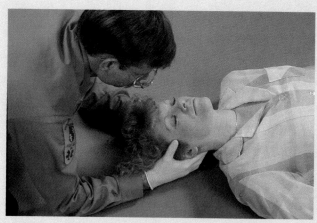

3. Maintain stabilization.

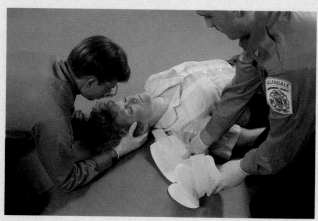

4. Set collar in place.

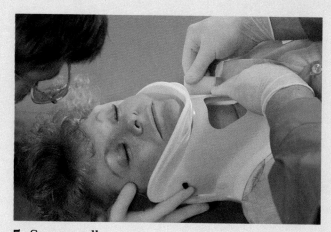

5. Secure collar.

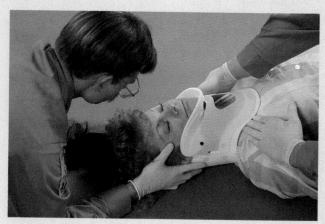

6. Continue to stabilize.

348

Spinal Injuries—
The Log Roll and the Long Spine Board

The Four-Rescuer Log Roll

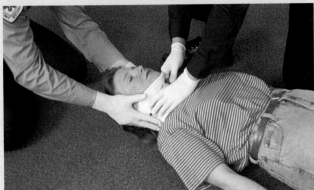

1. Stabilize the head and apply a rigid collar.

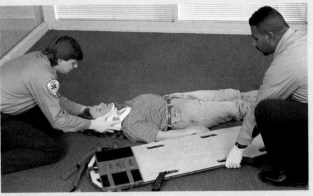

2. Place the board parallel to the patient.

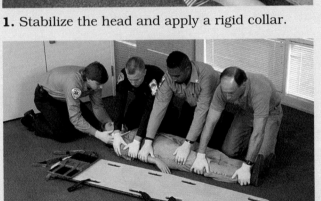

3. Three rescuers will kneel at the patient's side opposite the board, leaving room to roll the patient toward them. Place one rescuer at the shoulder, one at the waist, and one at the knee. One EMT will continue to stabilize the head. The rescuers will reach across the patient and take proper hand placement before the roll.

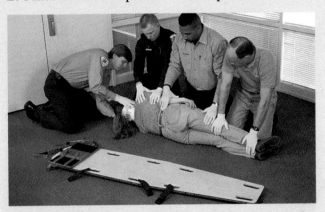

4. The EMT at the head and neck will direct the others to roll the patient as a unit.

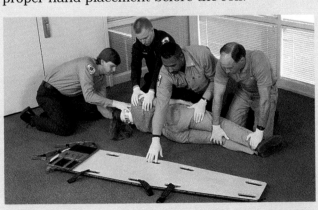

5. The EMT at the patient's waist will grip the spine board and pull it into position against the patient. (This can be done by a fifth rescuer.)

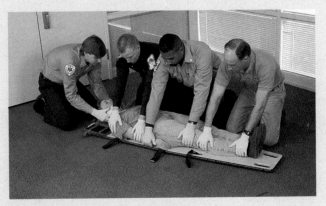

6. Roll the patient onto the board.

349

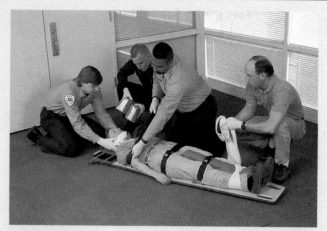

7. Secure the patient's body to the board.

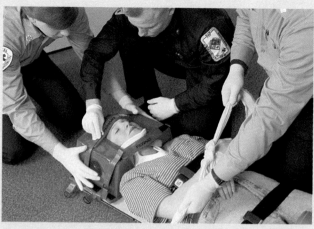

8. One rescuer will secure the patient's head to the board. Another rescuer will tie the patient's wrists. (See detail of head immobilization device below.)

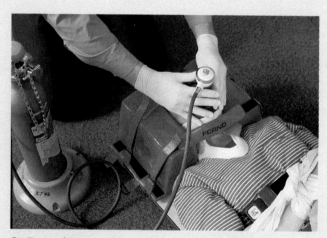

9. Provide oxygen and treat for shock.

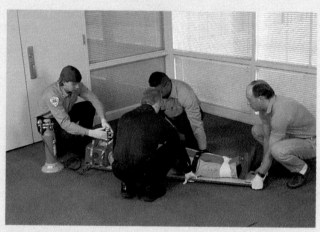

10. Prepare to transfer the patient.

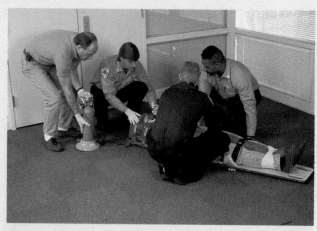

11. If necessary, have a bystander help carry equipment.

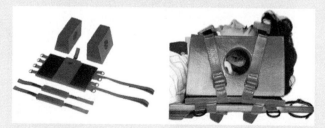

12.

Full Body Immobilization Devices

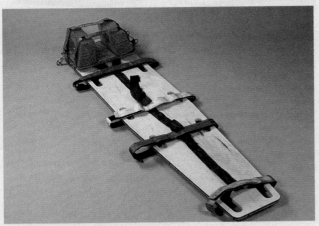

1. Long spine board with head immobilization and strapping devices

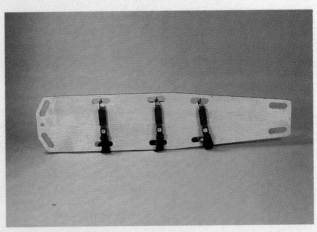

2. Long spine board with quick-hook straps

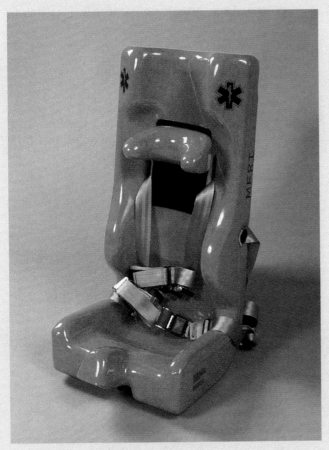

3. Pediatric immobilization

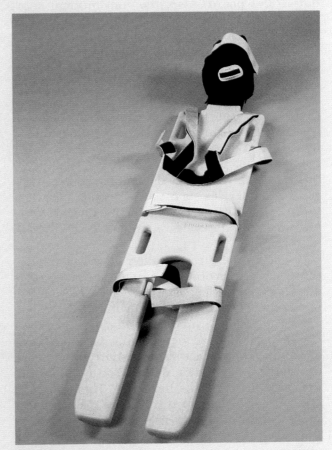

4. Miller board

Application of a Short Spine Board or Extrication Device

In some situations a patient with a possible spinal injury cannot be immediately secured to a long spine board. For example, the patient may be seated in a vehicle or, if lying down, may have to be moved into a seated position for extrication, or the patient may simply be in a confined space where a long spine board cannot be fitted.

In such situations the patient must be secured to a short spine board or extrication device that will immobilize the head, neck, and torso until the patient can be transferred to a long spine board or other full body immobilization device. First the patient's head and neck must be manually stabilized and a rigid collar applied. Then the patient is secured to the short spine board or extrication device.

A short spine board is just a shortened version of a long spine board. The original extrication device, it has been used for many years and is still often used. It is used less frequently now, not because of loss of popularity among users but by necessity. Today's automobiles have fewer bench-type seats and more bucket-type seats whose contoured backs do not accommodate a flat board. Also, the conventional short spine board is often too wide and too high to be used effectively in a small car.

A vest-style extrication device is a flexible piece of equipment useful for immobilizing patients with possible injury to the cervical spine. It can be used when the patient is found in a bucket seat, in a short compact car seat, in a seat with a contoured back, or in a confined space. It is also useful when the short spine board cannot be inserted into a car because of obstructions. A number of commercial vest-style extrication devices such as the Kendrick Extrication Device (KED) are available (Scan 12-6). You should use the devices approved by your EMS system.

The use of an extrication device eliminates many of the problems caused by a board's straps and buckles. The extrication device will immobilize the patient's head without the use of a confining chin strap (Figure 12-14).

A particular sequence must be followed in all applications, whether of a short spine board or a flexible extrication device. You must secure the torso first and the head last. This approach offers greater stability throughout the strapping process and may help prevent compression of the cervical spine. If the patient has suffered abdominal injuries or displays diaphragmatic breathing that prevents adequate securing of the torso, the torso straps will still be needed but care must be taken so as not to interfere with breathing.

There are eight special considerations when applying a short board to the patient.

1. Any assessment or reassessment of the back, scapulae, arms, or clavicles must be done before the device is placed against the patient.
2. The EMT applying the board must angle it to fit between, without striking or jarring, the arms of the rescuer who is stabilizing the head from behind the patient.
3. You must push a spine board as far down into the seat as possible. If you do not, the board may shift and the patient's cervical spine may compress during application of the board. To provide full cervical support, the top of the board should be level with the top of the patient's head. The uppermost holes must be level with the patient's shoulders. The base of the board should not extend past the coccyx.
4. Never place a chin cup or chin strap on the patient. Such devices may prevent the patient from opening his mouth if he has to vomit.
5. When applying the first strap to secure the torso, you must not apply the strap too tightly. This could aggravate existing abdominal injury or limit respirations for the diaphragmatic breathing patient.
6. Some short spine boards have buckles with release mechanisms that can be accidentally loosened during patient transfer operations. This is especially true of "quick-release"

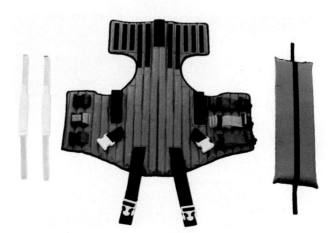

Figure 12-14 The Ferno KED (Kendrick Extrication Device).

buckles. These buckles must be taped closed after the final adjustment of the straps.

7. Do not allow buckles to be placed midsternum. Such a placement will interfere with proper hand placement should CPR become necessary.

8. Do not pad between collar and board. To do so will create a pivot point that may cause the hyperextension of the cervical spine when the head is secured. Instead, padding should be placed at the occipital region, but only enough to fill any void. This will help keep the head in a neutral position. Often if the shoulders are rolled back to the board, the head will come back to the board in vertical alignment.

The placement of straps for the short spine board is a little complex. (see Figure 12-15.) After applying the short spine board, the packaging of the patient will be completed as shown in Figure 12-16.

Immobilization for Removal From a Vehicle

The procedure for securing a patient to a short spine board or flexible extrication device before removal from a vehicle onto a long spine board requires three EMTs and one rescuer or bystander as a helper. In the steps that follow, they are designated as

EMT A—initially positioned outside the vehicle beside the patient

EMT B—initially positioned inside the vehicle behind the patient. EMT B is the team leader. The others must wait for his order before executing any move.

EMT C—initially positioned inside the vehicle on the seat beside the patient

Rescuer—holds the long spine board

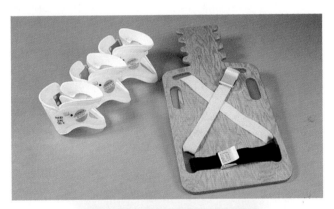

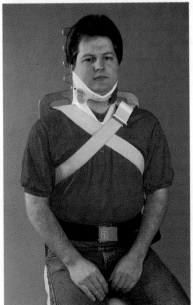

Figure 12-15 Short spine board.

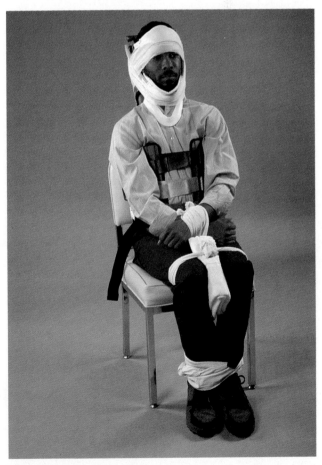

Figure 12-16 Finished application of a short spine board showing patient fully packaged and ready for removal.

The Kendrick Extrication Device (KED)

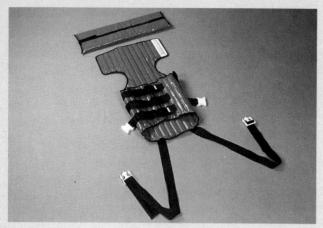

1. The KED.

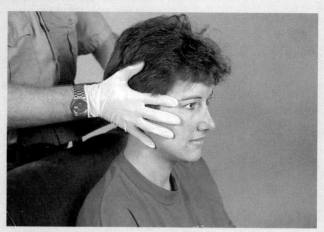

2. Stabilize the head and neck.

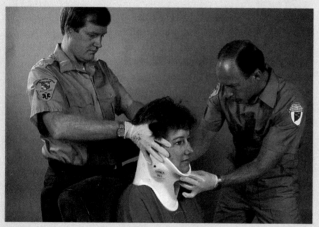

3. Measure and apply a rigid collar.

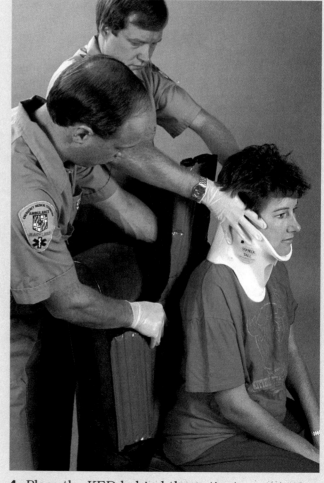

4. Place the KED behind the patient.

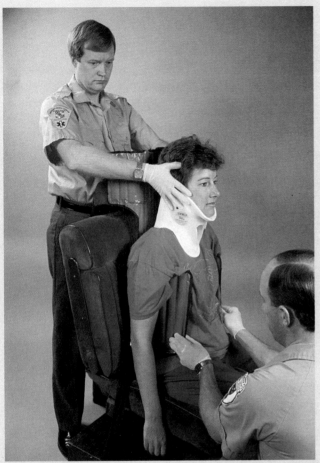

5. Align the KED and wrap the vest around the patient's torso.

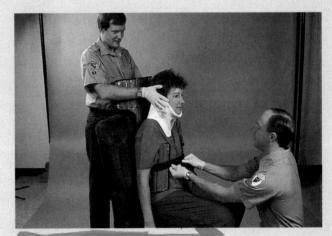

6. Secure the middle strap first.

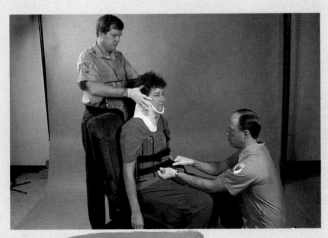

7. Secure the bottom strap next.

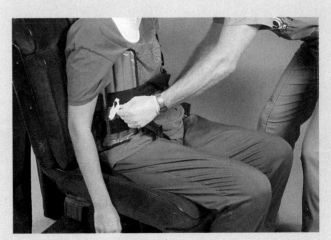

8. Connect each leg strap.

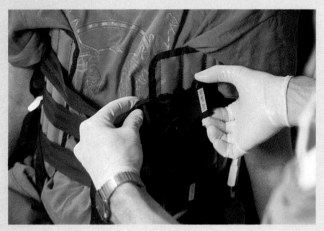

9. Secure the top vest strap last. (Some jurisdictions secure the top strap before the leg straps.)

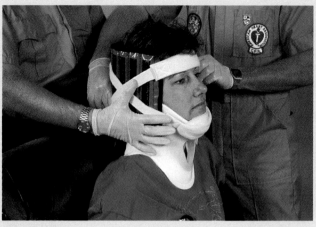

10. Secure the patient's head.

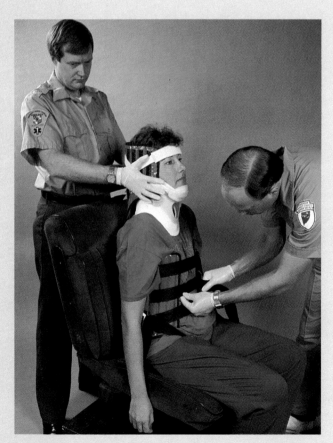

11. Recheck the snugness of the vest straps.

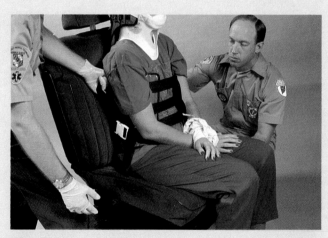

12. Secure the patient's wrists and legs and transfer to long board.

1. Stabilize the vehicle prior to anyone entering it. This will reduce movement that might further injure the patient.
2. Open *both* front doors of the vehicle to their widest limit of movement. This will enable the EMTs to have full access to the patient. If the doors need to be opened beyond their normal range, have the rescuers on the scene do it.
3. EMT B gets into the vehicle behind the patient to stabilize the head.
4. EMT A checks sensory and motor function in the extremities as well as the patient's AVPU.
5. EMT A applies a rigid collar to the patient.
6. EMT A moves the seat to its furthest rearward position.
7. EMT A places one hand on the farther side of the patient's hips and the other hand on the side next to himself. On command from EMT B, who continues to stabilize the head, EMT A slides the patient forward approximately 2 to 3 inches, making room to insert the spine board or extrication device.
8. EMT A places the spine board or extrication device between the arms of EMT B who is stabilizing the patient's head, making sure that the device is seated firmly at the base of the patient's coccyx. A vest device must be snug beneath the patient's armpits.
9. EMTs A and C secure the torso, legs, and head to the spine board or extrication device, as shown in Scan 12-6. If time permits it may be helpful to place a pad between the patient's knees and thighs, then tie the knees, ankles, and wrists with cravats.
10. The rescuer places the foot end of a long spine board over the edge of the seat next to the patient and holds it there.
11. EMTs A and C position themselves on each side of the patient and slide a strap under his thighs. Each EMT holds the strap in one hand and the other hand under the patient's armpit.
12. Together EMTs A and C lift on the strap and the patient's armpits and raise him just enough so that the rescuer can slide the board under the patient's buttocks until he is centered on it, then lower him to sitting position on the board.
13. Keeping the patient's knees bent, EMTs A and C rotate him so that his torso is aligned with the board, his back to the door. EMT A takes over stabilizing the patient's head while EMT B gets out of the car and positions himself behind the patient and resumes stabilizing the head.
14. As EMT B continues to stabilize the patient's head, EMTs A and C, with their hands under the patient's armpits, lower him to a supine position on the long spine board, knees still bent. This will prevent the head bandage or tape from coming loose. All three EMTs slide the patient, as a unit, along the board until his head is even with the head end as the rescuer steadies the board. At this point, the patient's legs can be lowered onto the board and the strap loosened as needed.
15. As the rescuer continues to steady the board, the EMTs strap the patient on securely.
16. The rescuer and the EMTs lift and carry the board to the stretcher, which is waiting nearby.

When, after the primary survey, the patient has been categorized as C (critical) or U (unstable) and the decision made to transport immediately, there may not be time to apply a short spine board or extrication device. For such situations, most EMS systems teach a variation on the normal extrication procedure in which the patient's head, neck, upper chest, and pelvis are stabilized manually as the patient is transferred to the long spine board. This procedure will be described in Chapter 29.

Extrication procedures must, obviously, be well practiced in advance to proceed quickly and smoothly and to provide continuous stabilization of the patient's head, neck, and torso.

KEY TERMS

You may find it helpful to review the following terms.

autonomic nervous system—the division of the nervous system that controls involuntary motor and visceral functions.

central nervous system (CNS)—the brain and spinal cord.

cerebrospinal (ser-e-bro-SPI-nal) **fluid (CSF)**—the fluid that surrounds the brain and spinal cord.

concussion—mild closed head injury without detectable damage to the brain. Complete recovery is usually expected.

contusion—in brain injuries, a bruised brain caused when the force of a blow to the head is great enough to rupture blood vessels.

cranial (KRAY-ne-al) **floor**—the inferior wall of the brain case; the bony floor beneath the brain.

cranium (KRAY-ne-um)—the bony structure making up the forehead, top, back, and upper sides of the skull.

epidural hematoma (ep-i-DU-ral he-mah-TOH-mah)—formed when blood from ruptured vessels flows between the meninges and the cranial bones.

intracerebral hematoma (in-trah-SER-e-bral he-mah-TOH-mah)—formed when blood from ruptured vessels pools within the brain.

laceration—in brain injuries, cuts into the brain itself that can occur as a result of a penetrating or perforating wound of the cranium.

LeForte fractures—three types of facial fractures. Type I is at the site of the maxilla and the hard palate, Type II from the palate upward across the nasal bone, Type III through the orbits to the temporomandibular joint, separating the face from the rest of the skull.

malar (MA-lar)—the cheek bone, also called the zygomatic bone.

mandible (MAN-di-bl)—the lower jaw bone.

maxillae (mak-SIL-e)—the two fused bones forming the upper jaw.

meninges (me-NIN-jez)—the three-layered membrane that surrounds the brain and spinal cord.

nasal bones—the bones that form the upper third, or bridge, of the nose.

orbits—the bony structure around the eyes; the eye sockets.

peripheral nervous system (PNS)—the nerves that enter and leave the spinal cord and that travel between the brain and organs without passing through the spinal cord (e.g. the optic nerve between the eye and the brain).

somatic nervous system—the division of the peripheral nervous system that transmits sensory information and controls voluntary movement.

spinous processes—the bony extensions of the posterior vertebrae.

subdural hematoma (sub-DU-ral he-mah-TOH-mah)—formed when blood from ruptured vessels flows between the brain and the meninges.

suture—where two bones of the skull articulate (join) to form an immovable joint.

temporal (TEM-po-ral) **bone**—bone that forms part of the lateral wall of the skull and the floor of the cranial cavity. There is a right and a left temporal bone.

temporomandibular (TEM-po-ro-man-DIB-u-lar) **joint**—the movable joint formed between mandible and temporal bone, also called the TM joint.

SUMMARY

The Axial Skeleton

The skull, spinal column, sternum, and ribs form the axial skeleton. The skull is made up of the cranium and the face. The spinal column is connected to the skull. That portion of the spine running through the neck is called the cervical spine. The ribs are attached to the thoracic spine. The midback contains the lumbar spine, while the sacral spine and coccyx are lower back structures. The brain is protected by the skull. The spinal column protects the spinal cord.

The Nervous System

The nervous system is divided into the central nervous system (the brain and spinal cord), the peripheral nervous system (the nerves that enter and leave the brain and spinal cord), and the autonomic nervous system, which controls involuntary motor and visceral functioning. Any injury that impairs an autonomic function can be life threatening.

Injuries to the Skull and Brain

Injuries to the skull include open head and closed head injuries. If the cranium remains intact, the injury is classified as a closed head injury. Open head injuries involve fractures of the cranium (skull fractures). There can be direct injury to the brain in open head injuries. Closed head injuries include indirect injuries to the brain, such as concussions and contusions. Cranial fractures may be obvious or difficult to detect. Always look for decreased consciousness, wounds to the head, pain or swelling, deformity of the skull, bruises behind the ear, unequal pupils, discolorations around the eyes, sunken eyes, or bloody or clear fluids flowing from the ears and/or nose.

Brain injury can occur with head injuries. Look for pain, a decrease in the level of consciousness, personality changes, vital sign changes, unequal pupils, doll's eye response, disturbances to vision, hearing, or equilibrium, vomiting, posturing, paralysis, or any sign of skull fracture or neurological impairment. When caring for a patient with injuries to the cranium or brain, you should immobilize the neck and spine and maintain an open airway using the jaw-thrust technique. Provide resuscitative procedures, if needed. Keep the patient at rest and talk to him. Control bleeding, but avoid pressure over the site of a fracture. Administer oxygen and manage for shock. Monitor vital signs. Be alert for vomiting.

Patients with no sign of neck or spine injury may be positioned with the head and torso elevated or supine, according to local protocols. Patients with possible neck or spine injury must be immobilized. Do not remove impaled objects, bone fragments, or any other objects from skull wounds. Stabilize impaled objects.

Signs of facial and mandible injury include blood in the airway, facial deformity, false bone movements, discoloration, swelling, loose teeth or bleeding around teeth, loss of lower jaw use, and difficulty of speech. Facial and mandible injuries often cause airway obstruction. You should maintain an open airway using the jaw-thrust technique. If there is possible spinal injury, immobilize the neck and spine.

Follow local protocols as to whether to remove a helmet. Study the special procedures for removal of a helmet, when indicated, while maintaining stabilization of the patient's head and neck.

Injuries to the Spine

Types of spinal injury include fractures, dislocations, ligament sprains, and disk injuries. Injury to the spine is always a possibility with any severe injury to the body. Certain mechanisms of injury also indicate possible spinal injury, including motor vehicle collisions, falls, and many sports accidents.

To detect spinal injuries, always consider the mechanism of injury, question the patient and bystanders about the accident, conduct a head-to-toe examination, and be alert for any of the signs or symptoms of spinal injury: pain without movement, pain with movement, tenderness or deformity along the spine, impaired breathing, priapism, posturing, loss of bowel or bladder control, paralysis, nerve impairment of the extremities, or severe (neurogenic) shock.

Care for possible spinal injury by first manually immobilizing the head and neck, then applying a rigid collar. If the patient is lying down, use a log roll technique to transfer the patient to a long spine board or other full body immobilization device. If the patient is standing, apply a long spine board, then lower the patient. Use a rope sling to pull a patient onto a long spine board from under an entrapment. Secure the patient to the long spine board, torso first, head last. Administer a high concentration of oxygen.

If the patient is in a vehicle or other confined space where a long spine board will not fit, you can secure the patient to a short spine board or flexible extrication device before transferring him to a long spine board.

CHAPTER 7

On the Scene

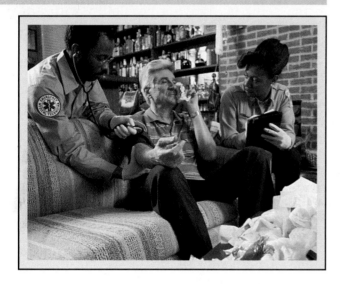

Tony Jacobsen is relaxing in his favorite chair, watching TV, when he feels a sneeze coming on. After the sneeze, he feels something trickle down his face. It's blood. "Not another nosebleed," Tony says to himself as he goes for a tissue. He sits back down in front of the television, but the bleeding doesn't stop. After five minutes, it's worse than before. Tony's wife glances into the living room and sees the blood. Since neither she nor Tony can stop the bleeding, she calls 911.

Your unit receives the call for a "nosebleed." On your arrival, you find Tony holding a blood-soaked washcloth to his nose.

You: *Mr. Jacobsen, I can see that you're bleeding a lot from your nose. Can you tell me how the bleeding started?*

Tony Jacobsen: *I just sneezed and felt blood coming from my nose.*

Mrs. Jacobsen: *He's been getting these a lot lately.*

You: *Mr. Jacobsen, I'd like you to lean forward and pinch your nostrils together. That should stop the bleeding.*

Tony Jacobsen: *Like this?*

You: *Yes, that's very good. We're just going to check your pulse, blood pressure, and respirations now.*

After Mr. Jacobsen pinches his nostrils together for several minutes, the bleeding reduces to almost nothing. During that time, you obtain vital signs and other information from Mr. and Mrs. Jacobsen.

Once the bleeding has stopped, Mr. Jacobsen doesn't want any further treatment. However, you know that nosebleeds can sometimes be a sign of a more serious condition. With a little help from his wife, you persuade Mr. Jacobsen to accept transport to the hospital.

Soft Tissues of the Head and Neck

Chapter Overview

In Chapter 9 you learned how to assess and care for soft tissue injuries, and in Chapter 12 you learned about injuries to the skull and spine. In this chapter you will draw on what you learned in those earlier chapters as you study special assessment and care procedures for soft tissue injuries of the head and neck.

Expected Outcome, Chapter 13: *You will be able to assess and care for soft tissue injuries of the scalp, face, and neck, including injuries to the eyes, ears, nose, and mouth.*

> **Warning:** Protect yourself from infectious diseases by using appropriate barrier devices such as a pocket face mask with one-way valve, face shield, or bag-valve mask; goggles or eye shield; and disposable gloves. Always conform to your local EMS system's infection exposure control plan.

Knowledge *After reading this chapter, you should be able to*

1. List the THREE exceptions to the rules for soft tissue injury care that apply to scalp and face injuries. (p. 363)

2. List the procedures for the emergency care of scalp wounds. (p. 363; Scan 13-1)

3. List the procedures for the emergency care of face wounds. (pp. 365-366)

4. Describe, step by step, the emergency care for a patient with an object impaled in the cheek. (pp. 366-367)

5. Cite the assessment and care procedures for foreign objects, contusions, abrasions, and lacerations of the eye. (pp. 369-371)

6. List the assessment and care procedures for puncture wounds and objects impaled in the eye. (pp. 369, 370, 371)

7. Describe the assessment and care procedures for THREE types of burns to the eye. (pp. 369, 370, 372-373)

8. Describe the assessment and care procedures for avulsions of the eye. (pp. 369, 370, 373)

9. Describe, step by step, the procedures for removing each of the four types of contact lenses. (pp. 373, 375-376; Scan 13-2)

10. Name the signs and symptoms that indicate skull fracture or injury to the inner ear. (pp. 376-377)

11. Describe the basic care for injuries to the external ear and what to do if you suspect internal ear injury. (p. 377)

12. Describe the emergency care procedures for injuries to the nose and nosebleeds. (pp. 378-379)

13. Describe the basic emergency care for injuries to the mouth, including dental injuries. (p. 380)

14. List FIVE signs of, and the care procedures for, blunt injury to the neck. (pp. 381-382)

15. Contrast the procedures used to control arterial bleeding from the neck to those used to control venous bleeding from the neck. (pp. 382-383)

Skills *As an EMT you should be able to*

1. Assess for types of soft tissue injuries of the head and neck.

2. Control bleeding and apply the proper dressing and bandage for a given injury to the scalp, face, eye, ear, nose, mouth, and neck.

3. Demonstrate the special emergency care procedures for
   - Impaled object in the eye
   - Impaled object in the cheek
   - Saving fully avulsed body parts
   - Severe bleeding from a neck vein
   - Severe bleeding from a neck artery

The following advice is so important that it will be repeated where appropriate throughout this chapter: Whenever you deal with *any* injury above the clavicles, you must be alert for

- Injury to the Cervical Spine—Assume spinal injury if the patient is unconscious or if the mechanism of injury is one that may produce spinal injuries.
- Airway Problems—Watch for any signs of difficult or compromised breathing that may indicate blockage of the airway.
- Bleeding and Shock—Whenever there is serious blood loss or the patient shows unstable or poor vital signs, take measures to control bleeding and care for shock, administering a high concentration of oxygen.

INJURIES TO THE SCALP AND FACE

The following text deals with injuries to the soft tissues of the scalp and face *except* for the eyes, ears, nose, and mouth, which will be covered specifically later in the chapter.

Patient Assessment— Scalp and Face Injuries

Of the many blood vessels in the scalp and face, quite a few are close to the skin surface. Wounds may bleed profusely even though a major vessel has not been severed. A minor laceration may initially have profuse bleeding. Usually, clotting is rapid and control is not a major problem. However, if an artery is cut, bleeding may be quickly fatal if no effort is made to control the flow of blood.

Severe trauma to the face also may produce skull fractures and possible airway obstruction. Many patients with head injuries also have neck injuries that may involve the spinal cord.

These conditions are especially likely in the case of facial injuries that result from vehicle collisions. Even with lap-and-shoulder belt in place, the patient's face may come in contact with the front post or windshield. If the plastic covering the post shatters and sharp points extrude, serious lacerations to the face can occur. If the head strikes the windshield, avulsions of the nose or even scalping of the patient may occur. The patient's mandible may strike the steering wheel, knocking out teeth or even causing a separation of the mandible or palate.

Patient Care— Scalp and Face Injuries

Manage most soft tissue injuries of the scalp and face as you would any other soft tissue injury (see Chapter 9). However, for scalp and face injuries there are three major EXCEPTIONS to the standard procedure.

☐ *Do not* attempt to clear or clean the surface of a scalp wound. To do so may cause additional bleeding and can cause great harm to the patient if there are skull fractures present.
☐ *Do not* apply finger pressure to the wound in an effort to control bleeding. Since there may be fractures to the skull, you will have to avoid any pressure that may force free bone edges or fragments into the brain.
☐ *Do* remove objects that are impaled in the cheek if they penetrate the cheek and exit into the oral cavity.

Patient Care—Scalp Wounds

Contamination occurs with every scalp wound. The hair may mat over the wound site. Foreign objects, such as glass fragments, pieces of metal, or bits of soil may be on the wound surface and in the wound itself. Dressing the wound will help prevent additional contamination.

Emergency Care Steps

To care for a scalp wound (Scan 13-1)

1. *Do not* clear the wound surface. *Do not* try to clean the wound. Wiping actions or irrigation with water could cause objects to be driven through breaks in the skull and contaminate the brain. Large pieces of loose gravel, dirt, or glass may have to be carefully picked from the hair or very gently brushed away from the wound with a cotton swab to allow for safe dressing and bandaging.
2. Control bleeding with a sterile dressing carefully held in place with gentle pressure. Avoid finger pressure if there is any indication that the skull is fractured.
3. Bandage the dressing in place. Strips of adhesive bandage do not work well in cases of scalp injury. Self-adherent roller bandage or gauze can be wrapped around the patient's head, or a cravat can be tied over the scalp in order to hold the dressing in place. An alternative way to hold a dressing on a scalp wound without applying excessive pressure is to use a triangular bandage. Remember that bleeding is to be controlled before a dressing is bandaged in place.
4. Keep the patient's head and shoulders raised to help control bleeding, provided that the patient survey, degree of trauma, and mechanism of injury do not indicate possible spinal injury or injury to the chest or abdomen. Do not put the unconscious trauma patient into a head-raised position even if he is secured to a long spine board. The patient may vomit and aspirate the vomitus.

Warning: Do not lift or attempt to wrap the head of a patient who is lying down if there are any signs of spinal injury or the mechanism of injury indicates a possible spinal injury. This will flex the neck and possibly worsen the injury.

Scan 13-1
Care for Scalp Wounds

WOUND TO FRONT OR SIDE OF HEAD

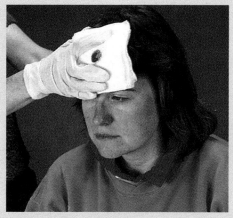

1. Apply a direct pressure dressing. Use gentle pressure.

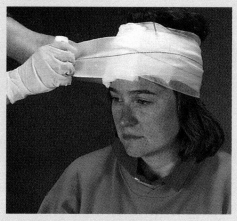

2. Secure the dressing in place with a roller bandage.

WOUND TO TOP OF SCALP

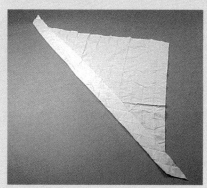

1. Prepare the cravat by making an initial fold at the base.

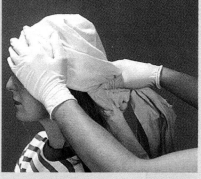

2. Lay cravat over dressing and anchor at bridge of nose and base of skull.

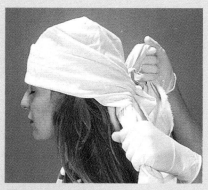

3. Secure the cravat at the base of the skull.

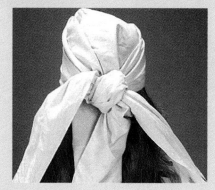

4. Take the tail and tuck it inside the knot.

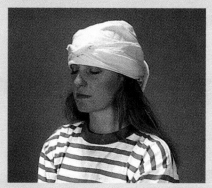

5. Secure the remaining cravat ends on the patient's forehead.

Patient Care—Face Wounds

Emergency Care Steps

When caring for a patient with face injuries, you must care for the following conditions.

- ☐ Possible neck or spinal injuries
- ☐ Airway compromise
- ☐ Breathing problems
- ☐ Bleeding
- ☐ Impaled objects

Specific care for these conditions is discussed below.

Possible Neck or Spinal Injuries Immobilize before treatment if such injuries are suspected or if the mechanism of injury makes such an injury possible. Protect the neck and spine during all procedures.

Airway Compromise With any facial injury there may be breathing problems caused by brain damage, broken facial structures, blood, debris, broken teeth or dentures, or the patient's tongue or loosened palate clogging the oral cavity and airway. In treating these problems, bear in mind the likelihood of an injury to the cervical spine and protect the spine before moving and positioning the patient to deal with airway and breathing problems. Monitor the patient to ensure an open airway (Figure 13-1).

Check the patient's mouth for foreign matter as you assess the extent of oral cavity dam-

age. Use your gloved fingers to carefully sweep the inside of the person's mouth clean of broken dentures and teeth, gum, vomitus, or other obstructions. (PROTECT YOUR FINGERS! Insert a bite stick or oral airway between the teeth.) Look to see if an external injury to the cheek may have perforated the cheek wall, thus opening into the oral cavity.

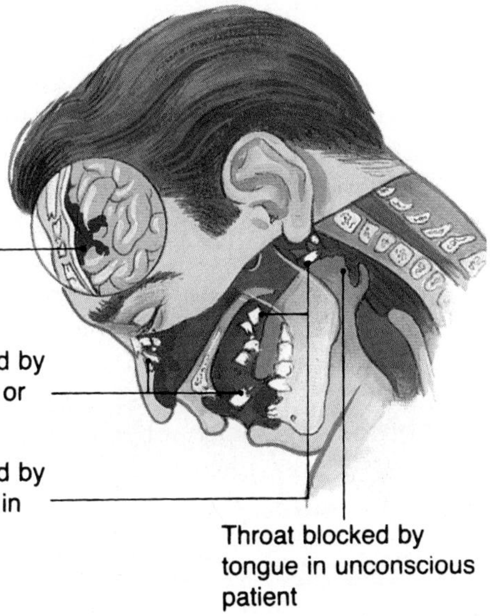

Breathing Problems Start artificial ventilation or CPR as required. Reposition the patient so that basic life support measures will be most effective after immobilizing the head, neck and spine if indicated. When injuries allow, a pocket face mask with a one-way valve or bag-valve mask unit with supplemental oxygen may have to be used to ventilate the patient. An airway adjunct will have to be inserted for all unconscious patients with head injury and no gag reflex; as long as the patient has no gag reflex, this airway can be left in (Figure 13-2).

Bleeding If bleeding is profuse, suction away blood, mucus, and vomitus. Position the patient in the lateral recumbent position, with the head tilted back and turned so the mouth tilts downward. SHOULD YOU SUSPECT INJURY TO THE CERVICAL SPINE, IMMOBILIZE THE PATIENT'S HEAD, NECK, AND SPINE BEFORE MOVING HIM TO A POSITION FOR DRAINAGE (see Chapter 12). Continue to suction the patient as needed.

Control bleeding by applying a bulky dressing over the wound; use only enough pressure to stop the flow of blood. Remember, there may be underlying facial fractures that are not obvious. Apply a dressing and bandage (Figure 13-3). You may need to use pressure point techniques to control bleeding. The temporal artery pressure point sites are useful (see Chapter 7), but be careful not to apply pressure over possible fractures. If blood vessels, nerves, tendons, or muscles have been exposed, they must be kept from drying out. Even a standard gauze dressing will offer some protection and is the choice of many EMS systems. A sterile dressing moistened with normal sterile saline (a commercial salt water solution) can be used to dress this type of open wound. You must be certain that the saline used is from a labeled, sterile source that has not been previously opened.

Partially avulsed facial skin can be returned to its normal position and dressings can be applied. Some systems use a sterile saline or water wash of the wound before repositioning the flap. Your instructor will tell you if this is

Brain damage resulting in loss of breathing stimulus

Airways blocked by injury to mouth or nose

Airways blocked by teeth and clots in throat

Throat blocked by tongue in unconscious patient

Figure 13-1 Injury-related breathing problems.

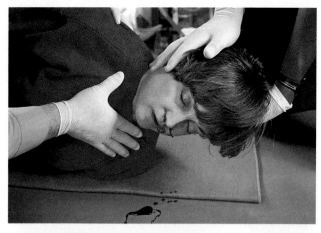

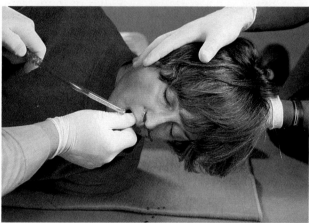

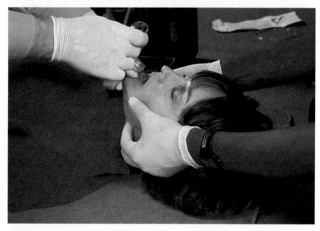

Figure 13-2 Correcting a breathing problem for a patient with facial injury (*and with no suspected spinal injury*). 1. Roll patient as a unit. 2. Suction airway. 3. Insert oropharyngeal airway if there is no gag reflex and ventilate with pocket face mask or bag-valve mask.

done in your area. Fully avulsed skin should be wrapped and secured in a dry dressing (or in a moist sterile dressing if allowed), covered with or bagged in plastic, labeled, kept cool, and transported with the patient.

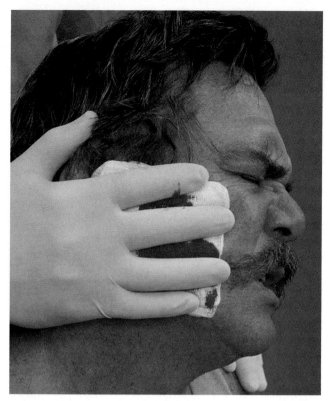

Figure 13-3 Care of soft tissue facial injury.

Impaled Objects A dangerous situation exists when the cheek has been penetrated by a foreign object. First, the object may go into the oral cavity and immediately become a possible airway obstruction, or it may stay impaled in the wall to work its way free and enter the oral cavity later. Second, when the cheek wall is perforated, bleeding into the mouth and throat may be profuse and interfere with breathing, or it may make the patient nauseated and induce vomiting. Simple external wound care will not stop the flow of blood into the mouth.

If you find a patient with an object impaled in the cheek, you should (Figure 13-4)

1. Gently examine both the external cheek and the inside of the mouth. Use your penlight and look into the patient's mouth. If need be, carefully use your gloved fingers to probe the inside cheek to determine if the object has passed through the cheek wall. This is best done with a dressing pad used to protect your fingers.
2. If you find perforation, carefully REMOVE THE IMPALED OBJECT by pulling it out in the direction that it entered the cheek. If

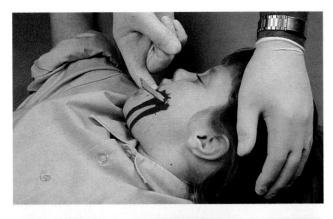

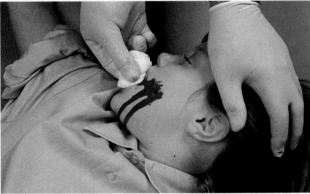

Figure 13-4 Procedure for removing an object impaled in the cheek.

this cannot be done easily, leave the object in place. Do not twist the object.

3. Make certain that you position the patient's head to allow for drainage (the possibility of spinal injuries may require you to immobilize the head, neck, and spine first). Keep in mind that an object penetrating the cheek wall also may have broken teeth or dentures, creating the potential danger for airway obstruction.

4. Once the object is removed, pack the inside of the cheek with rolled gauze between the cheek wall and the teeth. This also should be done in cases in which the perforating object cannot be removed. If this is the case, make sure that you stabilize the object on the external side of the cheek wall.

5. If the extent of injuries allows, keep the patient positioned to permit drainage. Provide suctioning as required. A lateral recumbent placement may be necessary during transport.

6. Dress the outside of the wound using a pressure dressing and bandage or apply a

sterile dressing and use direct hand pressure to control the bleeding.

7. Provide oxygen and care for shock. You may have to use a nasal cannula if constant suctioning is required. If any dressing materials are placed in the patient's mouth, use of standard face masks can be dangerous unless you leave 3 to 4 inches of the dressing outside of the patient's mouth.

Warning: Anytime you place something into a patient's mouth, you have taken on added responsibility for the patient. It is possible for objects such as rolled gauze to become airway obstructions. Should the patient vomit, objects in the mouth may trap vomitus, which may be aspirated by the patient. This usually does not happen, but the possibility exists. It is best to leave 3 to 4 inches of the dressing material outside the patient's mouth to allow for easy removal and so that it is visible to the next care provider. Keep a close watch on any patient with anything placed into the mouth. Remember, too, that a conscious patient may be able to monitor the dressings in his mouth, but he may not stay conscious. You will then have to hold the dressing in place with a gloved finger.

Transportation of a Patient With Face Injuries Some injuries to the face are relatively minor and require no special positioning of the patient. Since respiratory difficulty is often associated with this type of injury, the conscious patient may be transported in the lateral recumbent position with the head low or tilted to aid drainage (Figure 13-5).

If there are indications of spinal and/or neck injuries, fully immobilize the patient using a cervical collar and long spine board. The board can be propped on its side to assist with

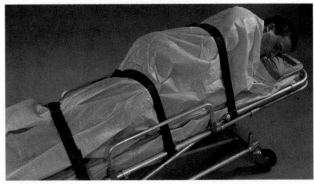

Figure 13-5 Transporting the conscious facial injury patient.

CHAPTER 13 Soft Tissues of the Head and Neck **367**

drainage. Continuous suctioning may be required. When the facial soft tissues are injured, there may be underlying facial bone fractures. Take care to transport the patient so that no unnecessary pressure is placed on facial injury sites. Monitor the patient and be alert for airway problems. (LeForte fractures, as discussed in Chapter 12, may cause airway management problems.)

INJURIES TO THE EYES

Before considering the various types of eye injuries and their appropriate care, it is important to know the major structures of the eye and how it functions (Figure 13-6).

Structure and Function of the Eye

The eye is a globular structure, situated in a bony depression of the skull called the **orbit**. Each orbit is made up of parts of the bones of the forehead, temple, and upper jaw. Any serious blow to these bones may transfer the trauma to the eyes. The typical eye is almost one inch in diameter, with over 80% of the globe hidden within the orbit.

The white of the eye is the **sclera** (SKLE-rah). This is a semirigid capsule of fibrous tissue that helps to maintain the shape of the globe and contains the fluids found inside the eye.

The colored portion of the external eye is the **iris**, which has an adjustable opening called the **pupil**. In dim light, the pupil dilates (expands) to allow more light to enter the eye while, in bright light, it contracts and restricts the amount of light entering the eye. Over the iris and pupil lies a clear portion of the sclera called the **cornea** (KOR-ne-ah). This structure protects the iris and pupil and helps to keep fluids inside the eye. In addition, the cornea is highly involved with the eye's function of focusing light.

A thin delicate membrane called the **conjunctiva** (kon-junk-TI-vah) covers the sclera, the cornea, and the undersurfaces of the eyelids. When irritated, its tiny blood vessels become swollen with blood, giving the eye a "bloodshot" or pink appearance. This is a sign of the condition known as conjunctivitis.

The internal eye is divided into an anterior cavity and a posterior cavity. The anterior cavity exists between the cornea and the lens. The **lens**

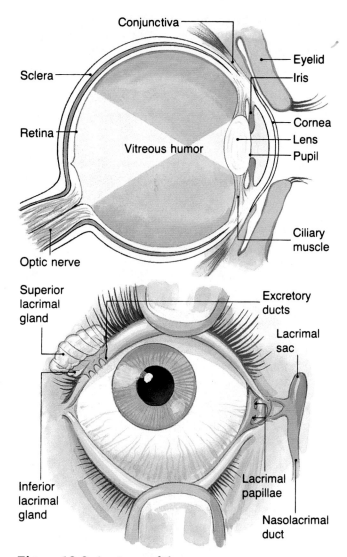

Figure 13-6 Anatomy of the eye.

is located behind the iris and pupil. This cavity is filled with a clear, watery fluid known as the **aqueous** (A-kwe-us) **humor**. In some penetrating eye injuries, this fluid will leak from the eye, but with time and proper care, the body can replace it. The entire posterior cavity is located behind the lens. It is filled with a transparent jelly-like substance called the **vitreous** (VIT-re-us) **humor**. This substance is very important in maintaining the shape and length of the globe. Normal lens function takes place with a certain amount of pressure exerted on it by the vitreous humor. This gel cannot be replaced, and it cannot be restored by the body.

Light rays pass through the cornea, the aqueous humor, and the lens. Muscular action can change the shape of the lens to focus the light on the **retina** (RET-i-na), or back of the eye.

The cells of the retina convert light into electrical impulses that are conducted through the **optic nerve** to the vision center in the **occipital** (ok-SIP-i-tal) **lobe** of the brain at the back of the head.

The eye is protected by the orbital bones and the eyelids. The inner surface of the eyelids and the surface of the eye are protected and moistened by tears produced by the **lacrimal** (LAK-re-mal) **gland**, or tear gland. Each time the eye blinks, the eyelids glide over the exposed surface, sweeping it clean of dust and other irritants. Tears are drained away through a lacrimal duct in the medial corner of the eye at the junction of the eyelids. This duct leads into the nasal cavity.

Types of Eye Injury

Commonly seen eye injuries include foreign objects in the eye, contusions, abrasions, lacerations, puncture wounds, burns, and avulsions.

Patient Assessment—Eye Injuries

Signs and Symptoms
Look for the signs and symptoms described below for these common eye injuries.

- ☐ Foreign Objects—Usually the patient complains of feeling the object and shows redness of the eye (the eye is "bloodshot"). The eye often waters heavily with tears.
- ☐ Contusions—When the eye is bruised, there may or may not be damage to the eyelids. The patient usually complains of pain. If the patient says that he is having trouble seeing out of the injured eye, or if he reports double vision, then the damage may be very serious. The eye may appear reddened or swollen. The iris may not be easily visible, or you may see blood between the cornea and the iris.
- ☐ Abrasions—Minor scratches to the surface of the eye can be caused by foreign objects. Such scratches are usually invisible. Look for major scratches on the cornea. These are very painful. The cornea should appear clear, smooth, and wet.
- ☐ Lacerations—Look for cuts in the eyelids and the sclera. Consider a lacerated sclera to be a serious situation since a deep cut may allow vitreous humor to escape.
- ☐ Puncture Wounds—Look for punctures, including eyelid perforations. Since the sclera tends to close itself on open wounds, a puncture may appear as an abrasion. You must consider the mechanism of injury and, when possible, gather information by interviewing the patient and/or bystanders. Take great care to look for embedded and impaled objects. Any puncture wound to the eye must be considered serious.
- ☐ Burns—The patient and bystanders usually are the source of information to tell you of a burn to the eyes. The scene also may give clues. Look for highly irritated or damaged tissues, including singed eyebrows or eyelashes. Burns to the eyelids indicate that there may be burns to the eyes.
- ☐ Avulsions—Look to see if the eyelids are torn or torn away and if the eyeball protrudes or is pulled from its socket.

Warning: Injury to the eye may mean that there are other head injuries, including brain damage. There also may be injuries to the cervical spine. Assume there are serious head injuries if

- ☐ There are any indications of fractures around the orbit.
- ☐ The sclera is red because of bleeding.
- ☐ One or both eyes cannot be moved.
- ☐ One pupil is larger than the other.
- ☐ Both pupils are unresponsive.
- ☐ One or both eyes protrude.
- ☐ The eyes cross or turn in different directions.

Patient Care—Eye Injuries

When caring for a patient with eye injuries, you will have to cover both eyes, even if only one eye is injured. Remember that when one eye sees something and moves, the other eye duplicates this movement. This action is called **sympathetic eye movement**. Explain to the patient why you must cover both eyes and maintain voice and touch contact with him to reduce his anxiety.

It is important to keep the eyelids of an unconscious patient closed. An unconscious person has no involuntary blinking action to sweep tears across the exposed portions of the eyes. An unprotected eye will dry out quickly and become damaged. This damage may be permanent. If the patient's eyes will not stay closed, place sterile dressings moistened with sterile saline over both eyes and bandage these dressings in place. If the patient is unconscious or has a low state of awareness, have someone attend to him at all times. This will help calm his fears should he regain consciousness or full awareness.

Emergency Care Steps

The following are general procedures for emergency care of eye injuries. Always follow local protocols which may differ from the procedures described here.

- ☐ Foreign Objects—Flush the eye with water.
- ☐ Contusions—Avoid using a cold pack which may contaminate or cause sudden changes in circulation. If injuries permit, transport in a semiseated position to reduce pressure in the eye.
- ☐ Abrasions and Lacerations—Cover with loose dressings or place a padding of dressings around the injured eye.
- ☐ Puncture Wounds and Impaled Objects—If there is no impaled object, cover with loose dressings. If an object is impaled in the eye, stabilize the object with gauze rolls or folded gauze pads and protect with a non-styrofoam disposable cup.
- ☐ Chemical Burns—Flush the eye with copious amounts of water for 20 minutes while en route to the hospital.
- ☐ Heat Burns—Apply a loose, moist dressing
- ☐ Light Burns—Cover the eyes with dark patches as they will be very sensitive to light.
- ☐ Avulsions—Shield an eye pulled from its socket with folded 4 x 4s. Cover torn eyelids with loose dressings. Follow local protocols for the care and transport of torn-away fragments.

These steps are discussed more fully below.

Foreign Objects Some EMS systems do not recommend that you wash a patient's eyes unless you are dealing with the problem of chemicals in the eye. Irrigation should not delay transport. Follow your local protocols in terms of the procedure and time spent at the scene. If you are permitted to wash objects from the eye, be certain that the globe of the eye has not been deeply lacerated or penetrated. The steps for washing the eye are shown in Figure 13-7. If an object remains on the inner lid surface and will

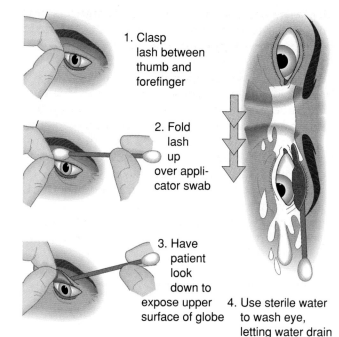

1. Clasp lash between thumb and forefinger

2. Fold lash up over applicator swab

3. Have patient look down to expose upper surface of globe

4. Use sterile water to wash eye, letting water drain down and away from eye.

Figure 13-7 Washing a foreign object from the eye. 1. Clasp the upper lash between your thumb and forefinger. 2. Fold the lash up over the applicator swab. 3. Have patient look down to expose upper surface of globe. 4. Use sterile water (or saline) to wash eye, applying water at the medial corner of the eye socket.

not wash away, use a sterile, moist applicator or gauze pad to carefully remove this foreign body. NEVER ATTEMPT TO REMOVE AN OBJECT ON THE CORNEA. Do not try to probe into the eye socket or remove embedded objects.

Even for cases in which debris is successfully washed from the eye, transport will be required. The patient must be seen by a physician.

Contusions Some patients will request a cold pack or ice pack for bruised eyes. This may help relieve discomfort; however, this procedure should not be done if the patient shows any symptoms or signs of serious eye or head injury. You do not want to increase the risk of additional contamination or cause rapid changes in circulation in the area of the injury. A cold pack will rapidly constrict blood vessels at and around the injury site. If cold is applied, do not use pressure.

Look at the iris. If it is not easily visible, or if you see blood between the cornea and the iris, the patient should be transported to a medical facility as soon as possible. If other injuries permit, position the patient in a semiseated position to help lower the pressure in the eye.

Abrasions and Lacerations If the eyelid is bleeding, do not apply a pressure dressing unless you are certain that there are no lacerations to the globe of the eye. Should the globe also have an open wound, cover the bleeding lid with loose dressings to aid clotting and prevent additional contamination. Do not touch the cornea or try to remove any foreign matter. Remember to cover both eyes.

In cases where there are no open wounds to the eyelid but the globe of the eye is bleeding or shows any other indication of an open wound, DO NOT APPLY PRESSURE. Use loose dressings. Remember to cover both eyes.

Remember: The jelly-like vitreous humor can be squeezed from an open eye wound. This substance cannot be replaced. Loss of vitreous humor may result in blindness.

An alternative method of care for a lacerated eyeball is similar to the care rendered for impaled objects in the eye. This method also is recommended for avulsed eyes. To provide care, you should

1. Close the injured eye.
2. Place folded 4 x 4s around the eye. The dressings must not touch the injured globe or lid.
3. Place a non-styrofoam disposable cup over the padding.
4. Set several gauze pads over the uninjured eye.
5. Hold the gauze pads and cup in place by self-adherent roller bandage. Have someone stabilize the cup and padding while you apply the bandage.

Puncture Wounds and Impaled Objects
Use loose dressings for puncture wounds with no impaled objects. If you find an object impaled in the eye, you should (Figure 13-8)

1. Place a roll of 3-inch gauze bandage or folded 4 x 4s on either side of the object, along the vertical axis of the head. These rolls should be placed so that they stabilize the object.
2. Fit a disposable drinking cup (do not use styrofoam) or paper cone over the impaled object and allow it to come to rest on the

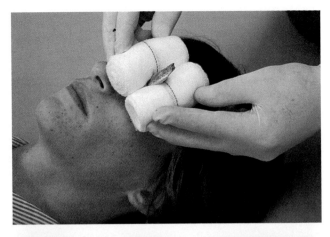

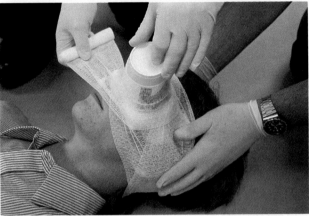

Figure 13-8 Managing a patient with an object impaled in the eye

dressing rolls. Do not allow it to touch the object. This will offer rigid protection and will call attention to the patient's problem.

3. Have another rescuer stabilize the dressings and cup while you secure them in place with self-adherent roller bandage or with a wrapping of gauze. Do not secure the bandage over top of the cup.
4. The uninjured eye should be dressed and bandaged to reduce eye movements.
5. Provide oxygen and care for shock.
6. Continue to reassure the patient and provide emotional support.

The above method can also be used as a pressure dressing to control bleeding in the area of the eye.

An *alternative* to the above method calls for the rescuer to make a thick dressing with several layers of sterile gauze pads or multi-trauma dressings (Figure 13-9). A hole is cut in the center of this pad, approximately the size of

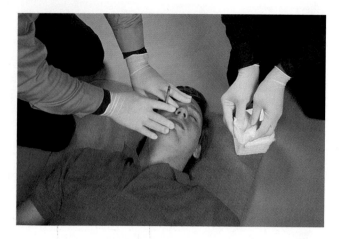
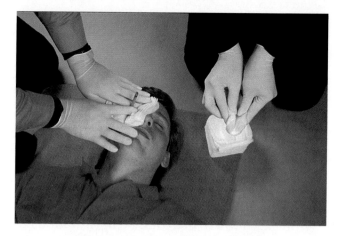
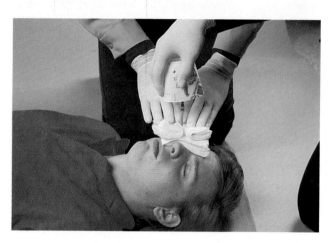
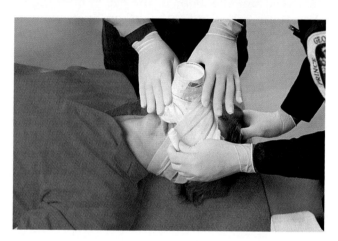

Figure 13-9 Alternative method of care for lacerated eyelid or injury to eyeball. 1. 4 x 4 sterile pads 2. Fold 2 or 3 sterile pads and cut a half moon in the fold. 3. Open gauze pad and place over injury. Cut and add pads as needed. 4. Place cup on pads and secure with roller bandage.

the impaled object. The rescuer then carefully passes this dressing over the impaled object and positions the pad so that the impaled object is centered in the opening. The rest of the procedure remains the same as previously described. If your EMS system has you use this technique, remember that you must take great care not to touch the object as the dressing is set in place.

Burns Burns to the eyes can be caused by chemicals, heat, or light (Figure 13-10).

- Chemical Burns—Turn the patient's head to the side so that you can flush the eyes with a steady stream of water. The pour should be from the medial (nasal) corner across the globe to the lateral corner. (This

prevents flushing the chemical into the other eye.) Use sterile water if it is available; otherwise, use tap water. For patients wearing contact lenses, remove the lenses while washing the eyes (see below). Some EMS systems are very specific on the time of the wash; however, the safest policy is to wash the eyes for 20 minutes or until transfer is made to the medical facility. For most chemical burns, it is best to start the wash as soon as possible and continue to irrigate the patient's eyes during transport to the medical facility. This will prevent transport delay and allow the patient to receive specialized care much sooner.

If the ambulance does not carry equipment for eye irrigation, use the rubber bulb syringe in the obstetric kit or an IV of nor-

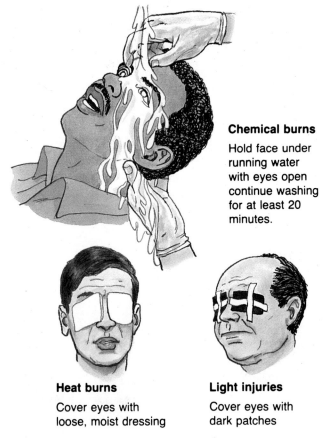

Chemical burns

Hold face under running water with eyes open continue washing for at least 20 minutes.

Heat burns

Cover eyes with loose, moist dressing

Light injuries

Cover eyes with dark patches

Figure 13-10 Managing burns to the eyes.

mal saline, using the tube for irrigation. When this bulb is used, control the flow so that it gently washes the eye. After washing, close the eyelid and apply a loose sterile dressing. If the patient complains of burning, remove the dressing and rewash.

- Heat Burns—In many cases, only the eyelids will be burned. Do not attempt to inspect the eyes if the eyelids are burned. With the patient's eyelids closed, apply a loose, moist dressing.
- Light Burns—Light injuries can be caused by a strong source of light or an ultraviolet light source. Light burns commonly occur from the flash of an arc welder or by the extreme brightness of the sun as it is reflected off sand or snow. These burns are generally very painful, with many patients saying that it feels as if there is sand in the eyes. The onset is usually slow, often taking several hours after exposure before symptoms develop. To make the patient more comfortable, close his eyelids and apply dark patches over both eyes. If you do not

have dark patches, apply a pad of dressings followed with a layer of opaque (light-blocking) material such as dark plastic or cardboard. Instruct the patient not to rub his eyes.

Avulsions An avulsed eye is an eye pulled from its socket. This is a very rare occurrence. Do not try to force the eye back in. Care for an avulsed eye the same as you would a lacerated eyeball (roll of gauze or folded 4 x 4s and rigid shield) or as you would an impaled object in the eye. Some EMS systems allow the initial dressing pads to be moistened with sterile water or saline, especially if transport is delayed or will take a long time to accomplish. Prior to its application, a sterile moist dressing may be added according to local protocol.

Lacerated and torn eyelids should be carefully covered with dressing materials. When the eyelid is torn off completely, the loose fragment should be recovered after proper wound care is completed on the remaining lid. Standard care is provided for the fully avulsed part, and it is kept cool and transported with the patient. Your EMS system's protocol may require that the part be placed in sterile dressings that have been soaked in sterile saline.

Removing Contact Lenses

Care of eye injuries (e.g. chemical burns) can be complicated by the presence of contact lenses. In some cases, when transport is delayed or will take a long time, the patient's contact lenses may be removed to avoid drying of the eyes and possible abrasive damage to the cornea. Most of the time, the lenses are left in place rather than delay the transport of an unconscious patient.

It is not recommended that you remove contact lenses if there is obvious injury to the eye. To do so may cause additional damage. Some EMS systems have guidelines as to when you can remove contact lenses. Be certain to follow the guidelines established in your area. Whenever you observe that a patient is wearing contact lenses, always report this fact to the medical facility staff.

Caring for patients wearing contact lenses is not as rare as you may think. Always ask the conscious patient if he or she is wearing contact lenses. Methods of removing contact lenses, which will be discussed below, are shown in Scan 13-2.

Removing Contact Lenses

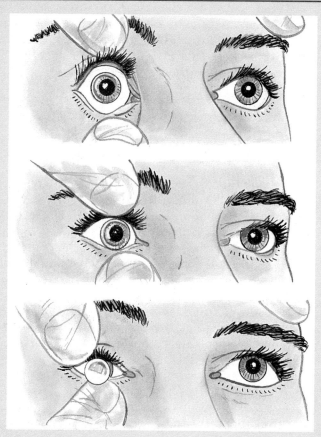

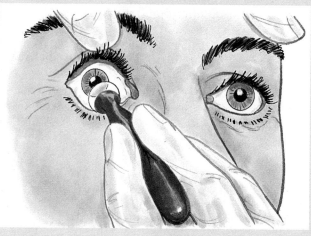

B. Using a moistened suction cup to remove a hard contact lens.

A. Removing a hard corneal contact lens.

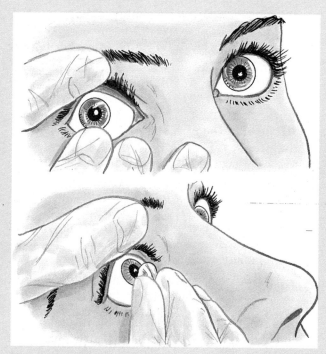

C. Removing flexible contact lenses.

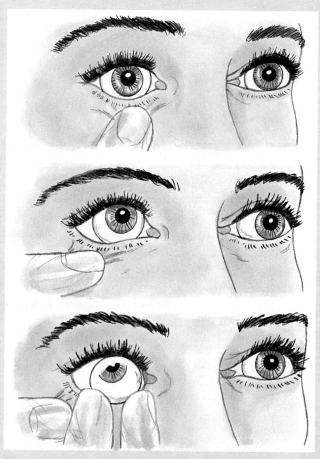

D. Removing a scleral lens

374

Types of Contact Lenses Four types of contact lenses are widely prescribed: hard, soft (flexible), extended wear, and scleral.

- Hard contact lenses are in wide use, even though soft lenses have become the most popular type of contact lens. When in place, this hard lens covers the cornea. It will appear to cover the entire iris. The typical size is about 0.3 inch in diameter (about the size of a shirt button).
- Soft contact lenses (flexible lenses) are very popular. A flexible lens is slightly larger than a dime (about 0.5 inch in diameter), covering the entire cornea and part of the sclera.
- Extended wear lenses or "perma lenses" are long-term wear lenses. They are gaining in popularity with the general public and also are worn by many postoperative cataract patients. In the field, you will not be able to distinguish these lenses from soft contact lenses.
- Scleral lenses are the least common contact lenses. They are about the size of a quarter, covering the cornea and a large portion of the sclera.

Removing Hard Lenses To remove hard corneal lenses, you should

1. With gloved hands, position one thumb on the upper eyelid and one thumb on the lower eyelid. Keep your thumbs near the margin (edge) of each lid.
2. Separate the eyelids and look for the lens over the cornea. The lens should slide easily with a gentle movement of the lids. If the lens is not directly over the cornea, slide it to that position with an appropriate movement of the eyelids.
3. Once the lens is over the cornea, open the eyelids further so that the margins of the lids are beyond the top and bottom edges of the lens. Maintain this opening.
4. Press both eyelids gently but firmly on the globe of the eye and move the lower eyelid to a position barely touching the edge of the lens.
5. Bring the upper eyelid margin close to the upper edge of the lens, keeping both lids pressed on the globe.
6. Press slightly harder on the lower lid, to move it underneath the bottom edge of the lens. This action should cause the lens to tip outward from the eye.
7. When the lens has tipped slightly, begin to move the eyelids together. The lens should slide out between the eyelids where it can be removed.

Remember: Never use force in removing a contact lens. If you see the lens but cannot remove it, gently slide it onto the sclera. The lens can remain there with greater safety until more experienced help is available.

Note: Special suction cups are available for the removal of hard contact lenses. They should be moistened with saline or sterile water before being brought into contact with the lens. The use of these cups is not recommended in cases of lacerated or chemically burned eyes.

Removing Soft or Extended Wear Lenses As a general rule, unless there are chemical burns, soft contact lenses are not removed in the prehospital setting. They are made of a special material that can be left in place for several hours. If you must remove a flexible contact lens, you should

1. With gloved hands, pull down on the lower eyelid, using your middle finger. Place your index fingertip on the lower edge of the lens.
2. Slide the lens down onto the sclera.
3. Compress the lens slightly between the thumb and index finger, using this pinching motion to cause the lens to double up.
4. Remove the lens from the eye.

Note: Some ambulances carry irrigating solutions to add to the eye before attempting to remove soft contact lenses. Such solutions should not be used if the eye is injured, particularly in cases of deep lacerations. Follow your local guidelines.

Removing Scleral Lenses To remove scleral lenses, you should

1. With gloved hands, position the index finger on the lower eyelid near the margin.
2. Slowly and carefully press the eyelid down until the bottom edge of the lens becomes visible. This requires more pressure than for the smaller corneal lenses. Be careful to avoid excessive pressure.
3. Maintaining gentle but firm pressure on the eyelid, move your finger in a lateral direction to pull the eyelid taut.
4. The eyelid margin should slide under the lower edge of the lens, lifting the lens to a position where it can be grasped.

After the contact lenses have been removed, place them in a container with a little water or saline and label the container with the patient's name. Soft lenses are best placed in normal saline. The patient may have a contact lens case with him. Use this case when possible, making certain that it is labeled with the patient's name and the right and left lenses are placed in their correct compartments.

For additional information, request a contact emergency care and instruction packet from the American Optometric Association, 243 N. Lindbergh Blvd., St. Louis, MO 63141.

INJURIES TO THE EARS

Injuries to the ear may go undetected by the EMT, or if detected they may be disregarded or treated lightly. Noting injury to the ear is very important since such an injury may be a sign of a more serious head injury. In addition, the internal structures of the ear may be damaged, leading to deafness and serious problems of balance.

Structure and Function of the Ears

The ear is actually two important organs housed in one anatomical structure (Figure 13-11). One is the mechanism for *hearing*, in which sound waves are converted into nerve impulses. The other is a major part of our *equilibrium* (system of balance), keeping track of head positioning and motion.

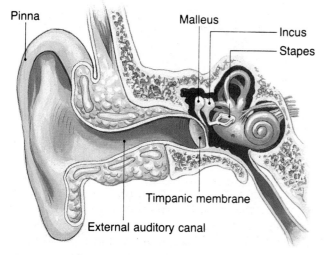

Figure 13-11 Anatomy of the ear.

The ear is divided into three parts: the external ear, the middle ear, and the internal ear. Most of the ear's structures are hidden from view, housed in the temporal bone.

The most prominent structure of the *external ear* is the **pinna** (PIN-nah) or auricle (AW-re-kl). Its shape is maintained by cartilage. The opening and canal that run from the pinna into the skull are called the **external auditory canal** (also called the external acoustic meatus, me-A-tus). This canal ends at the eardrum, known as the **tympanic** (tim-PAN-ik) **membrane**.

On the other side of the eardrum lies the *middle ear*, an air-filled chamber that connects with the nasal cavity by way of the **internal auditory canal** (eustachian tube). The middle ear contains three small bones, connected together to stretch from the drum to the inner ear.

The *inner ear* is a maze of fluid-filled chambers (hollowed out bone). Sound waves cause the eardrum to vibrate. These vibrations, carried by the middle ear bones to the inner ear, cause the fluids to vibrate and stimulate special nerve endings. These nerves send impulses to the auditory center of the brain to be interpreted as specific sounds. The inner ear also has receptors that react to the motion of fluids each time the head and body change positions. Impulses are sent to the brain so that body adjustments can be made to maintain balance.

Types of Ear Injuries

All three parts of the ear can be injured. Contusions and crushing injuries to ear cartilage are closed wounds of the ear. Lacerations, abrasions, and avulsions can occur to the external ear. Rupture of the ear drum is considered an external injury.

Patient Assessment—Ear Injuries

Injuries to the external ear are usually obvious, but you will not be able to tell if middle and inner ear structures are damaged. The same signs and symptoms can indicate either an injury to the internal ear or an injury to the bones of the skull.

Signs and Symptoms

All of these signs and symptoms *must* be considered to indicate either a possible skull fracture or an injury to the middle or inner ear.

The patient complains of
- ☐ Ringing in the ears
- ☐ Internal ear pain
- ☐ Excessive wetness in the ears
- ☐ Dizziness

You observe
- ☐ Blood coming from the ears
- ☐ Clear fluid coming from the ears
- ☐ Loss of balance as the patient attempts to position himself

Note: Bloody or clear fluids coming from the ear *must* be considered to be a sign of a possible skull fracture.

Patient Care—Ear Injuries

Emergency Care Steps

Follow these care procedures for injuries to the ear.

- ☐ Abrasions and Lacerations—Apply a sterile dressing, and bandage (Figure 13-12).
- ☐ Tears—Apply bulky dressings so that the torn ear rests between layers of dressing. Bandage in place.
- ☐ Avulsions—Return attached flaps to normal position. Apply bulky dressings and bandage in place. If the part is entirely avulsed and can be retrieved, it is to receive the same care as any other completely avulsed part, kept cool, and transported with the patient.

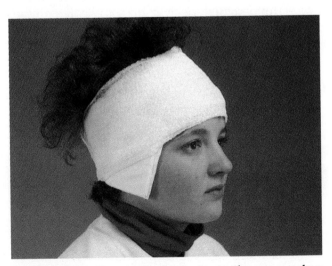

Figure 13-12 For external injuries to the ear, apply a dressing and bandage in place.

- ☐ Bleeding from the Ears—Do not pack the external ear canal. To do so may cause additional injury and serious problems if there is a skull fracture. Loosely apply dressings to the external ear and bandage in place.
- ☐ Clear Fluids Draining from the Ears—Do not remove any impaled objects. Do not pack the external ear canal. Apply loose sterile external dressings. Bandage the dressings in place.
- ☐ "Clogged" Ear and Objects in the Ear—When a patient complains of a clogged ear, this may be an indication that there is damage to the eardrum, fluids are in the middle ear, or foreign objects are in the ear canal. DO NOT PROBE INTO THE EARS. Prevent the patient from hitting the side of his head in an effort to free objects from the canal.

Note: If you obtain any of the signs or symptoms of middle or inner ear injury listed above, you *must* care for the patient as if there is a skull fracture. Care procedures for skull fracture were discussed in Chapter 12.

INJURIES TO THE NOSE

We inhale primarily through the nose, so airway obstruction can occur when there is a nasal injury. Injuries to the nose can also be associated with injuries to adjacent parts of the face, the back of the head, and the cervical spine.

Structure and Function of the Nose

The nasal cavity is divided into two chambers, right and left. Separating these two chambers is the **nasal septum**, which is made of cartilage. There are nasal bones between the eyes. Soft tissues complete the structure of the nose (Figure 13-13).

Types of Nasal Injuries

Injury can take place to the external nose and the internal nose (nasal cavity). The cartilage of the septum can be broken easily when struck with a blunt object, as can the nasal bones between the eyes. Contusions, abrasions, lacerations, puncture wounds, and avulsions can occur to the soft tissues of the nose. In addition, there may be foreign objects in the nose.

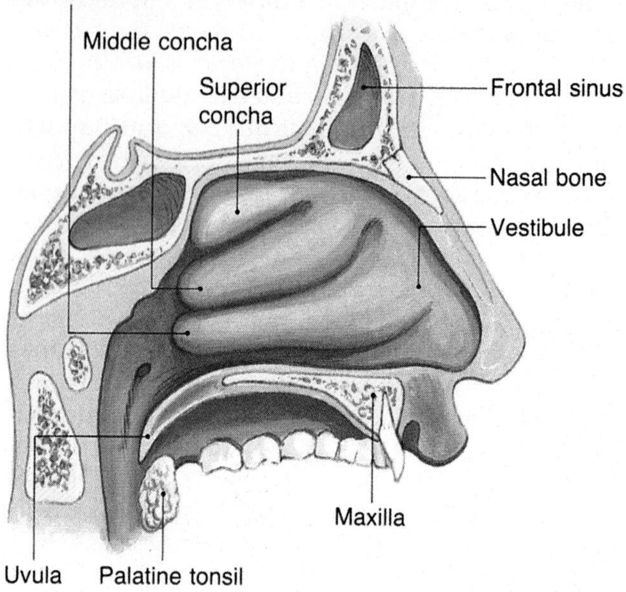

Figure 13-13 Anatomy of the nose.

Airway obstruction in the nasal cavity can occur with facial injury. Even though the mouth may be clear, blood and mucus released from nasal injuries can flow from the nose into the throat and cause a major airway obstruction.

Patient Assessment—Nasal Injuries

When you see damage to the soft tissues of the nose, realize that the following also may be injured.

- ☐ The nasal septum
- ☐ The nasal bones
- ☐ The bones of the upper jaw, the maxillae
- ☐ The bones of the lower jaw bone, the mandible
- ☐ The bones of the posterior head when the head has been forced back against something hard
- ☐ The cervical spine

Note: If the nasal injury patient is unconscious, or if the mechanism of injury or signs and symptoms indicate possible spinal injury, assume that there are spinal injuries.

Patient Care—Nasal Injuries

The care provided for nasal injuries is usually conservative, directed toward maintaining an open airway, controlling bleeding, and posi-

tioning the patient so that blood does not drain into the throat. Maintaining an open airway is the first priority.

Emergency Care Steps

Follow these care guidelines.

- ☐ Abrasions, Lacerations, and Punctures—Control bleeding, apply a sterile dressing, then bandage in place.
- ☐ Avulsions—Return attached flaps to their normal position, then apply a bulky dressing and bandage. Fully avulsed flaps of skin and any completely avulsed portions of the external nose (usually the tip) should be recovered and cared for the same as any completely avulsed part. It should be kept cool and transported with the patient.
- ☐ Foreign Objects—If the object protrudes, do not pull it free. It may have penetrated the septum or tissues high in the nose. Transport the patient without disturbing the object. If the object cannot be seen, do not probe for it. Have the patient gently blow his nose, keeping both nostrils open. Do not allow the patient to blow forcefully. If the object cannot be dislodged easily in this manner, transport the patient to a medical facility. Do not have the patient blow his nose if he is bleeding from the nostrils or has recently controlled a nosebleed.
- ☐ Nosebleeds—Position the patient for drainage of blood and mucus away from the throat, first immobilizing the neck and spine if spinal injury is a possibility. Pinch the nostrils for control of bleeding unless the presence of clear fluid indicates a skull fracture. (Care for nosebleeds is discussed more fully below.)

Care for Nosebleeds The medical term for a nosebleed is **epistaxis** (ep-e-STAK-sis). If there are no signs or symptoms of skull fracture, have the patient assume a seated position, leaning slightly forward to provide better drainage for blood and mucus. If a seated position is not practical, lay the patient back with the head elevated slightly, or simply turn the head to one side. Should the patient be unconscious, or if there are any indications of possible spinal damage, you *must* immobilize the neck and spine before positioning the patient and the board on its side for drainage. Suctioning may be required to keep the airway open.

There are three prescribed methods for controlling a nosebleed.

1. When the patient can do so, have him pinch his nostrils shut to control bleeding. If the patient cannot do this, you will have to do so, or have a bystander (with a gloved hand) help to allow you to attend to other patients (Figure 13-14). Pressure should be applied for at least 5 minutes. Pinching the nostrils is the simplest method and almost always works. *Do not* pack the patient's nostrils.
2. Place gauze pads under the patient's upper lip and hold in place until bleeding is controlled.
3. Place a cold pack on the bridge of the patient's nose. The cold will help to constrict the blood vessels to control bleeding.

As each of these methods is used, you may continue to pinch the patient's nostrils.

Warning: If there is clear fluid coming from the nose or ears, clear fluid in the ears, or a mix of blood and clear fluids draining from the nose or ears, the patient probably has a skull fracture. In this case, do not pinch the nostrils shut or attempt to stop the flow in any way. Do not blindly pass a suction catheter or nasal airway into the patient's nose.

Trauma-induced nosebleeds can range from minor to very serious. Often, the patient will swallow blood and vomit. Prolonged profuse nasal bleeding can cause a patient to develop shock.

Keep in mind that all nosebleeds are not the result of injuries related to accidents. High blood pressure can cause nosebleeds. So can infections and excessive sneezing. Such cases are usually easy to treat. If the patient has a bleeding disorder, however, bleeding can be difficult to control.

INJURIES TO THE MOUTH

Injury to the soft tissues of the mouth generally results from blunt trauma, as when the lips are forcefully compressed against the teeth. Common injuries to the mouth include lacerations of the lips, inner cheek wall, or tongue. Avulsions of the lips and tongue can also occur. Often associated with soft tissue damage in the mouth is damage to the teeth or dental appliances (Figure 13-15).

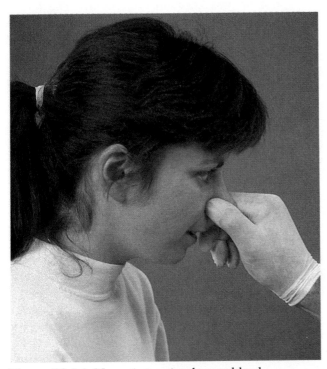

Figure 13-14 Managing a simple nosebleed.

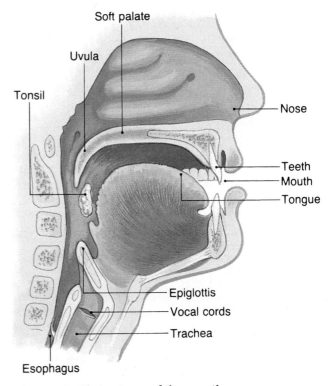

Figure 13-15 Anatomy of the mouth.

Patient Assessment—Oral Injuries

During the head-to-toe survey, using gloved fingers, search the mouth for any airway obstruction such as foreign objects, broken teeth, swollen tongue, blood and mucus, or vomit.

Patient Care—Oral Injuries

Emergency Care Steps

☐ Airway and Drainage—An open airway and proper drainage must be maintained throughout the care of the patient. (Procedures for clearing airway obstructions were discussed in Chapter 4.) If indicated, immobilize the neck and spine before opening the mouth or positioning the patient for drainage.

☐ Lacerated Lip or Gum—Control bleeding by placing a rolled or folded dressing between the lip and gum. If bleeding is profuse, position the patient to allow for drainage. Monitor so the patient does not swallow the dressing.

☐ Lacerated or Avulsed Tongue—Do not pack the mouth with dressings. Position the patient for drainage. If the tongue is fully avulsed (extremely rare), save and wrap the avulsed part and transport with the patient. Although rare, you may find a portion of fully avulsed tissue still in the patient's mouth. You must remove this tissue, provide the standard care for an avulsed part, keep it cool, and transport the part with the patient.

☐ Avulsed Lip—Return the flap to normal position, control bleeding with a pressure dressing, and position the patient for drainage. Do not bandage across the mouth. Save, wrap, label, and transport any fully avulsed tissues, keeping the part cool.

☐ Lacerated or Perforated Inner Cheek—External pressure dressings will not control bleeding in the case of perforations. Rolled dressings placed between the wound and the teeth should be used for perforations and lacerations. The patient must be positioned for drainage. Monitor the patient to prevent him from swallowing dressing materials or maintain internal pressure with your gloved finger. A conscious patient can assist by holding the dressing.

Patient Care—Dental Injuries

Problems involving teeth and dental appliances often occur with soft tissue injuries to the mouth.

Emergency Care Steps

☐ Dislodged Teeth, Crowns, and Bridges—With gloved hands, search for and remove any completely dislodged teeth, crowns, and bridges. Take great care in searching for dislodged teeth. There will be bleeding from the socket of a dislodged tooth. To control this bleeding, have the conscious patient bite down on a pad of gauze placed over the socket. In the case of the unconscious patient, you may have to place gauze into the socket. The less you disrupt the tissues of the socket, the better the chances a dentist will have to replace the dislodged tooth. Do not try to insert cotton packets into the socket.

Any dislodged tooth should be wrapped in moist dressings and transported with the patient. The tooth also can be kept moist by placing it in saline or milk, if available. Do not rub the tooth in order to clean it: doing so will destroy microscopic structures needed to replant the tooth. Inform the emergency department staff that you have the dislodged tooth. The sooner a dentist or oral surgeon can replant the tooth, the better the chances of success. Best results are seen if the procedure is carried out within 30 minutes of the incident.

☐ Dental Appliances—With gloved hands, remove loose dentures and the parts of broken dentures. Transport any dental appliance you remove, broken or intact, with the patient.

Be alert for adult patients with a unilateral partial appliance known as a Nesbit (commonly called a "spider"). This is typically a one- or two-tooth partial that is held in place at four points. Individuals have been known to swallow such devices. If you find one in the mouth of an injured or an unconscious patient, remove it. You must take care not to drop the appliance down the patient's throat. When practical, position the patient with his head turned to the same side as the Nesbit. To avoid the problems caused by blood, mucus, and saliva, grasp the Nesbit with a piece of gauze dressing. Transport the device with the patient.

INJURIES TO THE NECK

Injuries to the soft tissues of the neck can be classified as blunt or sharp. A blunt injury is any blow or collision with a blunt object. A sharp injury is from a sharp object such as glass or metal or a penetrating object such as an icepick, knife, or bullet. Both blunt and sharp injuries to the neck can be so life-threatening that only immediate surgical intervention can save the patient.

Any injury to the neck must be considered to be serious until proven otherwise. The neck contains many vital structures, including the cervical portion of the spinal cord, the larynx and part of the trachea, a portion of the esophagus, the **carotid** (kah-ROT-id) **arteries**, and the **jugular** (JUG-u-lar) **veins** (Figure 13-16).

Blunt Injuries to the Neck

Blunt injuries to the neck can occur in a variety of accident situations. In a vehicle collision, the driver may pitch forward and strike his neck against the steering wheel. Passengers often strike their necks on projections of the dashboard, arm rests, seatbacks, and objects being carried in the passenger compartment. However, you should realize that a person may receive a serious neck injury in nothing more than a simple fall should he strike his neck on some object.

Regardless of the cause, the major problem faced in blunt trauma to the neck is usually the collapse of the larynx or the trachea or swelling of their tissues, which creates a blocked airway. These are both rigid structures containing cartilage. Once they collapse or are crushed, they do not spring back to their original shape and resume normal function.

Patient Assessment—Blunt Injuries to the Neck

When a severe injury occurs to the neck, spinal injury also must be assumed.

Signs

For cases of blunt injury to the soft tissues of the neck (Figure 13-17), assess for

- ☐ Loss of voice or hoarseness
- ☐ Signs of airway obstruction when the mouth and nose are clear and no foreign body can be dislodged from the airway
- ☐ Contusions on or depressions in the neck
- ☐ Deformities of the neck
- ☐ Air or crackling sensations under the skin. This is known as subcutaneous emphysema, the result of air leaking into the soft tissues of the neck from a neck or airway injury or a pneumothorax in the superior portion of the lung (see Chapter 14).

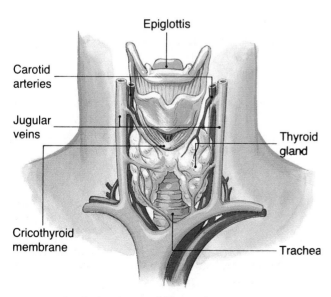

Figure 13-16 Anatomy of the neck.

Epiglottis

Carotid arteries

Jugular veins

Thyroid gland

Cricothyroid membrane

Trachea

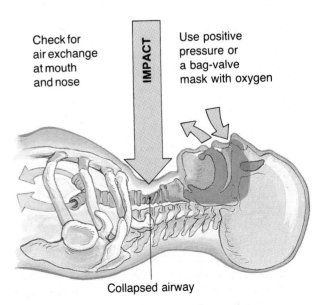

Figure 13-17 Blunt injuries to the neck.

Check for air exchange at mouth and nose

IMPACT

Use positive pressure or a bag-valve mask with oxygen

Collapsed airway

Patient Care—Blunt Injuries to the Neck

Remember: If the accident was serious enough to produce a blunt injury to the neck, it may have produced serious injury to the cervical spine. If basic life support measures must begin before immobilizing the neck, the jaw-thrust maneuver must be used and extreme care taken to move the patient's head no more than absolutely necessary. Aggravation of cervical spine injuries can lead to permanent paralysis or death.

Emergency Care Steps

☐ *If the injury is mild*, ensure an open airway, manually stabilize the head and neck, care for shock, administer a high concentration of oxygen, and apply cold packs to the site.

☐ *For serious blunt trauma injury*, manually stabilize the head and neck, apply a cervical collar, immobilize on a long spine board, and transport the patient to a medical facility without delay; emergency surgery may be needed to open the airway. Keep the patient calm and ask that he try to breathe slowly, if possible. Administer oxygen, using a bag-valve mask unit or other form of ventilation-assisted device if air must be forced past an obstruction. A cold pack should be applied to the injury site to reduce swelling.

Sharp Injuries to the Neck

The carotid arteries and the jugular veins pass through the neck, relatively close to the body's surface. Sharp injuries to these vessels (Figure 13-18) can produce catastrophic bleeding. A penetrating injury such as a gunshot wound can also cause a cervical fracture or spinal cord injury.

Patient Assessment—Severed Neck Vessel

Signs

A sharp injury to the neck that has severed a major artery or vein will produce these signs.

☐ *Arterial bleeding* will be profuse, with bright red blood spurting from the wound.

☐ *Venous bleeding* can be profuse with dark red to maroon-colored blood flowing steadily from the wound.

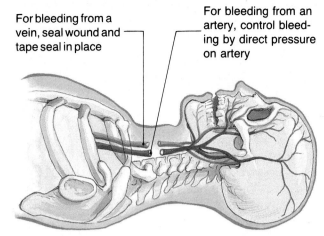

For bleeding from a vein, seal wound and tape seal in place

For bleeding from an artery, control bleeding by direct pressure on artery

Figure 13-18 Sharp injuries to the neck.

Patient Care—Severed Neck Artery

Emergency Care Steps

1. Manage arterial bleeding with direct pressure or pinching. Often direct pressure is not effective because it pushes the artery into the wound where it continues to bleed. If possible, grasp the exposed artery between your gloved thumb and index finger with a gauze pad. The pad will allow you to hold onto the artery while pinching it closed. When the bleeding has been controlled, cover the wound with an additional dressing and bandage. An alternative method would be to grasp the "bleeder" with a clamp, if authorized in your EMS system.
2. Assure an open airway.
3. Administer a high concentration of oxygen.
4. Care for shock.
5. Transport immediately.

Note: Bleeding from neck arteries is very difficult to control. Some EMS systems have now adopted the technique described below for both arterial and venous neck bleeding.

Patient Care—Severed Neck Vein

Bleeding from a large neck vein (Scan 13-3) usually cannot be controlled by direct pressure. Sometimes a large bulky dressing and firm hand pressure will control bleeding, but usually the ends of the veins pull away from

Severed Neck Veins — Occlusive Dressing

Dressing must be heavy plastic, sized to be no more than 2" larger in diameter than site.

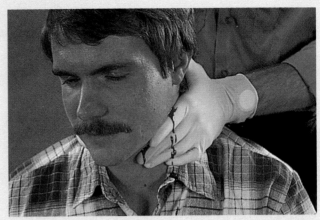

1. Do not delay! Place your gloved palm over the wound.

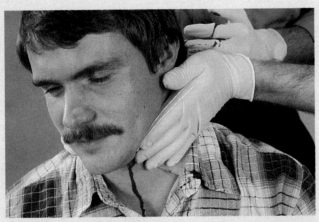

2. Occlusive dressing is placed over wound site.

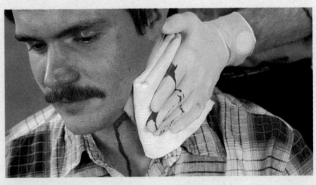

3. A dressing is placed over the occlusive dressing. (A roll of gauze can be placed between the trachea and the dressing to help keep pressure off the airway.)

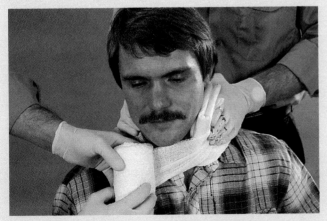

4. Start a figure-eight, bringing bandage over dressing.

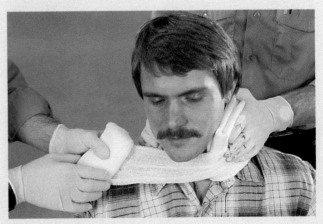

5. Cross over the shoulder.

Note: For demonstration purposes, patient is upright.

383

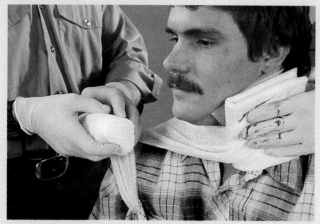

6. Bring bandage under the armpit. (Patient's arm can be extended and supported by an EMT while wrapping.)

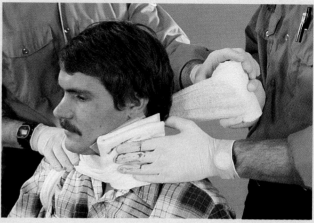

7. Cross back over shoulder and anchor several times to cover entire dressing. (If patient's arm was extended, lower it to pull pressure on the dressing.)

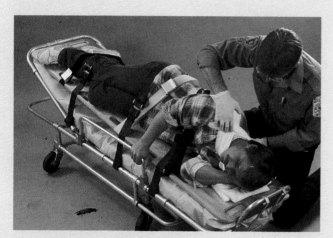

8. Place the patient on left side.

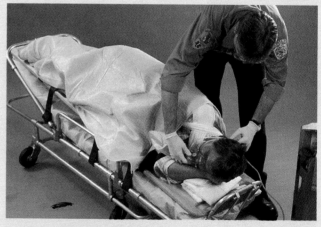

9. Care for shock and continue to administer a high concentration of oxygen.

Note: Bandaging should control bleeding without restricting breathing.

the wound site and bleed freely. In addition to the loss of blood, there may be the problem of air being sucked into the vein and carried to the heart as an air embolism. This is usually fatal.

Emergency Care Steps

To control bleeding from a neck vein, immediately cover the wound with a gloved hand, then apply an occlusive dressing. The problem with this procedure has always been bandaging the dressing in place. The blood on the skin and flowing from the wound prevents the effective use of tape. See Scan 13-3 for the correct procedure to use in applying an occlusive dressing to control bleeding from a severed neck vein. Note that this procedure allows for pressure to be applied over the site and usually above and below the injury.

CHAPTER REVIEW

KEY TERMS

You may find it helpful to review the following terms.

aqueous (A-kwe-us) **humor**—the fluid that fills the lens of the eye.

carotid (kah-ROT-id) **arteries**—the large neck arteries, one on each side of the neck, that carry blood from the heart to the head.

conjunctiva (kon-junk-TI-vah)—the delicate membrane that covers the sclera, cornea, and undersurfaces of the eyelids.

cornea (KOR-ne-ah)—the transparent portion of the sclera that covers the pupil and iris of the eye.

epistaxis (ep-e-STAK-sis)—a nosebleed.

external auditory canal—the opening of the external ear; the canal that runs from the external ear to the middle ear.

internal auditory canal—the canal that connects the middle ear with the nasal cavity.

iris—the colored portion of the eye in which the pupil is located.

jugular (JUG-u-lar) **veins**—the large neck veins, one on each side of the neck, that return blood from the head to the heart.

lacrimal (LAK-re-mal) **gland**—the tear gland.

lens—a cavity behind the iris and pupil of the eye.

nasal septum—the cartilage that separates the two chambers of the nose.

occipital (ok-SIP-i-tal) **lobe**—the posterior portion of the brain in which the vision center is located.

optic nerve—the nerve that carries impulses from the eye to the brain.

orbit—the bony depression in the skull in which the eye is situated.

pinna (PIN-nah)—the external ear, also called the auricle.

pupil—the adjustable opening that admits light to the eye.

retina (RET-i-na)—the back of the eye.

sclera (SKLE-rah)—the white of the eye.

sympathetic eye movement—the coordinated movement of both eyes in the same direction. If one eye moves, the other eye will carry out the same movement, even if it is covered or the eyelid is shut.

tympanic (tim-PAN-ik) **membrane**—the eardrum.

vitreous (VIT-re-us) **humor**—the fluid that fills the posterior cavity of the eye.

SUMMARY

For any injury above the clavicles, you must be alert for injury to the cervical spine, airway problems, bleeding, and shock.

Injuries to the Scalp and Face

Treatment of soft tissue injuries to the scalp and face is the same as treatment of other soft tissue injuries with three exceptions: For scalp wounds (1) do not try to clear the surface of the wound, and (2) do not apply finger pressure if there is any chance of skull fracture. (3) Do remove objects impaled through the cheek into the oral cavity.

Treat scalp wounds by controlling bleeding with dressings held in place by bandages, using bandaging strategies suitable for the head. Raise the head and shoulders of a conscious patient with no possibility of spinal injury.

For facial injuries, immobilize for potential neck or spinal injuries. Clear the mouth to establish an airway. Ventilate as necessary for breathing problems. Control bleeding with bulky dressings. If an impaled object has been removed from the cheek, pack the inside of the mouth with rolled gauze, but leave 3 to 4 inches of the dressing outside the mouth for visibility and easy removal. If possible, transport the patient with facial injuries in the lateral recumbent position with head low or tilted to aid drainage.

Injuries to the Eyes

To assess for eye injuries, listen to patient complaints of pain or irritation in the eye. Look for redness, swelling, major scratches to the cornea, or cuts or punctures to the eyelid. Listen to clues provided by the patient or bystanders to chemical, heat, or light burns.

When there are any indications of fractures around the orbit, red or bleeding sclera, immobility of the eyes, pupils that are unequal or unresponsive, or eyes that protrude, cross, or turn in different directions, assume serious head and spinal injuries and treat accordingly.

When one eye is injured, cover both eyes to prevent aggravation caused by sympathetic eye movement.

To remove foreign objects, flush the eye. For contusions, avoid cold packs and, if injuries permit, reduce pressure in the eye by transporting the patient in a semiseated position. For abrasions and lacerations, cover the eye with loose dressings or padding around the eye. Stabilize and protect any impaled object. For chemical burns, flush the eye with water; for heat burns, apply a loose, moist dressing; for light burns cover the eye with an opaque patch. Do not attempt to push in an avulsed eye, but shield it with loose dressings.

Ordinarily, leave contact lenses in the eye. If it is necessary to remove them, as when there is a chemical burn, use the special procedures for removing the four types of contact lenses: hard, soft (flexible), extended wear, and scleral lenses.

Injuries to the Ears

Dress and bandage abrasions, lacerations, tears, and avulsions to the external ear. Do not pack

the ear canal if there is bleeding or drainage of clear fluids. Do not probe for foreign objects and prevent the patient from hitting the side of his head to dislodge a foreign object.

Signs and symptoms of skull fracture or inner ear injury involve ringing in the ear, ear pain, a feeling of wetness in the ear, dizziness, blood or clear fluid coming from the ear, or loss of balance. If any of these indications is present, follow the care procedures for a skull fracture.

Injuries to the Nose

Apply dressings and bandage abrasions, lacerations, punctures, and avulsions of the nose. If the patient cannot dislodge a foreign object by gently blowing his nose with both nostrils open, make no other attempt to probe for or dislodge a foreign object but transport the patient to a medical facility. To control nosebleeds, if possible have the patient sit and lean slightly forward. Then use one of three methods to control the bleeding: (1) Pinch the nostrils, (2) place gauze pads under the upper lip, or (3) place a cold pack on the bridge of the nose.

Injuries to the Mouth

When there is an injury to the mouth, clear the mouth and maintain an open airway. For a lacerated lip or gum, place a rolled or folded dressing between lip and gum. For a lacerated tongue, do not pack the mouth but rather position the patient for drainage. Control bleeding from an avulsed lip or lacerated cheek with a dressing or bandage. Search for dislodged teeth, wrap them in moist dressings, and transport them with the patient. Remove loose dentures or parts of dentures or dental appliances.

Injuries to the Neck

Injuries to the neck can be blunt or sharp. Either must be considered serious.

Signs of blunt injury to the neck include loss of voice or hoarseness, signs of airway obstruction when the mouth and nose are clear, contusion, depression, or deformity to the neck, and air or crackling sensations under the skin of the neck. Treat by ensuring an open airway, if possible, and manually stabilizing the head and neck.

For sharp injuries to the neck in which a carotid artery has been severed (signaled by pro-

386   Trauma

fuse bleeding with bright red blood spurting from the wound), you may attempt to grasp and pinch or clamp the bleeding artery and, when bleeding is controlled, dress and bandage. When a jugular vein has been severed (signaled by possibly profuse bleeding with dark red to maroon-colored blood flowing steadily from the wound), apply an occlusive dressing. For all neck injuries, care for shock, administer a high concentration of oxygen, and transport as quickly as possible.

Any fully avulsed skin or parts such as an eyelid, tip of the nose, external ear, lip, or tongue should be retrieved, wrapped in a dry or moist sterile dressing (according to local protocols), kept cool, and transported with the patient.

CHAPTER 14

On the Scene

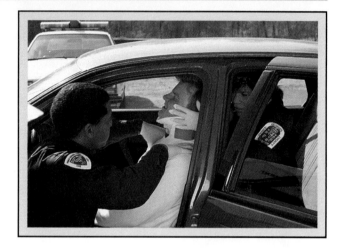

Twenty-three-year-old Ed Franklin is driving to work. It's a short trip he makes every day, so he doesn't bother with a seat belt. But on a curve, an oncoming vehicle pulls out to pass. There's no time to react. Ed's car is hit head-on.

The 911 dispatch center receives numerous calls for a "bad accident." Two ambulances and fire department rescue units are dispatched to the scene. Your ambulance is the second to arrive, and you are directed by the EMS command person at the scene to tend to Ed Franklin. You quickly explain to Ed who you are and obtain his consent to help.

Then . . .

You: There's going to be a person in the back seat behind you and he's going to hold your head still. Do you remember what happened?

Ed Franklin: Not exactly. Somebody hit me, I guess.

You (observing a severely bent steering wheel): Do you hurt anywhere?

Ed Franklin: My chest hurts a lot.

Ed appears pale. His breathing is rapid and labored. During a brief examination of his chest, you find no open wound, but you feel broken ribs and observe unequal chest expansion.

You (to your crew): Let's get a rigid collar on and prepare for a rapid extrication. (To your patient) Ed, we're going to be moving you from the car now and get you to the hospital. Here's how we're going to do it. . . .

Ed's signs of shock and the bent steering wheel were your first indications of a serious injury. Your examination of Ed's chest has led you to believe that there is air in the chest cavity, a pneumothorax. Since there is no open wound, and ribs seem to be fractured, you assume the air is coming from a punctured lung. You decide that Ed's status is critical, that he will need ventilatory assistance, and that he must be transported to the trauma center immediately.

The Chest, Abdomen, and Genitalia

Chapter Overview

Because the torso is the location of the body's vital organs, injuries to this portion of the body are often life threatening. In this chapter you will learn about injuries to the chest, abdomen, pelvis, and groin.

Expected Outcome, Chapter 14: *You will be able to assess and care for injuries to the chest, abdomen, pelvis, and groin.*

> **WARNING:** Protect yourself from infectious diseases by using appropriate barrier devices such as a pocket face mask with one-way valve, face shield, or bag-valve mask; goggles or eye shield; and disposable gloves. Always conform to your local EMS system's infection exposure control plan.

Knowledge *After reading this chapter, you should be able to*

1. Describe the anatomy and organs of the chest, abdomen, pelvis, and groin. (pp. 390-391; Chapter 2; Anatomy and Physiology Plates)
2. List THREE ways in which the chest can be injured. (pp. 390-391)
3. Define open chest wound and closed chest wound. (pp. 391-392)
4. Describe the general signs and symptoms associated with open and closed chest wounds. (p. 392)
5. Describe how to assess and care for possible open pneumothorax and tension pneumothorax. (pp. 392-395)
6. Describe how to assess and care for objects impaled in the chest, possible rib fractures, and flail chest. (pp. 395-399)
7. List and describe the common complications of chest injuries and basic emergency care for such complications. (pp. 399-401)
8. List the major signs and symptoms of abdominal injury. (pp. 402-403)
9. State the procedures used to care for open and closed abdominal injury. (pp. 403-404)
10. Describe how to assess and care for injuries to the urinary system. (p. 405)
11. Describe how to assess and care for injuries to the reproductive system. (p. 405; Scan 14-1)
12. Describe how to assess and care for an inguinal hernia. (p. 408)

Skills *As an EMT you should be able to*

1. Control bleeding and apply the proper dressing and bandage for a given open soft tissue injury to the chest, abdomen, pelvis, and genitalia.
2. Apply patient assessment and care techniques to possible
   • General open and closed chest injuries
   • Open pneumothorax
   • Tension pneumothorax
   • Impaled objects
   • Fractured ribs
   • Flail chest
   • Complications of chest injuries
   • Injuries to the abdomen
   • Injuries to the urinary system
   • Injuries to reproductive system
   • Inguinal hernia

Before or while you are studying this chapter on injuries to the chest, abdomen, pelvis, and groin, review the information in Chapter 2 on body cavities, abdominal quadrants, and major body organs. Also look over the Anatomy and Physiology Plates on the cardiovascular, respiratory, digestive, urinary, and reproductive systems at the end of this book.

INJURIES TO THE CHEST

The basic anatomy of the chest was presented in Chapter 10. Whenever you are assessing chest injuries, keep in mind that there may be injuries to the heart, great blood vessels, lungs, trachea,

liver, gallbladder, stomach, and spleen. Remember that there is a posterior portion of the thoracic cavity. Back injuries may involve chest structures, including the ribs, lungs, and heart (Figure 14-1).

Types of Chest Injuries

The chest can be injured in a number of ways, including

• Blunt Trauma—A blow to the chest can fracture the ribs, the sternum, and the costal (rib) cartilages. Whole sections of the chest may collapse. With severe blunt trauma, the lungs and airway can be damaged and the heart may be seriously injured.

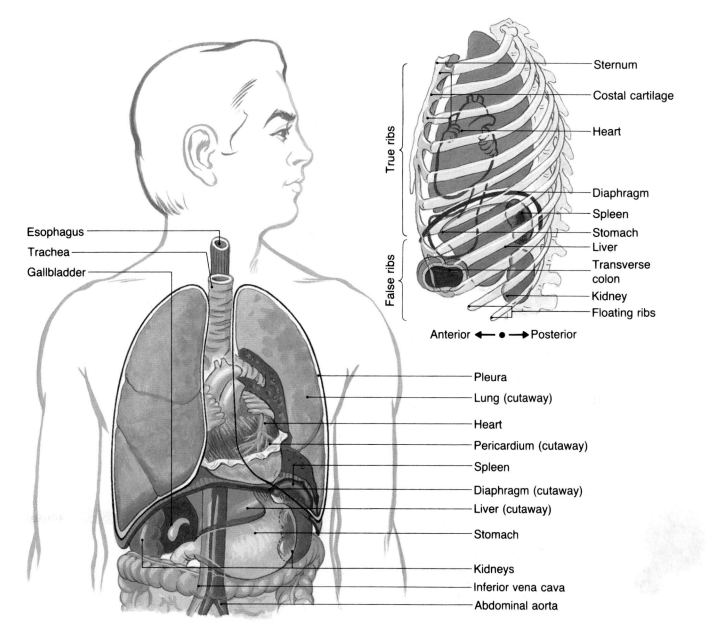

Figure 14-1 Anatomy of the chest and upper abdomen.

- **Penetrating Objects**—Bullets, knives, pieces of metal or glass, steel rods, pipes, and various other objects can penetrate the chest wall, damaging internal organs and impairing respiration.
- **Compression**—This is a severe form of blunt trauma in which the chest is rapidly compressed, as when the driver of a motor vehicle pitches forward after a head-on collision and strikes his chest on the steering column. The heart can be severely squeezed, the lungs can be ruptured, and the sternum and ribs can be fractured.

Chest injuries can be classified as OPEN or CLOSED.

- **Open**—When the skin is broken, the patient has an open wound. However, the term *open chest wound* usually means that the chest wall is penetrated, as, for example, by a bullet or a knife blade. An object can pass through the wall from the outside, or a fractured and displaced rib can penetrate the chest wall from within. The heart, lungs, and great vessels can be injured at the same time the chest wall is penetrated. It may be difficult to tell if the chest cavity has been penetrated by looking at the wound. *Do not* open the wound to determine its depth. Specific signs and symptoms will indicate possible open chest injury.

- Closed—The skin is not broken with a closed chest injury, leading many people to think that the damage done is not serious. However, such injuries, sustained through blunt trauma and compression injuries, can cause contusions and lacerations of the heart, lungs, and great vessels.

**Patient Assessment—
General Chest Injuries**

Signs and Symptoms

The most reliable sign of chest injury is

☐ An obvious wound (open chest injury)

When there is no such wound (closed chest injury), check for

☐ Pain at the injury site or on compression of the lateral chest wall
☐ Painful or difficult breathing
☐ Indications of developing shock, including rapid and weak pulse, indicating shock from blood loss; low blood pressure; and cyanosis, indicating oxygen deficiency
☐ Coughing up bright red frothy blood, indicating a possible punctured lung
☐ Distended neck veins
☐ Tracheal deviation—The trachea is pushed off to the uninjured side.
☐ Failure of the chest wall to expand and contract normally with respirations—Look closely for unequal chest movements.
☐ Unequal air entry
☐ **Subcutaneous emphysema** (SUB-ku-TA-ne-us EM-fi-SEE-mah)—Air has escaped from a puncture in the airway or the lung and has invaded the tissues of the thorax and neck. The patient may report "crackling" sensations under the skin, or you may feel this by placing your fingers over the injury site.

Recall how the above may be determined from a complete patient assessment.

Patient Care—General Chest Injuries

Basic cardiac life support may be the only course of action for the EMT. However, other care procedures can undoubtedly help save the patient's life in many situations. Such procedures are considered for each of the specific chest injuries described on the next few pages of this chapter.

Specific Open Chest Wounds

An open wound to the chest occurs when an object tears or punctures the chest wall, opening the thoracic cavity to the atmosphere. You must consider *all* open wounds to the chest to be life threatening.

Open chest wounds are usually puncture wounds, classified as *penetrating* or *perforating*. A penetrating puncture wound is one that penetrates the chest wall once; a perforating puncture wound has both an entrance and an exit wound as, for example, many gunshot wounds. Penetrating puncture wounds include pneumothorax and impaled objects, both discussed in more detail below. The object producing the wound may remain impaled in the chest, or the wound may be completely open.

Pneumothorax When the pleural sac is punctured and air enters the thoracic cavity, a **pneumothorax** (NU-mo-THO-raks) has occurred (Figure 14-2). The air can enter through an external wound, or the air may come out of a punctured lung, or both. If air is entering through an external wound, it is an **open pneumothorax**. The delicate pressure balance within the thoracic cavity is destroyed. Air enters the space between the pleura and the lung, and the lung no longer binds to the rib cage. This causes the lung on the injured side to collapse.

Patient Assessment—Open Pneumothorax

The term **sucking chest wound** is used when the thoracic cavity is open to the atmosphere. Each time the patient breathes, air can be sucked into the opening. This patient will develop severe **dyspnea** (difficult breathing).

Signs

☐ A wound to the chest

OPEN

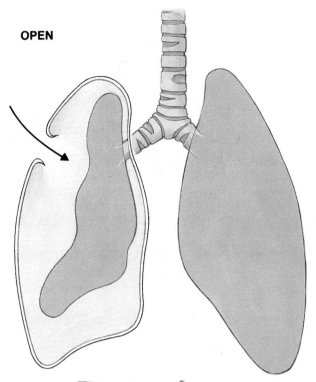

CLOSED

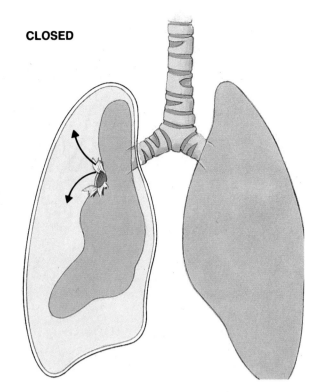

Figure 14-2 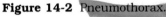 Pneumothorax.

☐ There may or may not be the characteristic sucking sound associated with a sucking chest wound.

☐ The patient may be gasping for air.

Be aware that the object that penetrated the chest wall may have seriously damaged a lung, major blood vessel, or the heart itself.

Patient Care—Open Pneumothorax

Open pneumothorax is a TRUE EMERGENCY that requires immediate initial care and transport to a medical facility as soon as possible.

Emergency Care Steps

1. Maintain an open airway. Provide basic life support if necessary.

2. Seal the open chest wound as quickly as possible. If need be, use your gloved hand. Do not delay sealing the wound to find an occlusive dressing.

3. Apply an occlusive dressing to seal the wound. When possible, the occlusive dressing should be at least two inches wider than the wound. If there is an exit wound in the chest, apply an occlusive dressing over this wound too.

There are two methods now in use. One approach, recommended in many local protocols, calls for taping the occlusive dressing in place, leaving a corner of the dressing unsealed (Figure 14-3). As the patient inhales, the dressing will seal the wound. As the patient exhales, the free corner will act as a flutter valve to release air that is trapped in the thoracic cavity.

A more traditional approach, still recommended in many local protocols, calls for sealing all four edges (Figure 14-4), the last edge being sealed when the patient forcefully exhales. If the seal is effective, respirations will be partially stabilized.

Follow local protocols as to the preferred type of dressing.

4. Administer a high concentration of oxygen.

5. Care for shock.

6. Transport as soon as possible. Unless other injuries prevent you from doing so, keep the patient positioned on the injured side. This allows the uninjured lung to expand without restriction.

On inspiration, dressing seals
wound, preventing air entry

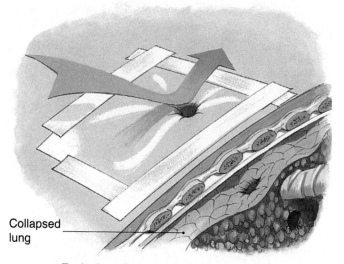

Collapsed
lung

Expiration allows trapped air to escape
through untaped section of dressing

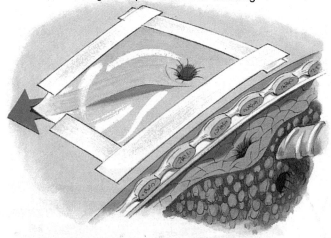

Figure 14-3 Creating a flutter valve to relieve pneumothorax.

7 Monitor the patient, making certain that the airway is open. Be prepared to suction blood from the oral cavity. Call ahead to alert the emergency department staff.

Note: Household plastic wrap is not thick enough to make an effective occlusive dressing for open chest wounds. If no other source for an occlusive dressing is available, this wrap can be used, but it must be folded several times to be of the proper thickness. Even then, it may fail. Most ambulances carry sterile disposable items that are wrapped in plastic. The inside surface of the plastic is sterile. If you do not have an occlusive dressing, use one of these wrappers or an IV bag. If there is no other choice, aluminum

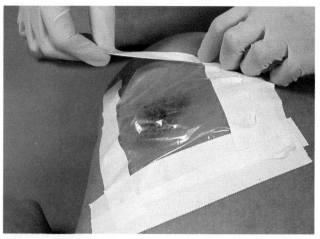

Figure 14-4 Applying an occlusive dressing for a pneumothorax, sealing all four sides.

foil can be used to make the seal. Be careful, however; foil edges may lacerate skin and may tear when lifted to release pressure.

Note: You may have to maintain hand pressure over the occlusive dressing en route to the hospital. The plastic dressings normally used are semipermeable and slowly allow air to enter. The tape also may not stick well to bloody skin or to skin that is sweaty from shock.

A complication can develop with an open pneumothorax that has been managed with the application of a sealed occlusive dressing. This complication is called **tension pneumothorax**.*

If a patient has a penetrating chest wound with a punctured lung, air will enter the thoracic cavity through the open wound in the chest wall and through the opening in the lung (Figure 14-5). If you seal off the chest wall opening, air will still flow from the punctured lung into the cavity with each breath. The air will not be able to escape and pressure will build in the cavity.

**Patient Assessment—
Tension Pneumothorax**

Signs

There are several signs of a possible tension pneumothorax.

___

* This condition also can occur if an open chest wound with a punctured lung seals itself or seals around an impaled object, or if the patient has a punctured or damaged lung with no open chest wound.

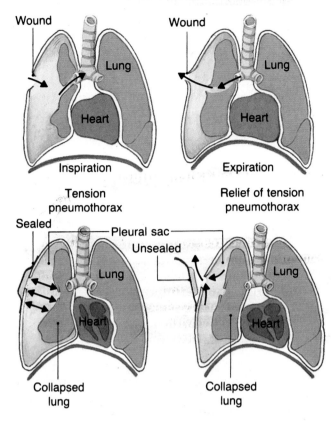

Pneumothorax with punctured lung

Wound — Lung — Heart

Inspiration

Wound — Lung — Heart

Expiration

Tension pneumothorax

Sealed — Pleural sac — Lung — Heart

Collapsed lung

Relief of tension pneumothorax

Unsealed — Lung — Heart

Collapsed lung

If patient's condition declines after sealing puncture wound, open the seal immediately

Figure 14-5 Tension pneumothorax may be a complication of open chest wound care.

- ☐ Increasing respiratory difficulty
- ☐ Indications of developing shock, including rapid, weak pulse, cyanosis, and low blood pressure due to decreased cardiac output
- ☐ Distended neck veins
- ☐ Tracheal deviation to the uninjured side
- ☐ Uneven chest wall movement
- ☐ Reduction of breathing sounds heard in the affected side of the chest (Listen with stethoscope.)
- ☐ Head, neck, and shoulders appearing dark blue or purple

Patient Care—Tension Pneumothorax

Tension pneumothorax is the reason why some medical authorities now recommend the flutter-valve occlusive dressing instead of the traditional occlusive dressing. If, instead, your local protocols recommend that you treat a

sucking chest wound with a traditional dressing sealed on all four sides and you find that the patient worsens rapidly, you will have to release hand pressure and lift a corner of the seal to let air escape. (The patient should respond almost immediately as pressure is released around the heart, great blood vessels, and uninjured lung.) Then you must reseal the wound and monitor the patient. You may have to unseal and reseal the wound again, continuing this process throughout care and transport.

Remember: Once the pneumothorax is sealed, you must continue to monitor the patient and stay alert for tension pneumothorax. Even if you use a flutter valve, you still must monitor the patient for this condition. The free corner of the dressing may stick to the chest or the dressing may be drawn into the wound, causing the valve to fail.

Impaled Objects Impaled objects were discussed in Chapter 9.

Patient Assessment—Impaled Objects

Assessment for an impaled object is generally not difficult. An object protruding from the chest is usually obvious.

Patient Care—Impaled Objects

An impaled object should be left in place. Follow the procedures below.

Emergency Care Steps

1. Stabilize the object with bulky dressings or pads (Figure 14-6).
2. Tape all dressings and pads in place. If blood or sweat prevents tape from sticking to the skin, hold the dressings or pads in place with wide cravats tied in place but not tied directly over wound sites. Make sure the object has not exited the other side of the patient's body before sliding cravats around the body.
3. If the object has passed through the patient's body from front to back, stabilize the object on the front side, then, when you roll the patient to check the back and place him on a long spine board, stabilize the object on the other side in the same manner.
4. *Do not* lay the patient on the side contain-

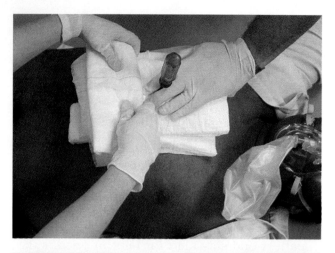

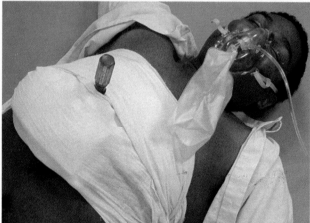

Figure 14-6 Stabilizing and dressing an object impaled in the chest.

ing the impaled object, and make certain that nothing touches the impaled object during transport. If the object has passed entirely through the body, transport the patient on his side.

Some impaled objects are much larger than shown in Figure 14-6. A motorcyclist may be propelled off his motorcycle and become impaled on a fencepost. A guard rail can penetrate the front of a car and literally pin the driver to his seat after penetrating his chest wall. Emergency care is basically the same, with the following additions.

1. Control bleeding as quickly and safely as possible while ensuring that the object does not move, nor the patient move in relation to the object, and cause further rupturing or tearing of organs or large blood vessels

2. The impaled object must be cut approxi-

mately 6 inches from where it enters the body, then stabilized.

3. If the object has passed completely through the patient, use the same procedures for both entry and exit wounds.

4. Remember that there will undoubtedly be great loss of blood, both internal and external. Treat for severe shock, administer a high concentration of oxygen, and transport as quickly as possible.

Specific Closed Chest Injuries

Closed chest injuries include rib fractures, flail chest (Figure 14-7), and compression injuries.

Rib Fractures Rib fractures usually result from blunt trauma or compression. The pain of a rib fracture can severely decrease the volume of air the patient is able to breathe in. In addition, if an intercostal artery is severed, it can quickly fill the chest cavity with blood (see the discussion of hemothorax later in this chapter).

Patient Assessment—Fractured Ribs

Often, you will not know for sure if a rib is fractured; however, some ribs are more susceptible to injury than others. The upper four pairs of ribs are rarely fractured because they are protected by the structures of the shoulder girdle. The fifth through tenth pairs of ribs are the ones most commonly fractured. The freedom of movement found in the "floating" ribs often prevents them from being fractured. A conscious, coherent person with fractured ribs can usually point out the exact injury site. Seldom is there any deformity associated with the injury.

Signs and Symptoms

The signs and symptoms of fractured ribs include

- Pain at the site of the fracture, with increased pain on moving and breathing
- Tenderness over the site of the fracture
- Shallow breathing, usually due to the pain associated with respiratory movements of the chest
- Sometimes the patient will report a crackling sensation (subcutaneous emphysema) at or near the site of fracture. You may be able to feel this by placing your fingertips over the injury site. This indicates a complication in the form of a pneumothorax.

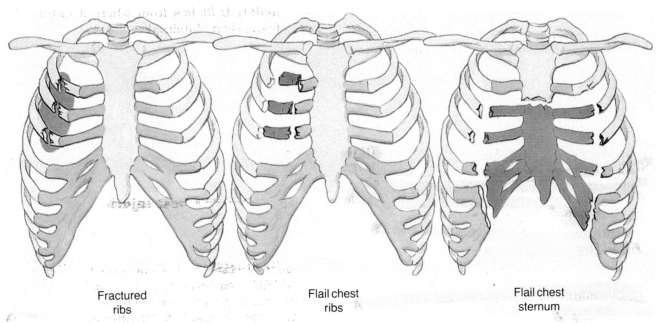

Fractured ribs   Flail chest ribs   Flail chest sternum

Figure 14-7 Rib fractures and flail chest.

☐ Characteristic stance, with the patient leaning toward the injured side and holding his hand over the fracture site (self-splinting)

Patient Care—Fractured Ribs

Always render care when the signs and symptoms indicate possible fractured ribs. Although a rib fracture may not be a serious injury, you will probably help to reduce the patient's pain and, since you will not be able to tell if the patient's injury is limited to a "simple rib fracture," you will want to provide protection for his lungs and the blood vessels that are located between the ribs (intercostal arteries and veins).

Emergency Care Steps

To provide care for possible fractured ribs

1. Position one cravat around the middle of the patient's chest. Place padding on the uninjured side and tie the cravat over top of the pad.
2. Position, pad, and tie a second cravat around the lower chest.
3. Secure a third cravat in the same manner around the upper chest.
4. Place the forearm of the injured side across the patient's chest. Apply a fourth cravat as a swathe to support the angle of the arm.

Note: Some EMS systems do not follow the above protocol. They have their EMTs apply a sling and swathe for patients with possible rib fractures (Figure 14-8). In a few localities, no action other than positioning for comfort and

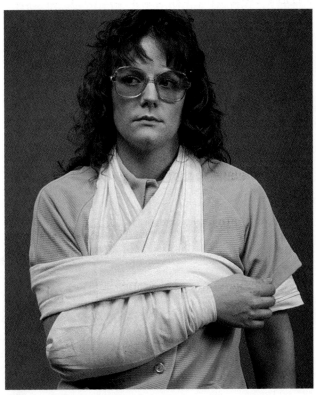

Figure 14-8 Care for fractured ribs. Apply sling and swathe to hold the arm against the chest.

transport is done for possible rib fractures. This is because some emergency department physicians fear that tied cravats will impair respiration. (Taping the chest also restricts respiratory movement.) If you use the tied cravat method, make certain that the patient is breathing comfortably.

Flail Chest There are two kinds of **flail chest**. (1) Flail chest usually occurs when three or more consecutive ribs on the same side of the chest are fractured, each in at least two places. (2) The second kind of flail chest occurs when the sternum is broken away from its cartilage attachments with the ribs.

Either kind of flail chest, of the ribs or the sternum, produces a section of chest wall that is unstable and will move independently of the rest of the chest wall. Often, this movement is in the opposite direction to the rest of the chest wall. This is known as **paradoxical motion** (sometimes incorrectly called paradoxical respirations). (Figure 14-9).

Patient Assessment—Flail Chest

EMTs see flail chest most often at motor vehicle collisions, usually caused by the patient being forced against the vehicle's steering wheel. The flail section usually occurs to the lateral chest wall or the sternum. Forceful blows to the back also may cause a flail chest, with damage usually being done to the lateral chest walls.

Signs and Symptoms

The signs and symptoms of flail chest include

- ☐ The signs and symptoms of fractured ribs. These are usually more pronounced with flail chest.
- ☐ The failure of a section of the chest wall to move with the rest of the chest when the patient is breathing. Typically, paradoxical motion is observed.
- ☐ The signs and symptoms of shock

Patient Care—Flail Chest

You must try to hold the flail section in place. Do not attempt to bind, strap, or apply tape directly to the injured section of ribs or the

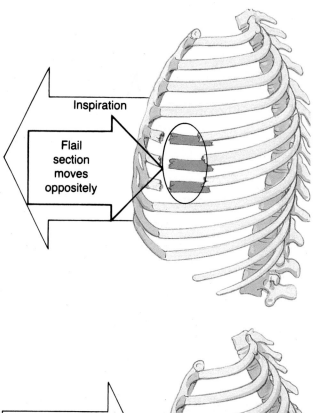

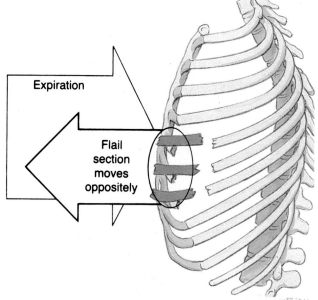

Figure 14-9 Paradoxical motion.

loose sternum. Instead, stabilize the flailed section.

Emergency Care Steps

To care for the flail chest patient, you should

1. Carefully locate the edges of the flail section by gently feeling the injury site.
2. Apply a thick pad of dressings over the site. This pad should be several inches thick. A small pillow can be used in place

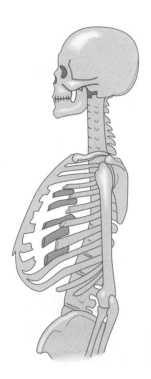

6. Monitor the patient, taking extra care to look for signs of heart, lung, or abdominal organ injury.

7. Transport as soon as possible with the patient in a semi-reclined position. If the patient cannot tolerate this position, gently place him on the injured side. This will help the flailed section move with the rest of the chest and reduce rubbing together of the broken ends of the ribs. The patient will be more comfortable and will be able to breathe more easily as the uninjured lung is free to rise and fall with respiration.

Warning: ALL cases of flail chest are very serious emergencies and must be viewed as life threatening. Even the patient who appears stabilized may rapidly develop severe respiratory problems and shock. Often the severity of other internal injuries is not immediately noticed. Closely monitor the flail chest patient.

Complications of Chest Injuries

In accidents involving the chest, the lungs, heart, and great vessels can be injured. Such injuries can result in serious complications, including hemothorax, hemopneumothorax, cardiac tamponade, traumatic asphyxia, closed tension pneumothorax, and spontaneous pneumothorax. Below are descriptions and assessment guidelines for each of these complications, followed by a set of care guidelines for them all.

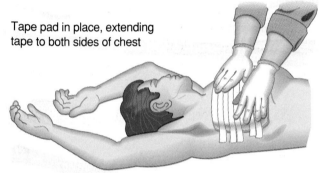

Tape pad in place, extending tape to both sides of chest

Figure 14-10 Care for flail chest.

of the pad of dressings, or other low-weight items can also be used, depending on the location of the flailed section and the position of the patient.

3. Use large strips of tape to hold the pad in place. (Place the tape as shown in Figure 14-10.) The tension on the tape bears down on the pad, which in turn depresses the flail section. If tape will not hold, do not be tempted to wrap the tape around the entire body, which will restrict respiration. Instead, hold the pad in place with light hand pressure from your gloved hand or place the patient on the injured side.

4. Administer a high concentration of oxygen. Assisted ventilation may be necessary.

5. Care for shock.

Hemothorax and Hemopneumothorax It is easy to distinguish these two complications from pneumothorax (Figure 14-11) if you remember that *pneumo* means "air" and *hemo* means "blood." In pneumothorax, there was a buildup of air in the thorax. In hemothorax and hemopneumothorax, blood creates or adds to the pressure buildup.

In **hemothorax** (HE-mo-THOR-aks), lacerations within the thoracic cavity can be produced by penetrating objects or fractured ribs. Blood will flow into the pleural space, the lung may collapse, and the heart may be forced against the uninjured lung. **Hemopneumothorax** (HE-mo-NU-mo-THOR-aks) is a combination of blood and air, usually producing the same results: a collapsed lung and pressure on the heart and uninjured lung.

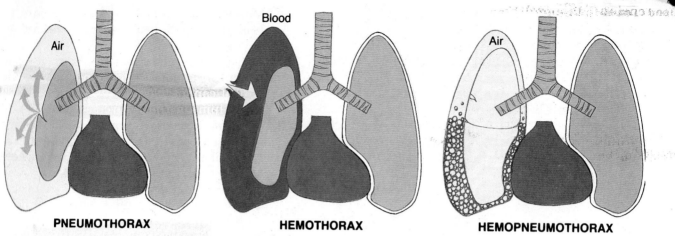

Figure 14-11 Conditions produced by chest injuries.

PNEUMOTHORAX **HEMOTHORAX** **HEMOPNEUMOTHORAX**

Patient Assessment— Hemothorax and Hemopneumothorax

Signs

☐ Hemothorax and hemopneumothorax usually present the same signs as pneumothorax, including dyspnea and a possible sucking wound.

☐ In addition, the patient may cough up frothy red blood, or flecks of blood may appear on the lips.

Cardiac Tamponade When a penetrating or blunt injury to the heart causes blood to flow into the surrounding pericardial sac, the condition produced is **cardiac tamponade** (CAR-de-ak TAM-po-NADE). The heart's unyielding sac fills with blood and compresses the chambers of the heart to a point where they will no longer fill adequately, backing up blood into the veins.

Patient Assessment—Cardiac Tamponade

Signs

☐ Distended neck veins
☐ Very weak pulse
☐ Profuse sweating
☐ Steadily decreasing **pulse pressure**. Pulse pressure is the difference between systolic and diastolic readings. When the two readings approach each other (systolic falling, diastolic rising or unchanging), it is a reliable sign of serious thoracic cavity injury. A pulse pressure below 15 mmHg is critical. This is life threatening, a TRUE EMERGENCY. Let the hospital know your estimated time of arrival.

Traumatic Asphyxia One aspect of what is known as acute thoracic compression syndrome is **traumatic asphyxia** (traw-MAT-ik a-SFIKS-e-ah). It is not a condition but a group of signs and symptoms that can be associated with sudden compression of the chest and, in some cases, the abdomen. When this occurs, the sternum exerts severe pressure on the heart, forcing blood out of the right atrium up into the jugular veins in the neck.

Patient Assessment—Traumatic Asphyxia

Signs and Symptoms

The signs and symptoms of traumatic asphyxia are shown in Figure 14-12. This is a TRUE EMERGENCY.

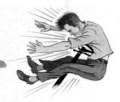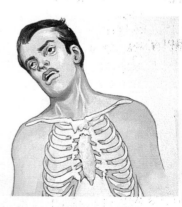

- Distended neck veins
- Head, neck, and shoulders appear dark blue or purple
- Eyes may be bloodshot and bulging
- Tongue and lips may appear swollen and cyanotic
- Chest deformity may be present

Figure 14-12 Signs and symptoms of traumatic asphyxia.

Closed Tension Pneumothorax Tension pneumothorax can arise in two ways. The first way was discussed above: In an *open chest injury*, air escapes from a punctured lung into the thoracic cavity and is trapped by an occlusive dressing. Tension pneumothorax can also occur in a second way: In a *closed chest injury*, a lung is punctured (e.g., by a fractured rib). Air builds up within the closed thoracic cavity, quickly impairing heart and lung function.

Patient Assessment—
Closed Tension Pneumothorax

Signs

The signs of closed tension pneumothorax include

- ☐ Increasing respiratory difficulty
- ☐ A weak pulse
- ☐ Cyanosis
- ☐ Low blood pressure as a result of decreased cardiac output
- ☐ Breath sounds possibly abnormal
- ☐ Unequal air entry
- ☐ Neck veins possibly distended
- ☐ Trachea possibly deviated to the uninjured side (a late sign)

Note: Closed tension pneumothorax cannot be relieved by releasing an occlusive dressing. There is no way for the air pressure to escape. This is a TRUE EMERGENCY.

Spontaneous Pneumothorax When a weakened section of the lung ruptures and releases air into the thoracic cavity, **spontaneous pneumothorax** results. This is usually a medical condition (see Chapter 15) but can also result from trauma.

Patient Assessment—
Spontaneous Pneumothorax

Signs

- ☐ Breath sounds will usually be decreased on the injured side.

Spontaneous pneumothorax is almost never life threatening, but it can become tension pneumothorax and require the same basic care.

Patient Care—
Complications of Chest Injuries

Except for flail chest, sucking chest wounds, and tension pneumothorax caused by an occlusive dressing, (the care for which was discussed earlier in this chapter), there is little the EMT can do for major chest injury complications such as hemothorax, hemopneumothorax, cardiac tamponade, traumatic asphyxia, closed tension pneumothorax, and spontaneous pneumothorax.

Emergency Care Steps

Realizing that most major chest injury complications are TRUE EMERGENCIES, provide the following care.

1. Provide immediate transport.
2. Administer 100% oxygen. It may be necessary to assist ventilations with a bag-valve-mask unit with a reservoir system. Use positive pressure when needed.

Providing the above basic life support measures may be all that you can do and may keep the patient alive until more advanced medical procedures can be delivered by the staff of the medical facility.

Warning: The use of positive pressure ventilation on patients with closed chest injuries requires approval by local medical control. Too great a pressure may cause a tension pneumothorax to develop or rapidly worsen an existing case of tension pneumothorax. Some EMS Systems have decided that the bag-valve-mask unit with an oxygen reservoir is more advisable than oxygen-powered breathing devices. Follow local guidelines.

INJURIES TO THE ABDOMEN

The more you know about the structures of the abdomen and their locations, the better able you will be to evaluate injuries in this region. Referred pain often originates with injuries or medical conditions in the abdomen. This means that pain may be felt in an area other than the site of injury. Damage to the appendix through disease or injury may be expressed as pain around the umbilicus. Injury or disease of the gallbladder may be felt as pain on the back of the right shoulder (see Chapter 16).

The abdominal organs can be classified as hollow or solid. Hollow organs are prone to bursting if they are full when abdominal compression takes place.The hollow organs are

- *Stomach*—where the initial chemical breakdown of foods begins
- *Small Intestine*—where chemical digestion is completed and absorption of foods take place
- *Large Intestine*—where the collection and removal of the wastes from digestion occurs. The large intestine includes the *colon, rectum,* and *anus.*
- *Appendix*—hollow fingerlike tube located at the beginning of the large intestine. It has no proven function.
- *Gallbladder*—a pear-shaped reservoir for bile, located on the posterior undersurface of the liver.

The solid organs are

- *Liver*—a large, multifunctional gland in the right upper quadrant, protected by the lower ribs. Its dome-shaped top presses against the diaphragm. Extremely vascular (containing many blood vessels), the liver is a delicate gland that can be easily torn by blunt impact or cut by penetrating objects. The resultant bleeding can be massive and quickly fatal. Injury may release bile into the abdominal cavity causing a severe reaction. The liver is essential to life.
- *Spleen*—a highly vascular organ located behind the stomach and protected by the lower ribs on the left side of the body. The spleen is involved with blood storage and the removal of old blood cells. It is vulnerable to rupture as a result of blunt trauma to the abdomen.
- *Pancreas*—an elongated, flat triangular gland located behind the stomach. It is involved with producing digestive juices and insulin. Serious injury to the pancreas is not common in accidents, but damage is seen in cases of kicking injuries, impacts with steering wheels, stabbings, and gunshot wounds. When injured, as in abdominal gunshot wounds, the pancreas can bleed profusely and release digestive juices into the abdomen. The pancreas is essential to life.

As you consider the names, functions, and locations of the organs and glands in the abdom-inal cavity, do not forget that this region has many blood vessels and nerves. In addition to these structures, there are many sensitive membranes in the cavity.

A large, fat-filled membrane attaches to the stomach and spreads downward like an apron over top of the intestine. It is called the *greater omentum* (o-MEN-tum) and may be seen as a yellowish, spongy tissue pushing out through open abdominal wounds.

The small and large intestines are attached to the posterior wall of the cavity by a membrane called the *mesentery* (MES-en-ter-e). This membrane is rich with blood vessels. A penetrating object may slide off the intestine, then lacerate many of the mesenteric blood vessels.

All these membranes are part of the major membrane that lines the abdominal cavity and covers the abdominal organs, the *peritoneum* (per-i-to-NE-um). This membrane is very susceptible to serious infection when the abdomen is opened or the intestines rupture. If bile or other digestive juices, partially digested foods, or free blood comes into contact with the peritoneum, a reaction of severe pain and abdominal wall muscle spasms usually occurs (*peritonitis*).

Types of Abdominal Injuries

Abdominal injuries can be open or closed, with closed injury usually due to blunt trauma. Internal bleeding can be severe if organs and major blood vessels are lacerated or ruptured. Very serious and painful reactions can occur when the hollow organs are ruptured and their contents leak into the abdominal cavity. *Penetrating wounds* to the abdomen can be caused by objects such as knives, ice picks, arrows, and the broken glass and twisted metal of vehicular collisions and structural accidents. Very serious *perforating wounds* can be caused by bullets (Figure 14-13), even when the bullet is of low caliber (small).

Patient Assessment—Abdominal Injuries

Although some persons believe otherwise, gunshot wounds without exit wounds can cause serious abdominal damage, just as those with exit wounds do. Another misconception about bullet wounds is that internal damage can be assessed easily. On the contrary, any projectile entering the body can be deflected, or it can explode and send out pieces in many directions. Do not believe that

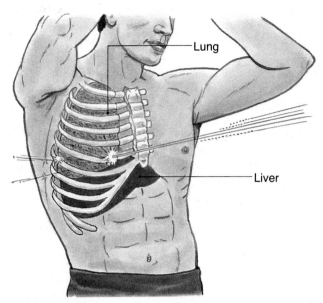

Figure 14-13 The damage done by gunshot wounds cannot be fully assessed in field emergency care.

only the structures directly under the entrance wound have been injured. Also, keep in mind that the pathway of a bullet between entrance wound and exit wound is seldom a straight line.

Complicating the problem even more is the fact that penetrating abdominal wounds can be associated with wounds in adjacent areas of the body. For example, a bullet can enter the thoracic cavity, pierce the diaphragm, and cause widespread damage in the abdomen. A complete patient survey is essential in determining the probable extent of injuries.

Remember: *Always* check for an exit wound.

Signs and Symptoms

The signs of abdominal injury can include

☐ Obvious lacerations and puncture wounds to the abdomen
☐ Lacerations and puncture wounds to the pelvis and middle and lower back or chest wounds near the diaphragm
☐ Indications of blunt trauma, such as a large bruised area or an intense bruise on the abdomen
☐ Indications of developing shock, including restlessness, delayed capillary refill, rapid shallow breathing, a rapid pulse, and low

blood pressure. (Sometimes patients with abdominal injury who are in extreme pain show an initial elevated blood pressure.)
☐ Coughing up or vomiting blood—The vomitus may contain a substance that looks like coffee grounds (partially digested blood).
☐ Rigid and/or tender abdomen—The patient tries to protect the abdomen (guarded abdomen).
☐ The patient tries to lie very still, with the legs drawn up in an effort to reduce the tension on the abdominal muscles.

The symptoms of abdominal injury can include

☐ Pain, often starting as mild pain then rapidly becoming intolerable
☐ Cramps
☐ Nausea
☐ Weakness
☐ Thirst

In Chapter 3, the methods used for palpating the abdomen were described. Remember to assess the patient for abdominal rigidity (firmness), tenderness, and distention.

Patient Care—Abdominal Injuries

Some emergency care steps apply to both closed and open abdominal injuries. Some additional care steps are necessary for open abdominal injuries.

Emergency Care Steps

For *both closed and open* abdominal injuries

1 Stay alert for vomiting and keep an open airway.
2 Place the patient on his back, legs flexed at the knees, to reduce pain by relaxing abdominal muscles.
3 Administer a high concentration of oxygen.
4 Care for shock.
5 Apply anti-shock garments if indicated and local protocols recommend
6 Give nothing to the patient by mouth. This may induce vomiting or pass through open wounds in the esophagus or stomach and enter the abdominal cavity.
7 Constantly monitor vital signs.
8 Transport as soon as possible.

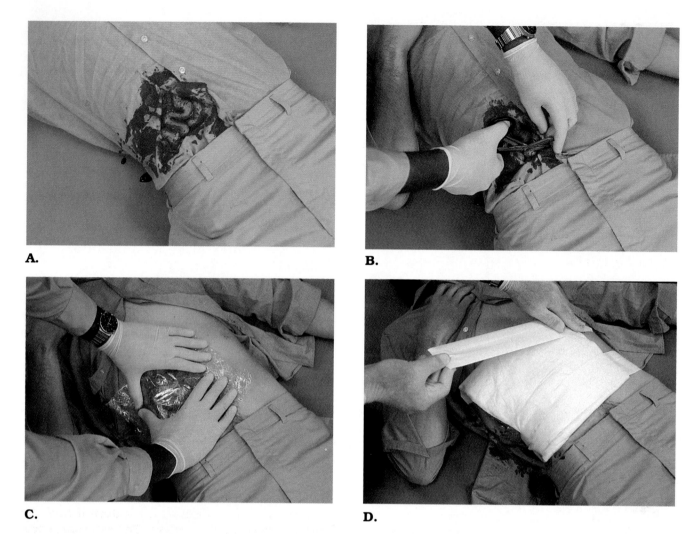

Figure 14-14 A. Open abdominal wound with evisceration. B. Cut away clothing from wound. C. Apply an occlusive dressing and tape in place. D. Cover occlusive dressing to maintain warmth. Secure covering with tape or cravats tied above and below position of exposed organ. *Note:* A saline-soaked dressing may be applied before the occlusive dressing if local protocols recommend.

In addition, for *open* abdominal injuries

1. Control external bleeding and dress all open wounds.
2. *Do not* touch or try to replace any **eviscerated**, or exposed, organs (Figure 14-14). If local protocols recommend it, apply a sterile dressing moistened with sterile saline over the wound site before you apply an occlusive dressing. Cover exposed organs with an occlusive dressing and maintain warmth by placing layers of bulky dressing or a lint-free towel over the occlusive dressing. (**WARNING:** *Do not* use aluminum foil. Aluminum foil occlusive dressings have been found to cut eviscerated organs.)
3. *Do not* remove any impaled objects. Stabilize impaled objects with bulky dressings that are bandaged in place. Leave the patient's legs in the position in which you found them to avoid muscular movement that may move the impaled object.

Note: If the patient has symptoms suggestive of heart attack, serious respiratory disorder, serious abdominal injury, or digestive disorder, you should assume that the patient has more serious problems, care for shock, and transport as soon as possible.

INJURIES TO THE PELVIS AND GROIN

The major structures housed in the pelvis include the urinary bladder, the end portions of the large intestine (including the rectum), and the internal reproductive organs. These structures are reasonably well protected, but they can be injured by intense blunt trauma, crushing injuries of the pelvis, the movement of fractured pelvic bones, and gunshot wounds and other penetrating injuries.

Injuries to the Urinary System

The urinary system (Figure 14-15) includes the *kidneys*, which filter out wastes from the bloodstream and make urine; the *ureters* (u-RE-ters), with one connecting each kidney to the urinary bladder; the *urinary bladder*, which serves as a reservoir for urine; and the *urethra* (u-RE-thrah), through which urine is expelled from the bladder.

The kidneys are not abdominal or pelvic organs. They are located behind the abdominal cavity (retroperitoneal). Severe blows to the back or abdomen can cause kidney damage.

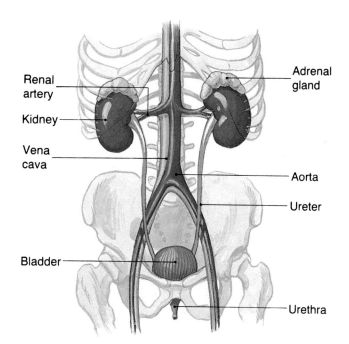

Figure 14-15 The urinary system.

Patient Assessment— Urinary System Injuries

Kidney damage cannot be determined by the EMT, even after a complete and proper patient survey. Likewise, damage to the urinary bladder, although severe, may not be evident to the EMT. The pain experienced by the patient cannot be specifically said to be from the kidneys or the bladder.

Signs and Symptoms

☐ Back or flank pain following blunt trauma indicates possible spinal injury and kidney damage.

☐ Blood in the urine indicates serious problems within the urinary system.

☐ Blood discharged from the urethra indicates a possible fractured pelvis.

Patient Care—Urinary System Injuries

If any of the signs or symptoms of spinal, kidney, or urinary system injury are present, manage care as if for a combination of spinal injury (see Chapter 12) and closed abdominal injury (above). If a fractured pelvis is suspected, treat accordingly (see Chapter 11).

Injuries to the Reproductive System

Injury can occur to both the external and the internal reproductive organs. The external reproductive organs are often referred to as the **genitalia** (jen-i-TAY-le-ah). More injuries occur to these structures than to the internal reproductive organs, because of the protection to internal organs offered by the bones of the pelvis. However, because of the location of the external reproductive organs, injuries are not common.

Patient Assessment— Reproductive System Injuries

See descriptions of injuries to the male and female reproductive systems in Scan 14-1.

Patient Care— Reproductive System Injuries

See Scan 14-1.

Note: Inappropriate management of genital injuries can be embarrassing to the patient. Approach the problem in a professional man-

The Reproductive System

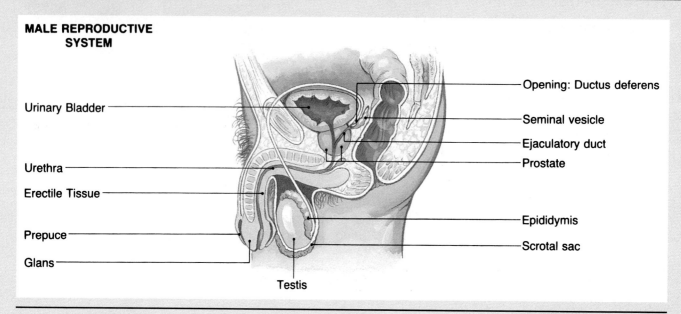

MALE REPRODUCTIVE SYSTEM

Urinary Bladder

Urethra

Erectile Tissue

Prepuce

Glans

Testis

Opening: Ductus deferens

Seminal vesicle

Ejaculatory duct

Prostate

Epididymis

Scrotal sac

STRUCTURE	INJURY	CARE
Scrotum (SKRO-tum) surrounds and protects the testes	Blunt trauma	Padded ice pack, transport.
	Lacerations and avulsions (rare)	Direct pressure, dressing, and triangular bandage applied like diaper. Keep avulsed parts moist, wrapped, and cool.
Testes (TES-tez) produce sperm cells and male hormone	Blunt trauma Lacerations and avulsions (rare)	Same as scrotum Same as scrotum
Spermatic (sper-MAT-ic) cords: suspend testes, contain blood vessels, nerves, and vas deferens (vas DEF-er-en's) which transport sperm.	Blunt trauma Lacerations (rare)	Same as scrotum Same as scrotum
Prostate (PROS-tat) gland: produces seminal fluids	Rare, usually gunshot wounds	Pressure dressing, treat for shock, oxygen, apply PASG when approropriate.
Seminal vesicles: store seminal fluids	Rare, usually gunshot wounds	Same as prostate
Penis Erectile organ containing the urethra	Blunt trauma Lacerations and avulsions (also called amputation), self-mutilation	Same as scrotum Same as scrotum
	Blunt trauma of the erect penis (known as "fracture")	Padded ice pack and transport.

FEMALE REPRODUCTIVE SYSTEM

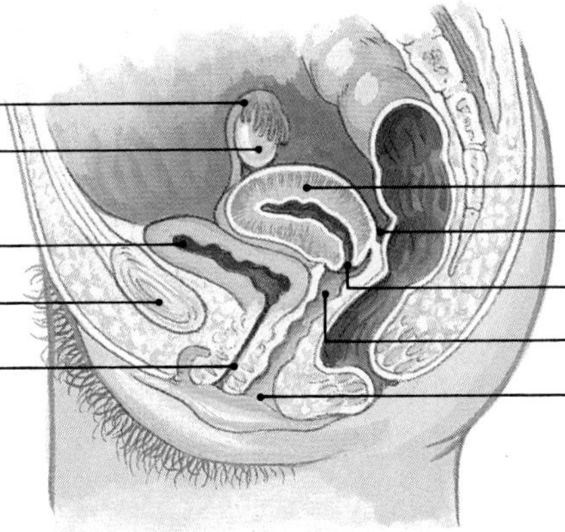

Fallopian (uterine) tube

Ovary

Bladder

Pubis

Urethra

Uterus

Pouch of Douglas

Cervix

Fornix

Vagina

STRUCTURE	INJURY	CARE
Vulva (VUL-vah); external genitalia	Blunt trauma	Padded ice pack, transport.
	Lacerations and avulsions	Sanitary napkin and triangular bandage applied like a diaper. Keep avulsed parts moist, wrapped, and cool.
Vagina (birth canal)	Lacerations (seen in rape, self-mutilation cases, abortion attempts)	External application of sanitary napkin and triangular bandage.
Uterus (U-ter-us) womb for the developing baby (fetus)	Rupture due to extreme blunt trauma or crushing injury	Unable to tell in field that specific organ is injured. Vaginal bleeding is often profuse. Treat as internal injury with internal bleeding; apply sanitary napkin and triangular dressing over vaginal opening. This is a **true emergency**. Apply PASG garment when appropriate.
	Lacerations (rare) usually due to gunshot or stab wound, abortion attempts	Treat as penetrating or perforating wound. Vaginal bleeding may or may not be seen. Apply PASG when appropriate.
Oviducts (O-vi-dukt's) or fallopian (fah-LO-pe-an) tubes: carry egg (ovum) from the ovary to the uterus	Lacerations (rare), usually due to gunshot wound	Treat as penetrating or perforating wound. Vaginal bleeding is usually not seen. Apply PASG when appropriate
Ovaries (O-vah-re's) produce female hormones and ova (O-vah) or eggs	Lacerations and puncture wounds (rare), usually due to gunshot or stab wounds	Treat as penetrating or perforating wound. Associated vaginal bleeding is not likely. Apply PASG when appropriate

407

ner. Decide on a course of action and then act with authority as a member of the professional health care team. Timid, hesitant movements will only add to the patient's embarrassment. Explain what you are going to do and why, then provide care with no hesitation. Protect the patient from the stares of onlookers. When emergency care measures are completed, cover the patient with a sheet.

Inguinal Hernia Commonly called a "rupture," the **inguinal** (IN-gwin-al) **hernia** occurs when abdominal membranes and part of the intestine bulge through a defect in the abdominal wall (Figure 14-16), usually as a result of severe muscle strain from an activity such as lifting, pushing, or jumping. The hernia may occur in the wall of the abdomen or in the groin area.

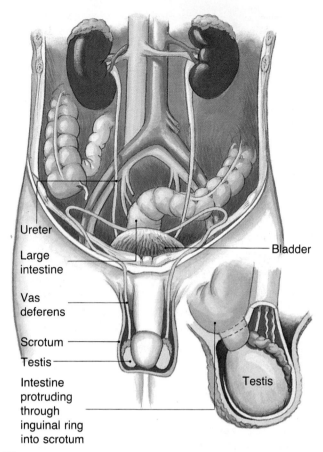

Figure 14-16 An inguinal hernia.

Patient Assessment—Inguinal Hernia

Signs and Symptoms

- ☐ Sharp pain
- ☐ A feeling of something giving way internally
- ☐ Possible nausea or vomiting
- ☐ Swelling at the site
- ☐ Tenderness at the site

Note: The patient may experience little or no pain or discomfort but may notice swelling at the site as the first sign.

Patient Care—Inguinal Hernia

Emergency Care Steps

1. *Do not* attempt to push the hernia back inside the abdominal wall. Internal injury could result.
2. Keep the victim lying quiet and still. Patient positioning is important to reduce pain. Let the patient assume a position that feels most comfortable. First suggest that he try lying on his back. Next, try to tilt the patient's body slightly so that he is in a head-low position. Should the pain remain too severe for the patient, try placing a pillow under his knees or let him draw his knees up. If pain is still intense, have the patient turn over onto his stomach and assume a knee-chest position by drawing the knees up until they rest against the chest.
3. Apply an ice pack wrapped in a towel to the site.
4. Monitor vital signs.
5. Since the blood supply to the intestine can be shut off due to constriction (strangulated hernia), transport is required for all hernia patients. (Keep in mind that the most favorable position for the patient's comfort may not be possible during transport to ensure patient safety.)

KEY TERMS

You may find it helpful to review the following terms.

cardiac tamponade (TAM-po-NADE)—condition when a penetrating or blunt injury to the heart causes blood to flow into the surrounding pericardial sac and compress the heart.

dyspnea (disp-NE-ah)—difficult breathing.

eviscerated (e-VIS-er-a-ted)—the condition of an intestine or other internal organ protruding through an incision or wound in the abdomen.

flail chest—injury in which usually three or more consecutive ribs on the same side of the chest are fractured, each in at least two locations. A flail chest also can occur when the sternum is fractured loose from its attachments with the ribs. This is sometimes referred to as a flailed sternum.

genitalia (jen-i-TAY-le-ah)—the external reproductive system.

hemopneumothorax (HE-mo-NU-mo-THOR-aks)—a combination of blood and air in the thoracic cavity.

hemothorax (HE-mo-THOR-aks)—blood in the thoracic cavity.

inguinal (IN-gwin-al) **hernia**—a soft tissue injury in which the abdominal membranes and part of the intestine bulge through a defect in the abdominal wall.

open pneumothorax (NU-mo-THOR-aks)—condition in which air is entering the thoracic cavity through an external wound.

paradoxical (pair-uh-DOKS-i-kal) **motion**—movement of a flailed section in the opposite direction to the rest of the chest during respirations.

pneumothorax (NU-mo-THO-raks)—condition resulting when air enters the thoracic cavity from an open wound or from a damaged lung or both. See also *open pneumothorax, spontaneous pneumothorax,* and *tension pneumothorax.*

pulse pressure—the difference between systolic and diastolic readings. When the two readings approach each other (systolic falling, diastolic rising or unchanging), it is a reliable sign of serious thoracic cavity injury.

spontaneous (spon-TAIN-e-us) **pneumothorax** (NU-mo-THOR-aks)—condition when a weakened section of the lung ruptures and releases air into the thoracic cavity.

subcutaneous (SUB-ku-TA-ne-us) **emphysema** (EM-fi-SEE-mah)—air under the skin. This is observed most frequently when a lung is punctured and air escapes into the surrounding tissues of the thorax.

sucking chest wound—an open wound to the chest that draws air from the atmosphere into the chest cavity. This is a form of pneumothorax.

tension pneumothorax (NU-mo-THOR-aks)—condition in which air is trapped in the thoracic cavity. In some cases, the air may enter through a sucking chest wound and be trapped as the wound seals itself shut. In *closed tension pneumothorax,* the air escapes from a damaged lung and there is no external wound through which it can escape. Tension pneumothorax may produce rapid death.

traumatic (traw-MAT-ik) **asphyxia** (a-SFIKS-e-ah)—a group of signs and symptoms associated with sudden severe compression of the chest and, in some cases, the abdomen. When this occurs, the sternum exerts severe pressure on the heart, forcing blood out of the right atrium up into the jugular veins in the neck.

SUMMARY

In studying injuries to the chest, abdomen, pelvis, and groin, it is important to be familiar with the anatomy of these areas and the locations of the major organs.

Injuries to the Chest

The chest can be injured by blunt trauma, penetrating objects, or compression. Chest injuries can be open or closed (with or without penetration of the chest wall). General signs and symptoms of chest injury include an obvious open wound and/or pain, breathing problems, shock, coughing up blood, distended neck veins, tracheal deviation, abnormal or unequal chest expansions, unequal air entry, or subcutaneous emphysema (air in the tissues of the thorax or neck).

Pneumothorax is air in the thoracic cavity. The air can come through an open wound (creating a "sucking chest wound" through which air is pulled in from the outside), from a damaged lung, or both. When the air comes from an open wound, it is an open pneumothorax. When the air cannot escape the thoracic cavity—whether because an occlusive dressing has blocked escape or because there is no opening to the outside through the chest wall—tension pneumothorax develops. Tension pneumothorax is a true emergency; it can lead quickly to death. For this reason, occlusive dressings over open chest wounds must either have a flutter valve at one corner or must be released by hand as necessary (according to local protocols) and, in either case, monitored carefully.

An object impaled in the chest must be stabilized in place with bulky dressings, never removed.

Fractured ribs can be indicated by pain, tenderness, shallow breathing, subcutaneous emphysema (a crackling sensation near the fracture), or self-splinting (the patient holds his arm or hand over the fracture). Depending on local protocols, fractured ribs may be treated with pads and cravats, a sling and swathe, or simply positioning the patient for comfort during transportation.

Flail chest is a section of ribs or the sternum that has broken free from the rest of the rib cage. In addition to the above signs and symptoms of fractured ribs, the flailed section will fail to move with the rest of the chest or will move in an opposite direction (paradoxical motion). There will be signs and symptoms of shock. A flail section is usually treated by holding it in place with padding secured over the site. The patient is given a high concentration of oxygen, monitored for shock and signs and symptoms of heart, lung, or abdominal injury, and transported.

Complications of chest injury include hemothorax (blood in the thoracic cavity), hemopneumothorax (blood and air in the thoracic cavity), cardiac tamponade (blood forced into the pericardial sac), traumatic asphyxia (a syndrome of signs and symptoms associated with severe compression injury, with blood forced out of the heart into the jugular veins), closed tension pneumothorax (in which there is no external wound through which air trapped in the thoracic cavity can escape), and spontaneous pneumothorax (pneumothorax resulting when a weakened section of lung ruptures spontaneously.

The signs and symptoms of such complications vary from those of pneumothorax to coughing up bloody froth, distended neck veins, cyanosis (bluish color), weak pulse, and signs of shock, among others.

The EMT can follow specific care procedures that include dressing and stabilizing open chest wounds, impaled objects, fractured ribs, and flail chest. For the other complications of chest injury, there is little the EMT can do beyond providing basic life support, administering oxygen and assisting ventilations if necessary, and providing immediate transport.

Injuries to the Abdomen

The signs of abdominal injury may include obvious wounds, bruises, signs of shock, coughing up or vomiting blood, rigid or tender abdomen, or legs drawn up. Symptoms can include pain, cramps, nausea, weakness, or thirst.

To provide emergency care for abdominal injuries, stay alert for vomiting and maintain an open airway. Place the patient in a supine position, knees flexed. Administer a high concentration of oxygen, and care for shock. Monitor vital signs and transport. For open abdominal injuries, also dress open wounds, cover eviscerated organs with an occlusive dressing, and stabilize any impaled objects.

Injuries to the Pelvis and Groin

Signs and symptoms of urinary system injuries include back or flank pain (indicating kidney damage) and blood in the urine. Blood discharged from the urethra indicates a possible fractured pelvis. Assume possible spinal injury and treat as if for a combination of spinal injury and closed abdominal injury. Treat for a fractured pelvis if indicated.

Most injuries to the genitalia (external reproductive organs) are blunt trauma injuries. Lacerations and avulsions are rare. Injuries to the internal reproductive organs usually result from gunshot or stab wounds or severe blunt trauma. In females, internal reproductive injuries may result from rape or abortion attempts. External injuries are dressed and cared for as for other soft tissue injuries. Internal injuries cannot easily be assessed by the EMT. Treat for shock, monitor vital signs, and transport.

Inguinal hernia (abdominal membranes or intestines bulging through a defect in the abdominal wall) may be indicated by pain and swelling or, at times, by swelling alone. Position the patient for comfort, apply a wrapped ice pack, monitor vital signs, and transport.

Remember: In treating injuries to the pelvis and groin, inappropriate management of genital injuries can be embarrassing to the patient. Approach the problem in a professional manner. Decide on a course of action and then act with authority as a member of the professional health care team. Timid, hesitant movements will only add to the patient's embarrassment. Explain what you are going to do and why, then provide care with no hesitation. Protect the patient from the stares of onlookers. When emergency care measures are completed, cover the patient with a sheet.

On the Scene

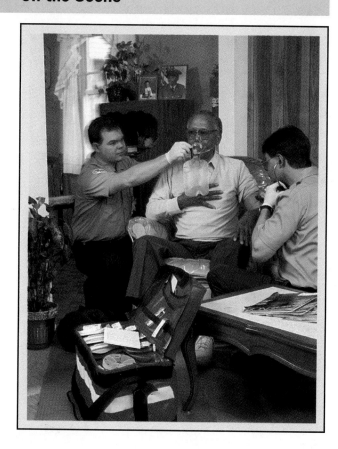

Your EMS unit is called to the home of a couple in their seventies. The elderly man, Jim Johnson, was watching television when he complained of bad indigestion. His wife, Ella, was concerned and called EMS.

When you arrive, Mr. Johnson is sitting in a chair. He tells you there is nothing really wrong with him and he doesn't know why his wife "bothered" the ambulance crew. You notice, however, that he is sweaty, clutching his chest, and has a bluish color to his lips. Mrs. Johnson is visibly upset. She is breathing deeply and rapidly, trembling, and pacing the room.

You: *Do you have pain in your chest, Mr. Johnson?*

Jim Johnson: *No. I just have a touch of indigestion.*

Ella Johnson: *Tell the truth, Jim. This is exactly what happened the last time, and you almost died!*

You: *Sir, you appear to be uncomfortable and maybe having some pain in your chest. I'm going to give you some oxygen and see if that helps you.*

Even though you have not yet performed a complete patient assessment, you have noted obvious signs and symptoms of a heart problem, possibly a heart attack. Mr. Johnson may be telling the truth when he says he has no chest pain, but you know that with a heart attack, chest pain may be absent, may appear in another part of the body, or may appear as indigestion. You and Mrs. Johnson talk Mr. Johnson into consenting to transport. You suspect that he is frightened and secretly glad to be talked into the ride to the hospital.

You and your partner have not forgotten, of course, that Mrs. Johnson must be cared for, too. As you tend to Mr. Johnson, your partner listens to Mrs. Johnson, explains to her everything that is happening, and offers her emotional support.

Cardiovascular and Respiratory Emergencies

You have just studied six chapters on injuries, also known as trauma. In this chapter and the next you will study medical emergencies. The term "medical emergencies" covers a wide variety of emergencies that are not related to trauma. As an EMT you will find that a large portion of your responses will be for medical emergencies.

By now you are familiar with the importance of the ABCs and know that any problem with a patient's airway, breathing, or circulation may be life threatening. Medical emergencies that involve the cardiovascular system (the heart and blood vessels) and the respiratory system (the airway and lungs) often fall into this critical category and are also among the medical emergencies you will most frequently encounter as an EMT. They are the subject of this chapter.

Expected Outcome, Chapter 15: *You will be able to assess and provide appropriate emergency care for common cardiovascular and respiratory disorders.*

Warning: Protect yourself from infectious diseases by using appropriate barrier devices such as a pocket face mask with one-way valve, face shield, or bag-valve mask; goggles or eye shield; and disposable gloves. Always conform to your local EMS system's infection exposure control plan.

WHAT ARE MEDICAL EMERGENCIES?

DISORDERS OF THE CARDIOVASCULAR SYSTEM
    The Nature of Cardiovascular Diseases
    Cardiovascular Disorders

DISORDERS OF THE RESPIRATORY SYSTEM
    Respiratory Distress
    Respiratory Disorders

Knowledge *After reading this chapter you should be able to*

1. Define *medical emergency.* (p. 414)

2. List the major signs, symptoms, and patient history facts associated with medical emergencies. (p. 415)

3. Relate coronary artery disease to specific changes in arterial walls. (pp. 417–419)

4. Compare and contrast the signs and symptoms of angina pectoris and acute myocardial infarction. (pp. 420, 422; Scans 15-1 and 15-2)

5. List the emergency care procedures for angina pectoris. (p. 420; Scan 15-1)

6. List the emergency care procedures for possible acute myocardial infarction. (pp. 422–423; Scan 15-2)

7. Define *congestive heart failure* and explain its signs and symptoms in terms of this definition. (p. 423)

8. Describe the emergency care for possible congestive heart failure. (p. 426)

9. Explain how the presence of implanted devices or a history of coronary bypass surgery affects patient care. (pp. 426–427)

10. List the signs and symptoms of stroke. (p. 427; Scan 15-3)

11. Describe the emergency care provided for stroke. (p. 427; Scan 15-3)

12. Define *dyspnea* and relate this term to respiratory distress. (p. 429)

13. List the signs and symptoms and sources of patient information for respiratory distress. (pp. 429–430)

14. Describe the emergency care procedures for respiratory distress. (p. 431)

15. Compare and contrast emphysema and chronic bronchitis in terms of signs and symptoms. (pp. 431–432)

16. Describe the emergency care procedures for chronic bronchitis and emphysema. (p. 432)

17. List the signs and symptoms of asthma. (p. 433)

18. Describe the emergency care procedures for asthma. (p. 433)

19. Describe the signs and symptoms and the emergency care procedures for hyperventilation. (pp. 433–434)

20. Define *spontaneous pneumothorax* and describe the signs, symptoms, and care for this condition. (pp. 434–435)

Skills *As an EMT you should be able to*

1. Assess patients and provide emergency care for disorders of the cardiovascular system.

2. Assess patients and provide emergency care for disorders of the respiratory system.

---

*I*n the basic EMT course, much emphasis is placed on injury. However, the EMT also is expected to provide care for medical emergencies. Sometimes you will know from the outset that the call is for a medical emergency, but don't forget that *any* patient may have or may develop a medical problem, even when an injury is his most obvious problem. As an EMT you must survey for medical problems in every prehospital situation.

WHAT ARE MEDICAL EMERGENCIES?

Medical emergencies are problems that the layperson would call illness or sickness. In emergency care, a medical emergency occurs as a result of one of the following factors.

- A defect in the structure or function of an organ or organ system. This can be present at birth (congenital) or acquired during life. Heart disease is an example.

- A disease caused by an infectious organism such as a bacterium or a virus. An example of this would be pneumonia.
- The effect of a harmful substance, such as a poison or a drug.

Medical problems fall into one of three classifications: chronic, episodic, or acute. A **chronic** medical problem is consistently present over a long period of time. Diabetes is an example of a chronic condition. A patient has diabetes for life. If the patient takes his medications, there may be few problems. If the diabetic patient forgets to take his medications or neglects to eat, however, suddenly there is a problem. The chronic condition has become an emergency.

An **episodic** problem affects the patient at irregular intervals and leaves him unaffected at other times. The patient expects the problems, but the onset may not be predictable. Asthma is an example of an episodic medical problem. The patient may not experience a problem for days or months. Suddenly, an asthma attack develops.

An **acute** medical problem is one that is sudden and severe, usually occuring for the first time. A heart attack is an example of an acute condition.

Patient Assessment—Medical Problems

The way the emergency presents—as chronic, episodic, or acute—may help you identify the type of medical problem.

Signs and symptoms are other indicators. Many of the signs and symptoms of medical emergencies seem minor in themselves but actually indicate a more serious underlying medical problem. The observations are often a matter of common sense. We have all seen a friend or family member who just "looked sick." Similar observations can be made of patients in the field.

The relative weight of the physical exam and the interview are different for a medical emergency than for trauma. A rule of thumb is that for trauma, the physical exam is 80% of the assessment and the interview 20%. With a medical emergency, it is the other way around: 20% physical exam and 80% interview.

The kind of information the patient can give you is also different with a medical emergency. The trauma patient can relate a specific incident to the injury: "I fell from the ladder and my leg hurts." Medical emergencies present differently. Often the patient experiences unusual but vague feelings that are difficult to describe other than to say that "something is wrong."

The following information will be helpful in assessing a medical problem.

Signs

- ☐ Altered states of consciousness
- ☐ Abnormal pulse rate and character. A pulse rate above 100 or below 60 beats per minute is abnormal for most adults.
- ☐ Abnormal breathing rate and character. A breathing rate above 28 or below 10 breaths per minute indicates an emergency for most adults.
- ☐ Abnormal skin temperature, condition, or color
- ☐ Unequal pupil size or abnormal eye response
- ☐ Abnormal color (pale, blue, gray, yellow) of the lips, tongue, nailbeds, ear lobes, or eyeballs
- ☐ Breath odors (i.e., acetone, fruity)
- ☐ Abdominal tenderness, distention, or rigidity
- ☐ Muscular spasms or paralysis
- ☐ Bleeding or discharges from the body

Symptoms

- ☐ Pain anywhere in the body
- ☐ Tightness or a crushing feeling in the chest
- ☐ Numbness or tingling sensations
- ☐ Dizziness or faintness
- ☐ Inability to move a body part or restricted movements
- ☐ Burning sensations
- ☐ An upset stomach
- ☐ Unusual bowel or bladder habits
- ☐ Unusual thirst or hunger
- ☐ Feelings of "temperature" or fever and chills

Medical History

- ☐ History of heart attack, heart disease, or angina pectoris
- ☐ History of stroke
- ☐ History of diabetes
- ☐ History of respiratory problems or chronic lung conditions
- ☐ Patient taking medications of any kind
- ☐ Patient currently under a doctor's care for any reason

A patient with an unknown medical condition may present the EMT with many signs, symptoms, and prior medical conditions to sort through. It is important to keep in mind that many medical emergencies have similar signs and symptoms. Your role as an EMT is not to diagnose but to assess the patient, provide initial care, and transport the patient to a medical facility so that a physician can make a diagnosis and provide definitive care. It is always best for the EMT to treat the whole patient rather than becoming focused on details.

The EMT should also realize that just because the patient has a chronic medical condition does not mean that *all* the patient's problems *must* be due to that condition. The patient who has chronic emphysema may have his chest tightness dismissed as an emphysema symptom but, in fact, be having a heart attack. The medical history is very important, but not the only information available to the EMT.

Also be aware that an underlying medical emergency may be hidden by trauma. Consider the patient who is found unconscious in a motor vehicle collision. Occasionally, a diabetic patient will become disoriented or unconscious while driving. EMTs arrive at the scene of a motor vehicle collision and find an unconscious person and assume that trauma is the cause of the unconsciousness. As another example, suppose that an elderly person falls down a flight of stairs. Did the patient slip, or did an underlying medical emergency cause the patient to feel dizzy? Many patients will not remember or realize this until asked. It is a classic question: "Which came first, the chicken or the egg?" Rewritten for EMS: "Which came first, the trauma or the medical emergency?"

Conversely, trauma or another stressful situation can bring on a medical emergency. Patients will survive a motor vehicle collision unscathed, but the stress of being in a collision or of seeing a friend or relative hurt may bring on chest pain, asthma, or other conditions. It is important that the EMT gather information from all available resources and not develop "tunnel vision" when dealing with any emergency.

Another problem that may be seen by the EMT is denial. Patients will often downplay or deny having symptoms of an illness, even though the symptoms are present. An observant EMT may note that the patient is having pain, discomfort, or difficulty breathing even when the patient denies it. This may be indicated by body positioning, facial expressions, and other signs. Although denying that you feel ill may seem irrational, remember that the patient is often experiencing a considerable amount of fear. He may fear death, hospitalization, or surgery. He may think back to what happened to a friend or family member who had similar pains and did not survive. Denial is a normal human response to many medical conditions.

To counteract the phenomenon of denial, treat any patient who appears sick or in pain as if there is a serious medical condition, even though the patient denies it. Often friends or family members may be enlisted to help the patient communicate his concerns and reduce the denial.

The information you gather during your assessment can help you determine what possible type of medical emergency is causing problems for the patient. As you study specific medical disorders in the rest of Chapter 15 and Chapter 16, you will get to know which signs and symptoms may indicate what specific diseases and disorders.

DISORDERS OF THE CARDIOVASCULAR SYSTEM

The **cardiovascular system** is made up of the heart (*cardio*) and the blood vessels (*vascular*) of the body and brain. Emergencies involving the cardiovascular system are a large percentage of the calls handled by the EMT. These emergencies include heart attack, heart failure, stroke, and other serious medical problems.

Before continuing with cardiovascular emergencies, it would be a good idea to review the basics of the cardiovascular system (Figure 15-1).

- The heart is a muscular organ, about the size of a clenched fist. It is located in the midportion of the thoracic cavity. The superior (top) surface of the heart lies directly behind the sternum, at about the level of the third rib. The inferior (bottom) portion of the heart extends into the lower left chest to a point near the fifth or sixth rib.
- The heart has four chambers. The two upper chambers are called atria, while the two lower chambers are called ventricles. A thick wall, or septum, divides the heart into a right side and a left side. The right side of the heart receives de-oxygenated blood from the body and sends it to the lungs to obtain oxygen and expel waste. The oxygenated blood from the lungs returns to the left side of the heart where it is pumped to the body.

- The circulation of the blood between the heart and the lungs is the pulmonary circulation. The blood pumped from the heart to the body is the systemic circulation. The functions of the left and right sides of the heart, and the pulmonary and systemic circulations, are important concepts to remember when we discuss heart failure.

- Blood leaves the heart by way of arteries. As blood continues toward the tissues, the arteries become smaller and smaller until they become arterioles. Arterioles lead into the capillary beds where the actual exchange of oxygen and carbon dioxide between blood and the tissues takes place. Venules take blood from the capillary beds to begin the return trip to the heart. Veins increase in size as the blood gets closer to the heart.

- The heart's contraction is initiated by a natural "pacemaker" which is located in the right atrium. This pacemaker sends electrical impulses throughout the heart which cause the physical contraction of the heart muscle. Disorders of this natural pacemaker and the cardiac conduction system are causes of some cardiac-related medical emergencies.

- The muscle of the heart is called the **myocardium** (*myo* = muscle, *cardium* = heart). The myocardium receives its oxygen through the **coronary arteries** (Figure 15-2). This is a system of arteries that have the sole function of supplying oxygen to the heart tissue. Diseases that affect the coronary arteries reduce or prevent blood flow to the myocardium. This is a leading cause of cardiac emergencies.

As additional background for this section, you may wish to review the diagram of the cardiovascular system in the Anatomy and Physiology Plates at the end of this book and the information on CPR, defibrillation, and oxygen therapy in Chapters 5 and 6.

The Nature of Cardiovascular Diseases

Most of the cardiovascular emergencies covered in this section are caused, directly or indirectly, by changes taking place in the inner walls of arteries. These arteries can be part of the systemic circulatory system, the pulmonary circulatory system, or the coronary system. Two conditions, atherosclerosis and arteriosclerosis, are involved in the changes found in these artery walls.

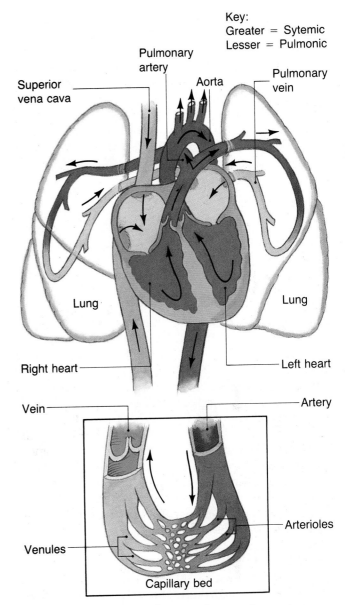

Figure 15-1 Anatomy of the cardiovascular system.

Atherosclerosis (ATH-er-o-skle-RO-sis) is a buildup of fatty deposits on the inner walls of arteries (Figure 15-3). This buildup causes a narrowing of the inner vessel diameter, restricting the flow of blood. Fats and other particles combine to form this deposit, known as **plaque**. As time passes, calcium can be deposited at the site of the plaque, causing the area to harden. In **arteriosclerosis** (ar-TE-re-o-skle-RO-sis), the artery wall becomes hard and stiff due to calcium deposits. This "hardening of the arteries" causes the vessel to lose its elastic nature, changing blood flow and increasing blood pressure.

Throughout the entire process of both ather-

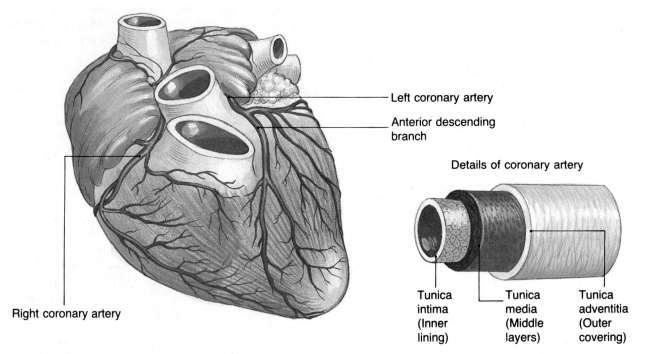

Left coronary artery

Anterior descending branch

Details of coronary artery

Right coronary artery

Tunica intima (Inner lining)

Tunica media (Middle layers)

Tunica adventitia (Outer covering)

Figure 15-2 The coronary artery system.

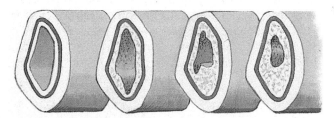

Figure 15-3 Atherosclerosis, the process of plaque formation.

osclerosis and arteriosclerosis, the amount of blood passing through the artery is restricted. The rough surface formed in the artery can lead to blood clots being formed, causing increased narrowing or **occlusion** (blockage) of the artery. The clot and debris from the plaque form a **thrombus** (THROM-bus). A thrombus can reach a size where it occludes (cuts off) blood flow completely, or it may break loose to become an **embolism** (EM-bo-liz-m) and move to occlude the flow of blood somewhere downstream in a smaller artery. In cases of partial or complete blockage, the tissues beyond the point of blockage will be starved of oxygen and may die. If this blockage involves a large area of the heart or brain, the results may be quickly fatal (Figure 15-4).

Another cause of cardiovascular system disorder stems from weakened sections in the arterial walls. Each weak spot that begins to dilate (balloon) is known as an **aneurysm** (AN-u-riz-m). This weakening can be related to other arterial dis-

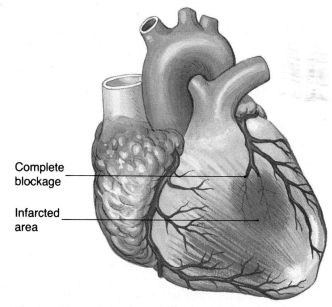

Complete blockage

Infarcted area

Figure 15-4 The relationship of arterial disease and heart disease.

eases, or it can exist independently. When a weakened section of an artery bursts, there can be rapid, life-threatening internal bleeding (Figure 15-5). Tissues beyond the rupture can be damaged because oxygenated blood they need is escaping and not reaching them. Tissues around the site often can be damaged by the pressure exerted on them by the blood pouring from the artery. If a major artery ruptures, death from shock (see

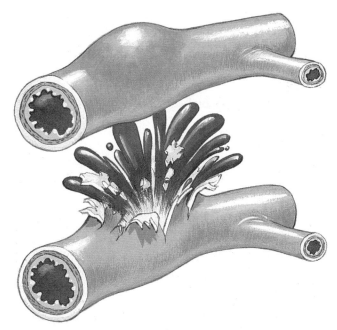

Figure 15-5 Formation and rupture of an aneurysm. A weakened area in the wall of an artery will tend to balloon out, forming a sac-like aneurysm, which may eventually burst.

Chapter 8) can occur very quickly. When an artery in the brain ruptures, a severe form of stroke occurs. The severity is dependent on the site of the stroke and the amount of blood loss.

Cardiovascular Disorders

Coronary Artery Disease While conditions such as atherosclerosis and arteriosclerosis can occur anywhere in the body, they are especially devastating in the heart.

As noted earlier, the heart is a muscle—a very active muscle. Like all other muscles, it needs oxygen to contract. When diseases cause blockage of the coronary arteries, blood flow is reduced, thereby reducing the amount of oxygen delivered to the heart. This might not be noticed when the body is at rest or at a low activity level. However, when the body is subject to stress or exertion, the heart rate increases. With the increased heart rate comes an increased need for oxygen. The arteries, narrowed due to plaque and calcium deposits, cannot supply enough blood to meet the demands of the heart.

Diseases affecting the arteries of the heart are commonly called **coronary artery disease (CAD)**. Coronary artery disease is a serious health problem that results in hundreds of thousands of deaths yearly in the United States.

There are factors that put a person at risk of

developing CAD. Some of these risk factors—such as heredity (a close relative who has CAD) and age—cannot be changed. However, there are also many risk factors that *can* be modified to reduce the risk of coronary artery disease. These include hypertension (high blood pressure), obesity, lack of exercise, elevated blood levels of cholesterol and triglycerides, and cigarette smoking.

Many patients have more than one of these risk factors. A positive note is that the damage caused by the latter list of risk factors may be reversed or slowed by changing behavior. Smokers return to the risk level of a non-smoker quickly after quitting. Medication and stress reduction programs can lower high blood pressure. Improved diet and exercise can help the other controllable factors. This is important information for the EMT as well as for his or her patients!

In the majority of cardiac-related medical emergencies, it is the reduced blood supply to the myocardium that causes the emergency. The most common symptom of this reduced blood supply is chest pain. Patients may have symptoms that range anywhere from mild chest pain to sudden death (the patient suddenly going into cardiac arrest). Angina pectoris (chest pain), acute myocardial infarction (heart attack), and congestive heart failure—all conditions that can be related to CAD—are discussed below.

Angina Pectoris **Angina pectoris** means literally "a pain in the chest." This condition is brought on by a reduced blood supply to the heart during times of exertion or stress (Figure 15-6).

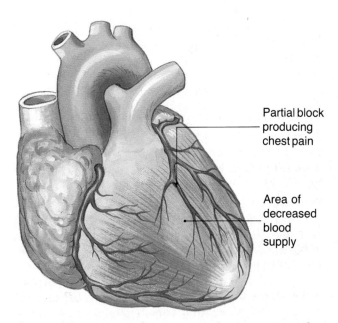

Partial block producing chest pain

Area of decreased blood supply

Figure 15-6 Angina pectoris produces pain in the chest that may be similar to that of a heart attack.

Coronary artery disease has caused a narrowing of the arteries that supply the heart. When the heart needs to beat faster due to some stress or exertion, more blood and oxygen are required. The narrowed coronary arteries cannot supply all the blood that is needed. As the heart works harder and doesn't get the oxygen it needs to do the work, the portion of the myocardium supplied by the narrowed artery becomes starved for oxygen. When the myocardium is deprived of the oxygen it needs, chest pain—angina pectoris—is the most frequent result. This pain is sometimes called an "angina attack."

Since the pain of angina pectoris comes on after stress or exertion, frequently the pain diminishes when the patient stops the exertion. As the oxygen demand of the heart returns to normal, the pain subsides. *Seldom does this painful attack last longer than 3 to 5 minutes.*

Patient Assessment—Angina Pectoris

The patient may be able to tell you that he has angina pectoris (often called simply "angina").

Another indication that the patient has a history of this condition is the if the patient has the medication nitroglycerin. Nitroglycerin is a medication that dilates the arteries of the body, especially the coronary arteries. Since this drug widens the arteries, more blood is allowed to reach the myocardium. Nitroglycerin is available in tablets that are placed under the patient's tongue to dissolve, and also in sprays and patches. The patches are affixed to the skin and gradually release nitroglycerin throughout the day.

Signs and Symptoms

A patient who complains of chest pain that lasts only a few minutes or that improves with rest may be suffering from angina pectoris. A complete list of the signs and symptoms of angina pectoris is given in Scan 15-1.

Note: Most angina patients are advised by their doctor to take nitroglycerin for their chest pain. Patients are usually told to rest and are allowed to take 3 nitroglycerin doses over a 10-minute period. If there is no relief of symptoms after that time they are instructed to call for help. As an EMT you may arrive after the patient has already taken nitroglycerin without relief. In this situation, you must assume that the patient is having an acute myocardial infarction, or heart attack (discussed later in this chapter).

Patient Care—Angina Pectoris

Emergency Care Steps

1. *Provide oxygen.* The primary field treatment for angina pectoris is oxygen. Patients with chest pain of any type should receive a high concentration of oxygen. Since the myocardium is oxygen starved, oxygen is an ideal treatment.
2. *Assist with medication.* If your EMS system allows, you may assist an angina patient in taking his nitroglycerin medication. Since nitroglycerin dilates arteries, do not allow patients with a systolic blood pressure below 90 mmHG to take the medication unless directed to do so by medical control. This may cause reduction of an already low blood pressure and lead to shock and unconsciousness.
3. *Position the patient.* Place the patient in a position of comfort and monitor him carefully. Attempt to reassure and calm the patient since stress will aggravate the chest pain.
4. *Transport.* Patients who experience chest pain should be transported to the hospital for evaluation and treatment. If an advanced-life-support unit has not been dispatched, arranged for an ALS intercept. Many patients who obtain relief from rest and nitroglycerin will not want to go to the hospital. Always attempt to convince these patients to go to the hospital. If a patient absolutely refuses to accept your transportation consult medical control and follow local protocols.

See Scan 15-1 for a complete list of emergency care steps.

Acute Myocardial Infarction The condition in which a portion of the myocardium dies as a result of oxygen starvation is known as **acute myocardial infarction (AMI).** Often called a **heart attack** by lay persons, AMI is brought on by the narrowing or occlusion of the coronary artery that supplies the region with blood. Rarely, the interruption of blood flow to the myocardium may be due to the rupturing of a coronary artery (Figure 15-7).

Angina Pectoris

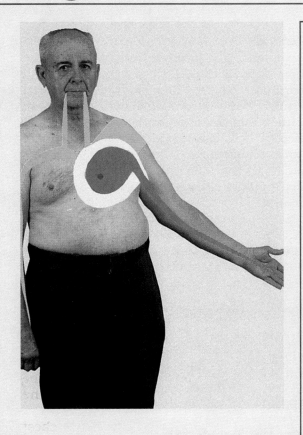

SIGNS AND SYMPTOMS may include

- Early symptoms are often mistaken for indigestion.
- As an attack worsens, pain originates behind the sternum and radiates to . . .
  - Either or both of the upper extremities (usually the left) with pain radiating to the shoulder, arm, and elbow. In some cases, the pain may extend down the limb to the little finger.
  - The neck, jaws, and teeth
  - The upper back
  - The superior, medial abdomen

  The pain may not originate under the sternum. Some patients have pain only in the jaw or teeth.
- Shortness of breath
- Nausea
- Pain lasts throughout the attack and is not influenced by movement, breathing, or coughing.
- Pain usually lasts 3 to 5 minutes.
- Patient usually remains still.
- Pain diminishes when physical or emotional stress ends or when nitroglycerin is taken.

Additional signs may include sweating, increased pulse rate, and, on rare occasions, a shock-level blood pressure. Patients who have taken repeated dosages of nitroglycerin may have low blood pressure as a result of blood vessel dilation.

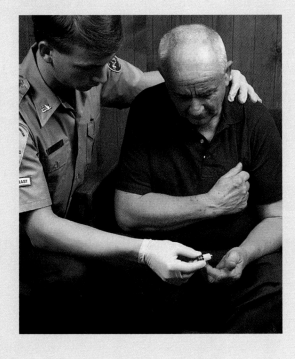

EMERGENCY CARE

1. Supply oxygen at a high flow rate as soon as possible.
2. Find out if patient takes nitroglycerin, when last dose was taken, and how much was taken over what period of time.
3. Contact medical facility and let them know
   - You have a patient with chest pain
   - When last medicated
   - Patient's vital signs and history
4. Assist the patient with prescribed dose of medication (nitroglycerin) if systolic blood pressure is above 90 mmHg.
5. Place the patient in a restful, comfortable position.
6. Provide emotional support—keep the patient calm and reassured.
7. Provide "quiet" transport and continue to monitor vital signs.

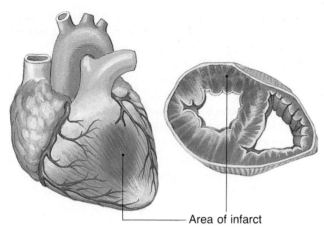

Figure 15-7 Cross section of a myocardial infarction.

The American Heart Association reports over a million cases of AMI in the United States each year. Hundreds of thousands of deaths annually are the result of cardiovascular disease. A major portion of these are cases of **sudden death**, a cardiac arrest that occurs within two hours of the onset of symptoms. In most cases, sudden death occurs outside of hospitals. The patient may have no prior symptoms of coronary artery disease. Nearly 25% of these individuals have no previous history of cardiac problems.

A variety of factors can cause an AMI. Coronary artery disease in the form of atherosclerosis is usually the underlying reason for the incident. However, for some patients, factors often regarded as harmless may trigger an AMI. These factors include chronic respiratory problems, unusual exertion, or severe emotional stress.

These patients may have an undetected, pre-existing disturbance in heart rate and rhythm known as **arrhythmia** (ah-RITH-me-ah). Arrhythmia (also known as dysrhythmia) occurs when the heart's natural pacemaker or any other part of the heart's electrical conduction system malfunctions. Some arrhymias are minor while others are lethal.

Most AMI victims experience some sort of arrhythmia. Some of the arrhythmias associated with AMI include

- *Asystole* (ah-SIS-to-le)—cardiac standstill, sometimes called "flatline"
- *Ventricular fibrillation* (ven-TRIK-u-lar fi-bri-LAY-shun)—when the ventricles no longer beat with a full, steady, symmetrical pattern. Instead of a producing forceful contraction, the heart muscle "quivers." This arrhythmia is common in adult AMI patients and may respond to defibrillation (see Chapter 5).

- *Bradycardia* (brad-i-KAR-de-ah)—when the heart rate is slow, usually below 60 beats per minute.
- *Tachycardia* (tak-e-KAR-de-ah)—when the heart rate is fast, above 100 beats per minute.

Another common complication seen with AMI is **mechanical pump failure.** A lack of oxygen has caused the death of a portion of the myocardium. The dead area can no longer pump and contract. If a large enough area of the heart dies, the pumping action of the whole heart will be affected. This can lead to cardiac arrest, cardiogenic shock (see Chapter 8), pulmonary edema (fluids "backing up" in the lungs), congestive heart failure (edema of lungs and other body organs—see later in this chapter), and cell death in various regions of the body due to oxygen starvation. A few AMI patients suffer cardiac rupture as the dead tissue area of the myocardium bursts open. This occurs days after an AMI.

Patient Assessment—AMI

You will not be able to diagnose a ruptured coronary artery or any other specific cause or complication of AMI in the field. As an EMT, however, you must be able to recognize the signs and symptoms of AMI.

Signs and Symptoms

The AMI patient often has chest pain; however patients can have an AMI and never experience this pain. When there is pain, it may not be relieved by rest or nitroglycerin. A list of the signs and symptoms of AMI appears in Scan 15-2. Note that there is a comparison of angina pectoris and AMI, which share some signs and symptoms. The Scan will help you recall the major differences between the two.

Warning: IF THERE IS ANY DOUBT WHETHER THE PATIENT IS SUFFERING FROM ANGINA OR AMI, SUSPECT AMI.

Patient Care—AMI

Cardiologists believe that many sudden deaths could be prevented if the victims receive prompt and efficient care in the early warning stages or CPR and defibrillation immediately after the cardiac arrest occurs. As an EMT you must be able to provide appropriate care for any possible AMI from first contact until advanced cardiac life support intervenes or you transfer the patient to the staff of a medical facility.

Emergency Care Steps

The treatment for both angina and AMI are very similar. If a patient has experienced chest pain serious enough for a call to EMS

1. *Provide oxygen.*
2. *Position the patient for comfort.* Attempt to reassure and calm the patient.
3. *Transport.*

A list of emergency care steps for a suspected AMI is given in Scan 15-2.

Warning: TREAT ALL SUSPECTED ANGINA AND AMI PATIENTS AS IF THEY ARE HAVING AN AMI. TRANSPORT THE PATIENT WITHOUT DELAY.

Remember: Transportation of a patient with a heart condition must be carried out in a thoughtful, calm, and careful fashion. A ride with siren wailing is likely to increase the patient's fear and apprehension, placing additional stress on the heart. The patient's condition could worsen and he could die due to complications brought about by improper transport. Speed is important; the patient must reach the hospital as quickly as possible. However, the judicious use of siren or horn must be balanced against the possibiliy of upsetting the patient.

Congestive Heart Failure **Congestive heart failure (CHF)** is a condition of excessive fluid buildup in the lungs and/or other organs and body parts. The fluid buildup causes edema, or swelling. The disorder is termed *congestive* because the fluids congest, or clog, the organs. It is termed *heart failure* because the congestion both results from and also aggravates failure of the heart to function properly. The congestion may also result from and aggravate failure of the lungs to function properly.

Congestive heart failure may be brought on by diseased heart valves, hypertension, or some form of obstructive pulmonary disease such as emphysema (discussed later in this chapter). CHF is often a complication of AMI. Congestive heart failure often progresses as follows.

1. A patient sustains an AMI. Myocardium in the area of the left ventricle dies. (Recall the function of the heart: The left is the side of the heart that receives oxygenated blood from the lungs and pulmonary circulation and pumps it to the rest of the body.)

2. Because of the damage to the left ventricle, blood backs up into the pulmonary circulation and then the lungs. Fluid accumulation in the lungs is called **pulmonary edema**. This edema causes a poor exchange of oxygen between the lungs and the bloodstream and the patient experiences shortness of breath or **dyspnea** (disp-NE-ah). Listening to this patient's lungs with a stethoscope may reveal crackling or gravelly lung sounds called **rales**. Some patients cough up blood-tinged sputum from their lungs.

3. Left heart failure, if untreated, commonly causes right heart failure. The right side of the heart (which receives blood from the body and pumps it to the lungs) becomes congested because the clogged lungs cannot receive more blood. In turn, fluids may accumulate in the dependent (lower) extremities, the liver, and the abdomen. Accumulation of fluid at the feet or ankles is known as **pedal edema**. The abdomen may become noticeably distended, a condition known as **ascites** (as-SI-tes). In a bedridden patient, fluids collect in the sacral area of the spine.

Patient Assessment—CHF

The swelling and breathing difficulties caused by fluid buildup are quick clues to congestive heart failure. Be alert to these and other signs and symptoms of CHF (Figure 15-8).

Signs and Symptoms

☐ Tachycardia (rapid pulse, 100 beats per minute or more)
☐ Dyspnea (shortness of breath)
☐ Normal or elevated blood pressure
☐ Cyanosis
☐ **Diaphoresis** (profuse sweating), or cool and clammy skin
☐ Pulmonary edema with rales, sometimes coughing up of frothy white or pink sputum
☐ Anxiety or confusion due to **hypoxia** (inadequate supply of oxygen to the brain and other tissues) caused by poor oxygen/carbon dioxide exchange
☐ Edema of the lower extremities
☐ Engorged, pulsating neck veins (late sign)
☐ Enlarged liver and spleen, with abdominal distention (late sign)

Acute Myocardial Infarction (AMI)

Signs and Symptoms may include

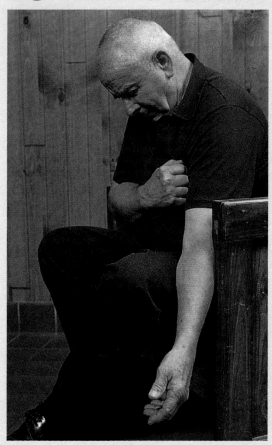

Respiratory
- Dyspnea—shallow or deep respirations
- Cough that produces sputum (rare)

Behavioral
- Feeling of impending doom
- Anxiety, irritability, inability to concentrate
- Depression
- Mild delirium, personality changes
- Fainting
- Occasional thrashing about and clutching of the chest
- Denial

Circulatory
- Pallor
- Profuse sweating (diaphoresis)
- Signs of shock
- Increased pulse rate, sometimes irregular. Some patients may have a slowed pulse rate.
- Reduced blood pressure in 50% of patients
  Normal blood pressure in 25% of patients
  Increased blood pressure in 25% of patients

Pain
- 15% to 20% are painless ("silent") attacks
- Marked discomfort that continues when at rest rather than a sharp or throbbing pain
- Usually not alleviated by nitroglycerin
- May last 30 minutes to several hours
- Usually originates under sternum and may radiate to arms, neck, or jaw

An AMI Can Lead To . . .
- Cardiac arrest (40% die before they reach the hospital)
- Mechanical heart failure with pulmonary edema
- Shock (usually within 24 hours)
- Congestive heart failure (immediately, or up to a week or more later)

Distinguishing Between Angina and AMI

Angina Pectoris
- Pain follows exertion or stress.
- Pain is relieved by rest.
- Pain is usually relieved by nitroglycerin (if not relieved after 3 doses in 10 minutes, assume AMI).
- Blood pressure is usually not affected.
- Short-term diaphoresis may be present.

AMI
- Pain is often related to stress or exertion but may occur when at rest.
- Rest usually does not relieve pain.
- Nitroglycerin may relieve pain.
- Pain lasts 30 minutes to several hours.
- Blood pressure is often reduced, but many patients have normal blood pressure.
- Diaphoresis is usually present.

AMI—Emergency Care

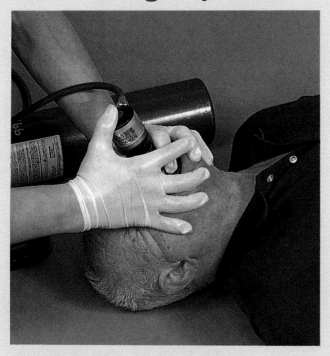

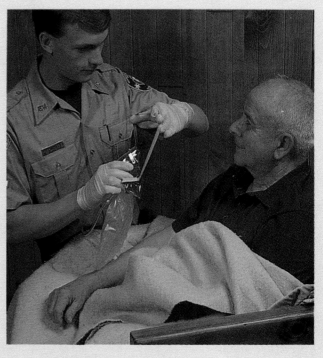

For The Unconscious Patient
1. Establish and maintain an airway.
2. Provide pulmonary resuscitation or CPR if needed (defibrillation if needed and if you are so trained). If respiratory or cardiac arrest develops, deliver oxygen with a bag-valve-mask unit or a demand-valve resuscitator.
3. Administer a high concentration of oxygen.
4. Loosen restrictive clothing.
5. Conserve body heat, but do not allow overheating.
6. Transport immediately—quiet transport (little or no use of siren). Arrange for an ALS intercept.
7. Monitor vital signs throughout care and transport.

For The Conscious Patient
1. Administer a high concentration of oxygen.
2. Keep the patient calm and still—do not allow patient to move himself to the ambulance stretcher.
3. Take history and determine vital signs.
4. Help patient with medication.
5. Conserve body heat.
6. Transport as soon as possible in a semireclined or sitting position. Provide quiet transport (little or no use of siren). Arrange for an ALS intercept.
7. Monitor vital signs throughout care and transport.

Emergency care may be complicated by many factors. If the patient is conscious, his irritability, restlessness, and feeling of impending doom may make him uncooperative and unwilling to settle down, even though it is vital that he do so. Some AMI patients will resist the placement of a face mask for oxygen delivery. If he resists after an explanation of the importance of oxgyen, use a nasal cannula at 6 liters/minute. Provide needed oxygen, but do not upset the patient.

Warning: TREAT ALL SUSPECTED ANGINA AND AMI PATIENTS AS IF THEY ARE HAVING AMIs.

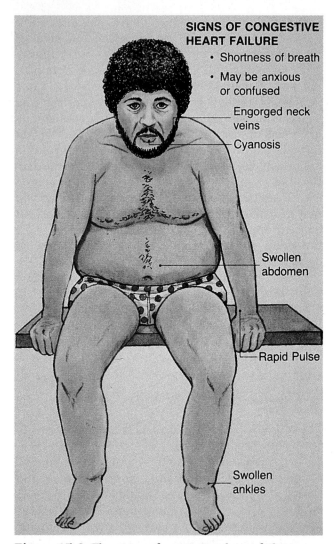

SIGNS OF CONGESTIVE HEART FAILURE
- Shortness of breath
- May be anxious or confused

Engorged neck veins

Cyanosis

Swollen abdomen

Rapid Pulse

Swollen ankles

Figure 15-8 The signs of congestive heart failure.

The CHF patient may be on medications for this condition. Often patients will tell you that they take a "water pill" for fluid buildup. This refers to a diuretic, a medication that helps remove fluid from the body system. Other medications may increase the strength of the cardiac contraction to counteract the heart failure.

Patient Care—CHF

The CHF patient's most severe immediate problem is probably difficulty in breathing because of his pulmonary edema. This is probably the problem that prompted the call for emergency aid. As an EMT your main emergency care objective is to help the patient breathe and get enough oxygen before and during transport.

Emergency Care Steps

1. *Place the patient in a position of comfort.* The patient will probably prefer to be in a seated or semireclined position, which allows for less labored respiration. The CHF patient will often experience severe dyspnea when lying supine.
2. *Give a high concentration of oxygen through a nonrebreather mask.* (See "Disorders of the Respiratory System," later in this chapter and see Chapter 6 on oxygen delivery to patients who may have COPD.)

Electronic Implants and Bypass Surgery

With the rapidly expanding medical technology available, the EMT may be presented with patients who have undergone surgeries or had special electronic devices implanted in the body. A general rule is that *all* patients, no matter what their prior medical history, are given a thorough primary assessment. The ABCs (including rescue breathing and CPR) and appropriate oxygen delivery will not change because of prior surgery or conditions. Some of the patients and devices you may observe in the field are

- Cardiac Pacemaker—When the heart's natural pacemaker does not function properly, an artificial pacemaker can be surgically implanted to perform the same function. This pacemaker helps the heart beat in a normal, coordinated function. The pacemaker will not prevent AMI, angina pectoris, or CHF. Care for patients with implanted pacemakers and signs of a cardiac emergency is the same as for those without a pacemaker. A pacemaker is often placed below the clavicles, is visible, and can be palpated. The fact that the patient has a pacemaker should be noted on your prehospital care report and reported to the hospital staff.

  Occasionally pacemakers malfunction. Although this situation is rare, it is possible. A malfunctioning pacemaker usually results in a slow or irregular pulse. The patient may have signs of shock due to the fact the heart isn't beating properly. If the patient with a pacemaker has angina, suspect pacemaker failure, even though this is a rare happening. Be aware that a pacemaker failure can be life threatening. Arrange for ALS intercept and transport immediately. *Do not defibrillate a pacemaker battery.*
- Implanted Defibrillators—Cardiologists are able to identify patients who are at a high

risk to develop ventricular fibrillation. These patients often receive a miniature defibrillator surgically implanted in the chest. When the patient develops this lethal cardiac rhythm, the implanted defibrillator identifies the rhythm and "shocks" the patient. These implanted devices are not as common as pacemakers but may be observed in the field. Since these defibrillators are directly attached to the heart, low energy levels are used for each shock. This should not pose a threat to the EMT. Emergency care and CPR for this patient are the same as for other cardiac patients.

- Cardiac Bypass Surgery—The coronary artery bypass has become a relatively common procedure in cardiac surgery. A blood vessel from another part of the body is surgically implanted to bypass an occluded coronary artery. This helps restore blood flow to a section of the myocardium. Should a patient with a suspected AMI tell you that he has had bypass surgery, or if you observe a midline surgical scar on the chest of an unconscious patient, provide the same emergency care and CPR as for any other patient.

Stroke Often thought of as a disorder of the brain, a stroke or **cerebrovascular** (SAIR-uh-bro-VAS-kyuh-ler) **accident (CVA)** begins as a problem of the cardiovascular system. In a CVA, an artery in the brain becomes occluded, preventing oxygenated blood from reaching the areas supplied by the occluded artery. The pathway of blood can also be disrupted by the rupturing of an artery, resulting in cerebral hemorrhaging. Cerebral hemorrhage not only prevents oxygenation of the areas supplied by the artery, it also sends blood into the brain. The brain itself is in a closed container (the skull). Since there is a limited amount of space available, blood escaping into the head can cause compression of the brain tissue which is also a serious problem.

Patient Assessment—Stroke

Age and physical condition influence the type of stroke suffered by a patient. This and the various sizes and locations of arteries involved give varied signs and symptoms. Sometimes the patient may have nothing more than a headache when first evaluated if the stroke is caused by bleeding from a ruptured vessel. Continued bleeding into the head or gradual death of brain tissue can cause the symptoms to worsen. However, headache is an unusual symptom. Most stroke patients do not experience headaches.

In many cases, you will find it difficult to communicate with the stroke patient because of the presence of **aphasia** (ah-FAY-zhah). This is a partial or complete loss of the ability to use words. The patient may be able to understand you but will not be able to talk, or will have great difficulty with speech. Sometimes, the patient will exhibit a special form of aphasia resulting from the stroke. He will understand you and know what he wants to say, but he will say the wrong words.

Signs and Symptoms

A list of signs and symptoms of stroke appears in Scan 15-3.

Patient Care—Stroke

Paralysis and aphasia are frightening to the patient. Paralysis may affect limbs and breathing ability. Do what you can to calm and reassure the patient.

Early transport is indicated. Place the patient in a semireclining position for transport and constantly monitor the airway. Avoid potentially upsetting high speeds and use of the siren. As with any patient with a cardiovascular emergency, administer a high concentration of oxygen.

When the patient has difficulty speaking or cannot speak, tell him not to be frightened. Let him know you understand what is happening. Tell the patient you will rely on his gestures and—as is sometimes possible even when the patient cannot speak—on his written messages. Always let the patient know when he has been understood. Realize that even patients who do not appear to be able to hear you may, in fact, hear and understand everything you say. Be sure to act and talk professionally at all times with these patients.

Emergency Care Steps

A list of emergency care steps for stroke patients appears in Scan 15-3.

Another type of cerebrovascular incident is a transient ischemic attack (TIA). This is a condition where a patient develops symptoms of a stroke, but they are transient (are present, then

Stroke—Cerebrovascular Accident

Causes of Cerebrovascular Accidents—Stroke

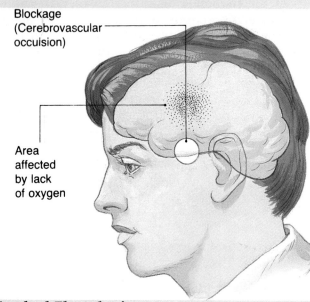

Blockage
(Cerebrovascular
occulsion)

Area
affected
by lack
of oxygen

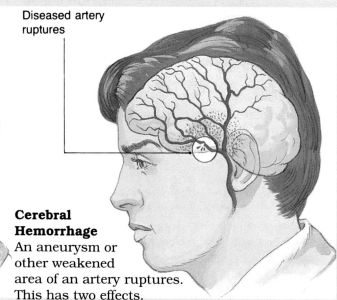

Diseased artery
ruptures

Cerebral Thrombosis
Blockage in arteries supplying oxygenated blood
will result in damage to affected parts of the
brain.

Cerebral Hemorrhage
An aneurysm or
other weakened
area of an artery ruptures.
This has two effects.

1. An area of the brain is deprived of oxygenated blood.
2. Pooling blood puts increased pressure on the brain, displacing tissue and interfering with function.

Cerebral hemorrhage is often associated with arteriosclerosis and hypertension (high blood pressure).

Signs and Symptoms of Stroke

- Confusion and/or dizziness
- Loss of function or paralysis of extremities (usually on one side of the body)
- Impaired speech
- Numbness (usually limited to one side of the body)
- Collapse
- Facial flaccidness and loss of expression (often to one side of the face)
- Headache
- Unequal pupil size
- Impaired vision
- Rapid, full pulse
- Difficult respiration, snoring
- Nausea and/or vomiting
- Convulsions
- Coma
- Loss of bladder and blowel control

Emergency Care of Stroke Patients

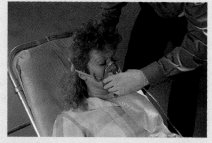

Conscious Patient
- Ensure an open airway.
- Keep patient calm.
- Administer high-flow oxygen.
- Monitor vital signs.
- Transport in semireclined position.
- Give nothing by mouth.
- Keep warm.
- Sit in front of the patient. Maintain eye contact, and speak slowly and clearly.

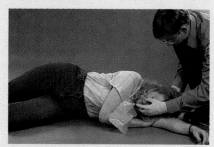

Unconscious Patient
- Maintain open airway.
- Provide high concentration of oxygen. Assist with ventilation as necessary.
- Monitor vital signs.
- Transport in lateral recombent position. Use protective padding.

disappear). Ischemia (is-KEM-e-ah) refers to a reduced oxygen level in body tissues. TIAs are characterized by a sudden onset of confusion, inability to speak, or the inability to move one or more body parts. Since TIAs are transient, the symptoms totally disappear within 24 hours. A patient experiencing a CVA will have similar symptoms, but the symptoms persist for a prolonged time. Patients with TIAs receive the same care as patients with CVAs.

Remember: TIA, even when symptoms disappear, means that the patient is at risk for a stroke. Patients who experience one CVA may be at risk for another. All patients who exhibit signs of stroke, whether transient or prolonged, should be transported to the hospital for evaluation.

DISORDERS OF THE RESPIRATORY SYSTEM

The **respiratory system** includes the airway and the lungs. Air moves into the lungs through the nose and mouth, pharynx, and trachea. From the inferior end of the trachea, right and left bronchi branch into the lungs. The primary bronchi branch into secondary bronchi which branch into bronchioles.

Some bronchioles are closed tubes. Air movement in them helps expand the lungs. Other bronchioles end in alveolar sacs. Pulmonary capillaries pass alongside the alveoli and, through their walls, the red blood cells take in oxygen, which has been breathed in, and give off carbon dioxide, which will be breathed out.

A respiratory disorder or condition is a malfunction or disease of any part or parts of the airway and/or lungs.

As additional background for this section, you may wish to review the diagram of the respiratory system in the Anatomy and Physiology Plates at the end of this book and the information on the airway, breathing, and oxygen therapy in chapters 4, 5, and 6.

Respiratory Distress

Respiratory distress is a combination of signs and symptoms that indicate a patient has a problem affecting the respiratory system. Respiratory distress is not a disease in itself; rather it is a series of indications that there is a problem with the patient's respiratory system.

Dyspnea (disp-NE-ah) means labored or difficult breathing and is one of the signs of respiratory distress. Dyspnea may be caused by a number of conditions including airway obstruction, pulmonary edema, emphysema, heart conditions, allergic reactions, pneumothorax, and carbon monoxide poisoning to name just a few. In most cases dyspnea occurs when a disease has caused some kind of interference with either the flow of air into and out of the lungs or with the exchange of oxygen and carbon dioxide within the lungs.

Adequate respiration is vital for the body to function properly. When something occurs to limit airflow or exchange, the body attempts to compensate for the lack of oxygen intake. The patient unconsciously begins to increase the rate and depth of respirations, under the direction of the respiratory center in the brain. If this increase does not provide enough oxygen to satisfy the needs of the body, dyspnea develops and the patient begins to feel short of breath. If the condition is prolonged, hypoxia (oxygen starvation) develops. As the intake of air or the efficiency of exchange in the lung decreases, the body will not be able to expel carbon dioxide. The respiratory centers will continue to increase the rate of respiration in order to control this problem. With time, this center is depressed and the breathing rate slows. If there is no improvement, **apnea** (the cessation of breathing) is the final result. Respiratory arrest leads to cardiac arrest and the death of the patient.

Patient Assessment—Respiratory Distress

Signs and Symptoms

☐ Increased rate and depth of respirations, followed by shortness of breath and possible gasping
☐ Additional signs and symptoms as shown in Figure 15-9

It is fairly obvious when a person is suffering from respiratory difficulty, as Figure 15-9 makes clear. But recognizing that the patient is in distress is only part of your assessment task. You must also try to find answers to the question, What is *causing* the distress? It is important to gain as much information as possible about the patient's condition, as this information will govern some aspects of care. For example, oxygen administration to certain patients with chronic obstructive lung disease can be dangerous and must be done with caution (see below), so it is important to try to find out if the patient has a history of chronic lung disorders. Use the following sources of information.

- The Patient Interview—What does the patient tell you about his condition? Ask about the onset, duration, and medications. Does the patient have a productive cough? Does he bring up mucus? If so what color is it? Mucus production may indicate chronic lung conditions or pneumonias. Can the patient speak in full sentences without feeling "out of breath?" Inability to speak in full sentences is a clear indication of respiratory distress. Does the patient sleep on several pillows or in a chair? Has the number of pillows increased recently? This is also an indication of respiratory distress. Does the patient have any other physical complaints? (Listen and probe for the symptoms listed in Figure 15-9.)

- The Physical Examination—How does the patient look? Is the patient cyanotic or using accessory muscles to breathe? Listen to the lungs with your stethoscope. Does the patient show signs of edema in the legs, feet, sacral spine area, or abdomen? (Look for the signs shown in Figure 15-9)

- Family members, Coworkers, Bystanders—Information from sources other than the patient may also be valuable. Be careful of medical terminology used to describe a patient's condition. A family member may tell you the patient has asthma when the patient actually has emphysema. This may be due to a lack of understanding of the different conditions and anxiety over the patient's illness.

- Medical identification devices and the prescription medicines being taken by the patient also can serve as sources of information. Do not try to determine what the medications indicate, but relay the names of the drugs to the emergency department physician. This must be done immediately if the patient has taken the medications and is still in distress.

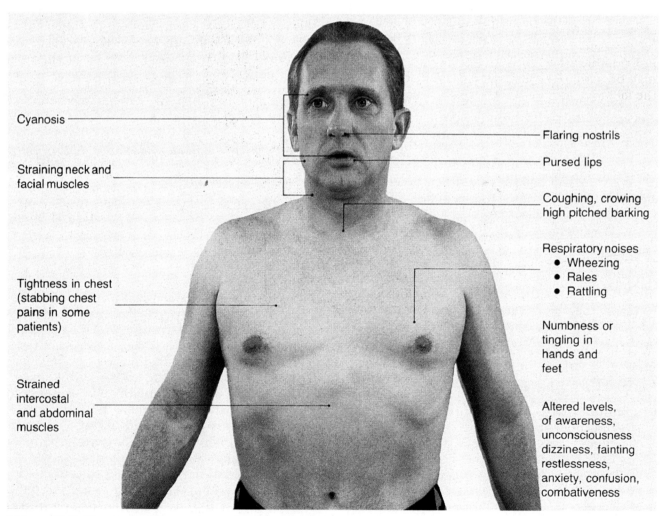

Cyanosis

Straining neck and facial muscles

Tightness in chest (stabbing chest pains in some patients)

Strained intercostal and abdominal muscles

Flaring nostrils

Pursed lips

Coughing, crowing high pitched barking

Respiratory noises
- Wheezing
- Rales
- Rattling

Numbness or tingling in hands and feet

Altered levels, of awareness, unconsciousness dizziness, fainting restlessness, anxiety, confusion, combativeness

Figure 15-9 The signs and symptoms of respiratory distress.

Patient Care—Respiratory Distress

Care for specific respiratory disorders will be discussed later in this chapter. Even if the specific disorder causing the respiratory distress cannot be determined, certain steps must be taken.

Emergency Care Steps

1. Ensure an open airway.
2. Treat for shock, administering a high concentration of oxygen.

   Note: There are some special considerations in administering a high concentration of oxygen to a patient with COPD. See the discussion of COPD later in this chapter.

3. Transport and arrange an ALS intercept.
4. Continue to monitor the patient carefully and be prepared to use a bag-valve mask and suction if the patient develops secretions or vomitus in the airway, respiratory depression or arrest.

If the specific disorder that is causing the respiratory distress is known or can be determined—such as COPD, asthma, or spontaneous pneumothorax—more specific courses of action may be taken. These disorders are discussed on the following pages.

Respiratory Disorders

Chronic Obstructive Pulmonary Disease (COPD) Chronic bronchitis, emphysema, black lung, and many undetermined respiratory illnesses that cause the patient problems like those seen in emphysema are all classified as **chronic obstructive pulmonary disease (COPD)**. Chronic bronchitis can be seen in children and teenagers; however, COPD is mainly a problem of middle-aged or older patients. This may be because these are disorders that tend to develop over a long period of time as reactions of tissues in the respiratory tract to smoking, allergens, chemicals, air pollutants, or repeated infections.

Chronic bronchitis and emphysema are compared in Figure 15-10.

In *chronic bronchitis*, the bronchiole lining is inflamed. Excess mucus is formed and released. The cells in the bronchioles that normally clear away accumulations of mucus are not able to do so. The sweeping apparatus on these cells, the cilia, have become paralyzed.

Usually the reason a COPD patient calls the ambulance is that a recent upper respiratory

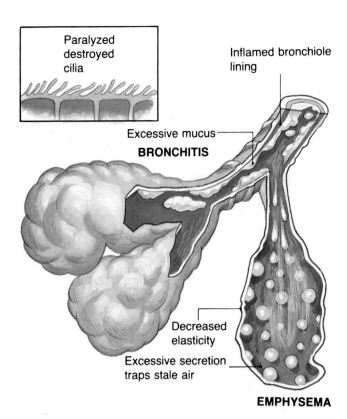

Figure 15-10 Chronic bronchitis and emphysema are chronic obstructive pulmonary diseases.

infection has caused an acute exacerbation of the disease.

Patient Assessment—Chronic Bronchitis

The typical chronic bronchitis patient will be an older person, usually a current or past heavy smoker. A patient with advanced chronic bronchitis who has cyanosis and edema is sometimes called a "blue bloater."

Signs and Symptoms

- ☐ Persistent cough
- ☐ Shortness of breath
- ☐ A tendency to tire easily
- ☐ Tightness in the chest
- ☐ Periods of dizziness (in some cases)

And in advanced cases . . .

- ☐ Cyanosis
- ☐ Edema of the lower extremities
- ☐ The patient wants to sit upright at all times.

Warning: It is important to protect yourself by wearing a mask and eye shield whenever a patient has a cough that produces mucus or spittle.

In *emphysema*, the walls of the alveoli break down, greatly reducing the surface area for respiratory exchange. The lungs begin to lose elasticity, and the alveoli and bronchioles secrete excess mucus. These factors combine to allow stale air to be trapped in the lungs, reducing the effectiveness of normal breathing efforts.

Patient Assessment—Emphysema

The typical emphysema patient is usually an older person who is a current or past heavy smoker or has been exposed to industrial smoke and gases. A patient with the signs of advanced emphysema is sometimes called a "pink puffer."

Signs and Symptoms

- ☐ The patient often has past history of respiratory problems or respiratory allergies.
- ☐ Signs that are the same as chronic bronchitis

And in advanced cases . . .

- ☐ Rapid pulse, occasionally irregular
- ☐ Breathing in puffs through pursed lips
- ☐ Barrel-chest appearance
- ☐ Wheezing

> **Note:** Even in advanced cases, blood pressure will usually be normal.

Patient Care— Chronic Bronchitis and Emphysema

In the prehospital setting, it is not necessary to distinguish the patient with chronic bronchitis from one with emphysema (the "blue bloater" from the "pink puffer"). The emergency care is essentially the same for both.

Emergency Care Steps

1. Ensure an open airway.
2. Monitor vital signs.
3. Allow the patient to assume the most comfortable position (usually sitting or semi-seated).
4. Administer oxygen as soon as possible. Patients who are in severe distress, have signs of shock, heart attack, or stroke should receive a high concentration of oxygen by mask. All COPD patients. who are given oxygen should be closely monitored (see below).
5. Loosen any restrictive garments.
6. Keep the patient warm but not overheated.
7. Do all you can to reduce stress.
8. Transport as soon as possible and ask for an ALS intercept.
9. Encourage coughing when necessary.

The method of oxygen delivery to the COPD patient is a difficult decision. A high concentration or flow rate of oxygen over a prolonged period of time will increase the blood concentration of oxygen. As discussed in Chapter 6, COPD patients may be in *hypoxic drive*. This means they have developed a tolerance to high carbon dioxide levels and, instead, their bodies determine the need to breathe based on decreased blood levels of oxygen. The higher oxygen levels that result from oxygen administration may signal the COPD patient to reduce breathing or even develop respiratory arrest. For this reason, some EMS systems recommend starting a patient who may have COPD on 24% oxygen by Venturi mask, then contacting medical control to see if the concentration should be increased.

In most cases, however, the hypoxic drive will not be a problem in the prehospital setting. The patient's need for oxygen will outweigh the risk involved with administration. If the patient has a possible heart attack or stroke, is developing shock, or has respiratory distress not related to the COPD, a higher concentration of oxygen will be required, in spite of the potential problems. IF OXYGEN IS REQUIRED BY THE COPD PATIENT, DO NOT WITHHOLD IT.

Constantly monitor the patient. If the patient dramatically slows his breathing or loses consciousness, be prepared to assist respirations with a bag-valve-mask and 100% oxygen. Realize that respiratory arrest will be easier to care for than the cardiac arrest that may develop from severe hypoxia (oxygen starvation). Do not decrease the oxygen delivered once you start administering it.

Transport the patient immediately and radio medical control for instructions. Always follow local protocols for oxygen administration.

Asthma Seen in young and old patients alike, **asthma** is an episodic disease. This is far different from chronic bronchitis and emphysema, both of which continually afflict the patient. Between episodes, the asthmatic patient can lead a normal life.

When an asthma attack occurs it may be triggered by an allergic reaction to something inhaled, swallowed, or injected into the body.

Attacks can be precipitated by insect stings, air pollutants, infection, strenuous exercise, or emotional stress. When an asthma attack occurs, the small bronchioles that lead to the air sacs of the lungs become narrowed because of contractions of the smooth muscles that make up the airway. To complicate matters, there is an overproduction of thick mucus. The combined effects of the contractions and the mucus cause the small passages to practically close down, severely restricting air flow.

The air flow is mainly restricted in one direction. When the patient inhales, the expanding lungs exert an outward force, increasing the diameter of the airway allowing air to flow into the lungs. During exhalation, the opposite occurs and the stale air becomes trapped in the lungs. This requires the patient to forcefully exhale the air, producing the characteristic wheezing sounds associated with asthma.

Patient Assessment—Asthma

Signs and Symptoms

The patient having an asthmatic attack will not usually have chest pain. The following signs and symptoms will usually be present.

- Wheezing (high-pitched) sounds that can frequently be heard without a stethoscope. There will be no doubt that the patient is having difficulty with expirations.
- An increased pulse rate, as high as 120 to 130 beats per minute. The rhythm of the pulse will be normal.
- Tenseness and anxiety. The patient is often obviously frightened.
- Distended (bulging) neck veins
- Shoulders hunched and chest pulled up by the effort to breathe
- Cyanosis (a late sign)
- Coughing

Patient Care—Asthma

Emergency care for the asthmatic patient is aimed at helping him breathe.

Emergency Care Steps

1. Try to reassure and calm the patient.
2. Assist the patient in taking any prescribed asthma medications.
3. Help the patient position himself so that he feels most comfortable.

4. Provide a high concentration of oxygen, humidified if possible. Asthma is not a disease associated with a hypoxic respiratory drive, so a high concentration of oxygen should not pose a problem. If you are unsure of the patient's actual disorder or if the patient is over 50 and a smoker, administer oxygen as discussed above for COPD patients.
5. Transport—Oxygen may provide only temporary relief.

Warning: All cases of asthma must be taken seriously since asthma can be fatal. Beware of the asthmatic who gets tired and quiet. He may be about to arrest.

In addition to the serious respiratory distress brought about by asthma, additional problems may develop. The asthma attack may have been set off by an allergen, and anaphylactic shock could develop. This must be considered a possibility any time you are caring for an asthma patient. Bronchospasms may occur before the patient develops anaphylactic shock.

Some patients develop prolonged asthma attacks that are life threatening (**status asthmaticus**). These patients can move only a small amount of air. For such patients, the chest is distended, the pulse rate is rapid, and breathing is obviously labored. So little air may be moved that the breathing sounds associated with asthma may not be heard. This is a TRUE EMERGENCY. Transport immediately and request ALS intercept. The status asthmaticus patient should be given a high concentration of humidified oxygen the same as for all asthma patients.

Hyperventilation Hyperventilation (HI-per-vent-i-LAY-shun) is a temporary condition in which respirations are too rapid and deep. This results in the body getting rid of too much carbon dioxide. Even though carbon dioxide is a waste product, reducing its level too much will adversely affect the patient.

Often hyperventilation will be brought on by fright or an emotionally upsetting experience. Once the patient begins to breathe rapidly, a series of events begins. The full, rapid breaths deplete the body's carbon dioxide levels. This brings on a variety of symptoms such as light-headedness, chest tightness, and numbness of the fingers and toes. These symptoms may cause the patient to feel he is having a heart attack. This causes breathing to speed up even more and the problem worsens.

Patient Assessment—Hyperventilation

Signs and Symptoms

☐ Breaths that are abnormally rapid and deep

☐ Some patients will have chest pain or other symptoms resembling an impending heart attack.

☐ Sensation in the upper extremity or the hands and feet and may display a cramping of the fingers.

Warning: The patient may tell you that he has attacks of hyperventilation. Even with this information, you should stay alert for changes in vital signs. The patient's problem in the past may have been simple hyperventilation, but this time it could be something more serious. Suspect hyperventilation only after considering more serious medical causes of rapid breathing, such as AMI, shock, and hypoxia.

Note: Hyperventilation is not only a condition, it can also be a sign. Patients with respiratory distress or AMI may also show hyperventilation brought on by the worry he has about the underlying condition. If the breathing is rapid, but *shallow* rather than deep, then the patient is not hyperventilating, Rapid, shallow breathing (tachypnea) *must* be considered to be a sign of more serious medical problems. Remember also that cyanosis usually indicates a problem more serious than hyperventilation (hyperventilation alone oxygenates the blood, whereas cyanosis indicates oxygen starvation). So cyanosis or its absence is a reliable clue that may help you to rule a more serious problem in or out.

Patient Care—Hyperventilation

Perhaps the best treatment for hyperventilation is to calm and reassure the patient. Tell the patient that his rapid breathing is what is causing him to experience dizziness, tingling, or chest pain. The patient may tell you that he has hyperventilated in the past.

A common treatment for the hyperventilating patient in the past was to have the patient breathe into a paper bag. The principle behind this was that the patient would rebreathe carbon dioxide that had been depleted. Recently, this procedure has come under scrutiny. If the patient has an underlying condition or if the patient is not actually hyperventilating, it may be harmful. Furthermore, harm may occur if the patient is allowed to breathe into the bag for too long. Most EMS systems no longer recommend this treatment.

Refer to your local protocols for treatments for hyperventilation. Some systems recommend oxygen in case there is an underlying problem. Still others recommend neither oxygen nor the paper bag. Calming, reassuring, and encouraging the patient to slow his respirations are sure to be helpful.

Spontaneous Pneumothorax Most cases of pneumothorax are associated with chest injuries (see Chapter 14). In rare cases, a weakened area of the lung ruptures without any associated trauma and releases air into the thoracic cavity. This is known as **spontaneous pneumothorax** (NU-mo-THOR-aks). It is most frequently seen as a problem in young, thin adult males and patients with COPD. The condition can be the result of congenital weakness, weakened scar tissue from previous injury or surgery, or certain types of lung cancer. When air enters the pleural space, the lung will collapse. If excessive pressure builds up in the pleural space, **tension pneumothorax** may result. This condition develops as the pressure increases and pushes the collapsed lung against the heart and the undamaged lung. Death may quickly follow.

Patient Assessment— Spontaneous Pneumothorax

The signs and symptoms of spontaneous pneumothorax include the pain of the rupture, the breathing difficulties caused by the pressure in the thoracic cavity and collapsed lung, and problems caused by pressure against the heart.

Signs and Symptoms

☐ Dyspnea

☐ Patients often report a sharp pain just before the dyspnea.

And if tension pneumothorax develops . . .

☐ Weak and rapid pulse

☐ Low blood pressure

☐ Uneven air entry into the lungs

☐ Distended neck veins

☐ The trachea may deviate to the side opposite the ruptured lung.

Patient Care—Spontaneous Pneumothorax

Warning: Pneumothorax is a serious condition. Tension pneumothorax is a TRUE EMERGENCY that may lead rapidly to death.

Emergency Care Steps

1. Administer a high concentration of oxygen.
2. Transport immediately and request ALS intercept.

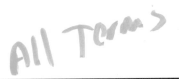

CHAPTER REVIEW

KEY TERMS

You may find it helpful to review the following terms.

acute—a medical problem with a sudden onset. Usually, the symptoms are severe and the critical stage of the problem is reached quickly.

acute myocardial infarction (ah-KUTE MY-o-KARD-e-ul in-FARK-shun) **(AMI)**—occurs when a portion of myocardium (heart muscle) dies when deprived of oxygenated blood; a heart attack.

aneurysm (AN-u-rizm)—the dilation, or ballooning, of a weakened section of an arterial wall.

angina pectoris (AN-ji-nah PEK-to-ris)—the sudden pain occurring when a portion of the myocardium is not receiving enough oxygenated blood.

aphasia (ah-FAY-zhah)—the complete loss or impairment of speech usually associated with a stroke or brain lesion.

apnea (ap-NE-ah)—the cessation of breathing.

arrhythmia (ah-RITH-me-ah)—a disturbance in heart rate and rhythm.

arteriosclerosis (ar-TE-re-o-skle-RO-sis)—"hardening of the arteries" caused by calcium deposits.

ascites (a-SI-tez)—the accumulation of excessive fluids in the abdomen.

asthma (AZ-mah)—a condition of respiratory distress caused when the bronchioles become narrowed and there is an overproduction of mucus causing a reduction in airflow on exhalation.

atherosclerosis (ATH-er-o-skle-RO-sis)—a build up of fatty deposits and other particles on the inner wall of an artery. This buildup is called plaque.

cardiovascular (CAR-de-o-VAS-kyu-ler) **system**—the system made up of the heart (*cardio*) and the blood vessels (*vascular*); the circulatory system.

cerebrovascular (SAIR-uh-bro-VAS-kyuh-ler)

accident (CVA)—a stroke; the blockage or rupture of a major blood vessel supplying the brain.

chronic—a medical problem that is consistently present over a long period of time.

chronic obstructive pulmonary disease (COPD)—a general classification for chronic bronchitis, emphysema, black lung, and many undetermined respiratory diseases that cause problems like those of emphysema.

congestive heart failure (CHF)—the failure of the heart to pump efficiently, leading to excessive blood or fluids in the lungs, the body, or both.

coronary (KOR-o-nar-e) **arteries**—blood vessels that supply the muscle of the heart (myocardium).

coronary artery disease (CAD)—the narrowing of a coronary artery brought about by atherosclerosis or arteriosclerosis. Occlusion (blockage) occurs in many cases.

diaphoresis (DI-ah-fo-RE-sis)—profuse perspiration.

dyspnea (disp-NE-ah)—difficult breathing.

embolism (EM-bo-liz-m)—a thrombus, or clot of blood and plaque, that has broken loose from the wall of an artery.

episodic—a medical problem that affects the patient at irregular intervals.

heart attack—an informal term for acute myocardial infarction (AMI).

hyperventilation (HI-per-vent-i-LAY-shun)—a temporary condition of rapid, deep breathing.

hypoxia (hi-POX-e-ah)—inadequate supply of oxygen to the body tissues.

mechanical pump failure—inability of the heart to funciton normally due to damaged tissues.

myocardium (mi-o-KAR-de-um)—heart muscle.

occlusion (uh-KLU-shun)—blockage, as in the blockage of an artery.

plaque (PLAK)—a fatty deposit on the interior walls of arteries.

pulmonary edema (PUL-mo-nar-e ed-EE-mah)—when the pulmonary vessels are engorged with blood and the alveoli contain excess fluids and foam. This may be associated with congestive heart failure.

rales (RAYLZ)—abnormal crackling or gravelly breathing sounds that can be heard in the lungs with a stethoscope, usually associated with fluids building up in the lungs.

respiratory system—the system made up of the airway (nose and mouth, pharynx, trachea, bronchi, and bronchioles) and the lungs.

spontaneous pneumothorax (NU-mo-THOR-aks)—when air enters the thoracic cavity through an opening in the weakened wall of a lung. The lung partially or completely collapses.

status asthmaticus (STAT-us az-MAT-i-kus)—a life-threatening prolonged asthma attack.

stroke—see *cerebrovascular accident*.

sudden death—a cardiac arrest that occurs within two hours of the onset of symptoms. The patient may have no prior symptoms or coronary artery disease.

tension pneumothorax—air pressure that builds within the thoracic cavity when air enters from a ruptured lung and has no means of escape.

thrombus (THROM-bus)—a clot formed of blood and plaque attached to the inner wall of an artery.

SUMMARY

What are Medical Emergencies?

Medical emergencies are illnesses that are not related to trauma. Chronic conditions are those that are constantly present over a long period of time. Episodic conditions are those that do not affect the patient every day but occasionally flare up. Acute illnesses are those that have a sudden onset.

The patient interview and physical examination are different for medical patients than for trauma patients. To evaluate for trauma, the EMT conducts a thorough hands-on survey for injuries. The medical patient is different. Although the physical exam is important, a majority of the information for the medical patient comes from the patient's interview and medical history, vital signs, medical identification devices, and family members or bystanders.

Signs and symptoms of medical emergencies may not seem serious in themselves but must be related to the underlying medical disorder.

Medical emergencies may be masked by other conditions such as trauma. A patient may lose consciousness and fall, injuring himself. EMTs are called for a fall. Unless the EMT realizes that the patient passed out before falling, a serious problem may be missed. It is important to find out which came first, the medical condition or the injury.

Disorders of the Cardiovascular System

The cardiovascular system includes the heart and the blood vessels. Coronary artery disease (CAD) is related to certain changes in the walls of the arteries of the heart. Atherosclerosis is a buildup of fatty deposits on the inner walls of arteries. The hardening of the arteries by calcium deposits is known as arteriosclerosis. When the coronary arteries become narrow or occluded, blood and oxygen do not reach the myocardium. This may lead to a variety of cardiac emergencies.

Angina pectoris is one of these emergencies. The onset of this condition usually occurs during stress or exertion. Chest pain or tightness is a classic symptom of angina. When the patient rests and takes nitroglycerin, the pain usually subsides.

An acute myocardial infarction (AMI) is what the lay person calls a heart attack. An occlusion of a coronary artery has caused a portion of the myocardium (heart muscle) to die. Depending on the size of the occlusion and the area of the heart affected, symptoms can range from chest pain to sudden death. The chest pains of AMI generally do not subside with rest. Additionally, the patient may have difficulty breathing, nausea, and sweating.

The treatment for angina pectoris and AMI are oxygen, careful monitoring, reassurance, and rapid transport, avoiding the use of the siren. Be prepared to provide rescue breathing using a bag-valve mask or to perform CPR (and defibrillation if you are so trained) if necessary.

Congestive heart failure (CHF) is usually related to a damaged or weakened heart that can no longer pump blood efficiently. Left heart failure causes pulmonary edema. Rales may be heard when a stethoscope is used to listen to the chest. Left heart failure eventually leads to right heart failure which often causes edema in the extremities and abdomen. Allow the congestive heart failure patient to sit in a position of comfort. Administer a high concentration of oxygen. If the patient has a history of COPD, be prepared for possible respiratory arrest, but do not withhold oxygen.

A patient with an implanted cardiac pacemaker or defibrillator or who has had cardiac bypass surgery can still suffer angina or an AMI. Treat these patients the same as you would treat any other patient with a cardiac problem.

A stroke or cerebrovascular accident (CVA) is caused by occlusion or rupturing of an artery supplying the brain. The conscious patient will usually be confused and have loss of extremity function (often to one side only), facial flaccidness, impaired speech, unequal pupil size, impaired vision, and a full, rapid pulse. A patient whose stroke results from a ruptured vessel may have a headache. Often the patient will have dyspnea and nausea. The patient may become comatose. If the stroke patient is conscious, maintain an open airway, keep him calm, administer oxygen, and transport in a semi-reclined position. Transport the unconscious patient in a laterally recumbent position and maintain the airway.

Disorders of the Respiratory System

Respiratory distress is caused when the flow of air in or out of the lungs is obstructed or when there is poor exchange of oxygen and carbon dioxide in the lungs. Dyspnea is difficult breathing, one of the signs of respiratory distress. Other signs and symptoms include altered levels of consciousness, anxiety, confusion or combativeness, cyanosis, flaring nostrils and pursed lips, straining neck and facial muscles, tightness or pain in the chest, strained intercostal and abdominal muscles, coughing, crowing, or barking, and rales or rhonchi heard with a stethoscope. Ensure an open airway, administer a high concentration of oxygen (with careful monitoring if the patient has a history of COPD), and transport.

Chronic obstructive pulmonary disease (COPD) is a general classificaton for diseases that include emphysema and chronic bronchitis. These diseases reduce the efficiency of gas exchange in the lungs. Signs and symptoms of both diseases include a persistent cough, shortness of breath, a tendency to tire easily, tightness in the chest, and sometimes dizziness. Patients with advanced chronic bronchitis may display cyanosis and edema of the extremities and may wish to remain upright at all times. Patients with advanced emphysema will usually have a normal blood pressure but may have a rapid, sometimes irregular pulse, will wheeze and breathe in puffs through pursed lips, and have a barrel-chested appearance.

Patient care for both chronic bronchitis and emphysema is the same, including administration of oxygen. Oxygen administration to COPD patients must be done with awareness that respiratory arrest is possible. COPD patients who show signs of shock, AMI, stroke, or respiratory distress that is not related to COPD should receive a high concentration of oxygen. NEVER WITHHOLD OXYGEN FROM ANY PATIENT WHO NEEDS IT!

Asthma is an episodic condition that causes restriction of the air passages. Reassure and calm the asthma patient. Administer a high concentration of oxygen and assist the patient with medications if allowed by local protocols.

Hyperventilation is a condition that may be a result of stress or fright but may also indicate a more serious underlying problem. Hyperventilating patients breathe rapidly and deeply. This causes a reduction in the carbon dioxide in the blood. Rapid, shallow respirations are most likely not hyperventilation. Patients who are hyperventilating will not display cyanosis. Calming the patient and encouraging him to breathe more slowly is the recommended treatment for hyperventilation.

Spontaneous pneumothorax is the collapse of a lung without obvious trauma. This condition requires immediate transport and oxygen with constant monitoring. This condition may turn into a tension pneumothorax in which air escaping from the damaged lung into the thoracic cavity builds up and puts pressure against the heart and the undamaged lung.

EMTs are frequently called to cardiovascular and respiratory emergencies. A firm knowledge of the many emergencies, with their symptoms, signs and treatments will help the EMT to handle these challenging calls.

16

On the Scene

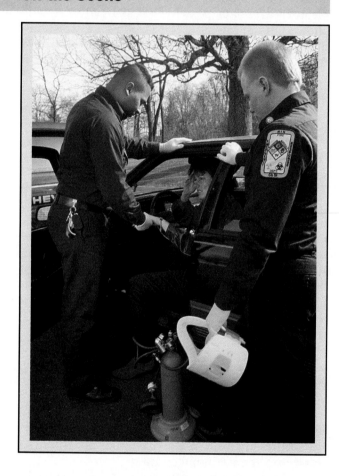

EMS response. When you arrive on the scene, the other motorist hurries forward to tell you that the driver who caused the accident is drunk. The police officer on the scene tells you that, while Rebecca is acting "off the wall," he is not sure what the problem is. "Check her out and let me know if you smell alcohol," he says.

You *(to Rebecca): Hello. (Pause) Hello, maam, we're from the ambulance.*

Rebecca Spicer: *I'm almost there. Two more blocks, and it'll be on the right.*

You: *Can you tell me your name?*

Rebecca Spicer: *Get out of the way! Can't you see I'm driving? How fast am I going?*

As Rebecca motions you away, you observe a bracelet on her wrist. It has the familiar shape of a medical identification bracelet. You ask Rebecca to see it. It confirms your suspicions that she is a diabetic. You advise the police officer of your findings and begin your treatment. Since she is able to swallow, you are able to persuade Rebecca to drink glucose mixed into some orange juice from a store up the street.

Twenty-five-year-old Rebecca Spicer begins to feel disoriented as she is driving. Before she knows it, she has run into the car in front of her. There isn't much damage, but as the driver of the other car comes back to see what happened, he notices that Rebecca appears intoxicated. "I knew it!" he mutters as he goes to call 911.

The 911 dispatcher calls for both police and

The change in Rebecca's behavior is rapid. As she begins to return to her normal orientation, she explains that she had taken her insulin but had forgotten to eat. She thanks you profusely for pulling her out of hypoglycemia. It's a dangerous condition, but a satisfying one to treat. Few emergencies in the field have provided you the opportunity to care for a patient with such immediate and rewarding results!

Diabetic and Other Medical Emergencies

As you learned in Chapter 15, medical emergencies are illnesses not related to injury or trauma. In that chapter you studied medical emergencies involving the cardiovascular system and the respiratory system.

Of course, there are many other kinds of medical emergencies. In this chapter you will study some of those that you will most commonly encounter as an EMT, including diabetic emergencies, seizure disorders, abdominal distress, communicable diseases, alcohol and substance abuse, and poisonings.

Expected Outcome, Chapter 16: *You will be able to assess and provide appropriate care for a variety of medical emergencies.*

> **WARNING:** Protect yourself from infectious diseases by using appropriate barrier devices such as a pocket face mask with one-way valve, face shield, or bag-valve mask; goggles or eye shield; and disposable gloves. Always conform to your local EMS system's infection exposure control plan.

MEDICAL CONDITIONS AND DISEASES
    Diabetes Mellitus
    Epilepsy and Other Seizure Disorders
    Acute Abdominal Distress
    Communicable Diseases

ALCOHOL AND SUBSTANCE ABUSE
    Alcohol Abuse
    Substance Abuse

POISONING
    Poison Control Centers
    Emergency Treatment for Poisoning

Knowledge *After reading this chapter, you should be able to*

1. Explain the "lock and key" mechanism of insulin and glucose. (p. 441)

2. Define *hyperglycemia* and *hypoglycemia* and compare and contrast their signs, symptoms, and emergency care. (pp. 442, 444; Scan 16-1)

3. List common causes of seizures. (pp. 444-445)

4. Describe two types of partial seizures and two types of generalized seizures, including the three phases of a tonic-clonic seizure. (pp. 445-446)

5. Describe patient assessment and care procedures for seizure disorders. (pp. 446-447)

6. List possible causes and the general signs and symptoms associated with acute abdominal distress. (pp. 447-448)

7. Describe the emergency care procedures for acute abdomen. (pp. 448-449)

8. List the general signs and symptoms of an infectious disease, kinds of infectious diseases, and appropriate means of protecting against contracting infectious diseases during EMT care. (p. 449)

9. Describe special problems faced when dealing with a patient under the influence of alcohol. (pp. 449-450)

10. Describe the signs and symptoms of alcohol abuse and alcohol withdrawal. (pp. 450-451)

11. Summarize the emergency care provided for the alcohol abuse patient. (p. 451)

12. Define *uppers*, *downers*, *hallucinogens*, *narcotics*, and *volatile chemicals*. (pp. 451-452)

13. Describe the signs and symptoms of drug abuse and drug withdrawal. (p. 453)

14. Summarize the emergency care provided for substance abuse patients. (pp. 453-454)

15. Define *poison* and state the four ways in which a poison can enter the body. (pp. 454-456)

16. Define *poison control center* and describe the role of such centers when you are pro-

viding emergency care for a poisoning patient. (pp. 456-457)

17. List the signs and symptoms of ingested poisoning and describe the appropriate emergency care. (pp. 457, 459; Scan 16-2)

18. List the signs and symptoms of inhaled poisoning and describe the appropriate emergency care. (pp. 460-462; Scan 16-3)

19. List the signs and symptoms of absorbed poisoning and describe the appropriate emergency care. (p. 462; Scan 16-4)

20. List the signs and symptoms of an injected poisoning (toxin) and describe the appropriate emergency care. (pp. 463, 465; Scan 16-5)

21. List the signs and symptoms of snakebite and describe the appropriate emergency care. (pp. 465-466)

22. List the sources and signs and symptoms of poisoning caused by marine life forms and describe the care for stings and punctures. (pp. 466-467)

Skills *As an EMT you should be able to*

1. Assess and provide emergency care for
   - Diabetic emergencies
   - Convulsive seizures
   - Acute abdomen
   - Possible communicable diseases

2. Protect yourself from communicable diseases.

3. Assess and provide emergency care for patients under the influence of alcohol or drugs and for patients suffering alcohol or drug withdrawal.

4. Assess obvious cases of ingested, inhaled, absorbed, and injected poisons (toxins) and communicate effectively with your local poison control center.

5. Receive and carry out instructions given by a poison control center.

6. Assess and provide emergency care for snakebites.

7. Assess and provide emergency care for marine-life-form poisonings.

Assessment of a medical emergency, as discussed in earlier chapters, differs from assessment of trauma. With trauma, the majority of your information will usually come from the physical exam; with a medical emergency, you will gain the majority of your information from the interview. Information about the current illness (such as time and circumstances of onset and detailed description of symptoms) is vital. For information about the patient's past medical history, you can use the AMPLE questions (see Chapter 3): (A—Allergies: *Are you allergic to anything?* M—Medication: *What medications are you taking?* P—Previous medical history: *Have you been having any problems? Seeing a doctor?* L—Last meal: *When did you eat last? What did you eat?* E—Events: *What led up to today's problems? What happened first? next?*) Information gained from the family and bystanders is also important.

Pain is a symptom of most medical emergencies, and the nature of the pain is an important clue. It is important to get the patient to describe it thoroughly. One method that helps to obtain a detailed description of pain is to ask the PQRST questions (see chapter 3): (P—Provocation: *What brought on the pain?* Q—Quality: *What does it feel like?* R—Region: *Where is the pain?* Referral: *Does the pain go anywhere?* Recurrence: *Have you had this pain before?* Relief: *Does anything make it feel better?* S—Severity: *On a scale of 1 to 10—if 0 is no pain and 10 is the worst pain you can imagine—how bad is the pain?* T—Time: *When did it start?*)

In addition, there are other important things to find out about pain. Remember that "pain" can include feelings of heaviness, tightness, and other sensations. Patients often do not realize this and will say "no" when asked if they have pain, but if questioned properly would tell the EMT about the crushing or squeezing feeling in their chest.

Keep your interviewing skills in mind as you read about the medical emergencies described in this chapter.

MEDICAL CONDITIONS AND DISEASES

Diabetes Mellitus

Glucose (GLU-kos), a simple sugar, is the body's basic source of energy. The complex sugars that a person eats are converted into glucose, which is then absorbed into the bloodstream. However,

this blood sugar cannot simply pass from the bloodstream into the body's cells. To enter the cells, **insulin** (IN-suh-lin), a hormone produced by the pancreas, must be present. Without insulin the cells can be surrounded by glucose but still starve for this sugar. The insulin/glucose relationship has been described as a "lock and key" mechanism. Consider insulin as the key. Without this "key," glucose cannot enter the "locked" cells (Figure 16-1).

When sugar intake and insulin production are balanced, the body can effectively use sugar as an energy source. If, for some reason, insulin production decreases, the glucose cannot be used by the cells. This glucose remains in circulation, increasing in concentration as more sug-

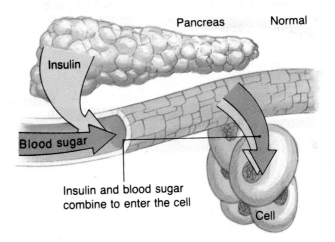

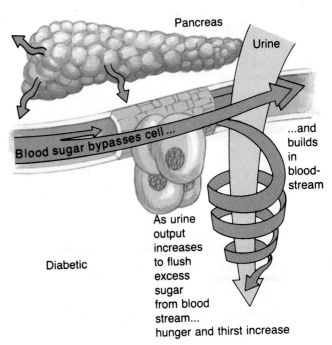

Figure 16-1. Insulin is needed for cells to take up sugar.

ars are digested by the person. The level of blood sugar climbs, eventually to be spilled over into the urine. The urine output of the body increases in an effort to rid the body of excess sugar. This, in turn, makes the patient abnormally thirsty.

The condition brought about by decreased insulin production is known as **diabetes mellitus** (di-ah-BEE-tez MEL-i-tus), or "sugar diabetes," often called just "diabetes." The person suffering from this condition is a diabetic.

There are two major classifications of diabetes mellitus. Type I, or insulin-dependent, diabetes occurs in individuals with little or no ability to produce insulin. This type of diabetes has been called "juvenile diabetes" since it tends to begin in childhood. The Type I diabetic must take daily doses of supplemental insulin. Type II, or noninsulin-dependent, diabetes occurs in individuals who have the ability to produce insulin but are unable to develop enough of it or to use it effectively. This disorder usually develops in adults and has been called "maturity-onset diabetes." Diabetes in adulthood is usually associated with obesity and is seen more often in older than in younger people. Type II diabetes can often be controlled without supplemental insulin through supervised diets and medications to lower their sugar.

The danger of undetected and untreated diabetes is severe. As the condition develops, the diabetic can become weak and lose weight even though he may increase his sugar and fat intake. Advanced diabetes is often associated with such complications as heart disease, kidney disease, and blindness.

Hyperglycemia and Hypoglycemia Two possible causes of medical emergencies for the diabetic are too much sugar in the bloodstream or not enough sugar in the bloodstream. Either situation can prove to be life threatening.

Hyperglycemia is also known as "*high* blood sugar." (*Hyper* means "more than normal" or "excessive.") This condition occurs because the diabetic does not produce enough natural insulin to take sugar out of the blood and into the cells, and because he

- Has not taken enough insulin to make up for this deficiency, or . . .
- Has forgotten to take his insulin, or . . .
- Has overeaten, or . . .
- Has an infection that has upset his insulin/glucose balance

With hyperglycemia, not only is there too much sugar in the blood, there is too little sugar

in the cells. The body attempts to overcome the lack of sugar in the cells by using other foods for energy, particularly stored fats. However, fats are not an efficient alternative to glucose, and the waste products of fat utilization, ketones (compounds that are in the same class as those used to make fingernail polish remover), begin to concentrate in the blood, turning the blood acid. The person will take in large quantities of water to offset the loss of fluids through excess urination. If allowed to go untreated, the acidity of the blood and the loss of fluids brought on by the high level of glucose in the blood eventually lead to **diabetic ketoacidosis** (KEY-to-as-i-DO-sis), which can lead to death.*

Hypoglycemia is also known as "*low* blood sugar." (*Hypo* means "less than normal" or "deficient.") This is caused when the diabetic

- Takes too much insulin
- Reduces sugar intake by not eating
- Overexercises or overexerts himself, thus using sugars faster than normal
- Vomits a meal

If there is too much insulin, it increases the rate at which sugar enters the cells. Not enough sugar remains in the bloodstream for the brain, which may lead to unconsciousness. Reducing sugar intake, overexercising, or vomiting will also cause a deficiency of sugar in the bloodstream with the same possible result, unconsciousness. Permanent brain damage can occur quickly if the sugar is not replenished.† Hypoglycemia can cause greater damage more quickly than hyperglycemia.

Patient Assessment—Diabetic Emergencies

Many students find that they confuse hyperglycemia and hypoglycemia. For this reason, the signs, symptoms, and procedures for care are presented side by side in Scan 16-1. For example . . .

☐ Onset—Note that hyperglycemia usually has a slower onset, while hypoglycemia tends to come on suddenly. This is because some sugar still reaches the brain in hyperglycemic (*high* blood sugar) states. With

---

*Diabetic ketoacidosis is sometimes called diabetic coma, but this is not an accepted medical term.

†Hypoglycemia is sometimes called insulin shock, but it is not a true form of shock, and this is not an accepted medical term.

Diabetic Emergencies

HYPERGLYCEMIA

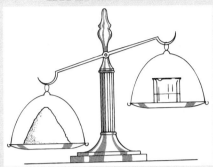

HYPOGLYCEMIA

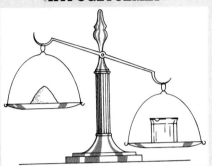

CAUSES
- The diabetic's condition has not been diagnosed and/or treated.
- The diabetic has not taken his insulin.
- The diabetic has overeaten, flooding the body with a sudden excess of carbohydrates.
- The diabetic suffers an infection that disrupts his glucose/insulin balance.

SIGNS AND SYMPTOMS
- Gradual onset of signs and symptoms, over a period of days
- Patient complains of dry mouth and intense thirst.
- Patient may appear to be intoxicated.
- Abdominal pain and vomiting common
- Gradually increasing restlessness, confusion, followed by stupor
- Coma, with these signs:
  - Signs of air hunger—deep, sighing respirations
  - Weak, rapid pulse
  - Warm, red, dry skin
  - Eyes that appear sunken.
  - Normal or slightly low blood pressure
  - Breath smells of acetone—sickly sweet, like nail polish remover

EMERGENCY CARE
- Administer a high concentration of oxygen.
- Immediately transport to a medical facility.
- Arrange for ALS intercept.

CAUSES
- The diabetic has taken too much insulin.
- The diabetic has not eaten enough to provide his normal sugar intake.
- The diabetic has overexercised or overexerted himself, thus reducing his blood glucose level.
- The diabetic has vomited a meal.

SIGNS AND SYMPTOMS
- Rapid onset of signs and symptoms, over a period of minutes
- Dizziness and headache
- Abnormal hostile or aggressive behavior, which may appear to be acute alcoholic intoxication
- Fainting, seizures, and occasionally coma
- Normal blood pressure
- Full, rapid pulse
- Patient intensely hungry
- Skin cold, pale, and clammy; perspiration may be profuse
- Copious saliva, drooling

EMERGENCY CARE
- Conscious Patient—Administer granular sugar, honey, Lifesaver or other candy placed under the tongue, orange juice, or glucose.
- Unconscious Patient—Avoid giving liquids; provide "sprinkle" of granulated sugar under tongue, or dab of glucose if protocols permit.
- Turn head to side or place in lateral recumbent (recovery) position.
- Provide a high concentration of oxygen.
- Transport to a medical facility.
- Arrange for ALS intercept.

SPECIAL NOTES: HYPERGLYCEMIA AND HYPOGLYCEMIA
When faced with a patient who may be suffering from one of these conditions . . .
- Determine if the patient is diabetic. Look for medical identification medallions, insulin in the refrigerator, or information cards; interview patient and family members.
- If the patient is a known or suspected diabetic, and hypoglycemia cannot be ruled out, assume that it is hypoglycemia and administer sugar.

Often a patient suffering from either of these conditions may simply appear drunk. Always check for other underlying conditions—such as diabetic complications—when treating someone who appears intoxicated.

hypoglycemia (*low* blood sugar) it is possible that *no* sugar is reaching the brain. *Seizures may occur.*

- Skin—Hyperglycemic patients often have warm, red, dry skin. Hypoglycemic patients have cold, pale, moist or "clammy" skin.
- Breath—The hyperglycemic patient often has acetone breath (like nail polish remover) while the hypoglycemic patient does not.
- Continue to make the comparison for yourself by studying Scan 16-1.

Although there appear to be clear-cut differences between the signs and symptoms of hyperglycemia and hypoglycemia, distinguishing between the two in the field may be difficult and is not really necessary since the emergency care for both (as discussed below) can be the same. In addition to noting signs and symptoms, always be alert for medical identification jewelry or cards, or insulin in the refrigerator. Seek information from the patient or bystander interviews that will alert you to the fact that the patient is diabetic.

Warning: Keep in mind that MANY HYPERGLYCEMIC PATIENTS AND SOME HYPOGLYCEMIC PATIENTS WILL APPEAR TO BE INTOXICATED. Always suspect a diabetic problem in cases that seem to involve no more than intoxication. Remember that the patient intoxicated on alcohol may also be a diabetic, with the alcohol breath covering over the acetone smell characteristic of diabetic ketoacidosis. The alcoholic diabetic is a good candidate for a diabetic emergency, because he tends to neglect taking insulin during the course of prolonged drinking and usually has a low blood sugar level.

Patient Care—Diabetic Emergencies

Emergency Care Steps

Since the primary cause of diabetic emergencies is an abnormal level of blood sugar, emergency care involves treating for this problem. The following procedures apply to both hyperglycemic and hypoglycemic patients.

- The Conscious Patient—Whenever you are in doubt as to whether a conscious patient is suffering from diabetic coma or insulin shock, give the patient instant glucose or orange juice and treat for insulin shock. The "glucose for everyone" policy is correct for conscious patients, since hyperglycemic patients will not be hurt by what you do provided they are transported, while hypoglycemic patients *need* sugar as soon as possible.
- The Unconscious Patient—Giving anything by mouth to an unconscious patient is a dangerous policy since it may lead to aspiration. A "sprinkle" of granulated sugar under the tongue is acceptable in some EMS systems, but no one advocates administering liquids by mouth to the unconscious patient. If you sprinkle sugar, do it from your fingers to avoid an accidental pouring. Provide just enough to be absorbed. Your EMS system may carry a commercially made thick glucose solution in a squeezable tube and may permit a small quantity of this substance to be placed under the unconscious patient's tongue. Follow local protocols. Keep the patient in a lateral recumbent position (recovery position) to avoid aspiration in case of vomiting.

Epilepsy and Other Seizure Disorders

If the normal functions of the brain are upset by injury, infection, or disease, the electrical activity of the brain can become irregular. This irregularity can bring about sudden changes in sensation, behavior, or movement, called seizures (also called fits, spells, or attacks by nonmedical people). Some seizures involve the uncontrolled muscular movements that are often called *convulsions.*

A seizure is not a disease in itself, but rather a sign of an underlying defect, injury, or disease. The most common causes of seizures include

- Brain Tumor—A brain tumor may occasionally manifest as a seizure.
- Congenital Brain Defects—Seizures due to congenital defects of the brain (defects one is born with) are most often seen in infants and young children.
- Febrile—Seizures with a high fever (febrile) are seen in children 6 months to 3 years of age, rarely in older children or adults.
- Idiopathic—Idiopathic seizures are those that occur spontaneously with an unknown cause.

- Infection—Swelling or inflammation of the brain caused by an infection (as with encephalitis) can cause seizures.
- Metabolic—Seizures can be caused by irregularities in the patient's body chemistry (metabolism).
- Toxic—Drug or alcohol use or abuse or withdrawal can cause seizures (*toxic* means "poisonous"; the drug or alcohol has worked as a poison).
- Trauma—Scars formed at the site of previous brain injuries may invite seizures.

In addition, convulsive seizures may be seen with

- Epilepsy
- CVA (stroke)
- Measles, mumps, and other childhood diseases
- Hypoglycemia
- Eclampsia in pregnancy (see Chapter 18)

Epilepsy is perhaps the best-known of the conditions that result in seizures. Some people are born with epilepsy while others develop epilepsy after a head injury or surgery. Conscientious use of medications allows most epileptics to live normal lives without seizures of any type. It is well for the EMT to remember that, while a patient with seizures may be an epileptic, epilepsy is only one condition that causes seizures.

Patient Assessment—Seizure Disorders

Not all seizures are alike. The activity and duration of the seizure may be determined by the underlying cause. The type of seizure most people associate with epilepsy and other seizure disorders is the generalized tonic-clonic seizure in which the person falls to the floor and has severe convulsions. However, this is only one of four common types of seizures in two classifications: partial seizures and generalized seizures. The characteristics of these classifications and types of seizures are described below.

Partial Seizures

☐ Simple Partial Seizure (also called focal motor, focal sensory, or Jacksonian)—There is tingling, stiffening, or jerking in just one part of the body. There may also

be an aura in which the person may experience sensations such as a smell, bright lights, a burst of colors, or a rising sensation in the stomach. There is no loss of consciousness. However in some cases the jerking may spread and develop into a generalized tonic-clonic seizure (see below).

☐ Complex Partial Seizure (also called psychomotor or temporal lobe)—Often preceded by an aura, this type of seizure is characterized by abnormal behavior that varies widely from person to person. It may involve confusion, a glassy stare, aimless moving about, lip smacking or chewing, or fidgeting with clothing. The person may appear to be drunk or on drugs, is not violent but may struggle or fight if restrained. Very rarely a complex partial seizure may result in such extreme behavior as screaming, running, disrobing, or showing great fear. There is no loss of consciousness but there may be confusion and no memory of the episode. In some cases the seizure may develop into a tonic-clonic seizure.

Generalized Seizures

☐ Tonic-Clonic (also called grand mal)—There is often no aura or other warning. The person may cry out before falling to the floor. This type of seizure is characterized by unconsciousness and major motor activity. The patient will thrash about wildly, using his entire body. The convulsion usually lasts only a few minutes and has three distinct phases.

1. Tonic phase—The body becomes rigid, stiffening for no more than 30 seconds. Breathing may stop, the patient may bite his tongue (rare), and bowel and bladder control could be lost.
2. Clonic phase—The body jerks about violently, usually for no more than 1 or 2 minutes (some can last 5 minutes). The patient may foam at the mouth and drool. His face and lips often become cyanotic.
3. Postictal phase—This begins when convulsions stop. The patient may regain consciousness immediately and enter a state of drowsiness and confusion, or he may remain unconscious for several hours. Headache is common.

☐ Absence (also called petit mal)—The seizure is brief, usually only 1 to 10 seconds. There is no dramatic motor activity and the person usually does not slump or fall. Instead there is a temporary loss of concentration or awareness. An absence seizure may go unnoticed by everyone except the person and knowledgeable members of his family. A child may suffer several hundred absence seizures a day, severely interfering with his ability to pay attention and do well in school. Absence seizures often stop before adulthood but sometimes worsen and become tonic-clonic seizures.

Warning: Partial and tonic-clonic seizures usually last no more than 1 to 3 minutes. When the patient has two or more convulsive seizures without regaining full consciousness and lasting 5 to 10 minutes or more, it is known as **status epilepticus**. Some systems consider all patients who are still seizing when EMS arrives on the scene to be status epilepticus. This is a TRUE EMERGENCY requiring immediate high priority transport and arrangement for ALS intercept. Do not try to restrain the patient, even if the convulsions appear to have ended. Keep in mind that the prolonged seizure activity may have caused hypoxia. The airway must be suctioned and a high concentration of oxygen should be administered at the scene and while en route.

As you can see from the above descriptions, seizures can vary widely in their characteristics.

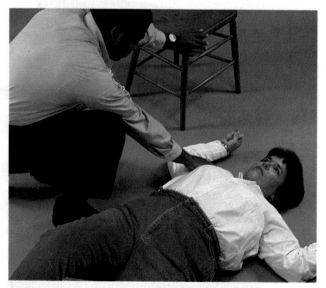

Figure 16-2. Protect the patient from injury.

As an EMT it is not your job to diagnose or classify a seizure. However it is very important to be able to describe it in detail to medical personnel. Always try to observe or to find out from bystanders the answers to the following questions.

- What was the person doing before the seizure started?
- Exactly what did the person do during the seizure—movement by movement—especially at the beginning? Was there loss of bladder or bowel control?
- How long did the seizure last?
- What did the person do after the seizure? Was he asleep (and for how long)? Was he awake? Was he able to answer questions? (If you are present, use the AVPU scale to measure level of consciousness.)

Patient Care—Seizure Disorders

Emergency Care Steps
If you are present when the seizure occurs, it is important to follow these steps.

For a Simple or Complex Partial Seizure

☐ Do not restrain the person; simply remove objects from his path and gently guide him away from danger.

For a Generalized Tonic-Clonic Seizure

1. Place the patient on the floor or ground. If possible, position for drainage from the mouth.
2. Loosen restrictive clothing.
3. Remove objects that may harm the patient.
4. Protect the patient from injury, but do not try to hold the patient still during convulsions (Figure 16-2).
5. After convulsions have ended, keep the patient at rest, positioned for drainage from the mouth. Suction the airway. Some patients become hypoxic (oxygen-starved) during a seizure, so be prepared to administer oxygen as soon as possible. Treat any injuries the patient may have sustained during the convulsions.
6. Take vital signs and monitor respirations closely.
7. Protect the patient from embarrassment. Ask onlookers to give the patient privacy.
8. Consider the cause of the seizure. If the patient does not have a history of epilepsy,

446 Medical Emergencies

consider fever (in children), hypoxia, hypoglycemia, and other possible causes. If these causes have a field treatment, consider undertaking that treatment (e.g., oxygen for hypoxia, sugar for hypoglycemia).

9 Transport to a medical facility, monitoring vital signs.

For an Absence Seizure

☐ Be aware that a seizure has occurred and provide missed information.

Note: *Never* place anything in the mouth of a seizing patient. Many objects can be broken and obstruct the patient's airway.

The epileptic is often very knowledgeable about his condition, medications, and history. Since seizures may be common for the patient, he may refuse transportation. The patient should be encouraged to accept transportation to a hospital for examination. Should the patient continue to refuse, he should not be left alone during the postictal phase of his seizure, and he must not drive. A competent relative or other responsible person must remain with the patient.

Acute Abdominal Distress

Acute abdominal distress, or **acute abdomen**, is the sudden onset of severe abdominal pain and discomfort. Acute abdomen may be the result of infection, inflammation, rupture, or disease to any of the abdominal organs.

Many abdominal problems start out as simple "indigestion" in the mind of the patient, and he waits for it to "go away." However, when pain does not go away, or it becomes so severe that it frightens the patient and his family, emergency medical services may be called to respond. Sometimes, after arrival at the hospital, it is determined that the cause of the pain *is* nothing more than indigestion. Other times it may prove to be such a problem as

- Appendicitis
- Gallbladder inflammation or gallstones
- Ectopic pregnancy (see Chapter 18)
- Intestinal obstruction
- An aneurysm
- Peritonitis (inflammation of the membranes lining the abdominal cavity)
- Perforated ulcers or another cause of internal bleeding

- Hernia (see Chapter 14)
- Kidney stones
- Inflammation of the pancreas
- Acute myocardial infarction (AMI—heart attack; see Chapter 15)

Patient Assessment—Acute Abdomen

The signs and symptoms of acute abdomen do not always help the EMT to figure out what the exact problem is. There are a large number of important organs in the same area, and pain may be felt in an area other than the site of its origin. Pain or discomfort from abdominal emergencies may be felt as far away as the shoulders and the legs (referred pain—Figure 16-3). So it is often difficult to differentiate among several abdominal emergencies. Remember, however, that definitive diagnosis is the physician's job, not the EMT's.

Look for any of the following signs and symptoms of abdominal distress.

Signs and Symptoms

☐ Pain—diffuse (generalized, widespread)
☐ Nausea and vomiting
☐ Diarrhea or constipation
☐ Rapid pulse (usually)
☐ Low blood pressure (sometimes high when the patient is in severe pain)
☐ Rapid and shallow breathing
☐ Fever and possible chills
☐ Distention of the abdomen
☐ Tenderness (local or diffuse)
☐ Rigid abdomen (a stiffness that cannot be relaxed on command)
☐ Abdominal wall muscle guarding
☐ An obvious protrusion seen or felt in the abdominal wall
☐ Signs of shock (from internal bleeding or severe infection)
☐ Vomiting blood (may appear as "coffee grounds" in the vomitus or as truly bloody vomitus)
☐ Unusual bowel movements (e.g., dark, tarry stools)
☐ Bleeding from the rectum, blood in the urine, nonmenstrual bleeding from the vagina
☐ Fear or apprehension

As you look for these indicators, consider the patient's overall appearance. Does he appear ill? Does he try to lie perfectly still in an effort to alleviate the pain? Does he try to

REFERRED AND ACTUAL PAIN AREAS

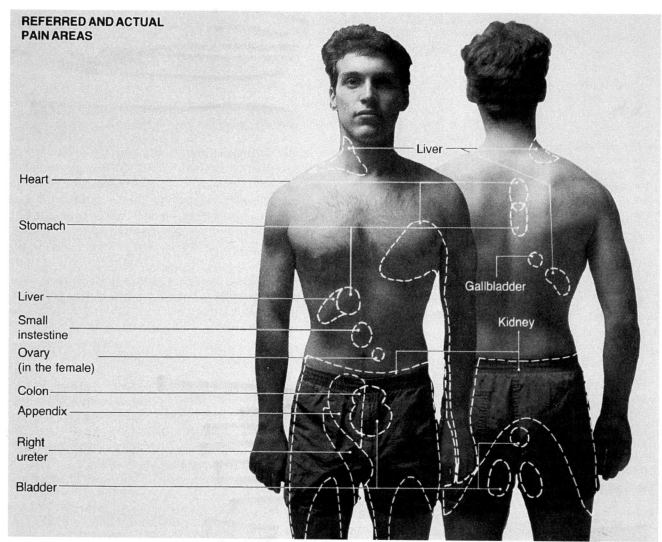

Heart

Stomach

Liver

Small instestine

Ovary (in the female)

Colon

Appendix

Right ureter

Bladder

Liver

Gallbladder

Kidney

Figure 16-3. Patterns of abdominal pain.

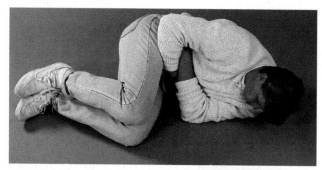

Figure 16-4. Posturing that is characteristic of severe abdominal distress.

draw his knees up against his abdomen (Figure 16-4)? Is he reluctant to move? Is he unable to find a comfortable position? Does he exhibit any of the signs of shock, including paleness, cool and clammy skin, and restless-

ness? All of these point to acute abdominal distress.

In the patient interview, attempt to collect information as to the time of onset of the pain, if it was gradual or sudden, the nature of the pain (stabbing, gnawing, sharp), when the patient last ate, what was consumed, and other information that can be elicited by using the AMPLE and PQRST questions listed at the beginning of this chapter.

Patient Care—Acute Abdomen

The signs and symptoms of acute abdominal distress should not be taken lightly. What you do and do not do can be critical for the patient. *Do not* try to guess the nature of the illness but follow the emergency care steps listed below for all cases of abdominal dis-

448 Medical Emergencies

tress. Field treatment centers largely around the prevention or treatment of shock plus transport.

Emergency Care Steps

1. Maintain an open airway and be on the alert for vomiting.
2. Provide care for shock.
3. Position the patient face up with the knees flexed, but stay on the alert for vomiting.
4. Reassure the patient . . . do not try to diagnose.
5. Administer oxygen if there is shallow breathing or other indications of respiratory difficulties.
6. Do not give anything to the patient by mouth.
7. Save all vomitus. Since the patient may have a communicable disease, avoid contact with ALL body fluids and discharges.
8. Transport the patient to a medical facility.

Communicable Diseases

As an EMT you may have to care for and transport a patient who has an infectious or communicable disease. *There may be no indications of infection*, or it may be noticeable when, upon assessment, the patient presents with

- Fever
- Diaphoresis (profuse sweating)
- Vomiting or diarrhea
- A rash or other lesions on the skin
- Headache, stiff neck, chest pain, abdominal pain
- Coughing or sneezing

Your role will be to transport, maintain an open airway, treat for shock, keep the patient warm, and give nothing by mouth.

EMTs often fear contracting an infectious disease in the course of their duties. Part of this fear stems from reading the long lists of diseases found in books and magazines designed for laypersons. Some of these diseases are very rare, are difficult to "catch" from simple exposure, or are no longer a problem. Others *are* of concern, particularly hepatitis, meningitis, and tuberculosis, which are serious and highly communicable diseases, and HIV, the virus that causes AIDS, which is not highly communicable but is deadly once contracted. Some other diseases can cause problems if you have never had them or been immunized specifically against them. Mumps is

an example. In addition to HIV, some other sexually-transmitted diseases (STDs) can occasionally be transmitted in ways other than through sexual contact. For example, genital herpes in its active stages produces lesions or sores in the genital area. Other varieties of herpes can appear as "fever blisters" on the lips or as lesions elsewhere on the body. Syphilis can be transmitted through contact with the patient's blood or other body fluids.

So your role is not only to care for the patient but to protect yourself and others. Review the information on infectious and communicable diseases and recommended means of protection under "Infection Control and the EMT" in Chapter 1. Use appropriate barrier clothing and devices including disposable gloves, and follow your agency's exposure control plan at all times.

If the presence of a communicable disease is a possibility, ask the emergency department physician if you need to do anything else or if you need special immunization or antibiotic treatment. Ask to be informed if the patient's disease is diagnosed as communicable. If so, you should be examined also. Make certain that you follow all local protocols to be sure that others helping at the scene (e.g., first responders, police, fire service personnel) are also notified.

ALCOHOL AND SUBSTANCE ABUSE

As an EMT you will see many patients whose conditions are caused, either directly or indirectly, by alcohol or substance abuse. Although these are often thought of as urban problems, the abuse of alcohol and other drugs crosses all geographic and economic boundaries.

Alcohol Abuse

While many persons consume alcohol without any problems, others occasionally or chronically abuse alcohol. Although alcohol is legal (for adults), it must not be forgotten that alcohol is a drug and has a potent effect on the central nervous system. Emergencies arising from the use of alcohol may be due to the effect of alcohol that has just been consumed, or it may be the result of the cumulative effects of years of alcohol abuse.

EMTs often do not take alcohol abuse patients seriously. This may be partially due to the belligerent or unusual behavior they often exhibit. In addition, frequent calls for intoxicated persons may cause the EMT to become callous toward them. The hygiene of many of these patients on the street leaves much to be desired. Some EMTs believe that alcohol abuse patients tie up ambulances so they are not available for patients "who really need them."

However, EMS system personnel believe that EMTs should provide care for the patient suffering from alcohol abuse the same as for any other patient. An alcohol problem is not looked on as a crime, but as a disease. Patients who appear intoxicated must be treated with the same respect and dignity as those who are "sober."

Further, you must not neglect your duty to provide medical care. Not only do alcohol abuse patients often have injuries from accidents and falls, but these persons are also candidates for many medical emergencies. Chronic drinkers often have derangements in blood sugar levels, poor nutrition, the potential for considerable gastrointestinal bleeding, and other problems. Experts now believe that the overuse of alcohol may contribute to some cancers. A person can be both intoxicated *and* having a heart attack or hypoglycemia. If the patient has ingested both alcohol and other drugs, this can also produce a serious medical emergency. When alcohol is combined with other depressants such as antihistamines and tranquilizers, the effects will be doubled or more than doubled and, in some cases, can be lethal.

Since EMT safety is a critical part of all calls, do not hesitate to ask for police assistance with any patient who appears intoxicated or irrational or exhibits potentially dangerous behavior. The nature of intoxication is such that a passive person may suddenly become aggressive. The EMT should always be prepared for this event. (See Chapter 21 for additional strategies for dealing with intoxicated patients and patients with special problems.)

Patient Assessment—Alcohol Abuse

Keep in mind that, while alcohol *may* be the patient's only problem, there may be another problem present. Conduct a proper survey and interview to assess for any medical emergencies. Remember that diabetes, epilepsy, head injuries, high fevers, hypoxia, and other medical problems may make the patient *appear* to be intoxicated. Also look for fractures or indications of other injuries. *Do not*

allow the presence of alcohol or the signs and symptoms of alcohol abuse to override your suspicions of other medical problems or injuries.

Since the interview of any patient who appears intoxicated will be difficult, your powers of observation and resourcefulness will be tested. Family members and bystanders may provide important information.

The signs and symptoms of alcohol abuse include those listed below.

Signs and Symptoms of Alcohol Abuse

- [ ] The odor of alcohol on the patient's breath or clothing. By itself, this is not enough to conclude alcohol abuse. Be certain that this odor is not "acetone breath" as with some diabetic emergencies.
- [ ] Swaying and unsteadiness of movement
- [ ] Slurred speech, rambling thought patterns, incoherent words or phrases
- [ ] A flushed appearance to the face, often with the patient sweating and complaining of being warm
- [ ] Nausea or vomiting
- [ ] Poor coordination
- [ ] Slowed reaction time
- [ ] Blurred vision
- [ ] Confusion
- [ ] Hallucinations, visual or auditory ("seeing things" or "hearing things")
- [ ] Lack of memory (blackout)
- [ ] Altered levels of consciousness or unconsciousness

The alcoholic patient may not be under the influence of alcohol but, instead, may be suffering from alcohol **withdrawal**. This can be a severe reaction occurring when the patient cannot obtain alcohol, is too sick to drink alcohol, or has decided to quit drinking suddenly. The alcohol withdrawal patient may experience seizures or **delirium tremens (DTs)**, a condition characterized by sweating, trembling, anxiety, and hallucinations. In some cases, alcohol withdrawal can be fatal.

Signs of Alcohol Withdrawal

- [ ] Confusion and restlessness
- [ ] Atypical behavior, to the point of being "mad" or demonstrating "insane" behavior
- [ ] Hallucinations
- [ ] Gross tremor (obvious shaking) of the hands
- [ ] Profuse sweating

- Seizures (common and often very serious)
- The signs and symptoms of shock due to fluid loss (rare). Initially, pulse, respirations, blood pressure, and skin temperature will be elevated.

Warning: Be on the alert for signs, such as depressed vital signs, that the patient's has mixed alcohol and drugs. When interviewing the intoxicated patient or the patient suffering from alcohol withdrawal, do not begin by asking the patient if he is taking *drugs*. He may react to this question as if you are gathering evidence of a crime. Ask if any *medications* have been taken while drinking. If necessary, when you are certain that the patient knows you are concerned about his well-being, you can repeat the question using the word "drugs."

Patient Care—Alcohol Abuse

Emergency Care Steps

To provide basic care for the intoxicated patient and the patient suffering alcohol withdrawal

1. Monitor vital signs, staying alert for respiratory problems. Be alert for changes in level of consciousness as alcohol is absorbed into the bloodstream.
2. Talk to the patient in an effort to keep him as alert as possible.
3. Help the patient during vomiting so that vomitus will not be aspirated. Have a rigid-tip suction device ready.
4. Protect the patient from self-injury. Use restraint only if authorized by your EMS system.
5. Provide care for shock.
6. Stay alert for seizures.
7. Be prepared to perform airway maintenance, suctioning, and positioning of the patient should the patient lose consciousness, seize, or vomit.
8. Transport the patient to a medical facility if indicated.

Note: In some systems, patients under the influence of alcohol who are not suffering from a medical emergency or apparent injury are not transported. They are given over to the police. This may not be wise since as many as 15% of patients having an alcohol-related emergency may die unless they receive addi-

tional care. In addition to this, the EMTs may have missed a medical problem or injury. Remember, too, that his condition may worsen as the alcohol continues to be absorbed by the patient's system. Be especially careful of patients with even minor head injuries, since subdural hematoma is common in alcoholics. If transport is refused or deemed unnecessary, do not leave the patient alone but make sure that he is in the care of a responsible adult. Document this in your prehospital care report. ALL PATIENTS WITH SEIZURES OR DTs MUST BE TRANSPORTED TO A MEDICAL FACILITY AS SOON AS POSSIBLE.

Substance Abuse

Substance abuse is a term that indicates that a chemical substance is being taken for other than therapeutic (medical) reasons. Many of the substances have legitimate purposes when used properly. When these same substances are abused, the results can be devastating.

Individuals who abuse drugs and other chemical substances should be considered to have an illness. They have the right to the same professional emergency care as any other patient.

The most common drugs and chemical substances that are abused and may lead to problems requiring an EMS response can be classified as uppers, downers, narcotics, hallucinogens, and volatile chemicals.

- **Uppers** are stimulants affecting the nervous system to excite the user. Many abusers use these drugs in an attempt to relieve fatigue or to create feelings of well-being. Examples are caffeine, amphetamines, and cocaine. Cocaine may be "snorted," smoked, or injected. Other stimulants are frequently in pill form.
- **Downers** have a depressant effect on the central nervous system. This type of drug may be used as a relaxing agent, sleeping pill, or tranquilizer. Barbiturates are an example, usually in pill or capsule form.
- **Narcotics** are drugs capable of producing stupor or sleep. They are often used to relieve pain and to quiet coughing. Many drugs legitimately used for these purposes (e.g., codeine) are also abused, affecting the nervous system and changing many of the normal activities of the body, often producing an intense state of relaxation or feeling of well-being. Illegal narcotics such as hero-

in are also commonly abused. Heroin is usually injected into a vein. Other narcotics are in pill form.

- **Hallucinogens** (huh-LOO-sin-uh-jens) such as LSD and PCP are mind-affecting drugs that act on the nervous system to produce an intense state of excitement or a distortion of the user's perceptions. This class of drugs has few legal uses. They are often eaten or dissolved in the mouth and absorbed through the mucus membranes.
- **Volatile chemicals** can give an initial "rush" and then act as a depressant on the central nervous system. Cleaning fluid,

glue, model cement, and solutions used to correct typing mistakes are commonly abused volatile chemicals.

Patient Assessment—Substance Abuse

As an EMT you will *not* need to know the names of the very many abused drugs or their specific reactions. It is far more important for you to be able to detect possible drug abuse at the overdose level and to relate certain signs to certain *types* of drugs and drug withdrawal. Table 16-1 provides some of the names of

TABLE 16-1   Commonly Abused Drugs

Uppers	Downers	Narcotics	Mind-Altering Drugs	Volatile Chemicals
AMPHETAMINE (Benzedrine, bennies, pep pills, ups, uppers, cartwheels)	AMOBARBITAL (blue devils, downers, barbs, Amytal)	CODEINE (often in cough syrup)	*Hallucinogenic*	AMYL NITRATE (snappers, poppers)
BIPHETAMINE (bam)	BARBITURATES (downers, dolls, barbs, rainbows)	DEMEROL	DMT	BUTYL NITRATE (locker room, rush)
COCAINE (coke, snow, crack)	CHLORAL HYDRATE (knock-out drops, Noctec)	DILAUDID	LSD (acid, sunshine)	CLEANING FLUID (carbon tetrachloride)
DESOXYN (black beauties)	ETHCHLORVYNOL (Placidyl)	FENTANYL (Sublimaze)	MESCALINE (peyote, mesc)	FURNITURE POLISH
DEXTROAMPHETAMINE (dexies, Dexedrine)	GLUTETHIMIDE (Doriden, goofers)	HEROIN ("H," horse, junk, smack, stuff)	MORNING GLORY SEEDS	GASOLINE
METHAMPHETAMINE (speed, meth, crystal, diet pills, Methedrine)	METHAQUALONE (Quaalude, ludes, Sopor, sopors)	METHADONE (dolly)	PCP (angel dust, hog, peace pills)	GLUE
METHYLPHENIDATE (Ritalin)	NONBARBITURATE SEDATIVES (various tranquilizers and sleeping pills: Valium or diazepam, Miltown, Equanil, meprobamate, Thorazine, Compazine, Librium or chlordiazepoxide, reserpine, Tranxene or chlorazepate and other benzodiazepines)	MORPHINE	PSILOCYBIN (magic mushrooms)	HAIR SPRAY
PRELUDIN		OPIUM (Op, poppy)	STP (serenity, tranquility, peace)	NAIL POLISH REMOVER
		MEPERIDINE (Demerol)	*Nonhallucinogenic*	PAINT THINNER
	PARALDEHYDE	PAREGORIC (contains opium)	HASH	TYPEWRITING CORRECTION FLUIDS
	PENTOBARBITAL (yellow jackets, barbs, Nembutal)	TYLENOL with Codeine (1,2,3,4)	MARIJUANA (grass, pot, tea, weed, dope)	
	PHENOBARBITAL (goofballs, phennies, barbs)		THC	
	SECOBARBITAL (red devils, barbs, Seconal)			

commonly abused drugs. Do not worry about memorizing this chart. Read it through so that you can place some of the more familiar drugs into categories in terms of drug type.

The signs and symptoms of substance abuse, dependency, and overdose can vary from patient to patient, even for the same drug or chemical. The problem is made more complex by the fact that many substance abusers take more than one drug or chemical at a time. Often, you will have to carefully combine the information gained from the signs, the symptoms, the scene, the bystanders, and the patient in order to be certain that you are dealing with substance abuse. In many cases, you will not be able to determine the substance involved.

When questioning the patient and bystanders, you will get better results if you begin by asking if the patient has been taking any medications. Then, if necessary, ask if the patient has been taking drugs.

Some significant signs and symptoms related to specific types of drugs include those listed below.

Signs and Symptoms of Drug Abuse

- ☐ Uppers—Excitement, increased pulse and breathing rates, rapid speech, dry mouth, dilated pupils, sweating, and the complaint of having gone without sleep for long periods. Repeated high doses can produce a "speed run." The patient will be restless, hyperactive, and usually very apprehensive and uncooperative.
- ☐ Downers—Sluggish, sleepy patient lacking typical coordination of body and speech. Pulse and breathing rates are low, often to the point of a true emergency.
- ☐ Hallucinogens—Fast pulse rate, dilated pupils, and a flushed face. The patient often "sees" or "hears" things, has little concept of real time, and may not be aware of the true environment. Often what he says makes no sense to the listener. The user may become aggressive or may withdraw.
- ☐ Narcotics—Reduced rate of pulse and rate and depth of breathing, often seen with a lowering of skin temperature. The pupils are constricted, often pinpoint in size. The muscles are relaxed and sweating is profuse. The patient is very sleepy and does not wish to do anything. In overdoses, coma is common. Respiratory arrest or cardiac arrest may develop rapidly.

- ☐ Volatile chemicals—Dazed or showing temporary loss of contact with reality. The patient may develop coma. The linings of the nose and mouth may show swollen membranes. The patient may complain of a "funny numb feeling" or "tingling" inside the head. Changes in heart rhythm can occur. This can lead to death.

Warning: When reading the above list, you should have noticed that many of the indications of drug abuse are similar to those for quite a few medical emergencies. As an EMT you must never assume drug abuse occurring by itself. You must be on the alert for medical emergencies, injuries, and combinations of drug abuse problems and other emergencies.

Signs and Symptoms of Drug Withdrawal

In addition to the effects of long-term drug use and overdose, you will have to deal with cases of severe drug withdrawal. As in reactions to the use of various drugs, withdrawal varies from patient to patient and from drug to drug. In most cases of drug withdrawal, you may see

- ☐ Shaking
- ☐ Anxiety
- ☐ Nausea
- ☐ Confusion and irritability (sometimes retreating from the persons at the scene)
- ☐ Hallucinations (both visual and auditory— "seeing things" or "hearing things")
- ☐ Diaphoresis
- ☐ Increased pulse and breathing rates

Patient Care—Substance Abuse

Your care for the drug abuse patient will be basically the same for all drugs and will not change unless you are ordered to do something by a poison control center with on-line medical control. When providing care for substance abuse patients, you should make certain that you are safe and identify yourself as an EMT to the patient and bystanders. The procedures for care may require you to

1. Provide basic life-support measures if required.
2. Call the emergency department and the poison control center in accordance with local policies.

[3] Monitor vital signs and be alert for respiratory arrest. Provide oxygen if needed.

[4] Talk to the patient to gain his confidence and to help maintain his level of consciousness. Use his name often, maintain eye contact, and speak directly to the patient.

[5] Protect the patient from self-injury and attempting to hurt others. Use restraint only if authorized by your EMS system.

[6] Provide care for shock.

[7] Assess closely for signs of fractures and internal injuries.

[8] Check carefully for head injuries.

[9] Look for gross tissue damage on the extremities resulting from the injection of drugs ("tracks"). Dress and bandage all such sites.

[10] Transport the patient as soon as possible, monitoring vital signs, staying alert for seizures, and being on guard for vomiting that could obstruct the airway.

[11] Continue to reassure the patient throughout all phases of care.

Warning: Many drug abusers may appear calm at first and then become violent as time passes. You are always to be on the alert and be ready to protect yourself. If the patient creates an unsafe scene and you are not a trained law enforcement officer, GET OUT and find a safe place until the police arrive. Be extra cautious if you suspect the patient has been using PCP. This drug may cause the patient to lose the understanding of right and wrong. Some PCP abusers will find nothing wrong in killing you! Have ample police support when dealing with substance abuse patients, especially if you suspect that a patient has used PCP.

Warning: When dealing with drug abuse, you must also protect yourself from the substance itself. Many hallucinogens can be absorbed through the skin and mucus membranes. Intravenous drug users may possess hypodermic syringes which pose a hazard of infectious disease transmission through accidental punctures. Use disposable gloves and other barrier devices and follow all infection exposure control procedures. *Never touch or taste any suspected illicit substance.*

POISONING

A **poison** is any substance that can harm the body, often seriously enough to create a medical emergency. In the United States there are more than a million cases of poisoning annually. Although some of these result from murder or suicide attempts, most are accidental. These accidents usually involve common substances such as medications, petroleum products, cosmetics, and pesticides. In fact, a surprisingly large percentage of chemicals in everyday use contain substances that are poisonous if misused.

We usually think of a poison as being some kind of liquid or solid chemical that has been ingested by the poisoning victim. This is often the case, but keep in mind that many living organisms are capable of producing a **toxin**, a substance that is poisonous to humans. Certain snakes, lizards, spiders, scorpions, insects, and some fish and other marine life forms produce a toxin called **venom**. Usually, the venom is injected into the victim by a bite or sting. Plants such as poison ivy contain toxins that cause reactions when they come into contact with the skin. There are also mushrooms and other common plants that can be poisonous if eaten. These include some varieties of house plants, including the rubber plant and certain parts of holiday ornamentals such as mistletoe and holly berries. Bacterial contaminants in food may produce toxins, some of which can cause a deadly disease (e.g., botulism).

A great number of substances can be considered to be poisons, with different people reacting differently to various poisons (Table 16-2). As odd as it may seem, what may be a dangerous poison for one person may have little effect on another person. For most poisonous substances, the reaction is far more serious in children and the elderly.

Once on or in the body, poisons can do damage in a variety of ways. A poison may act as a corrosive or irritant, destroying skin and other body tissues. A poisonous gas can act as a suffocating agent, displacing oxygen in the air. Some poisons are systemic poisons, causing harm to the entire body or to an entire body system. These poisons can critically depress or overstimulate the central nervous system, cause vomiting and diarrhea, prevent red blood cells from carrying oxygen, or interfere with the normal biochemical processes in the body. The actual effect and extent of damage is dependent on the nature of the poison, on its concentration, and sometimes on how it enters the body. These factors vary in importance depending on the victim's age, weight, and general health.

Poisons can be classified into four types, according to how they are taken in by the body: ingested, inhaled, absorbed, or injected (Figure 16-5).

TABLE 16-2   Common Poisons

Poison	Helpful Signs and Symptoms
ACETAMINOPHEN	Nausea, vomiting, heavy perspiration. The victim is usually a child. Possibly no symptoms of recent ingestion.
ACIDS	Burns on or around the lips. Burning in mouth, throat, and stomach, often followed by heavy vomiting.
ALKALIS (ammonia, bleaches, detergents, lye, washing soda, certain fertilizers)	Check to see if mouth membranes appear white and swollen. There may be a "soapy" appearance in the mouth. Abdominal pain is usually present. Vomiting may occur, often full of blood and mucus.
ARSENIC (rat poisons)	"Garlic breath," with burning in the mouth, throat, and stomach. Abdominal pain can be severe. Vomiting is common.
ASPIRIN	Delayed reactions, including ringing in the ears, rapid and deep breathing, dry skin, and restlessness.
CHLOROFORM	Slow, shallow breathing with chloroform odor on breath. Pupils are dilated and fixed.
CORROSIVE AGENTS (disinfectants, drain cleaners, household acids, iodine, pine oil, turpentine, toilet bowl cleaners, styptic pencil, water softeners, strong acids)	(See *Acids*)
FOOD POISONING	Difficult to detect since signs and symptoms vary greatly. Usually, you will note abdominal pain, nausea and vomiting, gas with loud, frequent bowel sounds, and diarrhea.
IODINE	Upset stomach and vomiting. If a starchy meal has been eaten, the vomitus may appear blue.
METALS (copper, lead, mercury, zinc)	Metallic taste in mouth, with nausea and abdominal pains. Vomiting may occur. Stools may be bloody or dark.
PETROLEUM PRODUCTS (some deodorizers, heating fuel, diesel fuels, gasoline, kerosene, lighter fluid, lubricating oil, naphtha, rust remover, transmission fluid)	Note characteristic odors on patient's breath, on clothing, or in vomitus.
PHOSPHORUS	Abdominal pain and vomiting. Vomitus may be phosphorescent.
PLANTS—Contact (poison ivy, poison oak, poison sumac)	Swollen, itchy areas on the skin, with quickly forming blister-like lesions.
PLANTS—Ingested (azalea, castor bean, elderberry, foxglove, holly berries, lily of the valley, mistletoe berries, mountain laurel, mushrooms and toadstools, nightshade, oleander, rhododendron, rhubarb, rubber plant, some wild cherries)	Difficult to detect, ranging from nausea to coma. Always question in cases of apparent child poisoning.

- **Ingested poisons** (poisons that are swallowed) can include many common household and industrial chemicals, medications, improperly prepared foods, plant materials, petroleum products, and agricultural products made specifically to control rodents, weeds, insects, and crop diseases.

- **Inhaled poisons** (poisons that are breathed in) take the form of gases, vapors, and sprays. Again, many of these substances are in common use in the home, industry, and agriculture. Such poisons include carbon monoxide (from car exhaust, wood-burning stoves, and furnaces), ammonia, chlorine,

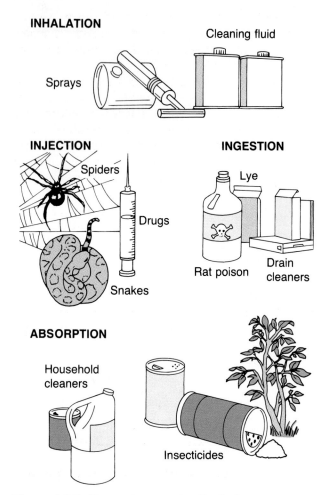

INHALATION

Cleaning fluid

Sprays

INJECTION

Spiders

Drugs

Snakes

INGESTION

Lye

Rat poison

Drain cleaners

ABSORPTION

Household cleaners

Insecticides

Figure 16-5. How poisons enter the body.

insect sprays, and the gases produced from volatile liquid chemicals (*volatile* means "able to change very easily from a liquid into a gas"; many industrial solvents are volatile).

- **Absorbed poisons** (poisons that are taken into the body through unbroken skin) may or may not damage the skin. However, most are corrosives or irritants that will injure the skin and then be slowly absorbed into body tissues and the bloodstream, possibly causing widespread damage. Included in this group are many insecticides and agricultural chemicals in common use. Contact with a variety of plant materials and certain forms of marine life can also damage the skin and possibly be absorbed into tissues under the skin.
- **Injected poisons** (poisons that are inserted through the skin, possibly into the bloodstream, for example by needle, snake fangs, or insect stinger) come from a number of sources. Insects, spiders, snakes, and cer-

tain marine forms are able to inject venoms into the body. The poison may be a drug or caustic chemical self-administered by way of a hypodermic needle. Rarely, industrial accidents also can cause caustics, acids, or industrial solvents to be forced into the body through open wounds.

Preventing poisoning is, of course, preferable to having to treat it. The EMT's own home and the squad building should be "child-proofed" against poisoning by keeping medications and other dangerous substances out of children's reach. The EMT can also share poisoning-prevention information with children and other members of the public during school visits and community outreach activities.

Poison Control Centers

Emergency care in poisoning cases presents special problems for the EMT. Signs and symptoms can vary greatly. Some poisons produce a characteristic set of signs and symptoms very quickly, while others are slow to appear. Those poisons that act almost immediately usually produce obvious signs, and the particular poison or its container is often still at hand. Slow-acting poisons can produce effects that mimic an infectious disease or some other medical emergency.

There will be times when you will not know the substance that caused the poisoning. In some of these cases, an expert may be able to tell, based on the combination of certain signs and symptoms. Even when you know the source of the poison, correct emergency care procedures may still be in question. Ideas about proper care keep changing as more research is done on poisoning. This constant change makes it impossible to print guides and charts for poison control and care that will be up to date when you use them. Even the information printed on labels of chemical containers may no longer be accurate at the time of the poisoning.

To overcome these problems, a network of poison control centers has been established throughout the country. In most localities, a poison control center can be reached 24 hours a day. The staff, through local EMS protocols and on-line medical direction, can tell you what should be done for most cases. You must know the telephone number for the center serving your area. Make certain to carry this number in your jump kit that you bring into the residence so that you don't have to run to the rig to get it!

To help the poison control center staff, note and report any containers at the scene of the poisoning. Let them know if the patient has vomited, and describe the vomitus. When possible quickly gather information from the patient or from bystanders before you call the center. An accurate description of signs and symptoms may be needed before the poison control center staff can tell you and the on-line medical direction what needs to be done for the patient.

Many people have the impression that the poison control center should be called only for cases of ingested poisonings. The center's staff can provide you with valuable care information for all types of poisoning.

Learning how to evaluate the effects of some poisons takes experience. Many can be learned through careful study. Your community may have special poisoning problems. Not every community is exposed to rattlesnakes, jellyfish, or powerful agricultural chemicals. Many EMS systems have compiled lists of special poisoning problems specific for their areas. Check to see if this has been done for the area in which you will be an EMT.

Emergency Treatment for Poisoning

Ingested Poisons Sometimes patients who have ingested poisons will require assisted ventilations. Direct mouth-to-mouth ventilations in such a case are dangerous, not only because of the usual danger of contracting an infectious disease but also because of possible contact with poisonous substances remaining on the patient's lips or in the airway or that may be vomited.

Warning: If intentional poisoning or attempted suicide is suspected, approach the scene with caution and have police backup if indicated. Use a pocket face mask with one-way valve, bag-valve-mask unit with supplemental oxygen, or positive pressure ventilation when providing ventilations to a patient who is suspected of ingesting a poison.

Patient Assessment—Ingested Poisons

You must gather information quickly in cases of possible ingested poisoning. If possible, do so while you are making a primary survey. Note any containers that may contain poisonous substances. See if there is any vomitus. Check if there are any substances on the patient's clothes or if the clothing indicates the nature of the patient's work (e.g., farmer, miner). Can the scene be associated with certain types of poisonings?

Question the patient and any bystanders. If the patient is a child, be on the alert for poisonous plant materials. These are commonly the source of poisoning when children "play house" or have "tea parties." Any poisoning related to plant materials requires immediate transport with care provided while en route. It is critical to reach medical control or the poison control center as soon as possible since there are no antidotes for many plant poisons.

Signs and Symptoms

☐ Burns or stains around the patient's mouth
☐ Unusual breath odors, body odors, or odors on the patient's clothing or at the scene.
☐ Abnormal breathing
☐ Abnormal pulse rate and character
☐ Sweating—often profuse
☐ Dilated or constricted pupils
☐ Excessive tear formation
☐ Excessive salivation or foaming at the mouth
☐ Pain in the mouth or throat, or painful swallowing
☐ Abdominal pain
☐ Abdominal tenderness, sometimes with distention
☐ Nausea
☐ Retching, vomiting
☐ Diarrhea
☐ Seizures
☐ Altered states of consciousness
☐ Any of the signs of shock

Patient Care—Ingested Poisons

To provide the proper emergency care for ingested poisons (Scan 16-2), follow the directions given to you by your medical control and the poison control center. In most cases of ingested poisoning, emergency care will consist of diluting the poison in the patient's stomach using one or two glasses of water or milk. *Never* attempt to dilute the poison if the patient is not fully alert. The directions given to you by the poison control center and the on-line medical control may vary depending on the patient.

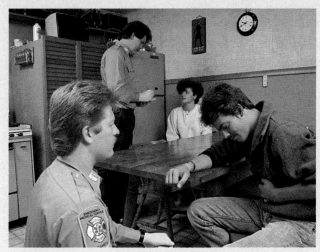

1. Quickly gather information, maintain an open airway, and transport immediately.

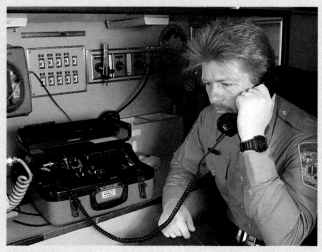

2. Call medical control or poison control while en route.

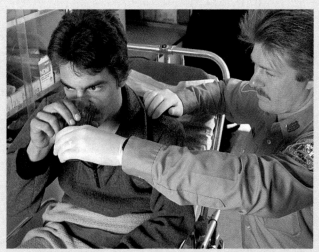

3. If directed, dilute the poison with water. (*Do not* give anything by mouth if the patient is having convulsions.)

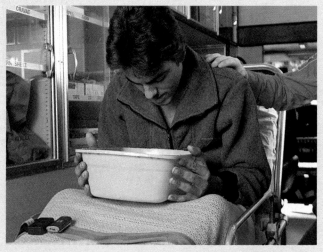

4. Position for vomiting, and save all vomitus. Have suction equipment ready.

Note: Some EMS systems will direct use of syrup of ipecac to induce vomiting and/or activated charcoal and water to bind the poison. Use these methods only if local protocols advise and you are so directed.

Warning: Even after dilution of the poison with water or milk, according to instructions from medical control, the patient may vomit. Vomiting of substances such as strong acids, alkali (including plant products such as strychnine), or petroleum products can cause damage to the esophagus and other tissues, especially if aspirated. Examples of these substances are oven cleaners, drain cleaners, toilet bowl cleaners, lye, ammonia, bleaches, kerosene, and gasoline (Figure 16-6). Aspirated vomitus containing petroleum products such as kerosene or gasoline can also cause severe, often lethal pneumonia. Always check for burns around the patient's mouth and the odor of petroleum products on the breath.

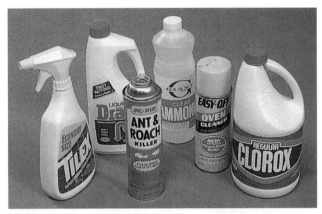

Figure 16-6. Examples of toxic household products.

Emergency Care Steps

1. Maintain an open airway and transport IMMEDIATELY.
2. While en route, CALL MEDICAL CONTROL OR THE POISON CONTROL CENTER.
3. For conscious patients, if directed by your medical control, dilute the poison by having the patient drink one or two glasses of water or milk unless otherwise directed by a physician or poison control center.
4. DO NOT GIVE ANYTHING BY MOUTH IF THE PATIENT IS HAVING A SEIZURE.
5. Position the conscious patient in a semi-recumbent position and monitor closely for vomiting. Have suction equipment with a rigid tip catheter ready. If he becomes unconscious, place him in a lateral recumbent position (recovery position) to help prevent aspiration of vomitus.
6. If transport is delayed, contact medical control or the poison control center for additional instructions.
7. Save all vomitus and transport it with the patient.

Note: Some EMS systems no longer permit administering syrup of ipecac to induce vomiting, but other systems do. Similarly, some systems do not recommend the use of activated charcoal mixed with water to "bind" the poison, while others do. Follow local guidelines and on-line instructions.

When possible, transport the poisoned patient as soon as possible, calling your medical control and the poison control center en route. Actions to dilute the poison are carried out during transport. Treat the patient for shock and administer oxygen as soon as it is practical to do so. Be prepared for vomiting, even after you have diluted the poison. Transport without delay is *critical* if the poisoned patient is unconscious.

Inhaled Poisons Remember that inhaled poisons are those that are present in the atmosphere and that you, as well as the patient, are at risk of breathing in.

Warning: If you suspect a patient has inhaled poison, approach the scene with care. Many EMS systems now include in EMT training the use of protective clothing and self-contained breathing apparatus to be used in a hostile environment (e.g., chlorine gas, ammonia, smoke conditions). Remember that many inhaled poisons can also be absorbed through the skin. Go only where your protective equipment and clothing will allow you to go safely to perform your mission, and only after you have been trained in the use of this equipment. *Do only what you have been trained to do and go only where your protective equipment will allow you to go safely. If you are underequipped, get someone there who is properly equipped.*

Carbon monoxide poisoning is a common problem, usually associated with motor vehicle exhaust and fire suppression activities (Figure 16-7). The number of cases has increased recently because of the carbon monoxide that can accumulate from the use of improperly vented wood-burning stoves and the unvented use of charcoal for heating and indoor cooking. Malfunctioning oil, gasoline, gas, and coal-burning furnaces and stoves can also be sources of carbon monoxide poisoning.

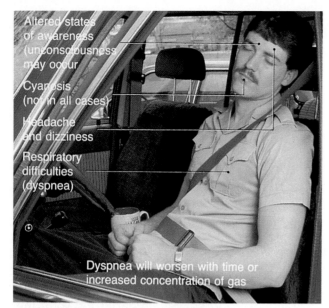

Altered states of awareness (unconsciousness may occur

Cyanosis (not in all cases)

Headache and dizziness

Respiratory difficulties (dyspnea)

Dyspnea will worsen with time or increased concentration of gas

Figure 16-7. Carbon monoxide poisoning.

Since carbon monoxide is an odorless and tasteless gas, you will not be able to directly detect its presence without special equipment. Look for indications of possible carbon monoxide poisoning, including wood-burning stoves, doors that lead to a garage or bedrooms above a garage where a vehicle has been kept running, closed garage doors where motor repair work is in progress, and any evidence that suggests that the patient has spent a long period of time sitting in an idling motor vehicle. When inhaled, carbon monoxide prevents normal carrying of oxygen by the red blood cells. Long exposure, even to low levels of the gas, can cause dramatic effects. Death may occur as hypoxia becomes more severe.

Other possible inhaled poisons include chlorine gas (often from swimming pool chemicals), ammonia (often released from household cleaners), spray agricultural chemicals and pesticides, and carbon dioxide (from industrial sources).

Patient Assessment—Inhaled Poisons

Before you enter the hostile environment to initiate rescue, be sure you are properly equipped and trained, gather information from the patient and bystanders without delay and assess the scene. Note if there are any indications of inhaled poisons, including broken or breached containers, distinctive odors, signs of fire or smoke, and poor ventilation. Possible sources of the poison can be automobile exhaust, stoves, charcoal grills, fire,

methane from vegetation decay, industrial solvents, and spray cans.

Signs and Symptoms

For carbon monoxide poisoning

☐ Headache
☐ Dizziness
☐ Breathing difficulties
☐ Nausea
☐ Cyanosis
☐ Unconsciousness (in the most severe cases)

Note: The cherry red skin color that is associated with carbon monoxide poisoning is a rare, late sign. This coloration usually develops after death.

For a variety of inhaled poisons

☐ Dizziness
☐ Shortness of breath
☐ Coughing
☐ Rapid or slow pulse rate
☐ Irritated or burning eyes.
☐ Burning sensations in the mouth, nose, throat, or chest.
☐ Burning or itching, often in the underarms, groin, and moist areas of the body
☐ Severe headaches
☐ Nausea and vomiting
☐ Changes in skin color (usually cyanosis)
☐ Blood-tinged sputum
☐ Excessive mucus production or tearing
☐ Spray paint or other substances found on the patient's face
☐ Unconsciousness or altered behavior (depression or euphoria)

Patient Care—Inhaled Poisons

Emergency Care Steps

The basic field emergency care for inhaled poisoning (Scan 16-3) is to

1. Remove the patient from the source of the inhaled poison. Avoid touching contaminated clothing.
2. Maintain an open airway.
3. Provide needed basic life support measures and administer a high concentration of oxygen, when possible by nonrebreather mask.
4. Remove contaminated clothing.
5. CALL MEDICAL CONTROL OR THE POISON CONTROL CENTER.

Inhaled Poisons

Warning: Protect yourself . . . do only what you have been trained to do and what your equipment allows.

Remember: Inhaled poisons can frequently be absorbed through the skin.

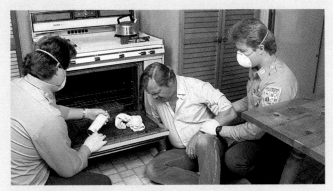

1. Remove patient from source.

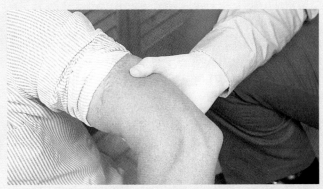

2. Avoid touching contaminated clothing and jewelry.

3. Remember: It is critical to establish and maintain an open airway.

4. Caution: Stay alert for vomiting. Properly position the patient and have suctioning equipment ready for use.

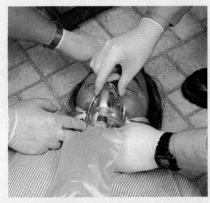

5. Administer a high concentration of oxygen.

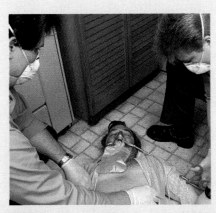

6. Remove contaminated clothing and jewelry.

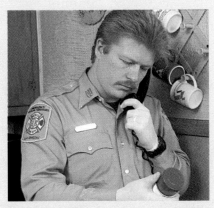

7. Call medical control or poison control . . . Follow directions.

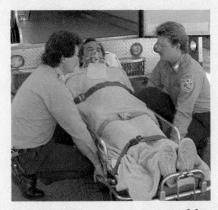

8. Transport as soon as possible.

Note: Masks shown on EMTs are used to filter large particulate matter. They will not protect the airway in a dangerous atmosphere.

Warning: Be careful to protect the rescuers and assure that the patient has been decontaminated by a "hazmat" team if exposure to a hazardous material has occurred.

6 Place the patient in the lateral recumbent position to reduce the chances of aspiration of any vomitus.

7 Transport as soon as possible.

Note: Ask others at the scene to find out if coworkers, family members, or others who live or work nearby have symptoms such as headaches, dizziness, or nausea and warn them that they, too, may need medical attention.

Warning: It may be necessary to remove contaminated clothing from the patient. Take care to avoid touching this clothing since the chemical may cause skin burns. Since some poisonous gases condense into liquids, you may have to care for the patient's chemical burns (see Chapter 19).

Remember: Unless you are trained to enter a scene having poisonous gases and have the proper equipment, do not try to provide care for a patient in a poisonous atmosphere.

Absorbed Poisons Absorbed poisons usually irritate or damage the skin. Some poisons can be absorbed with little or no damage done to the skin, but such cases are very rare.

Patient Assessment—Absorbed Poisons

The patient, bystanders, and what you observe at the scene will help you to determine if you are dealing with a case of absorbed poisoning. In the vast majority of cases, absorbed poisoning will be detected because of skin reactions related to chemicals or plants at the scene.

Signs and Symptoms

☐ Skin reactions (from mild irritations to chemical burns)
☐ Itching
☐ Irritation of the eyes
☐ Headache
☐ Increased relative skin temperature
☐ Abnormal pulse and/or respiration rates
☐ Anaphylactic shock (rare)

Patient Care—Absorbed Poisons

Emergency Care Steps

To provide emergency care for absorbed poisons (Scan 16-4)

1 Move the patient from the source of the poison while avoiding contact with the substance.

2 Use water to immediately flood all the areas of the patient's body that have been exposed to the poison. Dry chemicals should be brushed from the skin before washing. Be careful not to abrade the patient's skin as this will speed up absorption of the poison.

3 CALL THE ON-LINE MEDICAL CONTROL AND THE POISON CONTROL CENTER.

4 Remove all contaminated clothing (including shoes, jewelry, and watches) and wash the affected areas of the patient's skin a second time (the poison control center and on-line medical control may direct you to use soap and water for this wash). More specific directions for various chemical burns will be covered in Chapter 17.

5 Be on the alert for anaphylactic shock.

6 Transport immediately.

Injected Toxins Insect stings, spider bites, scorpion stings, and snakebites are typical sources of injected poisons, or toxins.

Commonly seen insect stings are those of wasps, hornets, bees, and ants. Insect stings and bites are rarely dangerous; however, 5% of the population will have an allergic reaction to the venom and a few people may develop shock. Those who are hypersensitive develop severe anaphylactic shock that is quickly life threatening (see Chapter 8).

All spiders are poisonous, but most species cannot get their fangs through human skin. Black widow and brown recluse ("fiddleback") spiders are two that can (Figure 16-8), and their bites can produce medical emergencies. Almost all brown recluse bites are painless, and patients seldom recall being bitten. The characteristic lesion appears in only 10% of cases, and then only after up to 12 hours have elapsed. EMTs are seldom called to respond for a brown recluse bite. Black widow bites cause a more immediate reaction.

Scorpion stings are common in the Southwest. They do not ordinarily cause deaths, but one rare species (Centroroides Exilcauda) is dangerous to humans and can cause serious medical problems, including respiratory failure, in children.

Snakebites are covered separately below. Poisons also can be injected into the body by way of a hypodermic needle. Drug overdose and drug contamination can produce serious medical emergencies, as discussed earlier.

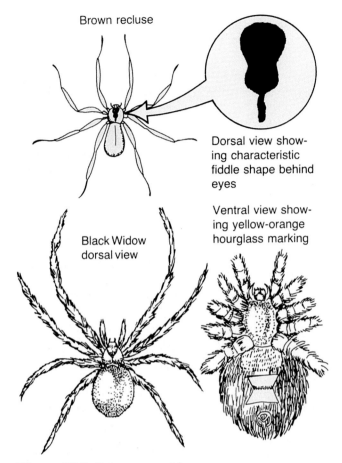

Brown recluse

Dorsal view showing characteristic fiddle shape behind eyes

Ventral view showing yellow-orange hourglass marking

Black Widow dorsal view

Figure 16-8. Poisonous spiders.

- [ ] Nausea and vomiting
- [ ] Muscle cramps, chest tightening, joint pains
- [ ] Excessive saliva formation, profuse sweating
- [ ] Anaphylaxis

Patient Care—Injected Toxins

As an EMT you are not expected to be able to classify insects and spiders as to their genus and species. Proper identification of these organisms is best left to experts.

If the problem has been caused by a creature that is known locally and is not normally dangerous (such as a bee, wasp, or puss caterpillar), the major concern will be anaphylactic shock. If anaphylactic shock does not appear to be a problem, care is usually simple.

If the cause of the bite or sting is unknown, or the organism is unknown, the patient should be seen by a physician. Call the emergency department or take the patient to a medical facility and let experts decide on the proper treatment for the patient.

If possible transport the stinging object or organism in a sealed container, taking care not to handle it without proper protection, even if it is dead. By sending this stinging object or organism to the emergency department with the patient, you may save precious minutes in identifying the toxin.

Emergency Care Steps

To provide emergency care for injected toxins (Scan 16-5)

1. Treat for shock, even if the patient does not present any of the signs of shock.
2. CALL MEDICAL CONTROL OR THE POISON CONTROL CENTER. This should be skipped only if the organism is known and your EMS system has a specific protocol for care.
3. Do not pull out bee and wasp stingers and venom sacs. To do so may inject another dose of venom. Instead, carefully scrape the site using a blade or a card.
4. Remove jewelry from any affected limbs. This should be done in case the limb swells, which would make removal more difficult later.
5. If local protocol permits, place a constriction band above and below the site if an

Patient Assessment—Injected Toxins

Gather information from the patient, bystanders, and the scene. Find out whatever you can about the insect or other possible source of the poisoning. The signs and symptoms of injected poisoning can include those listed below.

Signs and Symptoms

- [ ] Altered states of awareness
- [ ] Noticeable stings or bites on the skin
- [ ] Puncture marks (especially note the fingers, forearms, toes, and legs)
- [ ] Blotchy skin (mottled skin)
- [ ] Localized pain or itching
- [ ] Numbness in a limb or body part
- [ ] Burning sensations at the site followed by pain spreading throughout the limb
- [ ] Swelling or blistering at the site
- [ ] Weakness or collapse
- [ ] Difficult breathing and abnormal pulse rate
- [ ] Headache and dizziness

Scan 16-4
Absorbed Poisons

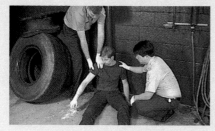

1. Remove patient from source or source from patient. Avoid contaminating yourself with the poison.

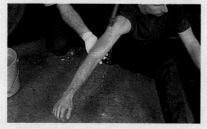

2. If appropriate, wash or brush the poison from the patient. Be careful not to abrade the patient's skin.

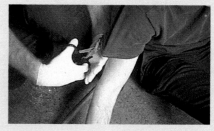

3. Remove contaminated clothing and other articles.

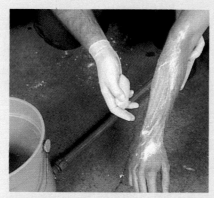

4. Call medical control or poison control. If appropriate, wash with soap and water.

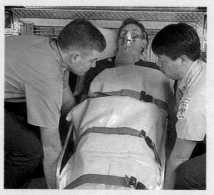

5. Be alert for shock and transport as soon as possible.

Warning: Be careful to protect the rescuers and assure that the patient has been decontaminated by a "hazmat" team if exposure to a hazardous material has occurred.

Scan 16-5
Injected Toxins (not snakebite)

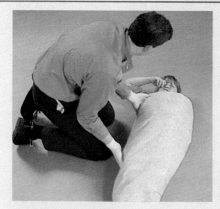

1. Care for shock. Call medical control or poison control.

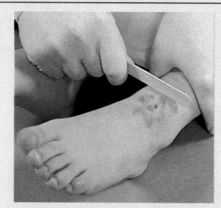

2. Scrape away stinger and venom sac. Apply constricting bands.

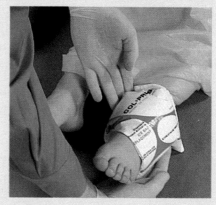

3. If protocols recommend, apply cold to site. Ready for transport.

extremity is the site of the sting. This is done to slow the spread of venom in the lymphatic vessels and superficial veins. The band should be made of ¾ to 1 ½ inch wide soft rubber or other wide, soft material. It should be placed about 2 inches from the wound (do not place the band around a joint). The band must be loose enough so that you can slide one finger underneath it; it should not cut off circulation to the limb.

6 Keep the limb immobilized. and the patient still to prevent encouraging distribution of the poison to other parts of the body.

Note: Some EMS systems recommend placing a cold compress over the bitten or stung area. Most EMS systems do not use cold for any injected toxin. Follow your local protocols.

Some patients sensitive to stings or bites carry medication to help prevent anaphylactic shock. Help all such patients to take their medications. Your EMT course may include training in how to administer injectable medications for cases when the patient cannot do so for himself. This is a serious legal question. Make certain that you follow local policies.

Remember: Be certain to look for medical identification devices that identify persons sensitive to certain stings or bites.

Snakebites Snakebites require special care. Nearly 50,000 people in the United States are bitten by snakes each year. Over 8,000 of these cases involve poisonous snakes, but on the average fewer than 10 deaths are reported annually (in the United States, more people die each year from bee and wasp stings than from snakebites). The signs and symptoms of snakebite poisoning may take several hours to develop. If death does result, it is usually not a rapidly occurring event unless anaphylactic shock develops. Most victims who will die survive at least one to two days.

In the United States there are two types of poisonous snakes, pit vipers (including rattlesnakes, copperheads, and water moccasins) and coral snakes. Up to 25% of pit viper bites and 50% of coral bites are "dry bites" without venom injection, but the venomous bite from a diamondback rattler or coral snake is considered very serious (Figure 16-9). Since each person reacts differently to snakebites, you should consider the bite from any known poisonous snake to be a serious emergency. Staying calm and keeping the patient calm and at rest is critical. There is time to transport the patient.

Patient Assessment—Snakebites

Unless you are dealing with a known species of local snake that is not considered poisonous, consider all snakebites to be from poisonous snakes. The patient or bystanders may say that the snake was not poisonous. They could be mistaken. The signs and symptoms of snakebite may include those listed below.

Signs and Symptoms

☐ A noticeable bite on the skin. This may appear as nothing more than a discoloration.

☐ Pain and swelling in the area of the bite. This may be slow to develop, from 30 minutes to several hours.

☐ Rapid pulse and labored breathing

☐ Progressive general weakness

☐ Vision problems (dim or blurred)

☐ Nausea and vomiting

☐ Seizures

☐ Drowsiness or unconsciousness

If the dead or captured snake is at the scene, your role as an EMT is not to identify the snake, but to provide care and to transport the

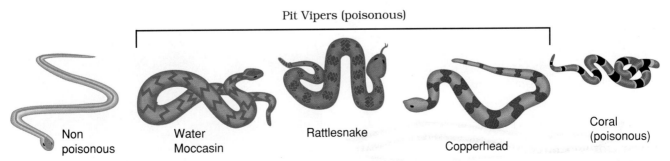

Pit Vipers (poisonous)

Non poisonous   Water Moccasin   Rattlesnake   Copperhead   Coral (poisonous)

Figure 16-9. Venomous snakes in the United States.

dead snake (in a sealed container) along with the patient. Arrange for separate transport of a live specimen. *Do not* attempt to transport a live snake in the ambulance.

Should you see the live, uncaptured snake, take great care or you may be its next victim. When possible, note its size and colorations. Getting close enough to look for details of the eyes or for a pit between the eye and mouth (the identifying feature of a pit viper) is foolish. How you classify a snake, whether it is dead or alive, will probably have little to do with subsequent care. The medical center staff will arrange to have an expert classify captured or dead specimen, and they have protocols to determine care if the snake has not been captured. Unless you are an expert in capturing snakes, do not try to catch the snake. Never delay care and transport in order to capture the snake.

Patient Care—Snakebites

Emergency Care Steps

1. CALL MEDICAL CONTROL OR THE POISON CONTROL CENTER.
2. Keep the patient calm.
3. Treat for shock and conserve body heat.
4. Locate the fang marks and clean this site with soap and water. There may be only one fang mark.
5. Remove any rings, bracelets, or other constricting items on the bitten extremity.
6. Keep any bitten extremities immobilized—the application of a splint will help. Try to keep the bite at the level of the heart or, when this is not possible, below the level of the heart.
7. Apply a light constricting band above and below the wound. (See more information on constricting bands below.)
8. Transport the patient, carefully monitoring vital signs.

Warnings: Do not place an ice bag or cold pack on the bite unless you are directed to do so by a physician. Do not cut into the bite and suction or squeeze unless you are directed to do so by a physician. *Never* suck the venom from the wound using your mouth. Instead, use a suction cup. Suctioning is seldom done.

Apply a constricting band above and below the fang marks (Figure 16-10). Each band should be about two inches from the wound, but never place the bands on either side of a joint, such as above and below the knee. The typical coral snake bite is to a finger or a toe, due to its small mouth. If so, one band may be placed above the site. If the bite is to a finger, the band can be applied to the wrist. The constricting bands should be from a snakebite kit or made of ¾ to 1 ½ inch wide soft rubber. If only one band is available, place it above the wound (between the wound and the heart). If no bands are available, use a handkerchief or other wide, soft material.

The purpose of the constricting bands is to restrict the flow of lymph, not of blood. They should be snug but not tight enough to cut off circulation. Monitor for a pulse at the wrist or ankle, depending on the extremity involved. Check to be certain that tissue swelling does not cause the constricting bands to become too tight.

Poisoning From Marine Life Forms Poisoning from marine life forms can occur in a variety of ways: from eating improperly prepared seafood or poisonous organisms, to stings and punctures. Patients who have ingested spoiled, contaminated, or infested seafood may develop anaphylactic shock. They should receive the same care as any patient in anaphylactic shock. During care, you must be prepared for vomiting. Most patients will show the signs of food poisoning. The care for seafood poisoning is the same as for all other food poisonings.

It is extremely rare for someone in the United States to eat a poisonous variety of marine life. Creatures such as puffer fish and paralytic

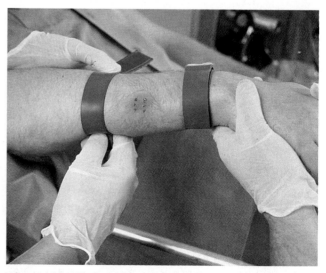

Figure 16-10. Care for snakebite.

shellfish are not readily available. For all cases of suspected poisoning due to ingestion, call your on-line medical control and the poison control center. Be prepared for vomiting, convulsions, and respiratory arrest.

Venomous marine life forms producing sting injuries include the jellyfish, the sea nettle, the Portuguese man-of-war, coral, the sea anemone, and the hydra. For most victims, the sting produces pain with few complications. Some patients may show allergic reactions and possibly develop anaphylactic shock. These cases require the same care as rendered for any case of anaphylactic shock. Stings to the face, especially those near or on the lip or eye, require a physician's attention. Swabbing the affected area with rubbing alcohol will reduce the pain of the sting.

Puncture wounds occur when someone steps on or grabs a stingray, sea urchin, spiny catfish, or other form of spiny marine animal. Although it is true that soaking the wound in hot water for 30 minutes will break down the venom, you should not delay transport. Puncture wounds must be treated by a physician and the patient may need an antitetanus inoculation. Remember, the patient could react to the venom by developing anaphylactic shock.

CHAPTER REVIEW

KEY TERMS

You may find it helpful to review the following terms.

absorbed poisons—poisons that are taken into the body through unbroken skin.

acute abdomen—inflammation in the abdominal cavity producing intense pain.

delirium tremens (DTs)—a severe reaction that can be part of alcohol withdrawal, characterized by sweating, trembling, anxiety, and hallucinations. Severe alcohol withdrawal with the DTs can lead to death if untreated.

diabetes mellitus (di-ah-BEE-tez MEL-i-tus)—also called "sugar diabetes" or just "diabetes," the condition brought about by decreased insulin production, which prevents the body's cells from taking the simple sugar called glucose from the bloodstream. The person suffering from this condition is a diabetic.

diabetic ketoacidosis (KEY-to-as-i-DO-sis)—a life-threatening condition resulting from loss of fluids and the build-up of ketones, which turn the blood acid; a complication of diabetes mellitus.

downers—depressants such as barbiturates that depress the central nervous system, often used to bring on a more relaxed state of mind.

epilepsy (EP-i-LEP-see)—an episodic medical disorder of sudden onset characterized by attacks of unconsciousness, with or without convulsions.

glucose (GLU-kos)—a simple sugar converted by the body from the complex sugars a person eats and required by the cells of the body as the basic source of energy. The presence of insulin is required for the body cells to take glucose from the bloodstream.

hallucinogens (huh-LOO-sin-uh-jens)—mind-affecting or -altering drugs that act on the central nervous system to produce excitement and distortion of perceptions.

hyperglycemia (HI-per-gli-SEE-me-ah)—too much sugar in the blood.

hypoglycemia (HI-po-gli-SEE-me-ah)—too little sugar in the blood.

ingested poisons—poisons that are swallowed.

inhaled poisons—poisons that are breathed in.

injected poisons—poisons that are inserted through the skin, possibly into the bloodstream, for example by needle, snake fangs, or insect stinger.

insulin (IN-suh-lin)—a hormone produced by the pancreas or taken as a supplement by many diabetics. Insulin must be present to enable the body cells to take glucose from the bloodstream.

narcotics—a class of drugs that affect the nervous system and change many normal body activities. Their legal use is for the relief of pain. Illicit use is to produce an intense state of relaxation.

poison—any substance that can harm the body by altering cell structure or functions.

seizure (SE-zher)—a sudden change in sensation, behavior, or movement, usually related to brain malfunctions that can be the result of diseased, infected, or injured brain tissue. The more severe forms produce violent muscle contractions called convulsions.

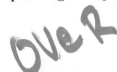

status epilepticus (STAY-tus or STAT-us ep-i-LEP-ti-kus)—a prolonged seizure or when a person suffers two or more convulsive seizures without regaining full consciousness. It is a true emergency, requiring immediate transport.

toxin—a poisonous substance secreted by bacteria, plants, or animals.

uppers—stimulants such as amphetamines that affect the central nervous system to excite the user.

venom—a poison (toxin) produced by plants or animals such as certain snakes, spiders, and marine life forms.

volatile chemicals—vaporizing compounds, such as cleaning fluid, that are breathed in by the abuser to produce a "high."

withdrawal—referring to alcohol or drug withdrawal, in which the patient's body reacts severely when deprived of the abused substance.

SUMMARY

Interviewing skills are critical in dealing with a medical emergency. Information about the current illness, including accurate descriptions of pain, and about past medical history are especially important.

Medical Conditions and Diseases

The body's cells need glucose, a simple sugar, as their basic source of energy but cannot take glucose from the bloodstream without the presence of insulin, a hormone produced by the pancreas. Diabetes mellitus is a condition in which the body does not produce enough insulin, thus depriving the cells of glucose and allowing a buildup of excess glucose in the bloodstream.

Two conditions can lead to diabetic emergencies: hyperglycemia and hypoglycemia. In hyperglycemia, there is too much sugar in the blood and too little in the cells. The body tries to compensate by metabolizing fats instead of sugars, but the waste products of this process allow a buildup of ketones (a substance similar to nailpolish remover) in the blood. The end result is diabetic ketoacidosis. In hypoglycemia, there is too little sugar in the blood. The brain is deprived of the sugar it needs. Both conditions are life threatening. The two conditions are difficult to distinguish in the field. A "glucose for everybody" policy of emergency treatment is advised, since the hyperglycemic patient will not be harmed by the extra sugar if he is transported to a medical facility, while the hypoglycemic patient *must* have sugar.

Seizures can be caused by a wide variety of injuries, defects, and medical conditions, including epilepsy. A tonic-clonic seizure has three phases: In the tonic phase, the body becomes rigid. In the clonic phase, the body jerks about violently. In the postictal phase, the patient recovers, regaining consciousness quickly or after several hours. If a convulsion occurs in your presence, help the patient to the floor, loosen restricting clothing, and protect the patient from injury without trying to hold him still. After the seizure, position for drainage from the mouth, suction the airway, and administer oxygen if indicated, monitor vital signs, consider treatment for underlying conditions that may have triggered the convulsion, and transport.

It is important for the EMT to observe or gather detailed information about any seizure to report to medical personnel. Be aware that status epilepticus—two or more seizures with no return of consciousness between them, and lasting 5 to 10 minutes or more—is a true emergency.

Acute abdominal distress (acute abdomen) may be the result of any of a variety of specific disorders such as appendicitis, peritonitis, or heart attack. The EMT should not try to diagnose the specific disorder but assess for the general signs and symptoms of acute abdomen (including pain which may be general or widespread, nausea, rapid pulse, diarrhea or constipation, fever, tenderness, abdominal guarding, or signs of shock). Maintain an open airway, be on the alert for vomiting (save all vomitus), care for shock, make the patient as comfortable as possible, administer oxygen if there are respiratory difficulties, and transport.

In dealing with a patient with a possible infectious or communicable disease, such as hepatitis, tuberculosis, mumps, genital herpes, HIV/AIDS, and others (some of which have obvious symptoms, some of which do not), protect yourself by using barrier clothing and devices and following your service's exposure control plan at all times.

Alcohol and Substance Abuse

Patients suffering from alcohol abuse are to receive the same level of professional care as any other patient. There may be another medical problem or injuries. Try to detect the odor of alcohol, slurred speech, swaying and unsteadiness of movement. Find out if the patient is nauseated. Be alert for vomiting. In cases of alcohol withdrawal, look for seizures and look for hand tremors and disoriented behavior that may indicate delirium tremens (DTs). In all cases of alcohol abuse or withdrawal, monitor vital signs and be alert for respiratory problems, vomiting, or shock. Transport if necessary or, if local protocols do not permit transport, leave the patient in the care of a responsible adult.

Drug abuse can show itself in many ways, depending on the drug, the patient, and whether you are dealing with withdrawal or overdose. Withdrawal from most drugs will produce shaking, anxiety, nausea, confusion and irritability, sweating, and increased pulse and breathing rates. Uppers usually speed up activity, speech, pulse, and breathing and tend to excite the user. Downers do just the opposite. Hallucinogens (mind-altering drugs) increase pulse rate, dilate the pupils, and cause the patient to "see" or "hear" things and to lose touch with reality. Narcotics reduce pulse and breathing rates. Pupils of narcotic patients usually will be constricted. The patient may appear sleepy and may not wish to do anything. Volatile chemicals act as depressants, causing the patient to be dazed. In cases of drug abuse or withdrawal, provide life-support measures as needed. Monitor vital signs and be alert for respiratory difficulties. Treat for shock. Assess and treat for any other medical conditions or injuries. Transport as soon as possible.

When dealing with alcohol abuse or drug abuse patients, remember to consider your own safety and request police support if necessary.

Poisoning

If you are dealing with a possible poisoning, always look for evidence at the scene that may indicate poisoning and the nature of the poison. In conjunction with your on-line medical control, learn to make use of your local poison control center.

There is a wide variety of signs and symptoms associated with ingested poisons. Always look for burns or stains around the patient's mouth and note any odd breath odors. Expect unusual breathing, pulse rate, and sweating. Abdominal pain, nausea, and vomiting are common. Be sure to save all vomitus. Inhaled poisons can cause shortness of breath or coughing. Often, the patient will have irritated eyes, rapid or slow pulse rate, and changes in skin color. Absorbed poisons usually irritate or damage the skin. Look for irritated eyes. Injected toxins sometimes cause pain and swelling at the site. Difficult breathing and abnormal pulse rate are often seen.

In ALL cases of poisoning, contact your on-line medical control and local poison control center. For conscious patients, you will usually be directed to dilute ingested poisons with water or milk. Transport the patient as soon as possible, positioned to reduce the chances of aspiration of vomitus.

With ingested poisons, be alert for vomiting, especially of petroleum products that may cause severe pneumonia if aspirated. In cases of inhaled poisons, make certain that you are safe, using protective clothing and gear, then remove the patient from the source. Provide basic life support measures as needed. It may be necessary to remove contaminated clothing. and jewelry, but be careful not to touch it. Continue to flood the exposed areas of the patient's skin, or wash with soap and water. When managing injected toxins other than snakebite, provide care for shock, scrape away stingers and venom sacs, and place a covered ice bag or cold pack over the stung area (if ordered to do so).

For snakebite, you should keep the patient calm, clean the site, and keep any bitten extremities immobilized. DO NOT APPLY COLD TO THE AFFECTED AREA. Provide care for shock. Apply a constricting band above and below the wound site but never on both sides of a joint. The bite of a coral snake requires one constricting band placed above the wound, since the bite is is usually on a finger or toe.

Poisoning by marine life forms can occur by eating contaminated seafood or seafood to which the patient is allergic. Some marine life forms will sting their victims. Puncture wounds can occur when spiny marine animals are grasped. In most cases, the major problem is possible anaphylactic shock from an allergic reaction. The care to provide will be the same as for any patient suffering anaphylactic shock.

17

On the Scene

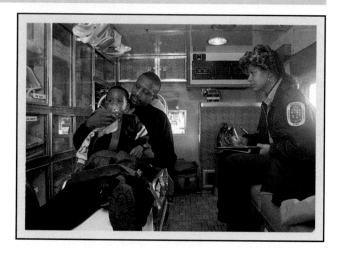

Three-year-old Danny Martin has a high fever. His parents noticed the fever as they were getting him ready for bed. When they looked in on him later, they found him sitting on the edge of his bed. Danny's fever had risen to 103 degrees Fahrenheit. His ribs were heaving, as if he was having to work hard to breathe. Mr. and Mrs. Martin were frightened and decided to call 911.

When you arrive, you immediately see that the child is in respiratory distress and drooling. Both of Danny's parents are nervous, and Danny can see that. You involve the parents by asking them to prepare clothes and coats and to introduce you to their child.

You: *Hi, Danny. My name is Carmen. I'm here to help you because your mommy and daddy tell me you don't feel well. (You pause a moment to observe his reaction and continue.) It looks like you're having some trouble breathing. I'll bet that's scary. You're a pretty brave guy!*

Danny: *(Nods his head yes but does not look at you. He seems more concerned with his breathing than with your presence in the room.)*

You: *Your daddy is going to carry you outside. We're going to take a ride in the ambulance to go see the doctor and help you feel better.*

You have enlisted Danny's father to carry him outside to minimize the stress of moving to the ambulance, which could make his condition worse. Once in the ambulance, Danny is allowed to sit on his father's lap. You prepare a pediatric nonrebreather mask and give it to Mr. Martin. Danny is afraid of the mask but tolerates his father holding it just in front of his face. You prepare a pediatric bag-valve mask and suction, just in case.

The receiving hospital is alerted to expect Danny's arrival and made aware that you suspect he is suffering from epiglottitis. At the hospital, you transfer Danny and his father to the emergency department staff. As you prepare to leave, you speak with the emergency physician. She says that your suspicion of epiglottitis was correct and compliments you on your observations and care.

Pediatric Medical Emergencies and Trauma

Chapter Overview

Emergencies involving children can be the most difficult for the EMT. We all react more intensely to the cries of infants and children and consider them special patients. We would like to be able to stop the pain and discomfort and correct all the problems. But it is necessary to control our emotions so we are not overwhelmed by cries of pain, expressions of fear, or the unnerving silence of the child who normally should be crying.

To manage children effectively, the EMT must have the knowledge, equipment, and skills to perform confidently in the field. This chapter will first review patient assessment for, then discuss management of, common pediatric medical situations and trauma.

Expected Outcome, Chapter 17: *You will be able to assess and care for children with medical emergencies or injuries.*

> **WARNING:** Protect yourself from infectious diseases by using appropriate barrier devices such as a pocket face mask with one-way valve, face shield, or bag-valve mask; goggles or eye shield; and disposable gloves. Always conform to your local EMS system's infection exposure control plan.

ASSESSING THE PEDIATRIC PATIENT
  Supporting the Parent
  The Primary Survey and Basic Life Support
  The Secondary Survey

MEDICAL EMERGENCIES COMMON TO CHILDREN
  Fever
  Hypothermia
  Seizures
  Respiratory Disorders
  Meningitis
  Acute Abdomen
  Diarrhea and Vomiting
  Poisonings
  Sudden Infant Death Syndrome

PEDIATRIC TRAUMA EMERGENCIES
  Managing Pediatric Trauma
  Head and Spine Injury
  Chest Injury
  Abdominal Injury
  Pelvic and Genital Injury
  Injuries to the Extremities
  Burns
  Trapped Extremities
  Transporting the Pediatric Patient
  The Abused Child

Knowledge *After reading this chapter, you should be able to*

1. State the age ranges for an infant and a child for basic life support, and describe developmental characteristics of the neonate, infant, toddler, preschool child, school age child, and adolescent in pediatric care. (p. 473; Table 17-1)

2. Describe how to support the parent during a pediatric emergency. (pp. 473-474)

3. Describe how to conduct a primary survey and basic life support on an infant and a child. (p. 474; Scan 17-1)

4. Describe appropriate methods of interviewing a child. (pp. 474, 478)

5. List the normal vital signs for the infant and child. (pp. 478-479; Table 17-2)

6. List in general the special problems searched for during the physical examination when the patient is an infant or a child. (pp. 480-482)

7. Describe the appropriate assessment and care for pediatric medical emergencies involving

   • Fever (p. 483)
   • Hypothermia (pp. 483-484)
   • Seizures (p. 484)
   • Croup (pp. 484-485)
   • Epiglottitis (pp. 485-486)
   • Bronchiolitis (p. 486)
   • Asthma (p. 486)
   • General respiratory disorders (pp. 486-487)
   • Meningitis (p. 487)
   • Acute abdomen (p. 488)
   • Diarrhea and vomiting (p. 488)
   • Poisoning (pp. 488-489)

8. Describe sudden infant death syndrome and the EMT's appropriate response before and after a doctor has declared the infant dead. (pp. 489-490)

9. Describe a general protocol for managing pediatric trauma, including assessment and care for airway, respiration, circulation, bleeding, shock, and neurological response. (pp. 490-493)

10. Describe the appropriate assessment and care for pediatric trauma emergencies involving

    • Head and spine injuries (pp. 493-494)
    • Chest injuries (p. 494)
    • Abdominal injuries (pp. 494-495)
    • Pelvic and genital injuries (p. 495)
    • Injuries to the extremities (pp. 495-496)
    • Burns (p. 496)
    • Trapped extremities (pp. 496-497)

11. Describe methods of transporting an infant or child. (p. 497)

12. Describe the signs of and care for physical and sexual abuse of a child and the appropriate conduct of the EMT in cases of child abuse and death of a child. (pp. 498-501)

Skills *As an EMT you should be able to*

1. Determine the general age category of the child (neonate, infant, toddler, preschool, school age, or adolescent).

2. Conduct a primary survey on infants and children and make a CUPS status decision.

3. Provide basic life support for both infants and children.

4. Conduct an interview of a child patient.

5. Conduct a physical examination of an infant or child, detecting atypical vital signs and assessing for possible medical problems or injuries.

6. Provide emergency care for pediatric medical emergencies.

7. Provide emergency care for pediatric trauma.

8. Provide emotional support to parents in cases of possible sudden infant death syndrome.

9. Act as a professional in cases of possible child abuse.

anaging a pediatric illness or injury is often like managing an adult illness or injury, because the principles of emergency care are basically the same. It can also be very different because children are *not* little adults. They have their own special characteristics. Moreover, the EMT will find that when a child is ill or injured, supportive care, if not emergency care, must be provided for the parents, family members, friends, and bystanders.

ASSESSING THE PEDIATRIC PATIENT

Medical practice considers a child to be in the pediatric category up to the age of 15. However, children often are treated by their pediatrician until they leave home for college, get married, or live on their own. For basic life support, the American Heart Association defines an infant as birth to 1 year, a child as 1 to 8 years, and an adult as anyone over 8. These age ranges do not always apply to the care of children in other medical or trauma cases. Even when guidelines are established, the EMT must often adjust care based on the physical size and the emotional reaction of the patient.

Table 17-1 shows common age-range categories for pediatrics that provide an understanding of the child's development and probable reaction to an emergency.

Supporting the Parent

Parents may react in one of several ways when their child suffers a sudden life-threatening injury or illness. Their first reaction may be one of denial or shock. Denial is a defense mechanism that protects us from having to deal with a bad situation at once. The numbness of shock enables us to grasp the full implications of a sit-

TABLE 17-1 Characteristics of Children

Neonate *Birth-1 month*	Problems are usually related to fetal development (congenital defects) or birth (prematurity or improper presentation); if ill, the neonate is either fussy or listless.
Infant *1 to 12 months*	The young infant follows movements with his or her eyes. The older infant is active, developing a personality, is anxious with strangers, cries for mom, is used to being undressed, and wants to be warm emotionally and physically.
Toddler *1 to 3 years*	Toddlers begin asserting their independence but do not like to be separated from parents, may not like having clothing removed or being touched, and tend to be uncooperative. They frighten easily, overreact, may understand more than they communicate, and want the comfort of a favorite toy.
Preschool *3 to 5 years*	Motor skills are being refined and preschoolers are very aware of their bodies. They may feel an injury is their fault. They are curious and communicative and cooperate if you take time to explain what you are going to do. They may still want to take along a favorite toy or blanket.
School Age *6 to 12 years*	This age group cooperates but likes explanations and wants their opinions considered. Allow them the responsibility of giving their history; but the emergency may cause the child to regress. They fear pain, punishment, and worry about being separated from parents. They do not like their bodies exposed and are concerned about death and disability.
Adolescent *13 to 18 years*	Adolescents feel they are indestructible. They vary in their emotional and physical development and may not be comfortable with their changing bodies. They are usually modest and embarrassed about being examined, need your respect, and want to be treated as adults but may need the support of a child.

uation slowly and get used to the idea. If parents react in this manner, be calm, reassuring, and supportive. Use simple language to explain what has happened and what is being done to and for their child.

Some parents will react by crying, screaming, or becoming angry. These parents are placed in a bad situation so quickly that their defense mechanism of denial doesn't have time to work before they react. Again, be calm, reassuring, and supportive.

Another common reaction is self-blame and guilt. Parents feel that if they can find a reason for this terrible situation, they will be able to deal with it more easily. If they blame themselves, listen and let them know that they did the right thing or that nothing they could have done would have made any difference, or that accidents can happen to anyone—whatever is true and believable as well as reassuring.

In some cases, an hysterical parent may interfere with your care of the child. This is a natural reaction to protect the child from further harm. Usually you can persuade the parent to assist you by holding the child's hand, giving you a medical history, or comforting the child. If, however, the parent is out of control and cannot or will not cooperate, have a friend or relative remove the parent from the scene.

At this point it should be noted that not all children live with two parents in a traditional nuclear family. The child may have a single parent or may be living with a grandparent or other relative or even with someone who is not related to the child. Whoever the child's fulltime caretaker or guardian is, that person is likely to have the same emotional responses in an emergency as any parent. The EMT should be sensitive to the fact that the child may or may not call this person "Mommy" or "Daddy" and may be upset if asked where his or her mother or father is. Tact is often required to find out who is responsible for the child and what the child calls that person. Keep this in mind as you read the rest of the chapter in which we will use "parent" or "mom and dad" to stand for any person or persons who act as parent, guardian, or principal caretaker to the child.

You need to gain the confidence and establish emotional control of all the people around the scene in order to be able to treat the child effectively. Your interactions with the child will show everyone present your concern, and the manner in which you provide care will show your professionalism.

The Primary Survey and Basic Life Support

The management of every patient, adult or child, begins with the primary survey. A child who is alertly watching your approach, squirming and able to talk with you, vigorously or even quietly crying, obviously has an airway, is breathing, has a pulse, and a blood pressure. If the child is quiet, appears to be sleeping deeply, or is unresponsive the child's airway, breathing, and circulation must be assessed and managed immediately. Details for the procedures used in the primary survey and basic life support for infants and children were presented in Chapters 3 through 8. Scan 17-1 is provided to review the steps of airway management, pulmonary resuscitation and CPR, controlling profuse bleeding, and treating shock. Be sure to make a CUPS status decision (see Chapter 3) before proceeding to the secondary survey.

The Secondary Survey

The Patient Interview You obviously will not be able to interview infants, and most toddlers are poor communicators. However, the parents or care providers who called for help can usually provide a history of the small child's illness or injury.

At the other end of the pediatric age range, adolescents should be able to tell you exactly how they feel and what happened. However, tact may be required to get information from an adolescent who is embarrassed, intimidated by the attention, or trying to hide the fact that he or she was doing something wrong.

In between are preschoolers and school-age children. Preschoolers can usually be interviewed if you take your time and keep your language simple. School-age children will be able to describe more clearly how they feel and what happened. They will talk with you honestly, but may feel that the injury or illness is a punishment for something they did. They must be reassured and told it's all right to feel this way or to cry. If parents, teachers, or care-providers are at the scene, talk with them but do not exclude the child. Seeing that familiar adults are being included gains the child's confidence if you follow up by talking directly to the child. If the parents are injured, you may not be able to get information from them, and the child needs to know that someone is caring for his or her parent as well.

The Primary Survey and Basic Life Support

- Act as a professional—control your emotions and facial expressions. This may help reduce the child's fear.
- Protect the head and spine. Remember, head and neck injuries are common because the head is proportionately large in a child.
- Always ensure an adequate airway. When needed, provide adequate ventilations.
- Carefully evaluate blood loss. Remember, even a small loss of blood may lead to shock.

CAUTION: The size and weight of the patient may be more important than age.

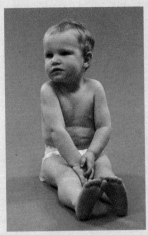 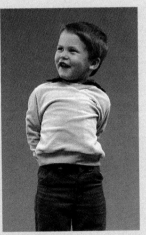

	INFANTS (Birth to 1 year)	CHILDREN (1 to 8 years)
Establishing Unresponsiveness	• The patient should move or cry when tapped and spoken to loudly. The patient should not be shaken in case there is spine injury.	
Airway	• Use the head-tilt, chin-lift or modified jaw thrust to provide an adequate airway. Do not use a head tilt if cervical spine injury is suspected. • Use the LOOK, LISTEN, FEEL approach. • If the patient is cyanotic or struggling to breathe, transport immediately. • Make certain that you have the proper head-tilt (neutral position for infants; neutral-plus for children). • If the patient is not breathing, use the mouth-to-mask technique to provide slow breaths—1 to 1½ seconds per breath. Watch for the chest to rise.	

Scan 17-1 (continued)

	INFANTS (Birth to 1 year)	CHILDREN (1 to 8 years)
Obstructed Airway	• If there is evidence of airway obstruction requiring attention:	
	• Make sure that you have not hyperextended or hyperflexed the neck. If so, reposition the infant's head and attempt to ventilate again. • Lay the infant face down along your forearm with the head lower than the trunk. Support the head by placing your hand around the jaw. Add support by resting your forearm on your thigh. Rapidly deliver up to 5 back blows using the heel of your hand. Strike forcefully directly between the shoulder blades. Place your free arm on the infant's back. Support the head with your hand and sandwich him between your two hands. Turn the infant over so his back is along your forearm. Place your forearm against your thigh again. The head should be lower than the trunk. • Rapidly deliver up to 5 quick chest thrusts as you would if providing external chest compressions for CPR. • If the airway remains obstructed, but the infant is conscious, continue back blows and chest thrusts. • If the airway remains obstructed but the infant becomes unconscious, place your thumb in the patient's mouth, over the tongue. Wrap your other fingers around the lower jaw and look for an obstruction. DO NOT attempt blind finger sweeps. When removing an obstruction, use your little finger. • If the infant is unconscious and the obstruction has not been dislodged, transport immediately. Provide two ventilations and repeat the procedures of back blows and chest thrusts, looking for and removing visible obstructions, and re-attempting ventilations.	• Reposition the child's head and attempt to ventilate again. • Place the heel of one hand on the midline of the child's abdomen above the navel but well below the rib cage and xiphoid process. Place your other hand on top of the first. Deliver 5 quick but separate and distinct upward thrusts. If you see the object, remove it. Repeat the series of 5 thrusts until the airway clears or the child becomes unconscious. • If the child becomes unconscious and the airway remains obstructed, place the child on his back on a hard surface. Provide support for the head and back as you move him. Place your thumb into the child's mouth, over the tongue. Wrap your other fingers around the lower jaw and look for an obstruction. DO NOT attempt blind finger sweeps. If you see the obstruction, sweep it out with your finger. • If the child is unconscious and the obstruction has not been dislodged, transport immediately. Attempt two ventilations and repeat the abdominal thrusts, looking for and removing visible obstructions and re-attempting ventilations.
Rescue Breathing	• Open the airway. • Use the mouth-to-mask technique to provide two slow breaths (1 to 1½ seconds per breath), noting the chest rise. Pause to take a replenishing breath after the first breath to be sure the second breath provides maximum oxygen, minimum carbon dioxide. • IF airway is clear and patient is still not breathing:	
	• Determine if there is a brachial pulse. • IF there is a pulse, provide one slow (1 to 1½ seconds), adequate breath every 3 seconds, or 20 breaths a minute. If air does not enter freely, reposition the infant's head or re-attempt to clear obstruction, or adust your breath volume or pressure.	• Determine if there is a carotid pulse. • IF there is a pulse, provide one slow (1 to 1½ seconds), adequate breath every 3 seconds, or 20 breaths a minute. If air does not enter freely, reposition the child's head or re-attempt to clear obstruction, or adust your breath volume or pressure.
	• Check for a pulse at the beginning of your assessment and frequently during airway assessment and rescue breathing. IF there is no breathing and no pulse, or if you cannot locate a pulse, wait no more than a few seconds before beginning CPR.	

	INFANTS (Birth to 1 year)	**CHILDREN (1 to 8 years)**
CPR	• Place the infant on his back on a hard surface (this can be your hand or forearm). • Apply compressions to the sternum, 1 finger-width below an imaginary line drawn between the nipples. Use the tips of 2 or 3 fingers. Use your other hand to support the infant's head in a position that will keep the airway open (unless you are using that arm to support the infant's body). • Depress the sternum ½ to 1 inch • Deliver compressions at a rate of at least 100/minute. • Deliver one ventilation, mouth to mask, EVERY 5 COMPRESSIONS. • Check for a brachial pulse every few minutes.	• Apply compressions to the sternum (place the heel of your hand 1 finger-width above the substernal notch). • Use the heel of one hand. Use the other hand to support the child's head in a position that will keep the airway open. • Depress the sternum 1 to 1½ inch • Deliver compressions at the rate of at least 100/minute. • Deliver one ventilation, mouth to mask, EVERY 5 COMPRESSIONS. • Check for a carotid pulse every few minutes.
Bleeding		• Use direct pressure as the primary method of controlling bleeding. • When necessary, use elevation, pressure points, or a BP cuff to maintain pressure over a dressing. • In rare instances, when a tourniquet must be used, a blood pressure cuff inflated to 100 mmHg used as a tourniquet will usually control the bleeding.
	• Consider a blood loss of 25 ml or more to be very serious.	• Consider a blood loss of 500 ml (½ liter or about 1 pint) or more to be very serious.
Shock		• No one sign is absolute, but consider the patient to be in shock if:
	• Blood loss is 25 ml or more. • Systolic BP is below 50 mmHg.	• Blood loss is 500 ml or more. • Systolic BP is under 50 mmHg for preschoolers, under 60 mmHg for children up to 12 years, or under 70 mmHg for teenagers. (Low BP is a late sign of shock.)
		• Capillary refill is delayed. • Consider shock to be more severe if there is evidence of dehydration (vomiting, diarrhea, exposures to high temperatures, overheating, high skin temperature), and if there is a rapid pulse. • Ensure adequate breathing, monitor pulse, and control serious bleeding. • Administer oxygen per local guidelines. • If there is no indication of head injury, spinal injury, or chest injury, elevate the lower extremities. • Prevent the loss of body heat. • Handle the child gently. • Give nothing by mouth. • Transport as soon as possible, monitoring vital signs.

All patients have some degree of fear at the emergency scene. Infants and children are usually more fearful than adults because they lack experience with illness and injury. In addition to this, the infant or child is easily frightened by the unknown. Since so many details of the emergency scene are unknowns, it is easy to see why emergencies can be scary for children. The elements associated with the emergency (pain, noise, bright lights, cold) can set off a panic reaction in infants.

A child lacks extensive communication skills. At an emergency, if the child feels he or she does not understand you, or believes that you do not understand in return, fear will increase. If the child is to communicate, he or she must remain calm. Putting the child at ease is a very important part of the care you must provide (Figure 17-1). Some children, when stressed, will regress and act like a younger child.

Any problems faced by the child will be intensified if the parents are not at the scene. Children find security by interacting with their parents when facing new problems or emergencies. Asking for mom or dad may be the child's first priority, even above that of having your help.

When dealing with pediatric patients you should

1. Identify yourself simply by saying "Hi, I'm Pat. What's your name?"
2. Let the child know that someone will call his or her parents.
3. Let the child have any nearby toy that he or she may want.

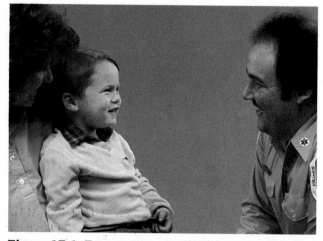

Figure 17-1 Emergencies are frightening for children. Take time to put them at ease.

4. Kneel or sit at the child's eye level. Assure that bright light is not directly behind you and shining into the child's eyes.
5. SMILE. This is a familiar sign from adults that reassures children.
6. Touch the child on the forehead or hold his or her hand. A child who does not wish to be touched will let you know. Do not force the issue; smile and provide comfort through your conversation.
7. Do not use any equipment on the child without explaining what you will do with it. Many children fear the medical items that are so familiar to the EMT, thinking they will cause pain.
8. Let the child see your face and have eye contact. (A child's inability or unwillingness to make eye contact is a key indicator of serious illness.) Speak directly to the child, making a special effort to speak clearly and slowly in words he or she can understand. Be sure the child can hear you.
9. Stop occasionally to find out if the child understands. Never assume the child understood you, but find out by asking questions.
10. Determine if there are life-threatening problems and treat immediately. If there are no problems of this nature, continue the patient survey and interview at a relaxed pace. Fearful children cannot take the pressure of a rapidly paced assessment and "meaningless" questions fired at them by a stranger.
11. Always tell the child what you are going to do as you take vital signs and do a physical exam. Do not try to explain the entire procedure at once. Instead, explain each step as you do it.
12. NEVER LIE TO THE CHILD. Tell him or her when the examination may hurt. If the child asks if he or she is sick or hurt, be honest, but be sure to add that you are there to help and will not leave. Let the child know that other people also will be helping.

Vital Signs The measuring of vital signs is an important part of assessment, but vital signs vary so much with the size of the patient and the patient's reaction to the situation that the EMT often finds it difficult to remember all the values. Table 17-2 gives ranges of vital signs you may expect to find in a quiet child with no fever, emotional stress, or physical injury. Keep in mind that the younger the child, the more rapid are the pulse and respiratory rates and the lower the blood pressure. As the child enters adolescence, the values approach those of adults. (Rather

TABLE 17-2 Vital Sign Ranges

Age Range	Respiratory Rate	Pulse Rate	Systolic Blood Pressure
Neonate *Birth–1 month*	30-50 min	120-160 min (avg/ 140)	50 to 80
Infant *1 to 12 months*	20-30 min	90-140 min (avg/120)	70 to 100
Toddler *1 to 3 years*	20-30 min	80-130 min (avg/100)	80 to 115
Preschool *3 to 5 years*	20-30 min	80-120 min (avg/100)	80 to 110
School Age *6 to 12 years*	20-30 min	70-110 min (avg/90)	80 to 110
Adolescent *13 to 18 years*	12-20 min	60-100 min (avg/80)	110 to 120

than memorizing these values, carry a copy of the chart in your pediatric kit.)

A quick formula can be used to determine a normal systolic blood pressure for a child over 1 year of age: 80 + (2 × child's age) = systolic pressure. Normally, the diastolic reading is about two-thirds of the systolic reading. A systolic blood pressure less than 70 + (2 x child's age) in a child over 1 year should be considered abnormal and may indicate shock.

Pediatric vital signs should always be taken in the field. Because they are so variable, it is important to get an initial set or baseline reading of vital signs as quickly as possible and monitor them frequently. This is the only way the EMT can determine whether the child is remaining stable or deteriorating. Children compensate for shock and appear well longer than adults, then decompensate and "go sour" far more rapidly than adults. So don't wait for the vital signs to indicate shock or spend time wondering if readings are within normal range. Always anticipate shock and treat by giving oxygen, maintaining body temperature, and positioning the patient appropriately.

The smaller child must first feel comfortable with you before you will be able to get him or her to sit still long enough for you to take a blood pressure and get respiratory and pulse rates. If the situation is not so serious that you feel you must transport immediately, take the time to let the child become familiar with the stethoscope and blood pressure cuff. Children are naturally curious and eager to help, even when ill or hurt. Let the child listen to your heart through the stethoscope while you sit quietly, then explain that you will listen as he or she sits quietly. To keep them quiet, show them how to look at your watch and let them say "when."

You may find it easier to count pulse and respiratory rates by listening through the stethoscope rather than watching for the rise and fall of the chest and abdomen and feeling for a peripheral pulse. You can also check for lung sounds at the same time. To get an estimate of the upper limit of a respiratory rate for a pediatric patient, subtract the child's age from 40. For example, a six-year old child should not be breathing faster than 34 breaths a minute.

An accurate blood pressure is hard enough to obtain in a child without being hindered with the wrong size cuff. Cuffs that are too large will give a falsely low reading and cuffs that are too small will give a falsely high reading. The width of the cuff should cover two-thirds of the upper arm; the bladder should not overlap when wrapped around the arm but cover at least two-thirds of the circumference. If an adult cuff is all that is available, take a reading on the thigh using the same measurement criteria for fitting the leg as for the arm. If the leg is used, it is the popliteal artery (the artery of the posterior leg behind the knee) that should be palpated or auscultated.

Note: There is one sign—capillary refill time greater than 2 seconds—that can be observed easily and help the EMT to quickly recognize a "shocky" child. You do not need to depress a nail bed, as in an adult. Just give a quick squeeze to the child's hand or foot, forearm or lower leg and observe how quickly the whitened area regains its pink color. If it takes longer than it takes you to say "capillary refill," the child is probably in shock. CHECK CAPILLARY REFILL TIME FREQUENTLY TO KEEP TABS ON WHETHER A CHILD IS GOING INTO SHOCK.

The Physical Examination The EMT normally performs the physical examination or body survey in head-to-toe order; but on alert infants and small children this is reversed. Starting with the toes and working your way toward the head will let the child get used to you and your touch before you, who after all are a stranger, attempt to touch them around the head and face. Playing with infants' feet often puts them at ease.

Always explain to parents or adults at the scene, as well as to the child of any age, what you are going to do before you do it, and why the physical exam is important (Figure 17-2). It also helps to explain to the child, who must endure these procedures, how long each step will take and that you will need his or her help. Warn the child if you think your exam may cause pain and for how long. Also have the child tell you if anything hurts when you touch it and how badly, from a little to a lot for smaller children, or on a scale of one to five for older children.

Unless there are possible injuries that indicate that the child should not be moved, the child should be held on the parent's lap.

Many EMS teams carry clean toys that can be given to the child during the physical exam. They can provide comfort to the child and allow you to explain the survey by using the toy as model. Point to an area on the toy to show the child where you must touch during the survey and where you will bandage when you need to provide emergency care. This type of one-to-one communication also helps build parent and bystander confidence, letting them know that a professional, compassionate EMT is caring for the child. (If you use a toy, then give it to the child to keep.)

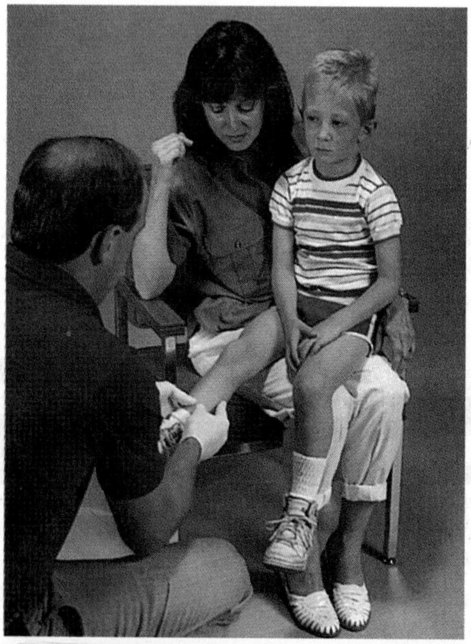

Most young children will suffer no embarrassment when clothing is removed or repositioned during the exam. Nonetheless, protect the child from the stares of onlookers. Many children around the age of 5 to 8 go through a stage of intense modesty. You may have to keep explaining why you must remove certain articles of clothing. Many parents, teachers, and day care personnel teach children that strangers should not remove their clothing or touch them. The children that you examine may not understand your intentions and may resist. Some children may become upset because they feel you are taking something away from them. Take your time and do not rush children into accepting all that is happening. Remember that children lose body heat rapidly, so if you expose them, quickly cover them with a blanket.

The young adolescent is often worried about the changes occurring to his or her body and uncertain if these changes are "normal." Handling the clothing of a teenager of the opposite sex can be awkward for the EMT as well as for the patient. In most cases, a simple description of the survey will set the patient at ease. However, you should make sure that both the adolescent and the parents understand what you are going to do and why it must be done. When possible, conduct the examination in the presence of an EMT of the same sex as the patient. Do not delay patient evaluation and care because you or the patient may be embarrassed. As a professional, you must put such feelings aside and act in a manner that will allow the patient to relax and understand that there is no need for embarrassment.

The survey of an infant or child is done to look for the same signs of injury and illness as in the case of the adult patient. However, you should take special care with the following (Figure 17-3)

- Head—Do not apply pressure to the "soft spots" (fontanelles) of an infant. The skin over the anterior fontanelle is normally level with the skull, or slightly sunken, and may

Figure 17-2 Explain to the child what you are going to do before you do it.

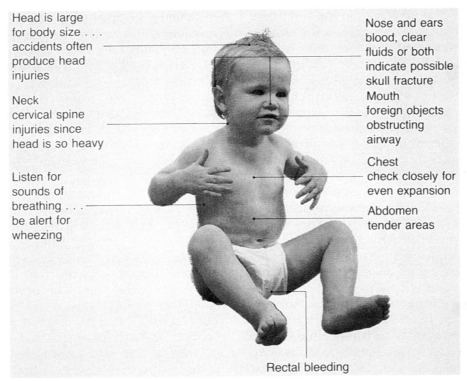

Head is large for body size . . . accidents often produce head injuries

Neck cervical spine injuries since head is so heavy

Listen for sounds of breathing . . . be alert for wheezing

Nose and ears blood, clear fluids or both indicate possible skull fracture

Mouth foreign objects obstructing airway

Chest check closely for even expansion

Abdomen tender areas

Rectal bleeding

AGE 1–2

Figure 17-3 The special areas to consider during the assessment of a child.

bulge naturally when the infant cries. Meningitis and head trauma cause the fontanelle to bulge due to increased intracranial pressure. Accidents involving infants and children can often produce head injuries.

Nose and Ears—Look for blood and clear fluids from the nose and ears. Suspect skull fractures if present. Children are nose breathers and mucus or blood clot obstruction will make it hard for them to breathe.

Neck—Children are more vulnerable to spinal cord injuries than adults. The head is proportionately larger and heavier than an adult's and has less support because muscles and bone structure are less developed. In medical emergencies, the neck may be sore, stiff, or swollen.

• Airway—Keep the infant's head in the neutral position and the child's head in the neutral-plus or sniffing position (chin thrust forward to maintain an open airway). If there is no suspicion of spinal injury, place a flat, folded towel under their shoulders to get the appropriate airway opening. Children's airways are more pliable and smaller than an adult's. Hyperextension or hyperflexion may close off the airway. For medical respiratory problems, the child may want to sit up.

• Chest—Listen closely for even air entry and the sounds of breathing. Be alert for rales and wheezes. Check for symmetry, bruising, paradoxical movement, and muscular retraction (pulling in) of the sternum or the muscles between the ribs. Remember that a child's soft ribs may not break, but there may be underlying injuries to the organs within the chest.

- Abdomen—Note any rigid or tender areas and distention. Because a child's abdominal organs (especially the spleen and liver) are large in relation to the size of the abdominal cavity, and because there is little protection offered by the still-undeveloped abdominal muscles, these organs are more susceptible to trauma than an adult's. Any injury that impedes the movement of the diaphragm will compromise a young child's breathing, as most children 8 years of age or younger are abdominal breathers.
- Pelvis—Check for stability of the pelvic girdle and bleeding or bloody discharge from the genital area.
- Extremities—Perform a neurological assessment with capillary refill and distal pulse check. With an infant or young child you do not have to press on a nail bed. You can quickly check capillary refill by squeezing a hand or foot, forearm or lower leg. Check for fractures, bruising, deformity, and wounds and bleeding. The bones of an infant or child are more pliable so they bend, splinter, and buckle before they fracture. The type of fracture common in children is a "greenstick" fracture (see Chapter 11). Injuries to the extremities should be checked for fractures at the distal ends in the area called the growth plate. Failure to identify and mismanagement of fractures in this area could result in bone and joint deformities or uneven growth.
- Vital signs—Children have faster pulse and respiratory rates and lower blood pressures than adults. Because chest and abdominal muscles are not fully developed, infants tire easily when there is respiratory distress and an elevated respiratory rate. Their smaller blood volume means that shock develops more quickly and from less severe wounds. Babies and young children have undeveloped temperature control mechanisms which may cause their extremities to feel cool to the touch and to appear mottled.

The neurologic evaluation often produces special problems. The "look test" is important here. Does the child make eye contact? Does the infant smile? Recognize his or her parents? Watch the infant carefully for responses to your touching, squeezing, and pushing. It is often necessary to treat all infants as if they were unconscious patients and test them for reaction to painful stimuli. Always note if the conscious infant's or child's eyes look in the direction of your hand or your face as you touch him or her. Children will normally follow your movements with their eyes. Notice if the patient stays alert, responds only when you call his or her name or speak loudly, or lapses quickly into a sleepy state. See if the patient will squeeze your fingers or reach for a toy. If you do not think spinal injuries are likely, continue to test the young child's neurologic reactions by simple childhood games such as "peek-a-boo." Holding your hand up to the young child's hand will often lead the patient to compare the size of his or her hand with yours. In doing so, the child will move his fingers and will press against your hand. If the child does not respond, see if he or she wants to play "pattycake," or hold an object that requires the use of both hands and eyes in coordination. The stethoscope or a clean stuffed animal is ideal for this purpose, provided the child shows no fear of the instrument or the toy.

Most infants and children can be comforted by a parent. Continued irritability is a sign that something is wrong with the child.

MEDICAL EMERGENCIES COMMON TO CHILDREN

Like adults, children can suffer a variety of medical problems from "belly ache" to heart conditions. Although emergency care measures for medical problems are generally the same for children as for adults, there are a few problems common to childhood that deserve special attention.

Fever

Above-normal body temperature is one of the most important signs of an existing or impending acute illness. Fever usually accompanies simple virus infections and ear aches as well as such childhood diseases as measles, mumps, chicken pox, mononucleosis, pneumonia, epiglottitis, and meningitis. The fever also may be due to heat stroke, any infection, or some other noninfectious disease problem.

Never regard a fever as unimportant. Parents may have an opinion about what they believe may be the problem, but the EMT is not qualified to diagnose or determine what is likely to happen over the next few hours.

Signs

Use relative skin temperature as a sign.

☐ Any child 1 to 5 years old with a body temperature (oral measurement) above 103°F must be evaluated at the hospital. When in doubt, transport.

☐ Any child from 5 to 12 with a body temperature above 102°F must be evaluated at the hospital. When in doubt, transport.

Note: An oral temperature is not normally done on a child under 5 years of age in the field; but taking a rectal temperature on a small, squirming child risks damaging delicate membranes. A high relative skin temperature is always enough reason to transport and seek medical opinion. Check your local protocols for taking temperature in the field.

Patient Care—Fever

Be aware that a mild fever can quickly turn into a high fever that may indicate a serious, if not life-threatening, problem.

Emergency Care Steps

☐ If the infant or child feels very warm to hot to the touch, then prepare the patient for transport.

Children can tolerate high temperature, and only a small percent will have a seizure due to fever (febrile seizures). It is the rapid rise in temperature rather than the temperature itself that causes seizures. Should you find an infant or child with high fever

1 Remove the child's clothing, but do not allow him or her to be exposed to conditions that may bring on sudden chills (hypothermia). If the child objects, let the patient keep on light clothing or underwear.

2 For heat stroke, cover the child with a towel soaked in tepid water. This will cool the child quickly.

3 Monitor for shivering and avoid hypothermia. This may develop quickly in children.

- *Do not* use rubbing alcohol to cool the patient (it can be absorbed in toxic amounts and is a fire hazard).

- *Do not* submerge the child in cold water, or cover with a towel soaked in ice water (which can cause hypothermia rapidly).

4 If local protocols permit, give the child fluids by mouth or allow him or her to suck on chipped ice. This may not prevent dehydration, but will increase comfort.

5 Transport all children who have suffered a seizure as quickly as possible, protecting the patient from temperature extremes.

Hypothermia

Children have a large surface area in proportion to their body mass, and exposure to cool weather and water can easily result in **hypothermia** (HI-po-THURM-i-ah), or cooling of the body temperature, a condition that is life-threatening if extreme or prolonged. Other causes of hypothermia in children include ingestion of alcohol or drugs that dilate peripheral vessels and cause loss of body heat; metabolic problems such as hypoglycemia; brain disorders that interfere with temperature regulation; and severe infection or sepsis.

Like adults, children lose heat more readily if their clothes are wet, if they are exposed to wind, or if they are submerged in cold water. The child's body attempts to compensate for a decrease in body temperature, but as these compensatory functions begin to fail, the core body temperature drops.

Patient Assessment—Hypothermia

Signs

As will be explained in more detail in Chapter 20, signs of hypothermia, from mild to extreme, include

☐ Shivering
☐ Slurred speech
☐ Incoordination
☐ Frostbite in the ears, nose, fingers, toes, hands, or feet
☐ Rigidity rather than shivering
☐ Low or falling respiratory and pulse rates (take vital signs for later comparison)
☐ Cyanosis

over

- Lethargy
- Unconsciousness
- Coma with dilated and fixed pupils
- Respiratory arrest
- Faint or no pulse
- Irregular heart rhythm

Patient Care—Hypothermia

Field care for children is the same as for adults with mild, moderate, or severe hypothermic conditions (see Chapter 20). Avoid rough handling and inserting anything in the mouth as these actions may cause ventricular fibrillation or cardiac arrest in the severely hypothermic child. Suction very gently if suctioning is necessary, being alert to the possibility of cardiac arrest.

If your protocols permit cooling of the feverish child, watch for shivering. If the skin becomes cool, stop cooling activities and cover the child with a light blanket to avoid hypothermia.

Seizures

High fever, epilepsy, meningitis, diabetic states, oxygen deficiency, poisoning, and head injury can bring on seizures. They are not usually life-threatening, unless prolonged. The child can generally tolerate a seizure for 20 minutes if the airway is maintained.

Patient Assessment—Seizures

Usually, you will arrive after the convulsion has passed.

1. Interview the patient as well as family members and bystanders who saw the convulsion. Ask them if the child has had seizures before, if they can tell you how long it lasted, what part of the body was twitching, and if the child is on any medication. Determine if the child has had fever.
2. Assess the child for symptoms and signs of illness or injury taking care to note any injuries sustained during the convulsion. All infants and children who have undergone a seizure require medical evaluation.

Note: Status epilepticus (prolonged or back-to-back convulsions without regaining consciousness—see Chapter 16) is a TRUE EMERGENCY requiring immediate transport.

Patient Care—Seizures

Emergency Care Steps

If the patient has a seizure in your presence, as well as during transport, provide the following care.

1. Monitor airway, breathing, and circulation.
2. Maintain airway with jaw thrust; do not insert airway or bitestick.
3. Be alert for vomiting; suction as necessary.
4. Provide oxygen by nonrebreather mask, but be ready to suction under the mask.
5. Protect from further injury.
6. Protect the head and splint injuries if trauma occurred.
7. Transport and monitor vital signs.
8. Provide comfort and emotional support.

Respiratory Disorders

Respiratory disorders are the most common cause of death in children. An infant or child can have the same breathing problems as an adult; however, certain additional problems are commonly seen with pediatric patients. These problems include croup, epiglottitis, bronchiolitis, and asthma.

Croup Croup (KROOP) is a group of viral illnesses that cause inflammation of the larynx, trachea, and bronchi (Figure 17-4). It is typically an illness of children 6 months to about 4 years of age that often occurs at night. This problem sometimes follows a cold or other respiratory infection. Tissues in the airway (particularly the upper airway) become swollen and restrict the passage of air.

Patient Assessment—Croup

Signs

During the day, the child usually will have

- Mild fever
- Some hoarseness

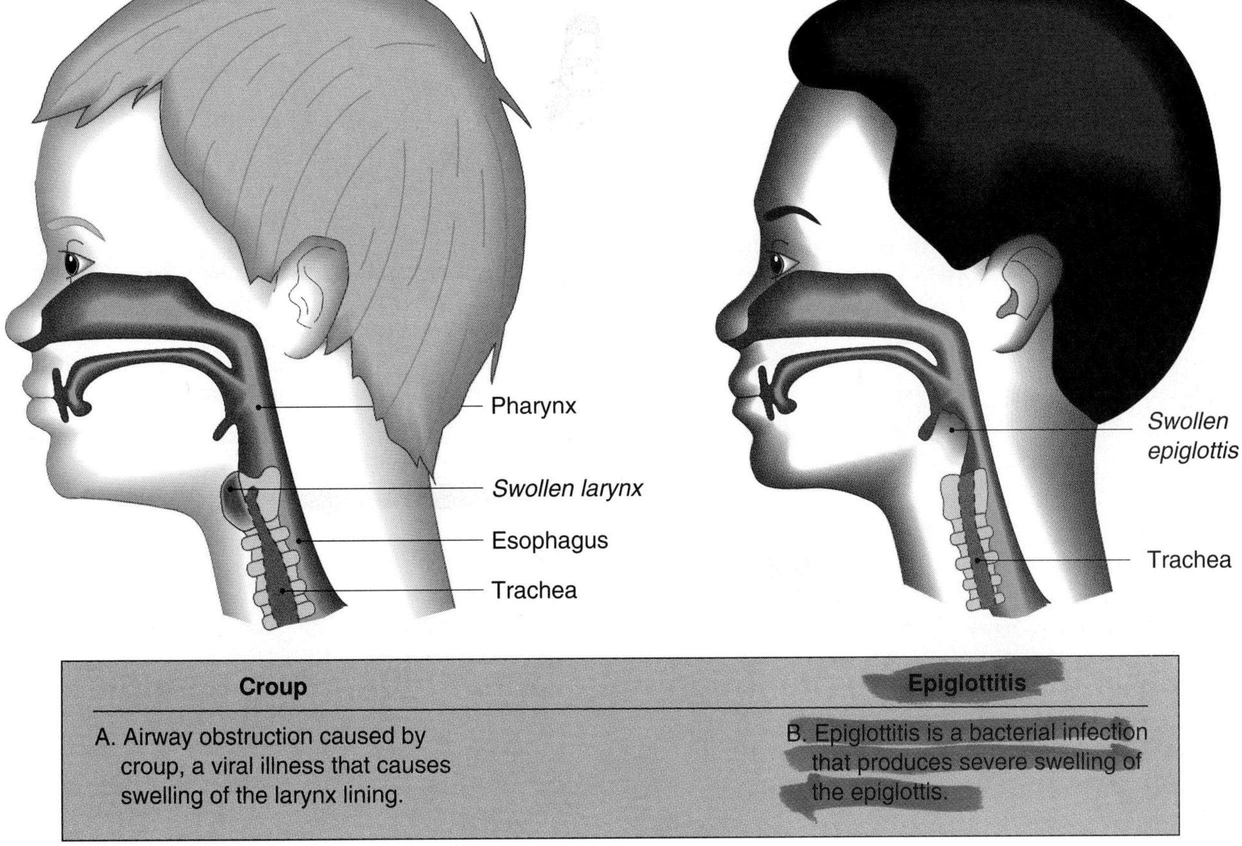
Pharynx
Swollen larynx
Esophagus
Trachea
Swollen epiglottis
Trachea
Croup
A. Airway obstruction caused by croup, a viral illness that causes swelling of the larynx lining.
Epiglottitis
B. Epiglottitis is a bacterial infection that produces severe swelling of the epiglottis.

Figure 17-4 Comparing the airway structures in croup and epiglottitis.

At night, the child's condition will worsen and he or she will develop

- A loud "seal bark" cough
- Difficulty breathing
- Signs of respiratory distress including nasal flaring, retraction of the muscles between the ribs, tugging at the throat
- Restlessness
- Paleness with cyanosis

Patient Care—Croup

Emergency Care Steps

1. Place the patient in a position of comfort (usually sitting up).
2. Administer a high concentration of oxygen. When possible, this should be from a humidified source.
3. Walking to the ambulance in the cool night air may provide relief as the cool air reduces the edema in the airway tissues.
4. Do not delay transport unless ordered to do so by the emergency department physician.

Epiglottitis **Epiglottitis** (epi-glo-TI-tis) is most commonly caused by a bacterial infection that produces swelling of the epiglottis and partial airway obstruction (Figure 17-4). The typical patient will be between 3 and 7 years old.

Patient Assessment—Epiglottitis

Signs

- A sudden onset of high fever
- Painful swallowing (the child often will drool to avoid swallowing)
- The patient will assume a "tripod" position, sitting upright and leaning forward with

the chin thrust outward and the mouth wide open (sniffing position) in an effort to maintain a wide airway opening.

☐ The patient will sit very still, but the muscles will work hard to breathe and the child can tire quickly from the effort.

☐ The child appears more generally ill than with croup.

Note: All cases of epiglottitis must be considered to be life threatening, no matter how early the detection.

Patient Care—Epiglottitis

Emergency Care Steps

1. Immediately transport the child, sitting on the parent's lap. This is a TRUE EMERGENCY.
2. Provide oxygen at a high concentration from a humidified source. Do not increase the child's anxiety. If he or she resists the mask, let the parent hold it in front of the child's face.
3. Constantly monitor the child for respiratory distress and arrest and be ready to resuscitate.
4. DO NOT PLACE ANYTHING INTO THE CHILD'S MOUTH, including a thermometer, tongue blade, or oropharyngeal airway. To do so may set off spasms along the upper airway (laryngospasms) that will totally obstruct the airway.
5. Notify the emergency department as soon as possible.

Note: The child will not want to lie down and you should not force him or her to do so. The child must be handled gently, since rough handling and stress could lead to a total airway obstruction from spasms of the larynx and swelling tissues.

Bronchiolitis Bronchiolitis (BRONG-ke-o-LI-tis) is an airway inflammation below the level of the trachea.

Patient Assessment—Bronchiolitis

Signs and Symptoms

Bronchiolitis has signs and symptoms that resemble asthma but is common in the child

of 1 or 2 years. Children under 1 year rarely have asthma. Signs may include

☐ Coughing
☐ Fever
☐ Wheezing and rales are sometimes heard.

Patient Care—Bronchiolitis

Emergency Care Steps

1. Provide oxygen from a humidified source.
2. Transport. Usually the patient will be most comfortable in a semisitting or sitting position.

Asthma Asthma (AZ-mah) is a sensitivity reaction to allergens that can cause the lower airways to obstruct. Even environmental, physical, and emotional stress and respiratory infections can stimulate an asthma attack.

Patient Assessment—Asthma

Like an adult, a child can have acute asthma attacks and status asthmaticus, showing the same signs, including wheezing (see Chapter 16).

Patient Care—Asthma

As with the adult, status asthmaticus is a life-threatening condition. Any first case of asthma must be cared for as if anaphylactic shock is a real possibility.

General Respiratory Disorders It is not easy to determine which respiratory problem the child may have. Many signs and symptoms are similar, and age ranges for occurrence overlap.

Patient Assessment— General Respiratory Disorders

DON'T TAKE THE TIME TO TRY TO DIFFERENTIATE SIGNS AND SYMPTOMS. If croup, epiglottitis, or asthma is possible, transport immediately. For other respiratory problems

1. Gather information quickly from the parents.
2. Do a rapid assessment of the child.

3 *Do not* put a tongue blade in the child's mouth to examine the airway. This may cause airway spasms that can totally obstruct the airway.

Patient Care— General Respiratory Disorders

ALL RESPIRATORY DISORDERS IN CHILDREN MUST BE TAKEN SERIOUSLY. Respiratory disease is the primary cause of cardiac arrest not due to trauma. If you treat the respiratory system, the heart will also respond. The EMT's primary concern when caring for infants and children with respiratory problems, whether medical or trauma related, is to establish and maintain an open airway. About one-third of all pediatric trauma deaths are related to mismanagement of airway.

Emergency Care Steps

1 *Do not* attempt to clear the airway of a foreign obstruction unless it is clear that this is the problem—the child has been observed ingesting a foreign object or the signs of such ingestion are clear (see Chapter 4). If the child is conscious or has a respiratory disorder, finger sweeps can can trigger airway spasms or gagging. The Heimlich maneuver is useless if the problem is a respiratory disorder with swollen and inflamed tissues.

2 If the patient appears to have partial obstruction of the airway and is breathing adequately, place the child in a seated position on the parent's lap, cover for warmth, provide oxygen (a humidified source is best, and the mask can be held in front of the child's face by the parent), and transport. Monitor the patient constantly during transport.

3 If the patient does not respond to oxygen or the obstruction is total, basic life support measures must be initiated. The unconscious patient without a gag reflex should receive a properly sized oropharyngeal airway, but *do not* use if epiglottitis is suspected.

4 *Do not* give the child anything by mouth as this could cause spasms or vomiting.

5 Transport immediately. All infants and children in respiratory distress or showing difficulty in breathing *must* be seen by a physician.

Meningitis

Meningitis (men-in-JI-tis) is caused by either a bacterial or a viral infection of the lining of the brain and spinal cord (the meninges). The majority of meningitis cases occur between the ages of 1 month and 5 years.

Patient Assessment—Meningitis

Signs and Symptoms

Signs and symptoms of meningitis include

- ☐ High fever
- ☐ Lethargy
- ☐ Irritability
- ☐ Headache
- ☐ Stiff neck
- ☐ Sensitivity to light
- ☐ In infants, the fontanelles may be bulging unless the child is dehydrated.
- ☐ Movement is painful and the child does not want to be touched or held.
- ☐ Sudden excitement may cause seizures.
- ☐ A rash may be present in the bacterial type infection.

Patient Care—Meningitis

It is most important to carefully follow all universal precautions for personal protection and disinfection.

Emergency Care Steps

1 Monitor airway, breathing, circulation, disability, and vital signs.
2 Provide a high concentration oxygen flow through nonrebreather mask.
3 Ventilate with a bag-valve-mask with supplemental oxygen if necessary.
4 Provide CPR if necessary.
5 Be alert for seizures.
6 Transport immediately. This is a TRUE EMERGENCY. *Do not* delay.
7 Observe respiratory precautions.

Acute Abdomen

Infants and children can develop abdominal pain for a variety of reasons: appendicitis, intestinal influenza, gas, indigestion, and bacterial infection of the bowels.

Patient Assessment—Acute Abdomen

You will not be able to tell one kind of abdominal problem from another, nor would EMT-level emergency care be different if you could. Any abdominal pain or cramp, even if intermittent, or any other sign or symptom of an abdominal problem must be considered serious in a child.

Signs and Symptoms

- ☐ Abdominal pain
- ☐ Abdominal cramps (perhaps intermittent)
- ☐ Reaction to pain or rigidity and tenderness on gentle palpation
- ☐ Marked distention (beyond the normal roundedness of a child's abdomen)
- ☐ Knees drawn up
- ☐ Fever
- ☐ Vomiting
- ☐ Blood in the stools
- ☐ "Lumps" in the abdomen
- ☐ The child may be dehydrated.
- ☐ In severe cases, signs of shock may be present.

Patient Care—Acute Abdomen

Emergency Care Steps

If any of the above signs or symptoms are present

1. Treat the child as you would an adult with acute abdomen (see Chapter 16).
2. Transport immediately.

Remember: You will have to provide much more emotional support than with an adult. If the parents cannot decide if they want their child to be transported, lead them away from the child and explain why it is important for the child to be seen by a physician.

Diarrhea and Vomiting

Diarrhea and vomiting are common in childhood illness.

Patient Assessment— Diarrhea and Vomiting

Both diarrhea and vomiting can cause dehydration that worsen whatever other condition the child may have and may lead to life-threatening shock. Infants are more susceptible to the effects of dehydration because, compared to adults, a greater percentage of their body proportion is water and their fluid maintenance needs are greater.

Patient Care—Diarrhea and Vomiting

Emergency Care Steps

For any pediatric patient with diarrhea or vomiting

1. If signs of shock are present, contact medical control immediately and transport.
2. If your protocols permit, offer the child sips of clear liquids or chipped ice as the child can tolerate without vomiting.
3. Monitor airway, breathing, circulation, disability, and vital signs.
4. Be prepared to provide oral suctioning
5. Provide oxygen.
6. Save a sample of vomitus and rectal discharge (e.g., a soiled diaper).

Poisonings

Children are often the victims of accidental poisoning, often resulting from the ingestion of household products or medications. Poisons can quickly depress the respiratory system and cause respiratory arrest and also can cause life-threatening conditions of the circulatory and nervous systems. The airway and gastrointestinal track can also be burned by corrosive substances on ingestion and with subsequent vomiting.

Patient Assessment—Poisonings

Review Chapter 16 for information on ingested, inhaled, absorbed, and injected poisons. This information applies to children as well as to adults. There are some special types of poisonings not often associated with adult patients, however. These special cases include

- ☐ Aspirin Poisoning—Look for hyperventilation, vomiting, and sweating. The skin may feel hot. Severe cases cause seizures, coma, or shock.
- ☐ Acetaminophen Poisoning—Many medica-

tions have this compound, including Tylenol, Comtrex, Bancap, Excedrin P.M., and Datril. The child may be restless (early) or drowsy. Nausea, vomiting, and heavy perspiration may occur. The loss of consciousness is possible.

☐ Lead Poisoning—This usually comes from ingesting chips of lead-based paint. It is often chronic (building up over a long time). Look for nausea with abdominal pain and vomiting. Muscle cramps, headache, muscle weakness, and irritability are often present.

☐ Iron Poisoning—Iron compounds such as ferrous sulfate are found in some vitamin tablets and liquids. As little as one gram of ferrous sulfate can be lethal to a child. Within 30 minutes to several hours, the child will show nausea and bloody vomiting, often accompanied by bloody diarrhea. Typically the child will develop shock but this may be delayed for up to 24 hours as the child appears to be getting better.

☐ Petroleum Product Poisoning—The patient will usually be vomiting with coughing or choking. In most cases, you will smell the distinctive odor of a petroleum distillate (e.g., gasoline, kerosene, heating fuel).

☐ Cyanide—Such seemingly innocent items as apple seeds contain cyanide.

Patient Care—Poisonings

Emergency Care Steps

☐ If directed by your medical control or poison control center, dilute the poison by giving water or milk.

Note: Some EMS systems will direct use of syrup of ipecac to induce vomiting and/or activated charcoal and water to bind the poison. Use these methods only if local protocols advise and you are so directed.

Note: VOMITING SHOULD NOT BE INDUCED FOR CORROSIVE SUBSTANCES OR FOR PETROLEUM PRODUCT POISONING (aspiration pneumonia is a serious problem with petroleum product poisoning). (Review Chapter 16.)

Remember: ALWAYS CARE FOR POISONINGS AS DIRECTED BY YOUR LOCAL POISON CONTROL CENTER AND ON-LINE MEDICAL CONTROL.

Sudden Infant Death Syndrome

In the United States, **sudden infant death syndrome (SIDS)**—the sudden unexplained death of an apparently healthy baby while it is sleeping—occurs to between 6,500 and 7,500 babies each year. These babies were usually receiving proper care and frequently have passed physical examinations within days of their sudden death. The problem is not caused by external methods of suffocation or by vomiting or choking. The problem may possibly be related to nerve cell development in the brain or the tissue chemistry of the respiratory system or the heart. Some relationships have been drawn to family history of SIDS and respiratory problems, but there is still no accepted reason why these babies die (Figure 17-5).

The cause of death in SIDS is often related to neurologic system immaturity, poor respiratory control, and respiratory failure. When asleep, the typical SIDS patient will show periods of cardiac slowdown and temporary cessation of breathing known as **sleep apnea** (ap-NE-ah). Exhaustion, respiratory disease, and overheating have been demonstrated as causing increased episodes of sleep apnea. Eventually, the infant will stop breathing and will not start again on its own. Unless reached in time, the episode can be fatal.

Patient Assessment—SIDS

Signs

☐ The infant may be found in an unusual position because of muscle spasms.
☐ The infant may have purple, mottled markings on the head and face—may appear to be bruised.
☐ Vomitus or blood-tinged or frothy fluids may be noted around the mouth and nose.

Patient Care—SIDS

Emergency Care Steps

For the possible SIDS patient

1 Provide basic respiratory and cardiac life support.
2 Be certain that the parents receive emotional support and that they believe that everything possible is being done for the child at the scene and during transport.

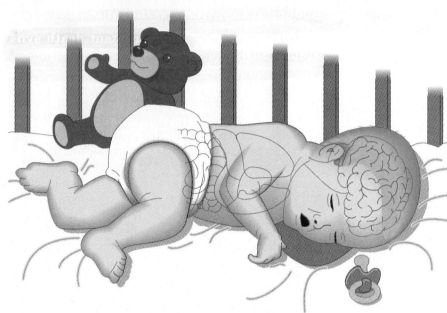

- Inadequate amounts of oxygen in the blood

- Undeveloped respiratory control and cardiac rhythm

- Irregular heart rhythm

- Altered brain activity

- Apnea

- Insufficient oxygen to tissues

- Deterioration of other body tissues

- Lividity of blood pooling

Figure 17-5 Causes of sudden infant death syndrome.

Parents who lose a child to SIDS often suffer intense guilt feelings from the moment they find the child. Whether or not the parents express such guilt, remind them that SIDS occurs to apparently healthy babies who are receiving the best of parental care. Do not be embarrassed to express your sorrow for their loss, but be sure to do so only after a physician has officially informed them of the child's death.

Remember: Speaking with a suspicious tone or asking inappropriate questions may only increase the parents' sorrow or guilt.

PEDIATRIC TRAUMA EMERGENCIES

When we think of trauma, injury from accidents usually comes to mind. This section will discuss assessment and management of accidental trauma as well as of the trauma caused by child abuse.

Many situations are traumatic to children because of their limited life experiences and their fear of the unknown. They are also curious and learning about their environment while exploring, which often leads to injury from accidental falls or things falling on them, burns, entrapment, crushing, and other mechanisms of injury.

When providing emergency care for the injured child, always tell him or her what you

are going to do before you do it. Making the child feel confident in you will help reduce their fear. If the child cries, let him or her know this is all right and you know he or she is trying to be brave, but everyone becomes scared when hurt.

Carry brightly colored adhesive bandages to hold dressings in place and let the child know these are especially for him or her as a reward for bravery. Other small "rewards" can be carried with you, like sheets of peel-off stickers. (Be sure the rewards are not small items that can be swallowed.)

Managing Pediatric Trauma

Assessment and injury management techniques are basically the same for children as for adults. There are some injuries that will require slightly different care, as will be discussed later.

When arriving on the scene, assure that it is safe and look for the mechanism of injury. You must always obtain information regarding the incident, perform a primary and secondary survey, and take initial vital signs. If a child is unable to provide a history, collect information from parents, care providers, bystanders, and from your own observations.

One common injury pattern found in preschoolers who wander into the street and are struck by a vehicle is the combination of femur, chest, and head injury. The bumper strikes the femur, the child's chest strikes the hood, and

490 Pediatrics and Childbirth

the child then lands on his or her head because of the size and weight of the child's head relative to body weight and size.

A Protocol for Pediatric Trauma Management Determine the mechanism of injury and always perform the following for every pediatric trauma patient. Apply this general protocol to all of the specific injuries that will be discussed on the following pages.

Primary Survey and Basic Life Support

1. Perform the ABCDEs: Assess and manage airway, breathing, circulation, and disability (neurological response), and expose the body to check for life-threatening wounds or injuries.
2. Insert an oral airway in the unconscious child with no gag reflex (nasal airways are not recommended as they may cause tissue damage and bleeding. Follow local protocols). Be prepared to suction the patient.
3. PROVIDE OXYGEN TO ALL PEDIATRIC TRAUMA PATIENTS—even if they are not in respiratory distress—by nonrebreather mask, or assist ventilations with bag-valve-mask with supplemental oxygen. Hyperventilate the head-injured child.
4. Perform CPR as necessary.
5. Seal open chest wounds and monitor for tension pneumothorax (see Chapter 14). Stabilize any flail segments or impaled objects.
6. Control bleeding and shock.
7. Make a CUPS status decision (see Chapter 3).

Note: See the more detailed discussions below under "Airway and Respiration," "Circulation," and "Disability."

Secondary Survey and Care for Injuries

1. Take an initial set of vital signs when the child is calm and quiet, then re-assess frequently.
2. Collect and record information regarding the incident.
3. Perform a head-to-toe exam (or toe-to-head for a young child), removing clothes as necessary; but protect the child's modesty and guard against hypothermia.
4. Recheck neurological responses, distal pulses, and capillary refill.
5. Be prepared to suction in the event of seizures and vomiting in head-injury patients. (Vomiting is especially common in children.)

6. Stabilize the head and neck in neutral alignment (you may have to place a folded towel under the child's shoulders) and apply a collar and appropriate immobilization for suspected head or cervical spine injury.
7. If there is no indication of head or cervical spine injury, place the child in the neutral or "sniffing" position.
8. Immobilize all fractures with the appropriate splinting techniques.
9. Transport all pediatric trauma patients.

Airway and Respiration Trauma can cause and be complicated by hypoxia due to blood loss, airway compromise, and neurological injury. The large size of the child's tongue in relation to the mouth and throat make airway obstruction by the tongue common. A child's airway passages are shorter and more narrow than in adults, and any pressure applied to the soft tissue of the throat during bag-valve-mask resuscitation can occlude the airway. Facial trauma can add to airway obstruction; and gastric distention from gulping air while crying inhibits chest expansion and limits oxygen intake.

Patient Assessment— Airway and Respiration

The crying child obviously has an open airway, is breathing, and has a pulse at this time. Wait until the child has calmed down before trying to get accurate vital sign values. Continue to monitor as blood, vomitus, tissue swelling, and broken teeth can obstruct the airway at any time. Expect respiratory problems at any time in any child with a head injury. Observe the patient for

☐ Use of accessory muscles (of the upper chest, clavicles, neck) to aid breathing
☐ Retraction (visible sinking) of the sternum or the muscles between the ribs with breathing
☐ Sounds of labored breathing

Patient Care—Airway and Respiration

The quiet or unconscious child or one who is struggling to breathe requires immediate airway management.

Emergency Care Steps

1 Open the airway with the appropriate

method; look, listen and feel for breathing; ventilate if necessary.

2 Listen for breath sounds in the axillary area, checking for airway obstruction sounds such as stridor, bubbling, or gurgling.

3 If you can't get control of the airway, transport immediately with spinal protection, supplemental oxygen, ventilation assistance, and suction as needed.

Note: It is important to aggressively manage the airway and ventilate with a high concentration of oxygen while protecting the cervical spine. Remember that the child's heart rate relates directly to the respiratory rate.

Circulation, Bleeding, and Shock The smaller the child, the less total blood volume he or she has. (An infant has about one soda can of blood; a preschooler has a six-pack.) Shock can develop in the small child who has a laceration to the very vascular scalp, or in the three-year old who loses as little as a cup of blood.

The child's body compensates for early shock by constricting arteries and veins and shunting blood to the central circulation. But as blood loss increases, this compensatory mechanism becomes less effective and the blood pressure begins to drop. Falling blood pressure is a late sign of shock and the child's condition is deteriorating rapidly.

**Patient Assessment—
Circulation, Bleeding, and Shock**

To assess the child's circulation and detect bleeding and signs of shock (Figure 17-6)

1 Look for obvious bleeding
2 Determine adequate circulation by observing color of skin, lips, mucus membranes, and nail beds (cool, pale, or mottled skin indicates circulation problems and shock).
3 Check capillary refill time. A refill time of more than 2 seconds indicates circulation difficulties and shock (hypothermia delays capillary refill time).
4 Assess for breathing and pulse rates that remain above the normal range, blood pressure below the normal range (see Table 17-2 for normal ranges).

Note: Symptoms of shock without external blood loss indicate internal bleeding. A child in hypovolemic shock will usually have a rapid respiratory rate.

**Patient Care—
Circulation, Bleeding, and Shock**

Emergency Care Steps

Care for bleeding and shock as in an adult.

1 Control bleeding, dress, and bandage.
2 Use an anti-shock garment where protocols allow; be aware that use of the anti-shock garment is controversial; if used, inflate the legs only—abdominal inflation will further compromise respiratory status.
3 Maintain body heat and administer a high concentration of oxygen.

Disability In the unconscious adult, we normally check for reaction to painful stimuli. In

SIGNS OF SHOCK IN A CHILD

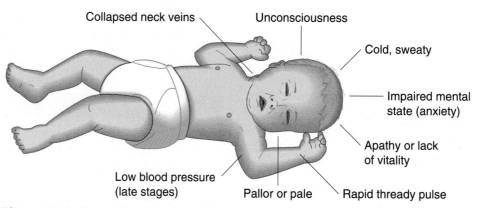

Figure 17-6 Signs of shock in a child.

the conscious adult we assess ability to identify our touch, return pressure, grip our hand, or wave a hand or foot. The same procedures can be used for pediatric patients. In children, altered consciousness levels normally result from hypoxia and head injury. If there is no improvement in mental status after providing oxygen, suspect a massive head injury or complications resulting from the injury.

Patient Assessment— Neurological Response

Use the AVPU or Glasgow Coma Scale, as described in Chapter 3, to assess neurological status. You may need help from the parent of a small child. Ask if the patient is normally this alert.

Patient Care—Neurological Response

Emergency Care Steps

If neurological response is impaired

1. Provide oxygen
2. Transport

Head and Spine Injury

Because of their larger heads, small necks, and weak cervical muscles, the possibility of cervical spine injury exists whenever a child receives a head injury. Head trauma is usually accompanied by multisystem trauma. The presence of head injury may hide injury to other body systems. Always suspect multisystem trauma and treat accordingly.

Patient Assessment— Head and Spine Injury

Signs and Symptoms

Signs and symptoms of head injury and central nervous system disfunction that will be revealed during the primary survey include

- ☐ Unconsciousness or drowsiness with the child being difficult to arouse
- ☐ Altered mental state

- ☐ Cool, pale skin with capillary refill of more than two seconds

In your secondary survey, look for

- ☐ Bulging fontanelles (infant—may indicate intracranial pressure)
- ☐ Obvious scalp, cranial, and facial injuries
- ☐ Irregular respiratory patterns
- ☐ Vomiting
- ☐ Clear or bloody fluids in the nose, ears, or both
- ☐ Problems with speech or the inability to talk
- ☐ Unequal pupils (a late sign)
- ☐ Convulsions
- ☐ Impaired neurological response and paralysis
- ☐ Any sign associated with head injury in the adult (e.g., raccoon eyes, Battle's sign)
- ☐ The child reports headache (often delayed)
- ☐ The child reports seeing double

Patient Care—Head and Spine Injury

Emergency Care Steps

1. Immobilize

   Note: Any child with trauma above the clavicles, altered level of consciousness, or neck pain should be immobilized as if there is spinal injury (see Chapter 12).

   Because of the small size of children, immobilizing them on the adult spine board may not be effective without additional padding between their body and the straps. The short spine board may be more appropriate for the smaller child, but you may still need to place rolled towels alongside the torso. Check the manufacturer's recommendations for using extrication vests for immobilizing children. Many car seats (if not damaged in the accident) will effectively immobilize the child if you stabilize the head and neck and pad the voids between the child, the sides of the seat, and beneath the torso straps (see "Transporting the Pediatric Patient" later in this chapter).

2. Assess ventilations and the need for assisted ventilation or hyperventilation if there is a head injury.

3 Transport.

Note: A stiff, sore neck occurring several days after open head injury indicates possible infection that may cause meningitis or possible unrecognized cervical injury and indicates immediate transport.

If the injury appears to be minor and the parents do not want you to transport the child, warn them that there are often hidden injuries and problems to be considered when a child has an accident. Tell them that it would be best if the child saw a physician.

Note: If the parents refuse transport, have them sign a release form and contact their physician.

Chest Injury

The bone and cartilage of a child's chest is very compliant. Blunt force trauma that would normally fracture adult ribs is, in children, transmitted to internal structures without causing fractures. Lung and heart contusions can occur without overlying fracture. Fortunately, the blood vessels are also compliant in healthy children and transection of the aorta will rarely occur. But the heart and major vessels can be compressed in tension pneumothorax. Hemothorax will also compress chest structures and cause hypovolemic shock and death without signs of external blood loss. A ruptured diaphragm will inhibit respiratory effort and allow abdominal organs to enter the chest cavity and further reduce lung capacity.

Patient Assessment—Chest Injury

Signs and Symptoms

When checking the chest, look for indications of blunt force trauma such as

- Swelling and bruising
- An asymmetrical chest wall
- Unequal chest expansion
- Respiratory distress

As indications of possible fractured ribs or flail chest, note

- Pain or tenderness
- Paradoxical motion

Patient Care—Chest Injury

Emergency Care Steps

1 Treat as for adult chest injuries (see Chapter 14).

2 If there is a penetrating injury, seal the opening immediately. Small penetrations may self seal and look minor, but it is still necessary to apply the appropriate dressing to seal the wound and monitor respiratory effort and quality. If symptoms worsen, temporarily unseal to be sure you are not turning an open pneumothorax into a tension pneumothorax (see Chapter 14).

3 Place the child on high-concentration oxygen as soon as possible and evaluate the need for ventilatory assistance.

4 Transport

Abdominal Injury

The solid organs are very vascular and in children are relatively large in relation to the size of the abdominal cavity. Their abdominal organs are also close together. Children have thin abdominal walls and weak, developing muscles that offer little protection from trauma. Blunt force trauma is readily transmitted to multiple organs causing bruising, rupture, and severe bleeding resulting in shock. Penetrating wounds, especially gunshot wounds with deflecting bullets and bullet fragments, can injure several organs at once.

Patient Assessment—Abdominal Injury

Signs and Symptoms

When you palpate the abdomen, check for

- Response to pain and tenderness on palpation
- Rigidity
- Distention

Note: Distention may be a result of the child gulping air when crying.

- Wounds indicating penetrating injury

Patient Care—Abdominal Injury

Provide care as for adult abdominal injuries, including dressing of any open abdominal wounds or eviscerations (see Chapter 14).

Pelvic and Genital Injury

Falls, straddle injury, and other blunt force and penetrating trauma can cause injury to the pelvic girdle, lower intestinal structures, and internal and external genitourinary organs.

Patient Assessment— Pelvic and Genital Injury

Signs and Symptoms

Palpate the pelvic girdle and note

- ☐ Response to pain and tenderness
- ☐ Whether the girdle is stable or unstable

Maintaining the patient's privacy as much as possible, check the genital and perineal areas for

- ☐ Bleeding, bruising, or swelling
- ☐ Loss of bowel or bladder control

Palpate the femoral pulses and note

- ☐ Femoral pulses that are weak or absent

Patient Care—Pelvic and Genital Injury

Emergency Care Steps

1. Apply a diaper type dressing or bulky padding to genital injuries or to control bleeding from the genital area.
2. Check local protocols for applying ice packs to reduce pain and swelling. (Never apply ice packs directly to the skin.)
3. Immobilize the pelvic injury by placing the child on a spine board or, if local protocols permit, in an anti-shock garment.

Injuries to the Extremities

The bones of children are more porous and flexible and tend to splinter, bend, or buckle more commonly than break. This increases the risk of soft tissue and neurovascular damage. Ligaments and tendons are strong in children and a child rarely suffers a sprain or strain.

Patient Assessment—Extremity Injury

Always remove or carefully cut away clothing from around the injury. The child may be con-

cerned about ruining clothing, but explain that his or her parents won't mind because they would want you to find out what is wrong. Examine the uninjured extremity first to show what you are going to do—to gain the child's confidence and so that pain is not the child's first experience when you touch him or her. When you examine the injured extremity, tell the child first what you will do and how long it will take. Let the child know if it will hurt, and that it is all right to cry if it does.

Signs and Symptoms

Note the following indications of an injured extremity.

- ☐ Pain—The child complains of pain in an extremity.
- ☐ Self-Splinting—A child will instinctively immobilize or self splint an injured arm or leg in a position that reduces pain. Observe the child's position and ask the child how the injury occurred before examining or moving the limb. If you suspect that an arm is broken, offer the child a toy to see which arm he or she uses to reach for it.
- ☐ Bruising or Swelling
- ☐ Puncture Wounds—Splintered bone may cause small open puncture type wounds making the injury an open fracture.
- ☐ *Severe* Pain—Severe pain may be an indication of **compartment syndrome**, an increase of pressure in the closed space of the muscle caused by bleeding and tissue swelling or a tight dressing. The forearm and leg are common sites for compartment syndrome to occur. In addition to severe pain, symptoms of include
  - Diminished pulses
  - Poor capillary refill time
  - Decreased sensation in the extremity

Since compartment syndrome can result from a tight dressing, watch for its signs and symptoms *after* the injury has been dressed and immobilized.

Patient Care—Extremity Injury

A child complaining of pain should be treated for fracture with special care and management of any injury in the area of the growth (epiphyseal) plate located at the ends of the long bones. Applying traction in this case may cause further damage to the growth plate.

Emergency Care Steps

1. If there are any open wounds, apply a dressing before splinting.
2. Gently place the fractured extremity on a splint and secure in place. Be sure to immobilize the joint above and below the fracture site. Some jurisdictions allow the EMT to straighten angulated fractures of long bones; others require splinting the extremity in the position found. Check local protocols.

Burns

Children are often the victims of burns resulting from contact with hot water, steam, cooking utensils, hot radiators, electrical cords, and the often disastrous results of playing with matches.

Patient Assessment—Burns

Assess burns thoroughly when caring for young children. Chapter 19 will deal with how to determine the type, extent, and severity of burns for infants and children as well as adults.

Be sure to assess the child for other injuries, including inhalation of smoke or fumes (see Chapter 19) and fractures or other injuries that may have caused or been caused by the burn emergency.

Patient Care—Burns

Principles of burn management for infants and children are basically the same as for adults.

Emergency Care Steps

1. Always assure that the environment is safe before you approach.
2. Stop the burning process as soon as possible by dousing with water or smothering with a blanket.
3. Remove any items that will hold the heat such as metal objects. Remove clothing and jewelry.
4. Cover the burn with the appropriate dressing (see Chapter 19) to prevent irritation of exposed nerve ends.
5. Wrap the child in a sheet and then a blanket, if necessary, to prevent hypothermia.

6. Treat for shock and provide oxygen as quickly as possible.
7. Transport is necessary to provide proper treatment for the burns and to make certain that the child did not receive any injuries due to smoke or toxic fume inhalation.
8. Carefully monitor respiratory status and give supplemental oxygen, especially if there is soot or signs of burns in the oral or nasal area.

Note: Use the "Rule of Nines" to estimate the extent of the burn, but do not let the burn direct your patient care. Assessment and management of other injuries is important and may take priority over burn care (see Chapter 19).

Trapped Extremities

Children often stick parts of their bodies into places where they become trapped. In some localities, specially trained personnel from the rescue squad or fire service are called to handle these situations, but occasionally an ambulance is dispatched and EMTs will be called upon to deal with the emergency.

Patient Assessment—Trapped Extremity

The fact that an extremity is trapped somewhere is usually obvious. Once the child is freed, conduct a patient assessment for injuries.

Patient Care—Trapped Extremity

Emergency Care Steps

1. Spend some time talking with and reassuring the child. The child may then be able to relax and slowly free him- or herself, with your help, from the entrapment. If this fails . . .
2. Use a lubricating substance to help slide the child free of the entrapment. If this fails . . .
3. Cut away the material that is holding the child. Explain what you are going to do step by step; then proceed with caution, making sure that the trapped part is well protected by padding and that the rest of the child's body is safe. Delay working if

the child becomes upset. It is important that the child not move around or struggle while you are cutting. Do not chop or tear away obstructions. Careful sawing is usually the best approach.

4 Once the child is freed, conduct a patient assessment and care for all injuries, usually minor abrasions and lacerations.

5 Transport, or advise the parents to see a physician, since an anti-tetanus injection may be required.

Transporting the Pediatric Patient

All children must be properly secured during transport whether they are injured or not. Total body immobilization is essential if head or spinal injury is suspected and if there are multiple fractures.

Federally approved car safety seats are ideal for transporting the under-4-year-old child in the ambulance. If the over-4-year-old child does not need to be transported on the backboard and cot, he or she should be strapped in a seat belt. Many car safety seats are designed so that they may be secured to either the car seat or to an ambulance cot. Car safety seats are crash tested facing front or rear. Do not buckle them sideways on the crew bench.

The infant who is in the car seat during the accident may remain and be immobilized in the seat if it is undamaged (Figure 17-7). Stabilize the head and place the appropriate size collar on the patient. If one is not available, place rolled towels on either side of the child's head and tape in place. Extend the tape over the forehead and maxilla (between upper lip and nose), across the towels, and attach behind the seat. Place additional towels on either side of the torso and, if necessary, a folded towel over the abdomen to assure that the harness will effectively secure the child in the seat. Place the towel so that you may monitor respiratory effort and heart sounds. Never use sandbags. They are too heavy and put unnecessary pressure on the chest and abdomen and inhibit respiratory effort.

The rest of the secondary survey can be performed while the child is in the car seat. Do not remove the child from the seat to check the back. This can be done at the hospital.

If the seat is damaged or the child was not in one, immobilize the child on either a long or short spine board as you would an adult, padding under the straps to effectively secure the child in place.

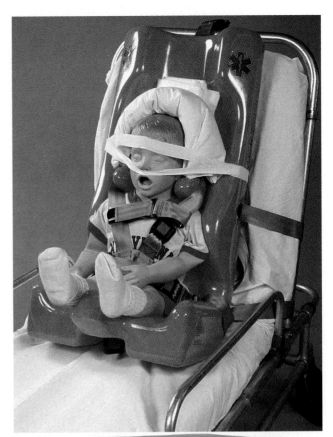

Figure 17-7 Infant immobilized in a car seat.

When transporting the child who is immobilized, make sure that the parents are seated where the child can see them so the child will not sustain further injury by struggling and moving his or her head to find mom and dad.

The Abused Child

At one time, people thought child abuse was a rare phenomenon; but it is a complex social and health problem that seems increasingly common, more often fatal, and more often the subject of media attention.

It is estimated that as many as 4 million American children are abused and neglected yearly, and as many as 5 thousand die as a result of physical abuse. In infants less than 6 months of age, physical abuse is a leading cause of death. Only SIDS and accidents are responsible for more deaths in infants and children. Emergency department physicians indicate on various surveys that 10% of ALL children under 5 years of age are physically abused. The younger the child, the higher the risk for abuse.

It is not certain how many children are victims of sexual molestation and abuse. However, it is believed that 10% of all boys and 20% of all girls are molested or abused sexually in some way before they reach the age of 18. At least 5% of all child physical abuse victims are also sexually abused.

The seeming worsening of the problem may be due to increased awareness and reporting. Even so, the problems of physical and sexual abuse are still thought to be more serious than the statistics indicate. Experts believe that for every abused child seen by the emergency or family physician, there are many more unreported cases who never receive care.

Child abusers are mothers, fathers, sisters, brothers, grandparents, stepparents, babysitters and other care givers, white-collar workers, blue-collar workers, and those who are unemployed, rich, or poor. There is no distinction as to race, creed, or ethnic background. There is no such person as a "typical" child abuser. In other words, ANYONE could be a child abuser, and the abuse can continue with increasing severity until death results.

Child abuse can take several different forms, often occurring in combination. These forms include

- Psychological (emotional) abuse
- Neglect
- Physical abuse
- Sexual abuse

A child's psychological problems and pathologic behavior are difficult to trace back to specific abuse, and this is not typically a problem directly in the realm of the EMT. What constitutes neglect is a serious legal question. As a child goes without proper food, shelter, clothing, supervision, and love, the effects surely will be seen, but seldom is this the major part of an emergency response. Physical and sexual abuse are the problems likely to be seen by EMTs.

Physical and Sexual Abuse The best way to describe the types of injuries that can be inflicted in child physical abuse cases is to say, "If it can happen to the body, it has been done by a child abuser." Physically abused children—often called "battered" children—are those who are beaten with fists, hair brushes, straps, electric cords, pool cues, razor straps, bottles, broom handles, baseball bats, pots and pans, and almost any object that can be used as a

weapon. Included in this group are children who are intentionally burned by hot water, steam, open flames, cigarettes, and other thermal sources. Battered children also include those who are severely shaken, thrown into their cribs or down steps, pushed out of windows and over railings, and even pushed from moving cars. The horror grows as we find children who are shot, stabbed, electrocuted, and suffocated.

The problems of sexual abuse range from adults exposing themselves to children, to adults touching children's genitals or having children touch their genitals (which does not result in physical injury), to sexual intercourse, oral sex, or sexual torture. Many of the cases reported are for adults exposing themselves to children. The other extreme, in which there is physical injury done to the child, also is usually reported. The cases in between, especially those in which emotional injury or minor physical injury were received, are usually not reported, and therefore are difficult to estimate.

Patient Assessment—Physical Abuse

Signs

In child physical abuse cases, you will find

☐ Slap marks, bruises, abrasions, lacerations, and incisions of all sizes and with shapes matching the item used. You may see wide welts from belts, in a looped shape from cords, or in the shape of a hand from slapping. You may find swollen limbs, split lips, black eyes, and loose or broken teeth. Often the injuries are to the back, legs, and arms. The injuries may be in various stages of healing, as evidenced by different-colored bruises.

☐ Broken bones are common and all types of fractures are possible. Many battered children have multiple fractures, often in various stages of healing, or have fracture-associated complications.

☐ Head injuries are common, with concussions and skull fractures being reported. Closed head injuries occur to many infants and small children who have been severely shaken.

☐ Abdominal injuries include ruptured spleens, livers and lungs lacerated by broken ribs, internal bleeding from blunt trauma and punching, and lacerated and avulsed genitalia.

☐ Bite marks may be present showing the teeth size and pattern of the adult mouth.

☐ Burn marks that are small and round from cigarettes; "glove" or "stocking" burn marks from dipping in hot water; burns on buttocks and legs (creases behind the knees and at the thighs are protected when flexed); and demarcation burns in the shape of an iron, stove burner, or other hot utensil are frequently found.

☐ Indications of shaking an infant include a bulging fontanelle due to increased intracranial pressure from the bleeding of torn blood vessels in the brain, unconsciousness, and typical signs and symptoms of head and brain injury.

There are times when you will treat an injured child and never think that he or she has been abused. The child relates well with the parents and there appears to be a strong bond between them. However, there are certain indications that abuse may be occurring in or outside the home, with the family feeling they must not admit to the problem. Be on the alert for

☐ Repeated responses to provide care for the same child or children in a family. Remember that in areas with many hospitals you may see the child more frequently than any one hospital.

☐ Indications of past injuries. This is why you must do a physical examination and why you must remove articles of clothing. Pay special attention to the back and buttocks of the child.

☐ Poorly healing wounds or improperly healed fractures. It is extremely rare for a child to receive a fracture, be given proper orthopedic care, and then show angulations and large "bumps" and "knots" of bone at the "healed" injury site.

☐ Indications of past burns or fresh bilateral burns. Children seldom put both hands on a hot object or touch the same hot object again (true, some do . . . this is only an indication, not proof). Some types of burns are almost always linked to child abuse, such as cigarette burns to the body and burns to the buttocks and lower extremities that result from the child being dipped in hot water.

☐ Many different types of injuries to both sides or the front and back of the body. This gains even more importance if the adults on the scene keep insisting that the child "falls a lot."

☐ Fear on the part of the child to tell you how the injury occurred. The child may seem to expect no comfort from the parents and may have little or no reaction to pain.

☐ The parent or care giver at the scene who does not wish to leave you alone with the child, tells conflicting or changing stories, overwhelms you with explanations of the cause of the injury, or faults the child may rouse your suspicions and cause you to assess the situation more carefully.

Pay attention to the adults as you treat the child.

☐ Do they have trouble controlling anger?

☐ Do you feel that at any moment there may be an emotional explosion?

☐ Do any of the adults appear to be in a deep state of depression?

☐ Are there indications of alcohol or drug abuse?

☐ Do any of the adults speak of suicide or seeking mercy for their unhappy children?

Parents or care givers who have called for help for the injured child may be reluctant to assist you with history of the injury and may even refuse transport. Take note of any parent who refuses to have their child sent to the nearest hospital or to a hospital where the child has been seen many times. This may indicate a fear of the staff remembering or seeing a record of past injuries that suggest possible abuse. (You can't transport without parental consent; however, you may be able to convince the parents the child needs to be seen by a doctor because of certain signs and symptoms that are "difficult to determine" in the field.) Be the child's advocate, but do not accuse the parent.

Patient Assessment—Sexual Abuse

Do your physical assessment and rearrange or remove clothing only as necessary to determine and treat injuries. This will help preserve evidence where possible. Examine the genitalia only if there is obvious injury or the child tells you of a recent injury. The child may be hysterical, frightened, or withdrawn and unable to give you a history of the incident. Be calm and as reassuring as possible.

Signs

- ☐ Obvious results of sexual assault, including burns or wounds to the genitalia
- ☐ Any unexplained genital injury such as bruising, lacerations, or bloody discharge from genital orifices (openings)
- ☐ Seminal fluid on their body or clothes or other discharges associated with sexually transmitted diseases
- ☐ In rare cases, the child may tell you that he or she was sexually assaulted.

Remain professional and control your emotions. Do not allow the child to become embarrassed. Do not say anything that may make the child believe that he or she is to blame for the sexual assault (many believe that they are). Tell the child that the people at the hospital will help and that he or she is not to be embarrassed.

Patient Care—Physical or Sexual Abuse

Emergency Care Steps

1. Dress and provide other appropriate care for injuries as necessary.
2. To preserve evidence of sexual abuse, if it is suspected
   - Discourage the child from going to the bathroom (for both defecation and urination).
   - Give nothing to the patient by mouth.
   - Do not have the child wash or change clothes.
3. Transport the child.

Note: You must plainly and clearly report to the medical staff any of your findings or suspicions that there has been physical or sexual abuse.

The Role of the EMT Remember that you are charged with providing emergency care for an injured child. You are not a physician trained to detect abuse, a police officer, court investigator, social worker, judge, or one-person jury.

Gather information from the parents or care giver away from the child without expression of disbelief or judgement. Talk with the child separately about how the injury occurred. As you assess the patient and provide appropriate care, control your emotions and hold back accusations. Do not indicate to the parents or other adults at the scene that you suspect child abuse. Do not ask the child if he or she has been abused. To do so when others are around could produce stress too great for the injured child to handle.

If you are suspicious about the mechanism of injury, transport the child even though the severity of injury may not warrant such action. Have the parents or care giver follow you to the hospital to keep them separate if necessary.

ALWAYS report your suspicions to the emergency department staff and in accordance with local policies. Every medical facility should take action to see if your fears are well founded. If you fear that the medical staff has not taken you seriously, then you must report your suspicions to the juvenile authorities of the local police department. This may not be a legal requirement in your state, but it is a professional obligation and you must be aware of reporting laws.

Keep accurate records of possible child abuse. State all your objective findings, but do not conclude that there is abuse. Draw a picture to indicate the size and location of all the child's injuries. Do not assume the cause of an injury (e.g., a cigarette burn). Instead, provide a detailed description of the injury site.

Maintain patient and family confidentiality. You cannot name the child or the family or give any details concerning the family to anyone other than the medical staff, the police, or your superior officer. Follow department requirements in reporting the problem.

Past responses can be checked and future responses noted in case a pattern develops to indicate possible abuse. However, even when talking to your partner, the hospital staff, the police, and your superiors, use the terms "suspicious" and "possible." Do not call someone a child abuser. If you break confidentiality, you could be sued. Keep in mind that the courts can deal harshly with those who provide patient care and then violate the confidentiality of the patient, the family, and the home. Keep in mind that rumors about abuse may, in the long run, cause mental or physical harm to your child patient.

It may be difficult, but keep in mind that the parent or care giver needs help also. Your actions, response, and concern directed toward the suspected abuser can help them recognize their problem and may encourage them to seek therapy and rehabilitation.

Infant death and child abuse are emotionally hard on EMTs. After providing basic life support, transporting the child, and doing all you can for the parents, take care of yourself. Talk with other EMTs. If your squad or service has a counselor, see this person for advice. You may think that you can handle the sorrow by yourself, but experienced EMTs know better. Unless you resolve the impact of an infant death or child abuse, the problems created will compound with others caused by the stress of being an EMT and could lead to "burn out." Contact your local Critical Incident Stress Debriefing team for assistance after incidents such as these.

CHAPTER REVIEW

KNOWALL

KEY TERMS

You may find it helpful to review the following terms.

asthma (AZ-mah)—a sensitivity reaction to allergens, to environmental, physical or emotional stress, or to respiratory infections that can cause the lower airways to obstruct.

bronchiolitis (BRONG-ke-o-LI-tis)—an airway inflammation below the level of the trachea.

compartment syndrome—an increase of pressure in the closed space of the muscle caused by bleeding and tissue swelling or a tight dressing, usually with an injury of the forearm or leg.

croup (KROOP)—a group of viral illnesses that cause inflammation of the larynx, trachea, and bronchi.

epiglottitis (epi-glo-TI-tis)—a potentially life-threatening condition most commonly caused by a bacterial infection that produces swelling of the epiglottis and partial airway obstruction.

hypothermia (HI-po-THURM-i-ah)—cooling of the body temperature, a condition that is life-threatening if extreme or prolonged.

meningitis (men-in-JI-tis)—a condition caused by either a bacterial or viral infection of the lining of the brain and spinal cord

sleep apnea (ap-NE-ah)—periods of cardiac slowdown and temporary cessation of breathing during sleep, often associated with sudden infant death syndrome.

sudden infant death syndrome (SIDS)—an unexplained sudden death of an apparently healthy infant while asleep.

SUMMARY

Assessing the Pediatric Patient

For CPR, an infant is anyone from birth to 1 year, a child is anyone from 1 to 8 years, an adult anyone over 8. In other pediatric medical and trauma situations, it may be helpful to consider children as neonates (birth to 1 month), infants (1 to 12 months), toddlers (1 to 3 years), preschool (3 to 5 years), school age (6 to 12 years), and adolescents (13 to 18 years).

The EMT can best support the parent of a child patient by being calm and reassuring, if possible involving the parent in the child's care. Remember that the child may have two parents, a single parent, or a guardian or caretaker who is a relative or unrelated.

For the steps of pediatric primary survey and pediatric basic life support, review Scan 17-1. Remember to make a CUPS status decision before doing the secondary survey.

Checking capillary refill time by squeezing an arm or leg is a quick way to determine if a child is in shock.

Take your time with the interview when the patient is a child. Talk to the parents, but also direct questions to the child. Show the child, the parents, and the bystanders that you are a concerned professional. Tell the child what you are going to do before you do it. Do not lie to the child. Tell him when he may experience pain. Apply the correct values for vital signs to infants and children (see Table 17-2). Do not use adult vital sign figures for infants and children.

When conducting a physical examination of a conscious infant or young child patient, use the toe-to-head approach. The older child is assessed by the head-to-toe approach. Take special care to look for head injuries, signs of skull fracture, cervical spine injuries, unusual breathing sounds, abdominal tenderness, and rectal bleeding. Always conduct a neurologic assessment. You may have to treat the infant as if he were an unconscious patient and depend on response to painful stimuli.

Medical Emergencies Common to Children

Do not underestimate the significance of fever, seizures, respiratory problems, diarrhea, vomiting, and abdominal pain in infants and children.

Croup usually occurs to young children, often following a cold or other respiratory infection. The patient will have a "seal bark" cough and respiratory distress. Oxygen (humidified) and transport are the major elements of care. Epiglottitis must always be considered to be a life-threatening emergency. The child will have a sudden onset of high fever and pain on swallowing (usually he will drool). The typical patient will assume a tripod position. Handle the patient gently, provide oxygen (humidified), and transport immediately. DO NOT PLACE ANYTHING IN THE CHILD'S MOUTH. Constantly monitor the child and be prepared for total airway obstruction and respiratory arrest. Bronchiolitis, asthma, and other respiratory disorders may share such symptoms as coughing, wheezing, and fever. Provide oxygen and transport. Notify the emergency department as soon as possible.

Meningitis may be indicated by high fever, lethargy, irritability, headache, stiff neck, sensitivity to light, bulging fontanelles (in an infant), pain on movement or being touched, seizures, or rash. This is a serious emergency. Transport immediately, providing a high concentration of oxygen. Be alert for seizures and ready to ventilate or provide CPR if necessary.

Remember that many children are accidental poisoning victims. Be on special alert for aspirin, acetaminophen, lead, iron, and petroleum product poisonings. Follow the instructions of your local poison control center and on-line medical command.

Sudden infant death syndrome (SIDS) victims must receive resuscitative measures. The parents will need strong emotional support. If they express feelings of guilt, tell them that SIDS occurs to thousands of apparently healthy babies each year. Even with the very best of care, these babies die. Do not be embarrassed to express your own sorrow after the physician has told them the infant is dead.

Pediatric Trauma Emergencies

Most assessment and care procedures for pediatric trauma are the same as for adults. Conduct a primary survey with special attention to airway and respiration; circulation, bleeding, and shock; and neurological assessment and make a CUPS status decision.

In cases of possible head or spine injury, chest injury, abdominal injury, pelvic or genital injury, injury to an extremity, or burn, assess as for the adult. In an infant, look for bulging fontanelles as a sign of increased intracranial pressure. When a child's extremity is trapped, help the child to relax, use lubricants, or carefully cut away the entrapping material.

Always take time to tell the child what you are going to do. When possible, allow the child to sit in a parent's lap or have the parent nearby and involved. If oxygen must be administered and the child fears the mask, allow the parent to hold the mask in front of the child's face. Transport the child in the parent's lap or, if injuries require immobilization, in a pediatric-sized carrying device, on a short spine board, or in an infant car seat. Monitor vital signs on arrival at the scene as well as during care and transport to detect changes in vital sign levels.

Always be on the alert for possible child abuse. Look for indications of injuries and behavior that may lead you to suspect physical or sexual abuse. Report all suspicions to the emergency department staff. Do a complete survey so that you will detect all obvious injuries and indications of past abuse. Remember to maintain patient and family confidentiality.

Do not hesitate to seek counseling for the sorrow or "burn out" you may experience as the result of encountering child abuse or infant death.

On the Scene

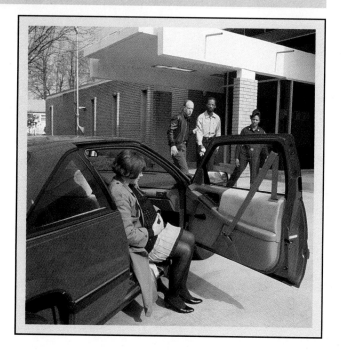

You: *I'm Joe Donaldson, and I'm a firefighter and EMT. What's your name?*

Marie: *Marie Walinsky. The baby's coming real soon.*

You: *Ok, Mrs. Walinsky. If it does, we'll be ready. Is this your first child?*

Marie: *Fourth. The last one came fast, too.*

You: *How far apart are your labor pains?*

Marie: *About two minutes.*

You: *Have you been getting checkups?*

Marie: *Yes . . . Oh, oh, a contraction . . . .*

You: *(You time the contraction and instruct Paul to help his wife with the breathing techniques they learned in Lamaze class.) One last question. Did your doctor expect any problems? A C-section, breech birth, or anything like that?*

Marie: *No, all my babies have been no problem at all. Here comes another contraction. . . .*

Thirty-three-year-old Marie Walinsky and her husband screech their car to a halt on the fire station ramp. Paul jumps out and explains to the nearest firefighter: Marie is five days overdue. Her water has broken, and her contractions are close together. She is sure the baby is going to be born before they can get to the hospital. Can the firefighters help?

Radio dispatch is instructed to respond an ambulance. Meanwhile, two firefighters help Marie to a couch. You approach and begin your evaluation.

While you have been talking with Marie, fellow firefighters have prepared your obstetric kit and arranged some screening around the couch for privacy. As you put on gloves, goggles, mask, and gown and prepare to position and drape the patient, you explain that you are going to check for crowning. When you check the vaginal area, you see the baby's head. The delivery of her baby girl does not wait for the ambulance or a trip to the hospital!

Two weeks later, the entire Walinsky family comes by the fire station to express their thanks. This is one the happiest experiences you have had as an EMT, and one that you will never forget.

Childbirth

Participating in the delivery of a baby is usually a wonderful and exciting event for the EMT. In most cases, you will be dealing with a natural event, not an emergency. In this chapter, you will learn how to help a mother deliver her baby.

Expected Outcome, Chapter 18: *You will be able to use correct terminology to describe the anatomy and physiology of pregnancy, and you will be able to assist in both normal and problem deliveries and prebirth emergencies.*

WARNING: Protect yourself from infectious diseases by using appropriate barrier devices such as a pocket face mask with one-way valve, face shield, or bag-valve mask; goggles or eye shield; and disposable gloves. Always conform to your local EMS system's infection exposure control plan.

THE ANATOMY AND PHYSIOLOGY OF CHILDBIRTH
    Pregnancy and Delivery
    Labor

NORMAL CHILDBIRTH
    The Role of the EMT
    The Normal Delivery

CHILDBIRTH COMPLICATIONS
    Complications of Delivery
    Abnormal Deliveries
    Predelivery Emergencies

Knowledge *After reading this chapter you should be able to*

1. Name and locate the anatomical structures of pregnancy. (p. 507)

2. List and describe the three stages of labor. (pp. 508-509)

3. Name the components of the sterile emergency obstetric pack and describe the uses for each item. (pp. 509-510)

4. Describe how to evaluate the mother before delivery. (pp. 510-511)

5. Define *supine hypotensive syndrome* and explain how to position the pregnant mother during transport to counteract it. (p. 511)

6. Describe how to prepare the mother, the delivery scene, and personnel prior to delivery. (pp. 511-512)

7. Describe, step by step, what the EMT should do to assist with delivery of the baby. (pp. 512, 514; Scan 18-1)

8. Explain how to assess the newborn infant. (pp. 514-515; Table 18-1)

9. Describe the care given to the infant after delivery, including airway and umbilical cord care. (pp. 515-518)

10. Describe the care given to the mother after delivery. (pp. 518-520)

11. List conditions that contribute to a high-risk pregnancy. (p. 520)

12. Explain the sequence of steps that should be followed to help a nonbreathing baby. (pp. 520-522).

13. Explain the procedure to follow when contractions are close together but delivery is prolonged. (p. 522)

14. List possible kinds of abnormal delivery and explain the assessment and care procedures for each. (pp. 522-527)

15. List possible predelivery emergencies and explain the assessment and care procedures for each. (pp. 527-532)

Skills *As an EMT you should be able to*

1. Evaluate a woman in labor and assist in the delivery of her child.

2. Provide postdelivery care for the newborn, including proper airway and umbilical cord care.

3. Provide postdelivery care for the mother, including emotional support, and provide care of the placenta.

4. Provide resuscitative measures for newborns in respiratory and cardiac arrest.

5. Provide emergency care and basic cardiac life support procedures for abnormal deliveries, including breech and premature birth.

6. Provide emergency care for predelivery emergencies, including excessive prebirth bleeding and miscarriage.

7. Record all vital information needed for the live birth or fetal death certificate.

Seldom is childbirth outside of a medical facility an emergency, except perhaps to an untrained attendant! Many people in our society presently believe that birth is meant to occur in a hospital delivery room. Although it is true that hospital care of mother and newborn does reduce the chance of problems and can correct most immediate complications, keep in mind that the vast majority of babies ever born on this planet were delivered away from any type of medical facility. This holds true today, for the majority of the world's women do not have access to modern medical facilities for the purpose of giving birth.

Birth is a natural process. The anatomy of the human female and the anatomy of the baby allow for the process to occur with few immediate problems. Nonetheless, EMTs need to know the procedures that can help mother and baby before, during, and after delivery, as well as the techniques that can be employed when complications arise.

THE ANATOMY AND PHYSIOLOGY OF CHILDBIRTH

Pregnancy and Delivery

The developing baby is called a **fetus** (FE-tus). During pregnancy, the fetus grows in its mother's **uterus** (U-ter-us), a muscular organ also called the womb (Figure 18-1). When the mother is in labor, the muscles of the uterus contract at ever-shortening intervals and push the baby through the neck of the uterus known as the **cervix** (SUR-viks). The cervix must dilate some 4 inches during labor to allow the baby's head to pass into the **vagina** (vah-JI-nah), or birth canal, so that delivery can take place.

More than just the fetus develops within the uterus during pregnancy. Attached to the wall of the uterus is a special organ called the **placenta** (plah-SEN-tah). Composed of both maternal and fetal tissues, the placenta serves as an exchange area between mother and fetus. Oxygen and foods (and drugs and alcohol) from the mother's bloodstream are carried across the placenta to the fetus. Carbon dioxide and certain other wastes cross from fetal circulation to maternal circulation. Since the placenta is an *organ of pregnancy*, it is expelled after the baby is born.

The mother's blood does *not* flow through the body of the fetus. The fetus has its own circulatory system. Blood from the fetus must be sent through the placenta and returned back into its body. This is done by way of the blood vessels contained in the **umbilical** (um-BIL-i-kal) **cord**. The umbilical cord, about 1 inch wide and 22 inches long at birth, is fully expelled with the birth of the baby and the delivery of the placenta.

While developing in the uterus, the fetus is enclosed and protected within a thin, membranous "bag of waters" known as the **amniotic** (am-ne-OT-ik) **sac**. This sac contains one to two quarts of liquid called amniotic fluid, which allows the fetus to float during development, cushions it from injury, and helps maintain a constant fetal body temperature. In the vast majority of cases, the amniotic sac breaks during labor and the fluid gushes from the birth canal. This is a normal condition of childbirth that also provides a natural lubrication to ease the infant's progress through the birth canal.

The nine months of pregnancy are divided into three three-month trimesters. During the first trimester the fetus is being formed. As the fetus remains quite small, there is little uterine growth during this period. After the third month, the uterus grows rapidly, reaching the umbilicus by the fifth month and the epigastrium (upper abdomen) by the seventh month. Other changes in a woman's body during this time include increased blood volume, increased cardiac output, and increased heart rate. The blood pressure is usually decreased slightly, and there is slowed digestion. One very important change is a

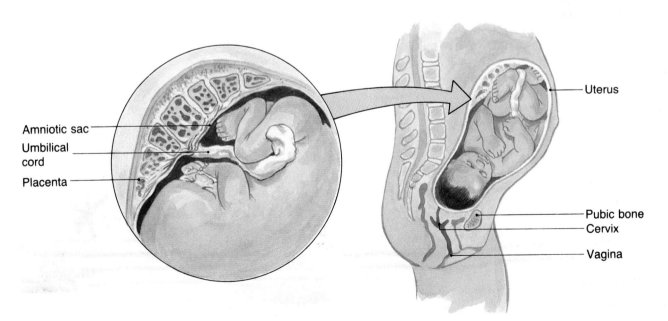

Amniotic sac

Umbilical cord

Placenta

Uterus

Pubic bone
Cervix

Vagina

Figure 18-1 The structures of pregnancy.

massive increase in vascularity (presence of blood and blood vessels) of the uterus and related structures.

Crowning occurs when the "presenting" part of the baby first bulges from the vaginal opening. The presenting part of the baby usually is the head. The normal head-first birth is called a **cephalic** (se-FAL-ik) **presentation** or *vertex* (VER-teks) *presentation*. If the buttocks or both feet of the baby deliver first, the birth is called a **breech presentation** or breech birth.

Labor

Labor is the entire process of delivery. There are three stages of labor (Figure 18-2).

- First Stage—starts with regular contractions and the thinning and gradual dilation of the cervix and ends when the cervix is fully dilated.
- Second Stage—the time from when the baby enters the birth canal until it is born.
- Third Stage—begins when the baby is born until the **afterbirth** (placenta, umbilical cord, and some tissues from the amniotic sac and the lining of the uterus) is delivered.

The first stage of labor is also called the dilation period. Picture the uterus as a long-neck bottle. In order to expel the contents, the neck of the bottle must be stretched to the size of a wide-mouth jar. Before the cervix can fully dilate, the long neck of the cervix must be shortened and thinned (this process is called effacement) to the wide-mouth-jar shape.

Sometimes, several days before the onset of actual labor, uterine muscles begin mild contractions and slight dilation occurs as the cervix begins to thin. When actual labor begins, the contractions of the uterus that occur during the first stage continue the thinning and dilation process, and the infant's head begins to move downward. The cervix gradually shortens and thins enough (wide-mouth-jar shape) to become flush with the vagina or fully open to the birth canal.

The cycle of contractions starts far apart and becomes shorter as birth approaches. Typically, these contractions range from every 30 minutes down to 3 minutes apart, or less. Labor pains may accompany the contractions.

As the fetus moves and the cervix dilates, the amniotic sac usually breaks. Normally, the

First stage: beginning of contractions to full cervical dilation

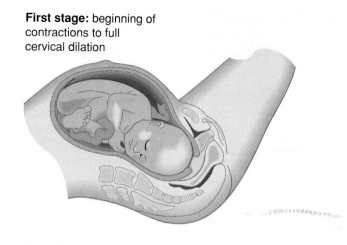

Second stage: baby enters birth canal and is born

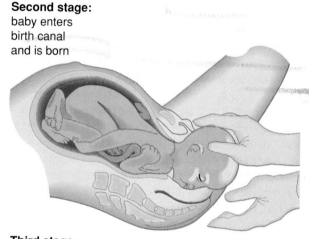

Third stage: delivery of the placenta

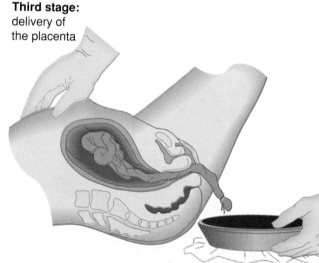

Figure 18-2 The three stages of labor.

amniotic fluid is clear. Fluid that is greenish or brownish-yellow in color may be an indication of fetal distress during labor and is called **meconium staining**. The full dilation of the cervix signals the end of the first stage of labor. Most women giving birth for the first time will remain in this first stage for an average of 16 hours. However, some women may remain in this stage for no more than 4 hours, especially if this is not the first child.

There may be a watery, bloody discharge (not bleeding) of mucus associated with the first stage of labor. Part of this initial discharge will be from a mucous plug that was in the cervix. This is usually mixed with blood and is called the "bloody show." It is not necessary to wipe it away. Watery, bloody fluids discharging from the vagina are typical for all three stages of labor.

The second stage of labor begins after the full dilation of the cervix. During this time, contractions become increasingly frequent. Labor pains may become more severe. In the second stage of labor, the cramping and abdominal pains associated with the first stage of labor still may be present, but most women report a major new discomfort, that of feeling they have to move their bowels. This is caused as the baby's body moves and places pressure on the rectum. The moment of birth is nearing and the EMT will have to decide whether to transport or to keep the mother where she is and prepare to assist with delivery.

Labor Pains The contractions of the uterus produce normal labor pains. Most women report the start of labor pains as an ache in the lower back. As labor progresses, the pain becomes most noticeable in the lower abdomen, with the intensity of pain increasing. The pains come at regular intervals, lasting from 30 seconds to one minute and occur at 2-to-3 minute intervals. When the uterus starts to contract, the pain begins. As the muscles relax, there is relief from the pain. Labor pains may start, stop for awhile, then start up again.

As an EMT you must time the following characteristics of labor pains.

- Contraction Time, or Duration—the time from the beginning of contraction to when the uterus relaxes (start to end).
- Contraction Interval, or Frequency—the time from the start of one contraction to the beginning of the next (start to start).

Some women experience **false labor**, or Braxton-Hicks contractions, complete with pain, at any time during pregnancy. The pain is caused by changes in the uterus as it adjusts in size and shape. False labor pains are usually different from true labor pains. In most cases, they are confined to the lower abdomen, with no back involvement, and do not show the regular interval pattern of true labor pains. Some women in false labor will have false labor pains that begin in the lower back.

NORMAL CHILDBIRTH

The Role of the EMT

Remember: EMTs do not deliver babies . . . mothers do! Your primary role will be one of helping the mother as she delivers her child.

Equipment and Supplies Assisting the mother and providing care is much easier if a few basic items are kept as part of the ambulance supplies. You will need a sterile obstetric kit that contains the items required for preparation of the mother, delivery, and initial care of the newborn (Figure 18-3). This kit should include

- Several pairs of sterile surgical gloves to protect from infection
- 5 towels or sheets for draping the mother
- 1 dozen 4 x 4 gauze pads (sponges) for wiping and drying the baby
- 1 rubber-bulb syringe (3 oz.) to suction the baby's mouth and nostrils
- 3 cord clamps or hemostats to clamp the umbilical cord (plus extra clamps in case of a multiple birth)
- Umbilical cord tape to tie the cord
- 1 pair of surgical scissors to cut the cord
- 1 baby blanket to wrap the baby and keep it warm
- Several individually wrapped sanitary napkins to absorb blood and other fluids

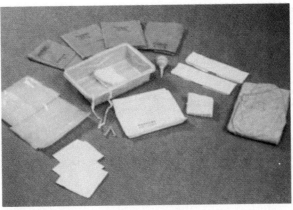

Figure 18-3 Contents of a sterile disposable obstetric kit.

In addition, you will find use for a stainless steel or plastic basin to catch the placenta, two large plastic bags for disposal of wastes and for packaging of the placenta, blood, and tissues to deliver with the mother to the hospital, as well as disposable masks, paper gowns, caps, and eye shields for self protection.

Occasionally, EMTs assist in the delivery of a baby without using a sterile delivery pack. Remember that most babies have been born without such packs. A few simple supplies are used to assist the mother.

- Clean sheets and towels to drape the mother and wrap the newborn
- Heavy flat twine or new shoelaces to tie the cord (do not use thread, wire, or light string since these may cut through the cord)
- A towel or plastic bag to wrap the placenta after its delivery
- Clean, unused rubber gloves and goggles. The lack of gloves and goggles will mean possible exposure to infectious diseases.

The Normal Delivery

Evaluating the Mother A simple series of questions, an examination for crowning, and determination of vital signs will allow you to make the decision for transport. However, do not let the "urgency" of this decision upset the mother. Your patient needs emotional support at this time. Your calm, professional actions will help her feel more at ease and assure her that the required care will be provided for both her and the unborn child.

To begin to evaluate the mother

1. *Ask her name and age and expected due date.*
2. *Ask if this is her first pregnancy.* The average time of labor for a woman having her first baby is about 16 to 17 hours. The time in labor is considerably shorter for each subsequent birth.
3. *Ask her how long she has been having labor pains, how often she is having pains, and if her "bag of waters" has broken.* Ask "Have you had any bleeding or bloody show?" At this point, with a woman having her first delivery, you may think that you can make a decision about transport. However, you should continue with the evaluation procedure. Also, you should begin to time the frequency and length of the contractions.

4. *Ask her if she is straining or if she feels as though she needs to move her bowels.* If she says yes, this usually means that the baby has moved into the birth canal and is pressing the vaginal wall against the rectum. Birth will probably occur very soon. The mother may tell you that she can feel the baby trying to move out through her vaginal opening. In such cases, birth is probably very near.
5. *Examine the mother for crowning* (Figure 18-4). This is a visual inspection to see if there is bulging at the vaginal opening or if the presenting part of the baby is visible. If part of the baby's head or presenting part is visible with each contraction, then birth is imminent.
6. *Feel for uterine contractions.* You may have to delay this procedure until the patient tells you she is having labor pains. Tell her what you are going to do, then, place the palm of your gloved hand on her abdomen, above the navel. This can be done over the top of the patient's clothing. You should be able to feel her uterus and its contraction. All contractions should be timed. Keep track of the duration and frequency of the contractions. The uterus and the tissues between this organ and the skin will feel more rigid as the delivery of the baby nears.
7. *Take vital signs at this time* if you do not have a partner to do it. Alert the medical facility staff if the mother's vital signs are abnormal.

Examining for crowning may be embarrassing to the mother, the father, and any required bystanders. For this reason, it is important that you fully explain what you are doing and why.

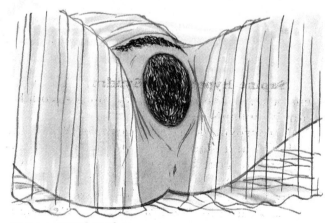

Figure 18-4 Crowning of the infant's head occurs in the second stage of labor.

Be certain that you protect the mother from the stares of bystanders. In a polite but firm manner, ask everyone who does not belong at the scene to leave. Carefully help the patient remove enough clothing to allow you an unobstructed view of the **vulva** (VUL-vah), or external genitalia.

Remember: A professional appearance coupled with a professional approach instills confidence in patients and bystanders alike.

If this is the woman's first delivery, she is not straining, and there is no crowning, there is little reason why she cannot be transported to a medical facility for delivery. On the other hand, if this is not her first delivery, and she is straining, crying out, and complaining about having to go to the bathroom, birth will probably occur too soon for transport. If the mother is having labor pains from contractions about 2 minutes apart, birth is very near. If the baby has crowned, do not transport until after the baby has been born.

You may find a patient who is afraid of transport because she believes that birth will occur along the way. Assure her that you believe there is enough time before delivery. Let her know that you are trained to assist with the delivery and that the ambulance is well equipped to handle her needs and care for the newborn should she deliver en route. If crowning occurs during transport, stop the ambulance and prepare for delivery.

If your evaluation of the patient leads you to believe that birth is too near at hand for transport, you and your partner should prepare to assist the mother with delivery. Remember, as part of the preparation, the patient will need emotional support.

Remember: Do not allow the mother to go to the bathroom, even though she says that she has to move her bowels. Birth is probably only a few minutes away. Do not allow the mother to hold her legs together or use any other "folkway" method to attempt to delay the delivery.

Supine Hypotensive Syndrome Near the time of birth, the weight of the uterus, coupled with the infant's weight, placenta, and amniotic fluid, approximates 20-24 pounds. When the mother is in a supine position, this heavy mass will tend to compress the inferior vena cava, reducing venous return to the heart and reducing cardiac output. This causes dizziness (vertigo) and a drop in blood pressure, a set of signs and symptoms known as **supine hypotensive syndrome**. The body begins to compensate when it senses the drop in blood pressure by contracting the uterine arteries and redirecting blood to the major organs. This can affect the fetus severely.

The drop in blood pressure signals shock, but the method of treating for shock by elevating the legs is not effective in this instance because it does not relieve pressure on the vena cava. To counteract or avoid the possible drop in blood pressure, all third trimester patients should be transported on their left side (left lateral recumbent position). A pillow or rolled blanket should be placed behind the back to maintain proper positioning.

A *severe* drop in blood pressure should alert the EMT to the possibility of internal hemorrhage (see "Ruptured Uterus" later in this chapter).

Preparing the Mother for Delivery When your evaluation leads you to believe birth is imminent, you must immediately prepare the mother for delivery. To do so, you should

1. *Control the scene* so that the mother will have privacy (her coach may remain). If you are not in a private room and transfer to the ambulance is not practical (crowning is present), ask bystanders to leave.
2. *In addition to surgical gloves, you and your partner should put on gowns, caps, face masks, and eye protection* since there is a high probability of splashing blood during delivery.
3. *Place the mother on a bed, sturdy table, or the ambulance stretcher.* Prop her on her left side with pillows supporting her back. Her left leg will be extended and slightly flexed. Her right leg will be flexed to keep her stabilized on her left side. This position keeps uterine weight off the vena cava. You will need about 2 feet of work space below the woman's buttocks to place and initially care for the newborn. Having the patient positioned on the stretcher may speed transport if complications arise.

Note: Do not delay positioning the patient. If time permits, and the mother is to be placed on a table or other hard surface, lay down a folded blanket, towels, or even newspapers with a sheet over them to make a cushion. If delivery is to be on a bed and time permits, firm up the mattress with plywood, table leaves, or other such rigid materials that can be placed between the mattress and the springs. Such firmness will tend to keep blood and other fluids from pooling in the work area. A rubber sheet, plastic bag, or newspapers placed under the sheet will help prevent the mattress from becoming soaked. However, do not leave the patient to find these materials.

4. *Remove any of the patient's clothing or underclothing that obstructs your view of the vaginal opening.* Replace your initial non-sterile surgical gloves with sterile gloves from the obstetric kit. Use sterile sheets or sterile towels to cover the mother as shown in Figure 18-5. Clean sheets, clean cloths, towels, or materials such as tablecloths can be used if you do not have an obstetric kit.

5. *Position your assistant*—your partner, the father, or someone the mother agrees to have assist you at the mother's head. This person should stay alert to help turn the mother's head should she vomit. As well, this person should provide emotional support to the mother, soothing and encouraging her.

6. *Position the obstetric pack* on a table or chair. All items must be within easy reach.

Note: If delivery is to take place in an automo-

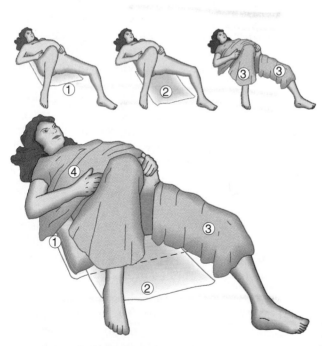

PLACEMENT OF SHEETS OR TOWELS
① One under the buttocks
② One under the vaginal opening
③ One over each thigh
④ One over the abdomen

Figure 18-5 Preparing the mother for delivery.

bile, position the mother flat on the seat. Arrange her legs so that she has one foot resting on the seat and the other foot resting on the floor.

Delivering the Baby Position yourself in such a way that you have a constant view of the vaginal opening. Be prepared for the baby to come at any moment.

Be prepared for the patient to experience discomfort. Delivering a child is a natural process, but it may be accompanied by pain. Your patient may also have intense feelings of nausea. If this is her first child, she may be very frightened. All these factors may cause your patient to be uncooperative at times. You must remember that the patient is in pain and she may feel ill. She will need emotional support.

During delivery, talk to the mother. Encourage her to relax between contractions. Continue to time her contractions from the beginning of one contraction to the beginning of the next. Encourage her not to strain unless she feels she must. Remind her that her feeling of a pending bowel movement is usually just pressure caused by the baby moving into her birth canal. Encourage her to breathe deeply through her mouth. She may feel better if she pants, although she should be discouraged from breathing rapidly and deeply enough to bring on hyperventilation. If her "bag of waters" breaks, remind her that this is normal.

Note: Unless there are signs of complications, consider the delivery to be normal if there is a cephalic presentation. Observe any unusual color in the amniotic fluid.

The steps for assisting the mother with a normal delivery are

1. *Continue to keep someone at the mother's head* to provide support, monitor vital signs, and be alert for vomiting. If no one is on hand to help, be alert for vomiting and check vital signs between contractions.

2. *Position your gloved hands at the mother's vaginal opening* when the baby's head starts to appear. *Do not* touch her skin.

3. *Support the baby's head.* Place one hand below the baby's head as it is delivered. Spread your fingers evenly around the baby's head (see Scan 18-1), remembering that the skull contains "soft spots" or fontanelles. Support the baby's head, but avoid pressure to these soft areas at the top and sides of the skull. A slight, well-distrib-

Normal Delivery

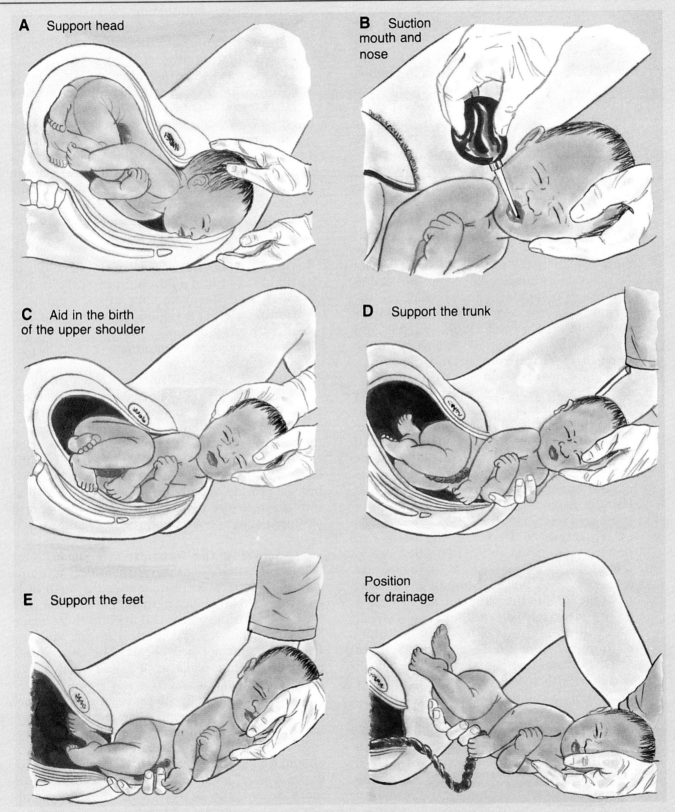

A Support head

B Suction mouth and nose

C Aid in the birth of the upper shoulder

D Support the trunk

E Support the feet

Position for drainage

Note: Assist the mother by supporting the baby throughout the birth process.

uted pressure may help prevent an explosive delivery. Keeping one hand on the baby's head and using the other hand to support the tissue between the mother's vagina and anus can help prevent tearing of this tissue during delivery of the head. DO NOT PULL ON THE BABY!

4. *Once the head delivers, check to see if the umbilical cord is wrapped around the baby's neck.* Tell the mother not to push while you check. If she can "pant," or take short quick breaths for just a moment, it may help relieve the urge to push while you check, then gently loosen the cord if necessary. Even though the umbilical cord is very tough, rough handling may cause it to tear. Try to place two fingers under the cord at the back of the baby's neck. Bring the cord forward, over the baby's upper shoulder and head. If you cannot loosen or slip the cord over the baby's head, the baby cannot be delivered. Immediately clamp the cord in two places using the clamps provided in the obstetric kit. Be very careful not to injure the baby. With extreme care, cut the cord between the two clamps. Gently unwrap the ends of the cord from around the baby's neck, and then proceed with the delivery.

5. *If the amniotic sac has not broken by the time the baby's head is delivered, use your finger to puncture the membrane.* Pull the membranes away from the baby's mouth and nose. The amniotic fluid should be clear. Meconium-stained amniotic fluid is caused by fetal feces released during labor, usually because of medical conditions of the mother or fetal stress. If the meconium is aspirated by the fetus, the baby can develop pneumonia or other infections.

6. *Check the baby's airway.* Most babies are born face down and then rotate to the right or left. Support the baby's head so that it does not touch the mother's anal area. When the entire head of the baby is visible, continue to support the head with one hand and, with the other hand, wipe the mouth and nose with sterile 4 x 4s. Use the rubber bulb syringe to suction the baby's mouth, then the nose.

Compress the syringe BEFORE placing it in the baby's mouth. Suction the mouth first, then the nostrils. Carefully insert the tip of the syringe about 1 to 1½ inches into the baby's mouth and release the bulb to allow fluids to be drawn into the syringe. Control the release with your fingers. With-

draw the tip and discharge the syringe's contents onto a towel. Repeat this procedure two or three times in the baby's mouth and once or twice in each nostril. The tip of the syringe should not be inserted more than ½ inch into the baby's nostril.

7. *Help deliver the shoulders.* The upper shoulder (usually with some delay) will deliver next, followed quickly by the lower shoulder. You must support the baby throughout this entire process. Gently guide the baby's head downward, to assist the mother in delivering the baby's upper shoulder. After the upper shoulder has delivered, if the lower shoulder is slow to deliver, assist the mother by gently guiding the baby's head upward.

8. *Support the baby throughout the entire birth process.* Once the feet are delivered, lay the baby on its side with its head slightly lower than its body. This is done to allow blood, fluids, and mucus to drain from the mouth and nose. Keep the baby at the same level as the mother's vagina until the umbilical cord stops pulsating

9. *Note the exact time of birth.*

Cautions: Babies are born with a protective coating called **vernix** (VER-nix) that makes them slippery. Make certain that you provide proper support. *Do not* attempt to clean off the protective vernix, although the baby should be dried off and wrapped to maintain warmth. Some deliveries are explosive. *Do not* squeeze the baby, but do provide adequate support. You can prevent an explosive delivery by using one hand to maintain slight pressure on the baby's head.

Assessing the Newborn The *vigor* of an infant should be assessed at 1 and 5 minutes after it is born. If you arrive after the birth, it is still your responsibility to make the assessments based on your first observations and those made 5 minutes later. Care for the infant and the mother should not be delayed. The assessment is meant to take place while these other activities are being performed.

Your system may call for a general or a specific evaluation protocol. A general evaluation usually calls for noting ease of respiration, crying, movement, and skin color. A newborn should be breathing easily, crying (vigorous crying is a good sign), moving its extremities (the more active, the better), and show blue coloration at the hands and feet only. Five minutes later, these signs should still be apparent, with breathing becoming more relaxed. The blue coloration may or may not disappear, but it should not spread to other parts of the body.

A specific evaluation usually employs the *Apgar scoring method* (developed by Virginia Apgar). This system has five scoring categories based on signs (Table 18-1). They are

1. Heart Rate—as determined with a stethoscope over the heart. Count for 30 seconds and multiply by 2. Some newborns can have a normal heart rate as high as 180 beats per minute. This is difficult to count. You are trying to determine if the heart rate is above or below 100 beats per minute. If the rate is below 100, you may be required to determine if it is below 80 beats per minute.
2. Respiration—a visual observation of the effort put forth by the baby as it breathes and cries
3. Muscle Tone—a visual observation to note if the newborn is limp, showing some flexion of the extremities, or is active by moving its limbs
4. Irritability—as determined by flicking the infant on the sole of its foot. Is there no response, some motion and crying, or vigorous motion and crying?
5. Skin Color—noting paleness, bluishness, or typical newborn color

Each sign is scored from 0 to 2 and a total is provided by adding the scores. The total score can range from 0 to 10. The higher the score, the more vigorous the infant. Most will score 7 to 9 at the first evaluation and 8 to 10 for the second. The signs are to be evaluated at 1 minute and 5 minutes following birth. Any baby scoring 7 or less after 5 minutes will need to be reassessed at 10 minutes.

A total Apgar score from 0 to 3 indicates severe distress. Basic life support measures may have to be initiated. Moderate distress is represented by scores from 4 to 6, and mild to no distress is noted by scores from 7 to 10.

To help remember the Apgar scale, many people use the mnemonic APGAR, where A = appearance (skin color), P = pulse (heart rate), G = grimace (irritability), A = activity (muscle tone), and R = respiration.

Caring for the Newborn Even with a normal delivery, each step in the care of the baby is essential for its survival. To care for the newborn, you should first place the baby on the bed or padded table surface, keeping the baby close to the level of the mother's vagina so that the infant's blood does not transfuse back into the placenta. *Do not* place the infant on the mother's abdomen at this time (not until the cord is clamped and cut—see below).

Caution: Keep the baby on its side, with the head positioned slightly lower than its body. This will help provide drainage from the nose and mouth.

Follow these steps for initial care of the newborn.

1. *Clear the baby's airway.* Use a sterile gauze pad to clear mucus and blood from around the baby's nose and mouth. (Figure 18-6).
2. *Keep the baby on its side* with the head

TABLE 18-1 The APGAR Scoring Method

Sign	0	1	2	Score 1 min	Score 5 min
Heart rate	Absent	Below 100	Over 100		
Respiration (effort)	Absent	Slow and irregular	Normal; crying		
Muscle tone	Limp	Some flexion— extremities	Active; good motion in extremities		
Irritability	No response	Crying; some motion; grimace	Crying; vigorous; cough; sneeze		
Skin color	Bluish or paleness	Pink or typical newborn color; hands and feet are blue	Pink or typical newborn color; entire body		
			TOTAL SCORE		

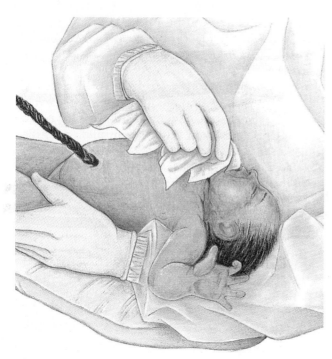

Figure 18-6 Use a sterile pad or clean handkerchief to clean blood and mucus from around the baby's mouth and nose.

slightly lower than the body and again suction the mouth, then the nose with a rubber bulb syringe. If necessary, you can cradle the baby in your arms. However, it is best to keep the baby on the cot or table surface (Figure 18-7).

Note: When the nostrils are suctioned, the baby may gasp or begin breathing and aspirate any meconium, blood, fluids, or mucus from its mouth into its lungs. That is why it is imperative to suction the mouth before the nostrils.

3. *Establish that the baby is breathing.* Usually the baby will be breathing on its own by the time you clear the airway. A newborn should begin breathing within 30 seconds. If it is not, then you must "encourage" the baby to breathe (Figure 18-8). Usually, a gentle but rigorous rubbing of the baby's back will promote spontaneous respiration. Should this method fail, snap one of your index fingers against the sole of the baby's foot. Do not hold the baby up by its feet and slap its bottom! Care of a nonbreathing

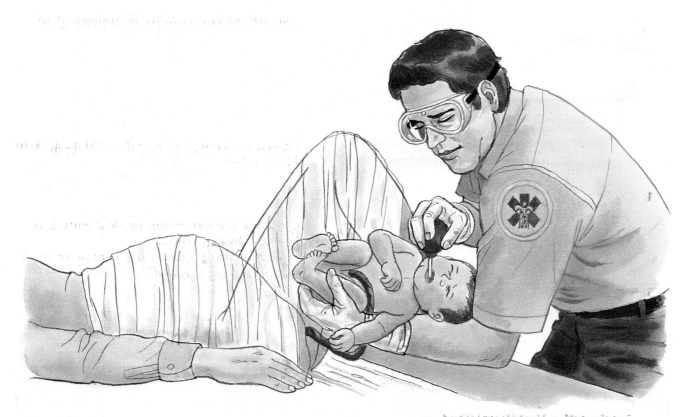

Figure 18-7 Suctioning the mouth of the newborn is accomplished by squeezing the bulb, then inserting the tip into the infant's mouth. The bulb is released to suction, then the tip is removed from the mouth and the bulb is squeezed to remove its contents.

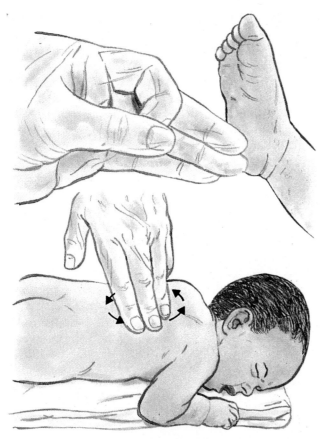

Figure 18-8 It may be necessary to encourage the newborn to breathe.

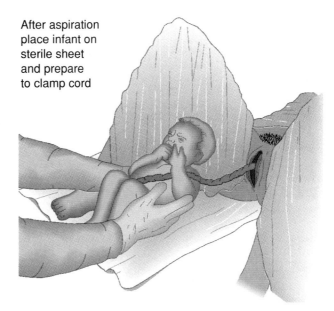

After aspiration place infant on sterile sheet and prepare to clamp cord

Figure 18-9 Placing the infant before clamping the umbilical cord.

infant will be covered later in this chapter. Do not become alarmed if the hands and feet of a breathing newborn appear slightly blue. It is not uncommon for this blue color to remain for the first few minutes. Check the difference in color at the first and second Apgar score reading.

4. *Keep the infant warm.* Dry off the baby and wrap it in a baby blanket or infant swaddler, clean towel, or sheet prior to clamping the cord (Figure 18-9). Keep the top of the baby's head covered to help reduce heat loss. Keep the ambulance warm.

5. *Prepare to clamp and cut the umbilical cord.* (See below.)

Do not wash the infant. Sometimes the mother may request you to do so, but it is best to leave the protective vernix coating on the infant until it reaches the medical facility.

Cutting the Umbilical Cord In a normal birth, the infant must be breathing on its own before you clamp and cut the cord. Before clamping and cutting the cord, palpate the cord with your fingers to make sure it is no longer pulsating. The general procedure for umbilical cord care is as follows.

1. *Use the sterile clamps or umbilical tape* found in the obstetric kit. If you do not have a kit, then use clean shoelaces. Use extreme care with any tying done to the cord, forming the knot slowly to avoid cutting the cord. Ties should be made using a square knot (right over left, then left over right).

2. *Apply one clamp or tie to the cord* about 8 to 10 inches from the baby. This leaves enough cord for intravenous lines to be used by paramedics or the staff at the hospital, if they are needed.

3. *Place a second clamp or tie* about 2 to 3 inches closer to the baby.

4. *Cut the cord between the clamps or knots using sterile surgical scissors* (Figure 18-10). Use caution and protect your eyes when cutting the cord as a spurt of blood is very common. *Never* untie or unclamp a cord once it is cut. The placental end of the cord should be placed on the drape over the mother's legs to avoid contact with expelled blood, feces, and fluids. Examine the fetal end of the cord for bleeding. *Do not* attempt to adjust the clamp or retie the knot. Should bleeding continue, apply another tie or clamp as close to the original as possible.

5. *Be careful when moving the baby* so that no

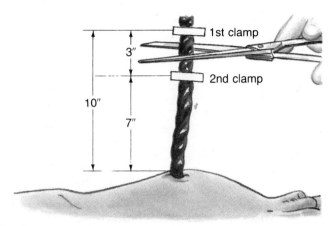

Figure 18-10 A newborn is separated from its mother by cutting the umbilical cord.

trauma is brought to the clamped cord. If the cord does not remain closed off completely, the baby may bleed to death from seemingly little blood loss. In most cases, the cord vessels will collapse and seal themselves.

Warning: *Do not tie, clamp, or cut the cord of a baby who is not breathing on its own, unless you have to do so to remove the cord from around the baby's neck during birth, or unless you have to perform CPR on the infant (see "The Nonbreathing Baby" later in this chapter). Do not cut or clamp a cord that is still pulsating.*

Note: Some EMS systems recommend that umbilical tape be used to tie the baby's clamped cord after it is cut. Tying is done with the obstetric kit's umbilical tape placed about one inch from the infant's body. The cord is slowly compressed with the tape and a square knot is tied. Both the tape and the clamp are left in place. Your instructor will tell you if this is the policy for your area.

If you are assisting at a birth when off duty, you will probably be able to find all the items you need to tie and cut the cord. If no clamps or tying devices are on hand, you may delay clamping and tying the cord if the infant will receive this care within 30 minutes. If you tie the cord and believe it will be some time before transport and transfer, you can soak scissors in alcohol for several minutes and use them to cut the cord. If the baby is still attached to the placenta when the organ is delivered, wrap the placenta in a towel and transport infant and placenta as a unit. The placenta should be placed at the same level as the baby, or slightly higher. Careful monitoring of the baby must be maintained.

Recording the Birth If adhesive tape is available, double face it (put the sticky sides together). Write the mother's last name and the time of delivery on a piece of the tape and loosely secure this tape around the baby's wrist. *Do not allow the adhesive to come into contact with the baby's skin.* Your partner should record the exact time of birth in accordance with local policy. Usually, this is done on a record of live birth. Any evaluation forms should be completed by this time.

It is critical that the baby be kept warm. Wrap the newborn in an infant swaddler and a warmed blanket or towel and let the mother hold the infant on her abdomen (Figure 18-11). Bubble wrap can also be used. It provides padded protection, warmth (pre-warm it), and allows visual monitoring of the infant. Be sure to cover the infant's head (but not the face). During the delivery of the placenta, have your partner hold the baby unless the mother insists otherwise.

Caring for the Mother Care for the mother includes helping her deliver the placenta, controlling vaginal bleeding, and making her as comfortable as possible.

- **Delivering the Placenta** The third stage of labor is the delivery of the placenta with its umbilical cord section, membranes of the amniotic sac, and some of the lining tissues of the uterus. (All of these together are known as the afterbirth.) Placental delivery begins with a brief return of the labor pains that stopped when the baby was born. You will notice a lengthening of the cord which indicates the placenta has separated from the uterus. In most cases, the placenta will be expelled within a few minutes after the

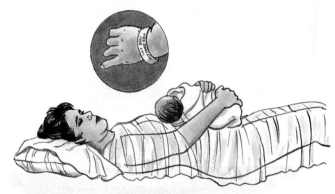

Figure 18-11 Wrap the baby and place it on the mother's abdomen.

baby is born. Although the process may take 30 minutes or longer, avoid the urge to put pressure on the abdomen over the uterus to hasten the delivery of the placenta. If mother and baby are doing well and there are no respiratory problems or significant uncontrolled bleeding, transportation to the hospital can be delayed up to 20 minutes while awaiting delivery of the placenta.

Save all afterbirth tissues (Figure 18-12). The attending physician will want to examine the placenta and other tissues for completeness since any afterbirth tissues remaining in the uterus pose a serious threat of infection and prolonged bleeding to the mother. Try to catch the afterbirth in a container. Place the container in a plastic bag, or wrap it in a towel, paper, or plastic. If no container is available, catch the afterbirth in a towel, paper, or a plastic bag. Label this material "placenta" and include the name of the mother and the time the tissues were expelled.

Remember: If the placenta does not deliver within 20 minutes of the baby's birth, transport the mother and baby to a medical facility without delay.

Note: Some EMS systems recommend transport without waiting for delivery of the placenta. There may be a condition in which the placenta does not separate from the uterine wall and it is important for mother and baby to get to the hospital. You can always stop the ambulance to deliver the placenta if it crowns en route.

- **Controlling Vaginal Bleeding After Birth** Delivery of the placenta is ALWAYS accom-

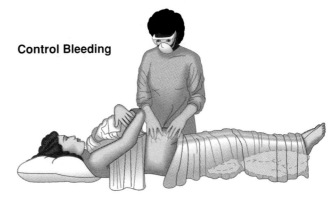

Control Bleeding

Figure 18-13 After delivery of the placenta, you will have to control vaginal bleeding.

panied by some uterine bleeding discharging through the vagina. Although the blood loss is usually around ½ pint, it may be profuse. To control vaginal bleeding after delivery of the baby and placenta (Figure 18-13), you should

1. Place a sanitary napkin over the mother's vaginal opening. Do not place anything in the vagina.
2. Have the mother lower her legs and keep them together. Tell her that she does not have to "squeeze" her legs together. Elevate her feet.
3. Massaging the uterus will help it contract. This will help control bleeding. Feel the mother's abdomen until you note a "grapefruit-sized" object. This is her uterus. Rub this area lightly with a circular motion. It should contract and become firm, and bleeding should diminish.
4. The mother may want to nurse the baby. This will aid in the contraction of the uterus. Check the baby's mouth first with your gloved finger to see if the palate (roof of the mouth) is complete. A cleft or split palate opens into the nasal cavity and will not allow the baby to swallow normally. Some pediatricians recommend the baby *not* nurse until a doctor has examined it.

The skin between the vulva and the anus is known as the **perineum** (per-i-NE-um). A slight tearing of tissue can occur in the perineum at the vaginal opening during the birth process. The mother may feel the discomfort from this torn tissue. Let her

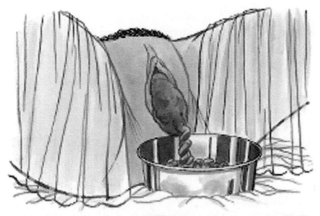

Figure 18-12 The placenta must be collected and transported with the mother and baby.

know that this is normal and that the problem will be quickly cared for at the medical facility. Treat the torn perineum as a wound. Dress by applying a sanitary napkin and applying some pressure.

- **Providing Comfort to the Mother** Keep contact with the mother throughout the entire birth process and after she has delivered. Your care for the mother does not end when you have completed your duties with the placenta and vaginal bleeding. Frequently take her vital signs. Be aware that she has just undergone a tremendous emotional experience and small acts of kindness will be appreciated and remembered. Childbirth is a rigorous task, and a woman is physically exhausted at the conclusion of delivery. Wiping her face and hands with a damp washcloth and then drying them with a towel will do wonders to refresh her and prepare her for the trip to the hospital. Replacement of blood-soaked sheets and blankets will make that trip more comfortable. Make sure that both she and the baby are warm.

    When delivery occurs at home, ask a member of the family or a trusted neighbor to help you clean up. You should clean up whatever disorder EMS care has caused in the house; however, you should not delay transport in order to complete these activities. In some areas, local protocol may have you return to the house after transport in order to complete the clean-up process. If you do, you will have to be accompanied by a member of the family.

    Remember: Birth is an exciting and joyous event. Talking to the mother and paying attention to her new baby are part of total patient care. A good rule to follow is to treat your patient as you would wish a member of your family to be treated.

CHILDBIRTH COMPLICATIONS

Complications of Delivery

Although most babies are born without difficulty, complications may occur during and after delivery. We have already considered three such complications: the cord around the neck, an unbroken amniotic sac, and infants who need encouragement to breathe. These problems can be handled by simple procedures. However, there are other complications that can threaten the life of both mother and newborn.

Conditions of High-Risk Pregnancy Risk of complications with delivery and immediately following the birth increases when the expectant mother

- Is a teenager
- Is over age 35
- Has first pregnancy
- Has had more than five pregnancies
- Has hypotension or hypertension (low or high blood pressure)
- Has signs or symptoms of toxemia (see "Pre-eclampsia and Eclampsia," later in this chapter)
- Has diabetes
- Has predelivery bleeding
- Has premature rupture of the membranes
- Has an infection or a communicable or sexually transmitted disease
- Is a substance abuser (drugs or alcohol)
- Is taking certain medications (lithium carbonate, magnesium, reserpine)
- Is involved in a major collision, fall, or abuse

A proper patient interview may be your only way of obtaining any of the above information. Take vital signs, including blood pressure, as you would for any medical patient.

Note: Certain infectious diseases of the mother's genitalia (e.g., genital herpes) may pose a serious risk to the baby while it is being born. If the woman reports that she has an infection, or you observe lesions on her vulva, call the emergency department physician for instructions. Remember, wear full protective clothing including gloves, mask, gown, cap, and eye protection.

The Nonbreathing Baby Remember that a newborn should begin breathing *within 30 seconds* after delivery.

**Patient Assessment—
The Nonbreathing Baby**

If the baby does not begin to breathe within the time it takes to place it on its side in a head-low position and suction the mouth and nose, intervention is needed.

Patient Care—The Nonbreathing Baby

Emergency Care Steps

Efforts to start the baby breathing should happen in this order.

1. *Gently but vigorously rub the infant's back.*
2. *If this fails, snap your fingers against the soles of the baby's feet as a stimulus to breathe.*
3. *If both efforts fail, establish an open airway, and suction as explained above.*
4. *If the infant does not start to breathe on its own, provide two <u>gentle</u> breaths with a pediatric BVM or mouth-to-mask that are enough to make the chest rise (Figure 18-14)*
5. *If there is a brachial pulse, but no breathing, begin pulmonary resuscitation immediately.* Protection from contact with the mother's blood and body fluids and the newborn's body fluids may be accomplished by using the mask from a pediatric bag-valve-mask device or a pediatric pocket face mask. Review and practice the use of a pocket face mask described in Chapter 6. Do not attempt to use a pocket face mask or pediatric bag-valve-mask unless you have been trained in these specialized skills.

   Rescue breathing efforts may initiate spontaneous breathing, but the infant still may be struggling to breathe. When this happens, you should provide a gentle breath each time the infant attempts to breathe in.
6. *If there is no brachial pulse for the non-breathing newborn, begin CPR immediately in accordance with American Heart Association guidelines.* Current recommendations call for the cord to be clamped and cut when a newborn requires CPR. The American Heart Association has established the following CPR guidelines for the newborn.
   - At the rate of 120 compressions/minute delivered midsternum with 2 thumbs, fingers supporting the back
   - Compress ½ to ¾ inch
   - 3 compressions: 1 adequate breath
7. *Transport the mother and baby to the hospital while you continue resuscitative efforts* until spontaneous heart and lung action begin, or until care is transferred to the staff of the emergency department. Extreme care must be taken when moving the mother and baby. Remember, the mother has yet to deliver the placenta, and she still carries a portion of the clamped umbilical cord.

   Moving the mother while providing CPR for the infant is difficult, if not impossible, for two rescuers. If police or additional EMS response can be achieved quickly (5 minutes or less), you may radio for help. When additional professional help is not on hand, or delay is not wise (which it seldom is when performing CPR), use bystanders to help with the move.
8. *If the infant begins spontaneous normal breathing, provide oxygen.* There is a danger in giving too much oxygen to a newborn baby, but if the time from birth to transfer at the medical facility is short (around 20 minutes or less), the benefits outweigh the dangers.

Do not blow a stream of oxygen directly into the baby's face. Often this causes an infant to hold its breath. Also, the rich oxygen supply can cause serious medical problems in the newborn if prolonged. (This is rarely seen in the prehospital setting—see Chapter 6.)

Make a tent above the infant's head (aluminum foil can be used to form the tent) and allow the oxygen to enter the tent (Figure 18-15). This will mix rich oxygen with room air and keep the concentration from exceeding 40%, thus preventing delivery of harmful levels of oxygen. When possible, use a humidified source of oxygen. You may be ordered by the emergency department physician to provide a higher concentration of oxygen by face mask if the infant's condition is considered to be critical.

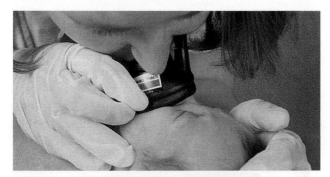

Figure 18-14 Pulmonary resuscitation of the newborn. Establish an adequate airway (do not overextend the neck). Provide breaths mouth-to-mask at the rate of 40 to 60 breaths per minute.

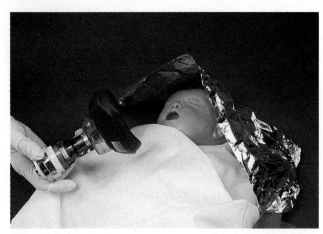

Figure 18-15 Make a tent over the baby's head in which the baby can breathe a mixture of oxygen and air.

Research by physicians who study newborns (neonatologists) indicate that withholding oxygen may be more damaging than delivering the wrong concentration for a short time period. It is difficult to attain the levels of oxygen that are harmful during typical EMT care and transport. Follow your local protocols for oxygen delivery to the newborn, but NEVER WITHHOLD OXYGEN FROM A SICK NEWBORN IN THE PREHOSPITAL SETTING.

If the infant is breathing but has a pulse rate below 80 beats per minute, its condition is considered severe. Some systems have as part of their basic EMT protocol the standing order to begin external chest compressions once the heart rate is below 80 and the infant has been on oxygen for several minutes. Most localities require their EMTs to obtain this order from the emergency department physician. Follow your local guidelines.

Do not give up hope! Newborn babies have been saved without brain damage even after 20 minutes of continued resuscitation. Be aware, however, that some babies are born dead, or **stillborn**. Under no circumstances should you attempt to resuscitate a stillborn that has obviously been dead for some time (see "The Stillborn Infant" later in this chapter). Turn your full attentions to the mother. She will need care that shows concern for her loss.

Note: Gas or oxygen-powered mechanical resuscitation devices should *never* be used on newborns. The technique for bag-valve-mask ventilation of an infant requires special training and practice.

Prolonged Delivery Closely spaced contractions (every 2 or 3 minutes) are a highly reliable sign that birth is imminent. If the baby is not delivered after 20 minutes of contractions that are 2 to 3 minutes apart, a **prolonged delivery** is indicated. Explain this to the mother and transport to a medical facility without delay.

Abnormal Deliveries

Whenever a patient has a breech presentation, a face or limb presentation, or a prolapsed umbilical cord, provide oxygen in high concentrations to the mother.

Breech Presentation Breech presentation is the most common abnormal delivery. It involves a buttocks-first or both-legs-first delivery. Through prompt and efficient emergency care, you can assist in the delivery of the baby. Should delivery not be possible, the care you provide can save the infant's life. Even though care at a breech birth is an EMT-level skill, keep in mind that this is a complicated emergency. Many hospitals have increased the number of cesarean sections in deliveries involving breech presentations. This is an indication that more problems have been associated with breech births than was once believed. Meconium staining often occurs with breech presentations.

Patient Assessment—Breech Presentation

If you evaluate a woman in labor and find the baby's buttocks or both legs presenting, rather than the head presenting, prepare the mother for delivery.

Patient Care—Breech Presentation

Emergency Care Steps

Follow these steps to assist in the delivery of an infant who presents in breech position.

1. *Allow the buttocks and trunk to deliver spontaneously.* Provide support as they emerge.
2. *Support the baby* by allowing the body to rest on the palm of your hand and letting the legs dangle astride your arm.
3. *Allow the head to deliver spontaneously.* If the head does not deliver within 3 min-

utes, special care procedures must be initiated immediately.

When the head does not deliver in 3 minutes, two things are happening that require special care. First of all, the umbilical cord is squeezed against the vaginal wall by the baby's head, reducing blood flow through the cord. Reduced circulation means reduced oxygen supply to the baby. Since oxygen flow through the cord is obstructed, spontaneous breathing is essential. However, when the baby attempts spontaneous breathing, the second problem occurs: The baby's face is pressed against the wall of the birth canal, obstructing the nose and mouth. In a breech presentation in which the head does not deliver within 3 minutes, quickly explain to the mother what you are going to do (Figure 18-16) and

1 *Carefully place your gloved hand in the vagina,* keeping your palm toward the baby's face. This will keep your hand in a position to support the head should the baby be delivered. Usually, the baby will be in a face-down position.
2 *Push the vaginal wall away from the baby's face.* Form a "V" with your fingers, placing the index finger on one side of the baby's nose and the middle finger on the other side. Push the vaginal wall away from the baby's face.

3 *Maintain the airway* until the head is delivered.
4 *Support the baby.* If the head delivers, support it and apply enough support along the baby's body to prevent an explosive delivery. After delivery, immediately wipe the infant's mouth and nose and then suction to clear the oral and nasal passages. Care for the baby, cord, mother, and placenta as in a cephalic delivery.

If the head is not delivered *within 3 minutes* of the established airway, maintain the airway and transport mother, child, and EMT as a unit. Administer oxygen to the mother. Take extreme care to maintain the airway being provided for the infant.

Remember: *Do not* attempt to deliver the baby by pulling on its legs.

Prolapsed Umbilical Cord Sometimes during delivery, the umbilical cord presents first (this is most common in breech births) and the cord is squeezed between the vaginal canal wall and the head of the baby. The cord is pinched, and oxygen supply to the baby may be totally interrupted. This occurrence is known as a **prolapsed umbilical cord**. It is a TRUE EMERGENCY, usually seen early in labor.

**Patient Assessment—
Prolapsed Umbilical Cord**

If, upon viewing the vaginal area, you see the umbilical cord presenting, the cord is prolapsed.

Patient Care—Prolapsed Umbilical Cord

Emergency Steps

1 *Keeping mother, child, and EMT as a unit, transport immediately to a medical facility.*
2 *Keep the mother in an exaggerated shock position* with a pillow or blanket under her hips (Figure 18-17) or in the knee-chest position (Figure 18-18).
3 *Provide the mother with a high concentration of oxygen* to increase the concentration carried over to the infant.
4 *Check the cord* for pulses and wrap the exposed cord, using a sterile towel from

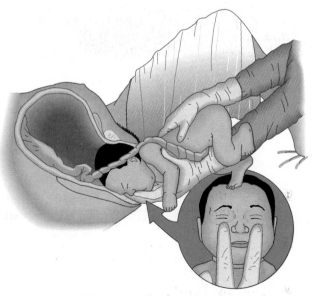

Figure 18-16 Procedures in a breech birth.

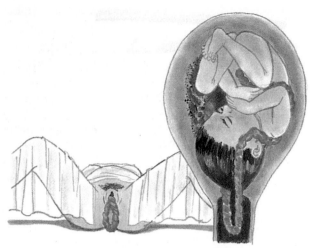

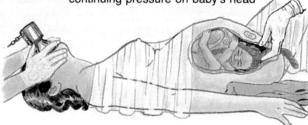

- Elevate hips, administer oxygen and keep warm
- Keep baby's head away from cord
- Do not attempt to push cord back
- Wrap cord in sterile moist towel
- Transport mother to hospital, continuing pressure on baby's head

Figure 18-17 Prolapsed umbilical cord.

the obstetric kit. The cord must be kept warm or spasms may occur and interrupt circulation. The best results are obtained if this towel is kept moist with *sterile saline*

and wrapped again with a dry towel to prevent evaporative heat loss.

5 *Insert several fingers of a gloved hand into the mother's vagina* so that you can gently push up on the baby's head or buttocks to keep pressure off of the cord. You will be pushing up through the cervix. This may be the only chance that the baby has for survival, so continue to push up on the baby until you are relieved by a physician. You may feel the cord pulsating when pressure is released.

Face or Limb Presentation In some presentations, the baby cannot be born without special assistance, possibly a cesarean section at the hospital. Presentation of the infant's face, brow, or chin may cause extreme hyperextension of the neck. If birth progresses, the neck will fracture. On rare occasions, a baby will have shoulders too large to fit through the pelvic bones (symphysis pubis) and the hollow of the sacrum. If one or more limbs present there is often a prolapsed umbilical cord. These are TRUE EMERGENCIES.

Patient Assessment— Face or Limb Presentation

When checking for crowning, you may notice the presentation of the infant's face, brow, or chin, or you may see (Figure 18-19) an arm, a leg, or an arm and leg together, or a shoulder and an arm. If one or more limbs present, there is often a prolapsed umbilical cord as well. Rarely, with symphysis pubis, you will find that the head has delivered but the shoulders have become wedged.

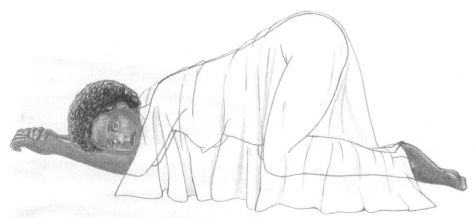

Figure 18-18 The knee-chest position can be used in the event of a prolapsed umbilical cord.

Patient Care— Face or Limb Presentation

Emergency Care Steps

When you discover a face or limb presentation or wedged shoulders

1. If there is a prolapsed cord, follow the same procedures as you would for any delivery involving a prolapsed cord. Remember, you have to keep pushing up on the baby until relieved by a physician. The baby must be kept off of the cord if it is to survive.
2. If the head delivers but the shoulders become wedged, wipe and suction the baby's mouth and be very careful not to aggravate the situation during transport.
3. Transport the mother immediately to a medical facility.
4. Keep the mother in a left lateral recumbent position with her feet slightly elevated or in the delivery position (follow local guidelines).
5. Administer a high concentration of oxygen.

Remember: For a limb presentation, *do not* try to pull on the limb or replace the limb into the vagina. If shoulders are wedged, *do not* pull on the baby's head. *Do not* place your gloved hand into the vagina, unless there is a prolapsed cord.

Multiple Birth When more than one baby is born during a single delivery, it is called a **multiple birth**. A multiple birth, usually twins, is not considered to be a complication, provided that the deliveries are normal. Twins are generally delivered in the same manner as a single delivery, one birth following the other.

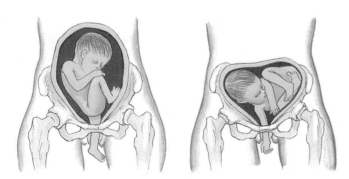

Figure 18-19 Limb presentation.

Patient Assessment—Multiple Birth

If the mother is under a physician's care, she will probably be aware that she is carrying twins. Without this information, you should consider a multiple birth to be a possibility if the mother's abdomen appears unusually large before delivery, or it remains very large after delivery of one baby. If the birth is multiple, labor contractions will continue and the second baby will be delivered shortly after the first. The second baby may present in a breech position, usually within minutes of the first birth. The placenta or placentas are delivered normally (Figure 18-20).

Patient Care—Multiple Birth

Emergency Care Steps

When assisting in the delivery of twins

1. Clamp or tie the cord of the first baby before the second baby is born.

Separate placentas

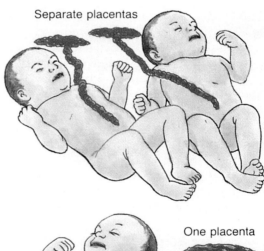

One placenta

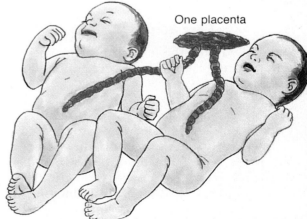

Figure 18-20 Multiple births.

2. The second baby may be born either before or after the placenta is delivered. Assist the mother with the delivery of the second baby.

3. Provide care for the babies, umbilical cords, placenta(s), and the mother as you would in a single baby delivery.

4. The babies will probably be smaller than in a single birth, so special care should be taken to keep them warm during transport.

When delivering twins, identify the infants as to order of birth (1 and 2 or A and B).

Premature Birth By definition, a **premature infant** is one that weighs less than 5½ pounds at birth, or one that is born before the 37th week or prior to the ninth month of pregnancy.

Patient Assessment—Premature Birth

Since you will probably not be able to weigh the baby, you will have to make a determination as to whether the baby is full-term or premature based on the mother's information and the baby's appearance. By comparison with a normal full-term baby, the head of a premature infant is much larger in proportion to the small, thin, red body. Sometimes they have respiratory problems.

Patient Care—Premature Birth

Premature babies need special care from the moment of birth. The smaller the baby, the more important is the initial care.

Emergency Care Steps

You should take the following steps when providing care for the premature infant (Figure 18-21).

1. *Keep the baby warm.* Once breathing, the baby should be dried and wrapped snugly in a warm blanket. Additional protection can be provided by an outer wrap of plastic bubble wrap (keep away from the face) or aluminum foil. Premature babies lack fat deposits that would normally keep them warm. Some EMS systems in cold regions

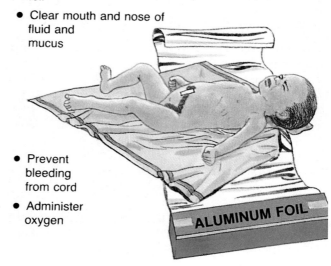

- Keep warm by wrapping in blanket and then in aluminum foil
- Clear mouth and nose of fluid and mucus
- Prevent bleeding from cord
- Administer oxygen

ALUMINUM FOIL

Figure 18-21 Premature infants need special care.

are using a plastic or bubble wrap or bag for the infant, covered by a blanket. This helps maintain warmth and allows for easier visual inspection of the clamped cord to check for bleeding. A stockinette cap should be placed on the baby's head to help reduce heat loss.

2. *Keep the airway clear.* Continue to suction fluids from the nose and mouth using a rubber bulb syringe. Keep checking to see if additional suctioning is required.

3. *Watch the umbilical cord for bleeding.* Examine the cut end of the cord carefully. If there is any sign of bleeding, even the slightest, apply another clamp or tie closer to the baby's body.

4. *Provide oxygen.* Deliver the oxygen into the top of an aluminum foil tent placed over the baby's head. Do not blow a stream of oxygen directly on the baby's face. If available, use a humidified source of oxygen. Remember, this procedure keeps the oxygen concentration below the harmful level for the time of transport.

5. *Avoid contamination.* The premature infant is susceptible to infection. Keep it away from other people. Do not breathe on its face.

6. *Transport the infant in a warm ambulance.* The desired temperature is between 90°F and 100°F. Use the ambulance heater to warm the patient compartment prior to transport. In the summer months, the air

conditioning should be turned off and all compartment windows should be closed or adjusted to keep the desired temperature.

7 *Call ahead and alert the medical facility.*

When a premature infant carrier is available, make certain that you are completely familiar with its use. Some require you to fill hot water bottles that are covered and placed in the carrier. The infant is to be wrapped in a blanket and aluminum foil or plastic wrap and a blanket. The carrier must be properly secured in the ambulance prior to transport. In some areas, a mobile intensive care unit or helicopter may be able to respond and transport the baby.

The Stillborn Infant Some babies die in the womb several hours, days, or even weeks before birth.

Patient Assessment—Stillbirth

When a baby has died sometime before birth, death is obvious by the presence of blisters, foul odor, skin or tissue deterioration and discoloration, and a softened head. At other times, a baby may be born in pulmonary or cardiac arrest but in otherwise good condition and with the possibility of being resuscitated.

Patient Care—Stillbirth

Emergency Care Steps

1 Stillborn babies who have obviously been dead for some time before birth are not to receive resuscitation.

2 Any other babies who are born in pulmonary or cardiac arrest are to receive basic cardiac life support measures.

3 When the baby is alive but death appears to be imminent, prepare to provide life support.

Nothing is quite so sad as a baby born dead or one that dies shortly after birth. It is a tragic moment for the parents and other family members. Your thoughtfulness may provide the distraught parents with comfort.

Do not lie to the mother. Many death-and-dying experts believe that she should be allowed to view her baby if she so desires. *Do not* stop her from seeing the dead baby if she desires to do so.

Christian parents may ask you to baptize the baby if death appears likely. This is acceptable practice for emergency personnel. Regardless of your own religious belief, you should comply with the parents' request. Ask the parents if they know the exact words of baptism for their denomination. Say exactly what they tell you. If they are not sure, simply sprinkle drops of water on the baby's head and say: "I baptize thee in the name of the Father, and of the Son, and of the Holy Spirit."

Needless to say, resuscitative efforts should be continued during and after the baptism and continued until transfer at the hospital. You must keep accurate records of the time of stillbirth and the care rendered for completion of the fetal death certificate. It is a good idea to note if the baby was baptized by EMS personnel.

Predelivery Emergencies

Excessive Prebirth Bleeding A number of conditions can cause excessive prebirth bleeding (Figure 18-22). One such condition is **placenta previa** (plah-SEN-tah PRE-vi-ah), a condition in which the placenta is formed in an abnormal location (usually low in the uterus and close to or over the cervical opening) that will not allow for a normal delivery of the fetus. As the cervix dilates, the placenta tears. Another is **abruptio placentae** (ab-RUP-she-o plah-SEN-ti), a condition in which the placenta separates from the uterine wall. This can be a partial or a complete abruption. In a complete abruption, the body of the placenta has separated from the uterine wall but the edges remain attached. Blood is trapped between the uterine wall and the placenta. Either placenta previa or abruptio placentae may occur in the third trimester and is life-threatening to the mother and fetus.

A pregnant woman does not have to be in labor to have excessive bleeding from the vagina. Bleeding in early pregnancy may be due to a miscarriage (see "Miscarriage and Abortion" later in this chapter). If the bleeding occurs late in pregnancy, it may be due to problems involving the placenta.

Patient Assessment— Excessive Prebirth Bleeding

Signs and Symptoms

☐ The main sign is usually simply profuse bleeding from the vagina.

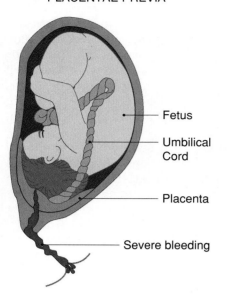

PLACENTAE PREVIA

Fetus

Umbilical Cord

Placenta

Severe bleeding

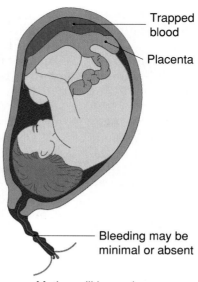

ABRUPTIO PLACENTAE

Trapped blood

Placenta

Bleeding may be minimal or absent

Mother will have signs and symptoms of shock

Figure 18-22 Difficulties with the placenta can cause excessive prebirth bleeding.

- In the case of placenta previa, there may be no pain or labor symptoms other than labor pain.
- With abruptio placentae with complete abruption, there may be no external blood loss. The signs of internal blood loss will be shock-like vital signs. The patient will have severe pain and a hard, rigid uterus. The patient may describe a tearing sensation.

Patient Care—Excessive Prebirth Bleeding

If a pregnant woman begins to have excessive bleeding from the vagina, you should (Figure 18-23)

1. Place the patient in a left lateral recumbent position and begin to treat for shock. *Do not* hold the patient's legs together.
2. Place a sanitary napkin over the vaginal opening. Note the time of napkin placement. DO NOT PLACE ANYTHING IN THE VAGINA.
3. Replace pads as they become soaked, but save all pads to use in evaluating blood loss.
4. Save all tissue that is passed.
5. Administer a high concentration of oxygen (non-rebreather mask, 8-15 liters per minute).
6. Transport as soon as possible.

You may be ordered to apply an anti-shock garment. In most cases, only the leg compartments are to be inflated. Follow the specific directions of the physician who orders the anti-shock garment to be applied.

Pre-eclampsia and Eclampsia Pre-eclampsia and eclampsia are stages of a condition known as *toxemia* ("poisoning" of the blood) of pregnancy. This problem is seen most often in young women having their first babies, usually without the benefit of medical care. Medical conditions of the mother that increase the risk for toxemia include diabetes, heart disease, kidney or renal problems, and hypertension.

In its early stages, toxemia of pregnancy is called **pre-eclampsia** (pre-e-KLAMP-se-ah). The advanced stage of toxemia of pregnancy is **eclampsia** (e-KLAMP-se-ah).

Patient Assessment—Pre-eclampsia and Eclampsia

Signs and Symptoms

Pre-eclampsia is recognized by

- Elevated blood pressure. The risk of abruptio placentae increases with the elevated blood pressure.

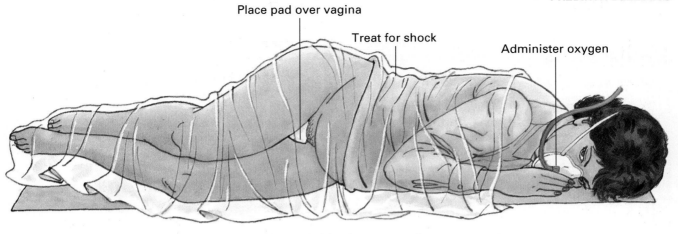

Place pad over vagina

Treat for shock

Administer oxygen

Figure 18-23 Attempt to control excessive prebirth bleeding. Immediate transport is required.

- Edema
- Excessive weight gain
- Extreme swelling of face, hands, and feet

When the condition is severe, the patient will complain of

- Headache
- Sensitivity to light
- Visual difficulties
- Pain in the upper abdomen
- Apprehension and shakiness

Eclampsia is distinguished from pre-eclampsia by

- The onset of convulsions or coma. At its worst, eclampsia can cause convulsions that are fatal for the mother. The risk of death for the fetus is high.

Consider all pregnant patients with elevated blood pressure to have pre-eclampsia; however, the blood pressure of a pre-eclampsia patient may be within normal range, since most women experience some blood pressure decline during pregnancy.

Patient Care—
Pre-eclampsia and Eclampsia

Emergency Care Steps

All patients with pre-eclampsia or eclampsia require

1. Transport.
2. Gentle handling at all times. Rough handling may induce a convulsion.
3. Avoidance of bright lights (dim the lights in the ambulance), and no siren when transporting unless absolutely necessary.

If the patient has a seizure, you should

1. Provide care as you would for any seizure patient, protecting her from harming herself.
2. Position the unconscious eclampsia patient on her left side to allow drainage and keep the tongue from blocking the airway. When she becomes conscious, keep the patient on her left side and elevate the head and shoulders.
3. Administer a high concentration of oxygen (non-rebreather mask, 8-15 liters per minute).
4. Keep her warm, but do not overheat.
5. Have suction ready.
6. Have delivery pack ready.

Warning: The use of lights and siren during transport may induce a convulsion in the pre-eclampsia or eclampsia patient.

Ectopic Pregnancy In normal pregnancy, the fertilized egg will begin to divide in the oviduct (fallopian tube) and eventually implant in the wall of the uterus. In an **ectopic** (ek-TOP-ik) **pregnancy**, implantation may take place in an oviduct, the cervix of the uterus, or in the abdominopelvic cavity. These areas or organs are not able to contain the growing embryo nor to support the developing fetus.

Patient Assessment—Ectopic Pregnancy

Signs and Symptoms

The problems related to this condition are seen early in pregnancy. Women with this type of pregnancy may have signs and symptoms including those indicating shock due to internal bleeding. Be alert to recognize signs before shock develops.

- ☐ Acute abdominal pain (most patients)
- ☐ Vaginal bleeding (most patients)
- ☐ A rapid and weak pulse (late sign—decompensated shock)
- ☐ Low blood pressure (late sign—decompensated shock)

An ectopic pregnancy can occur to a woman who does not know she is pregnant. Often, the patient associates her problems with menstrual irregularities. ANY female of childbearing age with acute abdominal pain, vaginal bleeding, or unexplained shock must be considered to have a possible ectopic pregnancy. The signs of shock may be out of proportion to any visible bleeding, vaginal or otherwise.

Patient Care—Ectopic Pregnancy

Emergency Care Steps

This is a TRUE EMERGENCY, requiring

1. Immediate transport
2. Positioning for shock
3. Care for shock
4. A high concentration of oxygen
5. Do not give the woman anything by mouth.
6. An anti-shock garment may be ordered by the emergency department physician.

Ruptured Uterus The uterus may rupture during labor, usually as a result of trauma. This is a very rare occurrence, but when it does happen it is a TRUE EMERGENCY, requiring transport without delay.

Patient Assessment—Ruptured Uterus

Be alert for this problem if the mother has had a cesarean section or any other surgery performed on her uterus. If the patient has had many full-term pregnancies, she may also be a candidate for a ruptured uterus. The previous pregnancies may have weakened the wall of the uterus. The uterus may rupture if the baby is too large for the pelvis or if labor is extended and forceful.

Signs and Symptoms

A patient may have a ruptured uterus if the following signs and symptoms are present.

- ☐ A tearing sensation in the patient's abdomen
- ☐ Constant pain
- ☐ Labor typically appears as if it is going to be extended. Contractions may start out being very forceful, then stop completely.
- ☐ There may not be any major vaginal bleeding, but internal bleeding may be severe.
- ☐ Decompensated shock may develop rapidly. Often, this is indicated by a marked drop in blood pressure.

Patient Care—Ruptured Uterus

Emergency Care Steps

1. Provide high concentration oxygen.
2. The emergency department physician may order the application of an anti-shock garment.
3. Transport the patient without delay
4. Care for shock.
5. You may have to provide resuscitative measures for the mother.

Miscarriage and Abortion For a number of reasons, the fetus and placenta may deliver before the 28th week of pregnancy—before the baby can live on its own. This occurrence is an **abortion**. When it happens on its own it is called a **spontaneous abortion**; the common term is **miscarriage**.

An **induced abortion** is an abortion that is the result of deliberate actions taken to stop the pregnancy. This may be done as a legal medical procedure (therapeutic abortion), or it may be an illegal attempt to stop the pregnancy (criminal abortion). Some women take excessive dosages of certain drugs, poisons, and other chemicals in an attempt to induce abortion. In some cases, women insert objects into the vagina to try to mechanically disrupt the pregnancy. This can result in internal as well as external bleeding.

Patient Assessment—
Miscarriage and Abortion

Signs and Symptoms

Women having a miscarriage that requires them to seek emergency care generally have

☐ Cramping abdominal pains not unlike those associated with the first stage of labor
☐ Bleeding ranging from moderate to severe
☐ There may be a noticeable discharge of tissue particles and blood from the vagina.

Ask the patient about the starting date of her last menstrual period. If it has been more than 24 weeks, be prepared with a delivery pack. Premature infants may survive if they receive rapid neonatal intensive care.

Women undergoing self-induced or non-medical abortions can show the same clinical picture as those having miscarriages. However

☐ The pain involved is usually much greater.
☐ Bleeding will be more severe.
☐ They may have high fever from infection.

Patient Care—Miscarriage and Abortion

Care is basically the same for both types of abortion: miscarriage (spontaneous abortion) and induced abortion.

Emergency Care Steps.

1. Provide a high concentration of oxygen.
2. Monitor and record vital signs.
3. Help control vaginal bleeding by placing a sanitary napkin over the vaginal opening. Do not pack the vagina.
4. Transport as soon as possible, positioning the patient for shock.
5. Care for shock.
6. Replace and save all blood-soaked pads.
7. Save all tissues that are expelled. Do not attempt to replace or pull out any tissues that are being expelled through the vagina.
8. You may be ordered to apply an anti-shock garment. Usually the order will be to inflate the legs only.
9. If the woman has tried to induce abortion by ingesting an overdose of drugs or poison, provide care as for any overdose or poisoning (see Chapter 16).
10. Emotional support is very important.

When speaking to the patient, her family, or where bystanders may hear you, ALWAYS use the term *miscarriage* instead of *spontaneous abortion*. Most people associate the word *abortion* with an induced abortion, not a miscarriage. On rare occasions, a patient who has tried to induce an abortion will be very uncooperative. It is essential to talk with the patient to gain her confidence and to allow you to provide emotional support.

Accidents Obviously the pregnant patient may sustain injury as any other accident victim. However, during the last two trimesters the uterus and fetus are also subject to injuries. Injuries to the uterus may be blunt or penetrating. In both cases the greatest danger to mother and baby is hemorrhage and hemorrhagic shock.

The most common cause of blunt trauma is automobile collisions but falls or beatings also account for many injuries. The uterus is well designed to protect the baby. The fetus is inside the uterus, a muscular chamber filled with water. The uterus acts as an efficient shock absorber. Thus most minor trauma to the abdomen, such as a blow or fall, does not harm the fetus.

Automobile collisions are a different story. The magnitude of forces is great. Because of its size and location, the uterus is frequently injured. Sudden blunt trauma to the abdomen during the later months of pregnancy may cause uterine rupture or premature separation of the placenta (abruptio placentae). Other blunt trauma injuries, such as ruptured spleen or liver, may also occur. Rupture of the diaphragm may occur with blunt trauma during later pregnancy. Multiple trauma with fractures of the pelvis can cause laceration or tearing of the vessels in the pelvis with massive hemorrhage. The common problem with most blunt injuries to the pregnant abdomen or pelvis is massive bleeding and hemorrhagic shock.

If a pregnant woman is injured in an accident, such as a motor vehicle collision or a fall, perform a patient assessment and treat her injuries as you would those of any other patient.

Patient Assessment—
Accident to a Pregnant Woman

Follow these patient assessment steps.

☐ Question the alert conscious patient to

determine if she received any blows to the abdomen, pelvis, or back.

☐ Examine the unconscious patient for abdominal injuries, remembering to consider the mechanism of injury.

☐ Ask the patient if she has had bleeding or rupture of fluids. When in doubt, examine the vaginal area for bleeding, being certain to provide privacy.

During your assessment, keep in mind that

☐ The pregnant patient has a pulse that is 10-15 beats per minute faster than the nonpregnant female. Vital signs may be interpreted as being suggestive of shock while they are normal for the pregnant female.

☐ A woman in later pregnancy may have a blood volume that is up to 48% higher than her nonpregnant state. With hemorrhage, 30-35% blood loss may occur before otherwise healthy pregnant females exhibit signs or symptoms.

☐ Although shock is more difficult to assess in the pregnant patient, it is the most likely cause of prehospital death from injury to the uterus.

Patient Care— Accident to a Pregnant Woman

Emergency Care Steps

Remember that maintenance of respiration and circulation and the control of bleeding are vital not only to the mother but also to the fetus. A developing fetus is critically dependent on the uninterrupted oxygenated blood supply that enters the placenta. What's good for the mother is good for the

baby. Since the mother-to-be may have undetected internal bleeding or the fetus may be injured

1 Provide resuscitation if necessary.

2 Provide a high concentration of oxygen. (Oxygen requirements of the woman in later pregnancy are 10-20% greater than normal. If in doubt, always give oxygen.)

3 Because of slowed digestion and delayed gastric emptying, there is a greater risk the patient will vomit and aspirate. Be ready with suction!

4 Transport as soon as possible. All pregnant women should be transported in the left lateral recumbent position unless a back injury is suspected. If so, first backboard the mother, placing a folded blanket or small pillow under her right hip to tip the uterus to the left, relieving pressure on the intra-abdominal organs. Be sure to monitor and record vital signs.

5 Provide emotional support. A pregnant woman who is an accident victim will naturally worry about her unborn child. Remind her that the developing baby is well protected in the uterus. Let her know that she is being transported to a medical facility that can take care of her needs and the needs of the unborn child.

If the mother dies in an accident and you begin CPR immediately, there is a chance of saving the life of the infant. CPR must then be continued until an emergency cesarean section can be performed. If CPR is delayed 5 to 10 minutes, chances of saving the baby are fair, while a 25-minute delay reduces the chances to almost zero. Continue CPR until you are relieved in the emergency department.

CHAPTER REVIEW

KEY TERMS

You may find it helpful to review the following terms.

abortion—spontaneous (miscarriage) or induced termination of pregnancy.

abruptio placentae (ab-RUP-she-o plah-SEN-ti)—a condition in which the placenta separates from the uterine wall; a cause of excessive pre-birth bleeding.

afterbirth—the placenta, membranes of the amniotic sac, part of the umbilical cord, and some tissues from the lining of the uterus that are delivered after the birth of the baby.

amniotic (am-ne-OT-ic) **sac**—the "bag of waters" that surrounds the developing fetus.

breech presentation—when the baby appears buttocks or both legs first during birth.

cephalic (se-FAL-ik) **presentation**—when the baby appears head first during birth. This is the normal presentation. Also called a *vertex presentation.*

cervix (SUR-viks)—the neck of the uterus that enters the birth canal.

crowning—when part of the baby is visible through the vaginal opening.

eclampsia (e-KLAMP-se-ah)—a severe complication of pregnancy that produces convulsions and coma.

ectopic (ek-TOP-ik) **pregnancy**—when implantation of the fertilized egg is not in the body of the uterus, occurring instead in the oviduct (fallopian tube), cervix, or abdominopelvic cavity.

false labor—contractions that occur at any time during pregnancy caused by changes in the uterus as it adjusts in size and shape; also called Braxton-Hicks contractions.

fetus (FE-tus)—the baby as it develops in the womb.

induced abortion—delivery of a fetus as a result of deliberate actions that are taken to stop the pregnancy.

labor—the three stages of delivery that begin with the contractions of the uterus and end with the expulsion of the placenta.

meconium staining—amniotic fluid that is greenish or brownish-yellow rather than clear; an indication of possible fetal distress during labor.

miscarriage—see *spontaneous abortion.*

multiple birth—when more than one baby is born during a single delivery.

perineum (per-i-NE-um)—the surface area between the vulva and anus.

placenta (plah-SEN-tah)—the organ of pregnancy where exchange of oxygen, foods, and wastes occurs between mother and fetus.

placenta previa (plah-SEN-tah PRE-vi-ah)—a condition in which the placenta is formed in an abnormal location (usually low in the uterus and close to or over the cervical opening) that will not allow for a normal delivery of the fetus; a cause of excessive prebirth bleeding.

pre-eclampsia (pre-e-KLAMP-se-ah)—a complication of pregnancy that can lead to convulsions and coma.

premature infant—any newborn weighing less than 5.5 pounds or being born before the 37th week of pregnancy.

prolapsed umbilical cord—when the umbilical cord presents first and is squeezed between the vaginal wall and the baby's head.

prolonged delivery—when birth is delayed more than 20 minutes after contractions are 2-to-3 minutes apart.

spontaneous abortion—when the fetus and placenta deliver before the 28th week of pregnancy; commonly called a *miscarriage.*

stillborn—born dead.

supine hypotensive syndrome—dizziness and a drop in blood pressure caused when the mother is in a supine position and the weight of the uterus, infant, placenta, and amniotic fluid compress the inferior vena cava, reducing venous return to the heart and reducing cardiac output.

umbilical (um-BIL-i-cal) **cord**—the fetal structure containing the blood vessels that travel to and from the placenta.

uterus (U-ter-us)—the muscular abdominal organ where the fetus develops; the womb.

vagina (vah-JI-nah)—the birth canal.

vernix (VER-niks)—the slippery protective coating that covers a baby when it is born.

vulva (VUL-vah)—the female external genitalia.

The Anatomy and Physiology of Childbirth

The fetus developing in the uterus is surrounded by the amniotic sac. While developing, the fetus receives nourishment and oxygen through the placenta. It is connected to the placenta by the umbilical cord.

The first stage of labor starts with contractions and ends with the full dilation of the cervix. The second stage of labor ends with birth. The third stage ends with the delivery of the placenta.

Normal Childbirth

Evaluate the mother to see if she is about to deliver. Consider if this is her first baby, how far apart the contractions are, if she feels pressure or feels as if she may have a bowel movement, if her "bag of waters" has broken, or if she feels the baby moving into her vagina. If birth is not imminent, place her in the left lateral recumbent position to relieve pressure on the inferior vena cava and prevent or relieve supine hypotensive syndrome.

If you believe that birth will occur shortly, provide the mother with as much privacy as possible. Position an assistant at her head. Position the mother on her back, with her buttocks elevated, her knees bent, feet flat, and legs spread apart. Remove any clothing obstructing your view of the vaginal opening. See if any part of the baby is visible or visible on contractions. This is crowning. If the head appears first, this is a normal cephalic presentation.

Assist the mother as she delivers her baby. Carefully support the head of the infant as it is born. Provide support for its entire body and head as birth proceeds. If you notice the umbilical cord around the baby's neck, gently loosen the cord with your fingers and slip the cord over the baby's head. When the cord will not loosen, you will have to clamp it in two locations and cut between the clamps. If the amniotic sac does not break, puncture it and pull it away from the baby's mouth and nose. Remember to record the exact time of birth and to assess the newborn at 1 and 5 minutes after it is born using the APGAR scoring method.

In caring for the newborn, clear the baby's airway by suctioning the mouth first, then the nostrils, and make certain that the baby is breathing. Always dry and wrap the newborn in a blanket to keep it warm. Assist the mother as she delivers the placenta and save all tissues for transport. Help control vaginal bleeding by placing clean pads over the mother's vaginal opening and massaging her abdomen over the site of the uterus. Remove all wet towels and sheets. Wipe clean the mother's face and hands. REMEMBER: Throughout the entire birth process, provide emotional support to the mother.

Be aware of the conditions of a high-risk pregnancy, including the mother's age (under 20 or over 35), number of pregnancies, medical conditions, medications, or substance abuse.

If it the baby is not breathing, gently but rigorously rub its back. Should this fail to produce spontaneous respirations, you will have to "encourage" the child to breathe by snapping your index finger on the soles of its feet. (Never lift and spank the baby.) For nonbreathing babies with a brachial pulse, provide mouth-to-mask resuscitation. If there is no pulse, provide CPR. If CPR is necessary, you will have to clamp and cut the cord. Do not tie, clamp, or cut a cord until the baby is breathing on its own and pulsations of the cord have stopped unless you have to remove the cord from the baby's neck or provide CPR for the infant.

Childbirth Complications

Be ready for complications during a delivery. If delivery is prolonged, transport the mother to a medical facility. When the buttocks or both legs appear first, this is a breech presentation. Provide an airway with your fingers. Maintain this airway until the baby is born or until you hand the mother over to trained professionals at a medical facility. Transport mothers with prebirth bleeding, prolapsed umbilical cords, or face or limb presentations to a medical facility as soon as possible. If there is a prolapsed cord, you will have to insert several fingers into the vagina to push the baby off the cord. Administer a high concentration of oxygen to all women having complications with birth.

Expect a multiple birth if contractions continue after a baby is born. Tie or clamp the umbilical cord of the first child before the next one delivers. Keep all premature babies warm, maintain a clear airway, monitor the cord for bleeding, provide oxygen to a tent over the baby's head, and protect from contamination. In cases of stillborns, remain professional and provide emotional support to the mother, father, and other family members. Unless there is evidence that the baby died several hours before birth, provide basic cardiac life support for all babies who are in cardiac arrest.

If there is severe bleeding before delivery, place a pad over the vaginal opening, treat for shock, administer a high concentration of oxygen, and transport as soon as possible. Patients with pre-eclampsia (swollen extremities, high blood pressure) or eclampsia (seizures) must be handled very gently, not exposed to bright light or sirens (unless they are actively seizing), and transported immediately. Patients with symptoms of ectopic pregnancy or ruptured uterus (intense abdominal pain, signs of shock), should be provided oxygen, treated for shock, and transported immediately.

In cases of miscarriage and abortion, be certain to provide emotional support to the mother. Place a pad over her vaginal opening if there is bleeding. Save all blood-soaked pads and any passed tissues. Care for shock and provide a high concentration of oxygen. If a pregnant woman has been in an accident, assess and treat as you would any accident victim and also check for vaginal bleeding. If the pregnant woman dies, begin CPR and transport immediately to attempt to keep the baby alive.

CHAPTER 19

On the Scene

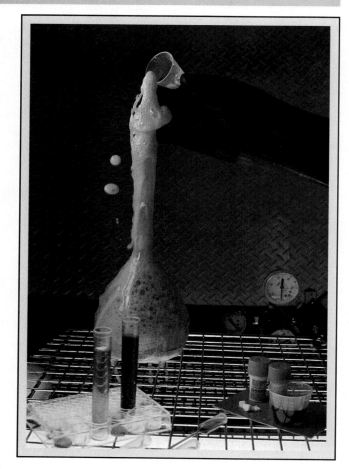

Twenty students are at work in the chemistry lab at Jefferson High School when an explosion takes place. On arrival you are designated the EMS command officer. The fire command officer, who is also acting as the incident commander (IC), advises you that there are approximately ten injured students who have apparently inhaled the unknown gas. Three also have injuries from the blast

itself. He advises you that the north parking lot and the softball field are upwind of the accident.

You radio a report to the EMS dispatcher.

You: *Dispatcher, this is EMS Command. I am declaring a multi-casualty incident. I will need seven additional ambulances to start. Have the responding ambulances stage in the north parking lot. The triage area will be set up on the softball field.*

You *(to your partner): Take the MCI and jump kits and begin triage. Wear the Triage Officer bib.*

Incident Commander: *We're about to make entry to check for any other victims. We've set up a decontamination area over here.*

You: *I'll call for our disaster van with extra supplies. Have you spoken with the teacher to get an idea of what chemicals were involved?*

Incident Commander: *We're doing it now. Parents are starting to show up. The police and the school will deal with them.*

The potential for a hazardous materials incident exists in every community. A successful resolution to a crisis such as this depends on pre-planning. In this situation, the fire department, EMS, and police have all worked together at drills in order to be prepared for an event like this one—training that will be invaluable today at Jefferson High.

Burns and Hazardous Materials

Chapter Overview

Environmental emergencies include those related to

- Fire
- Radiation
- Cold
- Electricity
- Explosions
- Water
- Chemicals
- Heat
- Ice

As you review this list, it will probably occur to you that environmental emergencies can be hazardous not only for your patients but also for you, the EMT. So protecting *yourself* is a major consideration in dealing with an environmental emergency.

This chapter provides a general introduction to environmental injuries, then deals with burns and other injuries related to the first five items on the list: fire, electricity, chemicals, radiation, and explosions. The remaining items—heat, cold, water, and ice—will be taken up in the next chapter.

Expected Outcome, Chapter 19: *You will be able to assess and care for burns and other injuries related to fire, electricity, chemicals, radiation, and explosions and to protect yourself at hazardous environmental emergency scenes.*

> **Warning:** Protect yourself from infectious diseases by using appropriate barrier devices such as a pocket face mask with one-way valve, face shield, or bag-valve mask; goggles or eye shield; and disposable gloves. Always conform to your local EMS system's infection exposure control plan.

ENVIRONMENTAL INJURIES
    The EMT's Responsibilities

BURNS
    Classifying and Evaluating Burns
    Treating Burns
    Smoke Inhalation

ELECTRICAL ACCIDENTS

HAZARDOUS MATERIALS
    On Arrival
    Sources of Information
    Rescue and Care Procedures

RADIATION ACCIDENTS
    Types of Radiation
    Effects of Radiation on the Body
    Types of Radiation Accidents
    On Arrival
    Rescue and Care Procedures
    Decontamination and Transport

EXPLOSIONS

Knowledge *After reading this chapter, you should be able to*

1. Explain the limits and the reasons for the limits to the role of the EMT at the scene of an environmental emergency. (p. 539)

2. List FIVE agents that cause burns. (p. 539; Table 19-1)

3. Define first-, second-, and third-degree burns. (p. 540)

4. State the factors used in determining the severity of burns. (pp. 540, 542-543)

5. Define the Rule of Nines (and fill out a body chart for both adult and child patients) and the Rule of Palm. (pp. 542-543)

6. List the factors used to distinguish among minor, moderate, and critical burns. (p. 543)

7. State the considerations in determining priority of care and transport for burn patients. (pp. 543-544; Table 19-2)

8. Describe emergency care for thermal and chemical burns. (pp. 544-547)

9. Describe assessment and emergency care procedures for smoke inhalation victims. (pp. 547-548)

10. Describe assessment and emergency care procedures for victims of electrical accidents. (pp. 548-550)

11. Describe the EMT's role in hazardous materials accidents. (pp. 550-552)

12. Describe rescue, assessment, and emergency care procedures for hazardous materials accidents. (pp. 552-553)

13. Describe types of radiation and types of radiation accidents. (pp. 554, 555)

14. Describe the EMT's duties and methods of self-protection at the scene of a radiation accident. (p. 555)

15. Describe rescue, assessment, and emergency care procedures—including decontamination and transport procedures—for radiation accidents. (pp. 555-557)

16. Describe assessment and emergency care procedures for victims of explosions. (p. 557)

Skills *As an EMT you should be able to*

1. Protect yourself while working at the scenes of hazardous accidents.

2. Assess and care for victims of thermal and chemical burns and smoke inhalation.

3. Assess and care for victims of electrical accidents, hazardous materials accidents, radiation accidents, and explosions.

The environment, of course, is everything around us. A safe and healthful environment sustains life and wellbeing. Yet nearly any element or combination of elements in the environment—elements that we encounter in our daily lives—*can* cause injury.

ENVIRONMENTAL INJURIES

The skin is the body's first line of defense against the environment. For this reason, many environmental emergencies involve injuries to the skin. The eyes also are particularly vulnerable. The airway opens the respiratory system to the outside, making the lining of the airway susceptible to damage from environmental factors. Respiratory injury can extend from the nasal membranes to the alveoli of the lungs.

The interior organs of the body and the body's chemical activities can also be altered by environmental factors. Radiation can affect cells deep within the body. Electricity can disrupt nerve, muscle, and heart actions. Many chemicals can destroy or alter the cells and tissues.

The effects of environmental emergencies are often complex. For example, a fire can burn the skin while heat from the fire alters the body's regulatory mechanisms and smoke damages the eyes and the airway. A person who falls into the water faces damage from excessive cold as well as the danger of drowning. The victim of electrocution will suffer burns and also changes to the body's vital chemical activities. Sometimes the injury process is rapid and dramatic; at other times it is slow and subtle.

As an EMT you must be prepared to provide care for a variety of environmental emergencies. Keep in mind that such emergencies can occur anywhere, at any time.

The EMT's Responsibilities

EMTs assess and provide care for patients with environmental injuries. However EMTs are not usually trained to handle all of the *sources* of environmental injuries or to control hazardous scenes except in a peripheral or preliminary way. For example, EMTs are usually able to control traffic and bystanders at an emergency scene, but not to fight fires, handle charged electrical wires, perform water rescues, or manage radiation accidents. Specially trained rescue and hazard personnel must handle such duties and assure the safety of everyone at the scene, including the EMTs.

Remember: Do only what you have been trained to do. "Heroic" efforts can place you and fellow rescuers in danger and may even delay proper care for the patient.

BURNS

Most people think of burns as injuries to the skin; but burns can do much more. Burn injuries often involve structures below the skin, including muscles, bones, nerves, and blood vessels. Burns can injure the eyes beyond repair. Respiratory system structures can be damaged, producing airway obstruction due to tissue swelling, even respiratory failure and respiratory arrest. In addition to the physical damage caused by burns, patients often suffer emotional and psychological problems that begin at the emergency scene and may last a lifetime.

When caring for a burn patient, always think beyond the burn. For example, a medical emergency or accident may have led to the burn. The patient may have had a heart attack while smoking a cigarette, and the unattended cigarette caused a fire. During the patient assessment, the EMT should detect the heart problem even though the burn may be the most obvious injury. Conversely, a fire or burn may cause or

aggravate another injury or medical condition. Someone trying to escape a fire may fall and suffer spinal damage and fractures. The EMT should detect not only the burn but the spinal damage and fractures as well.

Remember: The patient assessment should never be neglected in order to go immediately to burn care procedures.

Classifying and Evaluating Burns

The process of patient assessment, when there are burns, involves classifying then evaluating the burns.

> **Patient Assessment—Burns**
>
> Burns can be classified and evaluated in three ways.
>
> ☐ By agent and source
> ☐ By degree
> ☐ By severity

All are important in deciding the urgency and the kind of emergency care the burn requires. These classifications are discussed in detail below.

Agent and Source Burns can be classified according to the agent causing the burn (e.g., chemicals or electricity). Noting the source of the burn (e.g., hydrochloric acid or AC current) can make the classification more specific. You should report the agent and also, when practical, the source of the agent (Table 19-1). For example, a burn can be reported as "chemical burns from contact with hydrochloric acid."

TABLE 19-1 Agents and Sources of Burns

Agents	Sources
Thermal	Including flame; radiation; excessive heat from fire, steam, hot liquids, hot objects
Chemicals	Including various acids, bases, caustics
Electricity	Including AC current, DC current, lightning
Light (typically involving the eyes)	Including intense light sources, ultraviolet light (includes sunlight)
Radiation	Usually from nuclear sources; ultraviolet light can also be considered to be a source of radiation burns

Never assume the agent or source of the burn. What may appear to be a thermal burn could be from radiation. You may find minor thermal burns on the patient's face and forget to consider light burns to the eyes. Always gather information from your observations of the scene, bystanders' reports, and the patient interview.

Degree Burns involving the skin also can be classified as *partial-thickness burns* and *full-thickness burns*. Partial-thickness burns can involve the epidermis, or the epidermis and upper dermis, but they do not include burns that pass through the dermis to damage underlying tissues (see Chapter 9). A full-thickness burn will pass through epidermis and dermis, causing injury to the subcutaneous layers. Both partial- and full-thickness burns are described using an evaluation system employing the term *degree,* with burns involving the skin classified as first-, second-, or third-degree (Figure 19-1 and Scan 19-1). The least serious burn is the first-degree burn.

- **First-degree Burn**—This is a superficial injury that involves only the epidermis. It is characterized by reddening of the skin and perhaps some swelling. An example is a sunburn. The patient will usually complain about pain (sometimes severe) at the site. The burn will heal of its own accord, without scarring. Since the skin is not burned through, this type of burn is evaluated as a partial-thickness burn.
- **Second-degree Burn**—The first layer of skin is burned through and the second layer is damaged, but the burn does not pass through to underlying tissues. There will be deep intense pain, noticeable reddening, blisters, and a mottled (spotted) appearance to the skin. Burns of this type cause swelling and blistering for 48 hours after the injury as plasma and tissue fluids are released and rise to the top layer of skin. A second-degree burn is a partial-thickness burn. Intense pain will always accompany this type of burn. When treated with reasonable care, second-degree burns will heal themselves, producing very little scarring. Infection is an important concern with second-degree burns.
- **Third-degree Burn**—This is a full-thickness burn, with all the layers of the skin damaged. Some third-degree burns are difficult to tell from second-degree burns; however, there are usually areas charred black or areas that are dry and white. The

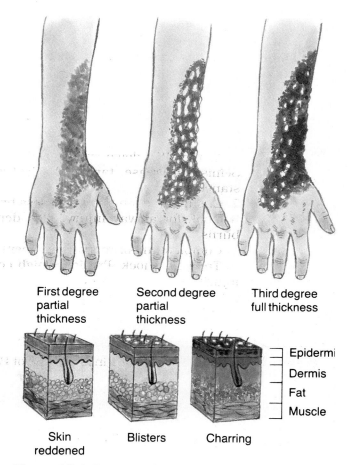

First degree partial thickness — Skin reddened

Second degree partial thickness — Blisters

Third degree full thickness — Charring

Epidermis
Dermis
Fat
Muscle

Figure 19-1 Degrees of burns.

patient may complain of severe pain, or if enough nerves have been damaged, he may not feel any pain at all (except at the periphery of the burn where adjoining second-degree burns may be causing pain). This type of burn may require skin grafting. As third-degree burns heal, dense scars form. Infection is a major concern with third-degree burns.

Severity When determining the severity of a burn, consider the following factors.

- **Agent or Source of the Burn**—The agent or source of the burn can be significant in terms of patient assessment. A burn caused by nuclear radiation may be minor but occasion other concerns about the effects of radiation on the body. Chemical burns are of special concern since the chemical may remain on the skin and continue to burn for hours or even days, eventually entering the bloodstream. This is sometimes the case with certain alkaline chemicals.

Scan 19-1
Care for Thermal Burns

STOP THE BURNING PROCESS!

1. Flame—Wet down, smother, then remove clothing.
Semisolid (grease, tar, wax)—Cool with water . . . do **not** remove substance.
2. Ensure an open airway. Assess breathing.
3. Look for airway injury: soot deposits, burnt nasal hair, and facial burns.
4. Complete the primary assessment.
5. Treat for shock. Provide a high concentration of oxygen. Treat serious injuries.

6. Evaluate Burns ⟨ Degree
Rule of Nines or Rule of Palm
Severity   Decide if special transport is needed.

Remove clothing, if necessary.

Type of Burn	Tissue Burned			Color Changes	Pain	Blisters
	Outer Layer of Skin	2nd Layer of Skin	Tissue Below Skin			
1st Degree	Yes	No	No	Red	Yes	No
2nd Degree	Yes	Yes	No	Deep Red	Yes	Yes
3rd Degree	Yes	Yes	Yes	Charred Black or White	Yes/No	Yes/No

7. Do not clear debris. Remove clothing and jewelry.
8. Wrap with dressing: Less than 9%, moisten; 9% plus, dry. (Follow local protocols.)
9A. Burns to hands or toes—Remove rings or jewelry that may constrict with swelling. Separate digits with sterile gauze pads. Moisten pads with sterile water. Apply loose dressings. Hand should be placed in position of function.
9B. Burns to the eyes—Do not open eyelids if burned. Be certain burn is thermal, not chemical. Apply moist sterile gauze pads to **both** eyes to prevent sympathetic movement of uninjured eye if only one is burned. If burn is chemical, flush eyes for 20 minutes en route to hospital.

FOLLOW LOCAL BURN CENTER PROTOCOL, AND TRANSPORT ALL BURN PATIENTS AS SOON AS POSSIBLE.

- **Body Regions Burned**—Any burn to the face is of special concern since it may involve injury to the airway or the eyes. The hands and feet also are areas of special concern because scarring may cause loss of movement of fingers or toes. Special care is required to reduce aggravation to these injury sites when moving the patient and to prevent the damaged tissues from sticking to one another. When the groin, buttocks, or medial thighs are burned, the chances for bacterial contamination present unusual problems that can be far more serious than the initial damage to the tissues.

  Circumferential burns (burns that encircle the body or a body part) can be very serious because they constrict the skin and, when they occur to an extremity, they can interrupt circulation to the distal tissues. The burn healing process can be very complicated with circumferential burns. This is particularly true when the burns occur to joints, the chest, and the abdomen where the encircling scarring tends to limit normal functions.

- **Degree of Burn**—The degree of the burn is important. In second- and third-degree burns, the outer layer of the skin is penetrated. This can lead to contamination of exposed tissues and the invasion of the circulatory system by harmful chemicals and microorganisms.

- **Extent of Burn Area**—It is important that you be able to estimate roughly the extent of the burn area. The amount of skin surface involved can be calculated quickly by using the "**Rule of Nines**" (Figure 19-2). For an adult, each of the following areas represents 9% of the body surface: the head and neck, each upper limb, the chest, the abdomen, the upper back, the lower back and buttocks, the front of each lower limb, and the back of each lower limb. These make up 99% of the body's surface. The remaining 1% is assigned to the genital region.

  The percentages are modified for infants and children, whose heads are much larger in relationship to the rest of the body than adults' heads are. The infant's or child's head and neck are counted as 18%; each upper limb, 9%; the chest and abdomen, 18%; the entire back, 18%; each lower limb, 14%; and the genital region, 1%. (This adds up to 101%, but it is only used to give a rough determination. Some systems count each lower limb as 13.5% to achieve an even 100%.)

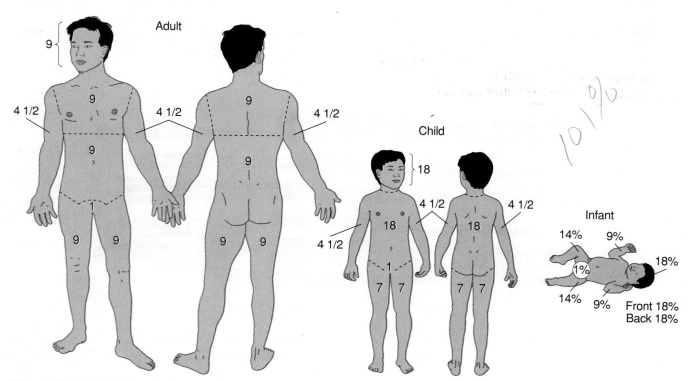

Figure 19-2 The Rule of Nines.

542 Environmental Emergencies

An alternative way to estimate the extent of a burn is the "**Rule of Palm**," which uses the *patient's* hand to approximate the surface area. The rule of palm can be applied to any patient—infant, child, or adult. Since the palm of the hand equals about 1% of the body's surface area, mentally compare the *patient's* palm with the size of the burn to estimate its extent (for example, a burn the size of five palms = 5% of the body). The rule of palm may be easier to apply to smaller or localized burns, the rule of nines to larger or more widespread burns.

- **Age of the Patient**—Age is a major factor in burn cases. Infants, children under age 5, and adults over age 60 have the most severe body reactions to burns as well as different healing patterns than other age groups. Burn intensity and body area involvement that would be classified as minor to moderate for a young adult may be fatal for the infant or an aged person. The infant and young child have a surface area that is much greater in proportion to the total body size when compared with the older child and adult. This factor means that a burn will produce a greater body fluid loss for the patient under age 5. In late adulthood, the body's ability to cope with injury is reduced by aging tissues and failing body systems. The ability of tissues to heal from any injury is lessened and the time of healing is increased. **Note:** An adult's reactions to a burn and the complications associated with burn injury healing increase significantly after age 35.

- **Other Patient Illnesses and Injuries**—Obviously, a patient with existing respiratory illnesses will be especially vulnerable to exposure to heated air or chemical vapors. Likewise, the stress of a fire or other environmental emergency will be of particular concern for patients with heart disease. Patients with respiratory ailments, heart disease, or diabetes will react more severely to burn damage. What may be a minor burn for a healthy adult could be of major significance to a patient with an existing medical condition. Similarly, the stress of a burn added to other injuries sustained during the emergency may lead to shock or other life-threatening problems that would not have resulted from the non-burn injuries or the burn alone.

Note: All burns are to be treated as more serious if accompanied by other injuries or medical problems. If you discover that the patient is hypotensive, always assume that he has other serious injuries. Attempt to determine the patient's problem through standard assessment techniques.

Classifying Severity Burns must be classified as to severity to determine the order of care, type of care, and order of transport and to supply the emergency department with as much information as possible. In some cases, the severity of the burn may determine if the patient is to be taken directly to a hospital with special burn care facilities. The following classification can be used.

Minor Burns

- Third-degree burns involving less than 2% of the body surface, excluding face, hands, feet, groin, or major joints.
- Second-degree burns that involve less than 15% of the body surface
- First-degree burns that involve less than 20% of the body surface

Moderate Burns

- Third-degree burns that involve 2% to 10% of the body surface, excluding face, hands, feet, groin, or major joints
- Second-degree burns that involve 15% to 30% of the body surface
- First-degree burns that involve 20% to 75% of the body surface

Critical Burns

- All burns complicated by injuries of the respiratory tract, other soft tissue injuries, and injuries of the bones
- Second- or third-degree burns involving the face, hands, feet, groin, or major joints
- Third-degree burns involving more than 10% of the body surface
- Second-degree burns involving more than 30% of the body surface
- First-degree burns involving more than 75% of the body surface

Treating Burns

Priorities for Burn Care A number of injuries and medical emergencies have priority over burns (Table 19-2), so the first care decision is where to place burn treatment in the

TABLE 19-2 Priorities for Emergency care

Highest Priority (Injuries)	Highest Priority (Medical Problems)
Airway obstructions	Heart attack
Severe breathing difficulties	Stroke
Burns involving the respiratory tract	Heat stroke
	Poisoning
Cardiac arrest	Abnormal childbirth
Severe bleeding	Diabetic emergencies
Shock	
Spinal injuries	
Severe head injuries	
Open chest wounds	
Open abdominal wounds	

Lower Priority (Injuries)

Burns not involving the respiratory tract
Others . . . .

sequence of emergency care. This holds true for deciding the sequence of care for the individual patient who has other injuries or medical conditions in addition to burns, as well as for deciding the order of treatment and transport at the multiple-patient scene.

Burns involving the respiratory tract are considered high-priority emergencies. This is the only burn that most EMS systems rate as highly as the other injuries and medical problems listed in Table 19-2.

Priorities for Transport Immediate transport for the individual burn patient is usually indicated for

- A patient whose burns can be classified as critical
- An infant, child, or elderly patient with deep or extensive second- or third-degree burns
- A patient with known chronic respiratory disease, heart disease, past history of stroke, or diabetes

If more than one patient is injured, transport is generally done in the order of estimated severity, with the following considerations taken into account.

- Respiratory and Cardiac Problems—Patients with respiratory tract injury, or complications involving respiration or heart action, are typically given first transport.
- Extent of Burns—Some systems next transport patients with burns covering 60% to 80% of the body surface—on the grounds that these patients have a higher chance of

survival if transported quickly than do those with burns over more than 80% of the body, for whom death is likely.

- Pain—Pain does not necessarily determine order of transport. Remember that third-degree burn patients will often have no pain due to the damage of nerve endings. While it may seem cruel to let a second-degree burn patient in pain wait, the third-degree burn patient has more serious injuries and should be transported first (if the severity is not so great that survival is unlikely).

Note: The order of patient care and transport varies according to locality. The above is only one example. Follow your local guidelines. More about the triage of patients (setting care priorities) will be discussed in Chapter 22.

Remember: If in doubt when evaluating a burn, overclassify. Should you be uncertain as to whether a burn is first-degree or second-degree, consider the burn to be second-degree. If you are uncertain as to whether a burn is second-degree or third-degree, consider it third-degree. The actual severity of some burns may not be known for several hours.

Patient Care—Thermal Burns

As an EMT you will have to care for thermal burns caused by scalding liquids, steam, contact with hot objects, flames, and flaming liquids and gases. On rare occasions, you may be called to care for sunburn, which can be severe when involving infants and young children. These patients may also have other heat-related injuries.

Emergency Care Steps

The steps for basic care of thermal burns are set forth in Scan 19-1.

Local protocols may vary somewhat. Some protocols have called for the use of a sterile burn kit that includes various-sized foam pads that can be placed over the burn area, then wrapped and held in place with clasps. A more advanced technique is the use of water-soluble gel that is applied directly to the burn area, both cooling and shutting off air to the wound. Either of these techniques is acceptable.

Another example of varying protocols: Some EMS systems state that all third-degree burns are to be wrapped with dry sterile dressing or a burn sheet., while some burn centers recommend moist dressings for partial-thickness burns to 9% or less of the body and dry dressings for more severe cases. The latter protocol is now being adopted by most EMS systems.

Table 19-3 is an example of a protocol for the field management of burn patients.

Note: EMTs must manage burns correctly until the patient can be transferred to the care of the staff of a medical facility. *Never* apply ointments, sprays, or butter (to do so would trap the heat against the burn site and the hospital staff would just have to scrape it off the burn surface). *Do not* apply ice to any burn (it can cause tissue damage). Keep the burn site clean to prevent infection. Keep the patient warm, as the temperature regulation function of the skin may be affected by the burn.

Warning: Do not attempt to rescue persons trapped by fire unless you are trained to do so and have the equipment and personnel required. The simple act of opening a door might cost you your life. In some fires, opening a door or window may greatly intensify the fire or even cause an explosion.

Patient Care—General Chemical Burns

Chemical burns require *immediate* care. It is hoped that people at the scene will begin this care before you arrive. At many industrial sites, workers and First Responders are trained to provide initial care for accidents involving the chemicals in use. Most major industries have emergency deluge-type safety showers to wash dangerous chemicals from the body. This will not always be the case. Be prepared for situations in which nothing has been done and there is no running water near the scene.

Emergency Care Steps

1 The primary care procedure is to WASH AWAY the chemical with flowing water. (One exception is dry lime. Brush it away. DO NOT WASH.) Simply wetting the burn site is not enough. Continuous flooding of the affected area is required, using a copious but gentle flow of water. Avoid hard sprays

TABLE 19-3 Maryland Protocol for Field Management of Burn Patients

1. Eliminate source of burn.
   a. Flame—Wet, smother, or remove smoldering clothing.
   b. Tar—Cool area until burning has stopped. Do not remove tar.
   c. Electrical—Remove from electrical source with nonconductive material.
   d. Chemical—Immediately wash area with copious amounts of water (for at least 10 to 20 minutes prior to transport). (Call engine company if necessary.)
2. Assess patient
   a. Airway (respiratory injury)—Look for singed nasal hairs, facial burns, soot in mouth, etc. (closed-space accident).
   b. Perform routine primary survey (be alert for associated trauma). Treat trauma as if burn did not exist. The use of PASG is appropriate when indicated for associated injuries.
   c. Obtain history (mechanism of injury and circumstances of injury).
   d. Determine depth and percent of body area burned ("rule of nines"—"rule of palm").

Note: If transfer to the Burn Center is desired, or if there is a question concerning treatment, contact Burn Center via EMS communications.

   e. Indications for transfer to Burn Center:
      (1) Second- and third-degree burns
         (a) Greater than 10% in patients under 10 or over 50 years old
         (b) Greater than 20% in other age groups
         (c) Burns of the face, hands, feet, or perineum.
      (2) Electrical burns.
      (3) Chemical burns.
3. Management
   a. Remove all jewelry and clothing necessary to evaluate burn.
   b. Wrap the patient in a clean, dry sheet.

Note: As an exception to the above, if the burn area is small (less than 9%), moist dressings for patient comfort are optional.

   c. After irrigation of chemical burns, cover with dry sheet.
   d. After initial cooling of tar, cover with dry dressings.
   e. For an inhalation injury, administer 100% oxygen per mask or nasal cannula.
4. Transport
   a. Maintain warm environment and continuously monitor vital signs.
   b. Utilize a helicopter if patient is more than 30 minutes from the Burn Center by ground.
   c. If patient has sustained an electrical injury, place patient on cardiac monitor and obtain consultation.

Special Warnings
1. Do not give patient with greater than 20% body surface area burns any fluid by mouth.
2. Do not give any medication intramuscularly, subcutaneously, or by mouth without consultation unless a cardiac emergency exists.
3. Do not place ice on any burn.

* *The Maryland Way, EMT-A Skills Manual.* Maryland Institute for Emergency Medical Services System, Baltimore, Maryland.

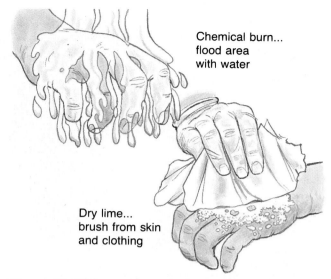

Chemical burn...
flood area
with water

Dry lime...
brush from skin
and clothing

Figure 19-3 Emergency care for chemical burns.

that may damage badly burned tissues (Figure 19-3). Continue to wash the area for at least 20 minutes, removing contaminated clothing, shoes, socks, and jewelry from the patient AS YOU APPLY THE WASH.

Warning: Protect yourself during the washing process. Wear rubber or latex gloves and control the wash to avoid splashing.

2 Apply a sterile dressing or burn sheet.
3 Treat for shock.
4 Transport.

When possible, find out the exact chemical or mixture of chemicals involved in the accident. Be on the alert for delayed reactions that may cause renewed pain or interfere with the patient's ability to breathe. Should the patient complain of increased burning or irritation, wash the burned areas again with flowing water for several minutes. Avoid removing dressings once they are in place.

Warning: Some scenes where chemical burns have taken place can be very hazardous. Always evaluate the scene. There may be large pools of dangerous chemicals around the patient. Acids could be spurting from containers. Toxic fumes may be present. If the scene will place you in danger, do not attempt a rescue unless you have been trained for such a situation and have the needed equipment and personnel at the scene.

Patient Care—Specific Chemical Burns

Some special chemical burn situations require specific care procedures.

Emergency Care Steps

☐ Mixed or Strong Acids or Unidentified Substances—Many of the chemicals used in industrial processes are mixed acids. Their combined action can be immediate and severe. The pain produced from the initial chemical burn may mask any pain being caused by renewed burning due to small concentrations left on the skin. When the chemical is a strong acid (e.g., hydrochloric acid or sulfuric acid), a combination of acids, or an unknown, play it safe and continue washing even after the patient claims he is no longer experiencing pain.

☐ Dry Lime—If dry lime is the burn agent, do not wash the burn site with water. To do so will create a corrosive liquid. Brush the dry lime from the patient's skin, hair, and clothing. Make certain that you do not contaminate the eyes or airway. Use water only after the lime has been brushed from the body, contaminated clothing and jewelry have been removed, and the process of washing can be done quickly and continuously with running water.

☐ Carbolic Acid (Phenol)—Carbolic acid does not mix with water. When available, use alcohol for the initial wash of unbroken skin, followed by a long steady wash with water. (Follow local protocols.)

☐ Sulfuric Acid—Heat is produced when water is added to concentrated sulfuric acid, but it is still preferable to wash rather than leave contaminant on the skin. An initial wash with mild soapy water can be used if the burns are not severe when you begin to provide care.

☐ Hydrofluoric Acid—Hydrofluoric acid is used for etching glass and in many other manufacturing processes. Burns from this acid may be delayed, so treat all patients who may have come into contact with the chemical, even if burns are not in evidence. First apply a bicarbonate of soda solution and then flood with water. If burning sensations are severe on your arrival, immediately begin the water wash. Do not delay care and transport to find neutralizing agents. (Follow local protocols.)

□ Inhaled Vapors—Anytime a patient is exposed to a caustic chemical and may have inhaled the vapors, provide a high concentration of oxygen (humidified, if available) and transport as soon as possible. This is very important when the chemical is an acid that is known to vaporize at standard environmental temperatures (e.g., hydrochloric acid or sulfuric acid).

Patient Care—Chemical Burns to the Eyes

A corrosive chemical can burn the globe of a person's eye before he can react and close the eyelid. Even with the lid shut, chemicals can seep through onto the globe.

Emergency Care Steps

To care for chemical burns to the eye (Figure 19-4), you should

1 IMMEDIATELY flood the eyes with water. Often the burn will involve areas of the face as well as the eye. When this is the case, you will have to flood the entire area. Avoid washing chemicals back into the eye or into an unaffected eye.

2 Keep running water from a faucet, low pressure hose, bucket, cup, bottle, rubber bulb syringe, IV setup, or other such source flowing into the burned eye.* The flow should be from the medial (nasal) corner of the eye to the lateral corner. Since the patient's natural reaction will be to keep the eyes tightly shut, you may have to hold the eyelids open.

3 Start transport and continue washing the eye for at least 20 minutes or until arrival at the medical facility.

4 After washing the eye, cover both eyes with moistened pads.

5 Wash the patient's eyes for 5 more minutes if he begins to complain about renewed burning sensations or irritation.

Warning: Do not use neutralizers such as vinegar or baking soda in a patient's eyes.

Note: For more about burns to the eyes, see Chapter 13.

*Some eye bath stations may run dirty water at first due to the age of the piping. Run water until clear.

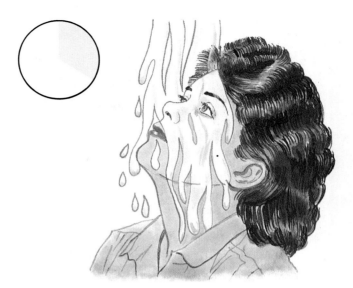

Figure 19-4 Care of chemical burns to the eyes.

Smoke Inhalation

Smoke inhalation is a serious problem associated with the scenes of thermal and chemical burns. The smoke from any fire source contains many poisonous substances. Modern building materials and furnishings often contain plastics and other synthetics that release toxic fumes when they burn or are overheated. It is possible for the substances found in smoke to burn the skin, irritate the eyes, injure the airway, cause respiratory arrest, and, in some cases, cause cardiac arrest.

Patient Assessment—Smoke Inhalation

As an EMT you will most likely find irritated (reddened, watering) eyes and, of far greater concern, injury of the airway associated with smoke.

Signs and Symptoms

Signs of an airway injured by smoke inhalation include

□ Difficulty in breathing
□ Coughing
□ Breath that has a "smoky" smell or the odor of chemicals involved at the scene.
□ Black (carbon) residue in the patient's mouth and nose. Be alert for this residue in any sputum coughed up by the patient.
□ Nose hairs singed from super-heated air

Patient Care—Smoke Inhalation

Emergency Care Steps

Smoke-caused irritations to the eyes may be treated by simple flooding with water. The first priority will be the patient's airway. In cases of smoke or toxic gas inhalation (Figure 19-5), you should

1. Move the patient to a safe area.
2. Do a primary survey and supply life support measures as needed.
3. Administer oxygen in a high concentration and continue this throughout transport. Use a humidified source if available. A nonrebreather mask is recommended.
4. Care for possible spinal injuries and any other injury or illness requiring care at the scene.
5. Provide care for shock. Most conscious patients are able to breathe more easily when kept in a semi-seated position.
6. Stay alert for behavioral changes. Some patients may try to jump up or push you aside as they recover from the effects of the smoke. Most patients become very restless. A few become violent.
7. Transport as soon as possible, monitoring the patient's vital signs.

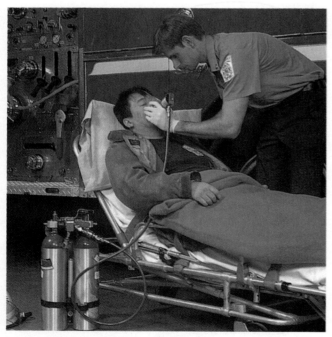

Figure 19-5 Care for smoke inhalation. Administering 100% oxygen.

Note: The body's reaction to toxic gases and foreign matter in the airway can often be delayed. Convince all smoke inhalation patients that they must be seen by a physician, even if they are not yet feeling the most serious effects.

ELECTRICAL ACCIDENTS

Warning: The scenes of injuries due to electricity are often very hazardous. Assume that the source of electricity is still active unless a qualified person tells you that the power has been turned off. *Do not* attempt a rescue unless you have been trained to do so and have the necessary equipment and personnel. For information about electrical hazards at the scene of a vehicle collision, see Chapter 29.

Electric current, including lightning, can cause severe damage to the body. The skin is burned where the energy enters the body and where it flows into a ground. Along the path of this flow, tissues are damaged due to heat. In addition, significant chemical changes take place in the nerves, heart, and muscles, and body processes are disrupted or completely shut down.

Patient Assessment—Electrical Injuries

Signs and Symptoms

The victim of an electrical accident may have any or all of the following signs and symptoms (Figure 19-6).

- Burns where the energy enters and exits the body
- Disrupted nerve pathways displayed as paralysis
- Muscle tenderness, with or without muscular twitching
- Respiratory difficulties or arrest (the tongue may swell and obstruct the airway)
- Irregular heartbeat or cardiac arrest
- Elevated blood pressure or low blood pressure with the signs and symptoms of shock
- Restlessness or irritability if conscious, or loss of consciousness
- Visual difficulties
- Fractured bones and dislocations from severe muscle contractions or from falling. This can include the spinal column.
- Seizures (in severe cases)

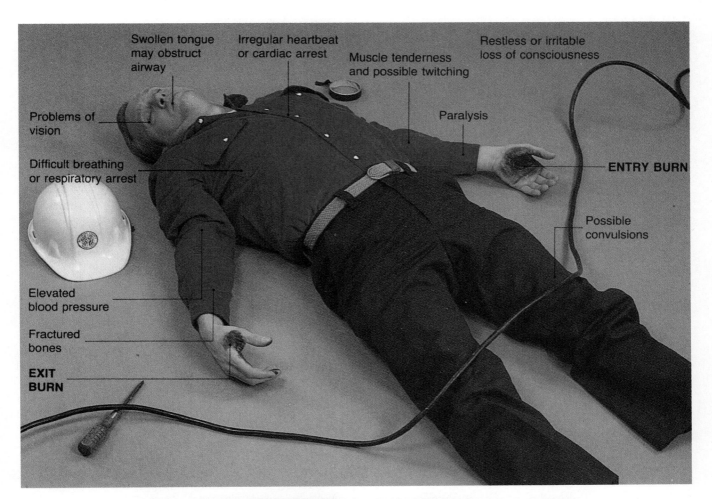

Swollen tongue may obstruct airway

Irregular heartbeat or cardiac arrest

Muscle tenderness and possible twitching

Restless or irritable loss of consciousness

Problems of vision

Paralysis

Difficult breathing or respiratory arrest

ENTRY BURN

Possible convulsions

Elevated blood pressure

Fractured bones

EXIT BURN

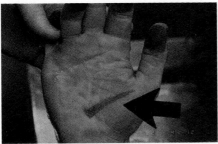
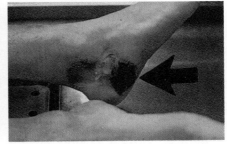

Figure 19-6 Injuries due to electrical shock.

Patient Care—Electrical Injuries

Emergency Care Steps

1. Make certain that you and the patient are in a SAFE ZONE (not in contact with any electrical source and outside the area where downed or broken wires or other sources of electricity can reach you).
2. Provide airway care (remembering that electrical shock may cause severe swelling along the airway).
3. Provide basic cardiac life support as required.
4. Care for spinal injuries, head injuries, and severe fractures.
5. Evaluate electrical burns, looking for at least two external burn sites: contact with the energy source and contact with a ground.
6. Cool the burn areas and smoldering clothing the same as you would for a flame burn.
7. Apply dry sterile dressings to the burn sites.

⑧ Care for shock and administer high concentration oxygen.

⑨ Transport as soon as possible. Some problems have a slow onset. If there are burns, there also may be more serious hidden problems. In any case of electrical shock, heart problems may develop.

Remember: The major problem caused by electrical shock is usually not the burn. Respiratory and cardiac arrest are real possibilities. Be prepared to provide basic cardiac life support measures.

HAZARDOUS MATERIALS

Warning: *Do not* attempt a rescue when an accident involves hazardous materials unless you have been trained to do so, have the needed equipment, and have the personnel necessary to ensure a safe scene. Many excellent courses are offered in hazardous materials. As an EMT you would do well to take a hazardous materials course as part of your continuing education. You should follow the guidelines set by the U.S. Department of Transportation (DOT), the Occupational Safety and Health Administration (OSHA), and the National Fire Protection Association (NFPA), as well as your community's emergency response plan for hazardous materials.

According to the DOT, a hazardous material is "any substance or material in a form which poses an unreasonable risk to health, safety and property when transported in commerce." One of the undesirable aspects of our modern world is the growing number of such materials (Table 19-4). They are needed for the industrial manufacturing of essential and beneficial products. Hazardous materials also can be the waste products of manufacturing. Even though safety procedures have been established and are followed for the most part, accidents involving hazardous materials do occur. They are especially likely to take place at factories, along railroads, and on local, state, and federal highways.

You must understand that as an EMT, you will be highly skilled in emergency care. However, without specialized training, you are still a layperson when it comes to hazardous materials. Special training is required to understand hazardous materials, to work at the scene of accidents involving these materials, and to render the scene safe. You cannot judge the state of a container or the probability of explosion without

TABLE 19-4   Examples of Hazardous Materials

Material	Possible Hazard
Benzene (benzol)	Toxic vapors; can be absorbed through the skin; destroys bone marrow.
Benzoyl peroxide	Fire and explosion.
Carbon tetrachloride	Damages internal organs.
Cyclohexane	Explosive; eye and throat irritant.
Diethyl ether	Flammable; can be explosive; irritant to eyes and respiratory tract; can cause drowsiness or unconsciousness.
Ethyl acetate	Irritates eyes and respiratory tract.
Ethylene dichloride	Strong irritant.
Heptane	Respiratory irritant.
Hydrochloric acid	Respiratory irritant; exposure to high concentration of vapors can produce pulmonary edema; can damage skin and eyes.
Hydrofluoric acid	Vapors can cause pulmonary edema and severe eye burns; vapors and liquid can burn skin; vapors can be lethal. There may be delayed reactions.
Hydrogen cyanide	Highly flammable; very toxic through inhalation or absorption.
Methyl isobutyl ketone (hexose)	Irritates eyes and mucus membranes.
Methylene chloride	Damages eyes.
Nitric acid	Produces a toxic gas (nitrogen dioxide); skin irritant; can cause self-ignition of cellulose products (e.g., sawdust).
Organochloride (Chlordane, DDT, Dieldrin, Lindane, Methoxychlor)	Irritates eyes and skin; fumes and smoke are toxic.
Perchloroethylene	Toxic if inhaled or swallowed.
Silicon tetrachloride	Water-reactive to form toxic hydrogen chloride fumes.
Tetrahydrofuram (THF)	Damages eyes and mucus membranes.
Toluol (toluene)	Toxic vapors; can cause organ damage.
Vinyl chloride	Flammable and explosive; listed as a carcinogen.

the benefit of specialized training. Do not believe that you can use safety equipment unless you have been trained in the care, field testing, and actual use of the equipment. With hazardous material accidents, you may be able to do nothing more than stay a safe distance away from the scene until expert help arrives.

On Arrival

As a responding EMT, you may be the first to recognize that a hazardous materials situation exists. For example, you may answer a call to a business where four employees are ill after being in the warehouse. When there are multiple medical victims, think "hazmat."

Should you arrive first at the scene of a hazardous materials accident, ESTABLISH A "DANGER ZONE" AND A "SAFE ZONE." Keep all people out of the danger zone, and try to convince them to leave the immediate area. Stay in the safe zone until expert help arrives and makes other areas safe to enter.

The safe zone should be on the same level as, and upwind from, the accident site. Avoid being downhill in case there are flowing liquids or gases that are burning or otherwise unsafe. Avoid any low-lying area in case fumes are escaping and hanging close to the ground. Avoid placing yourself higher than the accident scene so that you will not be in the path of escaping gases or heated air. Also be alert to the fact that a sewer system can rapidly spread the hazardous materials over a large area.

CALL FOR THE HELP THAT YOU WILL NEED. The support services required at the scene of a hazardous materials accident may include fire services, special rescue personnel, local or state hazardous materials experts, and law enforcement personnel for crowd control. If the accident has taken place at an industrial site or along a railway, the company experts in hazardous materials need to be notified. Much of this can be done by a single call to your dispatcher. (See also Table 19-5 and "Sources of Information," below.)

Local backup support will want to know certain facts, including

- Type of hazardous material: gas, liquid chemical, cooled chemical, dry chemical, radioactive liquid, radioactive gases, or solid radioactive materials
- Specific name of the material, or its identification number
- How much material is at the scene
- Current state of the material: escaping as a gas, leaking as a liquid, being blown into the air, in flames, or apparently still contained

TABLE 19-5 Hazardous Materials Hotlines

Organizations	24-Hour Hotline Numbers
CHEMTREC (Chemical Transportation Emergency Center, Washington, D.C.)	800-424-9300 202-483-7616
REAC/TS (Radiation Emergency Assistance Center/Training Site, Oak Ridge, Tennessee)	615-482-2441

- How long you estimate that the scene has been dangerous (when did the incident begin?)
- Other hazardous materials near the scene
- Estimated number of possible patients in the danger zone

Sources of Information

Vehicle drivers, plant and railroad personnel, and perhaps even bystanders may be able to tell you the name of the hazardous material. In many cases, there will be a colored placard (Figure 19-7) on the vehicle, tank, or railroad car. This placard will have a four-digit identification number. Older placards are usually orange and have an identification number preceded by the letters UN or UA. Your dispatcher may have access to the name of the material through this identification number. There also may be an invoice, shipping manifest (trains), or bill of lading (trucks) that can confirm the identity of the substance.

Figure 19-7 Hazardous materials placard.

Warning: *Do not* approach the scene to obtain this information. Placard information may be obtainable from a safe distance by observation with binoculars.

The Chemical Transportation Emergency Center (CHEMTREC) has been established in Washington, D.C. by the Chemical Manufacturers Association. They can provide your dispatcher or you with information about the hazardous material. They have a 24-hour, toll-free telephone number for the continental United States: 800-424-9300. In the Washington, D.C. area, the 24-hour number is 202-483-7616. CHEMTREC will accept collect calls in an emergency. When you call, keep the line open so that changes in the scene can be reported to CHEMTREC and the center can confirm that they have contacted the shipper or manufacturer. CHEMTREC will be able to direct you as to your initial course of action.

If there is no identification number and no one knows what is being carried, you may have no other choice than to wait for experts to arrive at the scene.

Warning: Recent studies by the Office of Technology Assessment have shown that some states report 25% to 50% of the identification placards have been found to be incorrect. These same studies indicate that many shipping documents also are inaccurate or incomplete. Do only what you have been trained to do, following the directions of hazardous materials experts.

Initial actions at the scene can be directed according to information sent to you by your dispatcher, hazardous materials expert, or CHEMTREC. Often, this initial action is based on the procedures presented in *Hazardous Materials, The Emergency Response Guidebook* (DOT P 5800.2), published by the United States Department of Transportation. When you call your dispatcher or CHEMTREC

1. Give your name and call back number.
2. Explain the nature and location of the problem.
3. Report the identification number if there is a safe way for you to obtain this information.
4. When possible, supply the name of the shipper or manufacturer.
5. Describe the type of container.
6. Report if the container is on rail car, truck, open storage, or housed storage.
7. Give the carrier's name and the name of the consignee.

8. Report local conditions, including the weather.
9. Keep the line of communication open at all times.

Rescue and Care Procedures

During the entire process, you must stay in a safe area. *Do not* walk in any spilled materials. *Do not* think that the scene is safe simply because the substance does not have any apparent color or odor. Keep people away from the scene.

As soon as possible, decide who will take charge of the scene. If this has not been decided in planning sessions prior to the incident, you or another professional at the scene should become the incident commander (IC) until experts arrive to take over responsibility.

After a safe zone is created, you may do the following, if trained to do so.

1. Put on 100% full-body protective clothing (Figure 19-8) and a self-contained breathing apparatus (you must know how to check out and properly wear such equipment).
2. Isolate the accident area and keep the safe zone clear of unauthorized and unprotected personnel.
3. Evaluate the scene in terms of possible fire or explosion (this takes special training).

Patient Assessment— Hazardous Material Injuries

Follow normal primary and secondary survey procedures, including patient and bystander interviews, to assess injuries. Do not overlook medical conditions and injuries that may be present in addition to burns and/or other immediate effects of the hazardous material.

Patient Care—Hazardous Material Injuries

As soon as it is safe to do so (expert judgment is required to determine this), begin assessment and care of patients.

Emergency Care Steps

1 Move any patients as quickly as possible if the scene is still potentially dangerous. Note that this is the kind of situation in which an emergency move of patients may need to be executed before assessment and

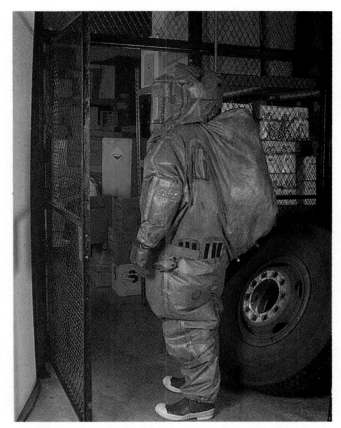

Figure 19-8 Special equipment and knowledge of its use are required at a hazardous material accident.

care can begin. (Such emergency moves are described in Chapter 25.) If, and only if, the experts assure you that the scene offers no immediate danger, begin life support measures within the danger zone.

2 Provide basic life support. For pulmonary resuscitation and CPR, use oxygen with a demand valve or a bag-valve mask and oxygen reservoir so that you do not have to take off your own protective gear.

3 Administer a high concentration of oxygen to any patient having difficulty breathing.

4 IMMEDIATELY flush with water the skin, clothing, and eyes of anyone who has come into contact with the hazardous material. Retain the run-off.

5 Remove clothing, shoes, and jewelry from all persons who have come into contact with the hazardous material. Continue flushing the person's skin with water for no less than 20 minutes, continuing to retain run-off.

6 Remove your protective gear as recommended by local guidelines.

7 Transport the patient(s) as soon as possible, providing care for shock, administering oxygen, and taking all steps necessary to maintain normal body temperature.

Warning: Do not neglect to decontaminate or to be sure others with the proper training have decontaminated the patient prior to transport. Otherwise the ambulance crew may be overcome en route and patient and EMTs can contaminate and even shut down the emergency department.

Remember: Some materials will allow you to act, while others will require experts to respond before you can gain access and provide care. This is why you need to provide your dispatcher with all the information available—so you can receive proper information about whether and when to proceed. Remember, you are an EMT, not an expert in hazardous materials.

RADIATION ACCIDENTS

Warning: An EMT is not expected to be an expert in radiation accidents. Do only what you have been trained to do. Every state has a procedure for emergency services to follow when radioactive substances are involved in an accident. All emergency care personnel must learn and understand these procedures, especially if duties are performed in heavily traveled transportation corridors.

Radiation is a general term that applies to the transmission of energy. This can include nuclear energy, ultraviolet light, visible light, heat, sound, and x-rays. When we speak of radiation accidents, we are referring to **ionizing radiation**. This radiation is from an atomic source and is used to generate electricity, provide isotopes for medicine and industry, and make nuclear weapons. Whenever atomic materials are made or used, there is a certain amount of waste material and contaminated material produced. The sources of radiation seen in accidents include not only radioactive materials in use but also radioactive waste materials.

In most cases of radiation accidents, industrial experts will be promptly available to provide you with instructions for your safety and the care of the patient. Away from the industrial site, local rescue experts or state and federal officials may direct your activities. When in doubt, call your dispatcher to secure directions. Advice on how to handle a radiation accident

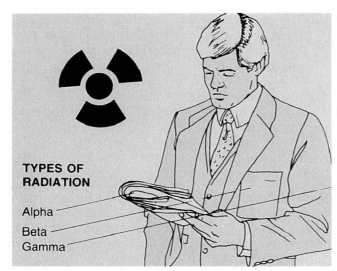
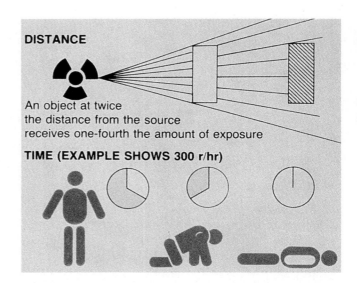

Figure 19-9 Factors determining radiation received.

can also be obtained by calling the Radiation Emergency Assistance Center/Training Site (REAC/TS) in Oak Ridge, Tennessee. Its 24-hour hotline number is 615-482-2441.

Types of Radiation

The three major types of ionizing radiation are alpha particles, beta particles, and gamma rays. Neutrons are a fourth type, but neutron radiation is primarily associated with nuclear reactor fuels and is rarely encountered.

- *Alpha particles* do little damage since they can be absorbed (stopped) by a layer of clothing, a few inches of air, paper, or the outer layer of skin. This is a low-energy source of radiation.
- *Beta particles* are higher in energy level and cannot be stopped by clothing (including turnout gear). The danger of exposure to alpha and beta radiation cannot be taken lightly. Irradiated dust particles and smoke can be inhaled into the lungs, particles can contaminate open wounds, and irradiated foodstuffs can be ingested. Once inside the body, they continue to cause cell damage until they are removed or until they decay.
- *Gamma rays and x-rays* can be considered the same thing. Gamma radiation is extremely dangerous, carrying high levels of energy able to penetrate thick shielding. The rays easily pass through clothing and the entire body, inflicting extensive cell damage.
- *Neutrons* can penetrate deep within the tis-

sues and cause serious tissue damage and death.

Since ionizing radiation cannot be seen, felt, or heard, some sort of detection instrument is needed to measure the radiation given off by a radiation source. The most commonly used device is the Geiger counter. The rate of radiation is measured in roentgens (RENT-gens) per hour (R/hr) or milliroentgens per hour (mR/hr) (1,000 mR = 1 R).

Effects of Radiation on the Body

Simply stated, ionizing radiation causes changes in the body cells. Gastrointestinal symptoms of nausea, vomiting, and/or diarrhea may present as the earliest symptoms. If enough radiation is absorbed, leukemia and other cancers may result. Certain extremely high dosages can cause death.

Determining exposure, absorption, and damage done by radiation requires highly specialized training. Look at the problem in a practical manner. If you are working for one hour in an area where the Geiger counter reading is 100 R/hr, you will probably tolerate the dose with no ill effects. Should your exposure be 200 R/hr, you may become ill. Increase this to 300 R/hr and you will become very ill. At 400 R/hr, you will probably die in a short time.

How much radiation a person receives depends on the source of radiation, the length of time exposed, the distance from the source, and the shielding between the person and the source (Figure 19-9). The amount of radiation at the patient's initial location may be 300 R/hr. If you are only exposed for 20 minutes, this is the same radiation equivalent as working one hour at a 100 R/hr scene. The amount of radiation may drop off quickly as the patient is decontaminated and as you move the patient away from his initial position. If you wear protective gear, the amount of radiation absorbed will be considerably less than the Geiger counter reading.

Keep in mind that if care requires 60 minutes at a scene of 300 R/hr, three EMTs can take turns providing the care, provided that they are under the direction of a radiation expert. Each EMT will be exposed for only 20 minutes, so the exposure per person does not exceed the equivalent of working for 1 hour at 100 R/hr.

Types of Radiation Accidents

As an EMT, you may respond to two types of radiation accidents: clean and dirty.

In the **clean accident**, the patient is exposed to radiation but is not contaminated by the radioactive substance, particles of radioactive dust, or radioactive liquids, gases, or smoke. If the patient has not been contaminated or is properly decontaminated before you arrive, there is little danger to you, provided that the source of radiation is no longer exposed at the scene. The body itself does not become radioactive.

The **dirty accident**, often associated with fire at the scene of a radiation accident, exposes the patient to radiation and contaminates him with radioactive particles or liquids. The scene may be highly contaminated, even though the primary source of radiation is shielded when you arrive. If you are the first to arrive, you may have to wait for technical assistance unless you have radiation detection instruments and know how to use them. Otherwise, what you consider to be a clean accident may actually be a dirty one.

On Arrival

To perform your duties at the scene, you should

1. Protect yourself from exposure.
2. Note any hazard labels that indicate there may be a radiation hazard.
3. Alert your dispatcher so you can obtain expert assistance.
4. Carry out those rescue procedures you are trained to do when appropriate equipment is at the scene.
5. Provide emergency care for the decontaminated patient.
6. Help prevent the spread of radiation through the control of contaminated articles.

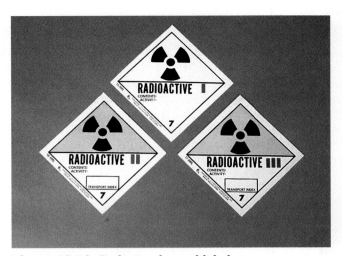

Figure 19-10 Radiation hazard labels.

When arriving at the scene, look for RADIATION HAZARD LABELS (Figure 19-10). These labels have a purple or black "propeller" on a yellow background. Notify your dispatcher immediately to inform the proper authorities and to send technical assistance to the scene. If your dispatcher tells you to leave the scene, or if a radiation expert tells you to leave, do so promptly and safely. Otherwise, park upwind, as far from the scene as practical, behind any shielding of considerable mass. Thick metal or concrete walls, earth banks, and even heavy vehicles and construction equipment offer some additional shielding.

Rescue and Care Procedures

You will have to wait for technical assistance unless you are trained to measure the radiation level and have the proper protective clothing and breathing equipment to allow a rescue. If you are trained to rescue the patient, remember to approach from upwind, avoiding when possible any dust clouds or smoke. If radiation levels are high, extricate the patient as quickly as possible, even when this means no survey, no immediate basic life support, and no splinting "where he lies." The rule is to "get in and out quickly." (Again, see the information on emergency moves in Chapter 25.)

Patient Assessment—Radiation Injuries

Determine if the accident is clean or dirty. If it is dirty, and until the patient has been decontaminated, carry out all assessment procedures while wearing full protective clothing.

Assessment will, of course, involve determining—with the help of on-the-scene experts—to what degree the patient has been contaminated with radioactive particles or liquids. However, do not neglect to do a complete patient assessment to detect any life-threatening conditions or additional medical conditions or injuries.

Patient Care—Radiation Injuries

If the accident is dirty, the patient must be decontaminated. While you are wearing full protective clothing

1. Move the patient to the edge of the ACCIDENT ZONE (this is determined by local standards).
2. Quickly remove the patient's clothing, shoes, and jewelry. If possible, place these articles in a plastic bag and place the bag in a metal container that has a tightly fitting lid.
3. If radioactive material remaining on the patient's skin exceeds local limits, *do not* remove your own protective clothing while you are caring for the patient.
4. Once the patient's contaminated clothing and jewelry has been removed and if you can be certain there is no contaminated material remaining on the patient's skin, you may remove your own protective garments and breathing apparatus. Bag these articles and place them in the container and close the lid. Some breathing apparatus may be too large to fit in this container. If this is the case, leave the apparatus next to the container. Make certain that someone guards this container so that it can be removed properly.

Whether the patient is or is not contaminated, do not delay care. Both before and after you are able to remove your protective clothing, carry out care procedures as indicated by your patient assessment as rapidly and carefully as you would in any emergency situation. Follow the guidelines for the four types of radiation accident patients described below.

☐ *Clean/patient received an external dose of*

radiation. THE PATIENT IS NO DANGER TO THE EMT.
☐ *Dirty/patient received an internal dose of radiation.* AFTER EXTERNAL CLEANSING, THE PATIENT IS NO DANGER TO THE EMT. Should rescue breathing be required before decontamination, use oxygen and a positive-pressure ventilator or a bag-valve mask unit with oxygen reservoir so that you do not need to remove any protective face- or headgear in order to provide breaths directly to the patient.
☐ *Dirty/patient externally contaminated.* THERE IS DANGER TO THE EMT. Basic life support and care for life-threatening problems, if needed, is both possible and mandatory. Keep on all of your protective clothing to avoid contact. Use oxygen with a positive-pressure ventilator or a bag-valve mask unit for rescue breathing.
☐ *Dirty/external surface contamination and wounds.* THERE IS DANGER TO THE EMT. Take care not to contaminate yourself during care. Use oxygen with a positive-pressure ventilator or a bag-valve mask unit if rescue breathing is required. Wounds should not be cleaned in the field. Dress the wounds.

Anytime that a patient is suspected of having received internal contamination, save all vomitus and body wastes for transport. Keep them in a sealed, properly labeled metal container. Label the container. Take nothing from the scene unless directed to do so by the radiation officer in charge.

Remember: NEVER SACRIFICE PATIENT CARE to decontaminating the patient. People rarely die from the effects of radiation; they die because their life-threatening injuries have been left unattended. Basic life support can usually be rendered before the patient is decontaminated if you keep your protective clothing on to avoid direct contact with the patient.

Decontamination and Transport

Before you transport a contaminated patient, he should be washed, if his medical condition permits. Ask for a safe area to do this that will be guarded in case of contaminated water runoff. Before transport, cover the ambulance stretcher mattress with a blanket. Wrap the patient in the blanket and fashion a head covering from a towel. Only the patient's face should show when he is ready for transport. Transport the patient to the medical facility in accordance with your local radiation accident plan. Radio ahead to alert the staff to the situation.

Decontamination or disposal of the equipment and clothing left at the scene will be done by those in charge of the radiation accident. Your ambulance, clothing, and supplies will be decontaminated by radiation experts. This is one reason why keeping an accurate ambulance equipment and supply inventory is so important. The experts must know what you used at the scene. You may be asked to help in the process, but you do not have the training to ensure a proper job by yourself.

This leaves the most important decontamination procedure—your own personal decontamination. Shower thoroughly or otherwise decontaminate yourself in accordance with your local radiation emergency plan. Have yourself checked by radiation experts and a physician.

Note: There is always some degree of risk when providing care at the radiation accident scene and when trying to provide care for the contaminated patient. BE CERTAIN TO FOLLOW ALL LOCAL GUIDELINES TO THE LETTER.

EXPLOSIONS

Fire and hazardous materials often lead to explosions. An explosion is defined as the rapid release of energy. The magnitude of an explosion depends on several factors, including the type of explosive agent, the space in which the agent is detonated, and the degree of confinement of the explosion.

The damage done is a result of the shock wave that is generated during the release of energy. As the wave extends outward in all directions, two types of pressure are generated. *Overpressure* is the pressure increase above the normal atmospheric pressure. Overpressure surrounds an object as the shock wave hits it and tends to crush the object inward. *Dynamic pressure* may be compared to a strong wind, striking each object in its path as the shock wave moves outward. Objects are pushed over or torn apart, and debris is picked up and propelled outward.

Patient Assessment—Explosion Injuries

Injury is usually related to the distance from the point of detonation. The closer the victim, the more injuries. Explosions generally cause blunt trauma from the shock wave. Penetrating trauma can result from flying shrapnel. When assessing the patient, be alert for the following typical explosion injuries.

- ☐ Ruptured ear drum
- ☐ Ruptured internal organs
- ☐ Internal bleeding
- ☐ Contusions of the lungs (due to rapid pressure changes)
- ☐ Burns
- ☐ Lacerations
- ☐ Impaled objects
- ☐ Fractures
- ☐ Crush injuries
- ☐ Severe respiratory system damage and thermal burns resulting from superheated air that can be produced by an explosion

Remember: Most of the major injuries typical of explosions can only be detected in the course of a thorough patient assessment. There may be a delay in the appearance of some serious injuries while transporting. Always assume that there are internal injuries.

Patient Care—Explosion Injuries

Basic life support is the first priority of care. Carry out other patient care and transport as indicated by your patient assessment and by local protocols for triage if the explosion is a multiple patient situation.

CHAPTER REVIEW

KEY TERMS

You may find it helpful to review the following terms.

clean accident—a radiation accident in which the patient is exposed to radiation but is not contaminated by any radioactive particles or liquids.

dirty accident—a radiation accident in which the patient is not only exposed to radiation but is also contaminated by radioactive particles or liquids.

first-degree burn—a burn involving only the epidermis.

ionizing radiation—the product of atomic decay, including alpha particles, beta particles, and gamma rays.

Rule of Nines—a method for estimating the extent of a burn. For an adult, each of the following areas represents 9% of the body surface: the head and neck, each upper limb, the chest, the abdomen, the upper back, the lower back and buttocks, the front of each lower limb, and the back of each lower limb. The remaining 1% is assigned to the genital region. For an infant or child the percentages are modified so that 18% is assigned to the head, 14% to each lower limb.

Rule of Palm—a method for estimating the extent of a burn. The palm of the hand, which equals about 1% of the body's surface area, is compared with the patient's burn to estimate its size.

second-degree burn—a burn involving the epidermis and the dermis but not penetrating through the dermis.

third-degree burn—a full-thickness burn with damage extending through the dermis.

SUMMARY

Environmental Injuries

Environmental injuries often include injuries to the skin, eyes, and airway, but also, in some circumstances, to the organs and cells of the body.

EMTs are not usually trained to control hazardous scenes and must wait for specially trained rescuers to do so. The EMT must not do more than he or she has been trained to do.

Burns

Burns can be caused by heat (thermal), chemicals, electricity, light, and radiation. As an EMT, you must be able to classify burns in terms of first-, second-, and third-degree. When in doubt, OVERCLASSIFY; consider a questionable first-degree burn to be second degree and a questionable second-degree burn to be third degree.

You must also be able to evaluate the severity of a burn, keeping in mind the agent and source, the body regions that are burned (burns to the face, hands and feet, and circumferential burns are especially serious), the degree of the burn, the extent of the burn area (using the Rule of Nines or Rule of Palm to estimate the percentage of the body that is burned), the age of the patient (burns are more serious for children and the elderly), and whether the patient may have other injuries or medical conditions. The severity of burns may be classified as minor, moderate, or critical.

Unless the burn involves the respiratory tract, a burn will usually have a lower priority for treatment than other life-threatening injuries and medical conditions. Among burn patients, those with the most severe burns are usually transported first with one exception: those whose burns are so extensive that they are likely to die will usually be transported after those with less extensive burns who are likely to survive with immediate transport.

In caring for a thermal burn, after stopping the burning process, ensure an open airway, assess breathing, complete the patient assessment, treat for shock, remove clothing and jewelry, dress the burn, and transport.

The primary care procedure for chemical burns is to wash away the chemical with flowing water for at least 20 minutes. An exception is dry lime which must be brushed, not washed, away. Carbolic acid (phenol) burns should first be washed with alcohol. Sulfuric acid burns may first be washed with mild soapy water. Hydrofluoric acid burns may first be neutralized with bicarbonate of soda. Patients who have inhaled chemical vapors should be provided a high concentration of humidified oxygen. When the chemical is mixed or unknown continue washing with water even after the patient no longer feels pain. For chemical burns to the eyes, flood the eyes with water, then cover with moistened pads.

Victims of smoke inhalation (signs include difficulty in breathing, coughing, breath that smells smoky or smells of the hazardous material that burned, black residue in the mouth or nose) should be provided a high concentration of oxygen, care for shock, and transport. Also assess for other injuries and stay alert for behavioral changes.

Electrical Accidents

For patients with electrical burns, your primary concern should be to assess and care for respiratory and cardiac difficulties. Look for at least two external burn sites, where the electricity entered and exited the body. Apply sterile or clean dressings, provide care for shock, and transport.

Hazardous Materials

Hazardous materials should be handled by experts. Learn to look for hazardous materials placards. Provide care only when safe to do so. If trained to do so, establish a safe zone and call for the help that you will need. When you can provide care, direct your attentions to basic life support and decontamination of the patient.

Radiation Accidents

Radiation accidents are generally those involving ionizing radiation, which is radiation from an atomic source such as nuclear materials or wastes. Four types of ionizing radiation involve alpha particles, beta particles, gamma rays or x-rays, and neutrons. Some radiation accidents are clean (the patients have been exposed to radiation but have not been contaminated with any radioactive particles or liquids) or dirty (the patients have been contaminated with radioactive particles or liquids, usually when there has been a fire or explosion).

Radiation accidents require expert assistance. Learn to look for radiation hazard labels. Alert your dispatcher and request the help that you will need. Park in a shielded area, wear protective clothing, and use a protective breathing apparatus. Once cleared to do so get in and out quickly. Remove the patient's jewelry and clothing and, when you are sure the patient is no longer contaminated, remove your contaminated gear. Place all contaminated items into a container with a tightly fitting lid. Provide assessment and care as you would for any patient. If rescue breathing is required for a contaminated patient, use oxygen and a positive-pressure ventilator or a bag-valve mask unit with oxygen reservoir so that you do not have to remove your protective gear. If possible, wash the patient to decontaminate him before transport. Follow local protocols to decontaminate yourself.

Explosions

Explosions can cause serious multiple injuries. Basic life support is the priority in care. A complete patient assessment is essential to detect possible multiple injuries and to provide the proper care.

On the Scene

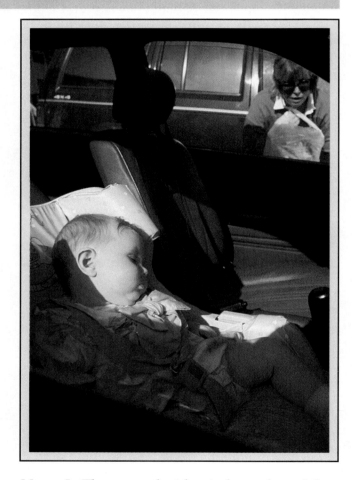

Mary Jo Thurman decides to leave her eighteen-month-old daughter Katie in the car while she runs into the market. Wanting to be careful, she parks near the door where she can see the car. Since it's a hot day, she also rolls the windows down "a crack." She doesn't intend to be gone long.

When she returns to the car and opens the door, she feels a burst of heat from inside the vehicle. Katie is asleep—or is she unconscious? Mary Jo tries to wake Katie, but the child doesn't respond. Mary Jo yells for help, and someone runs into the store to call 911.

As your ambulance pulls into the parking lot, Mary Jo runs to you, looking frantic.

Mary Jo: Help! Please help! My daughter is unconscious! The car got too hot. I didn't think it would get hot so fast.

Your small patient's skin is hot and dry to your touch. Realizing that this is most likely a heat-related emergency, you begin to act.

You (to Mary Jo): Yes, ma'am. We'll help your little girl. (To your partner) Turn on the air conditioning in the rig. I'll bring the child right over.

Mary Jo: Is she going to be all right?

You: We're going to get her into the cooler ambulance and check her out. Does she have any medical problems or conditions?

Mary Jo: No. No. Nothing.

You carefully lift Katie from the car, still in her car seat. You briefly observe her ABCs while removing her and find that she has deep respirations and a full, rapid pulse. At the ambulance, your partner has prepared lukewarm water to begin cooling the child. Mary Jo also climbs into the front of the ambulance for the trip to the hospital.

After Katie's temperature starts to drop, she begins to cry. So does her mother.

Heat, Cold, Water, and Ice

Chapter Overview

Our environment is the air—and occasionally the water or ice—around us. At times that environment is too hot or too cold for the body to sustain its normal internal temperature range. At the extremes, this can lead to death. Recreational and other activities in, on, or near the water or ice are also often associated with accidental injuries and medical problems.

Injuries or medical problems caused by or associated with excessive heat, excessive cold, water, or ice are environmental emergencies that EMTs must be able to recognize, assess, and treat in the prehospital setting.

Expected Outcome, Chapter 20: *You will be able to perform basic water and ice rescues and assess and provide emergency care for emergencies related to heat, cold, water, and ice.*

Warning: Protect yourself from infectious diseases by using appropriate barrier devices such as a pocket face mask with one-way valve, face shield, or bag-valve mask; goggles or eye shield; and disposable gloves. Always conform to your local EMS system's infection exposure control plan.

EMERGENCIES DUE TO EXCESSIVE HEAT
    Common Heat Emergencies

EMERGENCIES DUE TO EXCESSIVE COLD
    Local Cooling (Frostbite)
    General Cooling (Hypothermia)
    Other Cold-Related Emergencies

ACCIDENTS INVOLVING WATER
    Water-Related Accidents
    Drowning and Near-Drowning
    Water Rescues
    Emergency Care for Water-Related Accidents
    Diving Accidents

ACCIDENTS INVOLVING ICE
    Ice Rescues
    Emergency Care for Ice-Related Accidents

Objectives

Knowledge *After reading this chapter, you should be able to*

1. Distinguish between heat cramps, heat exhaustion, and heat stroke. (pp. 563-564; Scan 20-1)

2. List the steps in caring for heat-related emergencies. (p. 564)

3. State how to distinguish between frostnip, frostbite, and freezing. (pp. 566-567; Table 20-1)

4. Describe emergency care for frostnip, frostbite, and freezing. (pp. 567-568)

5. State the signs and symptoms of hypothermia. (pp. 568-569; Table 20-2)

6. Distinguish between mild, severe, and extreme hypothermia. (p. 569)

7. Describe the care procedures for mild, severe, and extreme hypothermia. (pp. 569-571)

8. Describe the signs and symptoms and compare care for chilblains and trench foot. (p. 571)

9. List the common types of injuries associated with swimming and diving accidents. (p. 572)

10. Distinguish between fresh water drowning and salt water drowning and between near-drowning and drowning. (p. 573)

11. List, in correct order, the methods to use when attempting to rescue someone from the water. (pp. 573-575)

12. Describe techniques for providing rescue breathing and care for possible spinal injuries in the water. (pp. 575-577; Scan 20-2)

13. State the basic order of care procedures for near-drowning patients who are out of the water. (p. 577)

14. Describe the basic assessment and care for diving board accident patients. (p. 577)

15. Describe two special types of problems people develop as a result of scuba diving accidents and describe the assessment and care for each type of problem. (pp. 578-579)

16. Describe basic ice rescue, assessment, and care procedures. (pp. 579-580)

Skills *As an EMT you should be able to*

1. Assess and care for problems associated with excessive heat.

2. Assess and care for problems associated with excessive cold.

3. Perform basic water and ice rescues.

4. Evaluate a patient who is the victim of a swimming or diving accident.

5. Apply resuscitation skills and other basic life support measures to the near-drowning patient and to the diving accident patient.

The body's chemical activities take place in a limited temperature range. They cannot occur with the efficiency needed for life if the body temperature is too high or too low. The body's own chemical processes generate heat, but the temperature and other characteristics of the environment also cause the body temperature to rise or fall. Air, water, and ice are environmental elements that can affect the body.

EMERGENCIES DUE TO EXCESSIVE HEAT

The body generates heat as a result of its constant internal chemical processes. A certain amount of this heat is required to maintain normal body temperature. Any heat that is not needed for temperature maintenance must be lost from the body, otherwise **hyperthermia** (HI-per-THURM-i-ah), an abnormally high body temperature, will be created. Unchecked, hyperthermia will lead to death.

Heat is lost by the body through the lungs or the skin. Mechanisms of heat loss include

Lungs
- Respiration—The air we exhale is warm. As the body overheats, respirations become more rapid as the body tries to rid itself of excess heat.

Skin
- Radiation—Heat is lost into the atmosphere in the form of rays.
- Evaporative Heat Loss—Perspiration is given off from glands in the dermis of the skin. As this perspiration evaporates, the skin is cooled and heat is lost in the process.
- Conduction—Heat is lost directly to the surrounding medium: air or water.

Consider what can happen to the body when it is placed in a hot environment. Air being inhaled is warm, possibly warmer than the air being exhaled. The skin may absorb more heat than it radiates. If high humidity is added, the evaporation of perspiration slows. To make things even more difficult, consider all this in an environment that lacks circulating air or a breeze that would speed up radiation and evaporative heat loss. Heat and humidity constitute the environment often associated with hyperthermia. This is why a "heat wave" greatly increases EMS responses for heat-related emergencies.

Since evaporative heat loss is reduced in a humid environment, moist heat can produce dramatic body changes in a short time. Moist heat usually tires people quickly, frequently stopping them from overexerting and harming themselves (although some people continue to engage in strenuous activity, running the risk of hurting themselves severely).

On the other hand, dry heat often deceives people. They continue to work or remain exposed to excess heat far beyond the point their bodies can tolerate. This is why you may see problems caused by dry heat exposure that are worse than those seen in moist heat exposure.

The same rules of care apply to heat-related emergencies as to any other emergency. You will still need to perform patient surveys and interviews and also be alert to problems other than those related to the heat. Collapse due to heat exposure may result in a fall that can fracture bones. A history of high blood pressure, heart disease, or lung problems may have hastened the effects of heat exposure. What may appear to be a problem related to heat exposure could be a heart attack. Age, diseases, and existing injuries all must be considered when evaluating the patient. Always consider the problem to be greater if the patient is a child or elderly, injured or having a chronic disease.

Common Heat Emergencies

There are three common emergencies brought about by prolonged exposure to excessive heat: heat cramps, heat exhaustion, and heat stroke.

Heat Cramps The emergency scene temperature does not have to be much greater than what would be considered "normal" for **heat cramps** to develop. The individual perspires heavily, often drinking large quantities of water. As the sweating continues, salts are lost by the body, bringing on painful muscle cramps. Researchers are trying to determine if the loss of water alone is enough to bring on heat cramps. Many medical authorities still believe that it is a combination of water and salt loss.

Heat Exhaustion The typical **heat exhaustion** patient is a healthy individual who has been exposed to excessive heat while working or exercising. **Heat exhaustion** is a form of shock brought about by fluid and salt loss. It is often seen among firefighters, construction workers, dock workers, and those employed in poorly ventilated warehouses. It is more of a problem during the summer and reaches a peak during prolonged heat waves. Heat exhaustion, which is commonly called "heat prostration," may develop into heat stroke.

Heat Stroke When a person's temperature-regulating mechanisms fail and his body cannot rid itself of excessive heat, **heat stroke** is brought about. This is a TRUE EMERGENCY. The problem is compounded when, in response to fluid and salt loss due to heat, the patient stops sweating, which prevents heat loss through evaporation. Athletes, laborers, and others who exercise or work in hot environments are common victims. The elderly who live in poorly ventilated apartments without air conditioning, and children left in cars with the windows rolled up, are common victims of heat stroke.

More cases of heat stroke are reported on hot, humid days. However, many cases occur from exposure to dry heat. Even though heat stroke is commonly called "sun stroke," it can be caused by excessive heat other than from the sun.

Heat cramps, heat exhaustion, and heat stroke are characterized and differentiated from each other by signs and symptoms involving the presence or absence of muscle cramps and characteristics of breathing, pulse, skin, perspiration, and feelings of weakness or loss of consciousness. The signs and symptoms of these three conditions are compared in Scan 20-1.

Patient Care—Heat-Related Emergencies

Care procedures for heat cramps, heat exhaustion, and heat stroke are detailed in Scan 20-1. Some elements of care require special consideration.

1. Cooling—*Rapid* cooling for heat stroke is recommended. Quickly move the patient to a cooler environment. Place cool compresses or ice packs on the head, neck, axilla, and groin. Immersion in a tub of cool water is another option. For school-age children, cooling is started using tepid (lukewarm) water. This water can then be replaced with cooler water at the recommendation of the emergency department physician.

2. Fluids—Patients with heat cramps or heat exhaustion should be given fluids containing electrolytes. Large volumes are usually required to prevent heat exhaustion from deteriorating into heat stroke. Follow the protocols established for your EMS system.

3. Transport—Transport immediately if
   * There are the signs and symptoms of heat stroke. (ALL cases of heat stroke are serious and the patient must be rapidly cooled and transported. Ice packs should be carried in the EMS unit during times of high environmental temperatures.)
   * There are the signs and symptoms of heat exhaustion.
   * The patient's condition worsens.
   * The patient does not respond to care.
   * You believe that the patient will return to the same environment and activity. A patient with heat cramps could become

a patient with heat exhaustion or heat stroke on your next run.
   * You believe that the patient may have other medical problems.

Beware of what you are told by some patients. They may not believe heat-related emergencies are serious. Many simply want to return to work. Nevertheless, interview the patient, take vital signs, and do the appropriate survey. If you have any doubts, tell the patient why he should be transported and seek his permission. You may have to spend a little time with some patients to gain their confidence.

EMERGENCIES DUE TO EXCESSIVE COLD

If the environment is too cold, body heat can be lost faster than it can be generated. The body attempts to adjust by reducing respirations, perspiration, and circulation to the skin. Muscular activity will increase in the form of shivering to generate more heat. The rate at which foods, which serve as fuel, are burned within the body increases to produce more heat. At a certain point, enough heat will not be available to all parts of the body, leading to damage of exposed tissues, a general reduction of body functions, or the cessation of a vital body function.

The body can lose heat by *conduction*, or direct transfer of heat from the body into the environment. When the body or clothing is wet, **water chill** is a problem, because water conducts heat away from the body 25 times faster than still air.

The body can also lose heat by *convection* as cool air passes over the body and carries away body heat. Thus the effects of a cold environment are worsened by **wind chill**. The more wind, the greater the heat loss. For example, if it is 10°F and there is a 20 mph wind, the amount of heat lost by the body is the same as if it were -25°F.

When evaluating the effects of cold temperatures on a patient, you must consider

☐ Temperature
☐ Wind chill
☐ Water chill

Heat-Related Emergencies

Condition	Muscle Cramps	Breathing	Pulse	Weakness	Skin	Perspiration	Loss of Consciousness
Heat cramps	Yes	Varies	Varies	Yes	Moist-warm No change	Heavy	Seldom
Heat exhaustion	No	Rapid Shallow	Weak	Yes	Cold Clammy	Heavy	Sometimes
Heat stroke	No	Deep, then shallow	Full Rapid	Yes	Dry-hot	Little or none	Often

1 HEAT CRAMPS

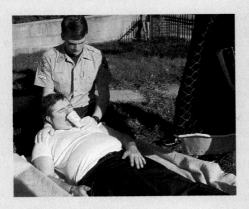

SIGNS AND SYMPTOMS

Severe muscle cramps (usually in the legs and abdomen), exhaustion, sometimes dizziness or periods of faintness.

EMERGENCY CARE PROCEDURES

- Move patient to a nearby cool place.
- Give the conscious patient fluids with electrolytes.
- Massage the cramped muscle to help ease the patient's discomfort. Massaging with pressure will be more effective than light rubbing. (Optional in some EMS systems)
- Apply moist towels to the patient's forehead and over cramped muscles.
- If cramps persist, or if more serious symptoms and signs develop, ready the patient and transport.

2 HEAT EXHAUSTION

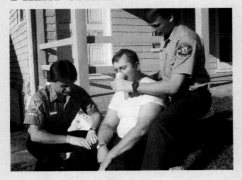

SIGNS AND SYMPTOMS

Rapid, shallow breathing; weak pulse; cold, clammy skin; heavy perspiration; total body weakness; dizziness; possible unconsciousness.

EMERGENCY CARE PROCEDURES

- Move the patient to a nearby cool place.
- Keep the patient at rest.
- Remove enough clothing to cool the patient without chilling him (watch for shivering).
- Fan the patient's skin.
- Give the conscious patient fluids with electrolytes. Do not try to administer fluids to an unconscious patient.
- Treat for shock, but do not cover to the point of overheating the patient.
- Provide high concentration oxygen.
- If unconscious, fails to recover rapidly, has other injuries, or has a history of medical problems, transport as soon as possible.

3 HEAT STROKE

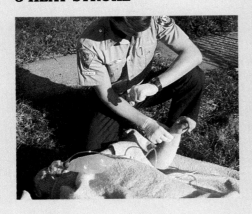

SIGNS AND SYMPTOMS

Deep breaths, then shallow breathing; rapid, strong pulse, then rapid, weak pulse; dry, hot skin; dilated pupils, loss of consciousness (possible coma); seizures or muscular twitching may be seen.

EMERGENCY CARE PROCEDURES

- Cool the patient—in any manner—rapidly. Move the patient out of the sun or away from the heat source. Remove patient's clothing and wrap him in wet towels and sheets. Pour cool water over these wrappings. Body heat must be lowered rapidly or brain cells will die!
- Treat for shock and administer a high concentration of oxygen.
- If cold packs or ice bags are available, wrap and place one under each armpit, one behind each knee, one in the groin, one on each wrist and ankle, and one on each side of the patient's neck.
- Transport as soon as possible.
- Should transport be delayed, find a tub or container. Immerse patient up to the face in cooled water. Constantly monitor to prevent drowning.
- Monitor vital signs throughout process.

- Exposed areas of the body
- Clothing
- Length of exposure
- Health of the patient
- Existing injuries
- Age
- How active the patient was during the exposure
- Possible use of alcohol or drugs

Patients with injuries or chronic illnesses will show the effects of cold much sooner than healthy persons. Those under the influence of alcohol or other substances tend to be affected more rapidly and more severely than others. The elderly will be more quickly affected. The unconscious patient lying on the cold ground or other cold surface is especially prone to rapid heat loss through conduction and will tend to have greater cold-related problems than one who is conscious and able to walk around.

Cold-related emergencies can be the result of local cooling or general cooling. *Local cooling* injuries are those affecting particular (local) parts of the body. They are grouped under the heading of **frostbite**. *General cooling* affects the entire body. This problem is known as **hypothermia** (HI-po-THURM-i-ah).

Local Cooling (Frostbite)

Local cooling is frostbite. Most commonly affected are the ears, nose, hands, and feet. When a part of the body is exposed to intensely cold air or liquid, blood flow to that particular part is limited by the constriction of blood vessels. When this happens, tissues do not receive enough warmth to prevent freezing. Ice crystals can form in the skin. In the most severe cases, gangrene (localized tissue death) can set in and ultimately lead to the loss of the body part.

There are three degrees of frostbite (Figure 20-1): incipient frostbite (called **frostnip**), superficial frostbite (called simply **frostbite**), and deep frostbite (called **freezing**).

As an EMT, you will need to know the symptoms, signs, and care procedures for all three degrees of frostbite (Table 20-1). As you read the following pages, notice how the signs and symptoms of frostbite are progressive. First, the exposed skin reddens, or in dark-skinned individuals, the skin color lightens and approaches a blanched (reduced color or

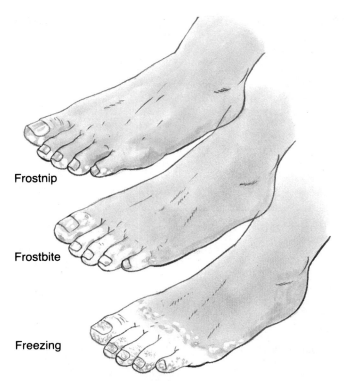

Figure 20-1 The three degrees of frostbite.

whitened) condition. Then, as exposure continues, the skin takes on a gray or white, blotchy appearance. Exposed skin surfaces become numb due to reduced circulation. If the freezing process is allowed to continue, all sensation is lost and the skin becomes dead white.

Frostnip Frostnip is *incipient* (the first stage of) *frostbite*, brought about by direct contact with a cold object or exposure of a body part to cold air. Wind chill and water chill also can be major factors. This condition is not serious. Tissue damage is minor and the response to care is good. The tip of the nose, the tips of the ears, the

TABLE 20-1 Exposure to Excessive Cold

Condition	Skin Surface	Tissue under Skin	Skin Color
Frostnip	Soft	Soft	Initially red, then white
Frostbite	Hard	Soft	White and waxy
Freezing	Hard	Hard	Blotchy, white to yellow-gray to blue-gray

upper cheeks, and the fingers (all areas generally exposed) are most susceptible to frostnip.

Patient Assessment—Frostnip

Patients are often unaware of the onset of frostnip until someone indicates that there is something unusual about their skin color.

Signs and Symptoms

- ☐ The affected area of the skin at first reddens, then blanches (becomes white). Once blanching begins, the color change can take place very quickly.
- ☐ The affected area feels numb to the patient.

Patient Care—Frostnip

Emergency Care Steps

Emergency care for frostnip is simple.

- ☐ Get out of the cold environment.
- ☐ Warm the affected area.

Usually, the patient can apply warmth from his own bare hands, blow warm air on the site, or if the fingers are involved, hold them in the armpits. During recovery from frostnip, the patient may complain about "tingling" or burning sensations, which is normal. If the condition does not respond to this simple care, begin to treat for frostbite.

Frostbite and Freezing In *superficial frostbite*, commonly called simply frostbite, the skin and subcutaneous layers become involved. Frostbite develops if frostnip goes untreated. In *deep frostbite*, or freezing, the subcutaneous layers, and the deeper structures of the body are affected. Muscles, bones, deep blood vessels, and organ membranes can become frozen.

Patient Assessment—Frostbite

Signs

- ☐ The affected area of the skin appears white and waxy.
- ☐ The affected area feels frozen, but only on the surface. The tissue below the surface must still be soft and have its normal resilience, or "bounce."

Do not squeeze or "poke" the tissue. The condition of the deeper tissues can be determined by gently feeling the affected area. Do the assessment as if the affected area had a fractured bone.

Patient Assessment—Freezing

Signs

- ☐ The skin turns mottled or blotchy. The color will turn to white, then grayish yellow, and finally a grayish blue.
- ☐ The tissues feel frozen to the touch, without the underlying resilience characteristic of superficial frostbite.

Patient Care—Frostbite and Freezing

Emergency Care Steps

Initial care for frostbite and for freezing (superficial and deep frostbite) is the same.

- ☐ *Transport to a medical facility without delay*, protecting the frostbitten area by covering it and handling it as gently as possible.
- ☐ *If transport must be delayed*, get the patient indoors and keep him warm. Do not allow the patient to smoke. Smoking causes blood vessels to constrict, decreasing circulation in the damaged tissues. Likewise, discourage the consumption of alcoholic beverages. Rewarm the frozen part as per local protocol, or request instructions from the emergency department physician (see below).

Important: Never listen to bystanders' myths and folktales about the care of frostbite. *Never* rub a frostbitten or frozen area. *Never* rub snow on a frostbitten or frozen area. There are ice crystals at the capillary level. Rubbing the injury site may cause these crystals to seriously damage the already injured tissues. DO NOT THAW A FROZEN LIMB IF THERE IS ANY CHANCE IT WILL BE REFROZEN.

Rewarming Frozen Parts Rewarming of frozen parts is seldom recommended; the chance of permanently injuring frozen tissues is too great. Consider rewarming only if local protocols recommend it, if you are instructed to do so by the emergency department physician, or if transport will be much delayed and you cannot reach the emergency department for instructions. If you are in a situation where you must attempt rewarming without instructions from a physician, follow the procedure described here.

You will need warm water and a container in which you can immerse the entire site of injury without the limb touching the sides or bottom of the container. If you cannot find a suitable container, fashion one from a plastic bag supported by a cardboard box or wooden crate (Figure 20-2). Proceed as follows.

1. Warm water to a temperature between 100° and 105°F. You should be able to put your finger into the water without experiencing discomfort.
2. Fill the container with the warm water and prepare the injured part by removing any clothing, jewelry, bands, or straps.
3. Fully immerse the injured part. Do not allow the frostbitten area to touch the sides or bottom of the container. *Do not* place any pressure on the affected part. When the water cools below 100°F, remove the limb and add more warm water. The patient may complain of moderate pain as the affected area rewarms or he may experience some period of intense pain. The presence of pain is usually a good indicator of successful rewarming.
4. If you complete rewarming of the part (it no longer feels frozen and is turning red or

blue), gently dry the affected area and apply a sterile dressing. Place pads of dressing material between fingers and toes before dressing hands and feet. Next, cover the site with blankets or whatever is available to keep the affected area warm. *Do not* allow these coverings to come in direct contact with the injured area or to put pressure on the site. It is best if you first build some sort of framework on which the coverings can rest.
5. Keep the patient at rest. Do not allow the patient to walk if a lower extremity has been frostbitten or frozen.
6. Make certain that you keep the entire patient as warm as possible without overheating. Cover the patient's head with a towel or small blanket to reduce heat loss. Leave the patient's face exposed.
7. Continue to monitor the patient.
8. Assist circulation according to your local protocols (some systems recommend rhythmically and carefully raising and lowering the affected limb).
9. Again, do not allow the limb to refreeze.
10. Transport as soon as possible with the affected limb slightly elevated.

General Cooling (Hypothermia)

The general cooling of the human body is known as systemic hypothermia. Exposure to cold reduces body heat. With time, the body is unable to maintain its proper core (internal) temperature. If allowed to continue, hypothermia leads to death. Be aware that hypothermia can develop in temperatures *well above* freezing.

Hypothermia is often a serious problem for the aged. During the winter months, many older citizens on small fixed incomes live in unheated rooms or rooms that are kept too cool. Failing body systems, chronic illnesses, poor diets, and a lack of exercise combine with this cold environment to bring about hypothermia.

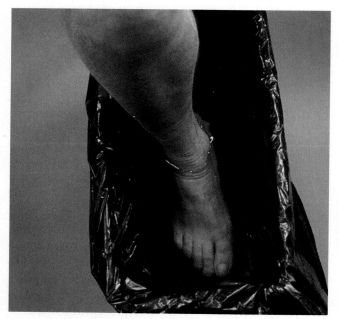

Figure 20-2 Rewarming the frozen part.

Patient Assessment—Hypothermia

Signs and Symptoms

The signs and symptoms of hypothermia (Table 20-2) include

☐ Shivering (early stages when body core temperature is above 90°F)
☐ Feelings of numbness

TABLE 20-2 Stages of Hypothermia

Body Temperature (core), °F	°C	Symptoms
99-96	37-35.5	Shivering.
95-91	35.5-32.7	Intense shivering. If patient is conscious, he has difficulty speaking.
90-86	32-30	Shivering decreases, is replaced by strong muscular rigidity. Muscle coordination is affected. Erratic or jerky movements are produced. Thinking is less clear. General comprehension is dulled. There may be total amnesia. The patient is generally still able to maintain the appearance of psychological contact with his surroundings.
85-81	29.4-27.2	Patient becomes irrational, loses contact with his environment, and drifts into a stuporous state. Muscular rigidity continues. Pulse and respirations are slow and patient may develop cardiac arrhythmias.
80-78	26.6-20.5	Patient becomes unconscious. He does not respond to the spoken word. Most reflexes cease to function. Heartbeat becomes erratic.

- Drowsiness and/or unwillingness or inability to do even the simplest of activities. A decreased level of consciousness may be observed.
- Slow breathing and pulse rates (seen in cases of prolonged hypothermia)
- Failing eyesight (seen in cases of prolonged hypothermia)
- Loss of motor coordination (the patient may stagger or be unable to hold things)
- Unconsciousness. Usually the patient has a "glassy stare" (seen in extreme cases)
- Freezing of body parts (seen in the most extreme cases). Action must be taken immediately, since the patient may be near death.

It is important to estimate the general severity of the patient's hypothermia. The hypothermia may be

- Mild—Shivering, perhaps some numbness or mild drowsiness
- Severe—Slow breathing and pulse, failing eyesight, coordination difficulties, drowsiness
- Extreme—Unconsciousness, absence of discernible vital signs, body very cold to the touch with core temperature possibly below 80°F, possible freezing of some body parts

Warning: It may be difficult to distinguish between mild and severe hypothermia. Do patient surveys and interviews to help you estimate the extent of the problem. If you are not sure, overestimate severity, since the care acceptable for mild hypothermia may be harmful to the patient with severe hypothermia.

Patient Care—Mild Hypothermia

Rewarming a patient with mild hypothermia in the field is allowed by some EMS systems but not all. This can prove to be a dangerous process if the patient's condition is more serious than believed. If you are allowed to rewarm a patient with mild hypothermia, do not delay transport. Rewarm the patient while en route.

Emergency Care Steps

For the patient with *mild* hypothermia, you should

1. Do patient surveys and interviews to determine the extent of the problem.
2. Keep the patient dry. Remove any wet clothing and replace the articles with dry items, or wrap the patient in dry blankets.
3. Use heat to raise the patient's core body temperature. This should be done during transport, but if transport is delayed, move

the patient to a warm environment if at all possible. Gently apply heat to the patient's body in the form of heat packs, hot water bottles, electric heating pads, hot air, radiated heat, and your own body heat and that of bystanders. DO NOT WARM THE PATIENT TOO QUICKLY. Rapid warming will circulate peripherally stagnated cold blood and rapidly cool the vital central areas of the body, possibly causing cardiac arrest.

The process used to rewarm the patient should be CORE REWARMING. This means that you must avoid rewarming the limbs. Heat should be applied to the lateral chest, neck, armpits, and groin. If the limbs are warmed first, blood will collect in the extremities due to vasodilation (dilation of blood vessels) and cause a fatal form of hypovolemic shock. If you rewarm the trunk and leave the lower extremities exposed, you can control the rewarming process and help prevent most of the problems associated with the procedure.

If transport must be delayed, a warm bath is very helpful, but you must keep the patient alert enough so that he does not drown. Again, do not warm the patient too quickly.

4 Keep the patient at rest. Do not allow the patient to walk. Such activity may set off severe heart problems, including ventricular fibrillation, as may rough transfer of the patient. Since the patient's blood is coldest in the extremities, exercise could quickly circulate this blood to lower the core temperature.

5 Provide care for shock and provide oxygen.

6 If the patient is alert, slowly give him warm liquids. When warm fluids are given quickly, circulation patterns change sending blood away from the core to the skin and extremities.

7 Except in the mildest of cases (shivering), transport the patient. During transport have the head lower than the feet. Continue to provide high concentration oxygen and monitor vital signs.

8 Never allow a patient to remain in, or return to, a cold environment. Hypothermia will probably recur.

Note: You will not be providing very much help to patients suffering from general cooling if you simply wrap them in blankets. Their bodies can no longer generate enough heat to make such

care useful. Provide external heat sources, but rewarm the patient slowly. Handle the patient with great care, the same as you would if there were unstabilized cervical spine injuries.

Patient Care—Severe Hypothermia

DO NOT TRY TO REWARM THE PATIENT WITH SEVERE HYPOTHERMIA. Even if you rewarm the patient slowly, you may cause the patient to develop lethal ventricular fibrillation.

Emergency Care Steps

For the patient with *severe* hypothermia, you should

1 Handle the patient as gently as possible. Rough handling may cause ventricular fibrillation.

2 Position the patient with his head lower than his feet. Make certain that he has an open airway.

3 Provide a high concentration of oxygen that has been passed through a warm water humidifier. If need be, the oxygen that has been kept warm in the passenger compartment can be used. If there is no other choice, oxygen from a cold cylinder may be used.

4 Wrap the patient in blankets. If available, use insulating blankets.

5 Transport *immediately*.

Patient Care—Extreme Hypothermia

In extreme cases of hypothermia, you will find the patient unconscious, with no discernable vital signs. (Take one minute to assess the carotid pulse. In hypothermia, the heart rate can slow to less than 10 beats per minute. If you detect a pulse during the period of a minute, do not start CPR.) The patient will feel very cold to your touch (the core temperature of the body may be below 80°F). *However, it is possible that the patient is still alive!**

Emergency Care Steps

1 If there is no detectable pulse, begin CPR immediately, keeping the head lower than the feet.

2 Transport immediately.

*The lowest temperature recorded for an accidental hypothermia patient who survived is 64.4°F.

The patient may not reach biological death for over 30 minutes. The staff at the emergency department will not pronounce a patient dead until after he is rewarmed as resuscitative measures are being applied. This means that you cannot assume that a severe hypothermia patient is dead on the basis of body temperature and lack of vital signs. As medical personnel point out, "You're not dead until you're warm and dead"!

Other Cold-Related Emergencies

Chilblains Lesions that occur from repeated prolonged exposures of bare skin to a dry, cool environment above freezing—between 32°F and 60°F—are called **chilblains**.

Patient Assessment—Chilblains

Signs and Symptoms

Chilblain lesions are areas that

- ☐ Are red and swollen
- ☐ Feel hot, tender, and itchy to the patient
- ☐ Are chronic; that is, they linger.

Patient Care—Chilblains

There is no emergency care procedure for chilblains other than to protect the injured area and try to prevent recurrence. Keep in mind that the role of the EMT does not include definitive diagnosis. Therefore, you should recommend that the patient be transported to a physician to receive the appropriate treatment and to make certain that the problem is, in fact, chilblains.

Trench Foot Sometimes called *immersion foot*, **trench foot** is a condition that develops when the lower extremities remain in cool water or a moist environment for a prolonged period.

Patient Assessment—Trench Foot

Signs and Symptoms

With trench foot, the affected part of the limb

- ☐ Becomes swollen
- ☐ Appears waxy and mottled
- ☐ Feels cold to the touch and to the patient

- ☐ May feel numb to the patient
- ☐ May give off a bad odor

Patient Care—Trench Foot

Emergency Care Steps

1. Remove wet shoes and stockings.
2. Do not open any blisters that may have developed.
3. Gently rewarm the extremity (it may become red and hot).
4. Place strips of sterile dressing between the toes and wrap the extremity lightly with sterile dressing.
5. Keep the limb slightly elevated.
6. Transport the patient (severe disability can occur with trench foot, so transport to a medical facility is necessary).

Protecting the Accident Patient from Cold The injured patient is more susceptible to the effects of cold. As an EMT you should begin to protect the patient who is in a collision vehicle or is entrapped in other accident debris or wreckage before extrication and throughout care and transport. The major course of action is to prevent additional body heat loss. Although it may be neither practical nor possible to replace wet clothing, you can at least create a barrier to the cold with blankets, a salvage cover, an aluminized blanket, a survival blanket, or even articles of clothing. A plastic trash bag can serve as protection from wind and water, and it will help prevent heat loss. Keep in mind that the greatest area of heat loss may be the head. Provide some sort of head covering for the patient.

When the patient's injuries allow, place a blanket between his body and the cold ground. Rotate warm blankets from the heated ambulance to the patient. If the patient will remain trapped in a collision vehicle or other wreckage for a period of time, plug holes in the wreckage with blankets or salvage covers. If available and safe, use a 500-watt incandescent lamp to supply external heat.

When administering oxygen to patients exposed to cold, keep the cylinder warm when possible. (Do not try to heat the cylinder, as overpressurization may occur.)

ACCIDENTS INVOLVING WATER

Warning: Do not attempt a rescue in which you must enter deep water or swim unless you have been trained to do so and are a very good swimmer. Except for shallow pools and open, shallow waters with uniform bottoms, the problems faced in water rescue are too great and too dangerous for the poor swimmer or untrained person to attempt. If this bothers you—having to stand by not being able to help—then take a course in water safety and rescue. Otherwise, if you attempt a deep water or swimming rescue, you will probably become a victim yourself rather than the person who rescues and provides care.

Water-Related Accidents

Drowning or near-drowning is the first thing people think of, and usually the first concern, in connection with water-related accidents. However, there are many types of injuries resulting from many types of accidents that can occur on or in the water. Boating, waterskiing, windsurfing, jet-skiing, diving, and scuba diving accidents can produce fractured bones, bleeding, soft tissue injuries, and airway obstruction. Even auto collisions can send vehicles or passengers into the water, resulting in any of the injuries usually associated with motor vehicle collisions as well as the complications caused by the presence of water.

Medical problems, such as heart attacks, can also cause or be caused by water accidents or can simply take place in, on, or near the water. Remember, too, that some water accidents happen far away from pools, lakes, or beaches, Bathtub drownings do occur. Adults, as well as children, can drown in only a few inches of water.

**Patient Assessment—
Water-Related Accidents**

Learn to look for the following problems when your patient is the victim of a water-related accident.

- ☐ Airway Obstruction—This may be from water in the lungs, foreign matter in the airway, or swollen airway tissues (common if the neck is injured in a dive). Spasms along the airway may be present in cases of near-drowning.
- ☐ Cardiac Arrest—This is often related to respiratory arrest or occurs before the near-drowning.
- ☐ Signs of Heart Attack—Through overexertion, the patient may have greater prob-

lems than obvious near-drowning. Some untrained rescuers are fooled into thinking that chest pains are due to muscle cramps produced during swimming.
- ☐ Injuries to the Head and Neck—These are expected to be found in boating, waterskiing, and diving accidents, but they are also very common in swimming accidents.
- ☐ Internal Injuries—While doing the patient survey, stay on the alert for fractured bones, soft tissue injuries, and internal bleeding (which may be missed during the first stages of care).
- ☐ Hypothermia—The water does not have to be very cold and the length of stay in the water does not have to be very long for hypothermia to occur (in some cases of near-drowning, the patient may have a better chance for survival in cold water).
- ☐ Substance Abuse—Alcohol and drug use are closely associated with adolescent and adult drownings. Elevated blood alcohol levels have been found in over 30% of drowning victims. The screening for drug use has not been as extensive as that done for alcohol, but research indicates that drugs are a contributory factor in many water-related accidents.
- ☐ Drowning or Near-Drowning—The patient may be or have been discovered under or face down in the water. He may be unconscious and without discernible vital signs or may be conscious, breathing, and coughing up water. (Drowning and near-drowning are discussed in detail, below.)

Drowning and Near-Drowning

The process of drowning begins as a person struggles to keep afloat in the water. He gulps in large breaths of air as he thrashes about. When he can no longer keep afloat and starts to submerge, he tries to take and hold one more deep breath. As he does, water may enter the airway. There is a series of coughing and swallowing actions, and the victim involuntarily inhales and swallows water. As water flows past the epiglottis, it triggers a reflex spasm of the larynx. This **laryngospasm** (lah-RING-go-spazm) seals the airway so effectively that no more than a small amount of water reaches the lungs. Unconsciousness soon results from hypoxia (oxygen starvation).

About 10% of the people who drown die from true **asphyxia**, or simply suffocation from

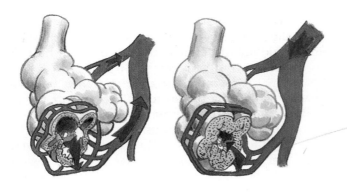

Figure 20-3 Salt water and fresh water have different effects on the body.

the lack of air. In the remaining victims, the person attempts a final respiratory effort and draws water into the lungs, or the laryngospasms subside with the onset of unconsciousness and water freely enters the lungs. What happens next depends on whether the victim is in fresh water or salt water.

In fresh-water drowning (Figure 20-3), the water washes away surfactant, a substance found on the inner surface of the alveoli. Surfactant is needed to maintain the elasticity of the lungs. As it is washed away, the alveoli collapse and air exchange is no longer possible (see *atelectasis*, Chapter 6). Ventricular fibrillation (or some other heart arrhythmia) occurs. This heart action is lethal and is probably the cause of death in many fresh-water drownings.

In salt-water drowning (Figure 20-3), water is taken from the bloodstream and moved into the lungs, causing massive pulmonary edema to develop. As much as one-fourth of the total blood volume may be lost as fluids move into the lungs. Death is due to hypoxia secondary to (resulting from) pulmonary edema. The victim basically suffocates in his own body fluids.

Patient Assessment— Drowning and Near-Drowning

As an EMT you should start using the term **near-drowning**. Obviously, if the patient is breathing and coughing up water, he has not drowned but nearly drowned. This is only part of what we mean by near-drowning. If a patient has "drowned" in layperson's terms,

he is not necessarily biologically dead. Resuscitative measures may be able to keep the patient biologically alive long enough for more advanced life support measures to be used to save the patient's life. Only when sufficient time has passed to render resuscitation useless has **drowning** truly taken place.

The phrase "sufficient time" has a different meaning today when applied to clinically dead patients. The concept of 4 to 6 minutes is not valid for some cases of cold-water near-drowning and hypothermia. We now know that patients in cold water can be resuscitated after 30 minutes or more in cardiac arrest. Once the water temperature falls below 70°F, biological death may be delayed. The colder the water, the better are the patient's chances for survival, unless hypothermia produces lethal complications. More will be said about this later in the chapter.

Patient Care—Near-Drowning

The initial care procedures will be the same regardless of whether the near-drowning has taken place in fresh or in salt water. Transport for the near-drowning patient should not be delayed. Care is discussed in more detail below under "Emergency Care for Water-Related Accidents."

Water Rescues

Unless you are a very good swimmer and trained in water rescue, *do not* go into the water to save someone. Such training is available from the American Red Cross and the YMCA in the form of water safety and rescue courses.

The following is the order of procedures for a water rescue (Figure 20-4)—most of which can be performed *short* of going into the water.

1. REACH
2. THROW and TOW
3. ROW
4. (as a last resort . . .) GO

Reach When the patient is responsive and close to shore or poolside, try to REACH him by holding out an object for him to grab; then pull him from the water. When doing this, your position must be secure to avoid being pulled into the water. Of all the items that could be used for such a rescue, line (rope) is considered the best choice. If no line is available, use a branch, fish-

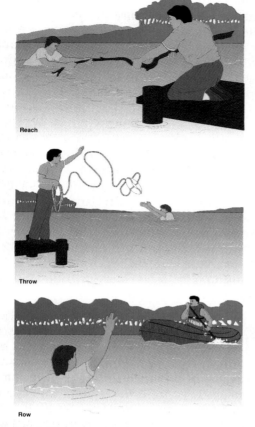

Reach

Throw

Row

Figure 20-4 First try to REACH and pull the patient from the water. If this fails, THROW him anything that will float and TOW him from the water. If this fails, ROW to the patient.

ing rod, oar, stick, or other such object. Remember that a towel, blanket, or even an article of your own clothing can work quite well.

In cases in which there is no object near at hand or conditions are such that you may have only one opportunity to grab the person (e.g., in strong currents), position yourself flat on your stomach and extend your hand or leg to the patient (not recommended for the nonswimmer). Again, make certain that you are working from a secure position.

Throw and Tow Should the person be alert but too far away for you to reach and pull from the water, THROW an object that will float (Figure 20-5). A personal flotation device (PFD or lifejacket), or ring buoy (life preserver) is best, if available. The primary course of action is to throw anything that will float and to do so as soon as possible. Buoyant objects that may be at the typical water-related accident scene include foam cushions, plastic jugs, logs, plastic picnic containers, surf boards, flat boards, large beach

balls, and plastic toys. Two empty, capped, plastic milk jugs can keep an adult afloat for hours. Inflatable splints can be used if there is nothing at the scene that will float.

Once the conscious patient has a flotation device or floating object to hold onto, try to find a way to TOW him to shore. From a safe position, throw the patient a line or another flotation device attached to a line. If you are a good swimmer and you know how to judge the water, wade out to no deeper than your waist should you find it necessary to cut down the distance for throwing the line. You must be wearing a personal flotation device and have a safety line that is secured on shore.

Row In cases in which the patient is too far from shore to allow for throwing and towing, or the patient is unresponsive, you may be able to ROW a boat to the patient. Do not attempt this if you cannot swim. Even if you are a good swimmer, wearing a personal flotation device while in the boat is *required*. In cases in which the patient is conscious, tell him to grab an oar or the stern (rear end) of the boat. You must exercise great care when helping the patient into the boat. This is even more tricky when in a canoe. Should the canoe tip over, stay with the canoe and hold onto its bottom and side. Most canoes will stay afloat.

If you take a boat to the patient and find that he is unresponsive, you can conduct a quick primary survey from your position in the boat and look for obvious signs of neck or spinal injury before trying to pull him from the water. Of course, this is a judgment call. Should conditions be such that you may lose the chance to grab the patient, then these assessment procedures must be delayed until after you have the patient safely in the boat.

Go Finally, when all other means have failed, you can GO into the water and swim to

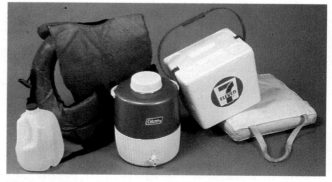

Figure 20-5 Throw the patient any object that will float.

the patient. *You must be a good swimmer, trained in water rescue and lifesaving.* Untrained rescuers can become victims themselves. Remember that "Go" is a last resort.

Emergency Care for Water-Related Accidents

You may initiate care when the patient is out of the water (already out when you arrive, or in the water when you arrive but rescued by others before you initiate care). At other times you may need and be able to initiate care—especially rescue breathing and immobilizing for possible spine injuries—*while the patient is still in the water.* Chest compressions will be effective only after the patient is out of the water.

Rescue Breathing In or Out of the Water If needed, rescue breathing should be begun without delay. If you can reach the nonbreathing patient in the water, you can provide ventilations as you support him in a semi-supine position (Scan 20-2). You can continue providing ventilations while the patient is being immobilized (see below) and removed from the water. If the patient is already out of the water, you can begin rescue breathing or CPR, if necessary, on the land.

Do not be surprised to find resistance to the ventilations you attempt to provide to the near-drowning patient. You will probably have to ventilate more forcefully than you would for other patients. Be sure that no foreign objects are in the patient's airway (obstruction may be due to laryngospasms). Remember, you must provide air to the patient's lungs as soon as possible.

A patient with water in the lungs usually will have water in the stomach. If there is enough water in the stomach, there will be added resistance to your efforts to provide rescue breathing or CPR ventilations. Since the patient may have spasms along the airway, or swollen tissues in the larynx or trachea, you may find that some of the air you provide will go into the patient's stomach. Remember, the same problem will occur if you do not properly open the airway or your ventilations are too forceful. However, American Heart Association guidelines do not call for you to attempt to relieve water or air from the patient's stomach. Doing so could drive materials from the stomach into the patient's airway and increase the chance of aspiration.

Humans have something in common with many other mammals: a process called the **mammalian diving reflex**. When a person dives into water, the body reacts to the submersion of the face. Breathing is inhibited, the heart rate slows (bradycardia), and a series of complex functions begin that shut off major blood flow to most parts of the body except the heart, lungs, and brain. Whatever oxygen remains in the blood supply is made available to the brain. The colder the water, the more oxygen we tend to divert to the brain. Therefore, a near-drowning patient should receive resuscitative care even if he has not been breathing for 10 minutes or more. Many such patients have been resuscitated. Recent studies have shown that some fresh-water near-drowning patients have been resuscitated, without brain damage, after 30 minutes or more without breathing. The colder the water, the better the patient's chances. Infants and young children have the best chance for survival.

Care for Possible Spinal Injuries In the Water Injuries to the cervical spine are seen with many water-related accidents. Most often, these injuries are received during a dive or when the patient is struck by a boat, skier, or ski. Even though cervical spine injuries are the most common of the spinal injuries seen in water-related accidents, there can be injury anywhere along the spine.

When a patient is unconscious, you may not be able to detect spinal injuries. In water-related accidents, you are to *assume* that the unconscious patient has neck and spinal injuries. Should the patient have head injuries, also assume that there are neck and spinal injuries. Keep in mind that a patient found in respiratory arrest or cardiac arrest will need resuscitation started before you can immobilize the neck and spine. Also, realize that you may not be able to carry out a complete survey for spinal injuries while the patient is in the water. Take care to avoid aggravating spinal injuries, but do not delay basic life support. Do not delay removing the patient from the water if the scene presents an immediate danger. When possible, keep the patient's neck rigid in a straight line with the body's midline. Use the jaw-thrust to open the airway.

If the patient with possible spinal injuries is still in the water and you are a good swimmer, able to aid in the rescue, secure the patient to a long spine board before removing him from the water. Assuring the integrity of the spine before removal from the water is critical in preventing permanent neurological damage or paralysis.

Water Rescue—Possible Spinal Injury

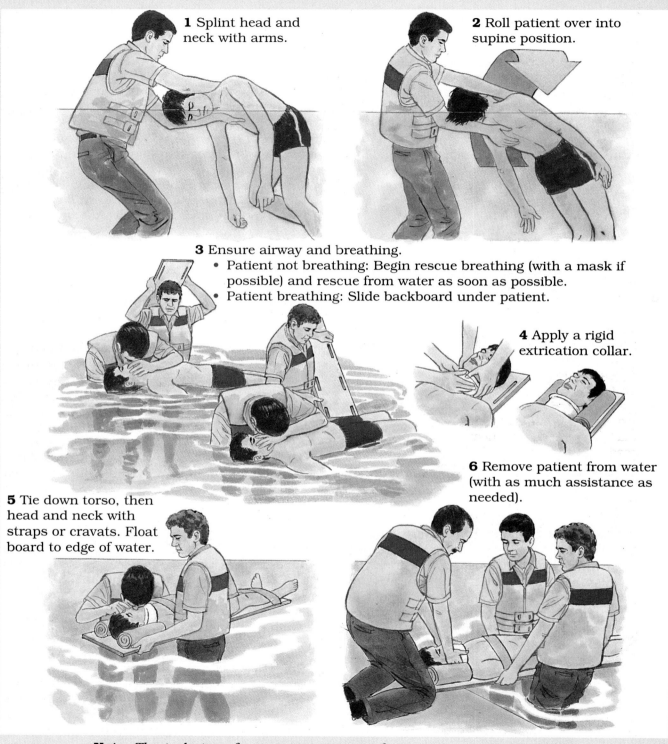

1 Splint head and neck with arms.

2 Roll patient over into supine position.

3 Ensure airway and breathing.
- Patient not breathing: Begin rescue breathing (with a mask if possible) and rescue from water as soon as possible.
- Patient breathing: Slide backboard under patient.

4 Apply a rigid extrication collar.

6 Remove patient from water (with as much assistance as needed).

5 Tie down torso, then head and neck with straps or cravats. Float board to edge of water.

Note: The technique for removing patients from water assuring integrity of the spine is critical. Interviews of paraplegics whose paralysis resulted from water-related accidents indicate that many were able to tread water after the injury and prior to being improperly removed from the water.

Steps for this procedure are shown on Scan 20-2. This type of rescue requires special training in the use of the spine board while in the water. This rigid device can "pop up" very easily from below the water surface. Make certain that you know how to control the board and how to work in the water.

Care for Patients Out of the Water In all cases of water-related accidents, *assume* that the unconscious patient has neck and spinal injuries. When the patient is rescued by others while you wait, or is out of the water when you arrive, you should

1. *Do a primary survey,* including the ABCDEs, protecting the spine as much as possible.
2. *Provide rescue breathing or CPR if needed.* Do not forget to check for airway obstruction. Protect yourself by using a pocket face mask with a one-way valve or bag-valve mask unit.
3. *Look for and control profuse bleeding.* Since the patient's heart rate may have slowed down, take a pulse for 60 seconds in all cold water rescue situations.
4. *Provide care for shock, administer a high concentration of oxygen, and transport the patient as soon as possible.*
5. *Continue resuscitative measures throughout transport.* Initial and periodic suctioning may be needed. The near-drowning patient receiving rescue breathing or CPR should be transported as soon as possible. For all other patients . . .
6. *If resuscitation and immediate transport are not required, cover the patient to conserve body heat and complete a secondary survey.* Uncover only those areas of the patient's body involved with the stage of the survey. Care for any problems or injuries detected during the survey, in the order of their priority. Stay on the alert for fluids in the mouth that will require suctioning. When transport is delayed and you believe that the patient can be moved to a warmer place, do so without aggravating any existing injuries. Do not allow the near-drowning patient to walk. Transport as necessary.

Information supplied to the dispatch or the medical center from the scene and during transport is critical in cases of near-drowning. The emergency department staff needs to know if this is a fresh- or salt-water drowning and if it took place in cold or warm water, and if it is related to a diving accident. You may be asked to transport the patient to a special facility or to a center having a hyperbaric chamber when decompression therapy (discussed later in this chapter) is needed.

Diving Accidents

Diving Board Accidents Water-related accidents often involve injuries that occur when individuals attempt dives or enter the water from diving boards. In the majority of these accidents, the patient is a teenager. Basically the same types of injuries are seen in dives taken from diving boards, poolsides, docks, boats, and the shore. The injury may be due to the diver striking the board or some object on or under the water. From great heights, injury may result from impact with the water.

**Patient Assessment—
Diving Board Accidents**

Most diving accidents involve the head and neck, but you will also find injuries to the spine, hands, feet, and ribs in many cases. Any part of the body can be injured depending on the position that the diver is in when he strikes the water or an object. This means that you must perform both the primary and secondary surveys on all diving accident patients unless you are providing life support measures. Do not overlook the fact that a medical emergency may have led to the diving accident.

Patient Care—Diving Board Accidents

Care for diving accident patients is the same as for any accident patient, if they are out of the water. Care provided in the water and in removing the patient from the water is the same as for any patient who may have neck and spine injuries. Remember, assume that any unconscious or unresponsive patient has neck and spinal injuries. There can be delayed reactions with patients having spinal injuries. Compression along the spine may cause a patient with no apparent injuries to suddenly exhibit indications of nerve impairment. Often this begins as a numbness or a tingling sensation in the legs.

Scuba Diving Accidents Scuba (Self-Contained Underwater Breathing Apparatus) diving accidents have increased with the popularity of the sport, especially since many untrained and inexperienced persons are attempting dives. Today, there are more than 2 million people who scuba dive for sport or as part of their industrial or military job. Added to this are a large number who decide to "try it one time," without the benefits of lessons or supervision. Well-trained divers seldom have problems. Those with inadequate training place themselves at great risk.

Scuba diving accidents include all types of body injuries and near-drownings. In many cases, the scuba diving accident was brought about by medical problems that existed prior to the dive. There are two special problems seen in scuba diving accidents. They are air emboli in the diver's blood and the "bends."

Patient Assessment—Air Embolism

Air embolism is the result of gases leaving a damaged lung and entering the bloodstream. Severe damage to the lungs may lead to a spontaneous pneumothorax. Air emboli (gas bubbles in the blood) are most often associated with divers who hold their breath because of inadequate training, an equipment failure, underwater emergency, or when trying to conserve air during a dive. However, a diver may develop an air embolism in very shallow water (as little as 4 feet). The onset is rapid, with many of the signs and symptoms of a cerebrovascular accident.

Signs and Symptoms

Expect to find any or all of the following.

- Blurred vision
- Chest pains
- Numbness and tingling sensations in the extremities
- Generalized or specific weakness—possible paralysis
- Frothy blood in mouth or nose
- Convulsions
- Rapid lapse into unconsciousness
- Sounds in the chest indicating gases are trapped outside the lungs, in the thoracic cavity
- Respiratory arrest
- Cardiac arrest

An automobile collision victim trapped below water may take gulps of air from air pockets held inside the vehicle. When freed, the patient may develop air emboli the same as a scuba diver.

Patient Assessment— Decompression Sickness

The "bends" are muscle and joint pains that are part of what is called **decompression sickness**, usually caused when the diver comes up too quickly from a deep, prolonged dive. The quick ascent causes nitrogen gas to be trapped in the body tissue, and this trapped nitrogen may find its way into the patient's bloodstream.

Bends in scuba divers takes from 1 to 48 hours to appear, with about 90% of the cases occurring within 3 hours of the dive. Divers increase the risk of decompression sickness if they fly within 12 hours of a dive. Because of this delay, carefully consider all information gathered from the patient interview and reports from the patient's family and friends. This information may provide the only clues that will allow you to relate the patient's problems to a scuba dive.

Signs and Symptoms

The signs and symptoms of decompression sickness include

- Personality changes
- Fatigue
- Deep pain to the muscles and joints (the "bends")
- Itchy blotches on the skin (mottling)
- Numbness or paralysis
- Choking
- Coughing
- Labored breathing
- Behavior similar to intoxication (e.g., staggering)
- Chest pains
- Collapse leading to unconsciousness
- Skin rashes that keep changing in appearance (in some cases)

Note: The well-trained scuba diver wears a preplanned dive chart. The chart may provide you with useful information concerning the nature and duration of the dive. This chart must be transported with the patient.

Patient Care—
Air Embolism or Decompression Sickness

Do not try to diagnose if the patient's problem is air embolism or decompression sickness. Follow the emergency care steps outlined below if the patient displays signs and symptoms of either condition.

Note: The National Diving Accident Network (DAN) was formed to assist rescuers with the care for underwater diving accident patients. The staff, available on a 24-hour basis, can be reached by phoning (919) 684-8111. Collect calls will be accepted for actual emergencies. DAN can give you or your dispatcher information on assessment and care and how to transfer the patient to a hyperbaric trauma care center (one with a special pressure chamber for treatment of such conditions).

Emergency Care Steps

1. Rapidly transport all patients with possible air emboli, decompression sickness, or possible pneumothorax.
2. Alert dispatch or the medical center for specific directions concerning where to take the patient. You may be sent directly to a hyperbaric trauma center.
3. Maintain an open airway.
4. Administer the highest possible concentration of oxygen by nonrebreather mask.
5. Manage shock, keeping the patient warm.
6. Positioning of the patient is critical, to avoid damage to the brain by gas bubbles in the blood (Figure 20-6). As noted under the care for neck vein wounds (Chapter 13), proper positioning will help trap gas bubbles in the right atrium. Place the patient on the left side in a head-down position (this should not be tried if there are any signs of neck or spinal injuries). Slant the entire body about 15 degrees rather than simply lifting the legs.

Continue to monitor the patient. You may have to reposition the patient to ensure an open airway.

ACCIDENTS INVOLVING ICE

Every winter many people die who fall through ice while skating or attempting to cross an ice-covered body of water. Often, the ice-related accident scene becomes a multiple-rescue problem as individuals try to reach the victim and also fall through the ice.

Ice Rescues

The number one rule in ice rescue is to protect yourself! Formal ice rescue training is available and needed to assist the EMT in making safer ice rescue attempts. A cold water submersion suit should be worn during any ice rescue attempt.

There are several ways in which you can reach a patient who has fallen through ice.

- Flotation devices can be thrown to the patient.
- A rope in which a loop has been formed can be tossed to the patient. He can put the loop around his body so that he can be pulled onto the ice and away from the danger area.
- A small, flat-bottomed aluminum boat is

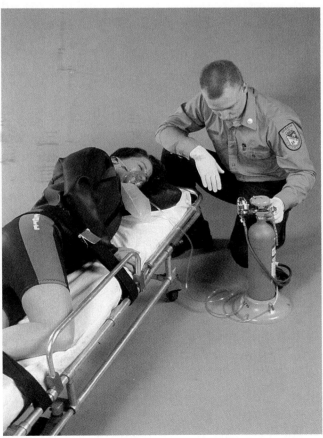

Figure 20-6 Positioning the patient after a scuba diving accident.

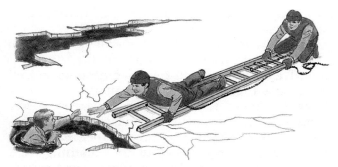

Figure 20-7 The safest way to perform an ice rescue is to work with others.

probably the best device for an ice rescue. It can be pushed stern (rear end) first by other rescuers and pulled to safety by a rope secured to the bow (front end). The primary rescuer will remain dry and safe should the ice break. The patient can be pulled from the water or allowed to grasp the side of the boat, although he may be unable to grasp or to hold on for long.

- A ladder is an effective tool often used in ice rescue. It can be laid flat and pushed to the patient, then pulled back by an attached rope. The ladder also can serve as a surface on which a rescuer can spread out his weight if he must go onto the ice to reach the patient. The ladder should have a line that can be secured by a rescuer in a safe position. Any rescuer on the ladder should have a safety line.

When attempting to rescue the patient, remember that he may not be able to do much to help in the process. The effects of hypothermia from the cold water may slow his mental and physical capabilities in a matter of minutes.

You should never enter the water through a hole in the ice in order to find the victim. Whenever possible, do not work alone when trying to perform an ice rescue. If you must work alone, do not walk out onto the ice, but throw a rope, or push a ladder to the patient. Never go onto ice that is rapidly breaking. Your best course of

action will be to work with others, from a safe ice surface or the shore (Figure 20-7). When there is no other choice, you and your fellow rescuers can elect to form a human chain to reach the patient. However, this is not the safest method to employ, even when all the rescuers are wearing personal flotation devices and using safety lines.

Emergency Care for Ice-Related Accidents

Emergency care for ice-related accidents is whatever is required for any suspected injuries plus care for hypothermia.

Patient Assessment—Ice-Related Accidents

Expect to find injuries to most patients who have fallen through the ice. Fractures to bones of the lower extremities are common. Hypothermia will almost certainly be a problem. Remember that blanket wraps are of little help to patients with mild hypothermia. They require the slow application of an external source of heat. Transport all patients who have fallen through ice. The patient with severe hypothermia should not be rewarmed in the field. There may be injuries that are difficult to detect and problems due to the cold that may be delayed.

Patient Care—Ice-Related Accidents

Emergency Care Steps

As required by your assessment of the patient's condition

1. Treat for near-drowning; provide basic life support.
2. Care for hypothermia (discussed earlier in this chapter).
3. Treat for shock.
4. Care for fractures and other injuries.
5. Transport as soon as possible.

CHAPTER REVIEW

KEY TERMS

You may find it helpful to review the following terms.

air embolism—gas bubbles in the bloodstream. The plural term is *emboli.*

asphyxia (as-FIK-si-ah)—suffocation from lack of air.

chilblains—lesions that occur from repeated prolonged exposures of bare skin to temperatures between 32°F and 60°F.

decompression sickness—a condition resulting from nitrogen trapped in the body's tissues caused by coming up too quickly from a deep, prolonged dive. A symptom of decompression sickness is "the bends," or deep pain in the muscles and joints.

drowning—death caused by changes in the lungs resulting from immersion in water. See also *near-drowning.*

freezing—*deep frostbite,* the third stage or the deepest of the three degrees of frostbite. The subcutaneous layers and the deeper structures of the body are affected; muscles, bones, deep blood vessels, and organ membranes can become frozen.

frostbite—the common term for *superficial frostbite,* the second stage or the middle of the three degrees of frostbite. Ice crystals form in the skin and subcutaneous layers. *Frostbite* is also used as the general term for all three degrees of frostbite (frostnip, frostbite, and freezing).

frostnip—*incipient frostbite,* the first stage or the least serious of the three degrees of frostbite. The skin reddens or whitens and becomes numb, but there is little or no tissue damage.

heat cramps—a condition characterized by muscle cramps and profuse perspiration, brought about by exposure to heat.

heat exhaustion—a form of shock characterized by rapid, shallow breathing, weak pulse, cold, clammy skin, and profuse perspiration brought about by exposure to heat; commonly called "heat prostration."

heat stroke—a life-threatening emergency that occurs when the body's temperature-regulating mechanisms fail during exposure to heat; characterized by deep, then shallow breathing, full, rapid pulse, hot, dry skin, and little or no sweating; commonly, and inaccurately, called "sun stroke."

hyperthermia (HI-per-THURM-i-ah)—an increase in body temperature above normal; life-threatening at its extreme.

hypothermia (HI-po-THURM-i-ah)—a generalized cooling that may reduce the body temperature below normal; life-threatening at its extreme.

laryngospasm (lah-RING-go-spazm)—spasm of the larynx that seals the airway, set off when water passes the epiglottis.

mammalian diving reflex—a reaction that occurs when the face is submerged in water. Breathing is inhibited, the heart rate slows, and major blood flow is sent to the brain, heart, and lungs.

near-drowning—the condition of having begun to drown. The near-drowning patient may be conscious, unconscious with heartbeat and pulse, or with no heartbeat or pulse but still able to be resuscitated. Only when sufficient time without breathing has passed to render resuscitation useless (sometimes 30 minutes or more if the patient has been in cold water) has *drowning* truly taken place.

trench foot—a condition characterizing by swelling, numbness, and waxy, mottled skin that develops when the lower extremities remain in cool water for a prolonged period; also called *immersion foot.*

water chill—chilling caused by conduction of heat from the body when the body or clothing is wet.

wind chill—chilling caused by convection of heat from the body in the presence of currents of cool air.

SUMMARY

Emergencies Due to Excessive Heat

Exposure to excessive heat can bring about heat cramps, heat exhaustion, or heat stroke. Heat cramps are seldom a serious problem. Some cases of heat exhaustion can turn serious. All cases of heat stroke are true emergencies. Review the signs and symptoms of all three conditions in Scan 20-1. You must be able to tell one condition from the others.

Care for heat cramps includes cooling the patient, giving fluids with electrolytes, and massaging cramped muscles. In cases of heat exhaustion, cool the patient, give fluids with electrolytes, administer oxygen if needed, and treat for shock.

For heat stroke, cool the patient as rapidly as possible. Do not delay transport . . . cool the patient en route. Use ice bags, cold packs, or soaked sheets, and additional cool water. Remember, *transport immediately*. This is a *true emergency*.

Emergencies Due to Excessive Cold

Exposure to cold can cause incipient frostbite (frostnip), superficial frostbite (frostbite), or deep frostbite (freezing). The signs for each of these conditions are given in Table 20-1.

Often, the patient can use his own body heat to warm frostnipped areas of the body. Frostbite and freezing require gentle handling of the affected part, keeping the patient warm, and transporting to a medical facility. If transport is delayed and instructions from a physician cannot be obtained, the affected area may be rewarmed by immersing it in water that is warm but still comfortable to your touch. The same basic care also applies to freezing.

Excessive cold can bring about hypothermia. Shivering, numbness, and drowsiness are most frequently noted in hypothermia. Care for mild hypothermia involves using external heat sources to raise the patient's body temperature slowly (follow local protocol). Hypothermia can be very serious. If the patient becomes unconscious, has problems with breathing, has a slowed pulse rate, has frozen body parts, or is in cardiac arrest, provide needed basic life support, wrap him in an insulated blanket, and transport as soon as possible. *Do not* try to rewarm the patient with severe or extreme hypothermia.

Chilblains are red, swollen, tender lesions that result from prolonged exposure of bare skin to cool or cold temperatures. No special treatment is required; however, the patient should be seen by a physician to be sure the lesion has no other cause. Trench foot is caused by prolonged immersion of the extremities in cool or cold water, characterized by swelling, numbness, a waxy and mottled appearance, and perhaps a bad odor. The extremity should be gently dried, rewarmed, dressed, and elevated, and the patient should be transported.

Injured patients entrapped in a collision vehicle or other wreckage are especially susceptible to the effects of cold and should be kept warm by blocking holes in the wreckage, removing wet clothing if possible, and covering the patient.

Accidents Involving Water

Drowning or near-drowning is the number one problem faced in all water-related accidents. However, injuries of all types do occur and medical problems may have caused the accident. Often associated with water and ice accidents are airway obstruction, cardiac arrest, heart attacks, head and neck injuries, internal injuries, and hypothermia.

In drownings, laryngospasms at first keep most water from entering the lungs. In later stages of drowning, water does enter the lungs. In fresh water drowning, surfactant is washed from the alveoli causing them to collapse and preventing further air exchange. Resulting heart arrhythmia is the usual cause of death. In salt water drownings, salt water in the lungs takes water from the bloodstream causing massive edema of the lungs. Death is due to resulting hypoxia.

Drowning occurs when breathing and heartbeat are stopped and successful resuscitation is no longer possible (often 30 minutes or more after cessation of breathing if the patient has been in cool or cold water). Near-drowning occurs when the patient does not lose consciousness, or does not lose heartbeat and breathing, or the patient is successfully resuscitated.

To rescue a patient who is in the water, first try to REACH him with an object and pull him out; if this fails, then THROW him something that will float and TOW him from the water; if this fails, ROW a boat to him; as a last resort, GO into the water and swim to the patient.

WARNING: DO NOT GO INTO THE WATER TO ATTEMPT A RESCUE UNLESS YOU ARE A GOOD SWIMMER AND HAVE BEEN TRAINED IN WATER RESCUE.

Consider any unconscious patient to have neck and spinal injuries and take care to protect the patient's neck and spine during care, both in and out of the water. Whenever possible try to support the patient's back and keep the neck rigid and in line with the midline of the body. When providing rescue breathing, use the jaw-thrust method to protect possible neck and spinal injuries.

If you are a good swimmer and have been trained in water rescue, you may be able to start rescue breathing, if needed, while the patient is in the water. If the patient in the water is unconscious, work to apply an extrication collar and to place the patient on a spine board for floating and lifting from the water.

Starting CPR while the patient is in the water will probably be ineffective. Get the patient onto land as quickly as possible if CPR must be instituted. Care for any patient already out of the water as required by your primary and secondary surveys and interviews.

All patients in water-related accidents should be managed for shock, kept as warm as possible without overheating, and given oxygen if needed. Do not allow the near-drowning patient to walk. Dispatch or the medical facility will need to know if the accident was in fresh or salt water and if it was a cold- or warm-water accident. Obtain directions for transport. You may have to take the patient to a special facility.

Diving accidents usually produce head, neck, and spinal injuries. The hands, feet, and ribs also are frequently injured. Scuba diving accidents may involve air embolism or decompression sickness. In either case, gas bubbles enter the blood. If the patient has been scuba diving, look for personality changes, distorted senses, convulsions, sudden loss of consciousness, and signs of air being trapped in the chest cavity, coughing, choking chest pains, and changes in the appearance of the skin (blotches or changing rashes). For decompression sickness, expect a delayed reaction and deep pains in the muscles and joints (the "bends"). For either air embolism or decompression sickness the treatment is the same: Place the patient on the left side, with the body slanted to keep the head in a slight downward position and maintain an open airway. Provide the highest possible concentration of oxygen, care for shock, and keep the patient warm. Find out if the patient is to be transported to a special care facility.

Accidents Involving Ice

If you must perform an ice rescue, you should be trained to do so and have the personnel and the equipment you will need. Try to throw a line or extend a pole to the patient. With the help of others, you may be able to reach the patient by sliding a boat onto the ice or crawling along a ladder. Treat the rescued patient for hypothermia and for any injuries he may have sustained.

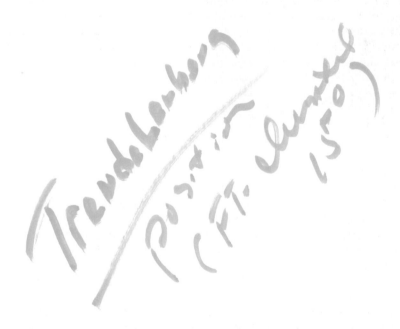

CHAPTER 21

On the Scene

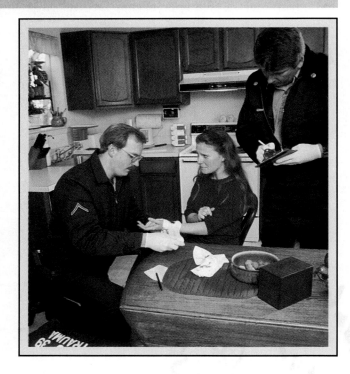

You: *That's a nasty cut, Miss Marks. How did it happen?*

Adele: *I was cutting up vegetables for dinner and my hand slipped. (You don't see any vegetables—only a bloody knife.)*

You: *Miss Marks, I see that you are upset, and I really want to help. I can help you better if you tell me more about what happened. Is it really true that you cut yourself cooking?*

Adele *(after a long pause, crying even harder): I've been depressed, and yesterday my boyfriend broke up with me. I tried to slit my wrists, and I couldn't even do that right. It probably sounds stupid to you.*

You: *No, it doesn't sound stupid, and I think we can get you some help. Thanks for telling me the truth. I'm sure it wasn't easy. Have you taken any medications today?*

Adele: *No. My psychiatrist prescribed pills for depression, but I haven't taken any for awhile. (crying harder) What'll I do now?*

You: *We'll take care of your arm and then take you to the hospital. There are some really good people over there who can help you.*

Adele *(still weeping): Okay.*

Adele Marks, 23 years old, summons your EMS unit for a laceration to her left wrist. The wound is approximately 5 cm long. There are several smaller scratches parallel to the largest wound. There is a small pool of blood on the floor, blood on the phone, and blood on Adele's clothes.

Adele is visibly upset and crying. Your survey reveals no further injuries. She is holding a towel over the wound, and bleeding has stopped. You observe a sheet of paper on the table near Adele. It looks like a note to someone. Adele quickly tucks it under a mat.

As you continue talking with Adele, you apply a dressing to the wound. Meanwhile, your partner is writing Adele's history and will gather up her medications to take along to the hospital.

What led you to believe that Adele Marks's wounds were not accidental? How has this changed your course of treatment? How has it affected scene safety? Your understanding of special patients has helped you work effectively in this situation.

Special Patients and Behavioral Problems

The more you work as an EMT, the more you will appreciate the variety of humanity. Of course, every patient is unique and special. In emergency care, however, *special patients* are those who require modified or special care procedures. Some of these special patients—such as children and substance abusers—have been discussed in earlier chapters.

In this chapter, you will learn care procedures for the elderly, the deaf, blind, and disabled, those who don't speak English, as well as patients who are suffering emotional problems, who are aggressive, who have attempted suicide, or who are victims of crime, including rape. You will also learn to care for *yourself,* when the job makes you vulnerable to violence or stress.

Expected Outcome, Chapter 21: *You will be able to modify and use special care procedures for patients with a variety of special problems, and to monitor and take care of your own well-being.*

Warning: Protect yourself from infectious diseases by using appropriate barrier devices such as a pocket face mask with one-way valve, face shield, or bag-valve mask; goggles or eye shield; and disposable gloves. Always conform to your local EMS system's infection exposure control plan.

MANAGING A CRISIS

COMMUNICATING WITH SPECIAL PATIENTS
    The Geriatric Patient
    The Deaf Patient
    The Blind Patient
    The Non-English-Speaking Patient
    The Physically Disabled Patient
    The Mentally Impaired Patient

DEALING WITH BEHAVIORAL PROBLEMS
    Stress Reactions
    Emotional and Psychiatric Emergencies
    Aggressive Behavior
    Attempted Suicide
    Victims of Crime

EMT STRESS SYNDROME

Objectives

Most special patients require special communications skills and emotional support. How you speak to a patient, what you say, how you express concern, how you listen, and how you indicate that you are listening are very important in special patient emergency care. Collectively, this is *personal interaction*, a skill that takes time to develop and experience with many different types of patients.

Personal interaction is of great importance when dealing with children, the elderly, deaf patients, blind patients, drug and alcohol abuse patients, patients with emotional emergencies, victims of crime and sexual abuse, and patients who have been injured by friends or members of their own families. Each of these patients may believe that the emergency they are experiencing is a crisis and that they are unable to control any aspect of the situation. In such a situation, personal interaction may be the key to effective total patient care.

MANAGING A CRISIS

When you are called to the scene of an accident or an illness, you consider the situation to be an emergency. To the patient, the situation may be a *crisis*, a crucial moment, or a turning point in his life. Bystanders may consider the emergency to be a crisis because they believe that what is happening is beyond their control and their ability to help.

Whenever there is a crisis, real or imagined, as an EMT you will have to initiate crisis management. Your professional attitude, your personal interaction skills, and the emergency care you provide will help the patient and the patient's family and friends to begin to deal with the crisis.

Simply put, a person in a crisis is upset, and emotional stress can steadily deteriorate the patient's physical and mental stability. Your emotional support can not only help the patient's mental well-being, it can also improve his physical well-being. You can not only keep

14. Describe the actions to be taken by the EMT if the patient is aggressive. (pp. 594-595)

15. Describe the actions to be taken by the EMT when caring for a patient who may attempt suicide. (pp. 595-596)

16. State the role of the EMT at the crime scene in relation to patient care and the chain of evidence. (p. 596)

17. Describe what special factors must be considered when providing care for the victim of assault or domestic violence. (p. 596)

18. Describe what special factors must be considered when providing care for the rape victim. (p. 596)

19. List the indications of EMT stress syndrome. (p. 597)

20. List some ways the EMT can relieve stress. (p. 597)

Skills *As an EMT you should be able to*

1. Use personal interaction with patients experiencing a crisis or having a stress reaction or an emotional or psychiatric emergency.

2. Initiate crisis management when appropriate.

3. Establish effective communication with elderly, deaf, blind, non-English-speaking, physically disabled, or mentally impaired patients.

4. Provide proper care for the aggressive patient and the patient about to attempt suicide, when your own safety is ensured.

5. Provide care at the controlled crime scene, helping to preserve the chain of evidence.

6. Provide proper care for crime victims, including victims of rape.

7. Apply stress reduction techniques to prevent EMT stress syndrome.

---

an emotional emergency from growing worse, you can help the patient relax and perhaps avoid developing serious shock.

At the scene of a crisis, remember to

- *Look and act like a professional provider of emergency care.*
- *React in a calm professional manner.* Be careful not to react to what may be meaningless insults or to overreact to what the patient may do or say. Remember, the patient in need of your care is not at his best.
- *Talk with the patient and listen to what he is saying.* Let him know that you are there to help. This tells the patient that he is important, that you are concerned, and that you recognize he truly has a problem.
- *Avoid improper conversation.* To the best of your abilities and training, answer the patient's questions and try to be positive about his situation, but do not lie. *Never* offer a simple solution to the patient's problem or tell him that everything is going to

be fine. Avoid comparing yourself with the patient or telling the patient your own problems. Don't confront the patient and tell him that he is wrong or not making sense.

- *Do something for the patient.* The idea that "actions speak louder than words" is very true in emergency care. Asking if the patient is in pain, controlling minor bleeding, or dressing a minor wound helps a patient deal with the emergency, even if he sees it as a crisis.

Be realistic in caring for patients. You do not have the time or the training to sit down with the patient and go through an entire crisis intervention procedure. The sooner you can calmly transport the patient to a medical facility, the sooner he will receive medical care and crisis management help from trained and experienced professionals. Your role with the patient is not a problem-solving role but one of providing some emotional support and taking the patient to where the patient care team can assess his needs and problems. Never think that because you are good at working with people or good at solving your own problems you can assess patients' abilities to handle crises and determine what they must do to solve their problems.

It is important for the patient to believe that you are concerned about him because he is a person, not just an emergency care problem for you to solve. Make certain that you use his name. When possible, do not just talk *to* the patient but have a conversation *with* him. Avoid spending most of the time talking with your partner. Some EMTs develop the habit of stopping conversation with the patient after the initial interview. They provide physical care, reserving conversation for other members of the EMS system. Don't lose sight of the fact that emotional support requires ongoing personal interaction with the patient.

When you arrive at the scene of injury, illness, or emotional crisis, make certain that you know why you are there and what you can do. Ask yourself, "What does this patient need?" and "What am I trained to do?" The patient may need many things, ranging from love and understanding to a solution for a family problem. You can't provide all of that, but you are trained to provide emotional support. And, in the midst of an emotional crisis, don't forget that the patient also needs professional emergency care for his physical injuries or medical problems!

There may be one more question you find yourself asking when you have been involved in the management of a crisis: "Did I make a difference?" Almost certainly you did. The reaction of the patient may not have been what you had hoped for, and there may not have been any "miracle" turnaround in the patient's emotional stress or demeanor, but you probably helped the patient deal with his stress at the scene and during transport, and the very fact that you transported the patient to a facility where he could gain access to total patient care must be considered a major helping factor. In addition, the emotional support you provided before transfer probably helped make the patient more receptive to the support offered by the patient care team at the medical facility.

COMMUNICATING WITH SPECIAL PATIENTS

All kinds of patients can sometimes be hard to talk with. However, EMTs often report special problems when interviewing children (see Chap-

ter 17), older patients, deaf patients, blind patients, patients who speak a foreign language, and patients who are mentally retarded, developmentally disabled, or confused.

Communication is any activity aimed toward understanding and making yourself understood. Communication can be verbal (oral or written), or nonverbal (using body language such as eye contact, gestures, posture, touching, physical proximity), or a combination of both.

To establish effective communications, remember to

- *Ensure that the patient is listening and understands you.* Never assume that you have established communications. Identify yourself, ask if you can help, and give the patient a chance to respond. You cannot develop rapport with a patient unless you are sure, verbally or nonverbally, that he is listening and understands what you are trying to express.
- *Be direct.* Let the patient know that you are taking responsibility for his care. Explain what you are doing and what you are looking for. Answer his questions honestly. Do not play down the fact that injury or medical problems exist. Do not give the false hope that nothing is wrong or that everything is or will be OK.
- *Communicate at the proper level.* Make certain that you are using terms that the patient understands. ("Are you having trouble breathing?" is more meaningful than "Do you have dyspnea?") Ask questions so that the patient may participate in his own care and you can assess his understanding of the situation.
- *Use nonverbal communication.* Squat or get down at their level. Keep eye contact with the patient. Realize that some people may feel threatened by eye contact and adjust such contact to suit the patient. Smile when appropriate. Stay relaxed enough so that the patient believes you have confidence in yourself and an interest in him and his problem. Allow the patient to be comfortable with you and your desire to help. Until then, give the patient his "space." Some people cannot tolerate the close physical proximity of another person until they have established some form of comfortable communication.

Remember: Patients expect you to be a competent EMT and may not notice that you are doing an efficient job. However, they will get upset if they feel you are not being nice to them.

The Geriatric Patient

Too often, we have preconceived notions of how certain people will act, think, and react. These are stereotypes. Many stereotypes are based on age: "Teenagers always do this," we think, and "Old people (geriatric patients) are like that."

Old age is nothing more than late adulthood, and people in this age category are individuals of all types and personalities, most of whom are as mentally competent as they ever were. A person is the total of all his experiences, and the average person in late adulthood probably has experienced more than the average person in early or middle adulthood. This means that you will find more variations with older patients. Having grown up in a different era than the one you grew up in, and perhaps undergoing some of the special experiences and problems associated with aging, however, you may find that many older patients do approach things differently than you do (Figure 21-1).

Keep the following ideas in mind as you care for the geriatric patient.

- *Address the older patient as you would any adult.* Identify yourself as an Emergency Medical Technician, trained to help. (While you may think that "all old people are alike," the older patient may think that all young people are alike . . . too inexperienced to help.) Ask the patient's name and use it frequently, never resorting to "old timer," "pops," "grandma," or other such

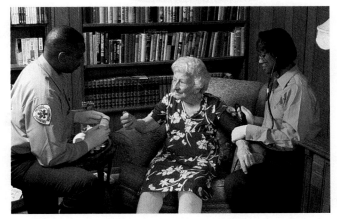

Figure 21-1 Let the geriatric patient set the pace of the interview.

terms. As with all adult patients, address the patient as Mr., Mrs., Miss, or Ms.—whatever is correct or the patient seems to prefer. If you can't discover the last name, use Ma'am or Sir, not the patient's first name, which is especially likely to offend an older person, unless the patient introduces himself that way. Talk to your patient as you would want another EMT to address your grandfather or grandmother.

- *Be aware that hearing may—or may not—be a problem.* As people age, hearing sometimes diminishes. Consider that a hearing problem may be the reason a patient is unresponsive, but do not assume it. Avoid shouting; remember that the older person who doesn't have a hearing problem will be insulted as well as irritated by being yelled at. A gentle tap on the arm may be all that is needed to alert an elderly patient to your presence. Maintain eye contact, speaking directly to the patient. (A common error in dealing with geriatric patients is to talk to the patient's younger relative rather than directly to the patient. This can be infuriating to the older patient, who will be quick to detect and resent any hint of being thought incompetent.) Begin by speaking in your normal voice. When in doubt, ask if the patient can hear you. If need be, speak directly into his ear.

- *Don't rush the conversation.* People in late adulthood spend more time thinking about what you say and what they are going to say in response. Younger people detect that the conversation is going more slowly than with someone their own age and assume that the older individual is thinking more slowly. Slowness in conversation has been shown to have nothing to do with the mind's slowing down. Older people, through experience, know that words carry a lot of weight. They spend more time in conversation simply because experience has taught them to place a high value on what is said. You will also find that many older people who live in isolation are simply out of practice in the art of conversation.

This is not to say that you will not sometimes encounter the older patient whose mind is deteriorating. Even when this is true, the best procedure is to talk with the person as patiently as possible.

- *Give the patient some control of the process.* Remember that the geriatric patient is an adult who has gone through other emergencies in his life. Older people know what works for them. After you are certain that there are no life-threatening problems, allow the older patient to have some control of the pace of the survey and interview.

- *Offer support to partners and friends.* If the patient's spouse or close friend is at the scene, think of yourself as having more than one patient. You may be caring for a husband while his wife of 30 years watches in total fear, believing that death will take him away. Provide emotional support to both individuals. Be watchful of elderly partners and friends, for the stress of the situation could set off a heart attack, convulsion, respiratory problem, or some other medical emergency.

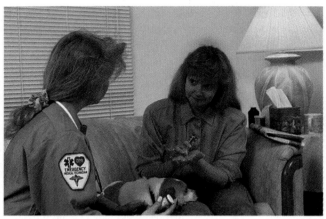

Figure 21-2 Communicate with the deaf patient through lip-reading, writing, gestures, or sign language.

The Deaf Patient

It is unfortunate, but most of us have little experience in communicating with the deaf and almost no skills to help us talk to them. This is true even though there are several million totally deaf people in our country, and many more who have some serious degree of hearing loss.

Seldom will you find a deaf person embarrassed about being deaf. Usually, it is the person with normal hearing who has this problem during a conversation with the deaf person. Even experienced EMTs find themselves embarrassed when trying to interview a deaf patient. The embarrassment usually comes from doing something you don't know how to do well. However, sometimes the uneasy feelings are due to guilt, as if the EMT had done something to cause the person's deafness. The deaf individual does not blame you for his deafness.

Follow these steps if you encounter or suspect deafness in your patient.

- *Find out if the patient is deaf.* Remember that any patient might not be able to hear you, even if he speaks clearly. In most cases, a deaf person will tell you that he is deaf or point to his ear and shake his head to indicate, "No, I cannot hear." Some patients may try to speak to you in sign, using their hands and fingers to communicate in gestures. When in doubt, write out, "Are you deaf?" on a card or paper.
- *Find a way to make yourself understood* (Figure 21-2). Once you are aware of the patient's deafness, write out or ask him, "Can you read lips?" When speaking to the

lip-reading deaf patient, make certain that your face is in bright light (shine a flashlight on your face if you have to) and speak slowly, but without distorting how you would normally form words. When you ask a question, point to your mouth to alert the person to the fact that he will have to read your lips. Never turn away from the person while you speak.

Many deaf people cannot read lips or find the process to be very difficult in an emergency. Your best methods of communication will be through writing and using gestures. If you point to an area on your body and make a face as if you are in pain and point back to the individual, he will usually understand your question. If you are examining the patient, point to your own body before you attempt to do something to his body.

- *Maintain physical contact.* Throughout the entire care of a deaf patient, try to remain face to face and keep direct physical contact (touching). Hold his hand, keeping one of your hands free to gesture or to gain his attention by a gentle tap on the shoulder. Point out the arrival of additional help or other events that may have gone unnoticed.
- *Ensure that you understand the patient.* Some deaf persons can speak clearly, some have speech that may take a little practice to understand, and others may not be able to speak at all. If the patient cannot speak, use written communication. Should the deaf patient be able to speak, listen very carefully to what he is saying. If you cannot understand something that has been said,

do not pretend to understand. This could be a serious mistake in gaining information and patient confidence. Always indicate that you do not understand by shaking your head in an obvious "no" gesture.

The Blind Patient

Blind people are seldom embarrassed by their blindness. Again, it is the inexperienced person trying to communicate with the blind who usually becomes embarrassed. Think for a moment: Why should it be difficult to converse with a blind person? After all, he can hear what you are saying and he is usually very aware of the world around him. Many EMTs claim that the survey and interview of blind patients are really not much different from those of sighted patients.

If you remember to tell the blind patient what you are going to do before you do it, if you keep voice and touch contact throughout the period of care, and if you keep the person informed of what is happening around him (e.g., the source of strange noises, the arrival of additional help), you will find little extra difficulty in caring for the blind patient.

Try to remember these things when dealing with the blind.

- *Do not shout or speak loudly.* Being blind does not mean the person cannot hear.
- *Do not change the words you would normally use in speaking to a patient.* People often become upset if they use the words "see" or "look" when they are with a blind person. Blind people also use these words. Your blind patients will know that you are not trying to embarrass them.
- *Keep in contact through speech or touch.*
- *When walking, let the blind person hold your arm* (Figure 21-3). Should you have to move a blind patient who can walk on his own, let him hold your arm, rather than you holding onto his arm. Position the patient slightly behind you, off to your side. Alert the blind patient of steps and other hazards. Never push or pull the blind patient, always lead him as he holds your arm.

The Non-English-Speaking Patient

Establishing patient confidence and carrying out a useful patient assessment can be extremely difficult if your patient does not speak English. In this situation, try these steps.

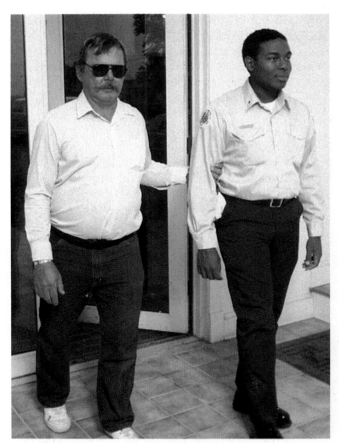

Figure 21-3 Lead a blind person as he holds your arm; never pull or push him.

- *Seek help from relatives or bystanders.* See if a relative or bystander can translate.
- *Identify yourself and your patient.* If no one is on hand to translate, point to yourself and say your name. Let the patient see your patch or badge. Try to find out your patient's name. Usually, if you point to yourself and say your name and then point to the patient, he will understand and respond with his name.
- *Use gestures.* Point to the part of a patient's body you need to touch or examine. Use gestures to indicate there may be pain or to ask if there is pain. Throughout the entire process, speak to the patient. He may understand more English than is at first apparent.

If you are an EMT whose service area includes communities of non-English-speaking individuals, learn a few phrases to help you gain patient confidence and provide emergency care. In many cases, those persons who live in the community would welcome the opportunity to help you and other EMTs learn their language as it applies to the emergency situation. In some areas the telephone company or hospital may have translators who are just a telephone call away.

The Physically Disabled Patient

The typical physically disabled patient has an orthopedic or neurologic disability. This type of patient can present special problems in assessment since it is difficult to determine injury to a body part that does not function properly or will not respond to neurologic tests. When caring for the physically disabled trauma patient

- *Assume injury.* You will have to assume injury, provide care accordingly, and transport so a physician can make the proper determination of the patient's problem.
- *Let the physically handicapped patient do what he can for himself.* If something is appropriate for the nonhandicapped patient to do, then it is appropriate for the handicapped patient who can do the task.
- *Communicate as you would with any other patient.* Do not avoid questioning the patient about his handicap. Use the terms "handicap" and "disability." Never use the terms "cripple," "crippled," or "lame."

The Mentally Impaired Patient

Not all handicaps involve body movement and functions. Some patients are handicapped by mental retardation or developmental disabilities. There will be times when this is easy to detect. At other times you may not be able to tell if these disabilities may be the cause of the patient's behavior or if you are dealing with a "normal" patient who is somehow confused. When dealing with a patient who is confused or may be mentally retarded or developmentally disabled, you should

1. *Begin by speaking to the patient as you would to any patient in his age group.*
2. *Ask questions and evaluate the patient's response.* Listen carefully to the patient, assessing his level of understanding, to help you determine
   - Patient understanding
   - If you are using terms at the appropriate level
   - If you need to re-explain anything that you have told the patient

3. *Slow the pace of the conversation.* This type of patient often gives delayed responses to questions and actions.

DEALING WITH BEHAVIORAL PROBLEMS

In an emergency, most patients will behave in a manner considered to be "normal" for the situation. However, the term *normal* implies certain medical and philosophical judgments about the behavior. It is more appropriate, as an EMT, to say that the patient is or is not behaving in a "typical" manner, or behaving "as expected." This also simplifies your assessment task. Based on your training and experience, you will be able to classify patients with simple statements such as that the patient is "behaving as expected" or "behaving in an unusual manner."

At the scene of accident or illness, you may have to provide care for a continuum of behavior ranging from typical stress reactions to emotional and psychiatric emergencies.

Stress Reactions

Most patients will display emotions such as fear, grief, and anger. These are typical *stress reactions* at the accident scene and common reactions to serious illness.

In the vast majority of cases, as you begin to take control of the situation and treat the patient as an individual, personal interaction will inspire confidence in your ability to help. The patient will begin to calm down and may even begin to feel that he can cope with the emergency.

Be as unhurried as you can. If you rush the survey and interview, the patient may think he has lost control of the situation. He also may believe that you are concerned about the problem, not him as an individual. Let the patient know that you are there to help.

Whenever you care for a patient who is displaying typical stress reactions

- Act in a calm manner, giving the patient time to gain control of his emotions.
- Quietly and carefully evaluate the situation.
- Keep your own emotions under control.
- Honestly explain things to the patient.
- Let the patient know that you are listening to what he is saying.
- Stay alert for sudden changes in behavior.

In so doing, you are applying *crisis management* techniques to help the patient deal with stress. If the patient does not begin to interact with you, or if he does not calm down, then you must assume that he is having a problem of a more serious nature than an expected stress reaction (see "Emotional and Psychiatric Emergencies," later in this chapter).

Sudden Death Any emergency involving patient death produces a great amount of stress for the patient's family, bystanders, and the EMTs. Death without warning due to trauma or medical causes can produce intense reactions from the patient's family. Be prepared to deal with intense expressions of grief, denial, guilt, or anger including crying, hysteria, or physical illness such as vomiting or fainting.

There may be little you can do for the family and bystanders since you will probably be initiating basic life support. Tell the family what you must do. Keep them informed of the care being provided. Do not offer false hope.

Watch for indications that the stress of the situation is affecting you or your partner (use the "buddy system"). Indications of immediate stress reactions you may notice in yourself or your partner include physical illness, feelings of helplessness, anger, guilt, or frustration, avoidance of the fact of death, using "gallows" humor, or taking a cold (hyperclinical) approach to the emergency (see "EMT Stress Syndrome" later in this chapter).

Terminal Disease The process of dying can produce even more stress on a family than the loved one's death. The patient and the family may display denial (the person is not going to die), bargaining ("If God lets him live I'll work for starving children), anger, or depression. Toward the end of the illness, the dying patient may reach a state of acceptance while his family or friends have not.

When providing care for the terminally ill, tactfully try to find out from the patient if he is prepared for death or if he wishes to speak to someone about death and dying. The emergency department staff should be informed of the request so that a referral can be made. The family should be asked the same questions. Do not isolate the family from the patient. Should death occur while the patient is under your care, and there is a "living will" or "DNR" (do not resuscitate) order, provide or withhold basic life support according to local protocol (see Chapter 1).

Emotional and Psychiatric Emergencies

Sometimes you will encounter a patient whose mental state seems to go beyond any expected or typical stress reaction. This patient may be having an emotional or psychiatric emergency.

In an *emotional emergency*, the patient may

- Display emotions beyond what is expected or typical, to a point where they interfere with his thoughts and behavior
- Seem far more frightened than most patients in a similar situation
- Be unable to calm his excited state after an accident and does not calm down during the interview and the beginning of care procedures, in spite of your efforts to establish some level of personal interaction
- Nevertheless remain within some bounds of behavioral control, responding to people around him and not showing any indications of being dangerous to himself or others

The patient in a *psychiatric emergency* is far more out of reach or out of control than the person in an emotional emergency. In a psychiatric emergency, the patient may

- Try to hurt himself
- Try to hurt others
- Withdraw, no longer responding to people or to his environment
- Continue to express rage and hostility
- Continue to act depressed, sometimes crying and expressing feelings of worthlessness
- Apparently wish to take no actions to help himself or to allow himself to be helped

Since you are not a doctor or a psychiatrist, you cannot diagnose what kind of emotional or psychiatric problem the patient may be having. As an EMT you only need to be able to rule out a typical or expected stress reaction, illness, or injury. You may say that "the patient is acting in an unusual manner" and "seems to be having some kind of emotional or psychiatric emergency." Use descriptive terms such as "excited," "fearful," "confused," "overactive," "unpredictable," "agitated," "aggressive," and "detached." Avoid diagnostic terms such as "mentally ill," "psychotic," "phobic," "paranoid," "manic," "neurotic," and "schizophrenic." And by all means avoid such terms as "crazy," "nuts," "wacko," "loony," and other nonprofessional terms.

Often, the patient having an emotional emergency simply needs more time to cope with the stress of an emergency, and personal interaction is your main course of action. Usually you will have to spend more time talking with him and listening than would be necessary for the patient undergoing a typical stress reaction. The patient may improve if he thinks that he has more control over the situation. Give him time to answer your questions. When appropriate, let him decide which arm will be used for the blood pressure determination and how he would like to be positioned for transport.

The assessment and care of the patient having a possible psychiatric emergency requires you to stay calm and to act in a strictly professional manner. Carefully observe the patient and listen to what he is saying. Detect whatever symptoms and signs are evident, making certain that throughout the entire process of care that you can eliminate the possibilities of head injury, stroke, insulin shock, drug reactions, high fever, and other such medical emergencies.

Again, personal interaction is your first line of action. Take extra time to talk to the patient and let him talk to you. Make certain that he knows that you hear what he is saying. Do not threaten the patient or argue with him. Try to provide reassurance by telling him that you are there to help. Speak in a calm, direct manner, keeping eye contact whenever possible.

You are the first professional to begin both the physical and mental health care of the patient. The more reassurance you can provide for the patient who is having an emotional or psychiatric emergency, the easier it will be for the emergency department staff to continue with his care.

Do not leave such a patient alone. Be alert to aggressive or potentially violent behavior (discussed below), and protect yourself from harm at all times.

Aggressive Behavior

Aggressive or disruptive behavior may be caused by trauma to the brain and nervous system, metabolic disorders, stress, alcohol, drugs, or psychological disorders. Sometimes you will know that you will be dealing with an aggressive patient from the information you receive from dispatch. Other times the scene may provide quick clues (e.g., drugs, unclean conditions, broken furniture). Neighbors, family members, or bystanders may tell you that the patient is dan-

gerous or that he is angry. The patient's stance or how he has positioned himself in the room may give you an early warning of possible violence. On rare occasions, you may start with an apparently calm patient who quickly turns aggressive.

When a patient acts as if he may hurt himself or others, YOUR FIRST CONCERN MUST BE YOUR OWN SAFETY.* In such cases

- *Alert the police.*
- *Do not isolate yourself from your partner or other sources of help.*
- *Make certain that you have an escape route.* Should a patient become violent, retreat and wait for police assistance.
- *Do not take any action that may be considered threatening by the patient.* To do so may bring about hostile behavior directed against you or others.
- *Always be on the watch for weapons.* Stay out of kitchens; they are filled with dangerous weapons. Stay in a safe area until the police can control the scene.
- *Do not try to restrain a patient unless it is legal for you to do so.* In most localities, an EMT cannot legally restrain a patient, move him against his will, or force him to accept emergency care. You cannot restrain a patient even when his family asks you to do so. The restraint and forcible moving of patients is within the jurisdiction of law enforcement officers; once the patient is under control, the police can order you to transport the patient to the appropriate medical facility or, in some states, the order can come from a physician. In some jurisdictions, a physician can order a patient to be restrained; however, the physician is not empowered to order you to do this if taking such actions may place you in danger.

Remember: Each EMS system has its own standard operating procedures for dealing with aggressive patients and patients who may hurt themselves or others. Always follow your local guidelines.

If you are authorized by police or a physician to assist in restraining a patient, DO NOT TRY TO ASSIST IN RESTRAINING A PATIENT UNLESS THERE ARE SUFFICIENT PERSONNEL TO DO THE JOB. You must be able to ensure your safety and the safety of the patient.

*WARNING: Some patients may act adversely to your uniform, believing that you are a law enforcement officer.

If you help the police or a physician restrain a patient, make certain that the restraints are humane restraints. Handcuffs and plastic "throwaway" criminal restraints should not be used because of the soft tissue damage they can inflict. Initially, the police may have to use such restraints; however, these types of restraints can be replaced with leather cuffs and belts (these are not authorized for use in all states). If authorized in your state and by local protocols, an ambulance should carry leather cuffs, a waist-size belt, and at least three short belts. Soft restraints for the wrists and ankles can be made from gauze roller bandage.

Do not remove police restraints until you and the police are certain that the gauze or leather restraints will hold the patient. Once soft restraints are placed on a patient, do not remove them, even if the patient appears to be acting rationally; the patient may display the same aggressive behavior after the restraints are removed. The removal of restraints is the responsibility of the emergency facility staff and the police.

Note: Never secure a patient to a stretcher in a position that will not allow the patient to be turned in case of vomiting. The patient must be secured so that his wrists and ankles remain secured but his body can be turned.

Attempted Suicide

Each year in this country, some 20,000 people commit suicide. Many more suffer both physical and emotional injuries in suicide attempts. Anyone may become suicidal if emotional distress is severe, regardless of age, sex, race, ethnic origin, or economic and social status.

People attempt suicide for many reasons, including depression, the death of a loved one, financial problems, a terminated love affair, poor health, loss of esteem, divorce, fears of failure, and alcohol and drug abuse. They attempt to end their lives by any of a variety of methods, most commonly with sedatives and hypnotic drugs, less commonly by hanging, jumping from high places, ingesting poisons, inhaling gas, wrist-cutting, self-mutilation, or stabbing or shooting themselves.

Whenever dealing with a patient who has attempted or is about to attempt suicide, YOUR FIRST CONCERN IS YOUR OWN SAFETY, then the safety and well-being of the patient.

In dealing with a patient who is threatening to attempt suicide or a conscious patient who has made an unsuccessful suicide attempt

- *Make certain that the scene is safe and the patient does not have a weapon.* Unless you are a trained law enforcement officer following standard operating procedures, you have no business dealing with someone who has a weapon. Should you see that a patient has a weapon, withdraw carefully, if you can. Do not frighten him with any sudden moves. Do not threaten him in any way. Above all, do not try to be a hero and attempt to seize the weapon.

  If you cannot withdraw to safety, your best course of action is to try to talk to the individual and keep him engaged in conversation until additional help arrives. Again, do not do anything foolhardy that will result in your getting hurt.

- *Establish personal interaction with the patient, and do not leave the patient alone.* Establish visual and verbal contact with the patient as soon as possible. If the scene is safe (there is no weapon and the patient is not displaying aggressive or violent behavior), approach the patient to talk with him in a normal manner; if the scene is not secure, try to talk with the patient from a safe distance. Talk in a calm, professional manner. Make no threats and offer no indication of using force. Do not argue with the patient or criticize him. Do not point out that he is not making sense or that he contradicts something he said earlier in the conversation. Never joke about the patient's situation.

  Unless there is a physical emergency that must be cared for, sit down and spend some time with the patient. Talk with him, but do not try to direct all the conversation. It is likely that the patient has a need to tell you his story. Provide reassurance rather than pity.

- *Conduct assessment and care procedures.* Ask if you can help. If he seems in doubt, tell him that you wish to help him. Ask if he is hurt or in pain. As you gain the patient's confidence, explain what questions he must answer and what must be done as part of the physical assessment. Let the patient know that you think it would be best if he went with you to the hospital. Tell him how you need his cooperation and help.

- *Back off if necessary.* If the patient indicates increasing fear or aggression, do not push the issues of the examination or transport. Instead, try to re-establish the conversation and give the patient more time before you tell him again that going to the hospital is a good idea.

Follow your state and local laws and protocols with regard to reporting any attempted suicide to the medical facility, police, or government agencies.

Victims of Crime

As in all aspects of emergency care, YOUR FIRST CONCERN MUST BE YOUR OWN SAFETY. If you arrive at the scene and a crime is in progress or the criminal is still active at the scene, do not attempt to provide care. Wait until the police arrive and they tell you that the scene is safe.

To provide care at the controlled crime scene, keep the following considerations in mind.

- *You must try to preserve the chain of evidence* that will go from the crime scene to the courtroom. Touch only what you need to touch. Move only what must be moved to protect the patient and to provide proper care. Do not use the telephone unless the police tell you that you may do so. Unless you have police permission, move the patient only if he is in danger or if he must be moved to provide proper care (e.g., to a hard surface for CPR).
- *When approaching a crime victim, clearly identify yourself* by name and state that you are an Emergency Medical Technician arriving to help. This may prove to be very important if you are the first person to see the victim since the crime. The patient may be very frightened and disoriented. He could think that you are the criminal still at the scene or returning to the scene.
- *Do not burden the patient with questions about the crime.* Keep to your duties involving the care of the patient, remembering that one of the most important things you can do when caring for the victim of a crime is to provide emotional support and reassurance. Be prepared for the patient to show outrage or disbelief. The patient may withdraw, become depressed, or display rage or hysteria. Severe reactions often are noted in cases of assault and attempted murder.
- *If called to the scene of a domestic dispute, wait for police assistance.* Domestic disputes are dangerous calls because the people involved often act unpredictably. The call to have you respond was probably placed because someone has been beaten or injured by some act of violence. If the violent person is still on the scene, he may turn his aggression toward you. Sometimes it is the victim of the aggressive act who will attack you because you are an outsider interfering with a family matter.
- *If the crime is rape, do not do, or encourage the patient to do, anything that will destroy evidence.* Do not wash the patient nor allow the patient to wash. Ask the patient not to change clothing, use the bathroom, or take any liquids or food. To do so may destroy evidence. Obviously, you may not physically prevent anyone from doing these things, but you can explain why such activities may break the chain of evidence. The patient will probably cooperate and follow your requests.

  Emotional support is a must in cases of rape. The privacy, comfort, and dignity of the patient must be considered from the beginning of care. A critical factor in rape is the loss of control the patient feels. Help the patient regain a sense of control by taking care to work with, not on, the patient, for example asking her permission before touching or treating her. Rape victims often feel more comfortable having a female attend to them, so the female crew member may be the right choice to be the primary care giver. The degree of future emotional problems faced by the rape victim may well depend on how the patient is initially treated by the professionals who respond to help.

Remember: As an EMT you may have a legal duty to report any situation in which injury is a possible result of crime—whether the patient is a victim, a bystander, or the possible perpetrator of the crime. In most localities, you should not leave the crime scene until the police give you permission to do so.

EMT STRESS SYNDROME

Caring for patients suffering from stress reactions and other behavioral emergencies can cause you to suffer delayed reactions to stress (post-traumatic stress disorder). This is commonly known as EMT stress syndrome. It is much the same as any stress syndrome, except that it is associated with the stress generated at accidents, medical emergencies, disasters (see Chapter 22), incidents involving child abuse (see Chapter 17), incidents involving death, crime scenes, and emotional and psychiatric emergencies. This syndrome can lead to "burnout."

Some of the indications of stress syndrome include

- Irritability
- Feeling unappreciated
- Fatigue
- Inability to concentrate
- Lack of enthusiasm, perhaps wanting to quit
- Insomnia or nightmares
- Loss of appetite and/or interest in sexual activities
- Decrease in social activities
- Alcohol or drug abuse
- Avoidance of change and new ideas
- Physiological reactions, such as nausea, symptoms and signs of ulcers, colitis, frequent headaches, and muscle aches

To help prevent, reduce, or stop the development of stress syndrome

- *Seek peer support.* Talk with other EMTs about situations that bother you.
- *Seek the support of family and friends.* Let them know the "what, how, and why" of any incident that was stressful. Be willing to show and accept your emotional reactions.
- *Seek the services of a Critical Incident Stress Debriefing (CISD) team* if one is available.
- *Seek professional counseling.* If your EMS system does not offer this service, see your family doctor. Since stress syndrome is a part of every level of health care, odds are that your physician will know how to help you or refer you to someone for help.
- *Assess the reasons why you became an EMT and why you have continued to be one.* Is being an EMT still what you want? Before deciding to leave the service, talk with a professional counselor about other solutions.
- *Take some time off.* Take a vacation from being an EMT. A little change in schedule or environment may help you sort out your problems and give you a better perspective of your role as an EMT.
- *Take advantage of continuing education to reestablish your confidence.*
- *Keep things in perspective.* Not everything about being an EMT is serious. Keep a sense of humor. Do not become hyperclinical.

Do not expect a great deal of help from your family if you have let being an EMT lead to family problems (e.g., letting them feel ignored or that they are a lower priority to you than your job, or letting family activities slip). The members of your family and your friends can be of help if you plan time to share with them and make certain that you do not place them at a lower priority than your career or your interest in emergency medical service. Let them share in what you do by inviting them to your station or squad (show off new equipment and procedures). Have them participate in social activities that are part of being an EMT. Tell them what you do and why you believe it is important to both you and the community. Help them receive training in first aid, basic life support, or first responder-level care or to become EMTs if they so desire.

Stress syndrome is best prevented by sharing your experiences with family and friends and with other health care providers who understand what you do.

CHAPTER REVIEW

SUMMARY

Managing a Crisis

Special patients are those who require modified approaches to care and special procedures designed for a specific problem. Often the EMT will find that these patients require an extra effort in terms of communication and emotional support.

What is an emergency to you may be a crisis for the patient. The patient sees the event as a crucial moment or a turning point in his life. For such situations, crisis management must be initiated by the EMT.

Your main method to employ in crisis management is personal interaction. You have to look and act professional, react calmly, talk with the patient and listen to what he says, and avoid improper conversation. As you provide emotional support, you must do something for the patient. Providing even the simplest of care measures is useful in helping to manage the crisis.

To communicate with the patient effectively, ensure that he is listening and understands you, be direct, communicate at the proper level, and use nonverbal communication skills.

Remember that you have been trained to provide professional-level emergency care. The patient may need many things, one of which is your professional help. Keep in mind that you do make a difference.

Communicating With Special Patients

Problems with communication can occur when providing emergency care. When dealing with elderly patients, remember that a patient in late adulthood may set a pace for the interview and examination different from yours. The older patient knows what works for him, so allow him some control. Never assume that an older patient cannot hear you or think clearly. Keep in mind that you will have to provide emotional support for the patient, family, and friends.

Always make certain that a patient is able to hear you. If the patient is deaf, establish this fact and then find out if the patient can read lips or if you will have to use writing and gestures for communication. Try to maintain face-to-face contact with the deaf person.

When dealing with blind patients, do not raise your voice. Talk as you would to any patient, and keep both verbal and physical contact with the patient throughout all stages of care.

Some of your patients may not speak English. Use the help of bystanders whenever you can. If there is a large community of non-English-speaking people in your locality, learn some of the basic words and phrases needed to help you provide emergency care.

Dealing With Behavioral Problems

Most patients will exhibit stress reactions during an emergency. They tend to calm down as you interact with them and begin care. In cases of sudden death, be prepared to deal with grief, denial, guilt or anger, crying, hysteria, or physical illness such as vomiting or fainting on the part of family or close friends. In cases of terminal illness, the patient and the family may display denial, bargaining, anger, or depression. Follow local protocols with regard to a living will or order not to resuscitate.

Emotional emergencies are those in which the patients have an atypical or unexpectedly severe emotional reaction to an emergency situation. Patients who act as if they wish to hurt themselves or others may be having a psychiatric emergency. This classification also applies to patients who continue to express withdrawal, rage, hostility, depression, or an unwillingness to take any action.

In cases of emotional emergency, patients often simply need longer to cope with the emergency than do most patients. For both emotional and psychiatric emergencies, personal interaction is your best approach as you provide care. Make certain that the problem is not due to an injury or medical emergency. You must eliminate the possibilities of head injury, stroke, insulin shock, drug reactions, high fever, and other problems.

If the patient is aggressive or violent, wait for police assistance. Never try to provide care for a patient who has a weapon. Do not try to illegally restrain or transport the patient.

In cases of attempted suicide, make certain that the scene is safe before you approach the patient. Establish contact and provide emotional support, exercising personal interaction with the patient. When you can safely approach the patient, provide assessment and care and try to persuade the patient to agree to be transported to a hospital.

Provide care for the victims of crime only when the crime scene is controlled and you are certain of your own personal safety. Preserve the chain of evidence whenever possible. Touch only what you need to touch, and move the patient only when care or safety requires him to be moved. Provide emotional support as well as physical care to all victims of crime but do not ask questions about the crime. In cases of domestic violence, wait for police assistance.

Emotional support is a must in cases of rape. The privacy, comfort, and dignity of the patient must be carefully considered from the beginning of care. Explain to the patient why she should not change clothing, wash, go to the bathroom, or take any liquids or food. Help the patient regain some feeling of control, for example by asking permission before touching or treating her.

As an EMT you may have a legal duty to report any attempted suicides and situations in which injury may be due to crime.

In all special care situations, your safety comes first.

EMT Stress Syndrome

Learn to recognize the indications of EMT stress syndrome, such as irritability, feeling unappreciated, fatigue, inability to concentrate, lack of enthusiasm, sleep problems, loss of appetite or interest in sexual activity, decrease in social activity, drug or alcohol abuse, avoidance of change, or physical problems. Try to keep perspective and interact with your peers, family, friends, and professional counselors to prevent this syndrome or to stop it before it can lead to burnout and other problems.

22

On the Scene

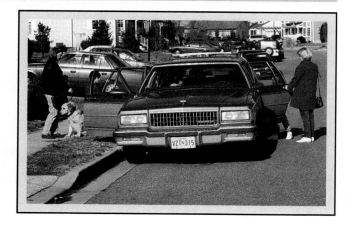

Marge Miller and Dot Henderson load up their three children and Dot's dog and set off for the park. Along the way, a squirrel runs into the road. An oncoming driver swerves into the path of Dot's car. Both cars go out of control and wind up in ditches on opposite sides of the road. Dazed, Dot struggles out of the car and to a house to call 911, then collapses.

You receive the call as a motor vehicle collision with an unknown number of injuries. As first to arrive, you spot the cars, observe a man and woman in one, the three children, a woman, and a dog inside the other.

You (as the senior EMT, to your partner): That woman is belted into the passenger seat. Where's the driver? I'll radio dispatch. You start triage.

Your Partner: Right. (He is already climbing into the car through the door Dot left ajar.)

You (over the radio to dispatch): Ambulance three-two-two to dispatch. We're on the scene at Garfield Road just south of Oak Lane. We have two cars off the road with six passengers inside, including three children. One driver is missing. Ambulance three-two-two is medical command. We're declaring an MCI [multiple-casualty incident]. Please dispatch four ambulances and a rescue truck. Have all units stage along the east shoulder of Garfield north of Oak. Can you advise where the call originated?

You slip into the bright orange command vest and prepare to direct incoming units. Your partner has determined that all the children, still belted into the back seat, are crying and so obviously have airway and breathing, but Marge Miller is not responsive. He has stabilized her head and is opening an airway. Dispatch relays the call's origin, and you direct one incoming EMT to that address to find the missing driver, Dot, while others tend to the children. The rescue crew gets to work on the other car, which is on its side and unstable. At one point you look around just in time to see a police officer placing Dot's dog into the squad car for safekeeping.

A few days later the local paper reports that all four adults, three kids, and the dog are fine thanks to good work by local EMS, rescue, and police.

Multiple-Casualty Incident and Disaster Management

Chapter Overview

You have been learning how to deal with individual patients at an emergency scene. But what if you are called to the scene of a multiple vehicle pile-up, airline crash, explosion, earthquake, or other situation in which there are many victims? In this chapter you will learn the basics of the EMT's role in such a situation.

Expected Outcome, Chapter 22: *You will understand the purpose and major elements of a community disaster plan and of the incident command system of organizing response to a multiple-casualty incident.*

Warning: Protect yourself from infectious diseases by using appropriate barrier devices such as a pocket face mask with one-way valve, face shield, or bag-valve mask; goggles or eye shield; and disposable gloves. Always conform to your local EMS system's infection exposure control plan.

DISASTER AND MULTIPLE-CASUALTY INCIDENT
OPERATIONS

SCENE MANAGEMENT
     Initial Triage
     Patient Identification
     Secondary Triage and Treatment

STAGING AND TRANSPORTATION
     Transportation Logistics
     Communicating with Hospitals

PSYCHOLOGICAL ASPECTS OF MULTIPLE-
CASUALTY INCIDENTS

Knowledge *After reading this chapter, you should be able to*

1. Define *multiple-casualty incident (MCI)* and *disaster* and explain how they differ. (p. 602)
2. Identify FOUR characteristics of a good disaster plan. (p. 603)
3. Explain the duties of the first EMTs to arrive at the scene of an MCI or disaster. (pp. 603-604)
4. Identify the FOUR priorities into which patients are categorized during triage. (p. 604).
5. Explain the limits to treatment that should be given to patients during initial triage and the reasons why treatment is limited at this stage. (pp. 604-605)
6. Explain the use of triage tags during primary and secondary triage. (pp. 605-606)
7. Define the responsibilities of the following EMS leaders at a multiple-casualty incident:
   - Medical/EMS command (p. 604)
   - Triage Officer (p. 605)
   - Treatment Officer (p. 605)
   - Staging Officer (p. 606)
   - Transportation Officer (p. 606)
8. Explain the proper methods of communicating with hospitals during an MCI or disaster. (p. 606)
9. Explain the basic approach an EMT should take to a psychologically stressed patient at an MCI or disaster. (p. 607)
10. Explain how an emotionally incapacitated EMT at the scene of an MCI or disaster should be managed. (p. 607)
11. Explain the role of a critical incident stress debriefing (CISD) team. (p. 607)
12. Explain how post traumatic stress disorder (PTSD) can affect rescue personnel. (p. 607)

Skills *As an EMT you should be able to*

1. Follow your community's disaster plan.
2. Initiate, carry out, or manage triage, transportation, and communications at the scene of an MCI or disaster.

Not every multiple-casualty incident is a disaster, and not every disaster is a multiple-casualty incident. It is wise to draw a distinction between the two types of events. By definition, a **multiple-casualty incident (MCI)** is any medical or trauma incident involving multiple patients (Figure 22-1). The numbers of patients required before an MCI can be declared varies in practice. Some jurisdictions will declare an MCI for as few as three patients on the grounds that practice with smaller-scale incidents will help prepare for larger ones. Other jurisdictions reserve the MCI designation for 5, 7, or more patients. Major MCIs, of course, can involve dozens or even hundreds of patients. A **disaster** is an emergency of such a magnitude as to severely overtax the capacity of an EMS system to deal adequately with the sick or injured.

What constitutes a disaster may often depend on the size of the community. A school bus accident with 30 patients may be a disaster for a small rural community, whereas a system such as that in New York City or Los Angeles would handle it as an MCI. Often sheer numbers of patients make an MCI a disaster. Sometimes the physical surroundings create a disaster even though the number of patients may be small. The important ingredient in a disaster is that, for whatever reason, the ability of the EMS system to respond to the situation is hampered by the situation itself. The experience of any major hurricane recently in the news demonstrates this well.

An example was Hurricane Andrew, which struck southern Florida in 1992. The fire department for the hardest-hit area had a disaster response team that was so good it had, at other times, been sent overseas to assist in foreign

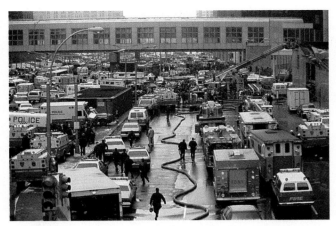

Figure 22-1 The scene of a multiple-casualty incident.

disaster operations. However, when Hurricane Andrew swept through the team's own backyard, the magnitude of the resulting damage far outpaced the availability of resources for many weeks. The fact that landmarks and street signs had been obliterated exacerbated the problem, making it extremely difficult to locate emergencies as they arose. Fire department personnel were on duty for as long as 36 hours at a time. Many had, themselves, suffered great losses in the hurricane and had to set aside personal worries to attend to other victims of the storm. The fire department was so overwhelmed with calls for service that its experienced disaster team was unable to function in accordance with their training and plans. Assistance from surrounding counties was essential.

The fundamental lesson of Hurricane Andrew and other similar events is that no service should expect to be able to manage a disaster on its own. Mitigating an emergency of this order requires interagency pre-planning and cooperation.

DISASTER AND MULTIPLE-CASUALTY INCIDENT OPERATIONS

Although the principles of managing MCIs and disasters are the same, disasters generally unfold over a longer period of time and require greater support from outside agencies. Well-trained and practiced EMTs can usually cope with MCIs pretty well. Experience has shown that even the best-trained EMTs have a difficult time managing in a disaster.

One way to minimize the operating difficulties of a disaster is for every EMT to be familiar with the local **disaster plan**. A disaster plan is a pre-defined set of instructions that tells a community's various emergency responders what to do in specific emergencies. While no disaster plan can encompass every eventuality, there are several features common to all good disaster plans. The plan should be

- Written to address the events that are conceivable for a particular location—Kansas needs to plan for tornadoes, not hurricanes.
- Well publicized—Each emergency responder should be familiar with the plan and how it is to be put into operation.
- Realistic—The plan must be based on the actual availability of resources.
- Rehearsed—Experience has proven that the only way to get a plan to work correctly is to exercise it and, in so doing, work out the unforeseen "bugs."

It is beyond the scope of this text to attempt to teach the new EMT to write a disaster plan or even to impart enough knowledge for the new EMT to be in charge of a disaster operation. However, it is important to understand the EMT's potential roles in the management of such an incident.

SCENE MANAGEMENT

The first EMTs on the scene of an MCI or disaster must be sure to initiate the **incident command system** that is in practice in their jurisdiction. This is the general plan for managing a multiple-casualty incident. The senior EMT will give a radio report on the nature of the emergency, its exact location, and their best estimate of the number of patients. This crucial information will be used by the dispatch center to send additional resources to the scene. The radio report should include a request for any special resources that the EMTs feel may be necessary.

If the disaster plan is to be put into operation, it is critical that other responding units be informed of this fact. The EMTs on the scene must take command of the scene until they are relieved. This will include telling other units what equipment to bring, what they should plan on doing once they arrive, how best to access the scene, and where to park. It is also important to keep uninjured people from becoming injured. This will probably require restricting access to the scene to only those personnel performing triage (explained below), extrication from wreckage, and/or patient care.

Usually the crew leader on the first arriving EMS unit will assume **medical** or **EMS command**. His or her role is to establish an EMS command post, to oversee the medical aspects of the incident and the safety of all personnel and to designate sector officers (i.e., triage, treatment, transport, staging), and to work closely with the fire commander and police commander. Most systems use brightly colored reflective vests that can be worn over protective clothing to make each incident sector officer easy to identify. Command may be transferred to higher-ranking EMS officers if and as they arrive on the scene. On larger incidents, EMS or medical command may have an aide to assist with communications as well as a safety officer and a public information officer.

Once medical/EMS command has been established, the next task is to quickly assess all the patients and assign each a priority for receiving treatment. This process is called **triage**, which comes from a French word meaning "to sort."

Initial Triage

The goal of the EMT, when faced with more than one patient, must be to afford the greatest number of people the greatest chance of survival. To accomplish this goal, the EMT must provide care to people according to the seriousness of their illnesses or injuries while keeping in mind that spending a lot of time trying to save one life may prevent a number of other patients from receiving the treatment they need.

To properly triage a group of patients, the EMT should quickly classify each patient into one of four groups.

- Priority 1: Correctable Life-Threatening Illness or Injuries—Examples include respiratory arrest or obstruction, suspected heart attack, severe bleeding, severe head injuries, cervical spine injuries, open chest or abdominal wounds, fractures without distal pulses, femur fractures, critical or complicated burns or burns involving respiratory complications, severe shock, tension pneumothorax.
- Priority 2: Serious But Not Life-Threatening Illness or Injuries—Examples include mod-

erate blood loss, moderate to critical burns without complications, open or multiple fractures (open increases priority), eye injuries, other medical emergencies including stable drug overdose.
- Priority 3: "Walking Wounded"—Examples include soft tissue injuries, simple fractures, sprains, minor to moderate burns.
- Priority 4 (sometimes called Priority 0): Dead or Fatally Injured—Examples include exposed brain matter, cardiac arrest (no pulse for over 20 minutes except with cold-water drowning or severe hypothermia), decapitation, severed trunk, incineration.

Patients in arrest are considered priority 4 (or 0) when resources are limited. The time that must be devoted to rescue breathing or CPR for one person is not justified when there are many patients needing attention. Once ample resources are available, patients in arrest become priority 1.

How triage is performed depends on the number of injuries, the immediate hazards to personnel and patients, and the location of backup resources. Local operating procedures will give the EMT more guidance on the exact method of triage for a given situation. Basic principles of triage are presented here.

The first triage cut can be done rapidly by using a bullhorn, PA system, or loud voice to direct all patients capable of walking (Priority 3) to move to a particular area. This has a two-fold purpose. One, it quickly identifies these individuals as having an airway and circulation. Two, it physically separates these patients from the others, who will generally need more care.

The EMT will need to rapidly assess each remaining patient, stopping only to secure an airway or stop profuse bleeding. It is important that the EMT *not* develop "tunnel vision"—spending time rendering additional care to any one patient and thus failing to identify and correct life-threatening conditions of the remaining patients. If Priority 3 patients are nearby and well enough to help, they may be employed to assist the EMT by maintaining an airway or direct pressure on bleeding wounds of fellow patients. Priority 3 patients who have been reluctant to leave ill or injured friends or relatives may be permitted to stay near them where they can be of possible help later.

Once all the patients have been assessed and treated for airway problems and severe bleeding, more thorough treatment can be initiated. The EMT will need to render care to the patients who are most seriously injured or ill but who stand the best chance of survival with proper treatment. This requires treating all the Priority 1 patients first, Priority 2 patients next, and Priority 3 patients last. Priority 4 patients do not receive treatment unless no other patients are thought to be at risk of dying or suffering long-term disability if their conditions go unattended.

Usually patients will be immobilized on backboards if necessary and carried by "runners" to the appropriate secondary triage sector or treatment sector (as described below). Extensive treatment does not occur at the incident site since it is in a hazard zone and since it could impede rescue and primary treatment of other patients.

Patient Identification

By now it should be clear that a system will be required to group and identify patients by treatment priority. A widely used system is to color-code patients according to their priority. For example, Priority 1 = red, Priority 2 = yellow, Priority 3 = green, Priority 4 = black or gray.

Different localities have different systems. It is important that you know and understand the system used in your area. It is equally important that different services in the same region use the same coding system. This is because many MCIs are multiple-agency events. If each agency were to use a different system, there would be no way to correctly coordinate the order in which patients receive care.

As an EMT moves among patients conducting initial triage, the EMT should affix a **triage tag** to each patient, indicating the priority group to which that patient has been assigned. Triage tags are color-coded and may have space in which limited medical information can be recorded (Figure 22-2).

There are some local variations of the triage tag. Some use adhesive-backed colored shipping labels. Others use colored surveyor's tape or duct tape to classify patients. Surveyor's tape can be quickly tied on as an arm band. Duct tape will stick to just about anything in any kind of weather. For this reason it is particularly useful in an MCI setting. It is also useful to have a laundry marker or wax pencil handy for wet conditions when a standard pen or pencil will not write well.

Whatever system is used, it is vital that the color coding be easily located and identified.

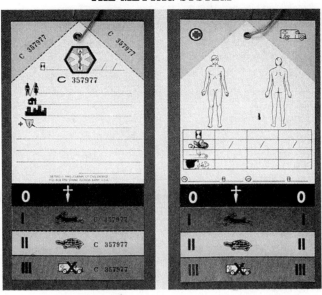

Figure 22-2 Typical triage tags used to identify Priority 1, Priority 2, Priority 3, and Priority 4 patients.

Properly done, this allows an EMT later to quickly identify which treatment group patients belong to and to institute treatment accordingly.

Secondary Triage and Treatment

As more EMTs arrive at the incident scene, they should be directed to assist with the completion of initial triage. If triage has been completed, these EMTs can initiate treatment.

Secondary triage generally begins at this point. In ideal triage systems, patients are gathered into a **triage sector** and, under the direction of the **triage officer**, are physically separated into treatment groups based on their priority level as designated by a triage tag. Some systems call for vehicles to carry red, yellow, and green tarps, which are used to designate these areas. An area to which patients are removed is referred to as a **treatment sector**. Each treatment sector should have its own **treatment officer**, an EMT responsible for overseeing the triage and treatment within that sector. The treatment officer should again triage the patients in that sector to determine the order in which they will receive treatment.

During secondary triage, it may be necessary to recategorize a patient whose condition has deteriorated or improved or who was incorrectly triaged to a higher or lower priority group than was medically warranted. This will necessi-

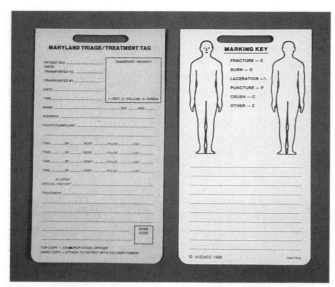

Figure 22-3 EMS disaster tag used during secondary triage.

tate moving the patient to the proper treatment sector, as resources permit. The treatment sector EMTs will need supplies and equipment from the ambulances such as bandages, blood pressure cuffs, and oxygen. Some systems use a different disaster tag during secondary triage on which more detailed information about the patient can be recorded (Figure 22-3).

STAGING AND TRANSPORTATION

Transportation Logistics

Once patients have been properly assessed and separated, and once treatment for the patients has been initiated according to their priority, consideration must be given to the order in which the patients will be transported from the scene of the MCI to a hospital. Again, this is done according to triage priority.

It is advisable to have a **staging sector** from which ambulances can be called to transport patients. The staging sector will be the responsibility of the **staging officer**. This person must keep track of the ambulance vehicles and personnel. In larger-scale incidents, the staging officer may need to arrange to meet human needs, such as restrooms, meals, and rotation of crews.

No ambulance should proceed to a treatment sector without having been requested by the **transportation officer** and directed by the staging officer. This EMT is responsible for communicating with each treatment sector to determine the number and priority of the patients in that sector. This information can then be used by the transportation officer to arrange for transport of patients from the scene to the hospital in the most efficient way.

It is vital that no ambulance transport any patient without the approval of the transportation officer. This is because the transportation officer is responsible for maintaining a list of patients and the hospitals to which they have been transported. This information is relayed from the transportation officer to each receiving hospital. (In a large-scale incident, the transport officer may actually have an aide who does nothing but speak to hospitals.) This way the hospitals know what to expect, do not receive patients they are incapable of handling, and do not receive a disproportionate share of patients. It is critical that the EMTs on ambulance comply with the instructions of the transportation officer, as failure to do so may result in patients being transported to the wrong facilities.

Once an ambulance has completed a run to a hospital, it will probably be directed to return to the staging area, perhaps bringing needed supplies, to await its next instructions from the staging officer.

Communicating with Hospitals

It is important that receiving hospitals be alerted to the nature of the MCI or disaster as soon as the magnitude of the incident is known. This allows the hospitals to call in additional personnel or to clear beds as necessary to accept the anticipated numbers of patients.

Because radio communication channels will be heavily used, the transportation officer, not individual EMTs, should communicate with the hospitals. This will keep unnecessary radio usage to a minimum. It will also ensure that the proper information is recorded at both ends of the ambulance ride. In large-scale MCIs, it is not necessary to give a patient report for each patient. This is because the transporting and treating EMTs will most likely be different and because there will generally be too many patients to allow EMTs to give a good patient radio report under the circumstances. In these instances, the hospital may only be told they are receiving a priority 1 patient with respiratory problems, for example.

PSYCHOLOGICAL ASPECTS OF MULTIPLE-CASUALTY INCIDENTS

During MCIs, EMTs often encounter another, frequently overlooked condition: psychologically stressed patients. While they may outwardly exhibit few signs of injury or emotional stress, people involved in MCIs have been subjected to devastating circumstances for which they are normally unprepared to cope. Proper early management of the psychologically stressed patient can facilitate later treatment and help ensure a faster recovery.

Adequately managing a patient during an MCI may require the EMT to administer "psychological first aid." This may take the form of talking with a terrified parent, child, or witness. The EMT *should not* attempt to engage in psychoanalysis and *should not* say things that are untrue in an attempt to calm a hysterical patient. A calm, caring, honest demeanor, however, will reassure a patient, as will listening to the patient and acknowledging his fears and problems. Often this is all the patient will need.

Patients are not the only ones subject to emotional stress during an MCI. So are the emergency responders. It is very important that EMTs understand that large-scale or horrific MCIs may affect rescuers as much as, if not more than, non-rescuers.

EMTs who become emotionally incapacitated should be treated as patients and removed to an area where they can rest without viewing the scene. These patients must be monitored by an EMS provider until a clinically competent provider can take over. These EMTs should not be allowed to return to duty without first being evaluated by someone professionally trained to do so.

Critical incident stress debriefing (CISD) teams are a resource that can provide the emotional and psychological support required by this type of incident. Intervention by a CISD team may help to prevent post-traumatic stress disorder.

As discussed in Chapter 21, it has become more widely recognized that EMT stress syndrome, also known as **post-traumatic stress disorder (PTSD),** can affect emergency responders days, weeks, or even months after an event. PTSD is manifest by loss of appetite, volatile mood swings, subtle changes in personality, depression, withdrawal, or alienation from peers. No rescuer is immune from the potential effects of PTSD. All personnel should be aware of the potential effects and prepared to refer EMTs who may be suffering from PTSD for expert help.

Remember that you can never fully predict how you will react to a stressful situation. Don't assume it will be another EMT who will be psychologically affected. It may be you. It can happen to anyone, and it is nothing to be ashamed of. If it does happen to you, the important thing is to seek the help you need to restore your emotional health.

CHAPTER REVIEW

KEY TERMS

You may find it helpful to review the following terms.

critical incident stress debriefing (CISD) teams—teams of counselors who provide emotional and psychological support to EMS personnel who are or have been involved in a multiple-casualty incident or disaster.
disaster—an emergency of such a magnitude as to severely overtax the capacity of an EMS system to deal adequately with the sick or injured.
disaster plan—a pre-defined set of instructions that tells a community's various emergency responders what to do in specific emergencies.
incident command system—a system used for the management of a multiple-casualty incident, involving assumption of responsibility for command and designation and coordination of such elements as triage, treatment, transport, and staging.
medical/EMS command—the senior EMS person on the scene who establishes an EMS command post and oversees the medical aspects of a multiple-casualty incident.
multiple-casualty incident (MCI)—any medical or trauma incident involving multiple patients.

post-traumatic stress disorder (PTSD)—adverse psychological effects resulting days, weeks, or even months after involvement in a stressful incident.

staging officer—the person responsible for overseeing and keeping track of ambulances and ambulance personnel at a multiple-casualty incident. The staging officer will direct ambulances to treatment areas at the request of the transportation officer.

staging sector—the area where ambulances are parked and other resources are held until needed.

transportation officer—the person responsible for communicating with sector officers and hospitals to prioritize and manage transportation of patients to hospitals from the scene of a multiple-casualty incident.

treatment officer—the person responsible for overseeing treatment of patients who have been triaged at a multiple-casualty incident.

treatment sector—the area in which patients are treated at a multiple-casualty incident.

triage—the process of quickly assessing patients in a multiple-casualty incident and assigning each a priority for receiving treatment according to the severity of their illness or injuries. From a French word meaning "to sort."

triage officer—the person responsible for overseeing triage at a multiple-casualty incident.

triage sector—the area in which secondary triage takes place at a multiple-casualty incident.

triage tag—color-coded tags indicating the priority group to which that patient has been assigned.

SUMMARY

A multiple-casualty incident (MCI) is any medical or trauma incident involving more than one patient. A disaster is any emergency that overtaxes the resources of an EMS system.

Disaster and Multiple-Casualty Incident Operations

A pre-planned disaster plan that coordinates the resources of a community's various emergency responders must be in place before a disaster strikes. A good disaster plan should be

- Written to address events conceivable for its location
- Well publicized
- Realistic
- Rehearsed

Scene Management

The first EMTs on the scene of an MCI or disaster must initiate the incident command system and radio to the dispatch center the nature of the emergency, its exact location, and their best estimate of the number of patients. They must tell other units what equipment to bring, what they will do on arrival, how to access the scene, and where to park. All units must be advised if the disaster plan is to be put into operation. Access to the scene must be restricted to those performing triage, extrication, or patient care.

The crew leader becomes medical or EMS command. Triage, a method of sorting patients into categories for receiving care and transportation, must be initiated immediately. The sorting is done based on the severity of the patients' illnesses and injuries. The categories are

Priority 1: correctable life-threatening illness or injuries

Priority 2: serious but not life-threatening illness or injuries

Priority 3: "walking wounded"—non-serious illness or injuries

Priority 4: dead or fatally injured

Treatment during initial triage is limited to care for immediately life-threatening conditions: airway blockage and profuse bleeding. Too much time spent on any one patient may prevent the EMT from identifying and correcting life-threatening problems of other patients. Priority 1 patients are treated first, Priority 2 patients second, and Priority 3 patients last. Priority 4 patients are not treated unless all others with life-threatening or serious injuries have been treated. Triage tags are used to identify the categories to which patients have been assigned and to record limited medical information.

During secondary triage, a triage officer oversees the movement of patients to treatment sectors corresponding to the priority they have been assigned. A treatment officer is in charge of each treatment sector. Patients are triaged again and reassigned if their conditions have deteriorated or improved since initial triage or if they were incorrectly categorized.

Staging and Transportation

The staging officer is responsible for overseeing ambulances and ambulance personnel in the staging sector. The transportation officer is responsible for communicating with triage officers and hospitals to prioritize and manage transport of patients to hospitals from the emergency scene. To avoid confusion, all communications with hospitals should be done by the transportation officer rather than by individual EMTs.

Psychological Aspects of Multiple-Casualty Incidents

An emotionally distraught patient can best be handled by talking with the patient in a calm, caring, honest manner and by listening to and acknowledging his fears and problems.

EMTs can also become emotionally incapacitated at an MCI or disaster scene. An EMT in emotionally unstable condition must be removed from the scene and not permitted to return to duty until professionally evaluated. Critical incident stress debriefing (CISD) teams can provide support for EMTs who have encountered a stressful situation. EMTs may also suffer from post traumatic stress disorder (PTSD), a delayed psychological reaction to severe stress. EMTs suffering from PTSD should be referred for expert help.

23

On the Scene

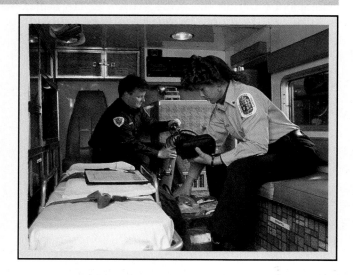

06:00 seems a little earlier than usual this particular morning. At the change of shifts for your ambulance squad, the two crews converse as they usually do. It's been a quiet night...only one minor call. As the night crew is about to exit, one of them says, "The rig should be in pretty good shape. We didn't use anything last night."

After placing your gear in its proper location and pouring a cup of coffee, you and your more experienced partner head for the garage.

Your Partner: *Sounds like the rig is in pretty*

good shape. Let's give it a quick wash and then grab some breakfast.

You: *You go ahead. I had a bite before I left home. I'll check the rig over.*

Your Partner: *You new kids. The night crew said it was OK. If you have to go through it, I'll help...but then we'll have a couple of those donuts I picked up on the way in.*

You: *Fair enough.*

While checking the rig, you find a few important things missing. The oxygen is empty, and there are no nonrebreather masks on board. Checking the ambulance turns out to have been a good idea, because before you and your partner can get to those donuts, a cardiac call comes in. If you hadn't insisted on checking the ambulance, the implications could have been severe!

Cleaning, restocking, and maintaining the ambulance are not, by far, the most glamorous parts of EMS, but the possible consequences of not doing it properly are too grim to contemplate. Imagine not having oxygen at a cardiac call, or finding a patient hemorrhaging and not having materials for a pressure bandage, or disposable gloves, mask, and goggles for infection control! You're glad you ignored the night crew's assurances and restocked the ambulance this morning. You know it won't be the last time you'll be glad you took the non-glamorous parts of your job seriously.

Preparing for the Ambulance Run

Chapter Overview

"Be prepared" is as good a slogan for EMTs as it is for Scouts. Time is so important at the emergency scene. Some patients have only moments to live without emergency resuscitative measures. Others require a quick and efficient full assessment, treatment, stabilization, and transport in order to receive hospital care within the "golden hour" after an injury or onset of serious illness. Time wasted running back and forth to the ambulance for supplies and equipment or, worse, discovering that needed supplies and equipment are not on hand, is inexcusable and could result in loss of life. An ambulance that is not in proper operating order can cause equally serious problems.

In this chapter you will study the preshift processes to prepare the ambulance for its run. In Chapters 24 through 28, you will learn about other aspects of the ambulance run.

Expected Outcome: You will be able to check supplies and equipment, replace what is missing, and organize the supplies and equipment for quick and efficient use—as well as check the ambulance and initiate needed repairs—before each shift.

Warning: Make sure the ambulance is stocked with barrier devices such as pocket face masks with one-way valve, face shields, and bag-valve masks; goggles or eye shields; and disposable gloves. Always conform to your local EMS system's infection exposure control plan.

THE AMBULANCE
    Ambulance Supplies and Equipment
    Organizing Supplies and Equipment
        for Immediate Use
    Ensuring That the Ambulance Is Ready
        for Service

Knowledge *After reading this chapter, you should be able to*

1. List and give uses for the items that should be included in each of the following categories of supplies and equipment.

   - Basic supplies (pp. 613-614)

   - Equipment for the transfer of patients (p. 614)

   - Equipment for airway maintenance, ventilation, and resuscitation (pp. 614-615)

   - Oxygen therapy equipment (p. 615)

   - Suction equipment (p. 615)

   - Equipment for cardiac compression (pp. 615-616)

   - Supplies and equipment for the immobilization of fractures (p. 616)

   - Supplies for wound care (p. 616)

   - Supplies and equipment for the treatment of shock (pp. 616-617)

   - Supplies for childbirth (p. 617)

   - Supplies and equipment for the treatment of acute poisoning (p. 617)

   - Special equipment for qualified EMTs, paramedics, and physicians (p. 617)

   - Miscellaneous and safety equipment (pp. 617-618)

2. List the steps that should be included in a preshift ambulance inspection. (pp. 618-620)

Skills *As an EMT you should be able to*

1. Identify and organize supply and equipment items carried on an ambulance.

2. Use the items carried on the ambulance during patient care activities.

3. Conduct a preshift ambulance inspection.

T he modern ambulance has come a long way from its primitive beginnings. It is far more than just a vehicle for transporting a patient to the hospital. Today's ambulance is a well-equipped and efficiently organized mobile pre-hospital emergency room and communications unit.

THE AMBULANCE

It is doubtful that anyone really knows when a wheeled conveyance was first used to move a sick or injured person from one place to another. "Body wagons" were used throughout medieval times, especially when thousands fell victim to a plague. As you can imagine, those conveyances were used to transport the dead, not the living.

During the Napoleonic Wars, hand-drawn and horse-drawn carts were given the designation "ambulance" and used for the singular purpose of transporting wounded soldiers. Military leaders decided that it would be better to transport wounded soldiers to safe places behind front lines rather than risk the lives of physicians in the midst of the fighting.

Ambulances evolved from horse-drawn wagons to motor vehicles in 1906, and motorized ambulances were extensively used on the battlefields of France and Flanders during World War I (Figure 23-1).

From the conclusion of World War I until the late 1960s, hearses were traditionally used as ambulances because they were the only vehicles in which a person could be transported lying down. It is likely that ambulances would still be built on long wheel base passenger car chassis if it were not for a report made in 1966 on the state of prehospital emergency care. In *Accidental Death and Disability: The Neglected Disease of Modern Society*, the need for ambulances better suited to the purpose of transporting sick and injured persons to medical facilities was detailed. The personnel of public and private agencies were inspired to establish and

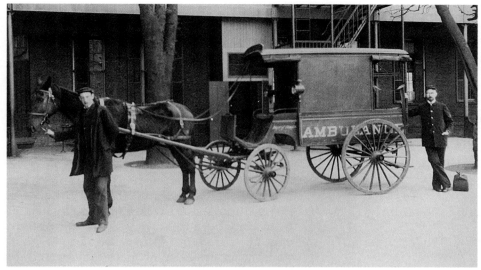

A.

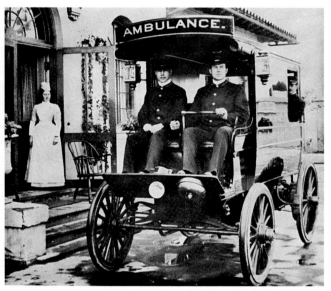

B.

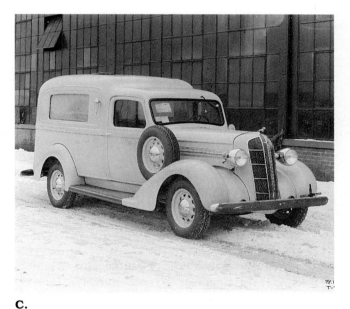

C.

Figure 23-1 Evolution of the ambulance
(A) A horse-drawn ambulance, 1893 (B) An early motorized ambulance (C) An ambulance from the 1930s.

refine design criteria, and from their efforts have come guidelines for the manufacture of modern ambulances.

Ambulance Supplies and Equipment

Even though it is especially designed and constructed, an ambulance is only another truck if it does not have the proper equipment for patient care and transportation.

Following are lists of supplies and equipment that should be carried in an ambulance so that EMTs can provide the correct care for a variety of illness and injuries. The lists are based on recommendations of the American College of Surgeons and the U.S. Department of Transportation.

Basic Supplies The ambulance should be provided with linens and blankets that serve not only to protect patients and keep them warm but also to reduce the possibility of contamination. There should be

- Two pillows
- Four pillow cases
- Four sheets
- Two spare sheets
- Four blankets (the number may vary according to local climactic conditions)

Certain items should be carried to assist in the care of a patient's personal needs.

- Six disposable emesis bags (for vomitus)
- Two boxes of tissues
- Disposable bedpan, urinal, and toilet paper
- Four towels
- A package of disposable drinking cups

Other basic supplies include

- One package of wet wipes
- Four liters of sterile water or saline
- Four soft restraining devices (upper and lower extremities)
- Packages of large and small red biohazard bags for waste or severed parts (according to Occupational Safety and Health Administration–OSHA–regulations)
- A package of large yellow bags for used linens or garbage (or otherwise color-coded or labeled according to local compliance with OSHA regulations for contaminated disposables)
- Disinfectant cleaner
- An empty plastic spray bottle with a line at the 1:100 level, a plastic bottle of water, and a plastic bottle of bleach for cleaning up blood spills. (Measure a mixture of 1 part bleach to 100 parts water; a weaker solution will not disinfect, a stronger solution may damage equipment.)

The following items should be carried for patient-monitoring activities.

- An adult sphygmomanometer kit with separate cuffs for average-sized and obese persons
- A pediatric sphygmomanometer kit with separate cuffs for children and infants
- An adult and a pediatric stethoscope
- Disposable thermometer and a hypothermia thermometer that goes down at least to 82 degrees

- A penlight
- A pulse oximeter (optional)

Equipment for the Transfer of Patients
The following carrying devices should be included.

- The *wheeled ambulance stretcher* is designed so that a sick or injured person can be transported in the Fowlers (head and torso up), supine, or Trendelenberg (supine with feet higher than head) position. Also called a cot or gurney, the wheeled stretcher should have a number of features. It should be adjustable in height. It should be adjustable so that a patient can be transported in a number of positions: with the head or foot end elevated for Fowlers or Trendelenberg positions. It should have detachable supports for intravenous fluid containers. Restraining devices should be provided so that a patient can be prevented from falling off the stretcher or sliding past the foot end or head end.
- A *Reeves stretcher* for carrying a patient who must lie supine down stairs when a conventional stretcher is too heavy or wide.
- A *folding stair chair* should be carried for times when a sick or injured person who can sit up must be moved down stairs or through hallways too narrow for conventional stretchers.
- A *scoop-style stretcher* (orthopedic stretcher) for picking up seriously injured persons with a minimum of body movement.
- A *Stokes, or basket, stretcher.* This stretcher comes with either a steel-wire-and-tubular frame or as a plastic basket with a reinforced aluminum frame. The plastic baskets are helpful for sliding patients in the snow. Either version is useful for long-distance carries, high-angle, or off-the-road rescues.
- A *child safety seat* (optional) for immobilizing and transporting infants or small children.

Carrying devices are discussed more fully in Chapter 25.

Equipment for Airway Maintenance, Ventilation, and Resuscitation A number of devices should be carried for maintaining an open airway.

- *Oropharyngeal airways* in sizes suitable for adults, children, and infants

- *Soft rubber nasopharyngeal airways* in sizes 14 through 30

The following devices should be carried for artificial ventilation efforts.

- Two *manually operated, self-filling, bag-valve-mask units* (one adult and one pediatric). The units should be capable of delivering 100% oxygen to a patient by the addition of a reservoir. Masks of various sizes should be carried. The masks should be designed to ensure a tight face seal and should have an air cushion. The masks should be clear so that an attending EMT can see vomitus and the clouding caused by exhalations during ventilation efforts.
- A *pocket face mask with one-way valve* should be available for times when oronasal ventilation is necessary but direct contact with the patient is either impossible or undesirable. The mask should have an oxygen inlet.
- A *commercially available jaw block* should be carried to prevent patients from biting EMTs' hands or airway tubes.

Airway maintenance devices are discussed more fully in Chapter 6.

Oxygen Therapy Equipment It is recommended that an ambulance be provided with two oxygen supply systems (one fixed and one portable) so that oxygen can be supplied to two patients, both at the scene of an emergency and during transportation to a medical facility.

- The *fixed oxygen delivery system* is provided to supply oxygen to a patient within the ambulance. A typical installation consists of a minimum 3,000-liter reservoir, a two-stage regulator, and the necessary yokes, reducing valve, non-gravity-type flowmeter, and humidifier. The oxygen delivery tubes, transparent masks, and controls should all be situated within easy reach of an EMT working at a patient's head. The system should be capable of delivering at least 15 liters of oxygen per minute, and the system must be adaptable to the bag-valve-mask units carried on the ambulance.
- The *portable oxygen delivery system* should have a capacity of at least 300 liters. It, too, must have the necessary hardware and masks of all sizes. The system should be capable of delivering at least 15 liters of oxygen per minute, and there should be a spare 300-liter cylinder. Many ambulances are equipped with portable units that can be used for resuscitation and suctioning as well as oxygen delivery.

The ambulance should also carry

- Six adult and pediatric nonrebreather masks
- Six adult and pediatric nasal cannuli
- Four adult Venturi masks (if used locally)
- Oxygen-powered positive pressure ventilation (local option)
- An *automatic transport ventilator* (ATV—optional)

Oxygen therapy is discussed more fully in Chapter 6.

Suction Equipment An ambulance should be provided with both a fixed suction system and a portable suction device.

- The *fixed suction system* should be sufficient to provide an air flow of over 30 liters per minute at the end of the delivery tube. A vacuum of at least 300 mmHg should be reached within 4 seconds after the suction tube is clamped. The suction should be controllable. The installed system should have a large-diameter, nonkinking tube fitted with a rigid tip. There should be a spare nonbreakable, disposable suction bottle, and a container of water for rinsing the suction tubes. There should be an assortment of sterile catheters. As with the oxygen delivery system, the suction tube and controls should be located within easy reach of an EMT working at a patient's head.
- The *portable suction unit* can be one of the many models powered by motor, hand or foot action, oxygen, vacuum, or compressed air. A portable unit should be fitted with a nonkinking tube that has a rigid tip, as well as spare large-bore Yankauer tips.

Suction equipment is discussed more fully in Chapter 6.

Equipment for Assisting with Cardiac Compression The short or long spine board that is generally carried on an ambulance for the immobilization of neck and back injuries can provide rigid support during CPR (cardiopulmonary resuscitation) efforts. A mechanical CPR compressor is an option in services with long transport time.

CPR is discussed more fully in Chapter 5.

Supplies and Equipment for the Immobilization of Fractures A well-equipped ambulance carries a variety of devices that can be used to immobilize skeletal injuries.

- *Traction splints* for the immobilization of fractured femurs
- A number of *padded board splints* for the immobilization of upper and lower extremities. Recommended are two 3 x 54-inch splints, two 3 x 36-inch splints, and two 3 x 15-inch splints.

Other devices that might be carried for the immobilization of injured extremities are

- *A variety of splints*: air-inflatable splints, vacuum splints, wire ladder splints, cardboard splints, canvas lace-up splints, soft rubberized splints with aluminum stays and Velcro fasteners, padded aluminum roll-up splints (for extremities), and splints that are inflated with cryogenic gas
- A number of *tongue depressors* to use to immobilize fractured fingers
- *Triangular bandages* for use with splints and for making slings and swathes
- Several rolls of *soft or Kling (self-adhering) roller bandage* for securing the various splints
- 6 *Chemical cold packs* for use on fractured extremities
- Two *long spine boards* for full-body immobilization, preferably with speed clips or Velcro straps. The long spine board can also be used for patient transfer.
- *Rigid cervical and extrication collars* in a variety of adult and pediatric sizes
- A *KED, XP1, or Kansas Board or LSP board* for persons who have possible spinal injuries
- Six 9-foot by 2-inch *web straps* with aircraft-style buckles or O-rings for securing patients to carrying devices
- A suitable *device for stabilizing the head* of a person who has a known or suspected cervical spine injury (such as a head immobilizer or rolled blanket)

The number and types of immobilizing devices carried on an ambulance are mostly decided by local policy on the recommendation of the unit's medical advisor.

Immobilization procedures are discussed more fully in Chapters 10, 11, and 12.

Supplies for Wound Care A variety of dressing and bandaging materials should be carried on an ambulance.

- *Sterile gauze pads* (2 x 2 inches and 4 x 4 inches)
- 5 x 9 inch *combine dressings*
- *Sterile universal dressings* (often called multitrauma dressings) approximately 10 x 36 inches when unfolded
- *Kling bandages* in 4- and 6-inch widths x 5 yards
- *Occlusive dressings* for the sealing of sucking chest wounds and eviscerations
- *Aluminum foil* (sterilized in separate package) for various uses such as occlusive dressing and also to maintain body heat or to form an oxygen tent for a newborn infant
- *Sterile burn sheets* or prepackaged *burn kit*
- *Adhesive strip bandages* for minor wound care (1 x ¾ inch and 1 x ½ inch), individually packaged (Band-Aids)
- *Hypoallergenic adhesive tape* (1- and 3-inch rolls)
- Large *safety pins* for the securing of bandages, slings and swathes
- *Bandage scissors*
- Box of *disposable gloves*—small, medium, and large

Control of bleeding and care of wounds and burns are discussed more fully in Chapters 7, 9, 13, 14, and 19.

Supplies and Equipment for the Treatment of Shock In the past the treatment for shock was usually limited to the elevation of a person's feet and the conservation of body heat. Today, EMTs are qualified to provide more definitive anti-shock measures; consequently, ambulances are equipped with the following:

- *Anti-shock garments* also known as pneumatic anti-shock garments (PASG) or military anti-shock trousers (MAST). These should be in sizes for adults and children.
- *Aluminum blankets* (survival blankets) for maintaining body heat

Treatment for shock is discussed more fully in Chapter 8.

Supplies for Childbirth A *sterile childbirth kit* should be carried. In some areas, ambulances carry kits provided by local medical facilities. In other areas, ambulances are provided with commercially available disposable obstetric kits. Whatever the source, an obstetric kit should contain the following items.

- A pair of surgical scissors
- Four umbilical cord clamps or umbilical tape
- A rubber bulb syringe (3 oz.)
- Twelve 4 x 4 inch gauze pads
- Four pairs of sterile disposable gloves
- Five towels
- A baby blanket (receiving blanket)
- Infant swaddler
- Sanitary napkins
- Two large plastic bags

In addition to the disposable gloves included in the obstetric kit, an ambulance should be provided with items that can be worn by EMTs to minimize contamination of the mother and baby during and after childbirth, including

- Two surgical gowns
- Two surgical caps
- Two surgical masks
- Two pairs of goggles with eye shields

Childbirth is discussed more fully in Chapter 18.

Supplies and Equipment for the Treatment of Acute Poisoning A number of *poison control kits* are available from emergency care equipment suppliers. Whether purchased intact or hand-made, a poison control kit should include these items.

- Drinking water that can be used to dilute poisons
- Syrup of ipecac (if allowed in your system)
- Activated charcoal (if allowed in your system)
- Paper cups and other equipment for oral administration
- Equipment for irrigating a person's eyes with sterile water
- Constriction bands for snakebites

Treatment for poisoning is discussed more fully in Chapter 16.

Special Equipment for Qualified EMTs, Paramedics, and Physicians Depending on state laws and local protocols, some ambulances are provided with *locked kits of supplies and equipment that can be used by paramedics or physicians*, especially in rural areas. This equipment may include supplies for

- IV fluid infusion
- Endotracheal intubation
- Chest decompression
- Drug administration
- Advanced airways such as the esophageal obturator airway (EOA), the esophageal gastric tube airway (EGTA), Combitube® airway, or pharyngo-tracheal lumen airway (PtL®)
- Tracheostomy or cricothyrotomy
- Cardiac monitoring and defibrillation

Miscellaneous and Safety Equipment Ambulances should also be provided with personal protective equipment for the EMTs, equipment for warning, signaling and lighting, hazard control devices, and tools for gaining access and disentanglement., including

- The U. S. Department of Transportation *Emergency Response Guidebook*
- Binoculars
- Clipboard and prehospital care report forms (PCRs)
- Ring cutter
- Portable radio
- Multiple casualty incident (MCI) kit with tags, command vests, and destination logs
- Eye shields or goggles
- Tyvec jumpsuits
- Disposable gloves
- Disposable masks and gowns
- Sharps containers
- Epinephrine pens (local option)
- Automated External Defibrillator (AED) and electrodes (local options—see Chapter 5) (**Note:** AEDs must be checked daily to be sure they are functioning correctly.)
- Mechanical CPR device, e.g. Thumper (local option)
- Flares
- Jumper cables
- Set of turnout gear (coat, helmet, eye shield, gloves) for each crew member

- Rescue tools for gaining access to the patient
- Glucose paste (for diabetic emergencies—local option)
- Portable kits (see the suggested types listed below). First-in kits come in all shapes and sizes with either hard cases or soft bags. When designing a first-in kit keep in mind the ABCDE steps of the expanded primary survey, aimed at detection and immediate treatment of life-threatening conditions, and include supplies and equipment for

A (Airway)—airways, suction, infection control, personal protective equipment

B (Breathing)—stethoscope, bag-valve mask, oxygen, oxygen delivery devices

C (Circulation)—blood pressure cuff, bandages and dressings, occlusive dressings, anti-shock garments, AED

D (Disability)—set of cervical collars, backboards, straps, penlight

E (Expose)—scissors, blanket

When you have an opportunity, compare the items listed in this chapter with the inventory of your ambulance. Learn where each item is stored so that you can reach it quickly in any emergency situation. Learn what every item is for and when it should be used. If the item is a mechanical device, learn not only what it is for and when it should be used but also how it works and how it should be maintained.

Organizing Supplies and Equipment for Immediate Use

The items on the preceding lists can be stored in compartments throughout the ambulance, but when emergency care items are stored in *kits*, they are immediately accessible. There is no need to go from compartment to compartment gathering up armloads of supplies and equipment. There are a variety of kits available from equipment vendors; however, you can make your own kits by fitting out readily available plastic or metal boxes and soft-sided bags.

A *first-in kit, or jump kit,* is the most useful of all the kits that might be carried on an ambulance. It should contain all the supplies and equipment that may be needed to initiate primary life-saving measures (see above).

An *airway maintenance and ventilation equipment kit* can carry airways, pocket masks and ventilation adjunct devices, bag-valve-mask units, and suction catheters. A *wound care kit* might include a variety of bandages and dressings, occlusive materials, tape, bandage shears, and related materials. Other supplies and equipment can be carried in an *obstetric kit*, a *burn kit*, a *rescue kit* of hand tools, and so on.

Ensuring That the Ambulance Is Ready for Service

The most modern well-equipped ambulance is not worth the room it takes up in a garage if it is not ready to respond at the time of an emergency. A state of readiness results from a planned preventive maintenance program that includes periodic servicing. Oil should be changed regularly, tires should be rotated, the vehicle should be lubricated, and so on. These are important steps, to be sure; but the one step that can ensure that an ambulance is continually ready for service is the *preshift inspection*. Each service should have a standard operating procedure for checking the vehicles and all equipment. The procedure should define how to handle equipment that needs repair. In addition, there should be a procedure defining how to handle vehicle failures or problems that occur on the road.

Let us say that you and your partner have just reported for duty. As soon as it is practical, speak with the crew members going off duty. Learn whether they experienced any problems with either the ambulance or the equipment during their shift. Make a thorough bumper-to-bumper inspection of the ambulance. Use a checklist if one is provided by your service.

Ambulance Inspection, Engine Off Following are inspection steps that can be taken while the ambulance is in quarters.

1. *Inspect the body of the vehicle.* Look for damage that could interfere with safe operation. A crumpled fender, for example, may prevent the front wheels from turning the maximum distance.
2. *Inspect the wheels and tires.* Remember that ambulance tires take a beating when they meet curbs, stones, and potholes. At accident scenes they may contact shards of glass and sharp pieces of metal and other

debris. Check for damaged wheels and damaged sidewalls. Look for signs of abnormal wear. Check the tread depth. Use a pressure gauge to ensure that all tires are properly inflated. Don't forget to inspect the inside walls of all tires.

3. *Inspect windows and mirrors.* Look for broken glass and loose or missing parts. See that mirrors are clean and properly adjusted for maximum visibility.

4. *Check the operation of the doors.* Ensure that every door will open and close properly and that all latches and locks are operational.

5. *Inspect the components of the cooling system.* (**Warning:** Allow the engine to cool before removing any pressure caps.) Check the level of the coolant. Inspect the cooling system hoses for leaks and cracks.

6. *Check the level of the other vehicle fluids,* including the engine oil and the brake, power steering and transmission fluids. Do not forget to check the level of the windshield washer fluid.

7. *Check the battery.* If the battery has removable fill caps, check the level of the electrolyte. If the battery is the sealed type, determine its condition by checking the indicator port. Inspect the battery cable connections for tightness and signs of corrosion.

8. *Inspect the interior surfaces and upholstery* for damage. See that interior surfaces are clean.

9. *Check the windows* for operation. See that the interior surface of each window is clean.

10. *Test the horn.*

11. *Test the siren* for the full range of operation.

12. *Check the seat belts.* Examine each belt to see that it is not damaged. Pull each belt from its storage spool to ensure that the retractor mechanisms work. Buckle each belt to ensure that latches work properly.

13. *Adjust the seat* for comfort and optimum steering wheel and pedal operation.

14. *Observe the dash-mounted indicator lights.* See that each is working.

15. *Check the fuel level.* An ambulance should be refueled after each run, however short. How much fuel was used on a run is less relevant than how much fuel may be needed for the next response.

Ambulance Inspection, Engine On The next steps require you to start the engine. Pull the ambulance from quarters if engine exhaust fumes will be a problem. Set the emergency brake, put the transmission in ""park," and have your partner chock the wheels before undertaking the following steps.

1. *Check the dash-mounted indicators again.* See if any light remains on to indicate a possible problem with oil pressure, engine temperature, or the vehicle's electrical system.

2. *Check dash-mounted gauges* for proper operation.

3. *Depress the brake pedal.* Note whether pedal travel seems correct or excessive.

4. *Test the parking brake.* Move the transmission lever to a drive position. Replace the lever to the ""park" position as soon as you are sure that the parking brake is holding.

5. *Turn the steering wheel from side to side.* Note whether the movement is smooth or jerky.

6. *Check the operation of the windshield wipers and washers.* The glass should be wiped clean each time the blade moves.

7. *Turn on the vehicle's warning lights.* Have your partner walk around the ambulance and check each flashing and revolving light for operation. Turn off the warning lights.

8. *Turn on the other vehicle lights.* Have your partner walk around the ambulance again, this time checking the headlights (high and low beams), turn signals, four-way flashers, brake lights, backup lights, side and rear scene illumination lights, and Interstate Commerce Commission marker lights.

9. *Check the operation of the heating and air-conditioning equipment.* While you check the operation of the equipment in the driver's compartment, have your partner check the equipment in the patient's compartment.

10. *Operate the communications equipment.* Test portable as well as the fixed radios and any radio-telephone communication equipment.

Return the ambulance to quarters, and while you are backing, have your partner note whether the backup alarm is operating (if the ambulance is so equipped).

Inspection of Patient Compartment and Emergency Supplies and Equipment Shut off the engine and complete your inspection by checking the patient space and equipment compartments.

1. *Check the interior of the patient compartment.* Look for damage to the interior surfaces and upholstery. Be certain that any needed decontamination has been completed and that the compartment is clean.
2. *Check emergency care supplies and equipment and rescue equipment.* See that the equipment listed on the inventory are in the ambulance and ready for use.

This last check should be more than merely a quick glance into storage cabinets and compartments. It should be an item-by-item inspection of everything carried on the ambulance, with findings recorded on a printed checklist.

Not only should items be identified during the ambulance inspection, they should also be checked for completeness, condition, and operation. The pressure of oxygen cylinders should be checked. Air splints should be inflated and examined for leaks. Suction and ventilation equipment should be tested for proper operation. Rescue tools should be examined for rust and dirt that may prevent them from working properly. Battery-powered devices should be operated to ensure that the batteries have a proper charge, and so on.

When you are finished with your inspection of the ambulance and its equipment, complete the inspection report. Correct any deficiencies, replace missing items, and if you can, repair nonworking items. Make your supervisor aware of any deficiencies that cannot be immediately corrected.

Finally, clean the unit if necessary for infection control (see Chapter 28) and appearance. Maintaining the ambulance's appearance enhances your organization's image in the public's eye. If you take pride in your work, show it by taking pride in the appearance of your ambulance.

CHAPTER REVIEW

SUMMARY

Ambulance Supplies and Equipment

A variety of supplies and equipment should be carried on an ambulance so that EMTs can cope with a wide range of injuries and illnesses.

Basic supplies and equipment should include items that an EMT can use to protect the patient and keep him warm, care for a patient's personal needs, and measure vital signs.

Equipment for patient transfer should include devices that EMTs can use to lift and carry sick or injured persons to the ambulance in a prone, supine, lateral recumbent, or sitting position.

Equipment for airway maintenance, ventilation, and resuscitation should include airways and artificial ventilation devices, fixed and portable *oxygen delivery systems*, fixed and portable *suction systems*, and *a spine board* that can be placed under a patient during CPR efforts.

Supplies and equipment for immobilizing fractures should include traction devices for lower extremities, padded board splints for both upper and lower extremities, other rigid and soft splints, long and short spine boards, web straps, triangular bandages and soft roller bandages, and head immobilization devices.

Supplies for wound care should include a variety of dressing and bandaging materials, occlusive dressings, tape, bandage shears, and safety pins.

Supplies and equipment for the treatment of shock should include pneumatic countershock devices and aluminum survival blankets.

Supplies for childbirth should include a sterile obstetric kit and sterile garments for the EMTs.

Supplies and equipment for the treatment of poisoning should include drinking water, syrup of ipecac (if used locally), activated charcoal, drinking water, and items for oral administration. Constriction bands for the care of snakebites should be carried.

Special advanced life support equipment should be carried when the ambulance will be staffed by a qualified EMT, paramedic or physician.

Miscellaneous other equipment should include *personal protective equipment, traffic and hazard control equipment,* and *rescue equipment.*

Organizing Supplies and Equipment for Immediate Use

Organize supplies and equipment in kits for immediate use. For example, set up a jump kit, an airway kit, a wound care kit, an obstetric kit, a shock kit, a rescue kit, and so on.

Ensuring that the Ambulance is Ready for Service

A thorough preshift inspection of an ambulance and its supplies and equipment should be made by EMTs to ensure that the unit is ready for service when the shift begins.

24

On the Scene

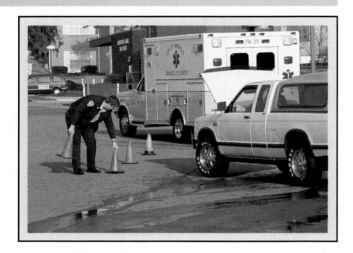

One afternoon, you receive a call for "disabled vehicle, unknown injuries" at a downtown location. As you round the corner, you come upon a truck with its hood up.

You: *Nobody inside. The driver must have gone somewhere to call 911.*

Your Partner *(who is operating the ambulance): Whoa! That looks like gas leaking from under there. I'm going to move the rig up out of the danger zone and call for police and fire department response.*

You: *OK. Get at least 100 feet away from that fuel. I'll put down some cones here to stop anything coming around that corner, and then I'll start marking off a bigger perimeter.*

As you begin to mark off the danger zone, police and fire units arrive. Meanwhile the dispatcher has helped your partner locate the driver inside a nearby delicatessen. She has already done a patient survey and is applying a rigid collar when you catch up with her. Leaving the care of the danger zone and disabled vehicle to the police and fire fighters, you and your partner transport the driver to the hospital.

Responding to the Call for Help

Objectives

Knowledge *After reading this chapter, you should be able to*

1. List FOUR advantages of the universal number for emergency reporting. (p. 625)

2. Explain the difference between basic 911 and enhanced 911 as shown in Figures 24-1a and b. (pp. 625-626)

3. List the FOUR key functions of the EMD. (p. 626)

4. List SEVEN questions that the EMD should ask every caller. (pp. 626-627)

5. List TWELVE questions that an EMD might ask a caller who is reporting a motor vehicle collision. (pp. 627-628)

6. List NINE things a safe ambulance operator must be or do. (pp. 628-629)

7. List FIVE privileges usually granted by state statutes to the operators of emergency vehicles. (p. 629)

8. Describe effects that a continuously sounded siren may have on other motorists, patients, and the ambulance crew. (p. 630)

9. List at least THREE suggestions as to the proper use of sirens. (p. 630)

10. Explain the proper use of the ambulance horn. (pp. 630-631)

11. Explain the proper use of the ambulance headlights, box lights, and four-way flashers. (p. 631)

12. Explain how the ambulance operator who is a defensive driver can affect perception distance, reaction distance, and braking distance. (pp. 631-633)

13. Explain the dangers of escorted and multiple-vehicle responses. (p. 633)

14. Explain how each of the following factors can affect an ambulance response.
    - Day of the week (p. 633)
    - Time of day (pp. 633-634)
    - Weather (p. 634)
    - Detours (p. 634)
    - Railroads (p. 634)
    - Bridges and tunnels (p. 634)
    - Schools and school buses (p. 634)

15. Explain the process of planning alternative routes. (p. 634)

16. List the observations that the attending EMT may make and the actions he might take during a response to a motor vehicle collision
    - As the ambulance leaves quarters and begins the run (p. 635)
    - As the ambulance nears the collision scene (p. 635)
    - When the ambulance is within sight of the scene (p. 635)
    - As the ambulance reaches the scene (p. 636)

17. Define the limits of the danger zone for each of the following situations.
    - When there are no apparent hazards (p. 636)
    - When fuel has been spilled (p. 636; Scan 24-1)
    - When a collision vehicle is on fire (p. 636; Scan 24-1)
    - When wires are down (p. 636; Scan 24-1)
    - When a hazardous material is involved (pp. 636, 638; Scan 24-1)

18. Describe the manner in which an ambulance should be parked
    - On a call to assist a sick or injured person (p. 638)
    - At the scene of a motor vehicle collision (p. 638; Scan 24-2)

Skills *As an EMT you should be able to*

1. Understand and respond to the Emergency Medical Dispatch system.

2. If you become an ambulance operator, drive safely, legally, and defensively.

3. If you are an attending EMT, make observations and take steps to ensure a safe trip.

4. Establish a danger zone around the scene of a collision.

*I*n many areas of the country, a person needs only to dial the **universal number**, 911, to access a community's ambulance service, fire department, rescue squad, police department, or other emergency service. A trained **Emergency Medical Dispatcher (EMD)** records information from callers, decides which service is needed, and alerts that service. (Always say *nine-one-one* when talking to community or school groups. Children can't find "eleven" on the phone dial or key pad.)

There are distinct advantages to the universal number concept.

- Citizens do not have to look for emergency service numbers in a telephone directory—if one is even available. Today few public telephone installations have directories.
- There is no need to decide which emergency service to call and no delay when the wrong service is called, as when a person calls the police department when he needs an ambulance.
- There is no chance that a telephone operator will misdirect calls.

- One-number emergency telephone centers are usually staffed by EMDs who are specially trained to elicit information from and give instructions to distraught and excited callers.

In some parts of the country two dispatch centers are provided, one for the police and the other for the fire, rescue, and ambulance services. Even though a caller may dial the police department when he needs an ambulance, the possibility of a delay in response is minimized because of cross-communication capabilities.

In still other areas of the country a request for emergency medical service may follow a roundabout route. A caller may reach a small dispatch center (which, in fact, may be someone's home or business), the ambulance garage, the local fire department, or the police department, depending on which of the many available numbers he dials. Valuable time is lost when calls for help have to be shuffled between agencies.

Figures 24-1a and b show variations of the emergency call system.

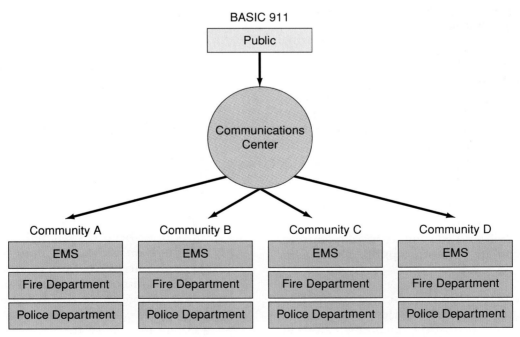

Figure 24-1a The basic 911 system utilizes a single access point for telephone exchange(s). The communications center dispatches EMS, Fire and Police for each community in the region.

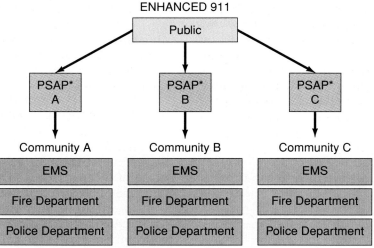

ENHANCED 911

* Public Safety Access Points

Figure 24-1b The enhanced 911 system utilizes multiple public safety access points (PSAP) which in turn dispatch EMS, Fire and Police for each of their respective communities. A feature of E911 is the ability to automatically identify the caller's phone number and to subdivide PSAPs within telephone exchange areas.

RECEIVING THE CALL FOR HELP

The Role of the EMD

Many cities and communication centers have implemented training and certification of Emergency Medical Dispatchers, or EMDs, based upon the medical dispatch priority card system, which originated through the vision and leadership of Jeffrey Clawson, M.D., in Salt Lake City in 1979. An EMD is trained in interrogation techniques, pre-arrival instructions, and call prioritization. The training course, a minimum of 24 to 40 hours, includes techniques of airway and hemorrhage control, CPR, Heimlich maneuver, and childbirth.

The four key functions of the EMD are

- To receive and process calls
- To provide medical instructions to patients and information to crews
- To dispatch and coordinate EMS resources
- To coordinate with other public safety agencies

Both the National Association of EMS Physicians and the American Heart Association's 1992 *Guidelines for Cardiopulmonary Resuscitation and Emergency Cardiac Care* take very strong positions in favor of the certification and training of EMDs.

Obtaining Routine Information

When answering a call for help, the EMD must obtain as much information as possible. Anything the EMD learns about the situation may be important to the responding crew. The questions the EMD should ask are

1. *What is the exact location of the sick or injured person?* The EMD must ask for the house or building number and the apartment number, if any. It is important to ascertain the street name with the direction designator (e.g., North, East), the nearest cross street, the name of the development or subdivision, and the exact location of the emergency.
2. *What is your call-back number? Stay on the line. Do not hang up until I (the EMD) tell you to.* In life-threatening situations, the EMD will offer instructions to the caller, after the units have been dispatched, that the caller or others on the scene should follow until the units arrive. It is also important to be able to contact the caller again if there is any question about the location given. This may be the case when several streets within a community have the same name or when you fail to learn whether the building is on North Main or South Main.
3. *What's the problem?* This will help the EMD

understand the caller's perception of the chief complaint. It will also help the EMD decide which line of questioning to follow and the priority of the response to send per preplanned medical response protocols.

4. *How old is the patient?* Most ambulances are set up to respond into the scene with a pediatric kit if the patient is a child rather than an adult. If pre-arrival CPR instructions are given, it will be necessary to distinguish between an infant (less than 1 year), a child (1 to 8 years), and an adult (over 8 years of age).

5. *What's the patient's sex?* This is asked if it is not already obvious.

6. *Is the patient conscious?* An unconscious patient will elicit a higher priority of response because of the potential that a serious illness or injury caused the unconsciousness.

7. *Is the patient breathing?* If the patient is conscious and breathing, the EMD will often ask many additional questions relative to the chief complaint to determine the appropriate level of response, for example first response, paramedics, or ambulance responding **COLD** (at normal speed—sometimes referred to as **Code 1** or **Priority 3**) or **HOT** (in emergency, lights-and-siren mode—sometimes referred to as **Code 3** or **Priority 1**). If the patient is not breathing, or the caller is not sure, the EMD will dispatch the maximum response and begin the appropriate pre-arrival instructions for a non-breathing patient, which may also involve telephone CPR if the patient is pulseless.

After the initial seven questions, the EMD will often ask additional, more specific questions by referring to the appropriate medical dispatch priority card.

Obtaining Information About a Vehicle Collision

If the chief complaint the EMD obtains is that there has been a traffic collision injury, a series of key questions must be asked to help determine the priority and amount of response. Any injury resulting from a collision involving a bicycle, motorcycle, or pedestrian should receive the highest priority of response because of the mechanisms of injury involved.

Key questions asked by the EMD will determine if the patient is alert, if any entrapment or vehicle submersion is involved, if the patient is breathing normally, and the location of the injuries. Typically, 50% of the collisions that are reported involve a personal injury and 1% involve a fatality.

1. *How many and what kind of vehicles are involved?* Many kinds of vehicles are involved in traffic collisions, and certain vehicles may require special attention from responding emergency service units. The EMD should determine, if possible, how many vehicles involved in the collision are passenger cars, buses, or trucks. If the EMD learns that a truck is involved, he will try to determine what type the truck is—for example, a box cargo truck, a tank truck, or a dump truck. Valid descriptions of collision vehicles help emergency service personnel plan their response and first-on-the-scene activities.

2. *How many persons do you think are injured?* A fact important to a response plan is information about injuries. When the EMD learns that some people have been injured in a traffic collision, he may assume that "some" means two or three and send a single ambulance. If he learns from the initial caller that five people have been injured, then he may deem it necessary or prudent to send two or three ambulances at the same time. Time, and perhaps lives, will be saved by knowing precisely the number of people injured in a vehicle collision.

3. *Do the victims appear trapped?* Rescue unit dispatch may be affected by this information.

With good interrogation of the caller, it may be possible for the EMD to appropriately dispatch one unit HOT and backup units COLD, which in turn will help prevent emergency vehicle collisions.

The EMD will also need to determine the exact location of the collision.

4. *What is the exact location of the collision?* If the collision has occurred in a built-up area, you should be able to learn a street address or the names of the nearest two streets that intersect. But if the collision has occurred in a rural area, there may be a problem learning the exact location, especially when the caller is not familiar with the area. The person reporting the collision

may say something like, "There's been a collision about three miles north of town." The EMD must try to pinpoint the location by asking questions about the nearest crossroad or the name of a nearby store, if there is one, or what landmarks are visible from the caller's point of view (e.g. mileposts, water towers, large silos, or radio antennas). Even if the caller cannot pinpoint his location, the telephone company should be able to provide the location of the phone, so, again, it is important to keep the caller on the line.

Next, the EMD should attempt to learn something about the scene by asking the caller these questions.

5. *Is traffic moving?*
6. *How many lanes are open?*
7. *How far is traffic backed up?*

If the EMD can inform responding units that all lanes of a particular road leading to the collision scene are blocked, operators can select alternative response routes.

Then the EMD should attempt to learn whether hazards have been produced by the collision by asking these questions.

8. *Are any of the vehicles on fire?*
9. *Are any of the vehicles leaking fuel?*
10. *Are any electrical wires down?*
11. *Do any of the vehicles appear unstable? Is any vehicle on its side or top?*
12. *Does a truck appear to be carrying a hazardous cargo?*

It takes a little time to gather this information, but what the EMD learns from a caller will enable him to alert the proper services, and what information he passes on will enable ambulance, fire, rescue, and other emergency service personnel to plan effective responses.

Transmitting Information to the Ambulance Service

This is how an EMD might dispatch an ambulance to the location of an injured person.

MEDCOM to Ambulance 621 and Medic 620, respond priority one to an unconscious male with breathing difficulty. The location is the Acme Paper Company at 123 Madison Street with Maple Avenue on the cross. Time now 16:45 hours.

The EMD will repeat the message to minimize any question as to its content, and give the time. The person receiving the message at the ambulance quarters should identify his station, note the information on a form provided for that purpose, and confirm the message.

OPERATING THE AMBULANCE

No textbook can fully prepare you for the task of driving an ambulance, nor can you become a good ambulance operator through experience alone. If you aspire to drive an ambulance, make every effort to attend a formal emergency vehicle operator training program that has both classroom and in-vehicle road sessions.

In the classroom you will learn how a vehicle operates, how it behaves on different types of roads, the proper use of audible and visual warning devices, laws regarding the operation of emergency vehicles, and so on.

On the driving range, you will learn, among other things, how to make a safe response, how to change lanes quickly and safely, how to recover from skids, and how to back the vehicle.

If you do not have an opportunity to attend a formal operator training course, attend the defensive driving course that is offered by local safety councils and law enforcement agencies. You will at least learn how to prevent collisions by staying alert for problems caused by other motorists, changing road conditions, and hazards. Then spend time behind the wheel driving under the guidance of a safe ambulance operator—one who practices defensive driving, cares about safety, and has a clean driving record.

Being a Safe Ambulance Operator

To be a safe ambulance operator, you must

- *Be physically fit.* You should not have any impairment that prevents you from turning the steering wheel, operating the gear shift, or depressing the floor pedals. Nor should you have any medical condition that might disable you while driving, such as a heart condition or uncontrolled diabetes or epilepsy.
- *Be mentally fit, with your emotions under*

control. Some emergency service personnel undergo personality changes when they drive an emergency vehicle, or when they are put in charge of an emergency situation. If you fit in this category, do not operate an ambulance.

- *Be able to perform under stress.*
- *Have a positive attitude about your ability as a driver,* but do not think that you are the best in the world.
- *Be tolerant of other drivers.* Always keep in mind that people react differently when they see an emergency vehicle. Accept and tolerate the bad habits of other drivers without flying into a rage. Appreciate the need for cooperation, and cooperate yourself.
- *Never drive while under the influence of drugs or alcohol* including "recreational" drugs such as cocaine, medicines such as antihistamines, "pep pills," or tranquilizers.
- *Never drive with a restricted license.*
- *Always wear your glasses or contact lenses* if required for driving.
- *Evaluate your ability to drive* based on personal stress, illness, fatigue, or sleepiness.

Understanding the Law

Every state has statutes that regulate the operation of emergency vehicles. Although the wording of the statutes may vary, the intent of the laws is essentially the same. Emergency vehicle operators are generally granted certain privileges with regard to speed, parking, passage through traffic signals, and direction of travel. However, the laws also clearly state that IF AN EMERGENCY VEHICLE OPERATOR DOES NOT DRIVE WITH DUE REGARD FOR THE SAFETY OF OTHERS, HE MUST BE PREPARED TO PAY THE CONSEQUENCES FOR HIS ACTIONS.

Following are some points usually included in laws that regulate the operation of ambulances.

- An ambulance operator must have a valid driver's license and may be required to have completed a formal emergency vehicle or defensive driver training program.
- Privileges granted under the law to the operators of ambulances apply when the vehicle is responding to an emergency or is involved in the emergency transport of a sick or injured person. When the ambulance is not on an emergency call, the laws that apply to the operation of non-emergency vehicles also apply to the ambulance.
- Even though certain privileges are granted during an emergency, AN AMBULANCE OPERATOR IS NOT RELIEVED FROM THE DUTY TO OPERATE THE VEHICLE WITH DUE REGARD FOR THE SAFETY OF ALL PERSONS. The privileges granted do not provide immunity to the operator in cases of reckless driving or disregard for the safety of others.
- Privileges granted during emergency situations apply only if the operator is using warning devices in the manner prescribed by law.

Most statutes allow emergency vehicle operators to

- Park the vehicle anywhere so long as it does not damage personal property or endanger lives.
- Proceed past red stop signals, flashing red stop signals, and stop signs. Some states require that emergency vehicle operators come to a full stop, then proceed with caution. Other states require only that an operator slow down and proceed with caution.
- Exceed the posted speed limit as long as life and property are not endangered.
- Pass other vehicles in designated no-passing zones after promptly signaling, ensuring that the way is clear, and taking precautions to avoid endangering life and property.
- With proper caution and signals, disregard regulations that govern direction of travel and turning in specific directions.

Remember: With these privileges come the responsibility to drive with due regard for the safety of all others.

Should you ever become involved in an ambulance collision, the laws will be interpreted by the court based upon two key issues. *Did you use due regard for the safety of all others?* and *Was it a true emergency?*

The requirement of due regard actually sets a higher standard for drivers of emergency vehicles than for the rest of the driving public. This is why it is not uncommon for there to be an investigation by the district attorney, as well as your ambulance service, following a collision.

Most states reserve the emergency mode of operation for a true emergency, defined as one in which the best information you have available to you is that there is a possibility of loss of life or limb. When dispatched to a call, there is often not much information to go on, so an "accident" will get an emergency response. However, once you arrive and find that your patient has only a fractured arm with no circulatory or nerve function damage, you have a stable patient and it is no longer a true emergency. A lights-and-siren, high-speed response to the hospital in such a situation would be ruled illegal in most states.

The privileges described here are just examples of those often granted to ambulance operators. Do not assume that they are granted in your state. Obtain a copy of your state's motor vehicle rules and regulations and study them carefully before you start to operate the ambulance.

Using the Warning Devices

Ambulance operators, like the operators of other emergency vehicles, sometimes become so obsessed with the idea that sirens and flashing lights will clear the roads that they overlook hazards and take chances. Audible and visual warning devices do serve a purpose; however, safe emergency vehicle operation can be achieved only when the proper use of warning devices is coupled with sound emergency and defensive driving practices.

It is important to note that studies have shown that other drivers do not see or hear your ambulance until it is within 100 feet of their vehicle. So never let the lights and siren give you a false sense of security.

The Siren Although the siren is the most commonly used audible warning device, it is also the most misused. Consider the effects that sirens have on other motorists, patients in ambulances, and ambulance operators themselves.

- Motorists are less inclined to give way to ambulances when sirens are continually sounded. Many feel that the right-of-way privileges granted to ambulances by law are being abused when sirens are sounded.
- The continuous sound of a siren may cause a sick or injured person to suffer increased fear and anxiety, and his condition may actually worsen as stress builds.
- Ambulance operators themselves are affected by the continuous sound of a siren. Tests have shown that inexperienced ambu-

lance operators tend to increase their driving speeds from 10 to 15 miles per hour while continually sounding the siren. In some reported cases, operators using a siren were unable to negotiate curves that they could pass through easily when not sounding the siren. Sirens also affect hearing, especially if used for long periods of time with the siren speaker over the cab. The best placement for the speaker is in the grille of the vehicle.

Many states have statutes that regulate the use of audible warning signals, and where there are no such statutes, ambulance organizations usually create their own operating procedures or policies. If your organization does not, you may find some of the following suggestions helpful when you think it is necessary to use the siren during an ambulance run.

- Use the siren sparingly, and only when you must. The more you use the siren, the greater the chance that other motorists will be indifferent to its sound.
- Never assume that all motorists will hear your signal. Buildings, trees, and dense shrubbery may block siren sounds. Soundproofing keeps outside noises from entering vehicles, and radios or tape systems also decrease the likelihood that an outside sound will be heard.
- Always assume that some motorists will hear your siren but ignore it.
- Be prepared for the erratic maneuvers of other drivers. Some drivers panic when they hear a siren.
- Do not pull up close to a vehicle and then sound your siren. Such action may cause the driver to jam on his brakes so quickly that you will be unable to stop in time. Use the horn when you are close to a vehicle ahead.
- Never use the siren indiscriminately, and never use it to scare someone.

Note: Some states require the use of the siren at all times when the ambulance is responding in the emergency mode. Other states require it only when the operator is exercising all of the privileges discussed above.

The Horn All ambulances must be equipped with a horn. Experienced operators find that in many cases the judicious use of the horn clears traffic as quickly as the siren. The guidelines for using a siren apply to the ambulance's horn as well.

Visual Warning Devices Whenever the ambulance is on the road, night or day, the headlights should be on. This increases the visibility of the vehicle to other drivers. In a number of foreign countries, it is required that the headlights be used all the time. In some states headlights are now required of all vehicles in low visibility conditions or whenever the window wipers are in use. Alternating flashing headlights should be used only if they are attached to secondary head lamps. In most states it is illegal to drive at night with one headlight out.

Probably the most useful light is the one in the cowling of the front vehicle hood. This is easily seen in the rearview mirror of another driver to get his attention if your siren has not yet alerted him. The lights on the front bumper in the grille are generally mounted too low to be effective. The large box lights found in the outermost corners of the box, or modular, should blink in tandem, or unison, rather than wigwagging or alternating. This helps the vehicle that is approaching from a distance identify the full size of your vehicle.

There is a lot of controversy about the use of strobes on ambulances. When planning the lighting package of an ambulance, check the research before making your decision. In general, it is wisest for the package to combine single beam bulbs and strobes rather than just one type of lighting system.

The four-way flashers and directional signals should not be used as emergency lights. This is very confusing to the public, as well as being illegal in some states. Drivers expect a vehicle with four-way flashers on to be traveling at a very slow rate of speed. Additionally, the flashers disrupt the function of the directional signals.

When the ambulance is in the emergency response mode, either responding to the scene or responding to the hospital with a critical or unstable patient, all the emergency lights should be used. The vehicle should be easily seen from 360 degrees.

In some communities fire department ambulances still use their emergency lights when returning to the station. This is a tradition that stems from the fact that, years ago, fire apparatus often carried firefighters on the back steps. The lights were kept on to alert the public of their presence. Today Occupational Safety and Health Administration (OSHA) regulations make it illegal to build a fire truck with a back step for personnel.

Basically the practice of keeping emergency lights on is very confusing to the public. Don't be surprised if other drivers do not pull over to the right when you are on an emergency run if they constantly see your ambulance at red lights and returning to the station—even responding to a standby at a neighboring department's headquarters, where the ambulance will just park on the ramp—with emergency lights on!

Remember: Audible and visual warning signals merely ask the drivers of other vehicles to give way to an emergency vehicle. They do not demand that drivers give way, and they certainly cannot physically clear the road.

SAVE THE USE OF LIGHTS AND SIREN FOR TRUE EMERGENCIES.

The Effect of Speed on an Ambulance Run

You are often told to drive slowly, as when visibility is poor and when the road surface is slippery. At this point you may be inclined to say something like, "How will I ever get a seriously ill or injured person to a hospital if I poke along?" We are not suggesting that you "poke along." But do drive with these facts in mind.

- Excessive speed increases the probability of a collision.
- Speed increases stopping distance and so reduces the chance of avoiding a hazardous situation.

Stopping distance is the number of feet that a vehicle travels from the instant that the operator decides to stop until the moment that the vehicle actually stops. It is dependent on several factors, including the speed and condition of the vehicle, road conditions, and the alertness of the operator.

Stopping distance is the total of **reaction distance** and **braking distance**. Reaction distance is the number of feet the vehicle travels from the moment that the operator decides to stop until his foot applies pressure to the brake pedal. Braking distance is the number of feet the vehicle travels from the start of the braking action until the vehicle comes to a complete stop. Table 24-1 shows stopping distances for a light truck, which is comparable to an ambulance. **Perception distance** is the number of feet traveled while the operator recognizes the

TABLE 24-1   Stopping Distances in Feet of a Light, Two-Axle Truck

Miles Per Hour	Driver Reaction Distance	Vehicle Braking Distance	Total Stopping Distance
10	11	7	18
15	17	17	34
20	22	30	53
25	28	46	74
30	33	67	100
35	39	92	131
40	44	125	169
45	50	165	215
50	55	225	280
55	61	275	336
60	66	360	426

Ambulance Accident Prevention Seminar, Student Workbook, 1988, New York State Emergency Medical Services Program

hazard and decides how to react. Perception distance does, of course, add to stopping distance but is usually not figured into stopping distance estimates because it varies so much with the individual.

What effect does speed have on an ambulance run? Consider a five-mile trip from an emergency scene to a hospital.

Assuming that you will not have to stop or slow down, at 60 miles per hour you will be able to cover the five miles in 5 minutes. At 50 miles per hour it will take 6 minutes to reach the hospital. At 60 miles per hour the ambulance will travel 426 feet before the operator can bring the vehicle to a complete stop once he reacts to a dangerous situation. But at 50 miles per hour the operator will be able to stop the ambulance in 280 feet.

The one minute gained in response time is not worth the risk of collision brought about by the 50% increase in stopping distance.

Driving Defensively

Ambulances, like all other vehicles, can become involved in a variety of collisions. The ambulance operator must drive defensively at all times. You must affect your perception distance by being aware and alert, keeping your eyes searching and scanning and your mind on your driving. You must favorably affect reaction distance, first by recognizing a potential hazard and covering the brake, and second by recognizing when the hazard becomes an actual threat and braking quickly. You must affect braking distance by maintaining a reasonable and prudent speed for

the conditions and by driving a safe vehicle that is frequently checked and adequately maintained.

The typical non-defensive driver often tries to rationalize his mistakes by saying, "Well it wasn't my fault," "I thought he was going to stop," or "That kid should have known better." It really does not matter who is at fault when the consequences are a serious injury or fatality. What does matter is doing everything you can to avoid your own driver errors and to watch out for the other driver.

One important defensive driving habit is covering the brake, that is, driving with your foot hovering over the brake pedal whenever you are driving under any potentially hazardous conditions.

Let's compare a non-defensive and a defensive ambulance operator in a potentially hazardous situation. Assume that both are experienced drivers who are in good physical and emotional condition, that the ambulance brakes have been well maintained, and that weather and road conditions are ideal.

The non-defensive ambulance operator is driving down a suburban street approaching three children playing ball close to the street—a potentially hazardous situation. He is not taking defensive driving precautions but, instead, is expecting the children to watch out for the ambulance.

Typically, this non-defensive driver is in the habit of keeping his foot on the accelerator while driving, even in a potentially hazardous situation. When the potential hazard turns into an actual threat, he must now move his right foot from the accelerator onto the brake pedal.

Suppose the ambulance is traveling at 30 miles per hour as he approaches the children. Suddenly a girl chases the ball into the street. The operator then recognizes the hazard and decides to apply the brake. While he is reacting, the ambulance travels 33 feet until the brakes are applied. At this point, the braking distance begins and the ambulance travels 67 additional feet before coming to a stop. The total stopping distance is 100 feet, or one-third the length of a football field. (A good exercise is to take out a tape measure and chalk, then mark off 100 feet on the street.)

Now let's consider an ambulance operator who has made defensive driving a habit. As soon as he sees the children playing, he recognizes the potential hazard and moves his foot from the accelerator to cover the brake. Since he has developed the habit of covering the brake in all "iffy" traffic situations, doing it in this situation is almost a reflex.

Like the non-defensive driver, our defensive driver is traveling at 30 miles per hour when he first sees the children. When the girl runs into the street, he is ready to brake. The ambulance would travel 9 feet until the brake is depressed, but covering the brake gave this operator an additional benefit because taking his foot off the accelerator slightly reduced the speed, bringing reaction distance down to about 8 feet. For the same reason, braking distance is reduced to about 66 feet. So the total stopping distance is 74 feet.

Take a moment and think about the results of this simple example. The defensive driver, by being alert and covering the brake, saved 26 feet, which in this case was enough to save a life!

During Escorted or Multiple-Vehicle Responses When the police provide an escort for an ambulance, the same dangers exist as during other driving situations, and new ones may be created. Too often, the inexperienced ambulance operator follows the escort vehicle too closely and is unable to stop when the lead vehicle(s) make an emergency stop. Also, the inexperienced operator may assume that other drivers know his vehicle is following the escort. In fact, other drivers will often pull out in front of the ambulance just after the escort vehicle passes.

Because of the dangers involved with escorts, most EMS Systems recommend no escorts unless the operator is not familiar with the location of the patient (or hospital) and must be given assistance from the police.

In cases of multiple vehicle responses, the dangers can be the same as those generated by escorted responses, especially when the responding vehicles travel in the same direction, close together.

In multiple-vehicle responses, a great danger also exists when two vehicles approach the same intersection at the same time. Not only may they fail to yield for each other; other drivers may yield for the first vehicle but not the second. Obviously, great care must be used at intersections during multiple vehicle responses.

Note: Be certain to follow your local protocols for the use of warning lights and sirens during escorts and multiple-vehicle responses. If everyone approaching the scene does not follow the proper protocols, the confusion may cause the vehicle operators and other motorists to make serious errors.

Factors That Affect Response

Movies and television programs often depict ambulance runs as effortless responses over straight, traffic-free roadways in good weather during daylight hours. Such an ambulance run is not always as trouble-free as it might seem. Studies show that the typical ambulance accident happens on a dry road, during daylight hours, in an intersection. Additionally, an ambulance response can be affected by several factors (see Figure 24-2).

Day of the Week Weekdays are usually the days of heaviest traffic flow because people are commuting to and from work. On weekends, commuter traffic generally diminishes, but traffic increases around urban and suburban shopping centers. Superhighways and interstate roads may be crowded on Friday and Sunday evenings. In resort areas, weekend traffic may be heavier than weekday traffic.

Time of Day There was a time when traffic patterns were quite predictable. During morning rush hours vehicles moved persons from sub-

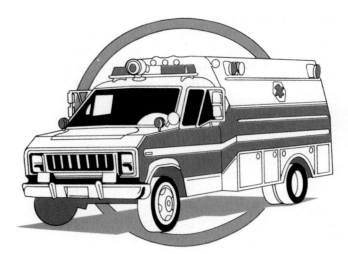

1. Day of the week
2. Time of the day
3. Weather
4. Detours
5. Railroads
6. Bridges and Tunnels
7. Schools
8. Alternate Routes

Figure 24-2 Factors that affect response.

urbs to cities, and in the evening the traffic pattern was reversed.

Today, downtown areas are still major employment centers, but so are suburban shopping malls, office complexes, and industrial parks. Accordingly, traffic over major arteries tends to be heavy in all directions during commuter hours. At these times, ambulance operators can expect blocked intersections, packed roads, and crawling vehicles regardless of the direction in which they must travel.

Weather Adverse weather conditions reduce driving speeds and thus increase response times. A heavy snowfall can temporarily prevent any response at all.

Detours The movement of vehicles can be seriously impeded by road construction and maintenance activities. A detour often affects the operation of emergency vehicles less than the closing of one or more lanes of a multi-lane highway. An ambulance can continue to travel over a detour, but when several lanes of a highway are merged into one, there is often no way for an ambulance to move around slow-moving or stopped vehicles or to pull off the road in favor of an alternative route. Thus there is no escaping the traffic jam. Neither siren-sounding nor light flashing can move vehicles out of the way when there is no place for them to go. Be aware of the road construction in your district and plan responses accordingly.

Railroads Although many road-grade crossings have been replaced with overpasses, there are still more than a quarter-million grade crossings in the United States. Thus there are still many opportunities for traffic to be blocked by long, slow-moving freight trains.

Bridges and Tunnels Bridges and tunnels are erected to allow the flow of vehicles over and under natural and artificial dividers. However, traffic over bridges and through tunnels slows during rush hours. When a collision occurs on a bridge or in a tunnel, the flow of vehicles, including emergency vehicles, may stop altogether. Collisions tend to occur when drivers forget that bridges freeze before roadways.

Schools and School Buses The reduced speed limits in force during school hours slow the flow of vehicles. Crossing guards also disrupt the flow of traffic, and drivers tend to slow down when an area is congested with children.

School buses also slow traffic. When a bus makes frequent stops along a two-lane road, traffic can back up behind the bus. Other vehicles cannot resume normal speed until the bus turns off or allows the traffic to pass. An emergency vehicle should never pass a stopped school bus with its lights flashing. Wait for the school bus driver to signal you to proceed by turning off the lights.

Remember: Emergency vehicles attract children, who often venture out into the street to see them. The operator of every emergency vehicle should slow down when approaching a school or playground.

When it appears that an ambulance will be delayed in reaching a sick or injured person because of these or other factors, the operator should consider taking an alternative route or requesting the response of another ambulance.

Selecting an Alternative Route

You must have a plan for times when changing conditions affect response. Obtain detailed maps of your service area. On the maps, indicate usually troublesome traffic spots such as schools, bridges, tunnels, railroad grade crossings, and heavily congested areas. Also indicate temporary problems such as road and building construction sites and long- and short-term detours.

Using another color, indicate alternative routes to areas where normal routes are often blocked. Indicate snow routes, and so on.

Hang one map in quarters and place another map in the ambulance. Then when you must travel past a problem area in response to an urgent call, you will be able to select an alternative route that will get you to your destination quickly and safely.

RESPONDING TO THE SCENE OF A VEHICLE COLLISION

Let us say that your ambulance has just been dispatched to the scene of a motor vehicle collision. Your partner is driving. If he is a good operator, one who concentrates fully on the driving task, he will spend every minute of the trip employing the special skills that are required for the safe response of an ambulance.

But what will you, as the attending EMT, do during the response? Here are some suggestions.

As you leave quarters and begin the run (Figure 24-3)

- *If necessary, confirm the location of the collision with your EMD.*
- *Ask whether there are any further details.* While you were preparing to leave quarters, the EMD may have been able to elicit additional important bits of information from the initial and subsequent callers.
- *Listen for other units on the radio.* If other units are responding, be watchful for them as you travel to the scene.
- *Listen for status reports.* Messages from first-arriving units often provide facts about the nature and severity of collisions, facts that will help you to formulate a plan of action even before you arrive on the scene.
- *Picture in your mind the location of rescue equipment on the unit.* The few seconds that you can save in acquiring rescue tools may mean the difference between life and death.

As you near the collision scene

- *When you near intersections, look and listen for other emergency service units approaching from side streets.* Remember that other units may be responding along with yours, or they may be responding to a different call. Remember also that in urban settings, sounds bouncing off of buildings can blend siren noises in such a way that you will not be able to determine the direction of an approaching emergency vehicle.
- *Look for signs of a collision-related power outage*—signs that will suggest that wires are down at the collision scene. During day-

light hours, look into the windows of stores and office buildings that would normally be lighted at the time. At night, suspect a power interruption when you see that dwellings and businesses are dark when you would expect them to be illuminated.

- *Observe traffic flow.* If there is no opposing traffic, suspect a blockade at the collision scene. Remember that all lanes of the road may be blocked for some distance from the crash site.
- *Look for smoke in the direction of the collision scene*—a sign that fire has resulted from the collision.

When you are within sight of the scene

- *Look at the involved vehicles.* If you see that a truck has been damaged, look for fumes or vapor clouds. If you see anything suspicious, stop the ambulance immediately. If you have binoculars on the ambulance, scan the vehicle for hazardous material warning placards. If you see such placards, notify your EMD and request advice, or consult the on-board reference book. If you elect to continue on, go directly to a safe place.
- *Look for collision victims on or near the road.* A person may have been thrown from a vehicle as it careened out of control, or an injured person may have walked away from the wreckage and collapsed on or near the roadway.
- *Look for smoke that you may not have seen at a distance*— indication of a developing fire.
- *Look for broken utility poles and downed wires.* At night, direct the beam of a spotlight or handlight on poles and wire spans as you approach the scene. Keep in mind that wires may be down several hundred feet from the crash vehicles.
- *Be alert for persons walking along the side of the road toward the collision scene.* ""Rubberneckers" (excited children in particular) are often oblivious to vehicles approaching from behind. Be especially watchful at night. You may not be able to see persons dressed in dark clothing until they are well within the stopping distance of your vehicle.
- *Watch for the signals of police officers and other emergency service personnel.* They may have information about hazards or the location of injured persons.

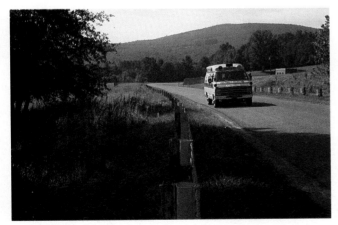

Figure 24-3 Prepare for the call while en route.

As you reach the scene

- *Sniff for odors.* The odor of gasoline or diesel fuel carries downwind for a considerable distance. An unusual odor may signal that a hazardous material has been released.
- *Note the direction and velocity of the wind by observing flags, pennants, smoke, and so on.* If you see that a vehicle is on fire, or if you suspect that a hazardous material has been released into the atmosphere, remember that you should park upwind and on the same level as the hazard.
- *Note the terrain.* If fuel or another liquid has been released from a ruptured tank, you should park uphill from the crash site, as well as upwind.

POSITIONING THE AMBULANCE

Far too many ambulance operators park their vehicles at collision scenes according to this formula: The closer the ambulance to the wreckage, the shorter the distance that equipment and people must be carried. This is not parking, this is merely stopping! Worse yet, it is stopping without regard for other vehicles that must use the road (including other emergency vehicles) and for any of a number of hazards that may be present.

Establishing the Danger Zone

A **danger zone** exists around the wreckage of every vehicle collision. The size of the zone depends on the nature and severity of collision-produced hazards (see Scan 24-1). An ambulance should never be parked within the danger zone.

When there are no apparent hazards

- Consider the danger zone to extend 50 feet in all directions from the wreckage. The ambulance will be away from broken glass and other debris, and it will not impede emergency service personnel who must work in or around the wreckage.
- If using highway flares to protect the scene, make sure that the person igniting them has been trained as to the proper technique and wears some type of protective clothing.
- Flares should have a wire stand rather than

the older-type spiked bottom. If you have the spiked type, after the flare has burned down and is out, remove the spike from the guardpost or asphalt so that it does not become a danger to children or the tires of passing vehicles.

When fuel has been spilled

- Consider the danger zone to extend a minimum of 100 feet in all directions from the wreckage. In addition to parking outside the danger zone, park upwind, if possible. Thus the ambulance will be out of the path of dense smoke if the fuel ignites. If fuel is flowing away from the wreckage, park uphill as well as upwind. If parking uphill is not possible, position the ambulance as far from the flowing fuel as possible. Avoid gutters, ditches, and gullies that can carry fuel to the ambulance.
- When personnel are available and conditions warrant it, have an EMT either divert the flow of fuel or form a dike using a hand shovel. Then have that EMT stand by with a fire extinguisher until the arrival of the fire department.
- Do not use flares in areas where fuel has been spilled. Under these conditions, use small orange traffic cones during daylight and reflective triangles at night.

When a collision vehicle is on fire

- Consider the danger zone to extend at least 100 feet in all directions even if the fire appears small and limited to the engine compartment. If fire reaches the vehicle's fuel tank, an explosion could easily damage an ambulance parked closer than 100 feet.

When wires are down

- Consider the danger zone as the area in which people or vehicles might be contacted by energized wires if they pivot around their points of attachment. Even though you may have to carry equipment and stretchers for a considerable distance, the ambulance should be parked at least one full span of wires from the poles to which broken wires are attached.

When a hazardous material is involved

- Check the Department of Transportation *Emergency Response Guide* for suggestions as to where to park, or request advice from

Scan 24-1
Hazards

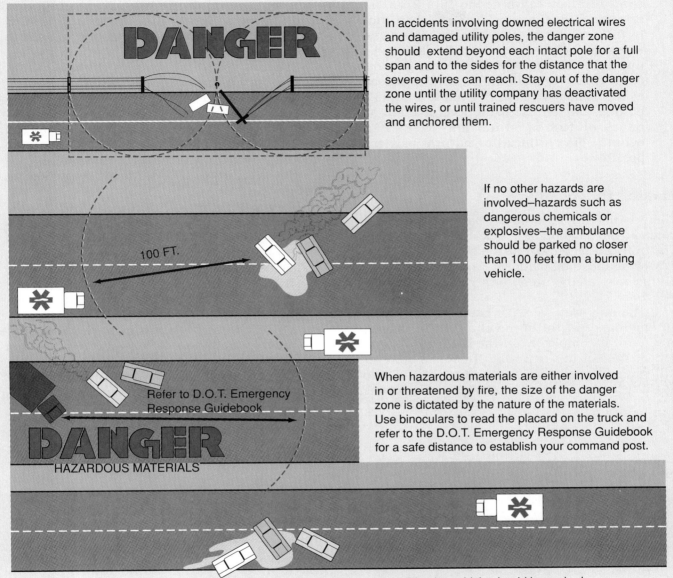

In accidents involving downed electrical wires and damaged utility poles, the danger zone should extend beyond each intact pole for a full span and to the sides for the distance that the severed wires can reach. Stay out of the danger zone until the utility company has deactivated the wires, or until trained rescuers have moved and anchored them.

If no other hazards are involved—hazards such as dangerous chemicals or explosives—the ambulance should be parked no closer than 100 feet from a burning vehicle.

When hazardous materials are either involved in or threatened by fire, the size of the danger zone is dictated by the nature of the materials. Use binoculars to read the placard on the truck and refer to the D.O.T. Emergency Response Guidebook for a safe distance to establish your command post.

The ambulance should be parked uphill from flowing fuel. If this is not possible, the vehicle should be parked as far from the fuel flow as possible, avoiding gutters, ditches, and gullies that may carry the spill to the parking site. Remember, your ambulance's catalytic converter is an ignition source over 1000 degrees.

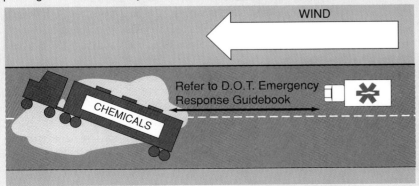

Leaking containers of dangerous chemicals may produce a health as well as a fire hazard. When chemicals have been spilled, whether fumes are evident or not, the ambulance should be parked upwind. If the hazardous material is known, seek advice from experts through the dispatcher or CHEMTREC.

an agency such as CHEMTREC. In some cases you may be able to park 50 feet from the wreckage, as when no hazardous material has been spilled or released. In other cases you may be warned to park 2,000 feet or more from the wreckage, as when there is the possibility that certain high explosives may detonate. In all cases, park upwind from the wreckage when you discover that a hazardous material is present at a collision site. Park uphill if a liquid is flowing, but on the same level if there are gases or fumes which may rise. Park behind some artificial or natural barrier if possible.

Parking the Ambulance

There is usually no problem parking the ambulance at the location of a sick or injured person. The unit can be parked at the curb or in a driveway or at a loading platform. The parking task is not so easy at the scene of a collision, however (see Scan 24-2).

The only way to really ensure the safety of an ambulance at the scene of a vehicle collision is to park it completely off the roadway, as on a service road or in a driveway. To do so, however, will severely reduce or even negate the ability of flashing and revolving warning lights to warn

approaching motorists before flares or other warning devices can be set out.

Studies have been done that show that red revolving beacons attract drunk or tired drivers. Consider pulling off the road, turning off your headlights, and using just amber rear sealed beam blinkers that blink in tandem or unison to identify the size of your vehicle.

There are two schools of thought about positioning an ambulance or other emergency vehicle on a road leading to a collision site. Some officials argue that the ambulance should be located beyond the wreckage (relative to the direction of traffic flow) to prevent an expensive ambulance from being struck by oncoming traffic. However, other officials favor the following procedure.

1. Place the ambulance at the edge of the danger zone between the wreckage and approaching vehicles. The unit's warning lights will help alert oncoming traffic to the hazard ahead, although it does not reduce the need for other warning devices. Side beacons can be used for scene lighting.
2. Once the ambulance is parked, set its emergency brake and firmly wedge wheel chocks under the tires in such a way that forward movement will be retarded if the ambulance is struck from behind.

CHAPTER REVIEW

KEY TERMS

You may find it helpful to review the following terms.

braking distance—the number of feet a vehicle travels from the start of braking action until it comes to a full stop.
COLD/Code 1/Priority 3—terms used throughout the United States to designate a non-emergency, normal-driving ambulance response mode.
danger zone—the area at the emergency scene in which rescue personnel, patients, and bystanders may be exposed to hazards such as fire, dangerous chemicals, explosion, downed electrical wires, or radiation.
Emergency Medical Dispatcher (EMD)—a person trained in interrogation techniques, pre-

arrival instructions, and call prioritization. An EMD's four key functions are to receive and process calls for help, to provide medical instructions to patients and information to crews, to dispatch and coordinate Emergency Medical Services (EMS) resources, and to coordinate with other public safety agencies.
HOT/Code 3/Priority 1—terms used throughout the United States to designate an emergency, lights-and-siren ambulance response mode.
perception distance—the number of feet a vehicle travels while the operator recognizes a hazard and decides how to react.
reaction distance—the number of feet a vehicle travels from the time the operator decides to stop until his foot applies pressure to the brake pedal.

Parking the Ambulance

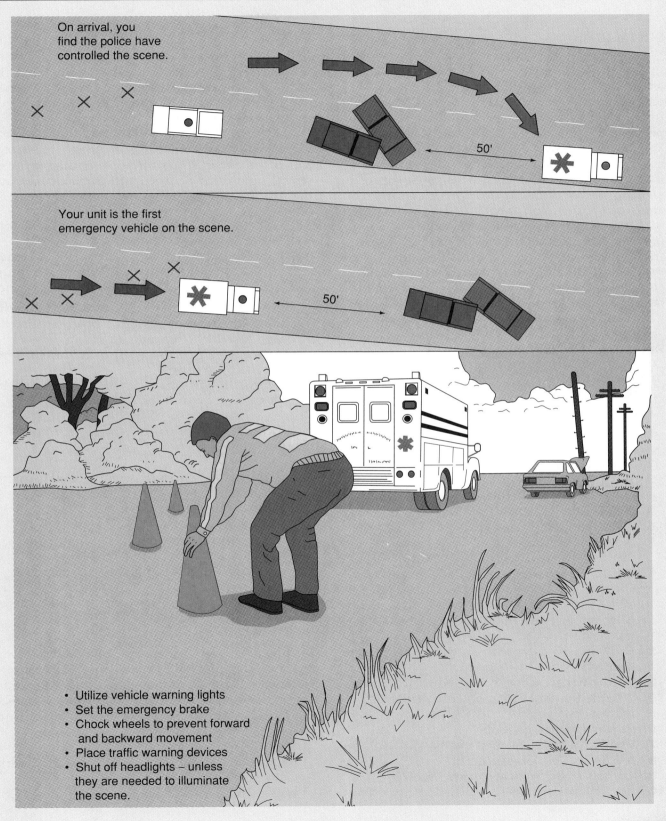

On arrival, you find the police have controlled the scene.

50'

Your unit is the first emergency vehicle on the scene.

50'

- Utilize vehicle warning lights
- Set the emergency brake
- Chock wheels to prevent forward and backward movement
- Place traffic warning devices
- Shut off headlights – unless they are needed to illuminate the scene.

stopping distance—the number of feet a vehicle travels from the moment the operator decides to stop until the vehicle actually stops. It is the total of reaction distance and braking distance.

universal number—the telephone number 911, used to gain access to the Emergency Medical Dispatch system.

SUMMARY

In some areas of the country, citizen requests for assistance go directly to universal number (911) emergency reporting centers where EMDs control the movements of fire, ambulance, rescue, police, and other emergency service units.

In other areas, citizen requests go to either a fire or police dispatch center. Delays in alerting and subsequent delays in response are possible but are usually minimal because of cross-communication capabilities.

In still other areas, citizen requests can go to a small dispatch facility, the fire department, the ambulance service, the rescue squad, the police department, or even a place of business or someone's home. Valuable time is often lost because of the misdirection of calls.

Receiving the Call for Help

EMDs should ask certain questions of a citizen requesting an ambulance for a sick or injured person. These questions should include

1. What is the exact location of the sick or injured person?
2. What is your call-back number?
3. What is the problem?
4. How old is the patient?
5. What is the patient's sex?
6. Is the patient conscious?
7. Is the patient breathing?

EMDs should ask these questions of someone who is reporting a motor vehicle collision.

1. How many and what kind of vehicles are involved?
2. How many persons do you think are injured?
3. Do the victims appear trapped?
4. What is the exact location of the collision?
5. Is traffic moving?
6. How many lanes are open?
7. How far is traffic backed up?
8. Are any of the vehicles on fire?
9. Are any of the vehicles leaking fuel?
10. Are any electrical wires down?

11. Do any of the vehicles appear unstable? Is any vehicle on its side or top?
12. Does any vehicle appear to be carrying a hazardous cargo?

Based on the information gained, the EMD will dispatch and coordinate ambulance, fire, rescue, and other services and transmit instructions to the caller and the ambulance crew.

Operating the Ambulance

A person who aspires to be an ambulance operator should

- Attend a formal emergency vehicle operators course that includes both classroom and in-vehicle instruction.
- Learn when to drive an ambulance, and when not to drive.
- Learn the laws that regulate the operation of emergency vehicles within his state.

During an ambulance run, a safe operator should

- Properly use the audible and visual warning devices.
- Drive at appropriate speeds.
- Drive defensively.
- Appreciate how certain factors affect response.
- Be prepared to select an alternative route.

Responding to the Scene of a Vehicle Collision

During a response to the scene of a motor vehicle collision, the attending EMT should make observations and take steps to ensure a safe trip. Thus the operator can concentrate on the driving task.

As the ambulance leaves quarters and begins the run, the attending EMT should

- Confirm the location of the collision with the EMD.
- Ask whether there are any further details.

- Listen for other units on the radio.
- Listen for status reports.
- Picture the location of rescue equipment on the ambulance.

As the ambulance nears the scene, the attending EMT should

- Listen and look for other emergency service units approaching from side streets.
- Look for signs of a collision-related power outage.
- Observe traffic flow.
- Look for smoke in the direction of the collision scene.

When the ambulance is within sight of the collision scene, the attending EMT should

- Look at the collision vehicles and assess the mechanisms of injury.
- Look for collision victims on or near the road.
- Look for smoke that might not have been seen at a distance.
- Look for broken utility poles and downed wires.
- Be alert for persons walking along the side of the road toward the collision scene.
- Watch for the signals of police officers and other emergency service personnel.

As the ambulance reaches the scene, the attending EMT should

- Sniff for odors characteristic of hazardous materials.
- Note the wind direction if a hazardous material has been spilled or released.
- Note the terrain.

Positioning the Ambulance

A danger zone should be established around every motor vehicle collision site. When there are no apparent hazards, the danger zone should extend for 50 feet in all directions from the wreckage. When fuel has been spilled, the minimum danger zone should extend for 100 feet in all directions. When a collision vehicle is on fire, the minimum danger zone should extend for 100 feet in all directions. When wires are down, the danger zone should include the area in which persons or vehicles might be contacted by broken wires if they rotate around their point of attachment. When a dangerous commodity has been spilled or released, the danger zone should be established on the basis of advice from the DOT *Emergency Response Guide* or other competent authority.

Most ambulance officials favor parking an ambulance at the edge of the danger zone between the wreckage and approaching traffic. Thus the unit's flashing and revolving lights will warn oncoming motorists and its side beacons will illuminate the collision scene.

25

On the Scene

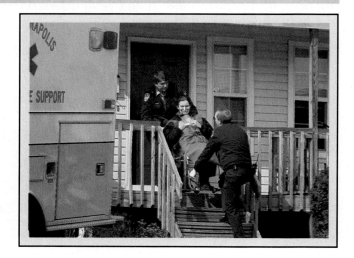

You have been dispatched to the second floor apartment of a 50-year-old woman. Mrs. Nagle has a history of cardiac problems. She tells you that she has had to sleep on an increasing number of pillows over the past month. "Last night the fluid in my lungs was so bad, I tried to sleep in this recliner." She awoke short of breath—the reason for her call for help.

Mrs. Nagle has been transported to the hospital many times in the past, and she begins to worry about having to lie down on a stretcher again. The anxiety seems to worsen her already labored breathing.

You: Mrs. Nagle, I realize it would be difficult for you to breathe if you lie down, so we have a special chair we can use to bring you down the steps.

Mrs. Nagle (with labored breathing): I could just walk down. I can't lie down, I just can't.

You: I can see how scared you are. Not being able to breathe is very scary. But you can sit up in this chair I told you about to move down the steps. And we can sit you straight up in the ambulance, too. I promise.

The choice of transportation devices is an important part of patient care. You have realized that transporting Mrs. Nagle in a reclining position would not only create additional anxiety but could worsen her condition. But what would you have done if Mrs. Nagle had fallen and required spinal immobilization? What if you had found her lying in bed or on the floor? What if she lived in a mobile home and had to be moved through a narrow corridor? Each patient situation requires a decision on methods of transfer to the ambulance.

Transferring the Patient to the Ambulance

Transferring a patient from the emergency scene to the ambulance may seem easy: Just put the patient on a stretcher and move him. But transfer is not so simple. The patient may be found in an awkward position. Dangerous circumstances or life-threatening conditions may necessitate moving an injured person before you can immobilize the spine, treat wounds or fractures, maybe even before you can assess his condition. The patient may have to be transferred from a confined space, through a narrow corridor, down a winding stairway, or lowered from a height.

In this chapter you will learn about moving and transferring a patient at the emergency scene.

Expected Outcome, Chapter 25: *You will be able to move a patient at the scene in both emergency and non-emergency situations and transfer the patient to an ambulance using a variety of carrying devices.*

WARNING: Protect yourself from infectious diseases by using appropriate barrier devices such as a pocket face mask with one-way valve, face shield, or bag-valve mask; goggles or eye shield; and disposable gloves. Always conform to your local EMS system's infection exposure control plan.

EVACUATING THE PATIENT
  Emergency and Non-Emergency Moves

TRANSFERRING THE PATIENT
  Conventional Patient-Carrying Devices
  Selecting the Proper Patient-Carrying Device
    —No Spinal Injury
  Selecting the Proper Patient-Carrying Device
    Possible Spinal Injury
  Packaging the Patient
  The Wheeled Ambulance Stretcher
  Folding Stair Chairs
  Scoop-Style (Orthopedic) Stretchers
  Basket-Style (Stokes) Stretchers
  Special Transfer Devices
  Moving the Patient Over Rough Terrain

Objectives

Knowledge *After reading this chapter, you should be able to*

1. Define *emergency move, non-emergency move,* and *transfer.* (pp. 644-645)

2. List TWO emergency and FOUR non-emergency situations that may necessitate evacuation of a sick or injured person before emergency care can be completed. (pp. 645-646)

3. List SIX rules for non-emergency moves. (p. 646)

4. List EIGHT steps for a correct lifting technique. (p. 646)

5. Describe FIVE one-rescuer moves, SIX one-rescuer drags, and THREE two-rescuer moves that can be used to evacuate persons. (pp. 646, 650; Scans 25-1 through 25-3)

6. List SIX steps for a three-rescuer move. (p. 650)

7. List the FOUR steps for transfer to the ambulance, regardless of the complexity of the transfer. (p. 650)

8. Describe these patient-carrying devices.
   - Wheeled ambulance stretcher (pp. 650-651)
   - Portable ambulance stretcher (p. 651)
   - Stair chair (p. 651)
   - Scoop (orthopedic) stretcher (p. 651)
   - Long spine board (pp. 651-652)
   - Basket (Stokes) stretcher (p. 652)

9. State what patient-carrying device or devices should be used in each of the following situations, assuming that the person does not have a possible spinal injury.
   - When movement to the ambulance is unrestricted (p. 652)
   - When the patient must be removed from a confined space or through a narrow opening or hallway (p. 652)
   - When the person must be carried down stairs (p. 652)
   - When the person must be moved from one level to another with a rope or ladder, or must be carried over debris or rough terrain, or moved uphill (p. 652)

10. State what patient-carrying device (or devices) should be used in each of the following situations, assuming that the person has a possible spinal injury.
    - When the person is on the ground or the floor of a structure (p. 652)
    - When the person has already been immobilized on a short spine board or in a vest (p. 652)
    - When the person must be moved from one level to another (p. 652)

On most ambulance runs you will be able to reach a sick or injured person without difficulty, assess his condition, carry out emergency care procedures where he lies, and then transfer him to the ambulance.

You will not always work under the best of conditions. At times you will have to work in darkness, in the rain, when it is cold, and in the presence of severe hazards, but you will be expected to care for and transfer the patient nonetheless.

EVACUATING THE PATIENT

There are three kinds of moves at an emergency scene. If a danger at the scene, such as fire, requires that you *evacuate* the patient, or move him quickly away from the place where you found him, this is known as an *emergency move.* Sometimes there are less urgent, but still valid, reasons to move the patient from where you found him, for example a patient with heat cramps who needs to be moved to a cooler envi-

11. Describe the procedures for packaging a patient. (pp. 652-653)

12. Describe the drawsheet method and the direct carry method for transferring a bed-level or ground-level patient to a wheeled ambulance stretcher. (p. 654; Scan 25-4)

13. Describe the end carry and the side carry methods of loading the patient into the ambulance. (p. 654; Scan 25-5)

14. Describe TWO methods of moving a patient into a stair chair. (pp. 654, 657)

15. Describe safe methods of moving a stair chair over level ground and down stairs. (pp. 657-658)

16. State the rules and procedure for use of a scoop-style (orthopedic) stretcher. (p. 658)

17. Describe THREE methods of transferring a patient with no possible spinal injury to a basket (Stokes) stretcher. (p. 659)

Skills *As an EMT you should be able to*

1. Perform the following:
   - One-rescuer assist
   - Piggyback carry
   - Cradle carry
   - Pack-strap carry
   - "Fireman's carry"
   - Shoulder drag
   - Foot drag
   - "Fireman's drag"
   - Incline drag
   - Blanket drag
   - Clothes drag

2. As an EMT working with a partner, you should be able to evacuate sick or injured persons from dangerous environments by means of the following:
   - Two-rescuer assist
   - Two-rescuer extremity carry
   - Two-rescuer chair carry

3. As an EMT working with a partner, you should be able to prepare each of the following patient-carrying devices for use, transfer a patient to the device, properly position the patient on the device, cover the patient, secure the patient, safely move the patient to the ambulance on or in the device, and load the patient into the ambulance.
   - Wheeled ambulance stretcher
   - Portable ambulance stretcher
   - Stair chair
   - Scoop (orthopedic) stretcher
   - Basket (Stokes) stretcher

ronment. This is known as a *non-emergency move*. The third kind of move at an emergency scene is taking the patient from the scene to the ambulance. This kind of move is called a *transfer* and is discussed later in this chapter.

Emergency and Non-Emergency Moves

There are times when you must move a patient quickly, using an emergency move. This type of move may have to take place before assessment can begin or be completed. You may not have had time to immobilize the spine or initiate basic life support, wound care, or splinting of fracture. Nevertheless, the move must be made without delay. An emergency move should be used when

- *The scene is hazardous.* Hazards may make it necessary to move a patient quickly in order to protect you and the patient. This may occur when there is uncontrolled traffic, fire or threat of fire, possible explosions, electrical hazards, toxic gases, or radiation.
- *Care of life-threatening conditions requires*

repositioning. You may have to move a patient to a hard, flat surface to provide CPR, or you may have to move a patient to reach life-threatening bleeding.

It may become necessary to perform a non-emergency move of a patient from where he was found before emergency care is completed or before you are ready to transfer him to the ambulance. Such a move may be called for when

- *Factors at the scene cause patient decline.* If a patient is RAPIDLY declining because of heat or cold, he may have to be moved. Should the patient appear to be allergic to something at the scene, he may have to be moved to reduce the chances of developing anaphylactic shock.
- *You must reach other patients.* When there are other assessed patients at the scene requiring care for life-threatening problems, you may have to move another patient to have the space needed to provide care. The patient being moved may need certain care procedures to avoid additional pain and injury before being moved.
- *Care of non-life-threatening conditions requires moving the patient.* This may happen when there are no injuries or severe medical problems, but the patient has a problem that can be relieved by moving him. Problems due to extreme heat or cold, such as heat exhaustion or hypothermia, are good examples.
- *The patient insists on being moved.* You are not allowed to restrain a patient. Explain to the patient why he should not move or be moved. If he tries to move himself, you may have to assist him. A patient may become so insistent that stress worsens his condition. If this type of patient can be moved, and the move is a short one, you may have to move him in order to reduce the stress and provide care.

Non-emergency moves should be carried out in such a way as to prevent additional injury to the patient and to avoid discomfort and pain. The following rules should be followed for a non-emergency move.

- The patient should be conscious.
- Patient assessment should be completed.
- All vital signs should be within normal range and stable.
- There should be no serious bleeding or wounds.

- There must be ABSOLUTELY no signs of spinal injury, no injuries associated with spinal injury, and the mechanism of injury should not indicate any chances of such an injury.
- All fractures must be immobilized or splinted.

Lifting Techniques Back injuries are the most common reason for permanent disabilities among EMTs. When moving patients, you must use correct lifting techniques in order to avoid lower back and knee injuries. Following the rules of correct lifting also will help you maintain your balance and prevent a fall that could injure you and your patient. When you must lift a patient, you should

1. Think through the move before attempting it. Know what you are going to do and how to prevent possible difficulties.
2. *Do not* attempt to lift or lower someone if you cannot handle and control the weight.
3. Start from a balanced position and stay aware of your balance. Hold heavy objects close to your body, not with arms extended, which will throw you off balance.
4. Start with firm footing and maintain this throughout the lift.
5. LIFT WITH YOUR LEGS, NOT YOUR BACK. Bend your knees, keeping one foot slightly in front of the other. Keep your back straight as you lift with your legs. You may want to consider using a lumbar support belt for lifting.
6. When possible, keep your back straight when carrying a patient.
7. Tighten your buttocks and move your pelvis forward to help you avoid using your back muscles.
8. Stay aware of your breathing. Do not hold your breath while lifting and carrying a patient.

Types of Moves In an emergency move, you will have to use the most efficient method for the amount of time you have to move the patient. The most commonly used moves, illustrated in Scans 25-1, 25-2, and 25-3, include

- **One-Rescuer Moves**
  One-Rescuer Assist—Patient is conscious and can walk with assistance.
  Piggyback Carry—Patient is conscious, can stand, and has no extremity fractures.
  Cradle Carry—Patient may be conscious or unconscious.

Emergency Moves—One Rescuer

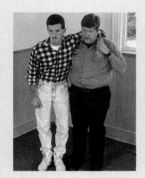

THE ONE RESCUER ASSIST

Place patient's arm around your neck, grasping his hand in yours. Place your other arm around patient's waist. Help patient walk to safety. Be prepared to change movement technique if level of danger increases. Be sure to communicate with patient about obstacles, uneven terrain, and so on.

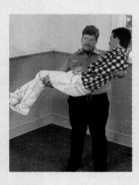

THE CRADLE CARRY

Place one arm across patient's back with your hand under his far arm. Place your other arm under his knees and lift. If patient is conscious, have him place his near arm over your shoulder. **Note:** This carry places a lot of weight on the carrier's back. It is usually appropriate only for very light patients.

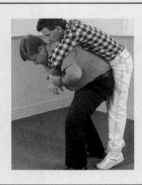

THE PACK STRAP CARRY

Have patient stand. Turn your back to him, bringing his arms over your shoulders to cross your chest. Keep his arms as straight as possible, his armpits over your shoulders. Hold patient's wrists, bend, and pull him onto your back.

THE PIGGY BACK CARRY

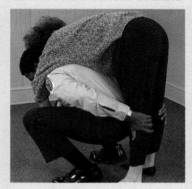

Assist the patient to stand. Place her arms over your shoulder so they cross your chest. Bend over and lift patient. While she holds on with her arms, crouch and grasp each thigh. Use a lifting motion to move her onto your back. Pass your forearms under her knees and grasp her wrists.

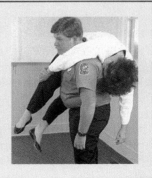

THE "FIREMAN'S CARRY"

Place your feet against her feet and pull patient toward you. Bend at waist and flex knees. Duck and pull her across your shoulder, keeping hold of one of her wrists. Use your free arm to reach between her legs and grasp her thigh. Weight of patient falls onto your shoulders. Stand up. Transfer your grip on thigh to patient's wrist.

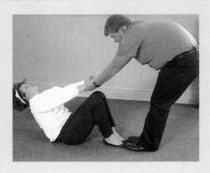

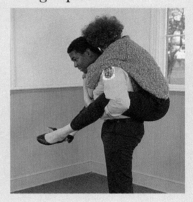

Emergency Moves—One-Rescuer Drags

Caution: Always pull in direction of long axis of patient's body. Do not pull patient sideways. Avoid bending or twisting the trunk if at all possible.

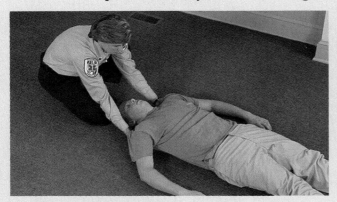

THE SHOULDER DRAG Be careful not to bump patient's head.

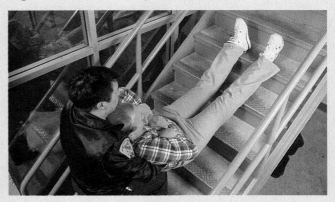

THE INCLINE DRAG Always head first

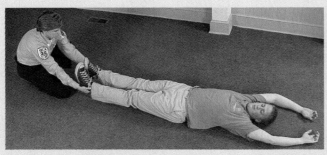

THE FOOT DRAG Be careful not to bump patient's head.

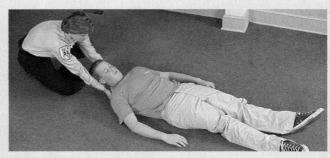

THE CLOTHES DRAG

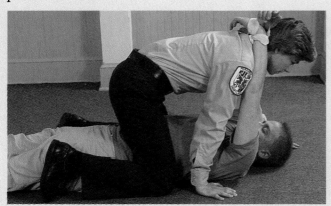

THE "FIREMAN'S DRAG" Place patient on his back and tie hands together with something that will not cut into his skin. Straddle the patient, facing his head; crouch and pass your head through his trussed arms and raise your body. This will in turn raise patient's head, neck, and upper trunk. Crawl on your hands and knees, dragging the person. During the drag, keep the patient's head as low as possible.

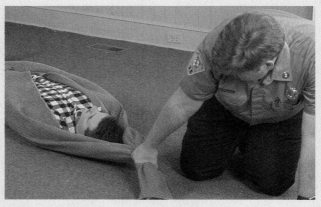

THE BLANKET DRAG Gather half of the blanket material up against the patient's side. Roll the patient toward your knees so that you can place the blanket under him. Gently roll the patient back onto the blanket. During the drag, keep the patient's head as low as possible.

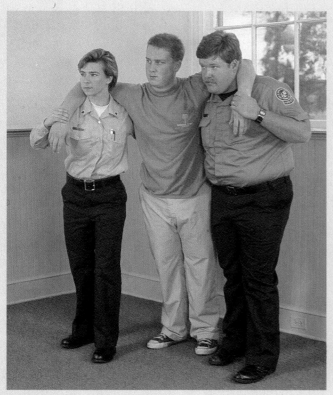

TWO-RESCUER ASSIST Patient's arms are placed around shoulders of both rescuers. They each grip a hand, place their free arms around patient's waist, then help him walk to safety.

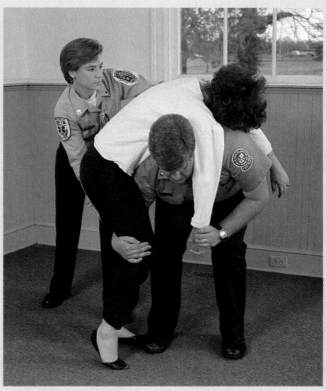

"FIREMAN'S CARRY" WITH ASSIST Have someone help lift patient. The second rescuer helps to position the patient.

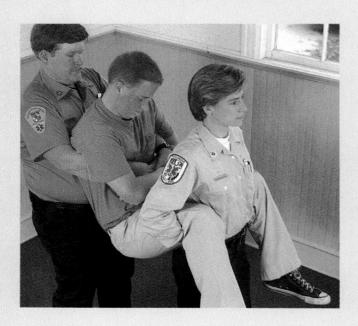

TWO-RESCUER EXTREMITY CARRY Place patient on back with knees flexed. Kneel at patient's head. Place your hands under his shoulders. Helper stands at patient's feet and grasps his wrists. Helper lifts patient forward while you slip your arms under patient's armpits and grasp his wrists. Helper can turn, crouch, and grasp patient's knees. Direct helper so you both stand at the same time and move as a unit when carrying patient.

649

"Fireman's Carry"—Patient is either conscious or unconscious with no fractures of the extremities.

Pack Strap Carry—Patient is conscious with no fractures of the extremities. This carry does not require any equipment.

One-Rescuer Drags—Patient is either conscious or unconscious with no fractures of the body part being held during the drag. There are six drags: the shoulder drag, the incline drag, the foot drag, the clothes drag, the "fireman's drag", and the blanket drag.

- **Two-Rescuer Moves**

  Two-Rescuer Assist—Patient is conscious and can walk with assistance.

  Extremity Carry—Patient is either conscious or unconscious with no fractures of the extremities.

  "Fireman's Carry" With Assist—Patient is either conscious or unconscious with no fractures of the extremities.

- **Three-Rescuer Moves**

  Three-Rescuer Carry—Patient is either conscious or unconscious, free of fractures of the extremities. If it is necessary to use a three-rescuer carry, use the following steps.

  1. Prior to movement, cross the patient's arms onto his chest and tie at the wrists using a soft bandage.
  2. Each EMT kneels on the knee toward the patient's feet. The EMT at the head of the patient slides one arm under the patient's head and shoulders, supporting the head. The other arm is under the patient's upper back. The middle EMT slides one arm under the patient's waist and his other arm under the patient's hips. The EMT at the patient's legs places one arm under the patient's knees and one arm under the patient's ankles.
  3. The head-end EMT directs all EMTs to lift the patient to their knees.
  4. The head-end EMT directs all EMTs to move to a standing position.
  5. On another signal, all EMTs roll the patient to their chests.
  6. Movement of the patient can take place by the rescuers either walking forward or sidestepping.

All of the above emergency move techniques can also be used for non-emergency moves, depending on the situation. If the rules for a non-emergency move are met, the one- or two-rescuer assist should be practical to use. A cradle carry or two-rescuer extremity carry may be useful in some cases.

Note: None of these moves provides adequate protection for the spine or an unsplinted fracture. However, of all these moves, drags that keep the patient flat and pull in the direction of the long axis of his body may do the least damage to the spine. The blanket drag provides some protection for the spine and the extremities.

TRANSFERRING THE PATIENT

Usually the transfer of a sick or injured patient involves little more than placing the patient on the wheeled ambulance stretcher and moving it a short distance to the ambulance. The process becomes more complicated when you believe the patient may have spinal injuries. For such cases, extrication collars and spine boards must be applied before the patient is placed on the stretcher (see Chapter 12). If a traction splint has been applied to a patient, special care must be taken to ensure that the splint will continue to immobilize the extremity and no additional injury occurs to the patient. When placing a patient with a traction splint into the ambulance, place him feet first to avoid having the traction splint hit the rear door. If he also needs oxygen or suction, which are likely to be on the front wall of the compartment and not extendible to the rear, use the portable oxygen and suction units.

Transfer to the ambulance is accomplished in four steps, regardless of the complexity of the operation.

1. Selecting the proper patient-carrying device.
2. Packaging the patient for transfer.
3. Moving the patient to the ambulance.
4. Loading the patient onto the ambulance.

Conventional Patient-Carrying Devices

Ambulances generally are provided with a number of different patient-carrying devices (Figure 25-1).

- *The wheeled ambulance stretcher* (gurney) may be a one-, two-, or multi-level device. Most can be adjusted so that a patient can be transported supine or in a Fowlers or semi-Fowlers position (seated or in a 45-

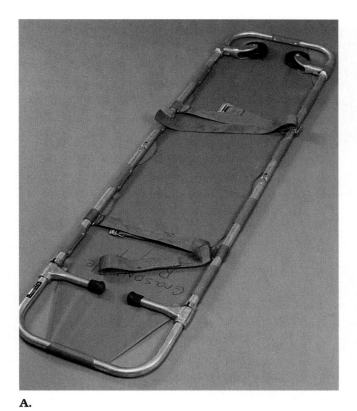

A.

B.

C.

Figure 25-1 Conventional patient carrying devices, all with straps for securing patient to the device: (A) a portable ambulance stretcher; (B) a stair chair; (C) a scoop stretcher or orthopedic stretcher.

degree-angle position) with or without the knees flexed, or in the Trendelenburg position (the foot end of the stretcher tilted up).

- A *portable ambulance stretcher* is usually carried so that a second nonambulatory patient can be carried in an ambulance. It becomes a necessity when space limitations or other factors prevent the transfer of a sick or injured person on the wheeled stretcher. Some portable stretchers are simply tubular metal frames with canvas or coated fabric bottoms and foldaway wheels and legs. Some models fold into easily stored units, and some have adjustable back rests.
- A *stair chair* is useful when a person must be carried down stairs or through hallways too narrow for conventional stretchers. This device is not recommended for use with unconscious or disoriented patients. Some stair chairs can be converted into full-length portable stretchers.
- A *scoop stretcher* (orthopedic stretcher) can be used to pick up a seriously injured person with a minimum of body movement. To use this type of stretcher effectively, you must have access to the patient from all sides. The scoop stretcher is *not* designed to be used as a primary spine immobilization device for suspected spinal injuries.
- A *long spine board* allows for the safe movement of a person with a suspected spinal injury. Some models are used with standard

9-foot straps; others have pins and speed clips which can be quickly connected. A number of head-restraint devices can be used with conventional wood spine boards.

- *A basket (Stokes) stretcher* is usually the device of choice when a sick or injured person must be moved from one level to another by ladder or rope. Newer-model wire or plastic basket stretchers are usually provided with four-point bridles, security straps, and adjustable foot rests. A tapered spine board should be used in conjunction with a Stokes stretcher. A Stokes is used for high-angle rescues. EMTs should *never* attempt high-angle rescues without the proper training.

Selecting the Proper Patient-Carrying Device—No Spinal Injury

Almost any of the conventional patient-carrying devices can be used to transfer a patient who has no spinal injury. Selection of the device is usually influenced by the condition of the pathway from the patient's location to the ambulance. As you approach the patient, evaluate your options and means of egress. Certain features, such as a narrow or winding staircase or a small elevator, will decrease your transport equipment options.

- Use the wheeled ambulance stretcher when there is an unrestricted pathway to the ambulance.
- Use the portable ambulance stretcher, stair chair, scoop stretcher, or long spine board when a person must be removed from a confined space, moved through a narrow opening, or carried through a narrow hallway.
- Use a stair chair when it is impossible to carry a person down stairs on a stretcher and when an elevator is too small for a stretcher.
- Use a basket (Stokes) stretcher to move a person from one level to another by rope or ladder.
- Use a basket (Stokes) stretcher when a person must be carried over debris, rough terrain, or uphill. Some Stokes stretchers can be fitted with a detachable wheel to facilitate movement over rough terrain.

Selecting the Proper Patient-Carrying Device—Possible Spinal Injury

When a person has a possible spinal injury, the patient-carrying device must provide straight-line neck and back immobilization. Selection of the device will be influenced by the location of the person and how the person must be moved.

- Use a long spine board when a spine-injured person is on the ground or the floor of a structure. In certain circumstances, it may be necessary to use a scoop stretcher for the initial short distance transfer of the patient to a long spine board. Once immobilized on the board, the patient can be carried directly to the ambulance or secured to the cot and wheeled there.
- Use a long spine board to immobilize a person who has already been immobilized with a short spine board or flexible, vest-type extrication device. Once a seated person has been immobilized on a short spine board or vest, he can be pivoted onto a long spine board.
- Use a long spine board to immobilize the person and then secure the board and patient in a basket (Stokes) stretcher when a spine-injured person must be moved from one level to another and movement cannot be made over stairs or by elevator. Then use a rope to lower the stretcher or to slide it down the beams of a ladder.

See Chapter 12 for more information on moving patients with possible spinal injuries.

Packaging the Patient

Packaging refers to the sequence of operations required to ready the patient to be moved and to combine the patient and the patient-carrying device into a unit ready for transfer. A sick or injured patient must be packaged so that his condition is not aggravated. Necessary care for wounds and fractures should be completed, impaled objects must be stabilized, and all dressings and splints must be checked before the patient is placed on the patient-carrying device. The properly packaged patient is covered and secured to the patient-carrying device.

Warning: Do not waste time packaging a badly traumatized patient. When a patient is categorized critical or unstable during the primary survey, transport quickly. A neatly packaged corpse has not received optimal care.

Covering the Patient Covering a patient helps to maintain body temperature, prevents exposure to the elements, and helps assure privacy. A single blanket or perhaps just a sheet may be all that is required in warm weather. A sheet and blankets should be used in cold weather. When practical, cuff the blankets under the patient's chin, with the top sheet outside. Do not leave sheets and blankets hanging loose. Tuck them under the mattress at the foot and sides of the stretcher. In wet weather, a plastic cover should be placed over the blankets during transfer. This can be removed once in the ambulance to prevent the patient from overheating.

If a scoop-style stretcher is used, you will have to fold a blanket once or twice lengthwise and carefully tuck the blanket under the patient. Cover the patient as best you can, place the patient and scoop-style stretcher on a wheeled ambulance stretcher, and then apply full covering. The same directions apply when using the long spine board. Do not move a patient with a possible spinal injury in order to tuck in a blanket.

When a basket (Stokes) stretcher is used, line the basket with a blanket prior to positioning the patient. If this is not done, cover the patient as you would in the case of the scoop-style stretcher.

Before seating a patient in the stair chair, place a sheet or blanket on the chair. This will facilitate transferring a nonambulatory patient later. Once seated on the chair, the patient should be covered. Have the patient sitting upright with his hands folded over his lap and his legs together. Drape a sheet and then a blanket over the patient's body and shoulders. Carefully tuck in the sheet and blanket all around.

In cold or wet weather cover the patient's head, leaving the face exposed. If the nature of the patient's injuries allows you to do so

1. Place a towel flat under the patient's head.
2. Pull the outermost edge of the towel up and over the patient's head so that it covers the forehead, but not the eyes.
3. Draw the corners of the towel diagonally to the patient's chest, allowing the towel to drape each side of the patient's head (Figure 25-2).
4. Always place an insulating blanket *under* the patient to prevent loss of body heat through conduction to the ground or a metal stretcher, such as a scoop.

Securing the Patient Many of today's devices used for the transfer and transport of patients should have a minimum of three straps holding the patient securely to the device. The

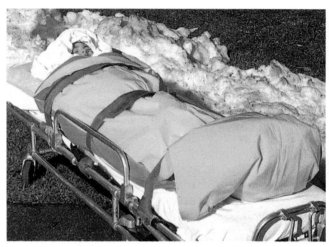

Figure 25-2 Covering the patient during normal, wet or cold weather conditions.

first strap should be at the chest level, the second at the hip or waist level, and the third on the lower extremities. Sometimes there is a fourth strap used if two are crossed at the chest.

All patients, including those receiving CPR, must be secured to the patient-carrying device before you attempt to transfer them to the ambulance.

If your patient is not on a carrying device such as a spine board but is just on the ambulance stretcher, some states, as a matter of policy, require shoulder harnesses that secure the patient to the stretcher to prevent him from sliding forward in case of a short stop.

The Wheeled Ambulance Stretcher

This is the most commonly used patient-carrying device. The principles of transfer that apply to this device also apply in general to all others.

Preparing the Stretcher Elevate the stretcher to bed-level if it is a two-level or multi-level device. Unfasten the safety straps; tuck them out of the way to make sure they do not become tripping hazards. Lower the rail on the loading side of the stretcher. Remove the blankets and the top sheet; place them on a clean surface nearby. Place the pillow in the appropriate position.

Transferring the Patient In some cases, a patient may stand and help place himself on the stretcher. When the patient with no spinal injury is in a vehicle, wreckage, or debris, you may have to adapt a standard patient moving technique to transfer him to the stretcher. An example would be to modify the cradle carry for someone seated and turned sideways in the front of an automobile. The patient *with* spinal injury should be secured to a long spine board before being transferred to the stretcher. The long board and the secured patient are lifted as a unit and secured to the wheeled ambulance stretcher.

The transfer of a bed-level or ground-level patient may require you to use special lifting techniques, the *drawsheet method* and the *direct carry method* shown in Scan 25-4. Regardless of the method used, protect yourself. Do not position yourself too far from the patient and do not strain to lift the patient. You must protect yourself from lower back strain and hernia. Also, you must be certain not to lose your balance and possibly injure yourself, your partner, or the patient. (Review the lifting techniques discussed earlier in this chapter.)

Covering and Securing the Patient The patient should be covered by a top sheet and blankets, as required by weather. The side rails should be locked in the up position and the body straps fastened.

Moving and Loading the Patient Whenever you move a conscious patient, explain what you are doing and what obstacles your are maneuvering around. This will help to comfort the patient, since most people find being moved an uncomfortable loss of control and independence.

Regardless of the method used to move a patient, you and your partner should walk naturally at a smooth, fairly slow pace. Use two hands on the bed of the stretcher, rather than just pulling on the handles, to roll and maneuver the stretcher at a safe, constant speed. Turn corners slowly and squarely to keep the stretcher level and minimize discomfort to the patient. Lift the stretcher over thresholds and rugs. Use caution when maneuvering the stretcher; bumps from a wheeled stretcher can cause unsightly and costly damage to walls and furniture.

The wheeled stretcher can be carried by the *end carry* method or the *side carry* method. The end carry is most widely used, with the side carry used to load the patient into the ambulance, as shown in Scan 25-5.

Often a stretcher is wheeled in the raised position by two EMTs, one at the head end and one at the foot. Be very careful *never* to leave a patient unattended on a wheeled stretcher in the raised position for even a few seconds, since the patient may shift position and the stretcher can easily be toppled over.

Folding Stair Chairs

These devices are useful in narrow corridors and doorways, small elevators, and stairways. *It is preferable not to use a stair chair for a patient who is unconscious or disoriented. A stair chair should not be used when a patient has a possible spinal injury or fractures of the lower extremities.* When a folding stair chair is not available, a strongly constructed desk chair may be used to move the patient. Do not use a patient's wheelchair when carrying the patient as it may break in your hands.

Preparing a Stair Chair The chair is unfolded and secured in the open position by positive locking devices (not on all chairs). The safety straps are unfastened and positioned so that they do not become tripping hazards.

Transferring the Patient The *direct carry method* (Scan 25-4) can be modified when a bed-level or ground-level patient must be moved into a stair chair. The first part of the technique is the same as for transfer of a patient to a wheeled stretcher. However, the foot-end EMT slides his arm under the patient's thighs rather than under the midcalf. This maneuver allows the lower part of the patient's legs to drop down into a sitting position as he is eased into the chair.

The *extremity transfer* (Figure 25-3) can be used to move a patient from the floor or ground to a stair chair or to any other patient-carrying device. This method is not to be used, however, when the patient has a spinal injury or extremity fractures. The procedure is as follows:

1. One EMT assumes a head-end position, while the other EMT takes the foot-end position.
2. The EMTs assist the patient to a sitting position.
3. The head-end EMT reaches under the patient's armpits and grasps the patient's wrists, holding the arms to the patient's chest.
4. The foot-end EMT flexes the patient's knees and slides his hands into position under the knees.
5. Simultaneously, on the command of the head-end EMT, both EMTs move to a standing position, lifting the patient.
6. They carry the patient to the chair and lower him onto it.

Scan 25-4
Wheeled Ambulance Stretcher—Transferring the Patient

Bed-Level Patient: Drawsheet Method

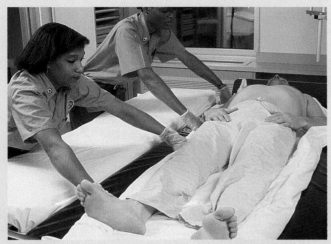

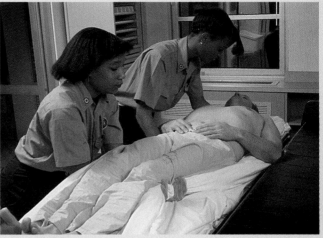

1. Bottom sheet of bed is rolled from both sides toward patient. The stretcher, rails lowered, is placed parallel to bed, touching side of bed. EMTs use their feet to lock the stretcher against the bed.

2. EMTs pull on drawsheet to move patient to side of bed. They each use one hand to support patient while they reach under him to grasp drawsheet. EMTs simultaneously draw patient onto stretcher.

Ground-Level Patient: Direct Carry Method

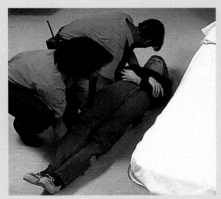

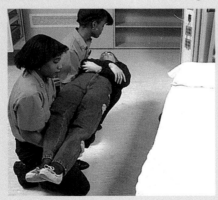

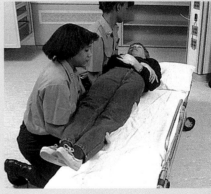

1. Stretcher is set in its lowest position and placed on opposite side of patient. EMTs drop to one knee, facing patient. The head-end EMT cradles patient's head and neck by sliding one arm under patient's neck to grasp shoulder, the other arm under the small of the patient's back. The foot-end EMT slides one arm under the patient's thighs and moves her arm from under patient's knees to a position under mid-calf area.

2. EMTs lift patient to their knees.

3. They stand and carry patient to stretcher, drop to one knee, and roll forward to place patient onto mattress.

Wheeled Ambulance Stretcher—Moving and Loading the Patient

Loading the Ambulance

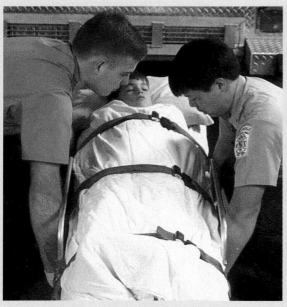

1. Clear interior of ambulance and lift rear step, if necessary. Move stretcher as close to ambulance as possible. Make sure stretcher is locked in its lowest level before lifting. EMTs position themselves on opposite sides of stretcher, bend at the knees, and grasp lower bar of stretcher frame.

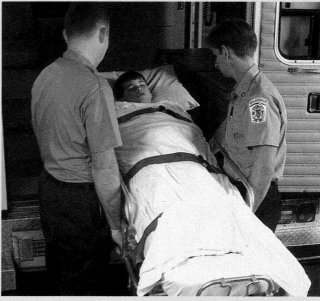

2. Both EMTs come to a full standing position with their backs straight. Oblique stepping movements are used to move stretcher onto ambulance.

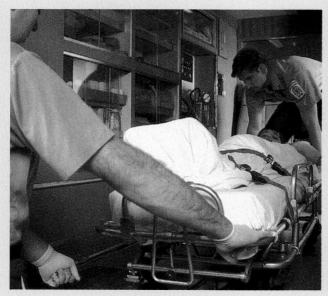

3. Stretcher is moved into securing device.

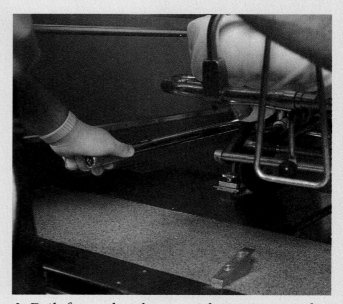

4. Both forward and rear catches are engaged to hold stretcher.

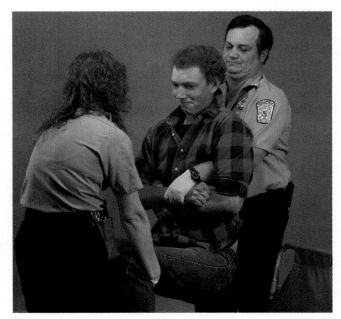

A. The EMTs assist the patient to a sitting position. On the signal from the head-end EMT, both lift the patient.

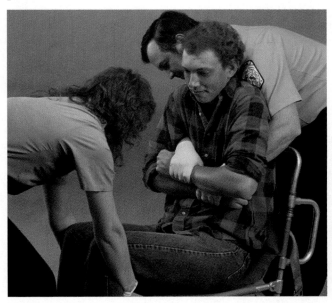

B. The EMTs lower the patient into the chair. Then the patient is secured and ready for transfer.

Figure 25-3 Extremity transfer to a stair chair.

7. The patient is draped with a sheet and a blanket is placed over his body and shoulders.
8. The patient is secured to the chair with three straps. One is fastened around the chest and the back of the chair. A second strap is placed across the thighs and around the seat of the chair. The third is fastened around the patient's legs and the lower portion of the chair.

Moving a Stair Chair A loaded stair chair is fairly easy to carry and maneuver, especially if the chair is on wheels. As with the ambulance stretcher, stair chairs should be rolled whenever possible; this reduces the risk of back strain for the EMTs and injury to the patient. However, the following procedure is suggested when a stair chair must be carried over level ground.

When the chair and patient are to be moved, one EMT must be behind the chair to tilt the chair back. Always warn the patient that you are going to tilt the chair. Tilt it carefully if the chair has wheels. The other EMT should stand at the patient's feet, with his back to the patient. As the chair is tilted back, he should crouch and grasp the chair by its legs. The two EMTs should lift the chair simultaneously and carry the patient to the wheeled stretcher. Be sure the patient's feet are on the bar, not below it, so you don't set it on his feet when you rest it on the ground. The patient should be transferred to the wheeled stretcher as soon as possible and before he is loaded onto the ambulance.

If the patient and chair must be carried down stairs, the foot-end EMT should face the patient while carrying the chair. A third person should support the foot-end EMT while the chair is being moved down the steps. If the chair has wheels, they should not be allowed to touch the steps (Figure 25-4). When you are carrying a

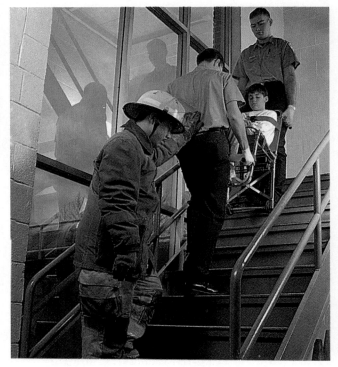

Figure 25-4 Moving a stair chair down steps.

patient down the stairs and feel you are going to fall, if you are at the head end sit down; if you are at the foot end lean into the stairs to save the fall from injuring anyone.

Scoop-Style (Orthopedic) Stretchers

The scoop-style stretcher can be used to lift and carry most patients; however, *in cases of possible spinal injury,* it should be used only to transfer a patient to a long spine board. A scoop-style stretcher should not be used to transport a patient with a possible spinal injury.

Preparing the Patient with Possible Spinal Injury An extrication or rigid collar should be secured to the patient as soon as possible. Someone should continue to support the head after the collar is applied and throughout the stretcher application procedure. The patient should be placed in a supine position, as anatomically straight as possible. His arms should be secured in place, with a cravat bandage applied to hold the wrists together (Figure 25-5).

Preparing the Stretcher ALWAYS adjust the length of the stretcher to fit the height of the patient. Separate the stretcher halves and place one half on each side of the patient. If the stretcher is the folding type, make sure the pins are properly set.

Applying the Stretcher Slide the stretcher halves under the patient one at a time. This may be difficult since the stretcher may snag on clothing, grass, or debris. If necessary, roll the patient as a unit to either side to allow for proper positioning of the parts. Mate the latch parts and make certain that the stretcher halves are securely locked together. Latching should be done from head to feet. Be careful not to pinch the patient when latching the two halves together—a common and uncomfortable mistake! Adjust the head support.

Covering and Securing the Patient The patient is covered with a blanket folded to size. A rolled blanket or a commercial head restraint is placed on each side of the patient's head and the head is secured to the stretcher by a cravat. Then the stretcher straps are fastened across the chest, hips, and legs.

The Velcro at the head end of folding scoop-style stretchers may not remain secure. To guard against this, tape the patient's head or tie securely with a cravat.

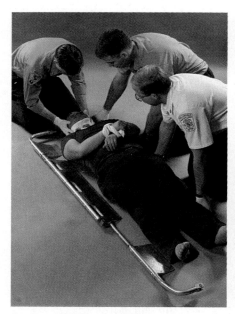 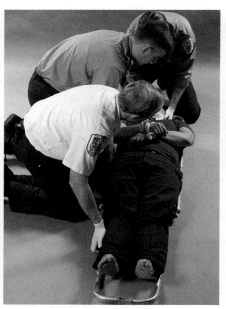 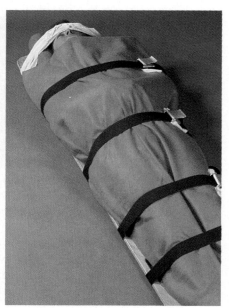

A. One EMT carefully supports the patient's head while half of the stretcher is positioned.

B. The stretcher halves are securely locked together and the head support is properly positioned.

C. A patient properly positioned, covered, and secured on a full spine board or a scoop stretcher.

Figure 25-5 Applying the scoop-style stretcher and covering and securing the patient for transport.

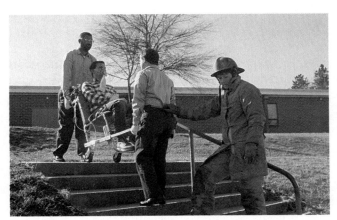

Figure 25-6 Keep the stretcher level, even when moving down steps.

Moving the Patient Lift the scoop-style stretcher by the end-carry method. The patient should be moved to a long spineboard as soon as possible. The patient and long spine board should be secured as a unit to the wheeled ambulance stretcher by using three straps. The stretcher must be kept level, even when moving down steps (Figure 25-6).

Basket-Style (Stokes) Stretchers

Warning: Do NOT attempt to move a patient in a basket (Stokes) stretcher by rope or ladder unless you have been specifically trained in the techniques used for such moves.

The basket stretcher can be used to move patients from one level to another or over rough terrain. The basket should be lined with blankets prior to positioning the patient.

Transferring the Patient to the Stretcher If the patient has no spinal injury, modifications of the direct carry and extremity transfer methods can be used by two EMTs to transfer a bed-level or ground-level patient to a basket stretcher. The drawsheet method also can be used to transfer a bed-level patient who has no spinal injury, provided the drawsheet can support the patient's weight while he is being lowered into the stretcher hammock-style.

Two additional techniques may be used to transfer a floor- or ground-level patient to a basket stretcher when he is heavy or when two EMTs cannot accomplish the transfer by themselves. Each technique requires additional personnel, however.

The three-rescuer lift is a modification of the lift that was used for the three-rescuer carry noted earlier. Prior to movement, cross the patient's arms onto his chest and tie at the wrists using a soft bandage. Each rescuer kneels on the knee toward the patient's feet. The EMT at the head of the patient slides one arm under the patient's head and shoulders, supporting the head. The other arm is under the patient's upper back. The middle EMT slides one arm under the patient's waist and his other arm under the patient's hips. The EMT at the patient's legs places one arm under the patient's knees and one arm under the patient's ankles. Once the patient is brought to knee level, he can be lowered into the basket stretcher.

The blanket lift is a procedure in which the blanket serves as the basket liner as well as the lifting mechanism. This lift can be done with four rescuers; however, it is best done with five. Four people can do the lifting, while the fifth one positions the stretcher. The following is the procedure for placing the patient on the blanket.

1. Gather half of the blanket material up against the patient's side.
2. Roll the patient toward your knees so the blanket can be placed under the patient.
3. Gently roll the patient back onto the blanket.
4. With two rescuers on each side, grasp the edge of the blanket and roll it in toward the patient.
5. Lifting by the rolled edges of the blanket, bring the patient to knee-level while the fifth rescuer positions the stretcher.

If the patient has a possible spine injury, first immobilize him on a backboard, then secure board and patient to the basket.

Special Transfer Devices

In showing the various patient transfer devices used by today's ambulance services, we would be remiss if we did not mention some of the additional stretchers used by many EMTs in the field (Figure 25-7).

- Miller board—used by many EMTs where a full spine board is needed when using a wire basket stretcher that has leg dividers. Also used in recovery from water accidents.
- Reeves stretcher—a canvas or synthetic rubberized material that has wooden slats sewn into pockets. It has six large lifting and carrying handles (three on each side),

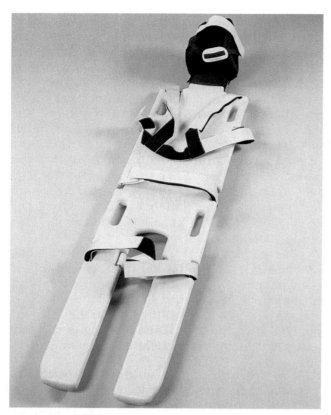

A. Miller board

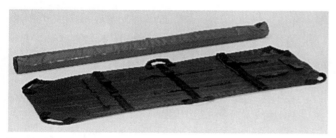

B. Reeves stretcher

Figure 25-7 Special Transfer Devices

making this a good stretcher for narrow and restricted hallways such as are found in mobile homes.

- Reeves sleeve—an envelope configuration into which a regular long spine board can be inserted. There are tabs with quick-hitch straps that encapsulate the patient, making him secure in almost any position in which you might need to carry him.
- SKED—a device that comes rolled in a package. When opened, this stretcher can be quickly assembled and used to rescue someone from a confined space, a height, or a snow or water emergency.

Moving the Patient Over Rough Terrain

At times a patient must be moved uphill or over debris or rough terrain. For example, he may have been thrown into a gully or may be lying in the debris of a building collapse. The stretcher must be kept level, even when the EMTs carrying it do not have a flat or firm footing. If the stretcher must be moved up a steep incline, a system of ropes and pulleys may be needed to assist in lifting the patient and stretcher.

The specific techniques for uphill or rough terrain moves will not be discussed here. Special training is required, and entry-level EMTs are not usually called upon to coordinate such moves.

CHAPTER REVIEW

SUMMARY

Evacuating the Patient

It will be necessary for you to quickly evacuate a sick or injured person whenever his life and yours are threatened by traffic, fire, explosion, electrical hazards, toxic gases, or radiation. At times you will have to move someone because there is no room for you to carry out life-saving patient care activities. Such moves are known as *emergency moves.*

Non-emergency moves are used in non-life-threatening situations when factors at the scene are causing patient decline, when necessary in order to reach other patients, when care requires moving the patient, or if the patient insists on being moved.

A *transfer* is taking the patient from the scene to the ambulance.

When you need to make an emergency move, do not just rush in, grab a person by the clothes or extremities, and drag him from the hostile environment. Choose an evacuation technique that will be least harmful. Also follow the rules for lifting that will protect you from back injury: Plan the move, do not attempt to lift a greater weight than you can handle, keep your balance, maintain a firm footing, lift with your legs instead of your back, keep your back straight, tighten your buttocks and move your pelvis forward, and do not hold your breath while lifting or carrying.

If the person can stand and walk, simply assist him to a safe place.

If there are no indications of extremity or spinal injury, use a piggyback carry, a cradle carry, a fireman's carry, or a pack strap carry.

One of a number of drags can be used to move a person who cannot be either assisted or carried: shoulder drag, incline drag, foot drag, clothes drag, "fireman's drag", or blanket drag.

A number of two-rescuer techniques can be used to move persons who have neither fractured extremities nor a spine injury. Assist an ambulatory person by supporting him between you and your partner, or use the extremity carry or the "fireman's carry" with assist.

A three-rescuer move can also be used. The patient's hands are tied across his chest. The three rescuers kneel, lift the patient onto their knees, rise, roll the patient to their chests, then carry the patient by either walking forward or sidestepping.

None of these moves offers adequate protection to the patient's spine or unsplinted fractures. Pulling the person in the direction of the long axis of the body may do the least damage to the spine. A blanket drag offers some support to the spine and extremities.

Transferring the Patient

Regardless of the complexity of the operation, four steps are usually followed in transferring the patient.

1. Selecting the proper patient-carrying device.
2. Packaging the patient for transfer.
3. Moving the patient to the ambulance.
4. Loading the patient onto the ambulance.

Use any of a variety of patient-carrying devices to transfer the patient to an ambulance. The devices that are usually carried on an ambulance are the wheeled ambulance stretcher, a portable ambulance stretcher, a stair chair, a scoop (orthopedic) stretcher, a long spine board, and, if space permits, a basket (Stokes) stretcher.

When your patient does not have a spinal injury, select a carrying device with regard to the pathway from the point of care to the ambulance.

- Use the wheeled stretcher when movement is unrestricted.
- Use a portable stretcher, stair chair, scoop stretcher, or long spine board when the person must be removed from a confined or through a narrow space.
- Use a stair chair to move a patient down a narrow stairway or small elevator.
- Use a basket (Stokes) stretcher when a person must be moved from one level to another by rope or ladder or over rough terrain.

When your patient has a spinal injury, select a carrying device suited to his location and situation.

- Once a seated person has been immobilized on a short spine board or vest, he can be pivoted onto a long spine board.
- When a spine-injured person must be moved from one level to another, first immobilize him on a long spine board. Secure the board in a basket stretcher, then lower the stretcher by rope or slide it down the beams of a ladder.

The patient may be transferred to a wheeled stretcher by the drawsheet method (if the patient is in bed, using the sheet under him to help move him) or by a direct carry method (when the patient is on the floor, lifting the patient to the EMTs knees, then transferring him to the stretcher). Once transferred to a carrying device, the patient must be packaged; that is, the patient must be covered and secured to the carrying device. An end carry is usually used to carry the stretcher, a side carry to load it into an ambulance.

Safe procedures must be followed for transferring a patient to and carrying a patient on a stair chair, a scoop-style (orthopedic) stretcher, or a basket-style (Stokes) stretcher. Additional carrying devices used by EMTs include the Miller board, the Reeves stretcher, the Reeves sleeve, and the SKED. Special training is required for moving patients uphill or over rough terrain.

On the Scene

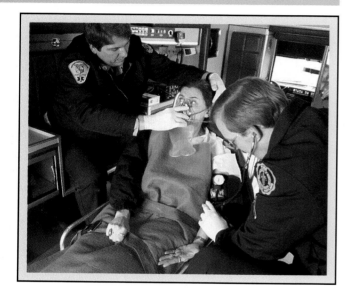

You have just transferred 50-year-old Mrs. Nagle into your ambulance. You suspected that she was in congestive heart failure, and because of this you chose to move her down the steps in the stair chair to relieve her breathing difficulty and her anxiety about lying down. You have allowed her to remain in a sitting position in the ambulance.

Often, EMTs feel that when they get the

patient into the ambulance their job is "almost over." In fact, it is less than halfway done.

You: Mrs. Nagle, how do you feel now that you are in the ambulance?

Mrs. Nagle: I'm still having trouble breathing.

You: Is it better, worse, or the same compared to when you were in your house?

Mrs. Nagle: A little better.

You: Good. I'm going to keep on giving you oxygen to help you breathe, and I'm going to take your pulse and blood pressure again, and then we'll be on our way. Is there anything else I can do to make you more comfortable?

Whenever you make any major change involving a patient, you should re-evaluate the patient. Even though Mrs. Nagle was carried to the ambulance, the movement may have been stressful. You are evaluating her condition now that she has been positioned in the ambulance, and you will continue to evaluate her frequently. You will provide care and continue to talk to her and reassure her all during the ride to the hospital.

Transporting the Patient to a Hospital

Chapter Overview

A common practice in the not-too-distant past was for ambulance attendants to load a sick or injured person into the patient compartment of an ambulance and then climb onto the front seat for the high-speed trip to a hospital. Patients, even seriously ill or injured ones, were often left to fend for themselves during transit.

In modern EMS systems, of course, this is no longer the procedure. EMTs provide continuous care en route to the hospital. The steps to follow while transporting the patient are the subject of this chapter.

Expected Outcome, Chapter 26: *You will be able to follow the correct procedures to prepare the patient for transport, care for the patient en route, communicate with the hospital emergency department while en route, and transfer the patient to the care of emergency department personnel when you arrive at the hospital.*

> **Warning:** Protect yourself from infectious diseases by using appropriate barrier devices such as a pocket face mask with one-way valve, face shield, or bag-valve mask; goggles or eye shield; and disposable gloves. Always conform to your local EMS system's infection exposure control plan.

PREPARING THE PATIENT FOR TRANSPORT

CARING FOR THE PATIENT WHILE EN ROUTE TO THE HOSPITAL

COMMUNICATIONS DURING TRANSPORT

TRANSFERRING THE PATIENT TO THE CARE OF EMERGENCY DEPARTMENT PERSONNEL

Knowledge *After reading this chapter, you should be able to*

1. List ELEVEN steps for preparing a sick or injured person for transportation to a medical facility. (pp. 664-666)

2. List TEN activities in which the attending EMT may have to engage during the transportation of a sick or injured person to a medical facility. (pp. 666-668)

3. Describe the procedure for caring for a patient who goes into cardiac arrest during transportation. (pp. 667-668)

4. List EIGHT essential elements of ambulance-hospital communication. (pp. 668-670)

5. Describe an orderly procedure for transferring a patient to the care of emergency department personnel. (pp. 670, 673; Scans 26-1 and 26-2)

Skills *As an Emt you should be able to*

1. Prepare a patient for transport in the ambulance.

2. Monitor a patient's vital signs and provide continuing care during transport.

3. Relay accurate and meaningful information by radio or cellular phone to emergency department personnel.

4. Complete an orderly patient transfer at the hospital.

Activities during transport include far more than just driving the patient to the hospital. A series of tasks must be undertaken from the time a patient is loaded into the ambulance until he is handed over to emergency department personnel.

PREPARING THE PATIENT FOR TRANSPORT

There are eleven steps that may be required to prepare a person for transport once he is in the ambulance.

Step 1: Ensure an Open Airway and Adequate Air Exchange

Make sure that a conscious patient is breathing without difficulty once you have positioned him on the stretcher. If the patient is unconscious with an airway in place, make sure he has an adequate air exchange once you have moved him into position for transport.

Step 2: Secure the Cot in Place in the Ambulance

Always ensure that the patient is safe during the trip to the hospital. Before closing the door, and certainly before signaling the ambulance operator to move, make sure that the cot is securely in place.

Patient compartments are equipped with positive locking devices that prevent the wheeled ambulance cot from moving about while the ambulance is in motion. It is unlikely, but in your haste you may engage the forward part of the cot in the hook of the fastener bar and fail to engage the rear hook completely. The fact that the cot is not secure might go undetected until the ambulance moves. An unfastened stretcher can create havoc in the patient compartment, and both you and your patient can be injured before the ambulance can be brought to a stop.

Step 3: Position and Secure the Patient

The need to move a patient from an upper floor or over rough terrain requires that he be firmly secured to a stretcher. Even an uncomplicated movement of the wheeled ambulance stretcher for a short distance may have to be accomplished with the patient in the supine position. This does not mean, however, that he must be transported to the hospital in that position. On the contrary, positioning should be dictated by the nature of his illness or injury.

- If he was not transferred to the ambulance in that position, shift an unconscious patient who has no potential spine injury, or one with an altered level of consciousness, into a position on his side that will promote maintenance of an open airway and the drainage of fluids.

- Position the security straps. Security straps applied when a patient is being prepared for transfer to the ambulance may tighten unnecessarily by the time he is loaded into the patient compartment. Adjust straps so they still hold the patient safely in place but are not so tight that they interfere with circulation or respiration or cause pain.

Step 4: Prepare for Respiratory or Cardiac Complications

It may be necessary to use a Reeves or long board to get the patient out of the house, but if the patient is suffering from respiratory distress or acute pulmonary edema, you must place him in the Fowler's (head raised) position. This will require removal from the backboard (as long as there is no spinal injury) or placing the patient on the stretcher, slipping the Reeves from under him, and then raising the head end of the stretcher.

If the patient is likely to develop cardiac arrest, position a short spine board or CPR board between him and the ambulance cot prior to starting on the trip to the hospital. Then if he does go into arrest, there will be no need to locate and position the board. Riding on a hard board may not be comfortable for a patient, but it is better that he suffer temporary discomfort than permanent injury or even death from delayed resuscitation efforts.

Step 5: Loosen Constricting Clothing

Clothing may interfere with circulation and breathing. Loosen ties and belts and open any clothing around the neck. Straighten clothing that is bunched under safety straps. Remember that clothing bunched at the crotch may be painful to the patient. Before you do anything to rearrange the clothing of a patient, however, tell him or her what you are going to do and why.

Step 6: Check Bandages

Even properly applied bandages can loosen during transfer to the ambulance, especially if there is considerable body movement. Check each bandage to see that it is secure.

Do not consider the problem of a loosened bandage lightly. Severe bleeding can resume when the pressure from a bandage is removed from a dressing, and if the wound site is covered with a sheet or blanket, bleeding may go unnoticed until the patient develops shock or is delivered to the hospital.

Step 7: Check Splints

Immobilizing devices can also loosen during transfer to the ambulance. Inspect the bandages or cravats that hold board splints in place. Test air splints with your fingertip to see that they have remained properly inflated during the transfer procedure and slightly re-inflate or deflate as necessary. Inspect traction devices to ensure that proper traction is still maintained.

Check the splinted limb for distal pulse, skin color and temperature at the fingertips or toes, capillary refilling, and neurologic activity.

Remember that the safe adjustment of splinting devices is virtually impossible when an ambulance is pitching about during the trip to a hospital, so be sure to complete this step before the ambulance moves unless immediate transport is required.

Step 8: Determine and Record Vital Signs

Once you have properly positioned the patient and adjusted straps, clothing, bandages, and splints, measure and record the patient's vital signs.

Step 9: Load a Relative or Friend Who Must Accompany the Patient

As a matter of policy, many ambulance services will not allow a relative or friend to accompany a sick or injured person to a hospital.

Consider the following guidelines if your service does not prohibit the transportation of a relative or friend with a sick or injured person: First, encourage the person to seek alternative transportation, if such is available. If there is just no other way the relative or friend can get to the hospital, allow him to ride in the passenger's seat in the operator's compartment—not in the patient's compartment where he may interfere with your activities. Make certain the person buckles his seat belt. If an uninjured child must come along, bring the family's child car seat and use it.

Step 10: Load Personal Effects

If a purse, briefcase, overnight bag, or other personal item is to accompany the patient, make sure it is placed and properly secured in the ambulance. If you load personal effects at the scene of a vehicle collision, be sure to tell a police officer what you are taking. Follow the policies and fill out the forms, if any, required by your local system for safeguarding of personal effects.

Step 11: Reassure the Patient

Apprehension often mounts in a sick or injured person after he is loaded in an ambulance. Not only is he held down by straps in a strange, confined space, but he may also be suddenly separated from family members and friends who have comforted him to this point. Say a few kind words and offer a reassuring hand.

Remember that a favorite toy such as a teddy bear can do much to calm a frightened child (Figure 26-1). Many ambulance units carry a sanitized, soft or padded brightly colored toy in a compartment just for frightened children. It is difficult at best to get information from a young child whose parents may have been injured and transported in another ambulance. Small children don't, as a rule, carry identification and you are a complete stranger in a hostile environment.

The crash scene, confusion, noise, injuries, possibly pain, disappearance of a parent, EMTs caring for injuries and gathering much needed information all lead to a hectic experience for a child. A female EMT or police officer may be helpful. Sometimes young children feel more comfortable talking to a woman. A smile and calm reassuring tone of voice are something that cannot be learned from a textbook, and they may be the most critical care needed by the frightened child.

Don't forget that an adult may be equally scared. Treat all patients as you would want an EMT to treat your mother! Hold the patient's hand and be honest and reassuring.

When you are satisfied that the patient is ready for transportation, signal the operator to begin the trip to the hospital.

Note: IF THIS IS A CRITICAL OR UNSTABLE PATIENT, MOST OF THE PREPARATION STEPS— LOOSENING CLOTHING, CHECKING BANDAGES AND SPLINTS, REASSURING THE PATIENT, EVEN VITAL SIGNS—CAN BE DONE EN ROUTE RATHER THAN DELAYING TRANSPORT.

Warning: Under no circumstances should you allow smoking in either the patient's compartment or the operator's compartment while oxygen is being administered. Oxygen itself is not flammable; it does, however, cause other combustible materials to burn vigorously. High concentrations of oxygen can develop in voids between articles of clothing and even under the cot linens and blankets. If a chance spark ignites clothing or bedding, the results can be disastrous. Weather permitting, ventilate the patient compartment well while oxygen is being delivered and once the ambulance is moving. (It is not a safe practice to idle with the rear door or windows open, as fumes may enter the patient compartment.)

CARING FOR THE PATIENT WHILE EN ROUTE TO THE HOSPITAL

Seldom will you be able to merely ride along with your patient. You may have to undertake a number of activities on the way to the hospital.

Step 1: Continue to Provide Emergency Care as Required

If life-support efforts were initiated prior to loading the patient into the ambulance, they must be continued during transportation to the hospital.

Maintain an open airway, resuscitate, administer to the patient's needs, provide emotional support, and do whatever else is required, including updating your findings from the initial patient assessment effort.

Step 2: Compile Additional Patient Information

If the patient is conscious and emergency care efforts will not be compromised, record patient information.

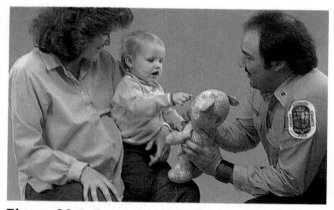

Figure 26-1 Reassuring the child patient with a teddy bear.

Compiling information during the trip to the hospital serves two purposes. First, it allows you to complete your report. Second, supplying information temporarily takes your patient's mind off his problems. Remember, however, that obtaining patient information is not an interrogation session. Ask your questions in an informal manner.

Step 3: Continue Monitoring Vital Signs

Keep in mind that changes in vital signs indicate a change in a patient's condition. For example, an unexplained increase in pulse rate may signify deepening shock.

Record vital signs on your report form and be prepared to relate changes in vital signs to an emergency department staff member as soon as you reach the medical facility.

Step 4: Check Bandages

Even though you checked bandages after loading the patient into the ambulance, check them again while in transit. Shifting of the patient in response to swaying of the ambulance may have caused bandages to loosen or tighten. Adjust them as required. If dressings and bandages become blood soaked, add fresh ones in a continuing effort to control bleeding. Remember that under no circumstances should you replace the blood-soaked dressings that are in contact with the skin.

If the fingers and toes of bandaged extremities become cool and blue tinged, loosen the bandage slightly; it may be interfering with circulation. Be careful not to disturb any impaled object while checking and adjusting bandages.

Step 5: Check Splints

Make both a visual and manual check to ensure that splinting devices have not shifted. Make adjustments if necessary. Ensure that circulation and nerve functions are not impaired. Check distal pulse, capillary refill, skin temperature and color, and distal neurologic activity.

Step 6: Collect Vomitus if the Patient Becomes Nauseated

If he is not already in position, arrange the patient so that the chance of his aspirating vomitus is minimized. Be prepared to apply suction. Place an emesis basin, bag, or pail by his mouth. When he has finished vomiting, place a towel over the container and deliver it to emergency department personnel when you hand over the patient. Examination of the vomitus may be important to treatment, especially in cases of poisoning.

Wear a mask and eye shield if your patient is vomiting.

Step 7: Talk to the Patient, but Control Your Emotions

Continued conversation is often soothing to a frightened patient. Occasionally, however, conversation may be difficult for you. Your patient may be a reeking, incoherent alcohol abuse victim, or a reckless driver who struck and killed a child before wrecking his own vehicle, or a drug addict with a life style completely alien to yours.

Regardless of the situation, do not allow your emotions or personal feelings to overshadow professional ethics and interest in your patient's welfare. If you find it difficult to converse in an ordinary manner, at least assure your patient that everything possible is being done to help him and that he will soon be at a medical facility.

Step 8: Advise the Ambulance Operator of Changing Conditions

No one likes a "back seat" driver. However, there will be times when you must ask the ambulance operator to adjust speed or alter his driving technique to suit the needs of your patient.

If, on the one hand, what began as a routine transport develops into an emergency run, you may have to ask the operator to accelerate. On the other hand, if you think that swaying because of high speeds and uneven streets is detrimental to a patient's condition, have the operator slow down or take an alternative route.

While the operator of an ambulance is responsible for his vehicle and the passengers carried in it, it is your responsibility to care for sick and injured persons; thus the operator should drive the ambulance according to your suggestions. The decision on use of lights and siren should always be made with the medical condition of the patient in mind.

Step 9: If the Patient Goes into Cardiac Arrest, Have the Operator Stop the Ambulance While You Initiate CPR

If cardiac arrest develops, have the operator stop the ambulance while you initiate CPR. Signal the operator to start up again once you have established CPR. Make certain that the emergency department is made aware of the arrest.

If you routinely position a rigid device between the back of high-risk patients and the cot mattress, you have only to drop the cot back to a horizontal position and start CPR. If not, you must position an object like a short spine board or CPR board so that chest compression efforts will be effective.

If you are trained in the use of an automated external defibrillator (AED), follow your medical director's protocols for the device. Local protocols may mandate intercept by an advanced-life-support team.

Note: You may want the ambulance operator to assist you with CPR while additional resources come to your aid. Use your judgment on this.

Step 10: Transmit Patient Information to the Medical Facility

Effective communications between ambulance and hospital are described in the next section.

COMMUNICATIONS DURING TRANSPORT

While ambulances have been equipped with two-way radios for quite some time, intercommunication capabilities were generally limited to dispatch centers and ambulances. If ambulance personnel needed to discuss anything with hospital staff members, it usually had to be done through a third party over a combination of telephone and radio links. The procedure was time consuming and error prone. With the development of efficient emergency medical service communication systems, however, EMTs now have the capability to talk directly with emergency department personnel.

Numerous protocols have been developed for ambulance-hospital radio or cellular phone communications. To be effective, messages from ambulances to hospitals should be brief but complete and transmitted without often-misunderstood and confusing codes.

An informational message from an EMT should include

- Hospital identification
- Ambulance designation
- Brief description of the chief complaint and status (CUPS—critical, unstable, potentially unstable, or stable)

- Facts learned during the subjective interview
- Facts learned during the objective examination (physical exam and vital signs)
- Your assessment of injuries or medical problems (what you "suspect")
- Emergency care provided thus far
- Your estimated time of arrival (ETA) at the medical facility

Step 1: Identify the Hospital in Your Initial Call

"Mercy Hospital . . ."

Complex EMS communication systems may have many hospitals in the network. Make sure that your message is immediately received by the proper hospital by identifying that facility at the start of your message.

Step 2: Identify Your Unit

". . . this is EMT Sanchez on ambulance six-two-one. How do you copy?"

Obviously there cannot be effective point-to-point communication unless both the message receiver and the originator are identified. Identify your unit, making sure that you clearly enunciate letters and numerals, thus minimizing misunderstanding. Keep in mind that persons who do not use two-way radios routinely often confuse words and phrases, especially when radio traffic or noise is considerable. For example "fifteen" may be mistaken for "sixteen." When there is a chance that your unit designation will be misunderstood, use the phonetic alphabet (if in use in your locality) and enunciate each numeral separately.

By giving your name and title, the emergency department staff may associate *you* with the voice and may pay more attention. Asking how the hospital is receiving your transmission will ensure that you are being received and will allow the hospital time to answer your call.

Step 3: Give a Brief Description of What Happened

"We are transporting a patient who has fallen approximately 10 feet from a ladder onto a concrete floor. His status is potentially unstable."

Remember that you have been taught to consider the mechanisms of injury when assessing an accident victim. When you briefly but accurately describe the incident to which you have responded, emergency department personnel can often visualize the mechanisms of injury.

Just as you were able to surmise that the man could have suffered long bone fractures, a head injury, a spinal injury, or abdominal insult by observing the mechanisms of injury, so, too, can emergency department personnel make a working diagnosis from your description of the incident. Your role is to "paint a picture" of the scene for them.

Be sure to state your patient's status on the CUPS scale, or using the format of your region. This helps the emergency department staff understand the severity of the complaint right away.

Step 4: State What You Learned in the Subjective Interview

"The patient is a 34-year old male who complains of a headache and moderate pain in the right leg. He was unconscious for a short time following the fall. He is a patient of Dr. Johnson."

Negative information learned in the interview, such as "the patient is not taking medication" or "the patient has no known allergies," can also be useful to the emergency department staff.

Step 5: State What You Learned From the Objective Examination and Vitals

"The patient is verbally responsive to my questions but is unable to tell me the date or his location. Vitals are respiration of 24 and regular, pulse of 86 regular and strong, BP of 140 over 90, and skin is pale and clammy. Positive findings are a contusion of the head in the occipital area and swelling and point tenderness over the right femur."

Start with your assessment of the patient's overall condition, follow with vital signs and then relate any positive findings or pertinent negatives from your objective examination.

When an accident victim has suffered multiple injuries, recite the major ones; do not bother with minor injuries, such as cuts and bruises.

Step 6: Report Your Assessment of Injuries or Medical Problems

"I suspect a fracture of the right femur and concussion."

The verb "suspect" does not cast doubt on your ability to assess a sick or injured person's condition. It simply underlines the fact that your assessment is tentative, based on subjective and objective information obtained at the scene of the accident. EMTs are sometimes criticized by emergency department personnel for making a "final diagnosis" at the time they arrive on the scene, only to have it proved wrong when the patient is examined at the medical facility. However, this possibility should not make you reluctant to report your assessment.

Step 7: Report What You Have Done for the Patient

"We have applied full spine immobilization and a traction splint and are providing 12 liters of oxygen by nonrebreather mask."

Again there is little need to relate what has been done for minor injuries, such as the application of a bandage to a small wound.

Step 8: Estimate Your Time of Arrival at the Medical Facility (ETA)

"Our ETA is 10 minutes."

Even though most emergency departments are ready to receive patients at any time, knowing when you will reach the hospital with the patient will assist them in making preparations to receive your patient. When you have a patient in critical condition and when the department is crowded with other patients, knowing the time of arrival is even more important to allow staff members to seek additional help, gather specialized equipment, and clear a treatment area.

Note: Studies show that EMTs often underestimate their ETA at the hospital. Knowing not only your area but your local traffic, road, and weather conditions will help improve the accuracy of your ETA.

Now . . . look at the entire message.

"Mercy Hospital, this is EMT Sanchez on ambulance six-two-one. How do you copy? [Pause for acknowledgment.] We are transporting a patient who has fallen approximately 10 feet from a ladder onto a concrete floor. His status is potentially unstable. The patient is a 34-year old male who complains of a headache and moderate pain in the right leg. He was unconscious for a short time following the fall. He is a patient of Dr. Johnson. The patient is verbally responsive to my questions but is unable to tell me the date or his location. Vitals are respiration of

24 and regular, pulse of 86 regular and strong, BP of 140 over 90, and skin is pale and clammy. Positive findings are a contusion of the head in the occipital area and swelling and point tenderness over the right femur. I suspect a fracture of the right femur and concussion. We have applied full spine immobilization and a traction splint and are providing 12 liters of oxygen by nonrebreather mask. Our ETA is 10 minutes."

Thus in about a minute you can transmit a wealth of information about a sick or injured person, information that will help emergency department personnel plan a course of definitive care even before they see the patient.

If your patient has an injury or illness that requires special emergency care procedures (as in cases of poisoning), you may request advice from the emergency department by radio or cellular phone.

TRANSFERRING THE PATIENT TO THE CARE OF EMERGENCY DEPARTMENT PERSONNEL

Definitive emergency care cannot be delivered by a single individual; it must come from a well-educated and competent team of Emergency Medical Dispatchers, EMTs, paramedics, nurses, physicians, administrators, and allied health personnel. Although the responsibilities of each team member may vary, each person plays an important part; failure of any team member to do his job may mean the difference between rehabilitation and disability, a short-term or long-term hospital stay, even life or death to the victim of a sudden illness or injury. It is therefore critical that all personnel responsible for some facet of life support and emergency care strive to provide optimum service at all times and in complete harmony with other persons within the system.

It is usually the emergency department nurse to whom the EMT most directly relates, either through the ambulance-hospital communication system or in face-to-face contact in the hospital.

The following are steps that you should take to see that the transfer of a patient to the care of emergency department personnel is accomplished smoothly and without incident. Brief as it may be, the transfer is a crucial step during which your primary concern must be the continuation of patient care activities. The steps of the transfer are illustrated in Scan 26-1.

Step 1: In a Routine Admission Situation or When an Illness or Injury is Not Life-threatening, Check First to See What Is to Be Done with the Patient

If emergency department activity is particularly hectic, as it is when several seriously injured accident victims are admitted at the same time, it might be better to leave your patient in the relative security and comfort of the ambulance while your operator determines where he is to be taken. Otherwise the patient may be subjected to distressing sights and sounds and perhaps be in the way. (If you do this, make sure an EMT remains with the patient at all times.) UNDER NO CIRCUMSTANCES SHOULD YOU SIMPLY WHEEL A NONEMERGENCY PATIENT INTO A HOSPITAL, PLACE HIM ON A BED OR A GURNEY, AND LEAVE HIM! This is an important point. Unless you transfer care of your patient directly to a member of the hospital staff, you may be open to a charge of abandonment.

Keep in mind that staff members may be treating other seriously ill and injured persons, so suppress any urge to demand attention for your patient. Simply continue emergency care measures until someone can assume responsibility for the patient. Remember, this is what you have been trained to do. When properly directed, transfer the patient to a hospital stretcher (Scan 26-2).

Step 2: Assist Emergency Department Staff Members as Required and Provide an Oral Report

Be sure to provide an oral report to the emergency department personnel taking care of your patient that is similar to the radio report discussed above, stressing any changes in condition you have observed.

EMTs should participate in the early emergency department care of sick and injured persons. Even when the emergency department staff has taken over completely, it is often beneficial for the EMTs to remain in the area to be of assistance. The experience not only promotes better patient care but also fosters improved communication and understanding between EMTs and emergency department personnel. Also important is the fact that working with the staff gives an EMT the opportunity to learn more about definitive care procedures while the staff can become comfortable with the EMT's abilities. This may not be possible in an EMS system with a high volume of calls where it is important to quickly prepare the ambulance for another call.

Transferring the Patient

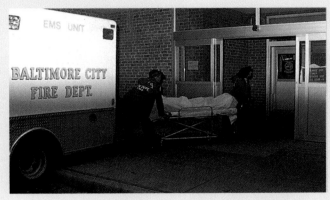

1. Transfer the patient as soon as possible. In a routine admission or when an illness or injury is not life-threatening, first check to see what is to be done with the patient. An EMT should remain with the patient until transfer is complete.

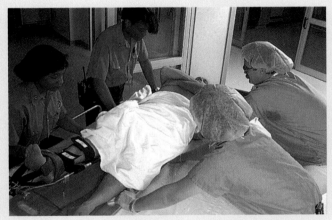

2. Assist the emergency department staff as required.

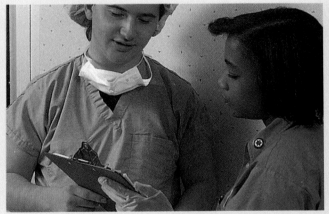

3. Transfer patient information as an oral report and a written prehospital care report.

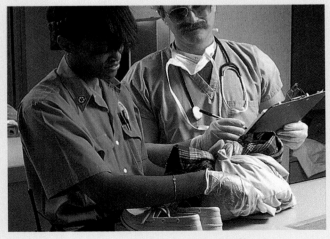

4. Transfer the patient's personal effects.

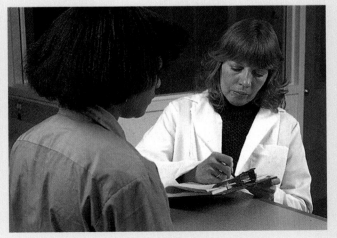

5. Obtain your release from the hospital.

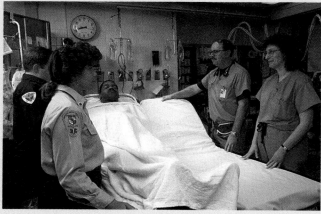

1. EMTs position raised ambulance cot next to hospital stretcher. Hospital personnel adjust stretcher (raise or lower head) to receive patient from ambulance cot.

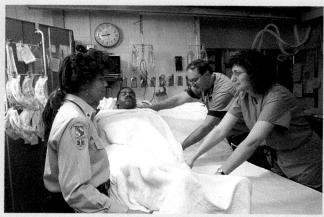

2. EMTs and hospital personnel gather sheet on either side of patient and pull taut in order to transfer patient securely.

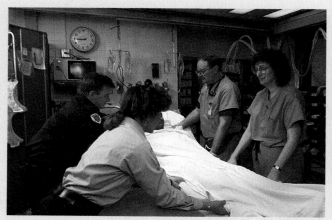

3. Holding gathered sheet at support points near shoulders, mid torso, hips, and knees, EMTs and hospital personnel slide patient in one motion to hospital stretcher.

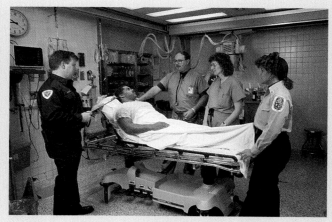

4. Assure patient is centered on stretcher. EMTs will exchange patient information with hospital personnel. **(Note:** Remember to raise stretcher rails before walking away from patient.)

Step 3: As Soon as You Are Free from Patient Care Activities, Prepare the Prehospital Care Report

Using your assessment card or notes and any additional changes in the patient's condition you have observed, you can now find a "quiet" spot and complete your prehospital care report. Preparation of a PCR will be discussed in Chapter 27.

Step 4: Transfer the Patient's Personal Effects

If a patient's valuables or other personal effects were entrusted to your care, transfer them to a responsible emergency department staff member. Some services have policies that involve obtaining a written receipt from emergency department personnel as protection from a charge of theft.

Step 5: Obtain Your Release from the Hospital

This task is not as formal as it sounds. Simply ask the emergency department nurse or physician if your services are still needed. In rural areas where not all hospital services are available, it may be necessary to transfer a seriously ill or injured person to another medical facility. If you leave and have to be recalled, valuable time will be lost.

CHAPTER REVIEW

SUMMARY

Preparing the Patient for Transport

Prepare a sick or injured person for transportation to a medical facility by ensuring an open airway, securing the cot, positioning the patient, allowing for respiratory or cardiac complications, loosening constricting clothing, checking bandages, checking splints, determining and recording vital signs, loading a relative or friend, loading personal effects, and reassuring the patient.

Caring for the Patient While En Route to the Hospital

During transportation, continue emergency care as required, compile additional patient information if possible, continue monitoring vital signs, transmit patient information to the medical facility, check bandages, check splints, collect vomitus if the patient becomes nauseated, talk to the patient, advise the ambulance operator of changing conditions, and administer CPR (and defibrillation, if you are trained in AED use and so authorized) if the patient goes into cardiac arrest.

Communications During Transport

When you transmit patient information to the medical facility, be sure to include (1) the hospital identification, (2) the ambulance designation, (3) a brief description of the patient's chief complaint, (4) facts learned from the subjective interview, (5) facts learned from the objective examination, (6) your assessment of the patient's problem, (7) the emergency care provided, and (8) your estimated time of arrival at the facility.

Transferring the Patient to the Care of Emergency Department Personnel

Ensure the smooth transfer of patient care to the hospital staff by first checking to see what is to be done with the patient, then assisting emergency department staff members, transferring accurate patient information, transferring personal effects, and checking to see if you are still needed before leaving the hospital.

27

On the Scene

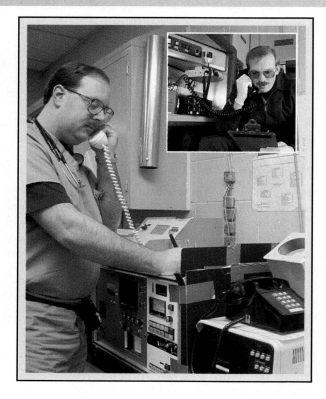

Mrs. Nagle, our "On the Scene" patient from Chapters 25 and 26, is having difficulty breathing. Your skills in face-to-face communication have helped to ease her fears and prevent stress from aggravating her condition unnecessarily. From the ambulance you radio the receiving hospital, speaking slowly and clearly.

You: Memorial Hospital, this is Ambulance 12. How do you copy?

Nurse Marilyn Wong: Ambulance 12, you're loud and clear. Go ahead.

You: Memorial Hospital, we are en route to your location with a 50-year-old female patient. Her chief complaint is difficulty breathing. Her status is potentially unstable. She is alert and oriented. Vital signs are respirations 28 and labored, pulse 104 and irregular, blood pressure 150 over 92. Our exam reveals rales in her lungs and edema in both ankles. I suspect congestive heart failure. She takes a "water pill" but is not sure of its name. We have the patient sitting up and a non-rebreather mask in place with oxygen running at 12 liters per minute. Our ETA is 15 minutes.

Mrs. Wong: Ambulance 12, we'll be expecting your arrival. Bring the patient directly to cardiac room number 2.

You: Cardiac room 2, message received.

During this brief transmission, important information was exchanged. You learned what the hospital expects you to do when you arrive. In turn, the hospital has learned enough about your patient to prepare for her arrival. You were careful to complete a "feedback loop" by checking to be sure the emergency department nurse understood you and by repeating her instructions.

Once at Memorial, you give an oral report to the physician on duty and turn over your written prehospital care report, containing several sets of vital signs and other observations. In your PCR you have noted that Mrs. Nagle could not sleep lying down and slept in a chair, important additional information.

Clear communication is essential. You have learned that the better your communications, the better the care your patient will receive.

Communications and Reports

According to the dictionary, *communicate* means "to give or exchange information, signals, or messages in any way, as by talk, gestures, or writing." In this chapter we will discuss three types of communications used in EMS: face-to-face oral and nonverbal communication, radio communication, and written communication.

Expected Outcome: *You will be able to communicate effectively with your patients and all others with whom you come in contact as an EMT.*

Warning: Protect yourself from infectious diseases by using appropriate barrier devices such as a pocket face mask with one-way valve, face shield, or bag-valve mask; goggles or eye shield; and disposable gloves. Always conform to your local EMS system's infection exposure control plan.

FACE-TO-FACE COMMUNICATION
    Oral Communication
    Tips for Improving Oral Communication
    Nonverbal Communication

RADIO COMMUNICATION
    The Emergency Radio Communication System
    Ambulance Communication Procedures
    Patient Condition Radio Reports

WRITTEN REPORTS
    Benefits of a Complete PCR
    Completing a Prehospital Care Report
    Other EMS Reports

Knowledge *After reading this chapter, you should be able to*

1. Define communication. (p. 675)

2. Define and compare verbal, nonverbal, oral, and written communication. (p. 676)

3. Explain what is meant by the communications feedback loop. (pp. 677-678)

4. List at least SIX ways to improve your oral communication skills. (pp. 677-679)

5. Give at least TWO examples each of good and bad body language. (pp. 679-680)

6. List SIX phases of a typical EMS radio communication sequence. (p. 680)

7. State the FOUR basic components of an emergency communications system. (pp. 680-681)

8. List at least FOUR ways in which a basic EMS communications system may be expanded. (p. 681)

9. Give TEN rules to follow in regard to EMS radio communications. (pp. 681-682)

10. Cite the information to include in an ambulance-to-hospital patient report. (p. 682-and review Chapter 26)

11. List some of the purposes served by prehospital care reports. (pp. 682-683)

12. Describe benefits for patient care, for legal protection of the EMT, and for the EMS system of preparing accurate, complete, and legible prehospital care reports. (pp. 687-688)

13. Explain how to document patient statements. (p. 688)

14. List at least TEN standard medical abbreviations that can be used when writing a prehospital care report. (p. 688; Table 27-1)

15. Explain how to list time on the prehospital care report using military time. (p. 688)

16. Describe the procedure for properly documenting a patient refusal. (pp. 689-690)

17. List at least THREE occasions when a special incident report might be appropriate. (p. 690)

Skills *As an EMT you should be able to*

1. Communicate effectively with patients, family members, bystanders, EMS personnel, and other medical professionals.

2. Conduct proper radio communications.

3. Present verbal reports in a professional manner.

4. Fill out a prehospital care report completely, accurately, and legibly.

A very important part of being a competent EMT is being able to communicate. Interpersonal skills can make the difference between gaining the confidence of your patient, control of bystanders, and the respect of other emergency services personnel or haphazardly muddling through a call and coming across as something less than a competent professional. Having a genuine interest in other people and a friendly, compassionate disposition are good starting points. Patients are not generally impressed by your EMT knowledge and skills, which they expect. They will be impressed by your demeanor, your kindness, and your ability to treat them with respect as you would someone in your own family.

People often confuse the words *verbal* and *oral*. *Verbal* means "with words." *Oral* means "spoken." Verbal communication can be either oral or written. *Nonverbal*, of course, means "without words" (e.g., gestures). We will discuss all of these kinds of communication on the next few pages.

FACE-TO-FACE COMMUNICATION

Face-to-face communication happens on every call, not only with your patient but with everyone you come in contact with as an EMT.

Oral Communication

The way you speak with people is usually the most important factor in determining the kind of relationship you establish with them.

With Your Partners From the moment you report to the station, you need to communicate with your partners. Some EMTs who work very closely with the same partner develop a rhythm that "clicks" on each call. You back each other up, know each other's strengths, and support each other's weaknesses.

Often as you work with the same partner and get to know each other well, there is less verbal communication because each of you knows what the other is doing. It is important not to take the nonverbal communication for granted, but rather to discuss the treatment with your whole crew so everyone is aware of your findings. Obviously a certain amount of common sense must be used in front of the patient.

With Your Patient The EMT needs to establish rapport with the patient and quickly gain his or her trust. It is best for one EMT to do the interview and physical examination while management and vital signs are delegated to the other EMTs. Explaining what you plan to do and giving patients choices, whenever possible, will help keep them informed and give them some sense of control. Remember, for the patients—such as one who just wrecked his new car—their world and emotions are often out of control. You are there to try to restore some stability to this volatile situation.

Along with gaining the patient's trust and listening to some very private information within the confines of the patient's home comes the EMT's responsibility to keep information and the patient's identity confidential, sharing information only with the professional personnel who need to know it.

With Other EMS Personnel On each call the EMT will need to communicate in a friendly but professional manner with other emergency services personnel such as the Emergency Medical Dispatcher (EMD), the firefighter, the police officer and other first responder or mutual aid agency personnel. It is courteous to report to those who were on the scene first before asking them for pertinent information and going about your business.

All too often, a routine call becomes an unsafe situation in which you will all need each other's support. If you have made a habit of cultivating a good working relationship with other emergency services personnel, it will make routine calls run more smoothly and may, in some situations, even save your life.

With Bystanders and Family Members The EMT must communicate with bystanders and family members to gain additional information about the patient and the incident itself. Be straight and professional with bystanders. If they are in the way, put them to work holding back the rest of the crowd. If the crowd becomes unruly, remove yourself and the patient as quickly as possible and request police backup. Some services have strict policies on not entering taverns or social clubs without a police backup because of the potential problems with unruly intoxicated crowds.

Family members may actually become additional patients if you are not careful to deal with their anxiety about the patient's illness or injury. This is especially true with the elderly or with parents of small children. They also know invaluable medical history about the patient, so they should not be shoved off into another room. Whenever possible, assign a crew member to interview and deal with the family members.

With Hospital Personnel Both on the radio and face-to-face in the emergency department, the EMT needs to communicate with the physicians, nurses, and other hospital professionals. You can be the smartest EMT in your class, with excellent skills, but if you do not refine your patient presentation skills and professional demeanor, emergency department personnel will develop an unfavorable first impression of you that will take a long time to overcome.

Practice presenting patients to other EMTs and use an assessment card to help you organize your thoughts. You will have some very important information about the patient and the environment you took them out of to pass along, so don't let poor communication block your message.

Tips For Improving Oral Communication

As an EMT you will need to polish your ability to talk with people. Here are some tips on improving this important skill.

- *Be aware of the "feedback loop."* When a message is sent, the person it is sent to may not be ready to listen or to interpret the message in the manner you expect. To assure that key information has been understood, always check understanding by creating a loop from person A to person B and back to person A. Whether you are person A, the sender, or person B, the receiver, you can achieve this by asking a question (*Do you copy?* or *Did you say "normal respirations"?*) or by repeating, or encouraging the listener to repeat, the message so it is clear how it has been interpreted (*Let me summarize what you have just told me to make sure I understand your complaint,* or *Can you repeat that back to me?*).

Remember the feedback loop when giving instructions to team members or when presenting a report to EMS personnel from another unit or to the emergency department. Sometimes emergency department (ED) personnel may be so busy they only "half hear" your information. If the loop has not been completed (you have not received confirmation that your information was properly listened to), be sure to "lobby for your patient" by repeating and emphasizing important information to the ED personnel, such as exactly how you found the patient or other important findings (*I just want to make sure you understand that although this patient looks stable now, when we found him his vehicle had been involved in a high speed collision and the engine was literally in the front seat!*).

Assuring the feedback loop is especially important when communicating on the radio because you cannot see the face of the receiver of your message or observe what else the receiver may also be doing while trying to listen to you. Whenever very important information is being passed on that could have life-threatening results if misinterpreted, create the feedback loop by checking for understanding of the information. Most EMS systems make a practice of repeating back to a physician on the radio any medical orders he or she has given. (e.g., Medical Control: *If the patient is conscious with a gag reflex, give him a small glass of orange juice with some sugar in it.* EMT: *To confirm: You are ordering orange juice and sugar.* Medical Control: *That's affirmative. Orange juice and sugar.*)

- *Be quiet and listen.* Hearing is passive; listening is active. You can hear sounds without really being aware of them. Listening involves conscious and deliberate interpreting and processing. To be an effective listener you need to understand the reason for listening, be attentive to the message, appropriately process the message, and then respond to the message.

Assessment, one of the most important skills in EMS, is often 90% based upon listening, so it is essential that the EMT develop listening skills. There are some pointers that can help improve your ability to listen.

First, learn the patient's name and use it. Remember that some patients resent being called by their first names. Many women feel they are being patronized when medical personnel, especially males, call them by their first name. Elderly patients, who grew up in a more formal era, may also prefer being respectfully addressed as Mr., Mrs., or Miss. Children, younger adults, and people of about your own age may feel better being called by their first name. Use tact and your intuition about this.

Eye contact with the patient can help improve your chance of receiving their message. Whenever possible, try to avoid doing multiple things while listening. Besides the patient seeing you are not paying attention to him or her, you can easily forget answers to the questions you asked. If extra distractions can be removed from the scene, it is helpful. Some EMS agencies respond with multiple units, police, and first responders. Once it is clear that all those rescuers are not needed, you may want to assign them other responsibilities outside the room, thank and release the extra help for another assignment, or move the patient into your "office" in the back of the ambulance where it is quieter and more conducive to a one-on-one conversation about the patient's complaints and medical history.

It is helpful to use an assessment card to write down a summary of what the patient has to tell you.

- *Don't tell the patient what to tell you.* Another part of being a good listener is to not put words into your patient's mouth. Good assessment questions are focused but open ended. Try not to ask questions that can be answered just "yes" or "no." Try asking questions that begin with "What" or "How" (e.g., *What happened that made you want to call the ambulance?* or *How did you happen to fall?*). Such questions allow patients to answer in their own words rather than saying what you want or expect to hear. Avoid providing words for the patient by saying, "Point to where the pain is and describe the pain," rather than "Is this crushing pain in the center of your chest?"

In life in general we would all be better off if we would simply think before we speak. Besides saying something you really did not mean or possibly offending someone, you can lose the patient's trust or make them unnecessarily anxious. For example, do not ask the patient, "Is this your first heart attack?" Instead, try asking, "Have you ever had pain like this before?"

- *Don't assume anything.* "Never assume" is said so often it is almost a cliche. It is, nevertheless, a very good rule for the EMT. Assuming gives an EMT "tunnel vision," which limits the possibilities severely. When we tunnel in on one problem that we assume is wrong with the patient, we can easily get caught off guard.

  This can be especially true with a chronic drinker or alcoholic whom you encounter often and begin to dismiss as "just a drunk." This patient may have called the ambulance many times while intoxicated and for "injuries" that turn out not to be real, but that does not mean that today's complaint is not valid. If this patient says he fell out the window and hurt his back, then check it out and treat him appropriately. The assumption that "he's just hallucinating again" could lead you to neglect a real injury. Remember that alcoholics are also more prone to gastrointestinal sickness and chronic subdural hematomas, so if they say they feel sick or hit their head, treat them for the worst potential illness or injury, not the least.

  Never, of course, assume that a person who appears to be intoxicated is just drunk. If you base your patient assessment on such an assumption, you may fail to treat a person who is actually suffering a diabetic emergency or other medical problem.

- *Remember that your tone can speak louder than your words.* It is sometimes hard to sound compassionately interested at 3 a.m. on your eighth call for the day when the patient has what seems to be a minor complaint. Although no one expects you to be artificially bubbly at such a time, it is important to maintain a professional tone that shows you are genuinely interested in the patient's complaint. Very quickly patients will sense whether you want to help them or not just by listening to your tone. This is especially true with children, who may not clearly understand your words but can readily sense your attitude towards them.

  Always remember that EMS is a service field, and you should be prepared to serve sick and injured (or even not-so-sick-or-injured) patients who are not always friendly or in control of their emotions. Sometimes it is helpful to ask yourself, "How would I feel or react if I were in the situation they are in?—going to the hospital with strangers, possibly in pain, out of control, with the world seeming to be falling down around me . . . and not knowing how I'm going to pay the bill!"

- *Use correct terminology.* Do not use laypersons' terms or slang when communicating with other EMS or medical personnel (e.g., use *fractured right femur* instead of *broken right thigh,* or *Observed grand mal seizure* rather than *Man had a fit*).

- *Don't use a term unless you know its meaning.* Although it is your responsibility to learn and use correct terminology, if you are unsure of a term it is better to use everyday language than to use the wrong term (e.g., use *adam's apple* if you can't remember *thyroid cartilage*).

- *Don't use medical jargon inappropriately.* Avoid using medical jargon when speaking to bystanders and patients, because they probably do not understand what you are talking about. Be aware of and ready to switch to the street names for certain conditions for clear communication with lay persons (e.g., use *miscarriage* rather than. *spontaneous abortion,* or *nosebleed* instead of *epistaxis*).

- *Use complete sentences and a calm, neutral tone.* The minute one person at an incident starts shouting or sounds anxious, everyone else gets nervous and begins raising voices. This only increases the tension and stress level of the incident for all involved and makes it almost impossible to understand you over the radio.

- *Remember that the patient is usually paying attention to you.* Don't drop your guard just because your patient seems unaware or is not looking directly at you. When presenting to the ED physician, speak of your patient as a human being, not a disease entity (e.g., say *This is Mrs. Woicek. Her chief complaint is . . .,* not *This one's a "rule out MI"*). The experts tell us that one of the last senses to go is hearing, so watch what you say, even when your patient becomes unconscious.

Nonverbal Communication

Your facial expressions, posture, and body position can give a strong message to the patient or bystanders. If you walk right up to someone and stare down at them, you may be giving off a message of superiority. Try squatting down next to a patient who is on the ground or in a chair or a patient who is a child. Move yourself down to their level so you can see eye to eye and do not seem as threatening or large.

Standing with your arms crossed shows that you are guarded or bored with the situation. If you make facial expressions like a frown or raised eyebrow to your partner, the patient may notice it and feel you are discounting or patronizing him or her. (It is difficult to confide in someone you feel might be laughing at you!) Show compassion and interest with your facial expressions and always respect the patient and his or her home in your actions. Sometimes showing concern by holding a patient's hand or giving a pat on the shoulder can be very reassuring providing it is not unnatural for you to do and you do not invade the patient's "personal space." You can develop an intuition about when a touch is welcome.

Use a slight leaning-in posture when interviewing a patient or bystander to suggest that you are interested and concerned. Use nonverbal "I'm paying attention" behaviors such as head nodding and reactive facial expressions.

If you want to be taken as a professional, then "look it" right down to the way you wear your uniform. Don't come across as a slouch who threw on a wrinkled shirt and unpressed pants. If your hair is long or very full, keep it neatly tied back. Wear the uniform with pride and good posture.

Be aware of the nonverbal signals you are sending. There will be fewer dissatisfied customers if EMS providers always send out signals of respect for themselves and their patients.

RADIO COMMUNICATION

Another form of verbal communication is radio communication (Figure 27-1). The radio communication sequence typically used on EMS calls consists of five to six phases.

1. The EMT is alerted to the call, usually by a paging system or portable radio.
2. The EMT acknowledges receipt of the call and obtains additional information about the priority of response and location of the assignment using EMT-to-dispatcher radio communications.
3. Throughout the call EMT-to-dispatcher communications are continued to keep the dispatcher apprised of the situation and the unit's status and to obtain additional information or backup units.
4. The EMT may need to communicate with

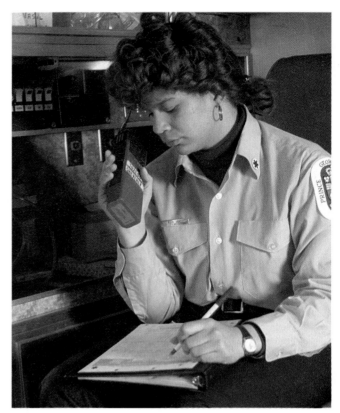

Figure 27-1 Communication from the ambulance can be by radio or cellular phone.

other responding units or supervisory personnel, usually through the EMT-to-dispatcher system, to upgrade or downgrade the response priority once an initial size-up of the scene and the patient's condition is done.

5. The EMT may need to communicate with other crew members on the scene and in the ambulance, perhaps by two-way radio or walkie-talkie, sometimes to obtain specific equipment from the ambulance.
6. The EMT communicates with the hospital emergency department through a direct ambulance-to-hospital communication link to present the patient's status and condition and the care being administered as the EMT transports the patient to their facility.

Below, we will discuss the radio communications system and some general considerations about its use.

The Emergency Radio Communication System

The basic emergency radio communication system includes the dispatcher's base station, the

EMS unit's mobile (transmitter/receiver) radio, the emergency department's remote center, and a telephone line backup. With these components the ambulance or EMS unit can send and receive messages from the dispatcher and the emergency department. This system is usually expanded to include many of the following enhancements.

- *Portable transmitter/receivers* are used by most EMS units to allow the EMT to communicate with the dispatcher from the patient's side. This is especially helpful when what was thought to be a safe scene turns violent. Some portables have emergency buttons alerting the dispatcher to an emergency transmission.
- *Multiple frequencies* are often used in cases where EMS units require a tactical or administrative frequency for radio transmissions that are not intended to go through the dispatcher and possibly interfere with normal emergency dispatch traffic. Many services have a second or third frequency in both their mobile and portable systems to advise incoming personnel of the situation or equipment needs.

  For multiple casualty incidents it is helpful for all the mutual aid ambulances to have a single separate frequency so they can talk to each other. It is helpful for EMS Command to communicate with the triage officer, treatment officer, transportation officer, and staging officer, all on a separate tactical frequency, while the incoming ambulances are advised to switch over to the multiple casualty incident (MCI) frequency and contact the staging officer for a location to which to respond. This helps to keep the regular dispatch frequencies clear for normal emergency traffic and the tactical frequency clear for command officer traffic.
- *Ambulance repeater stations or multiple towers* are used by many systems to retransmit between the two-way radios and the portable units, affording the low-powered portables a greater coverage range.
- *Biotelemetry* is the capability to send an electrocardiogram (ECG) over the radio to the hospital as it is being monitored from the patient. These units can make use of multiplex communications, meaning that the ECG and voice signals can be transmitted simultaneously on one channel.
- *Telephone patches* are sometimes used in systems where it is necessary for the dispatcher to receive a message by radio and

transmit it to a location over a phone line or receive a message by telephone and transmit it by radio.
- *Radio scanners* are frequently used by EMS units to monitor multiple frequencies. Multiple-band scanners can monitor hundreds of frequencies at once. The "band" refers to a small segment of the total frequency spectrum that has been assigned for a specific use by the Federal Communications Commission (FCC). For public safety use, the very high frequency (VHF) comprises the low band of 30-50 MHz (Megahertz or 1,000,000 cycles per second), the highband of 150-170 MHz, the ultra high frequency (UHF) band of 450-470 MHz, and the 800 radio bands. The FCC has set aside two UHF frequencies nationally for EMS dispatch use and eight for EMT-to-physician use.
- *Paging and alerting systems* are used to alert EMS crews in cases where they would not routinely be monitoring a portable radio. The latest technology has even developed a miniature-watch-pager system similar to the one in the old Dick Tracy comics.
- *Cellular telephones* are now commonly used throughout the country for ambulance-to-hospital communications and agency administrative purposes. It is also possible to transmit an ECG via cellular rather than the traditional UHF telemetry channels. In disaster situations there have been problems using cellular telephones, because the media use cellular telephones and may tie up all the cells.
- *Vehicle locator systems* are used by some sophisticated EMS systems. A constantly transmitting frequency on the ambulance gives the dispatcher an up-to-the-minute ambulance location. This location can then be plotted by computer to transmit instantaneously back to the ambulance a map showing the most direct route to the call location.

Ambulance Communication Procedures

For the frequencies allocated for emergency medical use, the FCC has ruled that, except for test transmissions, the ambulance radio is for official use only. Your calls are to relate to your duties, and they are to be carried out in a professional manner. When using the radio

- Do not try to transmit if other EMS personnel are using the channel or the EMD is speaking to you.

- Speak into the microphone using normal voice volume. Keep the tone of your voice neutral and slow your rate of speech.
- Speak clearly making an effort to pronounce each word distinctly.
- Be brief, using the correct terms and phrases needed to make your messages understood. Know what you are going to say before you transmit.
- Avoid using codes and abbreviations unless they are part of your system and will be understood by the person receiving them. Many systems have gotten away from codes and abbreviations in favor of plain English, which is more likely to be understood by everyone (e.g., describe exactly the patient's eye-opening, verbal, and motor responses, rather than saying *15 on the Glasgow Scale*).
- Receive a full message from the sender. Do not attempt to cut him or her off so that you can speak.
- Do not use slang or profanity.
- Do not use individuals' names or divulge confidential medical history that is not essential to the radio report (e.g., HIV status). Use unit, dispatch, and hospital identifiers.
- Do not use "please," "thank you," and other such terms. Politeness is *understood* to be a part of every radio transmission.
- Ask for a repeat if you do not understand something that is said while receiving. Never pretend to understand what was said.

Patient Condition Radio Reports

Most EMS systems routinely call the hospital to notify them that the ambulance is transporting a patient to their facility. In areas with a large amount of radio traffic, this is sometimes limited to the most serious patients so the hospital will be on standby for a medical or surgical emergency. It helps the emergency department prepare for the patient if they are alerted to what to expect. Some hospitals need the time to call staff down from the critical care units or surgical suite.

Although the manner of documenting a call is different for each agency, many services use an assessment card similar to the one in Figure 27-2 to obtain information from the patient and assist the EMT with a radio report to the hospital. Assessment cards can have reminders on questions to ask as well. They are often designed to follow the SOAP sequence.

S Subjective interview information
O Objective examination information
A Assessment (determination of "what's wrong")
P Plan for treatment

The actual completion of a prehospital care report can be done in a quiet room at the hospital ED rather than in the back of a moving ambulance.

Review the model ambulance-to-hospital report that was presented under "Communications During Transport" in Chapter 26.

WRITTEN REPORTS

The report that is completed by the EMT to document the assessment and treatment administered in the prehospital phase of each patient encounter is usually referred to as the prehospital care report, or PCR. Some localities still use traditional terms like "ambulance call report", "trip ticket," "trip sheet," or "run sheet."

Because a written report is routinely done on every call, the EMT must become proficient in complete and accurate documentation. When hospital personnel review your form, you will often not be there to fill in any gaps in the information. Therefore the story you have written must be as complete as possible.

The medical-legal experts all agree on one thing in respect to using PCRs: *If you didn't write it down, you will have difficulty proving you did it.*

A PCR could be a blank sheet of paper that is completed in a uniform manner on every call. However, most EMS systems use a standardized report that has spots in which to fill in the information needed on each run. The best forms have sections that prompt the EMT to use a standard patient approach and to document all the appropriate information on each patient encounter.

In the next section of this chapter, many of the essential sections of typical PCRs are discussed to help the student EMT learn about documentation. Good documentation skills do not come overnight. They take supervised practice and feedback by more experienced EMTs or EMS instructors. For that reason it is important that you practice completing your state's PCR, first in the classroom and then in the field. This text serves only as an introduction. You will need to receive specific instruction on how to complete the PCR your service uses.

Prehospital care reports shown in this

Assessment Worksheet

Patient Information:
Name _____
Address _____
_____
DOB _____ Age ____ Sex ____ Weight ____
MD _____ Run # _____

Chief Complaint:
Why EMS was called?
Degree of Distress

History:
Provocation
Quality
Radiation
Reoccurence
Relief
Severity
Time

Past Medical History:
Allergies
Medications
Past History
Last Meal

Vital Signs:

Time	P	BP	R	LOC	Pupils
		/			
		/			
		/			

Physical Assessment:
Head to Toes
Positive Findings
Pertinent Negatives
Lungs
EKG
SPO$_2$

Assessment:

Treatment Plan/Orders:
Treatment thus far
Orders Requested

Figure 27-2 Assessment card, Town of Colonie, New York.

chapter are examples from a number of different states that have a statewide database that provides management reports back to the ambulance services. It is important to note that there is no one best report style. The best reports try to balance the needs of the EMT, patient, hospital, service medical director, continuous quality improvement coordinator, emergency department staff, ambulance service management, and regional or state EMS system.

Different formats serve different needs. For example, research needs are best served by a form that is easily analyzed and input into a computer, such as the scannable forms used in Tennessee and Colorado. The EMT must carefully complete the scannable form without any stray marks that would cause the computer to reject or misread the form. Data can also be input from the EMTs by typing or keypunching it, but at a higher cost.

It is difficult to design a research form that

is easily input and that also allows the EMT to describe observations in a narrative form. To input data from a mostly narrative form is very time consuming, because each PCR needs to be read and interpreted by someone with at least the same training as an EMT. Yet narrative sections on forms are often more descriptive of the patient's condition, including observations and direct quotations from the patient. Thus is there is a conflict between the design requirements for a good research form versus those for complete documentation of observations and treatment. The PCRs used by Pennsylvania and Arizona combine a scannable side and a narrative side (Figure 27-3). PCRs used by New York, North Carolina, West Virginia, and Maine combine fill-in-the-box sections with narrative space (Figure 27-4). Missouri, New Hampshire, and New Mexico have each doubled the writing space to accommodate the many needs of the PCR.

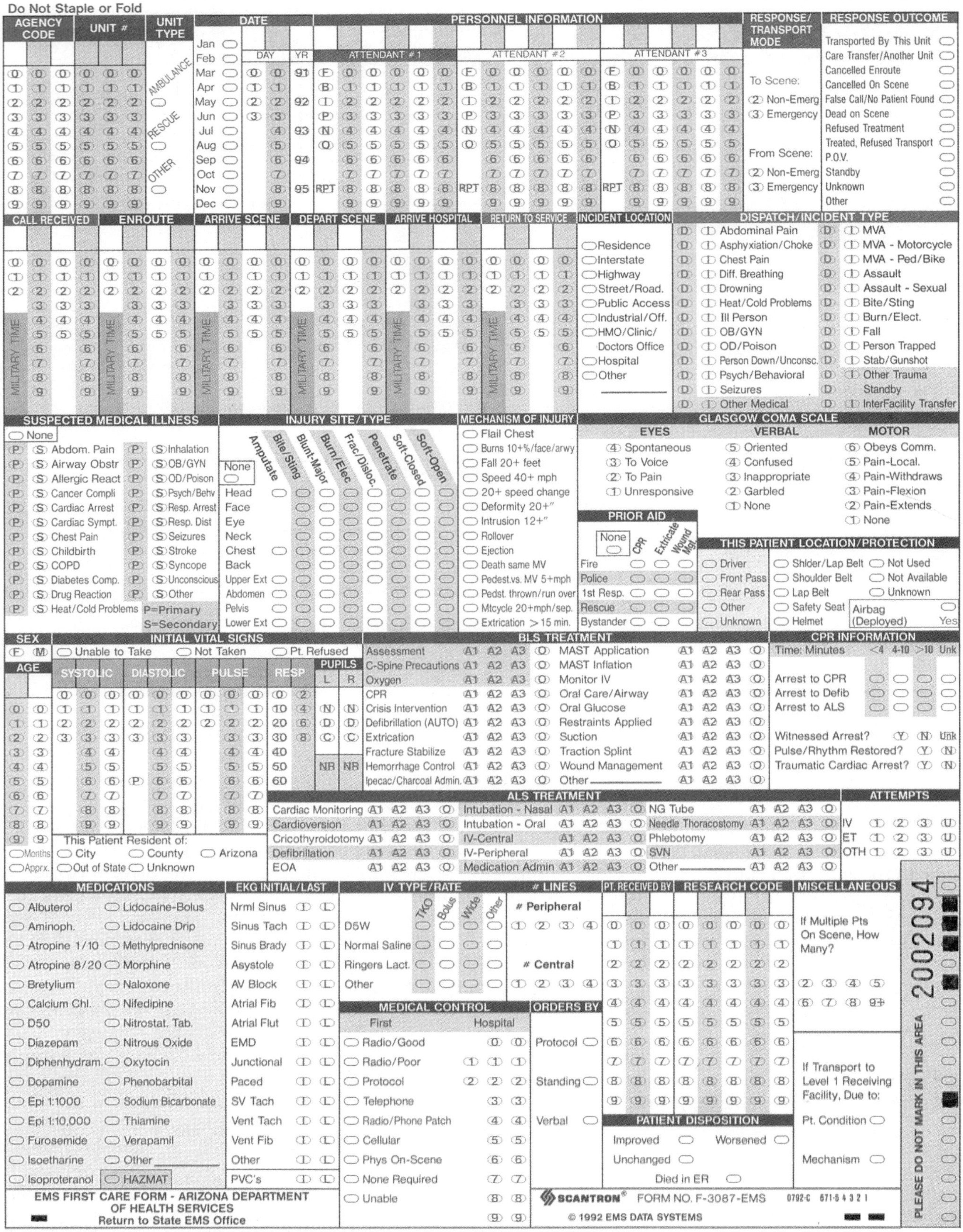

Do Not Staple or Fold

EMS FIRST CARE FORM - ARIZONA DEPARTMENT OF HEALTH SERVICES

AGENCY CODE	UNIT #	UNIT TYPE	DATE	PERSONNEL INFORMATION	RESPONSE/ TRANSPORT MODE	RESPONSE OUTCOME

UNIT TYPE: Ambulance, Rescue, Other

DATE: Jan, Feb, Mar, Apr, May, Jun, Jul, Aug, Sep, Oct, Nov, Dec — DAY — YR (91, 92, 93, 94, 95)

PERSONNEL INFORMATION: ATTENDANT #1, ATTENDANT #2, ATTENDANT #3

RESPONSE/TRANSPORT MODE:
To Scene: (2) Non-Emerg, (3) Emergency
From Scene: (2) Non-Emerg, (3) Emergency

RESPONSE OUTCOME:
Transported By This Unit, Care Transfer/Another Unit, Cancelled Enroute, Cancelled On Scene, False Call/No Patient Found, Dead on Scene, Refused Treatment, Treated, Refused Transport, P.O.V., Standby, Unknown, Other

CALL RECEIVED — ENROUTE — ARRIVE SCENE — DEPART SCENE — ARRIVE HOSPITAL — RETURN TO SERVICE (MILITARY TIME)

INCIDENT LOCATION: Residence, Interstate, Highway, Street/Road, Public Access, Industrial/Off., HMO/Clinic/Doctors Office, Hospital, Other

DISPATCH/INCIDENT TYPE: Abdominal Pain, Asphyxiation/Choke, Chest Pain, Diff. Breathing, Drowning, Heat/Cold Problems, Ill Person, OB/GYN, OD/Poison, Person Down/Unconsc., Psych/Behavioral, Seizures, Other Medical, MVA, MVA - Motorcycle, MVA - Ped/Bike, Assault, Assault - Sexual, Bite/Sting, Burn/Elect., Fall, Person Trapped, Stab/Gunshot, Other Trauma, Standby, InterFacility Transfer

SUSPECTED MEDICAL ILLNESS (P=Primary, S=Secondary):
Abdom. Pain, Airway Obstr, Allergic React, Cancer Compli, Cardiac Arrest, Cardiac Sympt., Chest Pain, Childbirth, COPD, Diabetes Comp., Drug Reaction, Heat/Cold Problems, Inhalation, OB/GYN, OD/Poison, Psych/Behv, Resp. Arrest, Resp. Dist, Seizures, Stroke, Syncope, Unconscious, Other

INJURY SITE/TYPE (Amputate, Bite/Sting, Blunt-Major, Burn/Elec, Frac/Disloc, Penetrate, Soft-Closed, Soft-Open): None, Head, Face, Eye, Neck, Chest, Back, Upper Ext, Abdomen, Pelvis, Lower Ext

MECHANISM OF INJURY: Flail Chest, Burns 10+%/face/arwy, Fall 20+ feet, Speed 40+ mph, 20+ speed change, Deformity 20+", Intrusion 12+", Rollover, Ejection, Death same MV, Pedest.vs. MV 5+mph, Pedst. thrown/run over, Mtcycle 20+mph/sep., Extrication >15 min.

GLASGOW COMA SCALE
EYES	VERBAL	MOTOR
(4) Spontaneous	(5) Oriented	(6) Obeys Comm.
(3) To Voice	(4) Confused	(5) Pain-Local.
(2) To Pain	(3) Inappropriate	(4) Pain-Withdraws
(1) Unresponsive	(2) Garbled	(3) Pain-Flexion
	(1) None	(2) Pain-Extends
		(1) None

PRIOR AID: None, CPR, Extricate, Wound Mgt — Fire, Police, 1st Resp., Rescue, Bystander

THIS PATIENT LOCATION/PROTECTION: Driver, Front Pass, Rear Pass, Other, Unknown; Shlder/Lap Belt, Shoulder Belt, Lap Belt, Safety Seat, Helmet; Not Used, Not Available, Unknown; Airbag (Deployed) Yes

SEX: F M — **AGE** (Months, Apprx.)

INITIAL VITAL SIGNS: Unable to Take, Not Taken, Pt. Refused — SYSTOLIC, DIASTOLIC, PULSE, RESP, PUPILS (L R: N, D, C, NR)

This Patient Resident of: City, County, Arizona, Out of State, Unknown

BLS TREATMENT (A1 A2 A3 O): Assessment, C-Spine Precautions, Oxygen, CPR, Crisis Intervention, Defibrillation (AUTO), Extrication, Fracture Stabilize, Hemorrhage Control, Ipecac/Charcoal Admin., MAST Application, MAST Inflation, Monitor IV, Oral Care/Airway, Oral Glucose, Restraints Applied, Suction, Traction Splint, Wound Management, Other

ALS TREATMENT (A1 A2 A3 O): Cardiac Monitoring, Cardioversion, Cricothyroidotomy, Defibrillation, EOA, Intubation - Nasal, Intubation - Oral, IV-Central, IV-Peripheral, Medication Admin, NG Tube, Needle Thoracostomy, Phlebotomy, SVN

CPR INFORMATION: Time: Minutes (<4, 4-10, >10, Unk), Arrest to CPR, Arrest to Defib, Arrest to ALS, Witnessed Arrest? (Y N Unk), Pulse/Rhythm Restored? (Y N), Traumatic Cardiac Arrest? (Y N)

ATTEMPTS: IV (1 2 3 U), ET (1 2 3 U), OTH (1 2 3 U)

MEDICATIONS: Albuterol, Aminoph., Atropine 1/10, Atropine 8/20, Bretylium, Calcium Chl., D50, Diazepam, Diphenhydram., Dopamine, Epi 1:1000, Epi 1:10,000, Furosemide, Isoetharine, Isoproteranol, Lidocaine-Bolus, Lidocaine Drip, Methylprednisone, Morphine, Naloxone, Nifedipine, Nitrostat. Tab., Nitrous Oxide, Oxytocin, Phenobarbital, Sodium Bicarbonate, Thiamine, Verapamil, Other, HAZMAT

EKG INITIAL/LAST: Nrml Sinus, Sinus Tach, Sinus Brady, Asystole, AV Block, Atrial Fib, Atrial Flut, EMD, Junctional, Paced, SV Tach, Vent Tach, Vent Fib, Other, PVC's

IV TYPE/RATE (TKO, Bolus, Wide, Other): D5W, Normal Saline, Ringers Lact., Other

 # LINES: # Peripheral, # Central

MEDICAL CONTROL: First, Hospital — Radio/Good, Radio/Poor, Protocol, Telephone, Radio/Phone Patch, Cellular, Phys On-Scene, None Required, Unable

ORDERS BY: Protocol, Standing, Verbal

PT. RECEIVED BY

RESEARCH CODE

PATIENT DISPOSITION: Improved, Worsened, Unchanged, Died in ER

MISCELLANEOUS: If Multiple Pts On Scene, How Many? If Transport to Level 1 Receiving Facility, Due to: Pt. Condition, Mechanism

EMS FIRST CARE FORM - ARIZONA DEPARTMENT OF HEALTH SERVICES — Return to State EMS Office

SCANTRON® FORM NO. F-3087-EMS 0792-C 671-5 4 3 2 1 © 1992 EMS DATA SYSTEMS

2002094

PLEASE DO NOT MARK IN THIS AREA

Figure 27-3 Arizona PCR combines a scannable side and a narrative side.

Incident Date ____/____/____   Incident Number _____

MEDS/EMSCOM/Private# _____   Billing# _____

Dispatcher _____   Call Received from _____

Provider Agency Name _____   City/Cnty Base _____

Unit Personnel & ID# _____   Additional Units _____

_____

Patient Name _____   Insurance/Medicare# _____

Address _____   Nearest Relative _____

Zip Code _____

Phone: _____ DOB ____/____/____   SSN _____

Family Doctor _____   Allergies _____

Medications _____

_____

Incident Location _____

Incident Description _____

Injury/Illness Description _____

_____

_____

_____

_____

_____

_____

_____

_____

_____

_____

_____

_____

_____

	TIME	DR	ORDERS

Vital Signs	Time							
	BP							
	Pulse							
	Resp							

I the undersigned have been advised of and understand my condition and the risks of refusing care.
If I refuse care I hereby release the above named Agency of all responsibility.

TIME	DOSE	MEDICATIONS

[ ] I CONSENT TO TREATMENT/TRANSPORT   [ ] I REFUSE TREATMENT/TRANSPORT

[ ] VERBAL [ ] IMPLIED [ ] INCOMPETENT   SIGNATURE _____

SIGNATURE CONSENT

WITNESSES _____   WITNESSES _____

DRUG BOX ISSUED# _____

MD OR RN RECEIVING PATIENT _____   PERSON FILING REPORT _____   ISSUED BY

1st Responder/Rescue Unit Only   Unit ID# _____

Personnel & ID# _____   Time Responded: _____

_____

5085

Care Transferred To: (Unit type and EMSCOM/MEDS ID#)

2002094

PATIENT'S RECORD

Figure 27-3 (continued) Arizona PCR, narrative side.

MAINE EMS

PRESS DOWN, YOU ARE MAKING THREE COPIES

RUN REPORT #	Mo.	Day	Year	M T W Th F S Sun	SERVICE NAME	SERVICE NO.	VEHICLE NO.	ALS ☐ Performed ☐ Back-up Called	SERVICE RUN NO.
746118									

NAME | BILLING INFORMATION

STREET OR R.F.D.

CITY/TOWN | STATE | ZIP

AGE / DATE OF BIRTH | ☐ Male ☐ Female | PHONE

INCIDENT LOCATION: ADDRESS | CITY/TOWN

TRANSPORTED TO: | TREATING / FAMILY PHYSICIAN | CREW LICENSE NUMBERS

TRANSPORTATION / COMMUNICATIONS PROBLEMS

☐ Medical
- ☐ Cardiac
- ☐ Poisoning/OD
- ☐ Respiratory
- ☐ Behavioral
- ☐ Diabetic
- ☐ Seizure
- ☐ CVA
- ☐ OB/Gyn
- ☐ Other ______

☐ Trauma
- ☐ Multi-Systems Trauma
- ☐ Head
- ☐ Spinal
- ☐ Burn
- ☐ Soft Tissue Injury
- ☐ Fractures
- ☐ Other ______

☐ Code 99

R	L	LUNG SOUNDS
☐	☐	CLEAR
☐	☐	ABSENT
☐	☐	DECREASED
☐	☐	RALES
☐	☐	WHEEZE
☐	☐	STRIDOR

TYPE OF RUN
- ☐ Emergency Transport
- ☐ Routine Transfer
- ☐ Emergency Transfer
- ☐ No Transport
- ☐ Refused Transport

TIME	CODE		ODOMETER
		Call Received	
		Enroute	
		At Scene	
		From Scene	
		At Destination	
		In Service	

☐ MEDICATIONS ☐ ALLERGIES

CHIEF COMPLAINT:

TIME	PULSE	RESP	BP	PUPILLARY RESPONSE	SKIN	VERBAL RESPONSE	MOTOR RESPONSE	EYE OPENING RESPONSE	CAPILLARY REFILL
			/			5 4 3 2 1	6 5 4 3 2 1	4 3 2 1	☐ Normal ☐ Delayed ☐ None
			/			5 4 3 2 1	6 5 4 3 2 1	4 3 2 1	☐ Normal ☐ Delayed ☐ None
			/			5 4 3 2 1	6 5 4 3 2 1	4 3 2 1	☐ Normal ☐ Delayed ☐ None

☐ MVA ☐ Concern AOB/ETOH SEAT BELTS: ☐ Used ☐ Not Used ☐ N/A ☐ Helmet Used

MUTUAL AID: Assisted/Assisted by Service # __________ Time Called: __________

PATIENT'S SUSPECTED PROBLEM: 746118

	Cleared Airway		Extrication
	Artificial Respiration/BVM		Cervical Immobilization
	Oropharyngeal Airway		KED/Short Board
	Nasopharyngeal Airway		Long Board
	CPR—Time:		Restraints
	Bystander CPR		Traction Splinting
	AED		General Splinting
	Suction		Cold Application
	Oxygen—LPMin___ ☐ Nasal ☐ Mask		MAST Inflated
	Pulse Oximetry		
	Autovent		

☐ Medication Administered | ☐ Defib Lic #______

☐ Monitor | ☐ Chest Decomp

☐ Pacing | ☐ Cricothyrotomy

MEDICAL CONTROL ☐ Written Order/Protocol ☐ Verbal Order/Protocol

IV — Total Attempts
- ☐ SUC LIC.# ______ ___
- ☐ UNSUC LIC.# ______ ___

EOA — Total Attempts
- ☐ SUC LIC.# ______ ___
- ☐ UNSUC LIC.# ______ ___

ET — Total Attempts
- ☐ SUC LIC.# ______ ___
- ☐ UNSUC LIC.# ______ ___

LIC #	EKG RHYTHM	TIME	MEDS / DEFIB / C-VERT	DOSE W/S	ROUTE

NAME OF E.D. TREATING PHYSICIAN SIGNATURE OF CREW MEMBER IN CHARGE

COPY 1 HOSPITAL

Figure 27-4 Maine PCR combines fill-in-the-box sections with narrative space.

Benefits of a Complete PCR

A complete PCR benefits the EMT in many ways.

Benefits for Patient Care A good PCR helps you standardize your approach to the patient and communicate your findings succinctly and in a manner that is easily understood by other medical professionals.

The usefulness of the PCR begins as soon as you arrive at the scene, providing a transition of documentation on care that was done prior to your arrival by bystanders, first responders, or other public safety agencies. Changes in the patient's vital signs, level of consciousness, circulatory or neurologic responses, or the patient's overall status should always be clearly documented on the PCR. It is not uncommon for the neurologist to ask questions about the manner in which a seizure progressed or the presence of movement of a spine-injured patient prior to arrival in the critical care unit. The trauma surgeon may want to understand the mechanism of injury involved in a motor vehicle collision or pertinent information like any entrapment, impingement of metal into the vehicle, or estimated speed of impact. These are important findings that EMTs may observe at the time of the call or gather from those who were first on the scene. If not documented on the PCR, this invaluable information can be lost forever.

Once EMT care is undertaken, the PCR can be a memory jogger to assure that the EMT asks the patient the most appropriate questions. For example the patient history portion of the PCR may remind the EMT to document information found in the acronym AMPLE, which stands for allergies, medications, past medical history, last meal, and events leading up to today's incident.

To assist in organizing a proper flow of information during the EMT's radio or face-to-face report at the hospital, many PCRs are set up with highlighted areas in a logical format, such as the SOAP sequence.

All medical professionals are trained to do assessments and document them. The nurse and physician in the ED begin an entirely new assessment when they see the patient. They should review the PCR to compare your findings to theirs, just as you may have compared your findings to the first responder's. This is good continuity of medical care from the first responder to the EMT to the advanced EMT (in some instances) to the nurse to the physician. A copy of the completed PCR should become a part of the patient's hospital chart. If your PCR and the face-to-face report you give is disjointed, illogi-

cal, or in need of being translated into medical terminology, the nurse and physician may lose respect for you as a professional and discount your information. So follow the PCR or an assessment card and fill it out to help you present your patient in an organized, complete, accurate, and professional manner.

Benefits for Legal Protection of the EMT Television programs such as *Emergency* or *Rescue 911,* in which the EMS system always operates smoothly and lives are almost always saved, have created very high expectations on the part of the public. This seems to have contributed to an increase in lawsuits when things don't have a perfect outcome.

Sometimes people will take a "shotgun approach" by suing every person and every agency that was even remotely involved in the incident, from the municipality where they tripped over a crack in the sidewalk to the EMS system that responded to immobilize the injured ankle and take them to the hospital. The legal system is often so slow that years may have passed since the call that you are being questioned about in court. The PCR will be your best memory jogger, as well as legal documentation, of what actually happened during that call. If, at the time of the call, you completed the PCR accurately, completely, and legibly, it can be a very helpful document to you. If not, it can be used to discredit your testimony.

Benefits for the EMS System The PCR also provides benefits to the EMS system. The legal benefits of complete and accurate documentation are just as beneficial to the system as they are to the individual EMT. Management reports obtained from PCR data can help services improve response time, prepare for the busy hours of the day or days of the week, and justify the need for additional resources. Management cannot plan for trends if they are unaware that they exist. Perhaps the responding units would be better off in different locations, or perhaps the addition of one unit during peak hours of the day would help decrease response times, especially to priority-one calls.

The data obtained from analyzing PCRs helps to document the extent of service to the community. This is often important for budgeting, fund raising, municipal contracts, or obtaining grants.

The PCR helps the EMS system document each EMT's experience and exposure to different types of patients. Skills can be documented so that underutilized skills can be practiced during continuing education inservice. Many services are able to tell EMTs how often they did specific skills listed on the PCR such as CPR, spinal immobilization, traction splinting, and emergency childbirth. The service medical director and continuous quality improvement coordinator will use the PCRs as means of identifying trends in service that require additional emphasis in the continuing education of EMTs as well as specific calls where the crew deserves a "pat on the back" for a job well done.

The PCR can also benefit the regional or state EMS system by providing statistical reports to evaluate trends of calls over many local services. These trends can lead to the development of new protocols or training programs. As the U.S. Department of Transportation develops the national standard EMT curriculum, it is able to take into consideration trends in prehospital care as revealed by such documentation and analysis at the state level.

In 1993 the federal government awarded a series of grants to Hawaii, Maine, Missouri, New York, Pennsylvania, Utah, and Wisconsin to match motor vehicle crash data with PCR data with in-hospital data to study the effects of seat belts and motorcycle helmets on the costs of health care. Your accuracy on the PCR can be very important to studies of this type which may have a considerable impact on shifting the emphasis of federal laws, regulations, or traffic safety dollars and human lives.

Completing a Prehospital Care Report

Do not delegate the documentation of the call to the person with the least training. If you ever get involved in a lawsuit, you will be sorry that your form was written by the least trained individual on the call! Use the SOAP format and document your professional observations within the scope of your training. If you document a statement from the patient, use quotation marks (e.g., *The patient stated, "I wanted to kill myself"* or *The patient said, "I drank about six beers"*). Document pertinent negatives that apply to the chief complaint (e.g., *Patient denies any loss of consciousness after striking his head*, or *Patient stated, "I didn't pass out."*).

Make sure the form is as accurate as possible. When documenting times, make sure your watch corresponds with the dispatcher's clock.

Just as important as knowing what to write is knowing what *not* to write. Write what you observed without making conclusions that you are not trained to make (e.g., write *The patient smelled of ETOH* rather than *Patient was drunk*). Do not write innuendoes, unprofessional language, slang, or derogatory statements. The "acid test" for a PCR is to ask yourself, "How would I feel if this was printed in the newspapers tomorrow?" or "What would the grand jury have to say about this PCR?"

Always give every member of the crew an opportunity to review and add comments to the PCR before handing it in.

Common Medical Abbreviations It is acceptable to use abbreviations on a PCR provided they are commonly used and known by all medical professionals who might read your documentation. Do not make up your own abbreviations, because only you will understand them and they will make your PCR unclear to others. Table 27-1 lists abbreviations and their meanings that are commonly used by EMTs and other medical professionals.

Sections of a Prehospital Care Report Here are some tips on how to fill out the various sections of a typical PCR.

- Call Dispatch Information—This section can be completed as you receive the assignment or at a later time in the call prior to turning in the PCR. Usually this section includes the priority, call type, location and cross street, special information, telephone instructions you were given, the date, agency name, vehicle or unit identification number, and the run number.
- Call Times—Most forms have a spot to fill in the time the call was received by the EMS unit, time en route to the call, time at the scene, time en route to the hospital, time of arrival at the hospital, and time your unit is back in service. Two other times are useful to analysis of the system response to the call but not always obtainable. They are the time the call was received by the dispatch center and the time of arrival at the patient's side. Only military time is used on PCRs. The EMT will need to learn how to convert regular time (in 12-hour spans) to military time (in 24-hour spans). There are a few tips to remember.

Midnight is 24:00
Noon is 12:00
All times after noon are the regular time plus 12 (ie: 1 p.m. = 13:00)
One minute after midnight is 00:01

TABLE 27-1 Common Medical Abbreviations

b.i.d.	twice a day
BP	blood pressure
CA	cancer
CAD	coronary artery disease
C/C or C.C.	chief complaint
CHF	congestive heart failure
c/o	complains of
CPR	cardiopulmonary resuscitation
COPD	chronic obstructive pulmonary disease
CVA	cerebral vascular accident
D.C.	discontinue
DOA	dead on arrival
Dx	diagnosis
EKG, ECG	electrocardiogram
ED	emergency department
ETOH	alcohol
Fx	fracture
GI	gastrointestinal
GU	genitourinary
Hg	mercury
Hx	history
IM	intramuscular
IV	intravenous
LOC	loss of consciousness
MI	myocardial infarction
MS	multiple sclerosis
NPO	nothing by mouth
OB	obstetrics
O.R.	operating room
p.o.	by mouth
pt.	patient
q	every
q.h.	every hour
q.i.d.	four times a day
R/O	rule out
Rx	treatment
S.C. or S.Q.	subcutaneous
S.L.	sublingual (under the tongue)
S.O.B.	shortness of breath
stat	immediately
t.i.	three times a day
V.S.	vital signs

- Patient Identification Information—This section of the PCR can be completed at the hospital after the call if patient care does not permit the time to complete it en route to the hospital. It includes the patient's name, address, age, date of birth, sex, phone number, physician, and insurance information. For unidentified patients, most systems use the race and sex (e.g., *unknown white male*).
- Mechanism of Injury—Some EMS systems collect information about the mechanism of injury (e.g., motor vehicle collision, fall, assault, etc.). Also the type of location where the injury occurred may be entered (work, home, road, recreational, etc). Other PCRs also designate if personal safety equipment was used for motor vehicle collisions (e.g., seat belts, airbags).

- Chief Complaint and Presenting Problems—The *chief complaint* is the reason why the ambulance was called, such as a motor vehicle collision. The *presenting problems* are usually more specific and often tied to local treatment protocols (e.g., respiratory distress, pain, cardiac arrest, burns, general body weakness, etc.). This information is the subjective information obtained from the patient describing his or her illness or injury.
- Past Medical History, Physical Exam, and Vitals—This is the objective information on the patient: the physical signs that the EMT observes and the vital signs that are taken. This section is very important and most PCRs have room for multiple sets of vital signs. Often this section will also include the Glascow Coma Scale, the trauma score, and a status determination such as CUPS (critical, unstable, potentially unstable, or stable). When listing medications, indicate clearly whether each is a medication that was taken or a medication the patient is allergic to. If you need additional space, use the narrative section.
- Treatments Given—There will be a list of treatments that may have been done in the field. What is on the list depends on whether the PCR is a form for BLS only or is a combined form for BLS and ALS (basic life support performed by EMTs, advanced life support performed by paramedics). Any treatment that is not listed with a check box should be clearly described in the narrative section.
- Narrative Section—Be sure to document all unusual incidents that happen on the call, such as a delayed response time caused by weather conditions. Document if there are changes in the patient's condition en route to the hospital and *any* special information that should be relayed to the hospital that the non-narrative sections did not allow you to cover. This is the section where it is important to quote the patient.
- Call Disposition—Every call has a disposition, and it should be documented on the PCR. Many systems use a numbering system for the hospitals you may have transported the patient to as well as other possible dispositions such as "cancelled," "gone on arrival," or "handled by another unit."

One disposition that is somewhat controversial is the refusal of medical aid or transportation (RMA). Make sure that your instructor clearly advises you of the local policy for documenting an RMA. The most important part of the process is that you clearly document what you did, exactly what you explained to the patient, how many times the patient was given the option to be taken to the hospital, and who witnessed what you said to the patient.

If your state's PCR has a section for the patient to sign, make sure it is read to him and witnessed when he signs it. Upon arrival at the hospital, some regions require a signature from the physician or nurse who receives the patient. This is done in busier hospitals for fear that a patient might not get turned over to a medical person when the ED staff is very busy. It should be a standard practice that no patient is left in the ED until turned over to a physician or nurse to whom you give your face-to-face presentation of the SOAP information on the patient.

- Agency, Unit, and Crew Identification—The PCR has a section to document your agency name, the unit number, and the names and training levels of the crew members who were on the call. Some forms designate who the driver was as well as who was in charge of the call.
- Other Useful Information—The PCR may also contain other useful details about the call such as an expanded section for insurance and billing information, if this is not on a supplemental form. Some forms have a spot to list the number of patients on this call as well as the means of communication with the hospital and if any transmission difficulties were encountered. A number of state PCRs now include information on the care that was being provided prior to the arrival of the EMS unit. This is especially important for CPR studies involving the use of bystander CPR. Another area that is beginning to show up on forms is the rea-

son for hospital selection (i.e., patient's choice, trauma center, protocol, etc.).

Your instructor will inform you of the distribution of the copies of the PCR. Most areas use a three part form where the original copy goes to the EMS agency and a copy goes to the patient's chart and a copy to the ED.

Other EMS Reports

Many states, such as New York and North Carolina, use a supplemental form for ALS calls or additional documentation for calls that were complex or involved (Figure 27-5).

Most agencies have a special incident report to document equipment failures, incidents such as a hazardous materials incident or a multiple casualty incident, or exposure of the crew to an infectious agent. These forms are usually agency specific rather than standardized statewide. An example of a special incident report from New York State's Town of Colonie EMS Department is shown in Figure 27-6.

Finally an example of a form that can be used by EMS agencies in the event that an EMS vehicle is involved in a collision is shown in Figure 27-7. There are often many forms used at the agency level, and the EMT should become familiar with their proper use.

The future of PCRs can be seen in some of the more innovative EMS systems that are already using notebook computers and pen computer devices. EMTs may receive their computer, enter their identifier, then read the day's messages, complete continuing education lessons programmed into the computer system, input all the day's PCR documentation, and then download the computer by telephone modem into the main computer that directly bills the patient's insurance. These technologies are new to EMS but not new to the transportation industry. Overnight package delivery companies have used handheld computers to document deliveries for many years.

CONTINUATION FORM
for the
Prehospital Care Report

Press Down Firmly. You're Making 4 Copies.

M	D	Y		RUN NO
DATE				

AGENCY CODE   VEH. ID.

Name	Agency Name	Enter PCR ID# (Top Center of PCR)	

ADDITIONAL HISTORY & PHYSICAL EXAM FINDINGS

Weight in Kilograms

R BREATH SOUNDS L	NECK VEINS	EDEMA	ABDOMEN
☐ Normal ☐	☐ Normal	☐ Pedal	☐ Normal
☐ Decreased ☐	☐ Distended	☐ Sacral	☐ Tender
☐ Absent ☐	TRACHEAL SHIFT	☐ Ascites	☐ Rigid
☐ Rales ☐		☐ Other	☐ Distended
☐ Rhonchi ☐	R ☐ L ☐		☐ Other
☐ Wheezes ☐			

SERIAL VITAL SIGNS, EKG, RHYTHMS, MEDICATIONS AND TREATMENT

TIME	RESP.	PULSE	B.P.	LEVEL OF CONSCIOUSNESS	EKG RHYTHMS	DEFIBRILLATION CARDIOVERSION	MEDICATIONS	DOSE	ROUTE
	Rate: ☐ Regular ☐ Shallow ☐ Labored	Rate: ☐ Regular ☐ Irregular		☐ Alert ☐ Voice ☐ Pain ☐ Unresp.	☐ NSR ☐ Brady. ☐ Asystole ☐ IVR ☐ V. Fib. ☐ V. Tach. ☐ PVC ☐ SVT ☐ Other		☐ Epinephrine ☐ Dopamine ☐ Naloxone ☐ Atropine ☐ Sodium Bicarb. ☐ Bretylium ☐ Dextrose ☐ Isoproterenol ☐ Nitroglyc. ☐ Lidocaine ☐ Lasix ☐ Other		☐ IV ☐ ET ☐ IM ☐ SL ☐ SQ ☐ PO ☐ Nebulizer
	Rate: ☐ Regular ☐ Shallow ☐ Labored	Rate: ☐ Regular ☐ Irregular		☐ Alert ☐ Voice ☐ Pain ☐ Unresp.	☐ NSR ☐ Brady. ☐ Asystole ☐ IVR ☐ V. Fib. ☐ V. Tach. ☐ PVC ☐ SVT ☐ Other		☐ Epinephrine ☐ Dopamine ☐ Naloxone ☐ Atropine ☐ Sodium Bicarb. ☐ Bretylium ☐ Dextrose ☐ Isoproterenol ☐ Nitroglyc. ☐ Lidocaine ☐ Lasix ☐ Other		☐ IV ☐ ET ☐ IM ☐ SL ☐ SQ ☐ PO ☐ Nebulizer
	Rate: ☐ Regular ☐ Shallow ☐ Labored	Rate: ☐ Regular ☐ Irregular		☐ Alert ☐ Voice ☐ Pain ☐ Unresp.	☐ NSR ☐ Brady. ☐ Asystole ☐ IVR ☐ V. Fib. ☐ V. Tach. ☐ PVC ☐ SVT ☐ Other		☐ Epinephrine ☐ Dopamine ☐ Naloxone ☐ Atropine ☐ Sodium Bicarb. ☐ Bretylium ☐ Dextrose ☐ Isoproterenol ☐ Nitroglyc. ☐ Lidocaine ☐ Lasix ☐ Other		☐ IV ☐ ET ☐ IM ☐ SL ☐ SQ ☐ PO ☐ Nebulizer
	Rate: ☐ Regular ☐ Shallow ☐ Labored	Rate: ☐ Regular ☐ Irregular		☐ Alert ☐ Voice ☐ Pain ☐ Unresp.	☐ NSR ☐ Brady. ☐ Asystole ☐ IVR ☐ V. Fib. ☐ V. Tach. ☐ PVC ☐ SVT ☐ Other		☐ Epinephrine ☐ Dopamine ☐ Naloxone ☐ Atropine ☐ Sodium Bicarb. ☐ Bretylium ☐ Dextrose ☐ Isoproterenol ☐ Nitroglyc. ☐ Lidocaine ☐ Lasix ☐ Other		☐ IV ☐ ET ☐ IM ☐ SL ☐ SQ ☐ PO ☐ Nebulizer
	Rate: ☐ Regular ☐ Shallow ☐ Labored	Rate: ☐ Regular ☐ Irregular		☐ Alert ☐ Voice ☐ Pain ☐ Unresp	☐ NSR ☐ Brady. ☐ Asystole ☐ IVR ☐ V. Fib. ☐ V. Tach. ☐ PVC ☐ SVT ☐ Other		☐ Epinephrine ☐ Dopamine ☐ Naloxone ☐ Atropine ☐ Sodium Bicarb. ☐ Bretylium ☐ Dextrose ☐ Isoproterenol ☐ Nitroglyc. ☐ Lidocaine ☐ Lasix ☐ Other		☐ IV ☐ ET ☐ IM ☐ SL ☐ SQ ☐ PO ☐ Nebulizer
	Rate: ☐ Regular ☐ Shallow ☐ Labored	Rate: ☐ Regular ☐ Irregular		☐ Alert ☐ Voice ☐ Pain ☐ Unresp	☐ NSR ☐ Brady. ☐ Asystole ☐ IVR ☐ V. Fib. ☐ V. Tach. ☐ PVC ☐ SVT ☐ Other		☐ Epinephrine ☐ Dopamine ☐ Naloxone ☐ Atropine ☐ Sodium Bicarb. ☐ Bretylium ☐ Dextrose ☐ Isoproterenol ☐ Nitroglyc. ☐ Lidocaine ☐ Lasix ☐ Other		☐ IV ☐ ET ☐ IM ☐ SL ☐ SQ ☐ PO ☐ Nebulizer
	Rate: ☐ Regular ☐ Shallow ☐ Labored	Rate: ☐ Regular ☐ Irregular		☐ Alert ☐ Voice ☐ Pain ☐ Unresp	☐ NSR ☐ Brady. ☐ Asystole ☐ IVR ☐ V. Fib. ☐ V. Tach. ☐ PVC ☐ SVT ☐ Other		☐ Epinephrine ☐ Dopamine ☐ Naloxone ☐ Atropine ☐ Sodium Bicarb. ☐ Bretylium ☐ Dextrose ☐ Isoproterenol ☐ Nitroglyc. ☐ Lidocaine ☐ Lasix ☐ Other		☐ IV ☐ ET ☐ IM ☐ SL ☐ SQ ☐ PO ☐ Nebulizer

COMMENTS:

MEDICAL FACILITY CONTACTED

CREW	ADDITIONAL NAME — CREW	ADDITIONAL NAME — CREW	ADDITIONAL NAME — CREW	ADDITIONAL NAME — CREW
	☐ EMS-FR ☐ EMT ☐ AEMT #	☐ EMS-FR ☐ EMT ☐ AEMT #	☐ EMS-FR ☐ EMT ☐ AEMT #	☐ EMS-FR ☐ EMT ☐ AEMT #

EMS 100A (11/86) provided by NYS-EMS PROGRAM

AGENCY COPY/**WHITE**   HOSPITAL PATIENT RECORD COPY/**PINK**   RESEARCH COPY/**BLUE**   EXTRA SERVICE COPY/**GREEN**

PAGE _____ OF _____

Figure 27-5 Supplemental form from New York State.

Special Incident Report

Town of Colonie
Department of Emergency Medical Services ——

EMERGENCY MEDICAL SERVICES
TOWN OF COLONIE

Date of Incident: _____   Time: _____   REMO #: _____

Town Run #: _____   Reported by: _____   Zone: _____

Type of Incident: ❑ MCI ❑ Rescue ❑ Personnel Matter ❑ Injury ❑ Accident with an EMS vehicle
❑ Infectious Disease Exposure ❑ Scene Conflict ❑ Other _____

Total # of Patients: ❑ #P-1: ____ ❑ #P-2: ____ ❑ #P-3: ____ ❑ #P-0: ____
Elapsed Scene Time: *(First unit arrival to last unit to hospital)* _____
Total Time of Incident: _____

Describe the Incident Below:
Attach any additional documentation such as news clippings and the pre-hospital care report.
Attach additional sheets if necessary.

_____
_____
_____
_____
_____
_____
_____
_____
_____
_____
_____
_____
_____
_____
_____
_____
_____
_____
_____
_____

Signature: _____   Date: _____

Office Use Only
This incident relates to: ❑ Day Operation: TOT   ❑ Night Operations: TOT: ❑ Administration: TOT:
_____   _____   _____

Disposition: _____
_____
_____   Date: _____

Notifications/Copies: ❑ Director   ❑ Deputy Director   ❑ Supervisors
❑ Deputy Supervisors ❑ Senior Medics   ❑ Zone Coordinator (s)
❑ Other _____   Zone: ❑ 2 ❑ 3 ❑ 4

Figure 27-6 A special incident report from New York State's Town of Colonie EMS Department.

On-The-Spot Ambulance Collision Report

Other Vehicle

Driver's/Owner's Name_____

Address_____

City_____ State_____

Driver's License Number_____ State_____

Make, Model, Year of Vehicle_____ License Plate Number_____

Witnesses

1 . Name_____

    Address_____ City_____ State_____

2 . Name_____

    Address_____ City_____ State_____

Note: If you cannot get the name of a witness, try to get a license plate number.

Passengers

1 . Name_____

    Address_____ City_____ State_____

    Injuries_____ Hospitalized? ☐ Yes ☐ No

2 . Name_____

    Address_____ City_____ State_____

    Injuries_____ Hospitalized? ☐ Yes ☐ No

3 . Name_____

    Address_____ City_____ State_____

    Injuries_____ Hospitalized? ☐ Yes ☐ No

4 . Name_____

    Address_____ City_____ State_____

    Injuries_____ Hospitalized? ☐ Yes ☐ No

If there were injuries, which patients were transported to hospital via ambulance?

Description of Events

Date_____ Time of Day_____

Location_____

Road conditions_____

Your approximate speed_____ Other vehicle_____

Did police investigate?_____ Department_____

Officer's name_____ Badge Number_____

Who received a ticket?_____

DOH-N2491 (12/88)

Figure 27-7 A sample EMS vehicle collision report, Ambulance Accident Prevention Seminar Student Workbook, New York State Emergency Services Program, 1988.

Complete description of collision (also complete diagram) _____
_____
_____
_____
_____
_____

Diagram of Collision

1. Number each vehicle and show direction of travel by arrow.

2. Use solid line to show path before collision, dotted line after collision.

3. Pedestrians shown by_____

4. Railroad shown by_____

5. Utility poles shown by_____

6. Motorcycle shown by_____

7. Follow dotted lines to draw outline of collision.

8. Identify streets and highways by name or number.

9. Draw an arrow in the circle on the diagram indicating north.

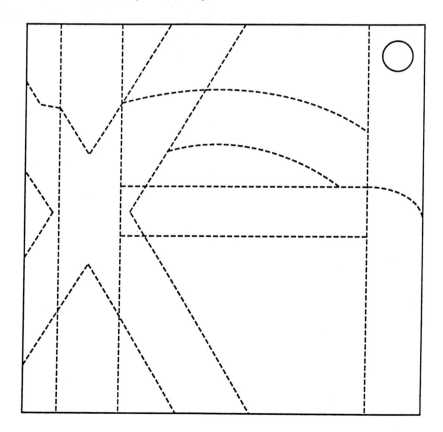

DOH-N2491 (12/88)

Figure 27-7 (continued)

SUMMARY

Face-to-Face Communication

Communication involves both verbal (oral and written) and nonverbal skills as well as face-to-face interpersonal skills. In communications involving EMT duties, be brief yet accurate and complete. Use the correct terminology, written or spoken, so that it can be understood. Communicate verbally in a calm professional manner.

Radio Communication

The basic components of an EMS radio communication system are the dispatcher base station, the ambulance radio, and the ED radio. Telephone backup should be a part of the system.

Radio communications should be limited to official use. Keep your transmission as brief and as accurate as possible. Make sure you know what you are going to say before you go on the air. Do not interrupt someone else when you transmit, including the dispatcher. Use codes only if they are a part of your system and the person you are communicating with understands the codes.

Written Reports

Correctly done PCR reports benefit patient care, protect the EMT and the EMS system in case of law suits, and benefit the entire EMS system in such tasks as allocating resources and improving EMT training.

Make your PCR and supplemental reports accurate and complete and finish them as soon as possible. Be sure all crew members are given the chance to review the PCR prior to turning it in to the hospital. Use correct medical abbreviations on PCRs and be very careful to document in a professional manner, keeping in mind that your form will become a permanent part of the patient's record.

On the Scene

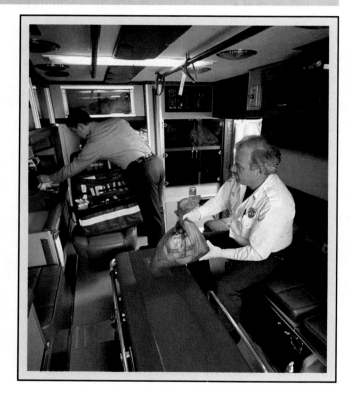

Walking from the hospital at the end of a particularly trying run, you and your partner, Bud Turley, return to your ambulance. The multiple trauma call you just finished has wreaked havoc with the patient compartment. Bud heaves a sigh as he opens the rear door of the ambulance. Inside, blood stains streak the usually clean floor and the equipment. In addition to the cleaning that will have to be done, a considerable amount of restocking is needed.

Bud: *It's going to take more than a "golden hour" to clean this up!*

You: *You got that right! Where do we start? Do you want to clean or put the kits back together?*

Bud: *I'll get the kits.*

You: *Don't forget to change the oxygen cylinders we emptied.*

Bud: *Yeah. And you be careful cleaning up in there. Don't forget to use infection control, just like with a patient.*

As the cleaning and restocking begin, you prepare by putting on a pair of heavy latex gloves. You locate the "red bag" labeled bio-hazard into which you will discard any potentially infectious wastes. You mix up some 1:100 bleach solution and begin cleaning the surfaces and soiled equipment. In the meantime, Bud has his hands full restocking kits, equipment, and supplies. As you do your separate tasks, you and Bud take advantage of the time to talk over and critique the run, something you always do, and one reason why you are such effective partners.

Terminating the run is similar to preparing for the run. The activities involved are far from exciting, but they are necessary nonetheless. An ambulance may not be placed in service without the proper equipment, and you and Bud, believers in "Murphy's Law," are sure that the piece of equipment you don't have is the one that will be needed on the next call!

Terminating the Run

Chapter Overview

An ambulance may receive another emergency call at any time—perhaps even before it can return from its current run. It is the responsibility of the EMTs to make the ambulance ready to respond to its next call as promptly and quickly as possible, with some actions toward this goal taken even before the return to quarters.

Expected Outcome, Chapter 28: *You will be able to undertake actions that will make the ambulance ready for its next run—at the hospital, during the return to quarters, and after the ambulance reaches quarters.*

Warning: Protect yourself from infectious diseases by using appropriate barrier devices such as a pocket face mask with one-way valve, face shield, or bag-valve mask; goggles or eye shield; and disposable gloves. Always conform to your local EMS system's infection exposure control plan.

AT THE HOSPITAL

EN ROUTE TO QUARTERS

IN QUARTERS

Knowledge *After reading this chapter, you should be able to*

1. List activities that should be undertaken at a medical facility to make the ambulance ready for immediate service. (pp. 698, 700; Scan 28-1)
2. List activities to make the ambulance ready for service that should be undertaken during the return to quarters. (p. 701)

3. List activities that should be undertaken in quarters to make the ambulance ready for service. (pp. 701, 704; Scan 28-2)

Skills *As an EMT you should be able to*

- Carry out procedures that will prepare the ambulance and its equipment for service when you are at the hospital, en route to quarters, and in quarters.

A
n ambulance run is not really over until the personnel and equipment that comprise the prehospital emergency care delivery system are ready for the next response.

The functions of EMTs in this final phase of activity include more than just changing the stretcher linen and cleaning the ambulance. A number of tasks must be accomplished at the hospital, during the return to quarters, and after arrival at the station.

AT THE HOSPITAL

While still at the hospital, the ambulance crew should begin making the ambulance ready to respond to another call. Time, equipment, and space limitations preclude vigorous cleaning of the ambulance while it is parked at the hospital. However, you should make every effort to quickly prepare the vehicle for the next patient (Scan 28-1).

1. Quickly clean the patient compartment while wearing rubber gloves according to Centers for Disease Control (CDC) and Occupational Safety and Health Administration (OSHA) guidelines. Follow biohazard disposal procedures according to your agency's exposure control plan. Examples

of biohazards are contaminated dressings and used suction catheters.

- Clean up blood, vomitus, and other body fluids that may have soiled the floor. Wipe down any equipment that has been splashed. Place disposable towels directly in a red bag.
- Remove and dispose of trash such as bandage wrappings, open but unused dressings, and similar items.
- Sweep away caked dirt that may have been tracked into the patient compartment. When the weather is inclement, sponge up water and mud from the floor.
- Bag dirty linens or blankets to be appropriately laundered.
- Use a deodorizer to neutralize odors of vomit, urine, and feces. Various sprays and concentrates are available for this purpose.

2. Prepare respiratory equipment for service.

- Clean and disinfect nondisposable used bag-valve-mask units and other reusable parts of respiratory-assist and inhalation therapy devices to keep them from becoming reservoirs of infectious agents that can easily contaminate the next patient. Disinfect the suction unit.
- Place used disposable items in a plastic bag and seal it. Replace the items with similar ones carried in the ambulance as spares.

Actions That Can Be Taken at the Hospital

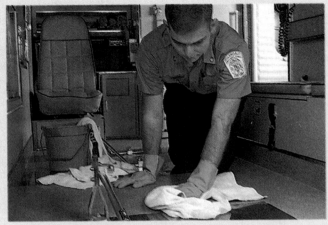

1. Clean the ambulance interior as required.

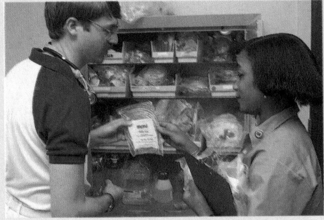

2. Replace respiratory equipment as required.

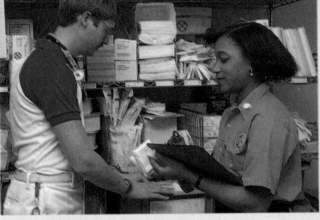

3. Replace expendable items according to local policies.

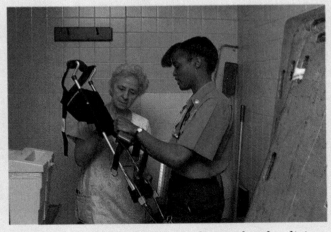

4. Exchange equipment according to local policies.

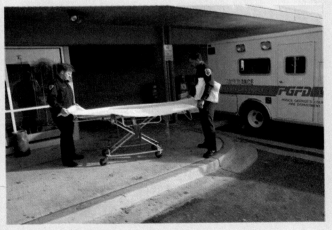

5. Make up the wheeled stretcher.

699

3. Replace expendable items.

- If you have a supplies replacement agreement with the hospital, replace expendable items from the hospital storerooms on a one-for-one basis—items such as sterile dressings, bandaging materials, towels, disposable masks, disposable gloves, sterile water, and oral airways.
- Do not take advantage of this exchange program. Keep in mind that the constant abuse of a supplies replacement program usually leads to its discontinuation. At the very least, abuse places a strain on ambulance-hospital relations.

4. Exchange equipment according to your local policy.

- Exchange items such as splints and spine boards. Several benefits are associated with an equipment exchange program: there is no need to subject patients to injury-aggravating movements just to recover equipment, crews are not delayed at the hospital, and ambulances can return to quarters fully equipped for the next response.
- When equipment is available for exchange, quickly inspect it for completeness and operability. Parts are sometimes lost or broken when an immobilizing device is removed from a patient.
- If you do find that a piece of equipment is broken or incomplete, notify someone in authority so the device can be repaired or replaced.

5. Make up the ambulance cot. The following procedure is one of many that can be used to make up a wheeled ambulance stretcher.

- Remove unsoiled blankets and place them on a clean surface.
- Remove the pillow case and place the pillow on a clean surface.
- Remove all soiled linen and place it in the designated receptacle.
- Raise the stretcher to the high-level position, if possible; this makes the procedure easier. The stretcher should be flat.
- Lower the side rails and unfasten straps.
- Clean the mattress surface with an appropriate detergent if necessary.
- Turn the mattress over; rotation adds to the life of the mattress.

- Center the bottom sheet on the mattress and open it fully. If a full-sized bed sheet is used, first fold it lengthwise.
- Tuck the sheet under each end of the mattress; form square corners and then tuck under each side.
- Place a disposable pad, if one is used, on the center of the mattress.
- Fully open the blanket. If a second blanket is used, open it fully and match it to the first blanket. This task should be done with an EMT at each end of the stretcher.
- Open a top sheet in the same way, placing it on top of the blanket. Fold the blanket(s) and top sheet together lengthwise to match the width of the stretcher; fold one side first, then the other.
- Tuck the foot of the folded blanket(s) and sheet under the foot of the mattress.
- Tuck the head of the folded blanket(s) and sheet under the head of the mattress.
- Place the slip-covered pillow lengthwise at the head of the mattress.
- Buckle the safety straps and tuck in excess straps.
- Raise the side rails and foot rest.
- Use the securing strap to hold the pillow.

The stretcher is now ready for the next patient. It must be reemphasized that this is one of many techniques for preparing a wheeled ambulance stretcher for service. Whatever the method, it should meet the following objectives.

- Preparation for the next call should be done as soon and as quickly as possible.
- All linens, blankets, and pouches should be stored neatly on the stretcher.
- All linen and blankets should be folded or tucked so that they will be contained within the stretcher frame.
- The cot must be replaced in the ambulance.
- Any nondisposable patient care items should be replaced.
- A check should be made for equipment left in the hospital.

Note: A neatly prepared stretcher inspires the patient's confidence. Don't use stained linen, even though it might be clean. Always make the presentation of your stretcher a matter of personal and professional pride!

EN ROUTE TO QUARTERS

Emphasis should be on a safe return. An ambulance operator may practice every suggestion for safe vehicle operation while en route to the hospital and then totally disregard those suggestions during the return to quarters. Defensive driving must be a full-time effort.

1. Radio the EMD that you are returning to quarters and that you are available (or not available) for service.

   - Valuable time is lost if an EMD has to locate and alert a back-up ambulance when he does not know that a ready-for-service unit is on the road. Be sure that you notify the EMD if you stop and leave the ambulance unattended for any reason during the return to quarters.

2. Air the ambulance if necessary.

   - If the patient just delivered to the hospital has a communicable disease, or if it was not possible to neutralize disagreeable odors while at the hospital, make the return trip with the windows of the patient compartment partially open, weather permitting. If the unit has sealed windows, use the air-conditioning or ventilating system to air the patient compartment.

3. Refuel the ambulance.

   - Local policy usually dictates the frequency with which an ambulance is refueled. Some services require the operator to refuel after each run regardless of the distance traveled. In other services the policy is to refuel when the gauge reaches a certain level. At any rate the fuel should be at such a level that the ambulance can respond to an emergency and then to a medical facility without fear of running out.

IN QUARTERS

When you return to quarters, there are many activities that need to be completed before the ambulance can be placed in service and before it is ready for another call.

With the emphasis today on protection from infectious diseases, you need to take every precaution to protect yourself. It is essential that you follow the infection control guidelines according to CDC and OSHA guidelines as discussed in Chapters 1 and 23 while handling contaminated linen, cleaning the equipment, handling the respiratory equipment and cleaning the ambulance interior (where there may be many hidden nooks and crannies where the patient's blood or body fluids could be).

Once in quarters, you are ready to complete cleaning and disinfecting chores (Scan 28-2).

1. Place contaminated linens in a biohazard container, noncontaminated linens in a regular hamper.

2. Clean any equipment that touched the patient.

   - Brush stretcher covers and other rubber, vinyl, and canvas materials clean, then wash them with soap and water.

3. Clean and sanitize used nondisposable respiratory-assist and inhalation therapy equipment in the following manner.

   - Disassemble the equipment so that all surfaces are exposed.
   - Fill a large plastic container with the cleaning solution outlined in your service's infection control plan.
   - Soak the items for 10 minutes, or as directed.
   - Clean the inner and outer surfaces with a suitable brush. Inner surfaces can be cleaned with a small bottle brush, while outer surfaces can be cleaned with a hand or nail brush. Make sure all encrusted matter is removed.
   - Rinse the items with tap water.
   - Soak the items in a germicidal solution. An inhalation therapist at a local hospital can suggest a germicide suitable for respiratory equipment. Follow directions for dilution, safe handling, and soaking time. Rubber gloves are recommended when using some germicides.
   - After the prescribed soaking period, hang the equipment in a well-ventilated clean area and allow it to dry for 12 to 24 hours.

4. Clean and sanitize the patient compartment.

   - Use a germicide to clean any fixed equipment or surfaces contacted by the patient or splashed with body fluids.

Termination of Activities in Quarters

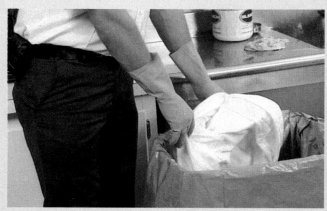

1. Place contaminated linens in a biohazard container, noncontaminated linens in a regular hamper.

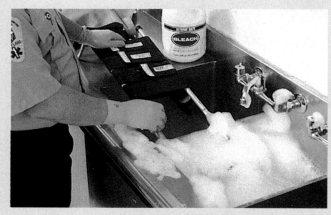

2. Remove and clean patient care equipment as required.

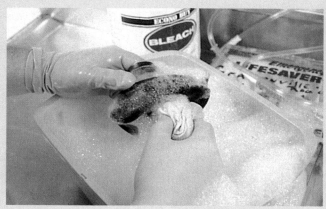

3. Clean and sanitize respiratory equipment as required.

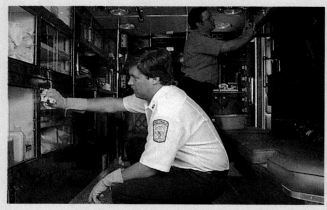

4. Clean and sanitize the ambulance interior as required. Any devices or surfaces that have come into contact with patient or his fluids must be cleaned with germicide.

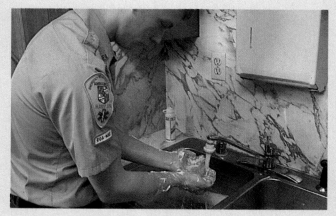

5. Wash thoroughly. Change soiled clothing. If exposed to communicable disease, this is first activity.

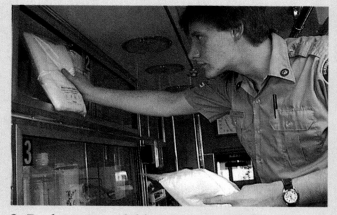

6. Replace expendable items as required.

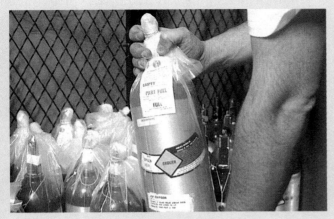

7. Always refill oxygen and air cylinders.

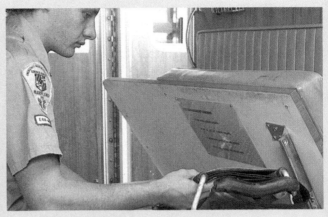

8. Replace patient care equipment as needed.

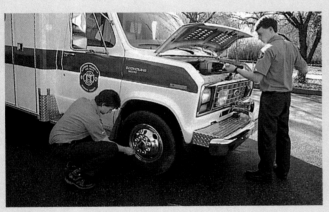

9. Maintain ambulance as required. Report problems that will take vehicle out of service.

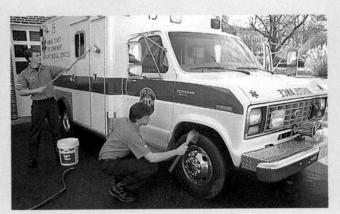

10. Clean ambulance exterior as needed.

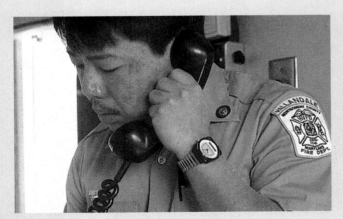

11. Report the unit ready for service.

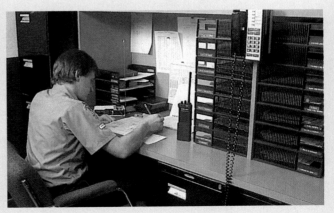

12. Complete any unfinished report forms as soon as possible.

5. Prepare yourself for service.

   - Wash thoroughly, paying attention to the areas under your fingernails. Remember that contaminants can collect there and become a source of infection not only to you but also to the persons whom you touch.
   - Change soiled clothes. Clean contaminated clothing as soon as possible, especially if you were exposed to someone with a communicable disease. It is a good policy to bring a spare uniform to work, and each EMS agency should have a washer and dryer. It is against OSHA regulations for soiled clothes to be taken home to be washed.

6. Replace expendable items with items from the unit's storeroom.

7. Refill oxygen cylinders even if only a small volume of gas was used.

8. Replace patient care equipment.

9. Carry out post-operation vehicle maintenance procedures as required. Check fluid levels, tire pressures, warning devices, lights, and so on. If you find something wrong with the vehicle, correct the problem or make someone in authority aware of it.

10. Clean the vehicle. A clean exterior lends a professional appearance to an ambulance. Check the vehicle for broken lights, glass and body damage, door operation, and other parts that may need repair or replacement.

11. Report the unit ready for service.

12. Complete any unfinished report forms as soon as possible.

SUMMARY

Termination activities begin at the hospital, continue during the return to quarters, and end when the ambulance is in quarters and completely ready for service. Disposable gloves should be worn by EMTs during any cleaning operation.

At the Hospital

Before leaving the hospital, clean the interior of the ambulance as necessary. Wipe blood, vomitus, and body fluids from the floor, equipment, and compartment surfaces. Remove any trash generated during the patient care effort. Replace disposable masks and other expendable items and exchange equipment according to local policy. Make up the ambulance stretcher.

En Route to Quarters

Radio the dispatcher that you are returning to quarters and that you can (or cannot) respond to calls. Air the ambulance (if necessary, and weather permitting) during the return to quarters. Refuel the ambulance, if necessary.

In Quarters

When in quarters, dispose of soiled linens, clean patient care and respiratory equipment, and clean and sanitize the patient compartment in accordance with your service's infection control plan. See Chapters 1 and 23 for more information on infection control procedures. Next, replenish oxygen cylinders, replace expendable items and patient care equipment, maintain and clean the ambulance, care for yourself, complete the report, and report the ambulance ready for service.

On the Scene

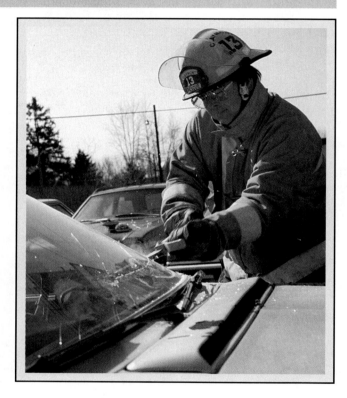

The sound of colliding metal wakes neighbors for several blocks. Your area's 911 dispatch center receives numerous calls for a "bad accident," and police, EMS, and fire-rescue units are simultaneously dispatched. Ini-

tial units arrive at the "T-bone" intersection collision and report a man trapped inside a vehicle.

Your ambulance arrives at the scene amidst the other emergency apparatus. A firefighter from the first response engine confirms that a man is trapped inside a car. You survey the scene, the vehicle, and—through the windshield—the man inside.

You: This patient appears to be unconscious with potential injuries. We have to get him out of there fast.
Fire Command: Let's get the roof off and you can do a rapid extrication vertically.

Under the Fire Command Officer's direction, one member of the fire-rescue team begins to cut out the windshield in preparation for cutting through the posts and removing the roof. Meanwhile, you and your partners put on protective clothing and prepare to conduct a rapid extrication of the patient as soon as the roof is out of the way.

With the combined efforts of the EMS and Fire Services, the man is quickly extricated and transported to a waiting trauma center in time for surgeons to save this patient's life.

Vehicle Rescue

Chapter Overview

Vehicle collisions are among the most difficult emergencies EMTs respond to. In addition to the injuries to your patient or patients, you will have to deal with the complexities and hazards of the collision scene itself. As in any hazardous situation, you must consider your own safety first.

Expected Outcome, Chapter 29: *While focusing your primary attention on your own safety and on the assessment and care of your patients, you will be able to manage hazards at the scene of a collision and to participate in the extrication of patients from a collision vehicle.*

> **WARNING:** Protect yourself from infectious diseases by using appropriate barrier devices such as a pocket face mask with one-way valve, face shield, or bag-valve mask; goggles or eye shield; and disposable gloves. Always conform to your local EMS system's infection exposure control plan.

SIZING UP THE SCENE

MANAGING COLLISION-PRODUCED HAZARDS
 Safeguarding Yourself
 Safeguarding Your Patients
 Managing Traffic
 Controlling Spectators
 Coping With Electrical Hazards
 Coping With Vehicle Fires
 Coping With Spilled Fuel
 Coping With Unstable Vehicles
 Coping With a Vehicle's Electrical System

EXTRICATING COLLISION VICTIMS
 Gaining Quick Access
 The Three-Part Extrication Procedure
 Normal and Rapid Extrication

Objectives

EMT roles in vehicle rescue vary from community to community. In some rural areas, fire departments have no rescue capabilities, and ambulance services are called upon to carry out vehicle rescue on their own. In areas where rescue and fire units are available, the ambulance may nevertheless arrive at the scene first. In this situation, time and lives can be saved if the EMTs—after calling for fire and rescue units, advanced life support, and additional ambulances if needed—are able to initiate hazard management and extrication procedures until the additional help arrives.

In any case, the main purpose of knowing extrication procedures, from the EMT's point of view, is to incorporate them into the patient care plan, to know what is involved in extricating a patient from a vehicle so that the EMT can communicate with the patient, anticipate untoward events, and initiate assessment and care as quickly as possible. No matter what is going on at a vehicle collision scene, as an EMT your primary responsibilities are always your own safety and the care of your patient.

SIZING UP THE SCENE

As you arrive on the scene of a collision, it is important to have a keen eye, because the first thing you need to do is evaluate hazards and calculate the need for additional backup: BLS and ALS (basic and advanced life support), police, fire, or rescue response, or special services such as power company representatives. Determine how many patients are involved, their priority, and the mechanisms of injury. If you think additional ambulances will be needed, call for them right away. You can always cancel them if they are not actually needed.

An important part of size-up is determining the extent of entrapment and the most appropriate means of egress for each patient. As soon as possible, evaluate if the patient is critical or stable, because the methods for removing these two categories of patient differ dramatically (see "Normal and Rapid Extrication" at the end of this chapter).

During the size-up, check to see if the vehicle is equipped with air bags. A car with an air bag has a large, rectangular steering wheel hub. Special steps should be followed if the air bag has not deployed (see "Step Three: Disentangle Occupants by Displacing the Front End" later in

this chapter). If the air bag has deployed, observers may have noticed "smoke" inside the vehicle during deployment. This is actually not smoke but dust from the cornstarch or talcum used to lubricate the bag as well as the seal and particles from within the bag. The powder may contain sodium hydroxide, which can irritate the skin. For this reason, it will be important to wear protective gloves and eye shields when you gain access to the passenger compartment and to protect to the patients from getting additional dust in their eyes or wounds.

Also during size-up, watch out for loaded bumpers. Most cars are equipped with 5 mph bumpers designed to absorb low-speed front and rear end collision damage. If the bumpers were involved in the collision, you may notice that the bumper shock absorber system is compressed, or "loaded." Never stand in front of a loaded bumper. If it springs out and strikes your knees, it will mostly likely break your legs! Some rescue teams are trained to unload the shock absorber or to chain it to prevent release.

MANAGING COLLISION-PRODUCED HAZARDS

Hazards at a collision scene can range from nuisances—such as broken glass and debris, a slippery road, inclement weather, or darkness—to severe threats to safety—such as downed wires, spilled fuel, or fire. Traffic and spectators can become hazards if they are not controlled. Some collision-related hazards must be managed, if not eliminated, before any attempt is made to reach injured persons in damaged vehicles.

Safeguarding Yourself

Collision sites can be dangerous workplaces. Jagged edges, flying glass, and fire are only a few of the hazards EMTs may deal with. Remember that you are no good as an EMT if you become a patient yourself. It is vital that you take the time to properly protect yourself prior to engaging in any rescue activities.

Human factors such as the following can also increase the potential for an EMT to be injured at a collision site.

- A careless attitude toward personal safety
- Lack of skill in tool use
- Physical problems that impede strenuous effort

Unsafe and improper acts also cause injuries.

- Failure to eliminate or control hazards
- Failure to select the proper tool for the task
- Using unsafe tools
- Failure to recognize mechanisms of injury and unsafe surroundings
- Lifting heavy objects improperly
- Deactivating safety devices designed to prevent injury
- Failure to wear highly visible outer clothing, especially when exposed to highway traffic

But the unsafe act that contributes most to collision scene injuries is

- Failure to wear protective gear during rescue operations.

Figure 29-1 shows two EMTs dressed for collision scene operations. The EMT on the left is dressed for a wide range of hazard management and extrication operations. The EMT on the right is dressed for situations where hazards are minimal.

Learn the value of protective gear, get your own if your service doesn't provide it (many states now require it on ambulances), and use it! Consider reviewing the following National Fire Protection Association standards when purchasing protective gear and uniforms: NFPA 1972 (Helmets for Structural Firefighting), NFPA 1973 (Gloves for Structural Firefighting), and NFPA 1975 (Station/Work Uniforms).

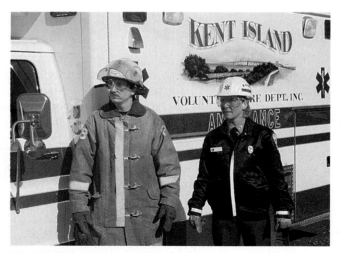

Figure 29-1 Two EMTs dressed for vehicle operations.

Following are descriptions of some kinds of personal protective gear that EMTs should use during rescue operations.

Headgear Good head protection is essential. Trendy baseball caps, uniform hats, and wool watch caps do little except protect against sunlight, identify the wearer as a member of an emergency service, or keep the head warm. Plastic "bump caps" worn by butchers and warehouse workers also do not provide adequate protection.

One good piece of headgear that does offer adequate protection is

- The *rescue helmet.* The model illustrated does not have the firefighter's helmet rear brim, which can be awkward in tight spaces, although many EMTs do prefer and use firefighters' helmets.

All helmets should be brightly colored with reflective stripes and lettering to make the wearer visible both day and night, and the Star of Life on each side to identify the wearer as an EMS worker. The level of training should also be indicated to make scene management easier when many EMS and rescue units are on hand.

Eye Protection Eye protection is vital. Hinged plastic helmet shields do not provide adequate protection; flying particles can strike the eyes from underneath or from the side. Two good forms of eye protection are

- *Safety goggles* with a soft vinyl frame that conforms to the face and indirect venting to keep them fog-free. These also suffice for infection-control eye protection.
- *Safety glasses* with large lenses and side shields. Yellow lenses make objects appear remarkably sharp on dull days or in low light.

Hand Protection Because EMTs stick their hands into all sorts of unfriendly places, every EMT should have optimal hand protection available. Good protection is afforded by

- *Firefighter's gloves*
- *Leather gloves*

Firefighter's gloves will protect an EMT's hands from a variety of sharp, hot, cold, and dangerous surfaces. They are bulky, but can be worn in most rescue situations. If greater dexterity is needed, intermediate weight leather gloves can be worn. Fabric garden or work gloves are too thin to offer adequate protection.

Body Protection An EMT will often protect his head, eyes, and hands and leave his body virtually unprotected. Light shirts or nylon jackets do little to protect from jagged metal, broken glass, or flash fires. Good upper body protection is offered by

- A *turnout coat*. A short coat is less cumbersome in tight spaces.
- A heavy-duty *EMS or rescue jacket* will protect from weather and minor injury.

As with helmets, bright colors and reflective materials make the wearer visible.

The following items offer good protection for the lower body.

- *Turnout pants* with cuffs wide enough to pull over work shoes
- *Fire-resistant trousers or jumpsuits*
- *High-top work shoes* with extended tops to protect the ankles

Protection Against Infectious Agents Any collision victim may be carrying an infectious disease. Accordingly, every rescuer should wear barrier protection whenever exposure to a collision victim's blood or other potentially infectious material is likely. For more information, see Chapter 1.

Safeguarding Your Patients

Your patients have been injured in the collision; it is imperative that further injuries not be inflicted during rescue operations. You can minimize the chance of such additional injuries by shielding the patient and exercising care. The following items (Figure 29-2) can protect the patient from heat, cold, flying particles, and other hazards.

- An *aluminized rescue blanket* offers protection from weather and, to a degree, from flying particles.
- A *lightweight vinyl-coated paper tarpaulin* can protect from weather and debris.
- A *wool blanket* should be used to protect from cold. Cover the wool blanket with an aluminized blanket or a salvage cover

whenever glass must be broken near a patient, since glass particles are just about impossible to remove from wool blankets.

- *Short and long wood spine boards* can shield a patient from contact with tools and debris.
- *Hard hats, safety goggles, industrial hearing protectors, disposable dust masks,* and *thermal masks* (in cold weather—and unless the patient is on oxygen) will protect a patient's head, eyes, ears, and respiratory passages.

Managing Traffic

Collisions almost always produce traffic problems. Often the wreckage blocks lanes of traffic. Even if it doesn't, backups are caused when drivers slow down to "rubberneck." Rescuers, firefighters, and police usually handle traffic control; but what if the ambulance EMTs are responding alone or ahead of other emergency service units?

Obviously, personal safety, rescue, and emergency care have priority. However, a two-person ambulance crew can still initiate basic traffic control, channeling vehicles past the scene.

Your ambulance with its warning lights will serve as the first form of traffic control; however, you should position other warning devices as soon as possible. Bad weather, darkness, vegetation, and curved or hilly roadways may keep approaching motorists from seeing your ambulance soon enough to stop safely.

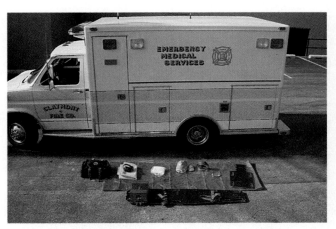

Figure 29-2 Supplies and equipment that can be used to protect the occupants of collision vehicles during rescue operations.

Using Flares for Traffic Control Although some argue that flares are unsafe, when used properly they are still a good device for warning motorists of dangerous conditions. Moreover, several dozen flares can be carried behind the front seat of an ambulance, while battery-powered flashing lights—an alternative to flares—take up valuable compartment space.

Scan 29-1 shows the proper positioning of flares at collision scenes, including a straight road, a curved road, and a hill. Keep in mind that the stopping distance for large trucks is much greater than for cars. When the road carries truck traffic, extend the flare strings beyond the distances shown.

Remember these points when you place flares.

1. Look for spilled fuel, dry vegetation, and other combustibles before you ignite and position flares, especially at a road edge.
2. Do not throw flares out of moving vehicles.
3. Position a few flares at the edge of the danger zone as soon as the ambulance is parked; they will supplement the ambulance warning lights.
4. Take a handful of flares and walk toward oncoming traffic.
5. Position the flares every 10 feet, if possible, to channel vehicles into an unblocked lane.
6. If the collision has occurred on a two-lane road, position flares in both directions.
7. Never use a flare as a traffic wand; flares can spew molten phosphorous, which can cause third degree burns to the skin.

Controlling Spectators

Spectators do more than just create problems for passing motorists. If allowed to wander freely, they will close in on the wreckage just to get a better view. They may get so close that they interfere with rescue and emergency care efforts.

Rescue squads, police, and fire units have personnel and equipment for crowd control; ambulances usually do not. However, an EMT can usually initiate some crowd-control measures. If local policies permit it, ask for assistance from one or more responsible-looking bystanders. Ask the persons you recruit to keep the spectators away from the danger zone. Give them a roll of barricade tape if you have one. Be sure not to put the recruited personnel in unsafe positions such as near spilled fuel or an unstable vehicle.

Coping With Electrical Hazards

Electricity poses many dangers at vehicle collision scenes. Keep these safety points in mind.

- High voltages are not as uncommon on roadside utility poles as people often think. In some areas, wood poles support conductors of as much as 500,000 volts.
- Assume that the entire area is extremely dangerous. Conductors may have touched and energized any part of the system, including electrical, telephone, cable television, and other wires supported by the utility pole, guy wires, ground wires, the pole itself, the ground surrounding the pole, and nearby guard rails and fences. Assume that severed or displaced conductors may be energizing every conductor and wire at the highest voltage present. Dead wires may be re-energized at any moment. Energized conductors may arc to the ground.
- Ordinary protective clothing does not protect against electrocution.

Note: When there is an electrical hazard, establish a danger zone and a safe zone. The danger zone should only be entered by individuals responsible for controlling the hazard, such as power company personnel or specialty rescue. The safe zone should be sufficiently far away to assure that an arcing or moving wire could not possibly injure any of the rescue personnel or bystanders.

Remembering these points and the following procedures may keep you alive at the scene of a collision where unconfined electricity is a hazard.

Broken Utility Pole with Wires Down A broken utility pole with wires down is very dangerous. You probably cannot work safely in the area until a power company representative assures you that the power is off and the scene is safe.

If you discover that a utility pole is broken and wires are down

1. Park the ambulance outside the danger zone.
2. Before you leave the ambulance, be sure that no portion of the vehicle, including the radio antenna, is contacting any sagging conductors.
3. Order spectators and nonessential emergency service personnel from the danger zone.

Positioning Flares to Control Traffic

Posted speed (mph)	Stopping distance for that speed*		Posted speed (in feet)		Distance of the farthest warning device
20 mph	50 feet	+	20 feet	=	70 feet
30 mph	75 feet	+	30 feet	=	105 feet
40 mph	125 feet	+	40 feet	=	165 feet
50 mph	175 feet	+	50 feet	=	225 feet
60 mph	275 feet	+	60 feet	=	335 feet
70 mph	375 feet	+	70 feet	=	445 feet

* Distances are given for passenger cars.

A. Flares are positioned according to a formula that includes the stopping distance for the posted speed plus a margin of safety.

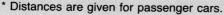
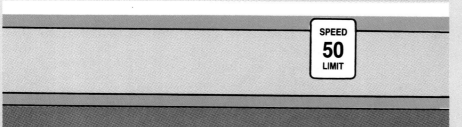

B. Flares positioned on a straight road. Approaching vehicles are moved into the correct lane before they reach the edge of the danger zone.

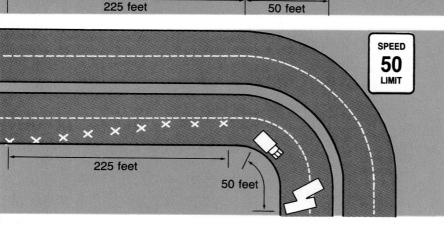

C. Flares positioned ahead of a curved section of road. The start of the curve is considered to be the edge of the danger zone.

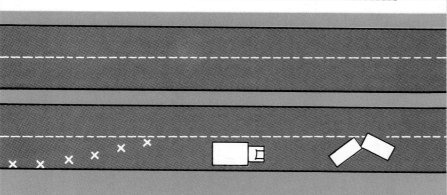

D. Flares positioned on a hill. The flares slow approaching vehicles and make them turn into the correct lane before they reach the top of the hill.

4. Discourage occupants of the collision vehicle from leaving the wreckage.
5. Prohibit traffic flow through the danger zone.
6. Determine the number of the nearest pole you can safely approach, and ask your dispatcher to advise the power company of the pole number and location.
7. Do not attempt to move downed wires. Metal implements will, of course, conduct electricity, but even implements that may not appear to be conductive, such as tools with wood handles or natural fiber ropes, may have a high moisture content that will conduct electricity and may cause a well-intentioned rescuer to become electrocuted.
8. Stand in a safe place until the power company cuts the wires or disconnects the power.

Be especially careful when approaching a collision located in a dark area such as a rural roadside at night.

1. As you walk from the ambulance, sweep the area ahead of you, to each side and overhead, with the beam of a powerful hand light. An energized conductor may be dangling just at head level.
2. If you discover that a wire is down, leave the area immediately and notify the power company.

Sometimes, especially in wet weather, a phenomenon known as ground gradient may provide your first clue that a wire is down. Voltage is greatest at the point where a conductor touches the ground, then diminishes with distance from the point of contact. That distance may be several inches or many feet. Being able to recognize and respond properly to energized ground can save your life.

1. Stop your approach immediately if you feel a tingling sensation in your legs and lower torso. This sensation means that you are on energized ground. Current is entering one foot, passing through your lower body, and exiting through your other foot. If you continue on, you chance being electrocuted!
2. Turn 180 degrees and take one of two escape measures. Bend one knee and grasp the foot of that leg with one hand. Hop to a safe place on one foot. Or shuffle away from the danger area with both feet together, allowing no break in contact between your two feet or between your feet and the

ground. Either technique helps prevent your body from completing a circuit with energized ground.

Broken Utility Pole with Wires Intact
Even if wires are intact, a broken utility pole is still dangerous. Conductors supporting the pole can break at any time, dropping pole and wires onto the scene. If you arrive to find such a situation

1. Park the ambulance outside the danger zone.
2. Notify your dispatcher of the situation.
3. Stay outside the danger zone until power company representatives can de-energize the conductors and stabilize the pole.
4. Keep spectators and other emergency service personnel out of the danger zone.

Damaged Pad-Mounted Transformer Pad-mounted transformers and underground cables supply electricity in many areas, instead of utility poles and overhead wires. When an above-ground transformer is struck and damaged, it poses a serious threat. In such a situation

1. Request immediate power company response.
2. Do not touch either the transformer case or a vehicle touching it, and warn other emergency service personnel not to.
3. Stand in a safe place until the power company de-energizes the transformer.
4. Keep spectators out of the danger zone.

Coping With Vehicle Fires

When you find a vehicle on fire, always request the response of firefighting units. Do not assume that someone else has called the fire department. In fact, an engine should always stand by at a vehicle rescue.

Extinguishing a vehicle fire is the responsibility of persons who are trained and equipped for the job: firefighters. Nonetheless, there are some measures that trained EMTs can take when they arrive before fire units (Scan 29-2).

For small fires, a 15- or 20-pound class A:B:C dry chemical fire extinguisher can extinguish virtually anything that may be burning in a vehicle, including upholstery, fuel, and electrical components. Only burning magnesium and other flammable metals cannot be extinguished by an A:B:C extinguisher.

Before you try to put out a fire, put on a full set of protective gear.

Extinguishing Fires in Collision Vehicles

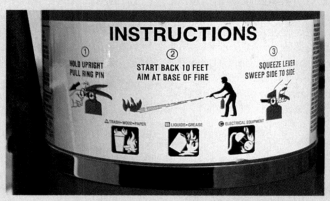

A. Markings that identify an extinguisher that can be used for Class A, B, and C fires.

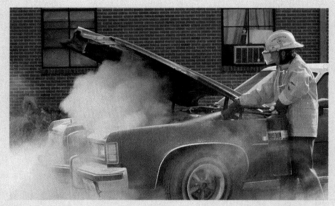

B. Extinguishing a fire in the engine compartment when the hood is fully open.

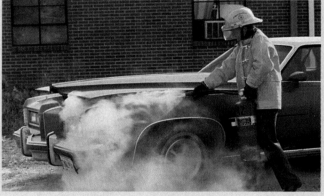

C. Extinguishing a fire in the engine compartment when the hood is partially open.

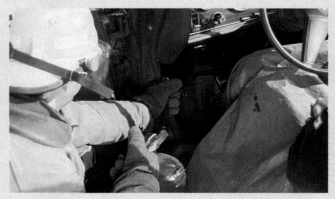

D. Extinguishing a fire under the dash. Care must be taken not to fill the vehicle's interior with a cloud of agent.

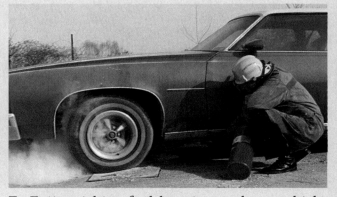

E. Extinguishing fuel burning under a vehicle. Flames are swept away from the vehicle.

Note: WEAR PROTECTIVE GEAR AND DO ONLY WHAT YOU ARE TRAINED TO DO.

In the Engine Compartment If the hood is fully open

1. Stand close to an A-post (front roof-supporting post) of the vehicle and, if possible, with your back to the wind to guard against the agent blowing back into your face or entering the passenger compartment. Dry chemical extinguishing agent irritates respiratory passages and may contaminate open wounds.
2. Sweep the extinguisher across the base of the fire with short bursts. Use no more than necessary to extinguish the fire. You will need what is left if there is a subsequent flare-up.

If the hood is open to the safety latch

1. To restrict air flow and deprive the fire of oxygen, do not raise the hood further.
2. Direct the agent through any opening to the engine compartment: between hood and fender, around the grill, or under a wheel well through a broken head lamp assembly. Again, use no more agent than what is needed.

If the hood is closed tight, let the fire burn under the closed hood, leaving its extinguishment to the fire department, and continue to get the patients out of the vehicle. The firewall should protect the passenger area long enough to get the patients out with rapid extrication techniques.

In the Passenger Compartment If the fire is under the dash or in upholstery or other combustibles

1. Carefully apply the agent directly to the burning material.
2. Apply sparingly to avoid creating a cloud of powder that may be harmful to occupants.

In the Trunk If there is fire in the trunk, as with fire under a closed hood, leave extinguishment to the fire department and continue working to get patients out of the vehicle.

Under the Vehicle Using a portable unit to extinguish burning fuel under a vehicle may be an exercise in futility when the spill is large. But when people are trapped in the vehicle, you must try.

1. Attempt to sweep the flames from under the passenger compartment as you apply the agent.

2. If you do extinguish the fire, be sure that sources of ignition are then kept away.

In a Truck An A:B:C extinguisher can also be used to combat truck fires. Be aware, however, that burning truck tires are especially dangerous; flames can quickly spread to the body of the vehicle and its cargo, or the tires can blow apart when heated by fire. NEVER stand directly in front of a truck wheel when there is a fire; approach from a 45-degree angle.

Remember: No matter how small the fire appears and how proficient you are with portable extinguishers, call for a fire department response as soon as you arrive and find that a vehicle is on fire.

Coping With Spilled Fuel

At times you will find that fuel is leaking from a damaged vehicle but is not on fire. If you discover that a fuel tank is leaking

1. Call for fire department response. The decision to continue the rescue effort should be governed by your perception of the danger. You should not be expected to continue rescue operations if gasoline is pooled under the vehicle or flowing toward a source of ignition.
2. Warn spectators away from flowing fuel to minimize possible sources of ignition.
3. Do not use flares near spilled fuel or in the path of flowing fuel.

Warning: Watch where you park your vehicle. The catalytic converter (usually located under front passengers' feet) often heats to over a thousand degrees and can ignite spilled fuel or other combustibles.

Coping With Unstable Vehicles

Unstable collision vehicles pose a hazard to rescuers and patients alike. Rescuers often fail to stabilize collision vehicles because they *appear* to be stable. Rather than taking the chance of incorrectly "reading" a collision vehicle's stability and having the vehicle move during rescue with disastrous results, you should consider *any* collision vehicle from which patients need to be extricated to be unstable and act accordingly.

Scan 29-3 shows methods for stabilizing a vehicle on its wheels, a vehicle on its side, and a vehicle on its roof.

Stabilizing Collision Vehicles with Cribbing

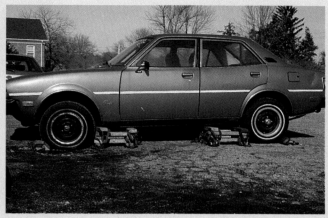

A. A car on its wheels can be stabilized by placing cribbing under the rocker panels to minimize rescuer-produced movements that may be harmful to the occupants. Deflate the vehicle's tires for maximum stability.

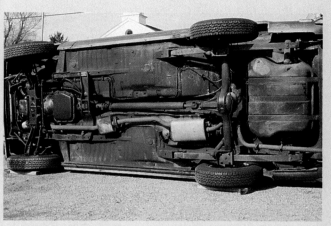

B. A car on its side can be stabilized by placing cribbing under the wheels, moving the car to the vertical position, and then . . .

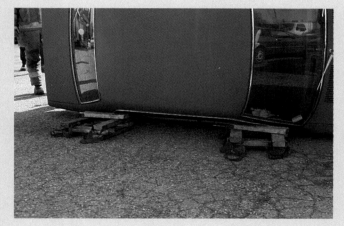

C. . . . placing cribbing under the A- and C-posts. Stabilizing in this manner allows EMTs to pull the roof down to expose the entire interior of the car.

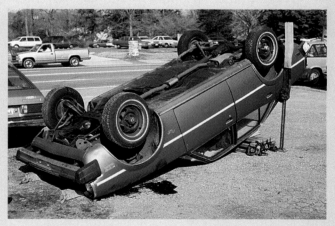

D. An overturned car can be stabilized by placing cribbing under the trunk, under the hood, or at both locations, depending on the position of the vehicle.

A Vehicle on Its Wheels A collision vehicle that is upright on four inflated tires looks stable. However, it is easily rocked up and down, side to side, and back and forth as rescuers climb into and over it. These motions can seriously aggravate occupants' injuries.

Cribbing (wood frameworking) placed at four points under the vehicle is the best method of stabilizing a vehicle on its wheels. If your ambulance is not equipped with cribbing, a degree of stabilization can be accomplished in the following manner.

1. If you have access to the passenger compartment, set the parking brake.
2. Prevent forward and rearward movement by placing wheel chocks ahead of one front wheel and behind the rear wheel on the same side.
3. Deflate all of the tires. Simply pull the valve stems from their casing with pliers. Then tell a police officer what you have done so investigators will not think that the tires are flat as a result of the collision. Give the valve stems to the police or rescue crew so the tires can be reinflated later to make vehicle removal easier.

A Vehicle on Its Side When a vehicle is on its side, there is a tendency for spectators to push it back onto its wheels. They fail to realize that this movement may injure, or more severely injure, occupants of the vehicle. Instead, the vehicle should be stabilized on its side.

There are many ways to stabilize a vehicle on its side, from using manpower alone to using hydraulic rams and pneumatic jacks. If your ambulance is equipped with stabilization equipment, you should attend a formal vehicle rescue course that includes basic stabilization procedures.

If the ambulance does not carry stabilization devices, or if you are not trained in their use, wait for a rescue squad to arrive before you try to make entry into the vehicle. For safety, place someone at each end of the vehicle to keep onlookers back until help and the proper equipment arrive.

A Vehicle on Its Roof A vehicle on its roof is likely to be in one of four positions.

- Horizontal, with the roof crushed flat against the body of the vehicle and both the trunk lid and hood contacting the ground
- Horizontal, resting entirely on the roof, with

space between the hood and the ground and space between the trunk lid and the ground
- Front end down, with the front edge of the hood contacting the ground and the rear of the car supported by the C-posts (rear posts)
- Front end up, with the trunk lid contacting the ground and much of the weight of the vehicle supported by the A-posts (front posts)

Cribbing and jacks are usually used to stabilize an overturned car. If your ambulance has these devices, use them in the manner you were taught. If the ambulance is not equipped, or if you are not trained, stand by until a rescue unit has stabilized the vehicle, even if roof posts are intact and the vehicle appears stable.

When the roof is crushed flat against the body, as when all the roof posts have collapsed, the car is essentially a steel box resting on the ground with the occupants completely trapped inside. Unless the vehicle is on a hill or perched precariously on debris or another vehicle, this is the one time when stabilization is unnecessary: the structure is rigid. It will have to be lifted or opened by the rescue crew.

Coping With a Vehicle's Electrical System

Many rescue units routinely disable the electrical system of every collision vehicle by cutting a battery cable. This was a reasonable practice years ago when vehicles had more combustible materials and when wiring did not have self-extinguishing insulation. Today, however, the situation is different. Unless gasoline is pooled under a vehicle or undeployed air bags need to be disabled, cutting the battery out of the electrical system may not only be a waste of time, it may actually hinder the rescue operation!

Remember that many cars have electrically powered door locks, window operators, and seat adjustment mechanisms. Being able to lower a window rather than breaking it eliminates the likelihood of spraying occupants with glass. Being able to operate door locks may eliminate the need to force doors open. And being able to operate a powered seat will create space in front of an injured driver.

If there is reason to disrupt the electrical system, disconnect the ground cable from the battery. In this way, you will not be likely to produce a spark that can drop onto spilled fuel or ignite battery gases. Such a spark can be created when the positive cable is pulled away from the battery terminal, or when a tool touches a metal component while in contact with the positive terminal or cable.

EXTRICATING COLLISION VICTIMS

Vehicle rescue prior to the mid 1960s is best described as crude. So-called "rescue" trucks were usually small walk-in step vans that carried more equipment for fire suppression and salvage than for rescue. The inventory of rescue equipment might have included some long pry bars, a few lengths of utility rope, a minimal hand tool kit, shovels and brooms, and—if the rescue unit was progressive—a 4-ton hydraulic jack kit. Personnel were poorly trained for rescue and, more often than not, victims were simply pulled through openings created by the collision.

The National Highway Safety Act of 1966 required states to improve prehospital emergency care capabilities. It was recognized that EMS personnel could not do much for collision victims who could not be extricated from vehicles in time for live-saving efforts to be effective. So vehicle rescue training courses were developed, and bigger and better-equipped rescue units were placed in service.

Training courses began to prepare EMS personnel for a wide range of collision scene rescue activities: unlocking and unlatching doors with commercially available and homemade tools, removing windshields and rear windows intact, using hydraulic rescue tools to open vehicle doors one at a time, and so on.

In the mid 1970s, smaller, more fuel-efficient cars were developed, but these created few problems for rescue personnel. Compact cars were simply small versions of large cars.

Problems did not start to plague the rescue services until the mid 1980s. Extrications were taking longer, powerful rescue tools did not seem to be working properly, and procedures that had worked well for years were no longer successful. The reason for this apparent backslide? Improved vehicle construction. For example, the Nader pin (named for Ralph Nader, the consumer advocate who lobbied for the device), is a case-hardened pin in an automobile door. In a collision, the cams in the door locks grasp the pin to keep the door from flying open. Prior to the Nader pin, rescue personnel could open a door with a crowbar. Subsequently, rescuers had to start using hydraulic spreader tools to peel the cams off the pins. Safety features designed to keep occupants inside wrecked vehicles were keeping rescuers out!

Vehicle rescue training was becoming complicated, and rescuers were being asked to learn dozens of techniques, some of which could be used only on certain models of cars. The need for simplified, effective procedures and new training courses became evident.

The next few pages will describe a three-part extrication procedure that can be used on virtually any car or light truck on the road today. If your ambulance usually arrives with or after fire and rescue units, you may not be called upon to participate in this procedure. If your ambulance often arrives long before other emergency units, your crew would be wise to consider the purchase of a lightweight but powerful hydraulic rescue tool and to become familiar with the use of hand tools as a backup.

Gaining Quick Access

First remember that, as an EMT, your responsibility is not the rescue of the vehicle but the rescue of the *patient*. You will usually assume that an occupant or occupants of the vehicle have sustained life-threatening injuries, and that at least one EMT needs to gain *quick* access to the patient, even while rescuers are working to gain a more wide-open access, create exitways, and disentangle occupants (described in the three-step procedure below).

If the vehicle is stable enough for an EMT to approach it safely

1. First see if a door can be opened or a window rolled down in the ordinary way.
2. Failing this, you may need to break a window to gain access even while the rescue crew is dismantling the vehicle for extrication of the occupants.

All automotive glass is one of two types: laminated or tempered. Windshields and some side and rear van and truck windows are *laminated* safety glass: two sheets of plate glass bonded to a sheet of tough plastic like a glass-and-plastic sandwich. Most passenger car side and rear windows are *tempered* glass. They are very resilient, but when they do break, rather than shattering into sharp fragments they break into small, rounded pieces.

You will usually try to gain access through a side or rear window as far as possible from the passengers. Use a center punch against a lower corner to break the glass. Punch out fingerholds in the top of the window and use your gloved fingers to pull fragments away from the window.

A flathead ax is usually required to break through a windshield. A windshield is usually not broken to gain access, but the rescue squad may need to remove it if they plan to displace the dash or steering column or remove the roof. Before the windshield is broken, passengers should be covered with aluminized rescue blankets or tarps, if possible.

There are some situations in which gaining quick access is more difficult.

- If a car has rolled over several times and come to rest on its wheels, the roof may be crushed and access through windows precluded. The roof may need to be raised with heavy-duty jacks before doors can be opened or the roof removed.
- If the vehicle is on its side, *do not* attempt to gain access before it is stabilized. While a car on its side may appear stable, simply climbing onto one side in an attempt to open a door may cause the vehicle to drop onto its roof or wheels. Moreover, you can be trapped under the vehicle when it topples. Once the vehicle is stabilized, if a door must be opened, tie it in the fully open position before you try to crawl inside.
- If the vehicle is resting on its roof, roof posts are intact, and the vehicle appears stable, it may be tempting to try to reach the vehicle's occupants by gaining access through window or door openings—immediately, and without stabilizing the vehicle. However, if the posts collapse, the vehicle may come crashing down, and woe to the EMT who is attempting to climb into the vehicle or who has an arm in a window opening. You must wait to gain access until the rescue crew has stabilized the vehicle.

  If the roof is crushed against the body of the vehicle, the vehicle is stable. It is, of course, impossible to gain access through a window, door, or the roof. However, it may be possible for the EMTs to cut through the floor pan and either crawl inside, if the opening is big enough or the EMT small enough, or to reach through the opening to touch and offer emotional support to the occupants until rescue personnel can lift or open the vehicle.

If the vehicle is unstable and cannot be safely approached by an EMT, get as close as possible so you can talk or signal to the occupants to reassure them that help is on its way

and begin getting an idea of their condition. Once an entry point is gained, at least one EMT should crawl inside the vehicle and immediately begin the primary survey and manual stabilization, while offering emotional support by talking to and reassuring the patient or patients.

The Three-Part Extrication Procedure

Following is a description of a three-part extrication procedure that can be accomplished by fire, rescue, and EMS personnel. The procedure is not vehicle specific; that is, it can be used on virtually any car or truck. The procedure does not include a lot of techniques that require special equipment. Personnel can be trained in a short course. And, most important to EMS personnel, there is no need to fill several compartments of the ambulance with rescue equipment.

Supplies and Equipment Figure 29-3 shows how an ambulance might be equipped both for gaining access and for disentanglement operations.

Two crates of 2 x 4 x 18-inch cribbing and six wood wedges are carried for vehicle stabilization. The wheel chocks that are carried on the ambulance can also be used for stabilization. The hand tool kit contains battery pliers, a 12-inch adjustable wrench for general disassembly operations, combination aircraft snips for cutting thin sheet metal, a 3- or 4-pound drilling hammer for times when striking force is needed, a manual or spring-loaded center punch for breaking tempered glass, two or three hacksaws for severing metal components, 10-inch locking-type pliers and 10-inch water pump pliers for

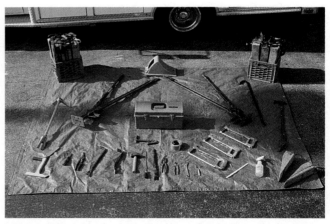

Figure 29-3 Supplies and equipment that might be carried on an ambulance for vehicle rescue operations.

facilitating grasp, two 12- to 15-inch flat pry bars for prying tasks, an 8-inch and a 12-inch flat blade screwdriver for disassembly operations, and a spray container of lubricant for cutting with the hacksaws. A 36-inch combination forcible entry tool and a 51-inch pinch bar can be used for a number of tasks where leverage is needed. Two large heavy duty jacks can be used for a number of tasks where leverage is needed. The two heavy duty jacks can be used for a number of stabilization and lifting operations.

A hydraulic tool and power unit are part of a new generation of rescue tools. The combination tool develops 12,000 pounds of spreading force, 10,000 pounds of pulling force, and 38,000 pounds of cutting force and weighs 36 pounds. The power unit develops a hydraulic pressure of 5,000 p.s.i. and weights 39 pounds.

Step One: Gain Access by Disposing of the Roof For more than 20 years, emergency service personnel have been trained to carry out a progression of procedures to reach the occupants of a wrecked vehicle: first try the doors; if that fails, unlock and unlatch the doors by nondestructive or destructive means; when all else fails, gain access through window openings. This multi-part procedure is time-consuming and requires a number of tools.

A quicker and far more efficient procedure is to dispose of the roof of a collision vehicle as soon as hazards have been controlled and the vehicle is stable. Disposing of the roof has two benefits.

- It makes the entire interior of the vehicle accessible. EMS personnel can stand beside or climb into the vehicle and pursue emergency care efforts while rescuers carry out disentanglement procedures.
- It creates a large exitway through which an occupant can be quickly removed when he has a life-threatening injury or when fire or another hazard is threatening the operation.
- It provides fresh air and helps cool off the patient when heat is a problem.

Scan 29-4 illustrates the procedure for folding a collision vehicle's roof back like the roof of a convertible. While this is the most commonly used procedure, it is not the only way to dispose of a roof. A roof can be folded forward after cutting both C- and B-posts (rear and middle posts), folded to either side after cutting the posts of the opposite side, or removed altogether after severing all of the roof posts. Lacking a hydraulic rescue tool, you can accomplish all of these procedures with ordinary hacksaws and a spray container of lubricant.

Step Two: Create Exitways by Displacing Doors and Roof Posts When rapid vertical extrication through the opened roof is not indicated, the next step is to open doors and displace roof posts. This step also has two benefits.

- EMS personnel can kneel beside the vehicle while carrying out patient care and immobilization procedures.
- Then the immobilized occupants can be easily rotated onto a long spine board or other patient-carrying device.

Scan 29-5 shows a team of EMTs using a combination hydraulic rescue tool to open doors that cannot be unlatched and pulled open in the usual manner, as when doors are damaged or locks and latches jammed.

Step Three: Disentangle Occupants by Displacing the Front End Most vehicle rescue training courses include procedures for displacing or removing seats, dash assemblies, steering wheels, steering columns, and pedals. A quicker and more efficient way to disentangle an injured driver and/or passenger from these mechanisms of entrapment is to displace the entire front end of the vehicle. While the task sounds difficult, it is not.

Scan 29-6 illustrates the procedure for displacing the front end of a passenger car with a combination hydraulic rescue tool. A dash displacement can also be accomplished with heavy duty jacks and hacksaws.

If the steering wheel hub is large and rectangular, the car probably has an air bag or bags (the passenger-side bag being in the glove compartment). If the bags have not deployed, they are not likely to deploy now unless extrication involves displacing the dash or steering wheel. If such displacement is to be done, air bag manufacturers recommend following these steps.

1. Avoid placing your body or objects against an air bag module or in its path of deployment.
2. Disconnect the battery cables.
3. Do not displace or cut the steering column until the system has been fully deactivated.
4. Do not cut or drill into an air bag module.
5. Do not apply heat in the area of the steering wheel hub.

Disposing of the Roof of a Car

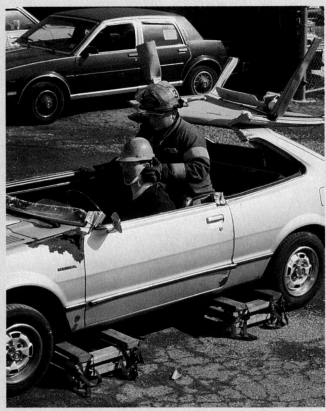

A. The traditional procedure for disposing of the roof is to sever the A- and B-posts, cut through the roof rails just ahead of the C-posts, and fold the roof back like the roof of a convertible. It is necessary either to remove or to cut the windshield, depending on the need for working space.

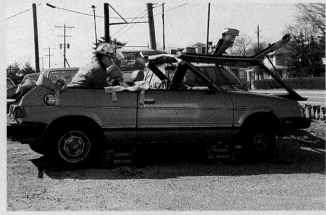

B. Folding the roof forward can be accomplished quickly when the C-posts are narrow. The roof is hinged either on the top or the bottom of the windshield, depending on the need for working space.

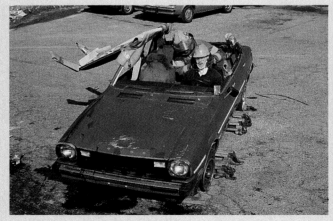

C. When a car has only one occupant, the roof can be folded to one side after severing the A-, B-, and C-posts of the opposite side.

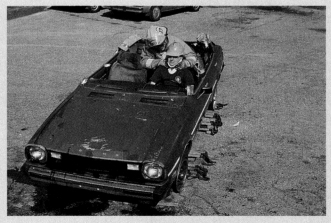

D. When a car has narrow C-posts, removing the roof altogether provides maximum working space.

Displacing Doors and
Roof Posts of a Car

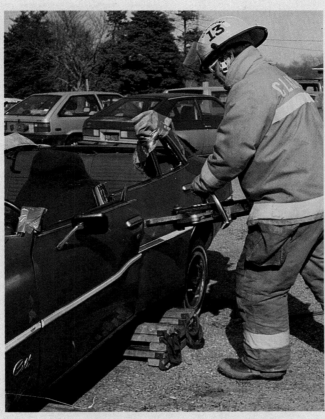

A. A collision vehicle's doors can be opened quickly with a hydraulic rescue tool. Doors can be opened at the latch or by breaking the hinges.

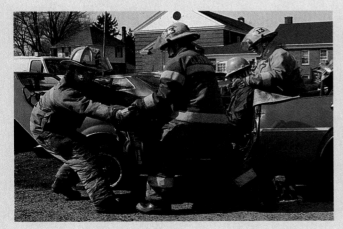

C. Once the front door has been opened, it can be moved beyond the normal range of motion by simply pushing on it. Seldom is there a need for removing a front door.

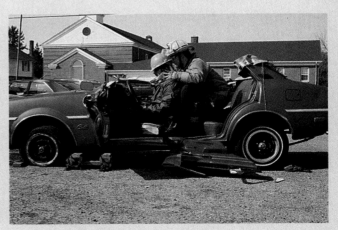

B. When the front doors of a four-door car have been opened at the latch side, the roof post and rear door can be pulled down simultaneously to expose the entire side of the vehicle.

Displacing the Front End of a Car

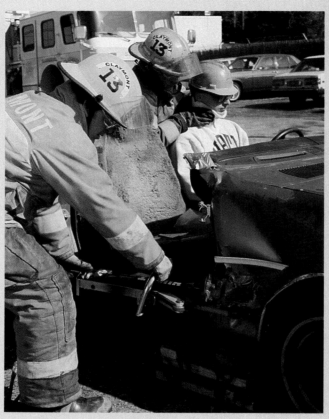

A. Relief cuts are made at the junction of the A-post with the rocker panel, and in the A-post between the door hinges.

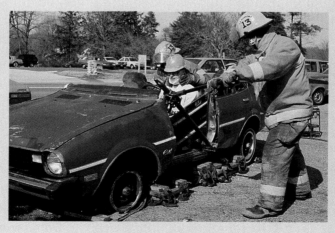

B. Heavy duty jacks are used to pivot the front end of the vehicle away from the relief cuts. Or . . .

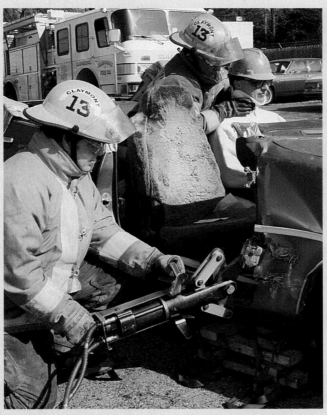

C. . . . the combination hydraulic tool can be used in the spreading mode to displace the front end.

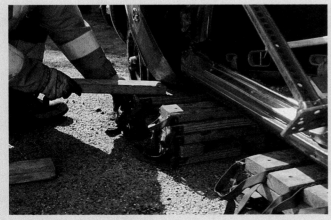

D. Displacing the front end will tend to lift the vehicle from the cribs. Cribbing must be added to the front cribs to prevent destabilization.

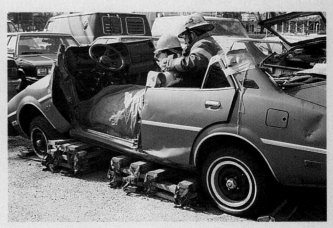

E. Displacing the front end creates working space by moving a number of mechanisms of entrapment away from front seat occupants.

Normal and Rapid Extrication

Must the three-part procedure just described be used for all extrication operations? Must the three procedures always be accomplished in the same order? Must all three procedures always be used?

Not at all! In some cases, it may be necessary only to force a door open to reach a single patient and create an exitway for his removal. In other cases, it may be prudent to open doors before disposing of the roof. In still other situations, there may not be a need to displace the front end of a collision vehicle.

During the initial size-up, you must be able to "read" a collision vehicle and develop a plan of action based on your knowledge of rescue operations and your evaluation of the patient's status.

A potentially unstable or stable patient (P or S on the CUPS scale) can wait for rescue personnel to force open the doors, then remove the roof and/or displace the front end. For such a patient, there is time to do a short board or vest immobilization and carefully transfer the patient to the stretcher using the long board. (This normal extrication technique is described in Chapter 12). If the patient is critical or unstable (C or U on the CUPS scale), it may make more sense to use a rapid extrication technique (Scan 29-7), whether for a vertical removal through the opened roof or for a horizontal removal through a doorway. The principles of spinal immobilization remain the same, but the requirements for speed of removal will dictate the specific technique you use.

CHAPTER REVIEW

SUMMARY

The extent to which you, as an EMT, will participate in vehicle rescue procedures depends on the role your EMS unit plays in vehicle rescue and whether or not your ambulance arrives ahead of fire and rescue units. The main purpose of knowing extrication procedures for the EMT is to incorporate them into the patient care plan.

Sizing Up the Scene

When you arrive on the scene of a collision, evaluate hazards and calculate the need for additional backup: BLS, ALS, police, fire, rescue, or special services. Determine if the car has airbags and, if they have deployed, be prepared to protect yourself and the vehicle occupants from air bag dust. Note if any bumpers are loaded and, if they are, stand clear.

Managing Collision-Produced Hazards

Safeguard your personal safety by availing yourself of training in rescue procedures, observing safety guidelines, and wearing appropriate protective gear at all times. Also safeguard collision victims from hazards at the scene and those generated by rescue procedures.

Police, firefighters, and others—not EMTS—usually manage hazards at a collision scene: traffic, spectators, electricity, fires, and unstable vehicles. An EMT's primary job is care of the injured. However, if the ambulance arrives first, EMTs may need at least to initiate hazard management.

Place flares (but not where fuel has been spilled) to channel traffic past the scene. Consider the start of a curve or the top of a hill to be an edge of the danger zone.

If local policies permit, ask willing bystanders to keep spectators away from the danger zone.

If wires are downed or a utility pole or a pad-mounted transformer is damaged, remain in a safe place and keep others away until power company workers make the area safe. Use a handlight to look for downed wires in a dark area. If you detect a tingling sensation that indicates you are on energized ground, carefully leave the area.

Use a portable fire extinguisher to combat vehicle fires only after you request fire department response and only after putting on a full set of protective clothing.

Rapid Extrication Procedure— For Critical or Unstable Patients Only

Note: In the photos, the roof of the vehicle has been removed to allow for easier illustration of the positions of the EMTs. In most cases, this procedure will be done and should be practiced with the roof intact.

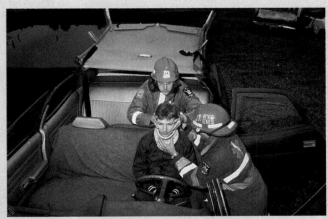

1. Manually stabilize the patient's head and neck and have a second EMT apply a rigid extrication collar.

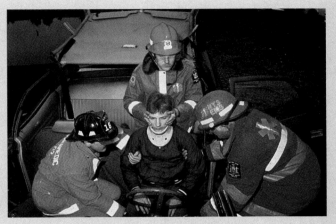

2. At the direction of the EMT stabilizing the head and neck, two EMTs each lift the patient by his armpits and buttocks/thighs just enough for a bystander or additional rescuer to slide a long spine board between the patient and the vehicle seat.

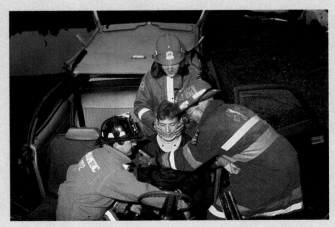

3. The EMTs reposition their hands so the EMT on the front seat inside the vehicle holds the patient's legs and pelvis while the EMT outside the vehicle holds the upper chest and arms.

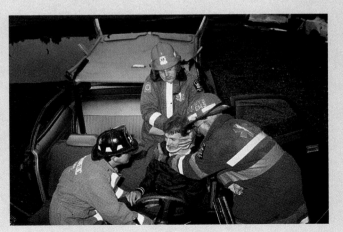

4. At the direction of the EMT holding the head and neck, carefully turn the patient a quarter turn so his back is facing the side door of the vehicle.

727

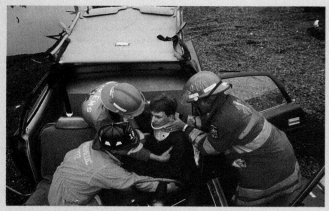

5. The EMT who was holding the pelvis temporarily holds the chest so the EMT who was holding the chest can take over head and neck stabilization. The EMT in the back seat can then reach over the seat and assist with the chest, and the EMT inside on the front seat can move his hands back to the pelvis.

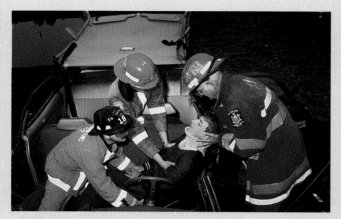

6. At the direction of the EMT at the head and neck, gently lower the patient to the spine board. **Note:** Sometimes it may be necessary to move the patient inside the vehicle a few inches so there is ample room to lay him down without touching the upper door opening.

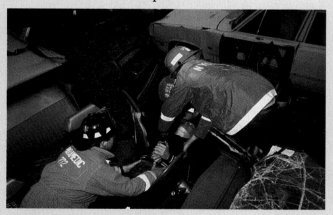

7. As a bystander or additional rescuer holds the end of the backboard, the EMTs slide the patient to the head end of the board.

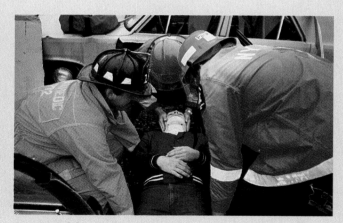

8. Quickly apply straps to the patient's chest, pelvis, and legs and remove the patient to a stretcher or the ground, under the direction of the EMT stabilizing the head and neck. **Note:** Since the patient's head is not yet fully immobilized (it is only being manually held stable by the EMT and collar), DO NOT walk more than a few steps with the patient. Once on stable ground or the stretcher, apply a head immobilizer or blanket roll and wide tape.

Note: The rapid extrication procedure is only for critical or unstable patients who must be moved in less time than would be required to apply a short spine board or extrication vest inside the vehicle before moving the patient to the long spine board. The normal extrication procedure using short spine board or vest is discussed in Chapter 12.

Photos by Robert Elling

Keep fire deprived of oxygen by discharging agent into the engine compartment through existing openings. Leave the extinguishment of fires in a closed engine compartment or trunk to firefighters while you work to remove patients. Apply the chemical agent sparingly inside the vehicle to avoid exposing occupants. Apply the agent to sweep fuel from under the vehicle. Never stand or walk directly in front of the tires of a burning truck; they may explode.

If fuel is leaking, call for fire department response.

Stabilize every collision vehicle from which patients need to be extricated to avoid aggravating cervical spine and other serious injuries and to protect rescue workers. Lacking any other equipment, stabilize a vehicle on it wheels by chocking the front and rear wheels of one side and then deflating all the tires. Do not attempt to enter a vehicle that has come to rest on its side or on its roof until it has been stabilized.

An intact electrical system allows operation of powered door locks, windows, and seats. So do not disable the electrical system unless there are undeployed air bags or danger of fire. If you decide it is necessary to disconnect the battery, disconnect the ground cable.

Extricating Collision Victims

In the past, emergency service personnel were required to learn dozens of procedures for hazard management, gaining access, and disentangle-ment. Today, many of those procedures cannot be accomplished because of stronger car construction and safety devices such as the Nader pin.

The primary responsibility of the EMT during extrication is rescue of the patient. Gain quick access through a door or window, if possible, so that you can begin the primary survey, manual stabilization, and emotional support—even while rescuers are proceeding with extrication operations.

A three-part extrication procedure has simplified vehicle rescue operations.

The first step of the procedure is to dispose of the roof of a collision vehicle in order to gain access to the occupants. The procedure has two major advantages. It enables EMS personnel to reach all of the occupants, and it creates an opening through which occupants can be removed quickly.

The second step is to displace doors and roof posts. This creates working space for EMS personnel at the side of the vehicle and exitways through which occupants can be safely moved.

The third step is to displace the front end of the vehicle. Front end displacement creates working space ahead of front seat occupants.

If a patient is stable, follow a normal extrication procedure by using a short board or vest to immobilize the spine, then moving the patient onto a long board after rescuers have completed removal of the roof, doors, and/or front end. If the patient is critical, follow a rapid manual extrication procedure and a vertical or horizontal removal, whichever is faster.

Advanced-Life-Support-Assist Skills

The chapters in this text have addressed the main knowledge and skills required of an EMT. However, there are several additional skills that complement basic EMT skills and can enhance your capabilities as a "team player" on calls where you will work with advanced life support personnel. The six most common of these **ALS-assist skills** are

- Assisting in ventilating with an endotracheal tube
- Assisting in trauma intubation
- Applying ECG electrodes
- Using a pulse oximeter
- Setting up an intravenous (IV) administration set
- IV maintenance

Your instructor will discuss with you which of these skills are or are not authorized by your medical director.

The information in this appendix is intended as an abbreviated overview. It is not an exhaustive treatment of each skill. The information provided here should be supplemented by your instructor as necessary.

VENTILATING A PATIENT WITH AN ENDOTRACHEAL TUBE

The "gold standard" for airway care is the endotracheal (ET) tube. All other airway devices are, at best, secondary to the ET tube. This is because the ET tube is directly inserted into the trachea, forming an open pathway for air, oxygen, or medications to be blown into the lungs.

In adult sizes, it has an inflatable cuff that will seal off the trachea so that stomach contents the patient may regurgitate cannot be aspirated into the lungs.

Patients who typically need to have an ET tube inserted are those in pulmonary or cardiopulmonary arrest, trauma patients in need of airway control or supplemental oxygen, and those in respiratory failure due to overdose, pulmonary edema, asthma, asphyxia (loss of consciousness caused by too little oxygen or too much carbon dioxide resulting from suffocation), or anaphylaxis (anaphylactic, or allergic, shock).

Intubation is usually done by a paramedic or EMT-Intermediate. This section will not teach how to do an intubation, but rather will discuss how an EMT can *assist* during intubation or assist in ventilating a patient whose trachea has been intubated with an ET tube.

Before the intubation, you may be asked to hyperoxygenate the patient for a minute or so with the bag-valve mask (give the patient an extra amount of oxygen to tide him through the intubation process). Then the paramedic will place the non-trauma patient in the "sniffing position" (neck elevated approximately 2 inches, chin and nose thrust forward, head tilted back) to align the mouth, throat, and trachea. Then he will pass the ET tube through the mouth (or, sometimes, the nose) into the throat and past the vocal cords into the trachea. The paramedic will usually remove the oral airway and use a laryngoscope to move the tongue and other obstructions out of the way and to see where the tube is going.

In order to maneuver the tube past the vocal cords correctly, the paramedic will need to see them. You may be asked to gently press on the throat to push the vocal cords into the paramedic's view and also to help prevent stimulating the gag or vomit reflex. You will do this by pressing your thumb and index finger just to either side of the medial throat over the cricoid cartilage, a ring-shaped cartilage just below the Adam's apple. This procedure is known as cricoid pressure, or Sellick's maneuver.

Once the tube is properly placed, the cuff is inflated with air from a 10cc syringe. While the tube is manually held in place, the paramedic uses a stethoscope to listen for lung sounds on both sides and over the epigastrium (the area just under the xiphoid process). If the tube has been correctly placed, there will be sounds of air entering the lungs, but no sounds of air in the epigastrium. If incorrect (ETs are occasionally erroneously placed in the esophagus, indicated by air sounds in the epigastrium), the tube position must be corrected immediately, or the patient will receive no oxygen. If correct, the tube is anchored in place with tape or a commercially made tube restraint. The entire procedure including the last ventilation, passing the tube, and the next ventilation should take less than 30 seconds.

When asked to ventilate a tubed patient, you should remember that the trachea is short, so very little movement can displace the tube. It is very important that, especially before the tube has been anchored or restrained, you hold the tube against the teeth, being careful not to push it in or pull it out. If the tube is pushed in, it will most likely go into the right mainstem bronchus, the easiest path for the tube to take. This complication, if unnoticed when listening to the lungs, can prevent any oxygen from going into the left lung. If the tube is pulled out, on the other hand, it can easily slip into the esophagus and all the ventilations will go directly into the stomach, causing severe gastric distention, increasing the chance of regurgitation, and denying the patient oxygen.

There are graduations on the side of the tube, and the typical adult male will be about 22 cm at the teeth when the tube is properly placed. If the tube moves, report this to the paramedic immediately. It is good practice to hold the tube with two fingers and the BVM with the other hand. A patient with an ET tube inserted offers less resistance to ventilations and may not require two hands squeezing the bag as a patient who is not intubated would. If you are ventilating a breathing patient, be sure to bag *with* his respiratory effort as much as possible

so he can take full breaths. It is also possible to assist the patient to increase his respiratory rate, if needed, by interposing extra breaths.

There are some cautions to remember.

- Pay close attention to what the ventilations feel like. One of the first signs of a tension pneumothorax is increasing resistance when bagging. Secretions in need of being suctioned can often be felt as well as seen or heard. A patient with COPD has a stiff chest and offers more resistance to ventilations. These patients are also prone to spontaneous pneumothorax, so you should note any changes in the resistance to ventilations.
- Whenever a patient is to be defibrillated, carefully remove the bag from the tube or else its weight may accidentally pull out the tube.
- Watch for any changes in the patient's level of consciousness. As the patient becomes more alert, he may need to be restrained to keep from pulling out the tube. An oral airway is generally used as a bite block to prevent the patient from biting the ET tube. If the patient's gag reflex returns along with an increased level of consciousness, you may need to pull the oral airway out a bit.

ASSISTING WITH A TRAUMA INTUBATION

Occasionally, you will be asked to assist in the endotracheal intubation of a patient who may have sustained a neck injury. Since placing the patient in the sniffing position risks aggravating a neck injury, some modifications to the normal procedure are necessary. You may be asked to provide manual in-line stabilization while a collar is being applied and throughout the intubation. Since the paramedic may sit at the patient's head with his or her thighs around the patient's head, it will be necessary for you to stabilize the front of the patient's neck with both hands while kneeling at the side of the patient's chest. The paramedic will use the laryngoscope and manipulate the jaw to bring the vocal cords into view, rather than manipulating the neck.

APPLYING ECG ELECTRODES

An electrocardiogram (ECG) is a reading of the electrical activity of the heart represented by lines on paper or an electronic screen. In the field, it is used to alert medical personnel to life-threatening dysrhythmias. This is a paramedic skill; basic-level EMTs do not take or interpret ECGs. (The closest you may come to this process as an EMT will be, if you are so trained and your jurisdiction permits, using an AED, or automated external defibrillator, which automatically reads heart rhythms and delivers or advises you to deliver a shock, as described in Chapter 5.) However, to save time you may be asked to assist the paramedic by applying the ECG electrodes.

In the field, three electrodes are placed on the patient's body to provide three different "views" of the heart's electrical activity. There are four steps to attaching the electrodes that you may be asked to carry out.

1. Turn on the ECG monitor.
2. Plug in the monitoring cables, also called "leads."
3. Attach the monitoring cables to the electrodes.
4. Apply the electrodes to the patient's body.

Make sure that the paramedics you work with review with you the ECG equipment they will be using and its special switches.

Prepackaged disposable electrode pads are the most commonly used in the field. Be sure to use fresh ones from a new package as loose ones dry out and produce poor ECG tracings. There are two types of electrodes: the smaller monitoring pads (designed specifically for monitoring, not for defibrillation) and the large defibrillator/monitoring pads (used for defibrillation, they can also be used for monitoring heart rhythms). The paramedic you are working with will make clear which type he wants to use. For patient comfort, attach the cable to the electrode snap before placing the electrode on the body, especially with the larger electrodes.

Next prepare the patient's skin for the electrode. The best connection is on dry, bare skin, so it may be necessary to dry off the area and shave excessive hair. Use a wash cloth to remove oil from the skin and consider using an antiperspirant on patients with very sweaty skin.

Become familiar with the monitoring configuration (where to place the electrodes) used by ALS personnel in your system. The most common setup is placing the negative (white) electrode under the center of the right clavicle, the positive (red) electrode on the left lower chest, and the ground (black or green) under the center of the left clavicle or the right lower chest.

There are a few pointers to remember when monitoring a patient.

- Do not neglect to monitor the patient's pulse as you ordinarily would just because there is an ECG present. The presence of an ECG does not mean that the patient has a pulse. Always check the patient's pulse yourself, and do not rely on the digital readout on an ECG monitor for the rate. The number on the monitor represents a sampling of the electrical activity of the heart, not the actual pulses generated by the heart.
- When cutting off the patient's clothing, be careful not to cut those expensive ECG cables!
- Most monitors have an ECG complex beep which is a useful tool but tends to make the patient and family nervous. Unless the paramedics request to hear the beeper, keep the sound volume low.
- Finally, don't become mesmerized watching the monitor screen. This, too, will worry the patient.

Remember: The ECG is just another tool. Treat the patient, not the monitor!

USING A PULSE OXIMETER

A pulse oximeter is a device that monitors oxygen saturation of the hemoglobin, known as SaO_2. In other words, it tells you if there is enough oxygen circulating in the blood. This technique, called oximetry, has made its way into the field because modern pulse oximeters are compact and portable (Figure A1-1). It consists of a small monitor and a sensing unit that simply clips onto the patient's finger. Light transmitted through a vascular bed in the finger senses the oxygen level. It should be used with all patients complaining of dyspnea or respiratory problems. It is useful in assessing the effectiveness of respirations, oxygen therapy, bronchodilator therapy, and manual ventilation.

The oximeter screen will display the percentage of oxygen saturation and also a pulse wave form. If a poor wave form is shown, try selecting another site for the probe. As a general rule, if the oxygen saturation is less than 95% with a good pulse wave form, increase the oxygen concentration being delivered to the patient and consider assisting the ventilations with a bag-valve-mask unit with a reservoir. If the SaO_2 reading is greater than 95%, continue the current oxygen therapy.

Warning: Oxygen should never be withheld from a patient whose condition or appearance indi-

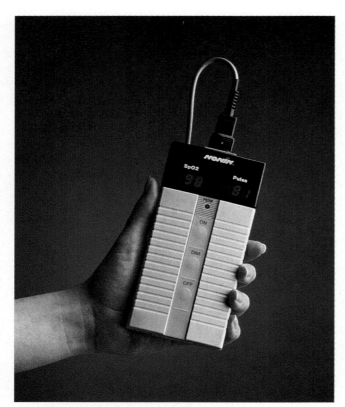

Figure A1-1. A pulse oximeter.

cates the need for oxygen, even if the oximeter shows a high reading.

It is important to note that

- Use of a pulse oximeter is helpful in "pushing" the EMT or advanced EMT to be more aggressive in oxygen therapy and ventilations of a patient, especially a conscious patient in respiratory distress.
- The measurement becomes inaccurate in hypothermic patients and patients in decompensated shock.
- The device will produce false "high %" readings in patients with carbon monoxide poisoning. This is because the carbon monoxide binds with hemoglobin in the blood more readily than oxygen, yet still produces the red color that the pulse oximeter reads. Also be aware that chronic smokers will normally have 10 to 15% more residual carbon monoxide in their blood than nonsmokers, so that smokers may have higher than normal readings while still requiring oxygen.

Remember: Monitor the pulse oximeter every five minutes as you would vital signs. As with all monitoring devices, this is just another tool to help you. Don't be hypnotized by the device. Treat the patient, not the oximeter!

SETTING UP AN IV FLUID ADMINISTRATION SET

An intravenous line (IV) is, essentially, a tube inserted into (intra) a vein (venous). Blood, fluids, or medications can be administered through an IV directly into the patient's circulation.

A blood *transfusion* is almost always given at the hospital. An *infusion* of other fluids or medications is a normal IV procedure in the field. For example, IVs are often set up to counter hypovolemic shock by introducing a fluid to help increase the volume in the circulatory system, to keep the vascular container full until the body can manufacture enough blood or regain control of heartbeat or vascular constriction and expansion (review Chapter 8 on shock). Fluids often used for this purpose in the field include Ringer's Lactate or NS (normal saline). Another fluid, D5W (5% dextrose in water), is commonly used to help keep a vein open for potential administration of medications.

IV therapy is an advanced life support procedure. In most cases, a paramedic will insert the IV catheter into the vein. However, an EMT may be enlisted to help set up the IV administration set while the paramedic is preparing the patient's vein.

You will need to be familiar with the following parts of an IV system.

- The Bag of Fluid—This is usually a clear plastic bag that collapses as it empties. Its collapsibility allows the use of a pressure infuser that will squeeze the bag and increase the flow when the patient's condition requires a greater flow.
- The Administration Set—This is the clear plastic tubing that will connect the fluid bag to the needle or catheter that has been inserted into the vein. The administration set, too, comes in a protective wrapping. There are three adjuncts to this tubing.
  1. The Drip Chamber—near the upper end, the end that will connect to the fluid bag. There are two basic types, the *mini drip* and the *macro drop*. The mini drip is used for children or for adults who require a minimal flow of fluid. It requires 60 small drops from

the tiny metal barrel in the drip chamber to equal 1 cubic centimeter (cc) or milliliter (mL). The macro drop is used when a high flow of fluid is needed, for example for a multi-trauma victim in decompensated shock. There is no little barrel in the drip chamber of the macro drop, and only 10 to 15 large drops equal 1 cc or mL.

2. The Flow Regulator—below the drip chamber. This is a stopcock that can be pushed up or down to start, stop, or control the rate of flow.

3. The Drug or Needle Port—below the flow regulator. This is an opening where medications, if needed, can be injected by the paramedic into the tubing to flow into the patient.

• An Extension Set—Extra tubing to lengthen the setup is often used with the micro drip set but should not be used with the macro drop set. The longer tubing has the benefit of being less likely to pull out of the patient's arm during movement. The drawback is that lengthening the tubing reduces the flow rate, which is contrary to the purpose of the macro drop. (Some services store the extension set, micro drip set, and D5W wrapped together.)

To set up the IV while the paramedic is preparing the patient's vein, you will

1. Take out and inspect the fluid bag. The bags come in a protective overwrap to keep them clean. If you are setting up the IV, you must remove the overwrapping, then inspect the bag (Figure A1-2) to be sure it contains the fluid that has been ordered and that the fluid is clear and free of particles. Squeeze the bag to be sure it is free of leaks. (Rarely, the fluid comes in a bottle. If so, be sure it is free of cracks.). If anything is wrong, report the problem and take another bag or bottle.

2. Select the proper administration set. Uncoil the tubing, and do not let the ends touch the ground.

3. Connect the extension set to the administration set, if an extension set is to be used.

4. Make sure the flow regulator is closed. To do this, roll the stopcock away from the direction of the fluid bag (Figure A1-3).

5. Remove the protective covering from the port of the fluid bag and the protective cov-

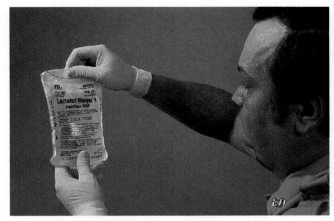

Figure A1-2. Inspect the IV bag to be sure it is the solution that was ordered, for clarity, leaks, and to be sure it has not expired.

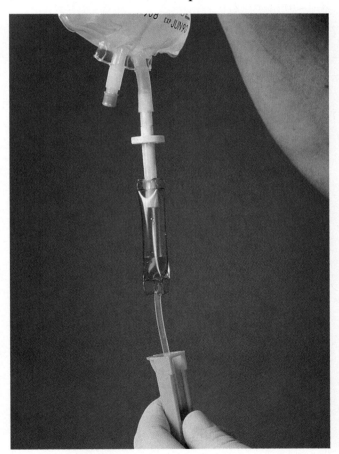

Figure A1-3. The extension tubing is joined to the administration set, and the flow regulator valve is closed.

ering from the spiked end of the tubing (Figure A1-4). Insert the spiked end of the tubing into the fluid bag with a quick twist. Do this carefully to protect the "bayonette's" sterility.

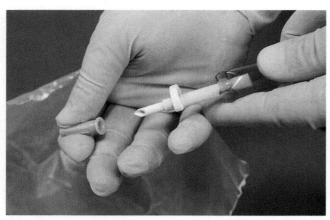

Figure A1-4. The protective covering is removed from the port of the fluid bag, and the protective covering is removed from the spiked end of the infusion tubing.

6. Hold the fluid bag higher than the drip chamber. Squeeze the drip chamber a time or two to start the flow and fill the chamber to the marker line, approximately one-third full.

7. Open the flow regulator and allow the fluid to flush all the air from the tubing. You may need to loosen the cap at the lower end of the tubing to get the fluid to flow. Maintain the sterility of the tubing end and replace the cap when you are finished. Most sets can be flushed without removing the cap. Be sure that all air bubbles are flushed from the tubing to avoid introducing a dangerous air embolism into the patient's vein.

Make sure the setup stays clean while waiting for the paramedic to do the venipuncture (insertion of the needle and catheter into the vein) and request the tubing. The paramedic will remove the needle and connect the IV tubing to the catheter left inside the patient's vein.

Occasionally, the paramedic will draw blood from the vein for various samples before inserting the IV. You may be asked to assist by placing the blood in sample tubes and labeling the tubes as your local hospitals require.

MAINTAINING AN IV

In some states, EMTs are allowed to maintain IVs. Maintaining an IV means keeping it flowing at the proper rate once it has been inserted into the vein.

There are a number of problems that may come up which you should be prepared to resolve

if you are charged with maintaining an IV. Any of the following may interrupt the flow of the IV.

- The flow regulator may be closed.
- A clamp may be closed on the tubing.
- The tubing may kink.
- The tubing may get caught under the patient or backboard.
- The constricting band or tourniquet that was used to raise the vein for insertion of the needle may have been mistakenly left on the patient's arm, perhaps covered by a sleeve.
- The tubing may have pulled out of the vein.
- The position of the IV or of the patient's arm may need to be adjusted. Some IVs are "positional," meaning that they only flow when the patient's arm or IV site is in a certain position. Adjusting the arm position or even splinting the arm (Figure A1-5) may be helpful as long as the splint is not too tight. Since the IV's flow usually depends on gravity, be sure that the IV bag is held well above the IV site and the patient's heart.

Insufficient flow can cause blood to clot in the catheter. This can be prevented by adjusting the flow to an adequate "keep the vein open" or KVO rate. The KVO rate varies but is usually about 30 drops per minute for a micro drip and 10 drops per minute for a macro drop administration set. If the drip chamber is overfilled, clamp the tubing, invert the drip chamber, and pump some fluid back into the bag. An IV with a flow rate that is too fast is called a "runaway IV" and can rapidly fluid-overload the patient. If the patient is in acute pulmonary edema, the last

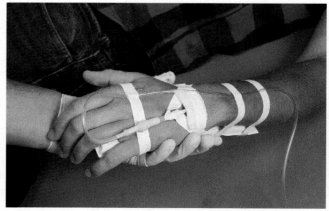

Figure A1-5. The insertion site is covered with a sterile dressing; the catheter is taped in place, and the arm is secured to an arm board if the flow rate is positional.

thing he needs is a runaway IV to fill up his lungs!

IVs are not supposed to hurt after the initial puncture of the skin and vein. If the patient complains of pain at the IV site, it is usually because the IV has *infiltrated*. An infiltrated IV is one where the needle has either punctured the vein and exited the other side, or the needle or catheter through which the fluid is flowing has pulled out of the vein. In either case, the fluid is flowing into the surrounding tissues instead of into the vein. An unnoticed infiltrated IV can be very dangerous if the paramedic is administering certain high concentration medications such as 50 ccs of 50% dextrose (25 grams), which will kill the surrounding tissue into which it leaks. In addition to complaints of pain, there is usually swelling at the site which is noticeable except in some obese patients. If EMTs are so authorized in your state, you must stop the flow and discontinue the IV according to your local protocols. If not so authorized, report the problem immediately to the paramedic or the medical control.

If you learn how to help advanced life support personnel start an IV, run through an administration set, label blood tubes, and maintain an IV, valuable time can be saved at the scene and during transport.

Optional EMT Skills

Five additional skills have been included in Appendix 2 that are, in most states, considered **optional EMT Skills**. These are skills that are practiced by EMTs in some, but not all, jurisdictions. These are invasive skills (skills that involve "invading" the interior of the patient's body). They involve the use of

- An esophageal obturator airway (EOA)
- An esophageal gastric tube airway (EGTA)
- A pharyngo-tracheal lumen airway (PtL®)
- A Combitube®
- An epinephrine pen

Your instructor will discuss with you which of these skills are or are not practiced by EMTs in your state and are or are not authorized by your medical director.

The information in this appendix is intended as an abbreviated overview. It is not an exhaustive treatment of each skill. The information provided here should be supplemented by your instructor as necessary.

INSERTING AN ESOPHAGEAL OBTURATOR AIRWAY (EOA) OR ESOPHAGEAL GASTRIC TUBE AIRWAY (EGTA)

It is often necessary to establish a better airway than can be achieved by manual means or by inserting an oro- or nasopharyngeal adjunct, which merely help to prevent the tongue and other structures from falling into and obstructing the airway. Endotracheal intubation (described in Appendix 1) is considered an advanced skill, requiring use of a laryngoscope to see where the endotracheal tube is going and precise placement of the tube between the vocal cords and into the trachea. As noted earlier, it is easy to miss the trachea and place the tube into the esophagus, sending air into the stomach instead of the lungs. It is also easy to push the tube in too far so that it lodges in the right mainstem bronchus, depriving the left lung of air. For these reasons, endotracheal intubation requires considerable training and frequent practice and is currently considered a skill that is beyond the EMT level.

Remember: During discussion of airway adjuncts, it is important to recall that the trachea is the passageway into the lungs and the esophagus is the passageway into the stomach. The trachea passes through the anterior throat, the esophagus through the posterior throat.

For over twenty years, alternative methods of intubating the patient using the esophageal obturator airway (EOA) and it close cousin the esophageal gastric tube airway (EGTA) have also been available. They can be passed "blindly" into the pharynx, eliminating the need to use a laryngoscope to visualize the process as it is happening, and they do not need to be maneuvered between the vocal cords into the trachea. They are thus considered to be within the skill level of the EMT in many states.

The ease of use and simplicity of both these devices have probably been overemphasized. It is true that they are easier to insert than the endotracheal tube. Nevertheless, they are invasive procedures, and the EMT using either device must be well versed in its complications, indications, and contraindications.

The major feature of the EOA or EGTA is an inflatable cuff that allows the trachea to be open but closes off the esophagus. The device is usually used during CPR or rescue breathing to "seal the meal," or prevent regurgitation (bringing up stomach contents that can be aspirated into the lungs) and prevent gastric distention (blowing air meant for the lungs into the stomach, which in turn tends to cause vomiting or regurgitation).

Both the EOA and the EGTA are usually connected to a bag-valve-mask unit which blows air or oxygen through the mask port. (As noted above, the EOA or EGTA tube doesn't go into the trachea, but since the esophagus is sealed off by the inflatable cuff, the only place for the ventilation to go is into the trachea and the lungs.) The EOA or EGTA is only effective as a ventilation tool in the hands of a one or two competent BVM operators who can seal the mask against the face and squeeze the bag hard enough to provide an adequate ventilation volume.

Although the EOA or EGTA is less often misplaced than an endotracheal tube, it does sometimes get pushed into the trachea instead of the esophagus. When this happens—if the error is not quickly recognized through listening for lung sounds—it can be fatal, since the result will be to seal off the trachea and provide no air to the lungs while sending air into the stomach instead.

There are certain contraindications to the use of the EOA or the EGTA. Neither should be used in

- A patient who is alert, verbally responsive, or who responds to painful stimuli and also still has a gag reflex. Vomiting and aspiration are likely.
- A patient who is under the age of 16 or who is less than 5 feet tall. The devices come in only one size and are too long for the anatomy of a small patient
- A patient who has ingested a corrosive substance. A corrosive could perforate the tip of the device, or may weaken the esophagus so that the device could perforate the esophagus wall.
- A patient with a known esophageal disease such as cancer or esophageal varicose, which weaken the wall of the esophagus and increase the chance for a ruptured esophagus
- A patient with significant upper airway bleed-

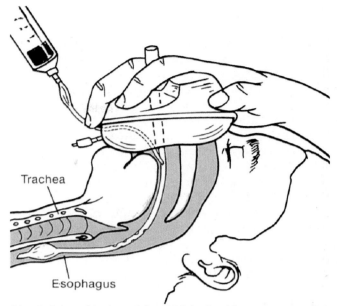

Trachea

Esophagus

Check the positioning of the EOA by hooking an oxygen line to it or blowing air into it, watching for bilateral expansion of the chest and auscultating for bilateral breath sounds. If the chest does not rise on both sides and breath sounds are not heard, withdraw the tube and reinsert it. When the tube is correctly positioned, the cuff will lie below the carina of the trachea. To avert possible esophageal rupture, inflate the cuff. Use no more than 35 ml air.

Figure A2-1. The esophageal obturator airway (EOA).

ing. Blood flowing from the nose or mouth will pass directly into the lungs once the inflated cuff has closed off the esophagus.

Although the EOA and EGTA have much in common, the differences are important to learn. Both have an air-cushion-inflatable mask and a 16-inch tube with a 35cc inflatable air cuff on the distal end. The EOA has a closed distal end to the tube and series of air holes on the proximal end of the tube. As air is ventilated into the tube with the mask sealed against the face, the air exits the holes into the pharynx. Since the tube has a blind end and the cuff is inflated after insertion, no air gets into the esophagus. (Figure A2-1).

The EGTA has an open end to the tube, or a valve at the end through which a tube can be inserted into the esophagus and the stomach. In this way, stomach contents can be suctioned or medications administered to the stomach. Ventilations are not blown through the tube port (indeed, this port is designed so that a BVM coupling will not fit, thus avoiding ventilating the stomach by mistake). Instead, the ventilations enter through a second port which, like the first and only EOA port, is a standard 15 mm ventilation device adapter. These ventilations, of course, do not travel through the tube at all but flow freelying under the mask and into the mouth and pharynx on the outside of the tube. In other words, the EGTA provides access to the stomach while still protecting the trachea, while the EOA only protects the trachea.

To attach the mask to the tube of either device, insert the tube into the port 180 degrees from the desired normal anatomical position, then twist the tube 180 degrees until it snaps into place in the mask. To detach the mask from the tube, simply squeeze the plastic tips that protrude through the mask and pull out the tube from the opposite direction from which it was inserted. Both devices should be stored in the position of function. They should never be stored flat or rolled into a coil as the shape of the tube will be lost and will decrease your chances of correctly intubating the esophagus.

To insert either device, you will first need to assemble all the correct supplies.

- An EOA or EGTA tube with the proper mask (*the masks are not interchangeable* and will fit only the correct tube)
- A water-soluble lubricant, such as K-Y jelly, Lubifax, or Surgilube. (A silicone-based lubricant or a petroleum-based lubricant such as Vaseline must not be used because it will cause aspiration pneumonia should the tube be inadvertently placed in the trachea.)
- A BVM with reservoir
- A stethoscope
- A suction unit and rigid Yankauer tip
- A supply of 4 x 4 gauze pads
- A 35cc syringe
- Gloves, goggles, and mask

Then perform the following procedures.

1. One EMT hyperoxygenates the patient with the BVM. Meanwhile . . .
2. A second EMT lubricates the tube with the water-soluble lubricant.
3. Stop the resuscitation momentarily and lift the jaw and tongue straight upward without hyperextending the neck. This is best accomplished with the neck in the neutral or slightly flexed position.
4. Pass the tube following the pharyngeal curvature until the mask is seated against the face (Figure A2-2).
5. Give one ventilation with the BVM and watch for the chest to rise. This is the way to check

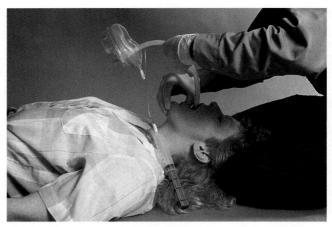

Figure A2-2. Advance airway carefully behind tongue and into pharynx and esophagus.

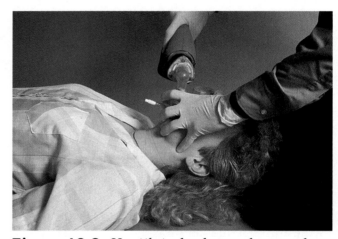

Figure A2-3. Ventilate by bag-valve mask or positive-pressure ventilator.

that the tube has been correctly placed in the esophagus and has not been incorrectly inserted in the trachea (which would block off the trachea and air passage into the lungs). Once you are certain that the tube is correctly placed in the esophagus . . .
6. Inflate the cuff using the 35 cc syringe. (You must be certain the tube is in the esophagus. Inflation of the cuff in the trachea could cause serious damage.)
7. Use the stethoscope to listen to both lung fields (sounds of air intake into the lungs should be present) and the epigastrium. Having assured correct placement of the device . . .
8. Ventilate the patient using the BVM or a positive-pressure ventilator.

Note: The key point to remember is that the EOA or EGTA mask must be sealed in the same manner as a BVM mask (Figure A2-3). In fact, the American Heart Association Emergency Cardiac Care Guidelines recommend that ventilation with a mask be a two-person, four-handed skill: two hands on the mask attending to the seal, two hands squeezing the bag. Otherwise, a sufficient ventilation tide is unlikely to be delivered. * Remember, for adequate ventilation to occur, your technique must be flawless.

When working with the EOA or EGTA, keep the following considerations in mind.

- Remove the bag from the mask prior to each defibrillation to prevent its weight from pulling out the tube.
- Be alert for vomitus in the airway and the need for suction, since regurgitation *can* occur even with the EOA or EGTA in place. If you need to suction, temporarily remove the mask from the tube.
- If a CPR board is used, which has an indentation to hyperextend the neck, be especially careful as hyperextension can increase the changes of misplacing the EOA or EGTA in the trachea. To guard against this possibility it is wise to place a towel under the back of the patient's head to put it in the neutral or flexed position. THE IMPORTANCE OF LISTENING TO LUNG SOUNDS TO CONFIRM CORRECT PLACEMENT CANNOT BE OVEREMPHASIZED.

If the patient becomes conscious, you must remove the tube. REMEMBER THAT EXTUBATION IS LIKELY TO CAUSE VOMITING OR REGURGITATION. Follow these guidelines for removing the EOA or EGTA.

- Always have the suction unit with a rigid Yankauer tip standing by.
- Do not deflate the EOA or EGTA cuff until the patient has resumed breathing and an endotracheal tube has been inserted and its cuff is inflated in the trachea. If you are using an EGTA, a gastric tube can be inserted through it to decompress the stomach or evacuate its contents to reduce the chances of regurgitation or vomiting.
- Provided there is no possibility of a spinal

injury, or if the patient is secured to a spine board, turn the patient on his side, insert the syringe into the one-way valve, and withdraw air slowly from the EOA or EGTA cuff.
- Carefully remove the tube, staying alert for vomiting.

Warning: Whenever an EOA or EGTA is inserted or extubated, gloves, mask, and goggles should be worn to protect the EMT from the potential spraying of body fluids.

INSERTING A PHARYNGO-TRACHEAL LUMAN AIRWAY (PTL®)

One problem with airway devices such as the endotracheal tube, the EOA, and the EGTA is that they must be correctly placed into the intended passageway, the trachea or the esophagus. The Pharyngo-tracheal Lumen Airway (PtL®) has been constructed to get around this problem. It can easily be inserted into either the trachea or esophagus with minimum skill, and it will work no matter which passageway it is in.

The PtL® has two tubes (lumens), one inside the other, and for this reason it is sometimes referred to as a double-lumen airway. A long tube endotracheal-type tube is located within a short, large-diameter tube. The long tube can be inserted into either the trachea or the esophagus, while the shorter tube opens into the pharynx above the epiglottis. Both tubes have low-pressure cuffs at their distal ends. On the long tube, the cuff, when inflated, provides a seal for the trachea or esophagus, depending on which of the two passageways it is resting in. On the short tube, the larger-volume cuff, when fully inflated, seals off the oropharynx.

When the long, inner tube of the PtL® is placed in the esophagus and its cuff is inflated to seal off the esophagus, air delivered through the short outer tube is diverted into the trachea and the lungs. When the long, inner tube is placed in the trachea, air is delivered through that tube, not the short outer tube, to the lungs. Whether it is in the esophagus or the trachea, the longer tube's cuff prevents air from leaking into the esophagus and stomach.

The PtL® also solves the problem of needing extra hands to provide a seal for a face mask. The cuff on the short, outer tube seals the pharynx and prevents delivered air from escaping through the mouth and nose, as well as preventing blood and debris from entering the airway

*A 1983 study showed that experienced EMTs had difficulty using a single hand to seal the BVM mask while achieving an adequate tidal volume with a single-handed BVM bag squeeze: Elling, R., Politis J., An evaluation of emergency medical technicians' ability to use manual ventilation devices., *Annals of Emergency Medicine,* 1983; 12:765-768.

from above. Both tubes of the PtL® have a 15 mm adaptor to which a BVM or other positive-pressure ventilator can be attached.

The PtL® also includes inflation lines so that the cuffs can be inflated. A metal stylet is provided to facilitate guiding the tubes into position. A plastic bite block prevents the patient's teeth from occluding the airway. A neck strap secures the airway to the patient's head.

As with the EOA or EGTA, the PtL® should *not* be used on

- A conscious patient or one with an active gag reflex
- A patient under the age of 16
- A patient who has swallowed a corrosive substance.
- A patient with a known esophageal disease.

The procedure to insert the PtL® starts with preparing the equipment. Ensure that both cuffs are fully deflated, that the long, clear, inner #3 tube (see Figure A2-4) has a bend in the middle, and that the white cap is securely in place over the deflation port located under the #1 inflation valve. Lubricate the long #3 tube with a water-soluble lubricant such as K-Y jelly, Lubifax, or Surgilube. Do not use a silicone or petroleum-based jelly as it can cause an aspiration pneumonia if it gets into the lungs.

If the patient has facial trauma, quickly sweep out the mouth with your gloved fingers and remove any broken teeth, dentures, or other debris that could damage the air cuffs or interfere with passing the tube.

When the patient and the airway are ready, insertion should be accomplished quickly between ventilations.

1. Open the airway. In a patient with potential spinal trauma, have a partner stabilize the head in a neutral position while you pass the airway with minimal cervical manipulation. Use a thumb-in-mouth jaw-lift or tongue-lift method to open the airway. If you have ruled out spinal trauma, hyperextend the patient's head with one hand, insert your thumb deep into the patient's mouth, grasp the tongue and lower jaw between your thumb and index finger, and lift straight upward.
2. Hold the PtL® in your free hand so that it curves in the same direction as the natural curvature of the pharynx. Then insert the tip of the airway into the patient's mouth and advance it carefully behind the tongue until

the teeth strap contacts the lips and teeth. (Positioning the airway in this manner with the teeth strap against the lips and teeth is proper for an average-sized adult. If the patient is very small, it may be necessary to withdraw the airway so that the teeth strap is as much as one inch from the teeth. When the patient is very large, it may be necessary to insert the airway beyond the normal depth so that the teeth strap is actually inside the patient's mouth, past the teeth.)

3. When the tube is at the proper depth, flip the neck strap over the patient's head and tighten it with the hook-and-tape closures located on both sides of the strap.
4. Inflate the small cuff that seals either the esophagus or the trachea and the large cuff that seals the oropharynx, first making sure that the white cap is in place over the deflation port located under the inflation valve. To inflate both cuffs simultaneously, deliver a sustained ventilation into the inflation valve. Failure to inflate the cuffs properly can be detected by the failure of the exterior pilot balloon to inflate or by hearing or feeling air escaping from the patient's mouth and nose. In this case one of the cuffs, probably the large one, may be torn. Quickly remove the airway and replace it with a new one. When you see by the pilot balloon that the two cuffs are inflated, deliver puffs of air to increase pressure in the cuffs and improve the seal.
5. Is the long, clear #3 tube in the esophagus or the trachea? Determine its location by ventilating the short, green #2 tube. If the chest rises, the long tube is in the esophagus and air is, obviously, being diverted through the trachea into the lungs. In this case, deliver ventilations with breaths or with air or oxygen delivered from a BVM or positive-pressure ventilator through the short, green #2 tube.
6. If the chest does not rise when the short, green #2 tube is ventilated, the long, clear #3 tube is probably in the trachea. In this case, remove the stylet and deliver ventilations through the #3 tube. Verify proper delivery of ventilations by listening to both lung fields (for sounds of air entering both lungs) and the epigastrium (where there should be *no* sounds of air entering the esophagus and stomach). Also verify chest rise with each breath.
7. Continue ventilations through the airway

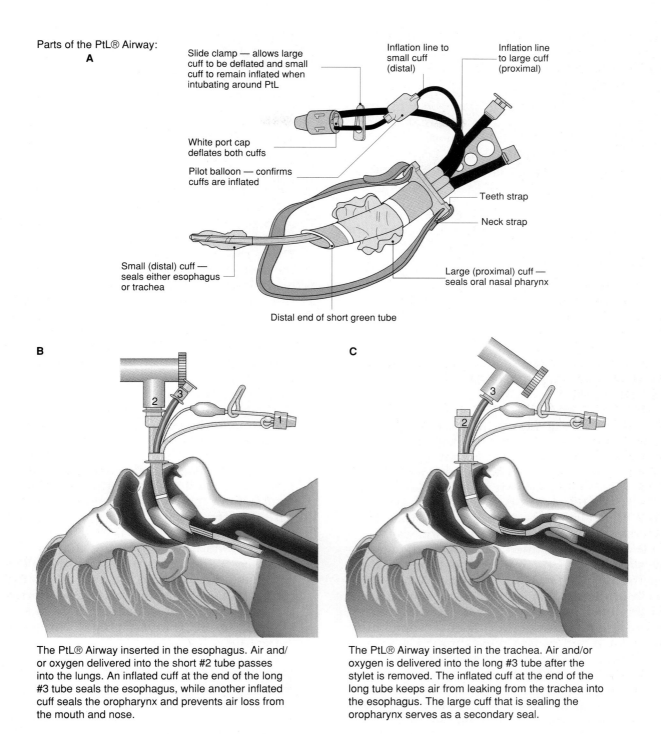

Parts of the PtL® Airway:
A

Slide clamp — allows large cuff to be deflated and small cuff to remain inflated when intubating around PtL

White port cap deflates both cuffs

Pilot balloon — confirms cuffs are inflated

Small (distal) cuff — seals either esophagus or trachea

Inflation line to small cuff (distal)

Inflation line to large cuff (proximal)

Teeth strap

Neck strap

Large (proximal) cuff — seals oral nasal pharynx

Distal end of short green tube

B

C

The PtL® Airway inserted in the esophagus. Air and/or oxygen delivered into the short #2 tube passes into the lungs. An inflated cuff at the end of the long #3 tube seals the esophagus, while another inflated cuff seals the oropharynx and prevents air loss from the mouth and nose.

The PtL® Airway inserted in the trachea. Air and/or oxygen is delivered into the long #3 tube after the stylet is removed. The inflated cuff at the end of the long tube keeps air from leaking from the trachea into the esophagus. The large cuff that is sealing the oropharynx serves as a secondary seal.

Figure A2-4. The PtL® in place in (a) the esophagus or (b) the trachea.

until the patient regains consciousness or protective airway gag reflexes return, or the patient is delivered to the emergency department.

Continually monitor the appearance of the pilot balloon during ventilation efforts. Loss of pressure in the balloon will signal a loss of pres-sure in the cuffs. If you suspect that a cuff is leaking, increase cuff pressure by blowing force-fully into the #1 inflation valve, or replace the airway. Repositioning the PtL® to ensure that the teeth strap is snug against the patient's teeth is another way of reducing leakage.

As with the EOA or EGTA, if the patient becomes conscious, you must remove the PtL®.

REMEMBER THAT EXTUBATION IS LIKELY TO CAUSE VOMITING OR REGURGITATION. Follow these guidelines for removing the PtL®.

- If there is no possibility of trauma, or if the patient is secured to a spine board, turn the patient onto his side and make sure that the stomach has been decompressed and that gastric contents have been evacuated. This can be accomplished by passing a #18 French Levine suction catheter into the non-airway tube.
- Remove the white cap from the deflation port to simultaneously deflate both cuffs.
- Carefully withdraw the airway and discard it.
- Stay alert for vomiting.

Warning: Whenever a PtL® is inserted or extubated, gloves, mask, and goggles should be worn to protect the EMT from the potential spraying of body fluids.

ESOPHAGEAL TRACHEAL "COMBITUBE®"

The most recent alternative to the EOA, EGTA, and PtL® airways is called the esophageal tracheal combitube or, more commonly, "Combitube®." Like the PtL® airway, the Combitube® is a double lumen airway and functions very much like a PtL®. With the Combitube®, however, one lumen is not inside the other. Rather, the two lumens are separated by a partition wall.

In one lumen of the Combitube®, the distal end is sealed and there are perforations in the area that would be in the pharynx. When the tube is in the esophagus, ventilations are delivered through this tube. The sealed end prevents the ventilations from entering the esophagus and stomach and diverts them through the perforations into the pharynx from which they flow into the trachea and the lungs.

In the other lumen of the Combitube®, the distal end is open. When the tube is in the trachea, ventilations are delivered through this tube.

The Combitube® has a distal cuff that inflates to seal the esophagus or trachea, depending on which passageway it is in. (When the trachea is sealed, the cuff prevents stomach contents from being aspirated, but does not prevent ventilations from entering the trachea via the tube that passes through the cuff.)

There is also a pharyngeal balloon that, as with the PtL® seals the pharynx, preventing air from escaping the mouth and nose and blood and debris from entering the airway.

As with the EOA or EGTA, the PtL® should *not* be used on

- A conscious patient or one with an active gag reflex
- A patient under the age of 16
- A patient who has swallowed a corrosive substance.
- A patient with a known esophageal disease.

Follow these steps to insert the Combitube®.

1. Insert the device blindly, watching for the two black rings on the Combitube® that are used for measuring the depth of insertion. These rings should be positioned between the teeth and the bony cavities where the teeth have their roots.
2. Use the large syringe to inflate the pharyngeal cuff with 100 cc of air. On inflation, the device will seat itself in the posterior pharynx behind the hard palate.
3. Use the smaller syringe to fill the distal cuff with 10cc to 15 cc of air.
4. Usually the tube will have been placed in the esophagus. On this assumption, ventilate through the esophageal connector. It is the external tube that is the longer of the two and is marked #1. As with the PtL®, you must listen for the presence of breath sounds in the lungs and the absence of sounds from the epigastrium in order to be sure that the tube is, in fact, placed in the esophagus.
5. If there is an absence of lung sounds and presence of sounds in the epigastrium, the tube has been placed in the trachea. In this case, change the ventilator to the shorter tracheal connector, which is marked #2. Listen again to be sure of proper placement of the tube.

An advantage of the Combitube® over the PtL® is no stylet that must be withdrawn from the open-ended esophageal lumen before suctioning of the stomach can take place, making this process quicker. Another advantage is the automatic seating of the pharyngeal cuff.

The biggest advantage of the Combitube® is that rapid intubation is possible independent of the position of the patient, which is helpful for trauma patients requiring limited cervical spine movement.

As with the EOA, EGTA, or PtL®, if the patient becomes conscious, you must remove the Combitube®. REMEMBER THAT EXTUBATION IS LIKELY TO CAUSE VOMITING OR

REGURGITATION. Have suction equipment ready. Follow the same guidelines as for removal of the other airway devices.

Warning: Whenever a Combitube® is inserted or extubated, gloves, mask, and goggles should be worn to protect the EMT from the potential spraying of body fluids.

ASSISTING PATIENTS WITH SELF-ADMINISTERED EPINEPHRINE

For years, physicians have prescribed epinephrine (EP-uh-NEF-rin) in the form of "bee sting kits," AnaKits, or EpiPens® for patients who are susceptible to severe allergic reactions called anaphylaxis. When such reactions occur, due to insect stings or bites, shellfish ingestion, drugs, or other allergens, epinephrine can save a life by reversing the respiratory distress, cardiovascular collapse, and airway swelling anaphylaxis brings about. It quickly acts to counter vasodilation (blood vessel expansion) and the increased vascular permeability which leads to hypotension (low blood pressure). It also relaxes the bronchial smooth muscles, thus alleviating dyspnea and wheezing.

In some jurisdictions, EMTs may be authorized by their medical director to help patients experiencing an anaphylactic reaction administer the epinephrine they carry or use an EpiPen®, which is a preloaded epinephrine auto-injector. The EpiPen® was originally developed for the military and the National Aeronautics and Space Administration.

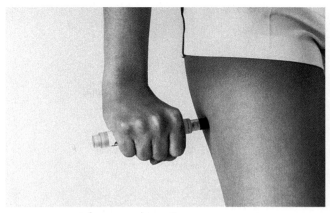

Figure A2-5. The EpiPen®.

Since the dose for a child of 0.15 mg 1:2000 is different from the adult dose of 0.3 mg 1:1000, the EpiPen® comes in two different strengths. The device is designed to be simple to use with no visible needle, which minimizes fear and resistance to self injection. To activate the EpiPen®, you remove the cap and push the pen against the thigh (Figure A2-5) until it auto-injects the medication, and then remove the needle from the skin. Once administered, in addition to relief of symptoms, expect the patient's pulse to increase.

Warning: Epinephrine should be used cautiously, if at all, in patients with hypertension, hyperthyroidism, ischemic heart disease, or cerebral insufficiency. Follow local protocols. If you have any questions, do not hesitate to contact medical control for instructions.

Reference Section

Musculoskeletal System
Skeleton

The skeleton is a living framework made by the joining of bones. It serves to provide support, body movement powered by muscular contractions, protection for the vital organs and other soft structures, blood cell production, and storage for essential minerals. There are 206 bones in the adult body, forming the two divisions of the skeletal system. The axial skeleton is comprised of skull, vertebrae, rib cage, and sternum. The upper and lower extremeties and the shoulder and pelvic girdles form the appendicular skeleton.

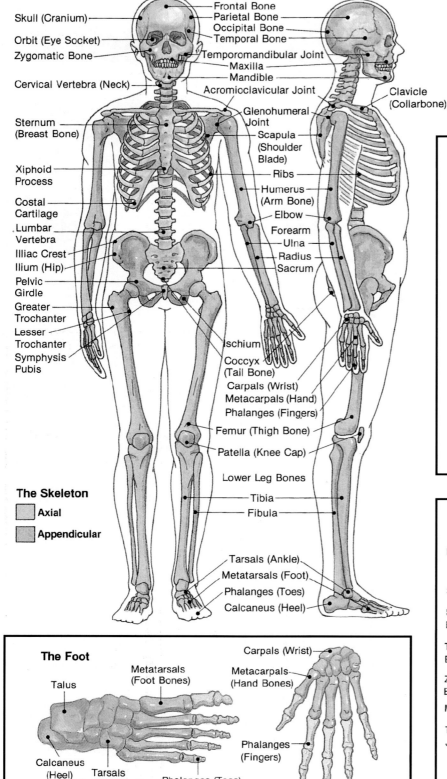

Skull (Cranium)
Orbit (Eye Socket)
Zygomatic Bone
Cervical Vertebra (Neck)
Sternum (Breast Bone)
Xiphoid Process
Costal Cartilage
Lumbar Vertebra
Illiac Crest
Ilium (Hip)
Pelvic Girdle
Greater Trochanter
Lesser Trochanter
Symphysis Pubis

Frontal Bone
Parietal Bone
Occipital Bone
Temporal Bone
Temporomandibular Joint
Maxilla
Mandible
Acromioclavicular Joint
Glenohumeral Joint
Scapula (Shoulder Blade)
Ribs
Humerus (Arm Bone)
Elbow
Forearm
Ulna
Radius
Sacrum

Clavicle (Collarbone)

Ischium
Coccyx (Tail Bone)
Carpals (Wrist)
Metacarpals (Hand)
Phalanges (Fingers)
Femur (Thigh Bone)
Patella (Knee Cap)
Lower Leg Bones
Tibia
Fibula
Tarsals (Ankle)
Metatarsals (Foot)
Phalanges (Toes)
Calcaneus (Heel)

The Skeleton
- Axial
- Appendicular

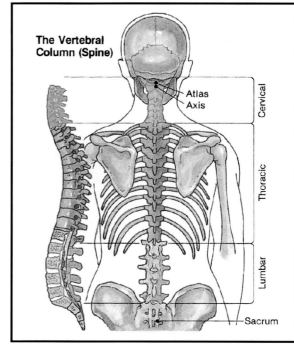

The Vertebral Column (Spine)

Atlas
Axis
Cervical
Thoracic
Lumbar
Sacrum

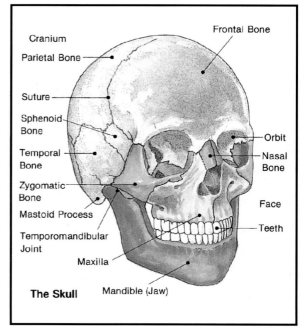

The Skull

Cranium
Parietal Bone
Suture
Sphenoid Bone
Temporal Bone
Zygomatic Bone
Mastoid Process
Temporomandibular Joint
Maxilla
Mandible (Jaw)
Frontal Bone
Orbit
Nasal Bone
Face
Teeth

The Foot
Metatarsals (Foot Bones)
Talus
Calcaneus (Heel)
Tarsals (Ankle Bones)
Phalanges (Toes)

Carpals (Wrist)
Metacarpals (Hand Bones)
Phalanges (Fingers)
The Hand

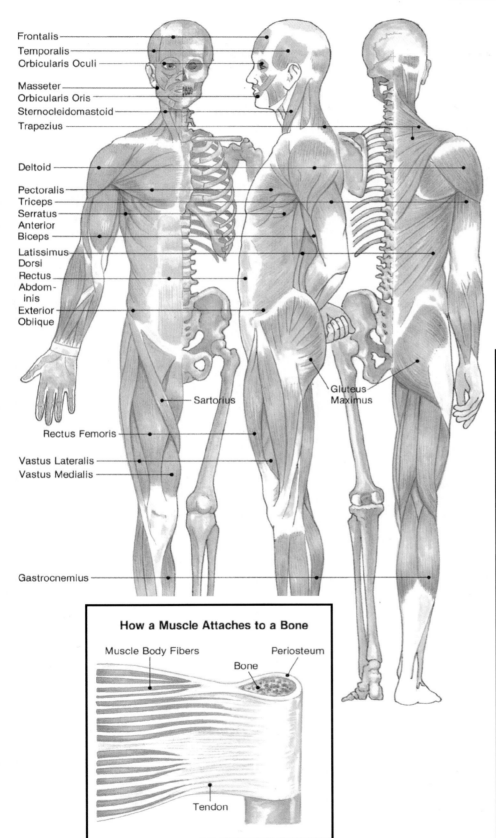

Frontalis
Temporalis
Orbicularis Oculi
Masseter
Orbicularis Oris
Sternocleidomastoid
Trapezius
Deltoid
Pectoralis
Triceps
Serratus Anterior
Biceps
Latissimus Dorsi
Rectus Abdominis
Exterior Oblique
Sartorius
Rectus Femoris
Vastus Lateralis
Vastus Medialis
Gluteus Maximus
Gastrocnemius

The tissues of the muscular system comprise 40 to 50% of the body's weight. The skeletal muscles of the body are voluntary muscles, subject to conscious control. They exhibit the properties of excitability; that is, they will react to nerve stimulus. Once stimulated, skeleton muscles are quick to contract and can relax and very quickly be ready for another contraction. There are 501 separate skeletal muscles that provide contractions for movement, coordinated support for posture, and heat production. Muscles connect to bones by way of tendons.

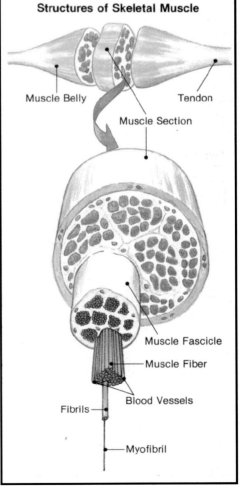

Structures of Skeletal Muscle

Muscle Belly
Tendon
Muscle Section
Muscle Fascicle
Muscle Fiber
Blood Vessels
Fibrils
Myofibril

How a Muscle Attaches to a Bone

Muscle Body Fibers
Periosteum
Bone
Tendon

Nervous System

Brain and Spine

The nervous system includes the brain, spinal cord, and nerves. Structures within the system may be classified according to divisions: central, peripheral, and autonomic divisions of the nervous system. The central nervous system includes the brain and spinal cord. The sensory (incoming) and motor (outgoing) nerves make up the peripheral nervous system. The autonomic nervous system has structures that parallel the spinal cord and then share the same pathways as the peripheral nerves. This division is involved with motor impulses (outgoing commands) that travel from the central nervous system to the heart muscle, blood vessels, secreting cells of glands, and the smooth muscles of organs. The impulses will stimulate or inhibit certain activities.

The Brain

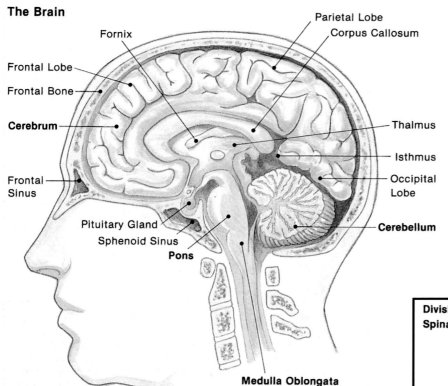

- Fornix
- Frontal Lobe
- Frontal Bone
- **Cerebrum**
- Frontal Sinus
- Pituitary Gland
- Sphenoid Sinus
- **Pons**
- Parietal Lobe
- Corpus Callosum
- Thalmus
- Isthmus
- Occipital Lobe
- **Cerebellum**
- **Medulla Oblongata**

The Spinal Cord

- Sympathetic Trunk
- Spinal Ganglion
- Pia Mater
- Dura Mater
- Body of Vertebra
- Intervertebral Disk
- Spinal Cord
- Posterior Root
- Anterior Root
- Arachnoid
- Spinous Process of Vertebra
- Spinal Nerves
- Sympathetic Ganglion
- Transverse Process of Vertebra

Divisions of the Spinal Cord

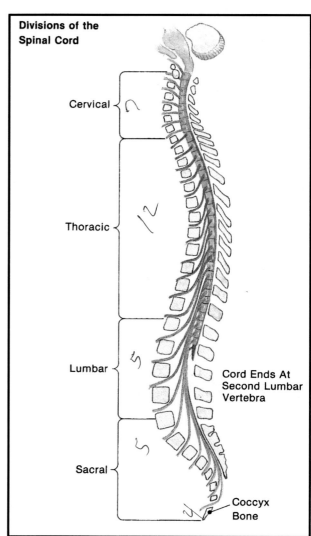

- Cervical
- Thoracic
- Lumbar
- Sacral
- Cord Ends At Second Lumbar Vertebra
- Coccyx Bone

Nervous System

Nerves

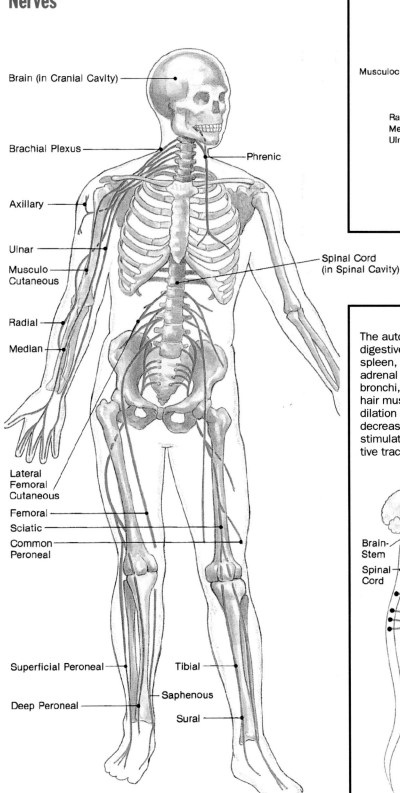

- Brain (in Cranial Cavity)
- Brachial Plexus
- Phrenic
- Axillary
- Ulnar
- Musculo Cutaneous
- Radial
- Median
- Spinal Cord (in Spinal Cavity)
- Lateral Femoral Cutaneous
- Femoral
- Sciatic
- Common Peroneal
- Superficial Peroneal
- Tibial
- Deep Peroneal
- Saphenous
- Sural

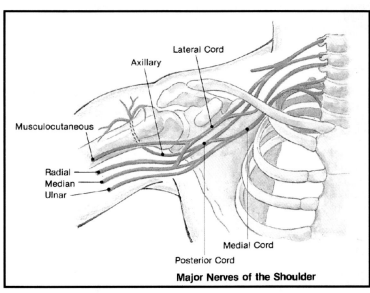

- Lateral Cord
- Axillary
- Musculocutaneous
- Radial
- Median
- Ulnar
- Medial Cord
- Posterior Cord

Major Nerves of the Shoulder

Autonomic Nervous System

The autonomic nervous system affects the heart, blood vessels, digestive tract, salivary and digestive glands, pancreas, liver, spleen, anal sphincter, kidneys, urinary bladder, urinary sphincter, adrenal glands, thyroid gland, gonads, genitalia, nasal lining, larynx, bronchi, lungs, iris and ciliary muscles of the eyes, tear glands, and hair muscles. Impulses can increase or slow heart rate, stimulate dilation or constriction of blood vessels, cause glands to secrete or decrease secretion, initiate or inhibit contractions in the bladder, stimulate or decrease a wave of muscle contraction along the digestive tract, and many other essential body activities.

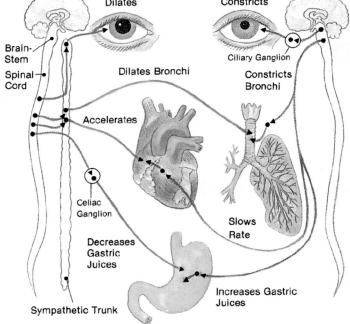

Sympathetic (partial representation) **Parasympathetic**

- Dilates
- Constricts
- Brain-Stem
- Spinal Cord
- Ciliary Ganglion
- Dilates Bronchi
- Constricts Bronchi
- Accelerates
- Celiac Ganglion
- Slows Rate
- Decreases Gastric Juices
- Sympathetic Trunk
- Increases Gastric Juices

Cardiovascular System

Heart

The heart is a hollow, muscular organ that pumps 450 million pints of blood in the average lifetime. Its superior chambers, the atria, receive blood. Both atria fill and then contract at the same time. The inferior chambers are the ventricles. They pump blood out of the heart. Both ventricles fill and then contract at the same time. When the atria are relaxing, the ventricles are contracting.

The right side of the heart receives blood from the body and sends it to the lungs (pulmonic circulation). The heart's left side receives oxygenated blood from the lungs and sends it out to the body (systemic circulation).

The heartbeat originates at the sinoatrial node (pacemaker) and spreads across the atria to stimulate contraction. After a slight delay, the impulse is sent from the atrioventricular node, down the bundles of His, and out across the ventricles. This stimulates the ventricles to contract while the atria are relaxing.

The heart muscle (myocardium) receives its blood supply by way of the right and left coronary arteries. These vessels are the first branches of the aorta.

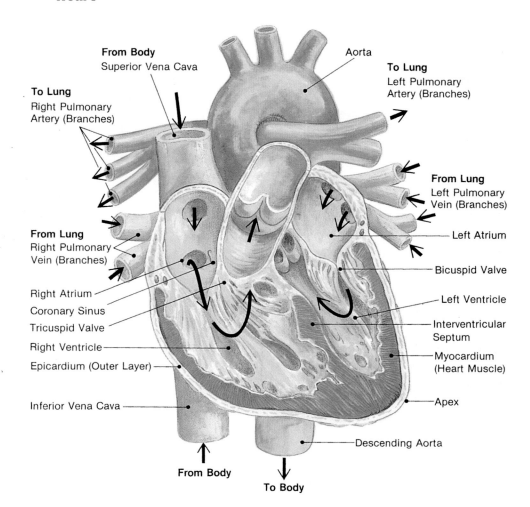

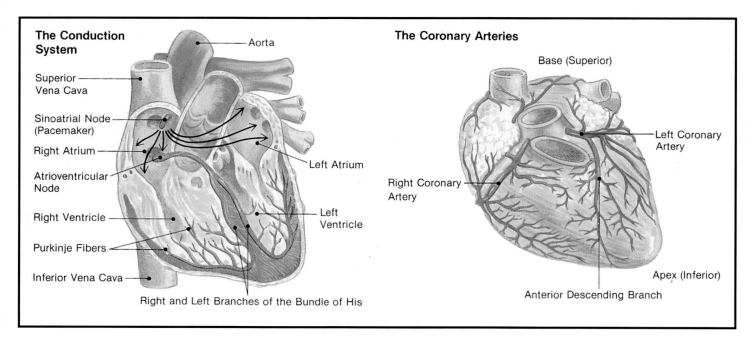

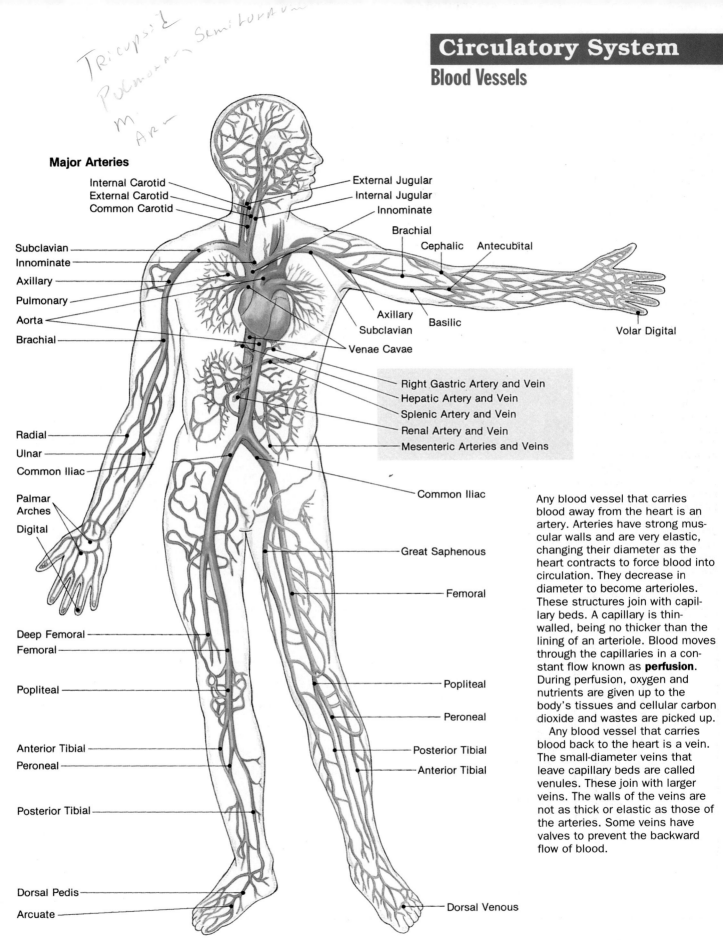

Tricupsid
Pulmonary Semilunar
m.
Ar.

Major Arteries

Internal Carotid
External Carotid
Common Carotid

External Jugular
Internal Jugular
Innominate

Brachial
Cephalic   Antecubital

Subclavian
Innominate
Axillary
Pulmonary
Aorta
Brachial

Axillary
Subclavian
Basilic

Venae Cavae

Volar Digital

Right Gastric Artery and Vein
Hepatic Artery and Vein
Splenic Artery and Vein
Renal Artery and Vein
Mesenteric Arteries and Veins

Radial
Ulnar
Common Iliac

Common Iliac

Palmar
Arches
Digital

Great Saphenous

Femoral

Deep Femoral
Femoral

Popliteal

Popliteal

Peroneal

Anterior Tibial
Peroneal

Posterior Tibial
Anterior Tibial

Posterior Tibial

Dorsal Pedis
Arcuate

Dorsal Venous

Any blood vessel that carries blood away from the heart is an artery. Arteries have strong muscular walls and are very elastic, changing their diameter as the heart contracts to force blood into circulation. They decrease in diameter to become arterioles. These structures join with capillary beds. A capillary is thin-walled, being no thicker than the lining of an arteriole. Blood moves through the capillaries in a constant flow known as **perfusion**. During perfusion, oxygen and nutrients are given up to the body's tissues and cellular carbon dioxide and wastes are picked up.

Any blood vessel that carries blood back to the heart is a vein. The small-diameter veins that leave capillary beds are called venules. These join with larger veins. The walls of the veins are not as thick or elastic as those of the arteries. Some veins have valves to prevent the backward flow of blood.

Respiratory System

The airway consists of structures involved with the conduction and exchange of air. Conduction is the movement of air to and from the exchange levels of the lungs. Air enters through the nose (primary) and mouth (secondary) and travels down the pharynx to enter the larynx. After passing through the larynx, air enters the trachea. At its distal end, the trachea branches into the left and right primary bronchi. These bronchi branch into secondary bronchi, which then branch into the bronchioles. Some of the bronchioles end as closed tubes. Air movement in them helps the lungs expand. The rest of the bronchioles carry the air to the exchange levels of the lungs.

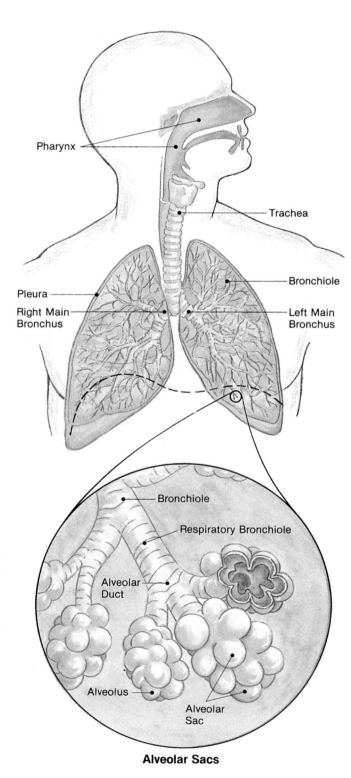

Alveolar Sacs

The respiratory bronchioles turn into alveolar ducts. These form alveolar sacs that are made up of the alveoli. Gas exchange takes place between the alveoli and the capillaries in the lungs.

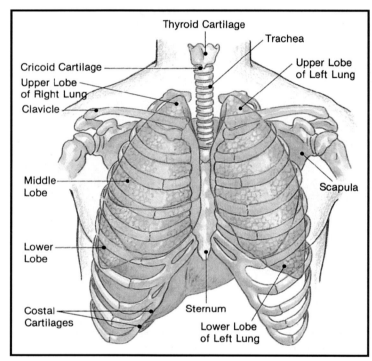

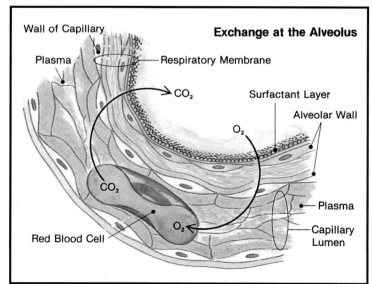

Exchange at the Alveolus

The digestive system includes the digestive tract and various supportive structures and accessory glands. The tract begins at the oral cavity with the teeth and tongue. The salivary glands release saliva into the mouth to moisten food for swallowing. The tract continues down the throat to the esophagus, through the cardiac sphincter, and into the stomach. Acid and digestive enzymes are added to the food to produce chyme. The chyme passes through the pyloric sphincter to enter the small intestine. Digestive enzymes from the pancreas and bile from the liver are added to the chyme. The processes of digestion and absorption are completed in the small intestine. Wastes are carried through the ileoceccal valve into the large intestine. The wastes are moved to the rectum, from where they can be expelled through the anus.

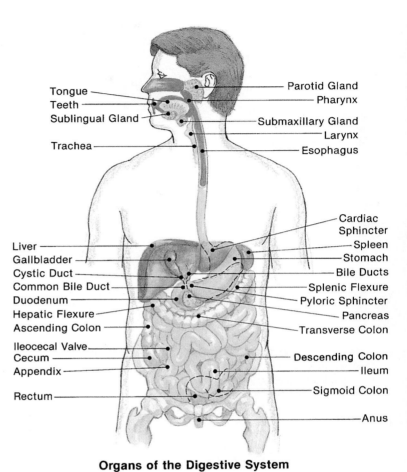

Organs of the Digestive System

Liver, Stomach, and Pancreas

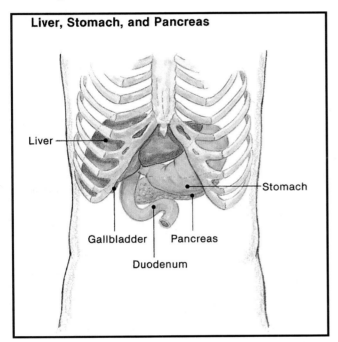

Small Intestine

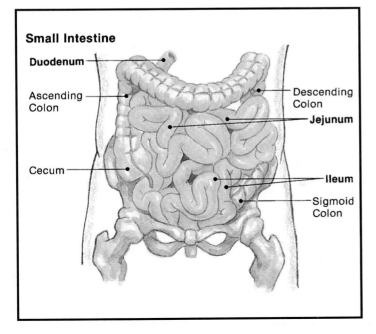

Large Intestine

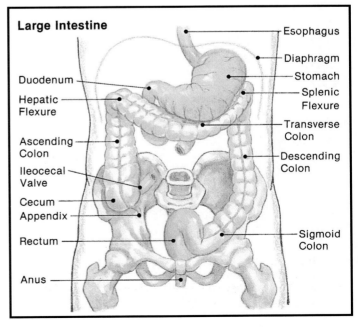

Urinary System

Organs of the Urinary System

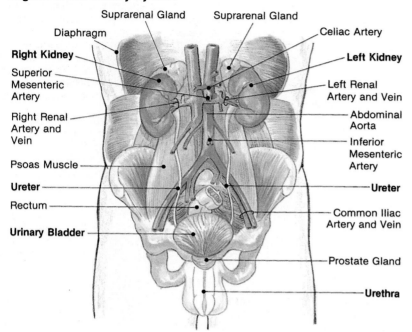

- Suprarenal Gland
- Suprarenal Gland
- Celiac Artery
- Diaphragm
- **Right Kidney**
- **Left Kidney**
- Superior Mesenteric Artery
- Left Renal Artery and Vein
- Right Renal Artery and Vein
- Abdominal Aorta
- Inferior Mesenteric Artery
- Psoas Muscle
- **Ureter**
- **Ureter**
- Rectum
- Common Iliac Artery and Vein
- **Urinary Bladder**
- Prostate Gland
- Urethra

The urinary system is part of the body's excretory structures (urinary system, lungs, sweat glands, and intestine). The kidneys remove the wastes of chemical activities (metabolism) in the body. These wastes are removed from the blood to produce urine. At the same time, the kidneys remove certain excess compounds, regulate the blood pH (acid–base balance), and the concentration of sodium, potassium, chlorine, glucose, and other important chemicals.

The Nephron

Each kidney is made up of microscopic nephrons. Both wastes and needed chemicals are filtered from the blood. As these materials are passed through the nephron, the needed compounds (including water) are sent back into the blood. Wastes are collected as urine.

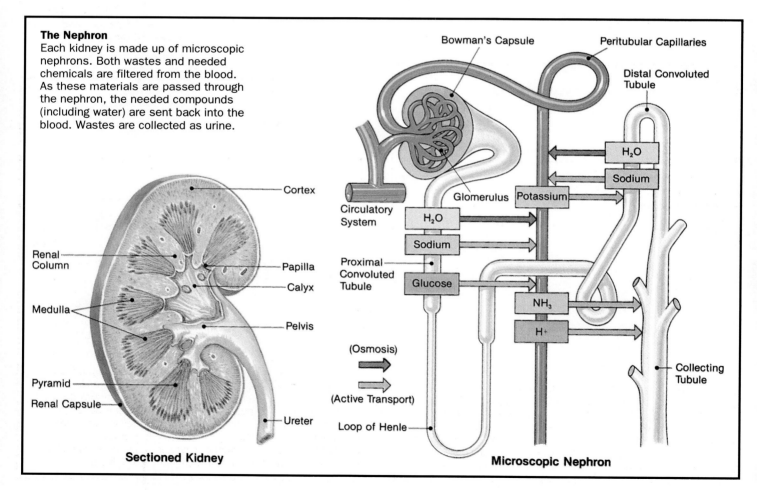

- Bowman's Capsule
- Peritubular Capillaries
- Distal Convoluted Tubule
- H_2O
- Sodium
- Glomerulus
- Potassium
- Circulatory System
- H_2O
- Sodium
- Proximal Convoluted Tubule
- Glucose
- NH_3
- H^+
- (Osmosis)
- (Active Transport)
- Loop of Henle
- Collecting Tubule

Microscopic Nephron

- Cortex
- Renal Column
- Papilla
- Calyx
- Medulla
- Pelvis
- Pyramid
- Renal Capsule
- Ureter

Sectioned Kidney

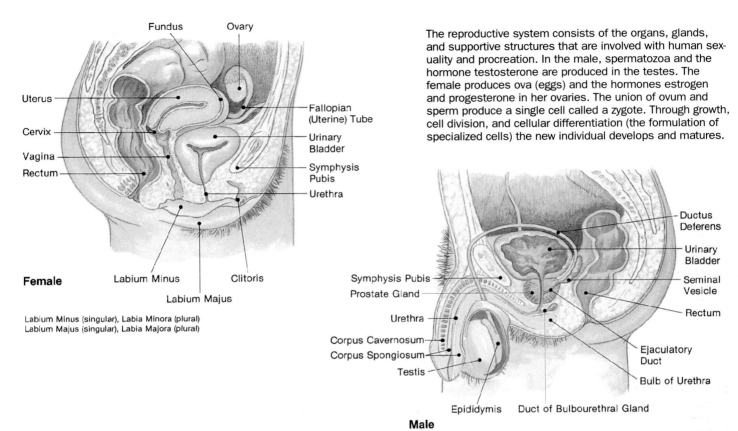

Female

Labium Minus (singular), Labia Minora (plural)
Labium Majus (singular), Labia Majora (plural)

The reproductive system consists of the organs, glands, and supportive structures that are involved with human sexuality and procreation. In the male, spermatozoa and the hormone testosterone are produced in the testes. The female produces ova (eggs) and the hormones estrogen and progesterone in her ovaries. The union of ovum and sperm produce a single cell called a zygote. Through growth, cell division, and cellular differentiation (the formulation of specialized cells) the new individual develops and matures.

Male

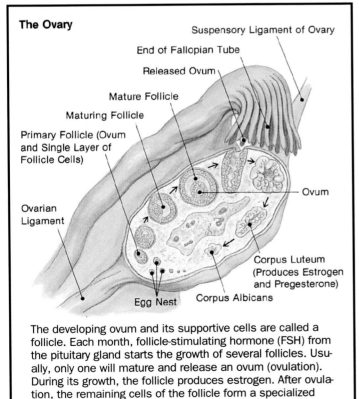

The Ovary

The developing ovum and its supportive cells are called a follicle. Each month, follicle-stimulating hormone (FSH) from the pituitary gland starts the growth of several follicles. Usually, only one will mature and release an ovum (ovulation). During its growth, the follicle produces estrogen. After ovulation, the remaining cells of the follicle form a specialized structure that produces both estrogen and progesterone.

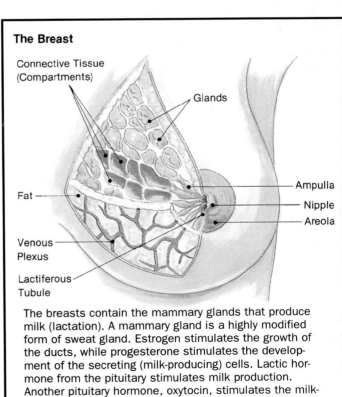

The Breast

The breasts contain the mammary glands that produce milk (lactation). A mammary gland is a highly modified form of sweat gland. Estrogen stimulates the growth of the ducts, while progesterone stimulates the development of the secreting (milk-producing) cells. Lactic hormone from the pituitary stimulates milk production. Another pituitary hormone, oxytocin, stimulates the milk-producing cells to eject their milk into the ducts.

The Skin

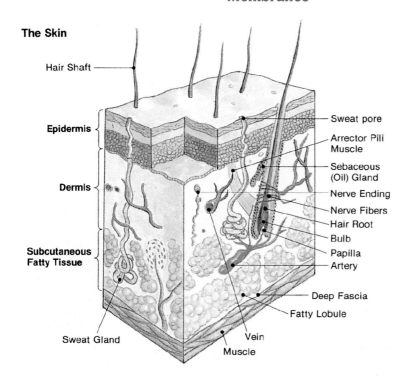

Hair Shaft

Epidermis

Dermis

Subcutaneous
Fatty Tissue

Sweat Gland

Sweat pore
Arrector Pili Muscle
Sebaceous (Oil) Gland
Nerve Ending
Nerve Fibers
Hair Root
Bulb
Papilla
Artery
Deep Fascia
Fatty Lobule
Vein
Muscle

The skin is the largest organ of the body. In the adult the skin covers about 3000 square inches (1.75 square meters) and weighs about 6 pounds. It is involved with protection, insulation, thermal regulation, excretion, and the production of vitamin D.

The Peritoneum

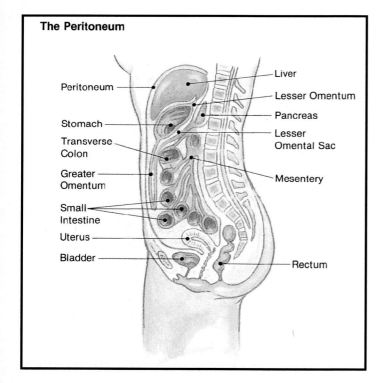

Peritoneum

Stomach

Transverse Colon

Greater Omentum

Small Intestine

Uterus

Bladder

Liver
Lesser Omentum
Pancreas
Lesser Omental Sac
Mesentery
Rectum

Membranes

Membranes cover or line body structures to provide protection from injury and infection. There are four major classes of membranes. Mucous membranes line those structures that open to the outside world (for example, the mouth, the airway, digestive tract, urinary tract, and vagina). Serous membranes line the closed body cavities and cover the outsides of organs. The cutaneous membrane is the skin. Synovial membranes line joints to reduce friction during movement.

A serous membrane that covers an organ is called a visceral layer. The term parietal layer is used for the part of the serous membrane that lines a cavity. The serous membrane in the thoracic cavity is called pleura (for example, the parietal pleura lines the chest cavity). In the abdominal cavity, it is called peritoneum (for example, the parietal peritoneum). A double layer of peritoneum is called mesentery. The membrane that lines the sac surrounding the heart is pericardium.

Synovial Joint

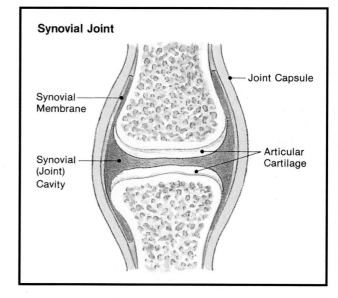

Synovial Membrane

Synovial (Joint) Cavity

Joint Capsule

Articular Cartilage

The Pleura

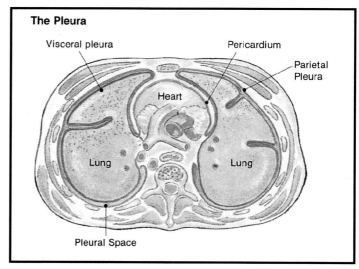

Visceral pleura

Pericardium

Parietal Pleura

Heart

Lung

Lung

Pleural Space

The Eye

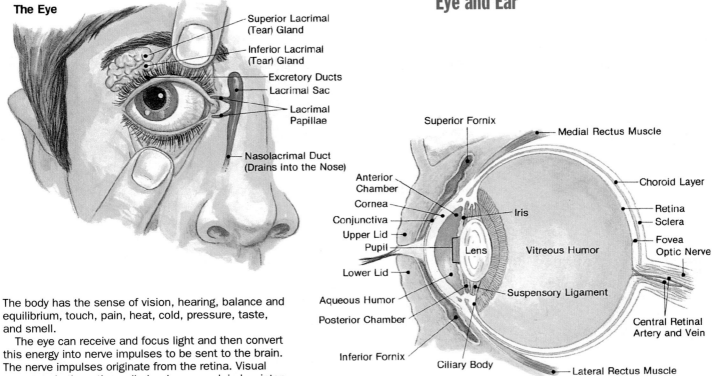

Superior Lacrimal (Tear) Gland

Inferior Lacrimal (Tear) Gland

Excretory Ducts
Lacrimal Sac
Lacrimal Papillae

Nasolacrimal Duct (Drains into the Nose)

Superior Fornix
Medial Rectus Muscle
Anterior Chamber
Cornea
Conjunctiva
Upper Lid
Pupil
Lower Lid
Aqueous Humor
Posterior Chamber
Inferior Fornix
Ciliary Body
Iris
Lens
Vitreous Humor
Suspensory Ligament
Choroid Layer
Retina
Sclera
Fovea
Optic Nerve
Central Retinal Artery and Vein
Lateral Rectus Muscle

The body has the sense of vision, hearing, balance and equilibrium, touch, pain, heat, cold, pressure, taste, and smell.

The eye can receive and focus light and then convert this energy into nerve impulses to be sent to the brain. The nerve impulses originate from the retina. Visual receptors in the retina called rods can work in low intensity light. They have no color function. The visual receptors called cones operate in high intensity light and do receive colors.

The ear's functions include hearing, static equilibrium (balance while standing still), and dynamic equilibrium (balance when moving). The outer and middle ear are responsible for sound gathering and its transmission. The inner ear has the nerve endings for hearing and equilibrium.

The Ear

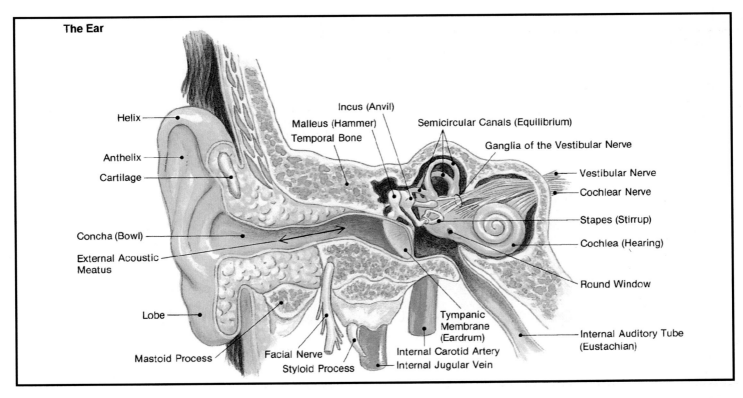

Helix
Anthelix
Cartilage
Concha (Bowl)
External Acoustic Meatus
Lobe
Mastoid Process
Facial Nerve
Styloid Process
Incus (Anvil)
Malleus (Hammer)
Temporal Bone
Semicircular Canals (Equilibrium)
Ganglia of the Vestibular Nerve
Vestibular Nerve
Cochlear Nerve
Stapes (Stirrup)
Cochlea (Hearing)
Round Window
Internal Auditory Tube (Eustachian)
Tympanic Membrane (Eardrum)
Internal Carotid Artery
Internal Jugular Vein

Atlas of Injuries

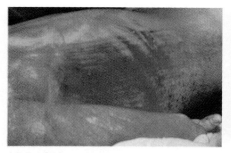
ABRASION (Gravel Roadway)

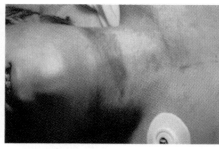
ABRASION (Rope or Cord)

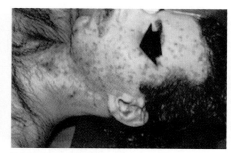
PITTED ABRASION

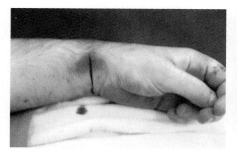
INCISION

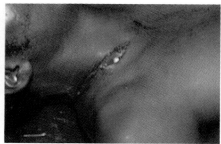
INCISION

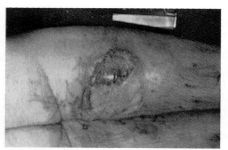
LACERATION (Jagged Margins)

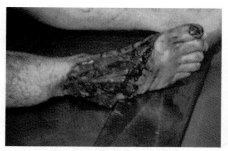
LACERATION (Tendons Still Intact)

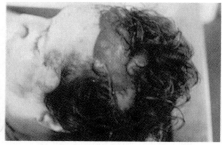
SCALP LACERATION (With Skin Separation)

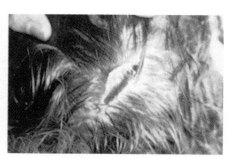
SCALP LACERATION (Minor)

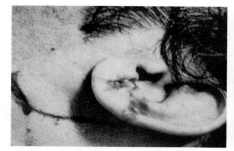
PUNCTURE WOUNDS (Stab Wounds)

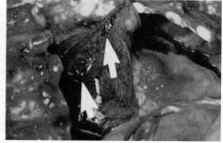
PUNCTURED LUNGS – FROM STAB WOUNDS (Autopsy)

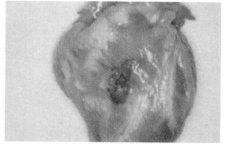
PERFORATED HEART (Bullet Wound)

ALL PHOTOGRAPHS ON THIS PAGE ARE FROM:
Dr. Lee J. Abbott, PO Box 1285, Laxahatchee, FL 33470

Atlas of Injuries

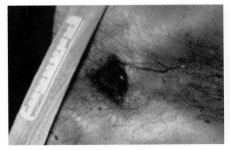

ENTRANCE WOUND (Bullet)

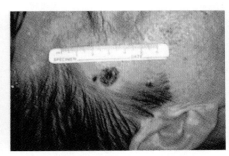

ENTRANCE WOUND (Bullet – Close Range)

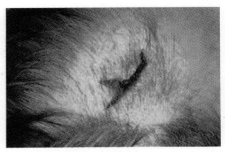

EXIT WOUND (Bullet)

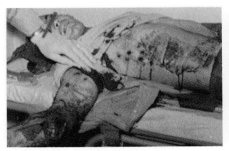

SHOTGUN WOUND

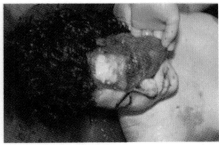

FACIAL AVULSION

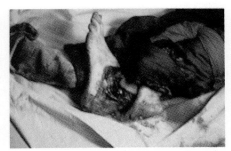

SKIN AVULSION (All Layers)

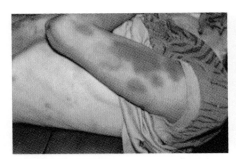

CONTUSIONS

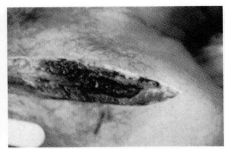

CONTUSION (Opened to Show Blood Accumulation)

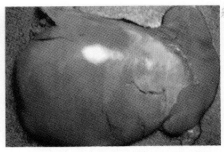

LACERATED LIVER (Abdominal Trauma)

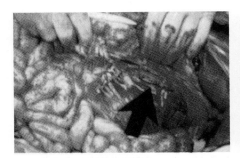

LACERATED SPLEEN

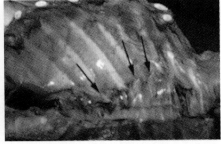

FRACTURED RIBS (Death due to Blood Loss from Lacerated Lungs)

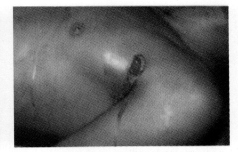

PERFORATED CHEST (Sucking Chest Wound)

ALL PHOTOGRAPHS ON THIS PAGE ARE FROM:
Dr. Lee J. Abbott, PO Box 1285, Laxahatchee, FL 33470

Atlas of Injuries

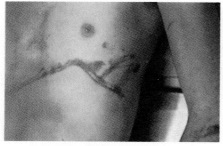

BLUNT TRAUMA TO CHEST

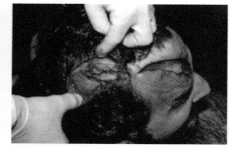

OPEN HEAD WOUND – SKULL FRACTURE

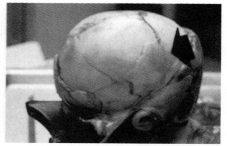

RADIATING SKULL FRACTURE (Blunt Trauma)

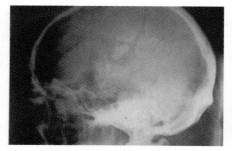

MULTIPLE SKULL FRACTURES (X-ray)

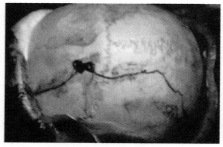

DEPRESSED SKULL FRACTURE (Force from Small Object)

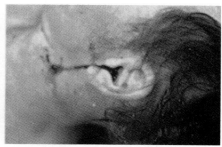

BLEEDING FROM EAR (Possible Skull Fracture)

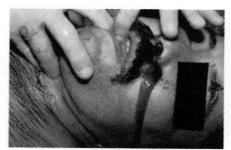

BLEEDING FROM NOSE (Possible Skull Fracture)

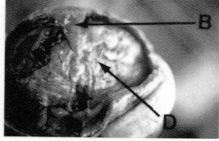

EPIDURAL HEMATOMA (D = Dura, B = Bone Fragment)

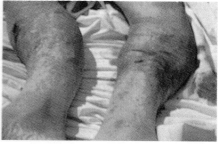

EXTENSIVE BILATERAL INJURY – LOWER EXTREMITIES (Impact with Car)

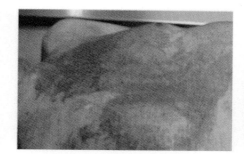

FIRST-DEGREE BURN

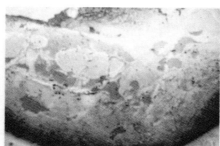

SECOND-DEGREE BURN

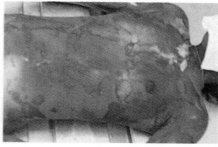

THIRD-DEGREE BURN

ALL PHOTOGRAPHS ON THIS PAGE ARE FROM:
Dr. Lee J. Abbott, PO Box 1285, Laxahatchee, FL 33470

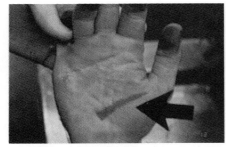

ELECTRICAL BURN
(Contact with Source)
LJA

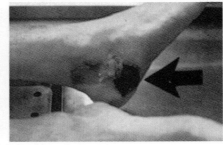

ELECTRICAL BURN (Exit)
LJA

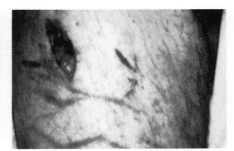

OPEN FRACTURE (Femur)
UT

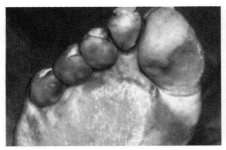

FROSTBITE

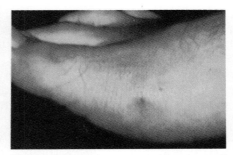

SNAKEBITE
UT

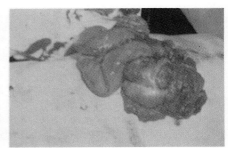

BOWEL EVISCERATION

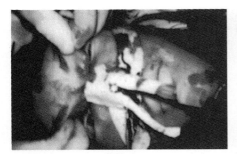

ORBITAL EDEMA

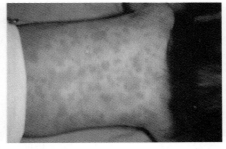

HIVES
AFIP Neg. No. 65-6982-4

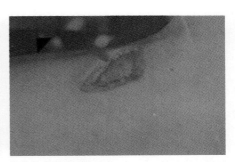

DOG BITE (Leg)
AFIP Neg. No. 62-12291

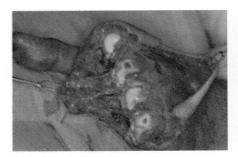

AMPUTATION (Fingers)
AFIP Neg. No. 75-20914

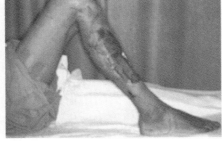

LACERATED LEG
AFIP Neg. No. 68-15269

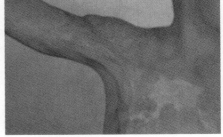

BURN (Hot Water)
AFIP Neg. No. 64-8320

LJA = Dr. Lee J. Abbott   AFJP = Armed Forces Institute of Pathology
UT = University of Tennessee, Memphis, Division of Forensic Pathology

Medical Terminology

As an EMT, you will probably never have to use more than a few medical terms in the course of your prehospital emergency care activities, and most of them will probably deal with parts of the body. Physicians and nurses prefer EMTs to speak in other than medical terms. But if you are an avid reader, much of what you read is likely to be freely sprinkled with medical terms, and if you cannot translate them, you may not understand what you are reading.

Medical terms are comprised of words, word roots, combining forms, prefixes, and suffixes—all little words, if you will, and each with its own definition.

Sometimes medical terms are made up of two whole words. For example, the word SMALL, is joined with the word POX to form the medical term SMALLPOX, the name of a disease. Would that it were all so simple!

Word roots are the foundations of words and are not used by themselves. THERM is a word root that means heat; to use it alone would make no sense. But when a vowel is added to the end of the word root to make it the combining form THERM/O, it can be joined with other words or word roots to form a compound term. THERM/O and METER (an instrument for measuring) combine to form THERMOMETER, an instrument for measuring heat or temperature.

More than one word root or combining form can be joined to form medical terms; ELECTRO-CARDIOGRAM is a good example. ELECTR/O (electric) is joined to CARDI (heart) and the suffix -GRAM (a written record) to form the medical term that means a written record of the heart's electrical activity.

Prefixes are used to modify or qualify the meaning of word roots. They usually tell the reader what kind of, where (or in what direction), or how many.

The term -PNEA relates to breathing, but it says nothing about the quality or kind of breathing. Adding the prefix DYS- qualifies it as difficult breathing.

ABDOMINAL PAIN is a rather broad term; it gives the reader no clue as to exactly where the pain is located either inside or outside the abdomen. Adding the prefix -INTRA to ABDOMINAL pinpoints the location of the pain, for INTRA-ABDOMINAL PAIN means pain within the abdomen. -PLEGIA refers to paralysis of the limbs. The prefix QUADRI informs the reader as to how many limbs are paralyzed. QUADRIPLEGIA means paralysis of all four limbs.

Suffixes are word endings that form nouns, adjectives, or verbs. Medical terms can have more than one suffix, and a suffix can appear in the middle of a compound term affixed to a combining form. A number of suffixes have specialized meanings. -ITIS means inflammation; thus ARTHRITIS means inflammation of a joint. -IAC forms a noun indicating a person afflicted with a certain disease, as for example, HEMOPHILIAC.

Some suffixes are joined to word roots to form terms that indicate a state, quality, condition, procedure, or process. PNEUMON*IA* and PSOR*IASIS* are examples of medical conditions, while APPENDECTOM*Y* and ARTHROSCOP*Y* are examples of medical procedures. The suffixes in each case are underlined.

Some suffixes combine with word roots to form adjectives, words that modify nouns by indicating quality or quantity or by distinguishing one thing from another. GAST*RIC*, CARD*IAC*,

FIBROUS, ARTHRITIC, and DIAPHORETIC are all examples of adjectives formed by adding suffixes (underlined) to word roots.

Some suffixes are added to word roots to express reduction in size, -OLE and -ULE, for example. An ARTERIOLE is smaller than an ARTERY, and a VENULE is smaller than a vein.

When added to word roots, -E and -IZE form verbs. EXCISE and CATHETERIZE are examples.

Finally, some of what are commonly accepted as suffixes are actually the combination of a word root and a suffix. -MEGALY (enlargement) results from the combination of the word root MEGAL (large) and the suffix -Y (which forms the term into a noun). CARDIOMEGALY means enlargement of the heart.

STANDARD TERMS

The following terms are used to denote direction of movement, position, and anatomical posture.

ABDUCTION: movement away from the body's midline.

ADDUCTION: movement toward the body's midline.

AFFERENT: conducting toward a structure.

ANTERIOR: the front surface of the body.

ANTERIOR TO: in front of.

CAUDAD: toward the tail.

CEPHALAD: toward the head.

CIRCUMDUCTION: circular movement of a part.

CRANIAD: toward the cranium.

DEEP: situated remote from the surface.

DISTAL: situated away from the point of origin.

DORSAL: pertaining to the back surface of the body.

DORSIFLEXION: bending backward.

EFFERENT: conducting away from a structure.

ELEVATION: raising a body part.

EXTENSION: stretching, or moving jointed parts into or toward a straight condition.

EXTERNAL: situated outside.

FLEXION: bending, or moving jointed parts closer together.

INFERIOR: situated below.

INTERNAL: situated inside.

LATERAD: toward the side of the body.

LATERAL: situated away from the body's midline.

LATERAL ROTATION: rotating outward away from the body's midline.

LEFT LATERAL RECUMBENT: lying horizontal on the left side.

MEDIAD: toward the midline of the body.

MEDIAL: situated toward the body's midline.

MEDIAL ROTATION: rotating inward toward the body's midline.

PALMAR: concerning the inner surface of the hand.

PERIPHERAL: away from a central structure.

PLANTAR: concerning the sole of the foot.

POSTERIOR: pertaining to the back surface of the body.

POSTERIOR TO: situated behind.

PRONATION: lying face downward or turning the hand so the palm faces downward or backward.

PRONE: lying horizontal, face down and flat.

PROTRACTION: a pushing forward, as the mandible.

PROXIMAL: situated nearest the point of origin.

RECUMBENT: lying horizontal, generally speaking.

RETRACTION: a drawing back, as the tongue.

RIGHT LATERAL RECUMBENT: lying horizontal on the right side.

ROTATION: turning around an axis.

SUPERFICIAL: situated near the surface.

SUPERIOR: situated above.

SUPINATION: lying face upward or turning the hand so the palm faces forward or upward.

SUPINE: lying horizontal, flat on the back and face up.

VENTRAL: the front surface of the body.

PLANES

A plane is an imaginary flat surface that divides the body into sections.

CORONAL OR FRONTAL PLANE: an imaginary plane that passes through the body from side to side and divides it into front and back sections.

MIDSAGITTAL PLANE: an imaginary plane that passes through the body from front to back and divides it into right and left halves.

SAGITTAL PLANE: an imaginary plane parallel to the median plane. It passes through the body from front to back and divides the body into right and left sections.

TRANSVERSE PLANE: an imaginary plane that passes through the body and divides it into upper and lower sections.

WORD PARTS

Prefixes are generally identified by a following dash (AMBI-). Combining forms have a slash and a vowel following the word root (ARTHR/O). Suffixes are generally identified by a preceding dash (-EMIA).

A- (not, without, lacking, deficient); *afebrile*, without fever.

AB- (away from); *abduct*, to draw away from the midline.

-ABLE, -IBLE (capable of); *reducible*, capable of being reduced (as a fracture).

ABDOMIN/O (abdomen); *abdominal*, pertaining to the abdomen.

AC- (to); *acclimate*, to become accustomed to.

ACOU (hear); *acoustic*, pertaining to sound or hearing.

ACR/O (extremity, top, peak); *acrodermatitis*, inflammation of the skin of the extremities.

ACU (needle); *acupuncture*, the Chinese practice of piercing specific peripheral nerves with needles to relieve the discomfort associated with painful disorders.

AD- (to, toward); *adduct*, to draw toward the midline.

ADEN/O (gland); *adenitis*, inflammation of a gland.

ADIP/O (fat); *adipose*, fatty; fat (in size).

AER/O (air); *aerobic*, requiring the presence of oxygen to live and grow.

AF- (to); *afferent*, conveying toward.

AG- (to); *aggregate*, to crowd or cluster together.

-ALGESIA (painful); *hyperalgesia*, overly sensitive to pain.

-ALGIA (painful condition); *neuralgia*, pain that extends along the course of one or more nerves.

AMBI- (both sides); *ambidextrous*, able to perform manual skills with both hands.

AMBL/Y (dim, dull, lazy); *amblyopia*, lazy eye.

AMPHI-, AMPHO- (on both sides, around both); *amphigonadism*, having both testicular and ovarian tissues.

AMYL/O (starch); *amyloid*, starchlike.

AN- (without); *anemia*, a reduced volume of blood cells.

ANA- (upward, again, backward, excess); *anaphylaxis*, an unusual or exaggerated reaction of an organism to a substance to which it becomes sensitized.

ANDR/O (man, male); *android*, resembling a man.

ANGI/O (blood vessel, duct); *angioplasty*, surgery of blood vessels.

ANKYL/O (stiff); *ankylosis*, stiffness.

ANT-, ANTI- (against, opposed to, preventing, relieving); *antidote*, a substance for counteracting a poison.

ANTE- (before, forward); *antecubital*, situated in front of the elbow.

ANTERO- (front); *anterolateral*, situated in front and to one side.

AP- (to); *approximate*, to bring together; to place close to.

APO- (separation, derivation from); *apoplexy*, sudden neurologic impairment due to a cardiovascular disorder.

-ARIUM, -ORIUM (place for something); *solarium*, a place for the sun.

ARTERI/O (artery); *arteriosclerosis*, thickening of the walls of the smaller arteries.

ARTHRIO (joint, articulation); *arthritis*, inflammation of a joint or joints.

ARTICUL/O (joint); *articulated*, united by joints.

AS- (to); *assimilate*, to take into.

AT- (to); *attract*, to draw toward.

AUDI/O (hearing); *audiometer*, an instrument to test the power of hearing.

AUR/O (ear); *auricle*, the flap of the ear.

AUT/O (self); *autistic*, self-centered

BI- (two, twice, double, both); *bilateral*, having two sides; pertaining to two sides.

BI/O (life); *biology*, the study of life.

BLEPHARIO (eyelid); *blepharitis*, inflammation of the eyelid.

BRACHI/O (upper arm); *brachialgia*, pain in the upper arm.

BRADY- (slow); *bradycardia*, an abnormally slow heart rate.

BRONCH/O (larger air passages of the lungs); *bronchitis*, inflammation of the larger air passages of the lungs.

BUCC/O (cheek); *buccal*, pertaining to the cheek.

CAC/O (bad); *cacosmis*, a bad odor.

CALC/O (stone); *calculus*, an abnormal hard inorganic mass such as a gallstone.

CALCANE/O (heel); *calcaneus*, the heel bone.

CALOR/O (heat); *caloric*, pertaining to heat.

CANCR/O (cancer); *cancroid*, resembling cancer.

CAPIT/O (head); *capitate*, head-shaped.

CAPS/O (container); *capsulation*, enclosed in a capsule or container.

CARCIN/O (cancer); *carcinogen*, a substance that causes cancer.

CARDI/O (heart); *cardiogenic*, originating in the heart.

CARP/O (wrist bone); *carpal*, pertaining to the wrist bone.

CAT-, CATA- (down, lower, under, against, along with); *catabasis*, the stage of decline of a disease.

-CELE (tumor, hernia); *hydrocele*, a confined collection of water.

CELI/O (abdomen); *celiomyalgia*, a pain in the muscles of the abdomen.

-CENTESIS (perforation or tapping, as with a needle); *abdominocentesis*, surgical puncture of the abdominal cavity.

CEPHAL/O (head); *electroencephalogram*, a recording of the electrical activity of the brain.

CEREBR/O (cerebrum); *cerebrospinal*, pertaining to the brain and spinal fluid.

CERVIC/O (neck, cervix); *cervical*, pertaining to the neck (or cervix).

CHEIL/O, CHIL/O (lip); *cheilitis*, inflammation of the lips.

CHEIRIO, CHIR/O (hand); *cheiralgia*, pain in the hand.

CHLOR/O (green); *chloroma*, green cancer, a greenish tumor associated with myelogenous leukemia.

CHOL/E (bile, gall); *choledochitis*, inflammation of the common bile duct.

CHONDR/O (cartilage); *chondrodynia*, pain in a cartilage.

CHROM/O, CHROMAT/O (color); *monochromatic*, being of one color.

CHRON/O (time); *chronic*, persisting for a long time.

-CID- (cut, kill, fall); *insecticide*, an agent that kills insects.

CIRCUM- (around); *circumscribed*, confined to a limited space.

-CIS- (cut, kill, fall); *excise*, to cut out.

-CLYSIS (irrigation); *enteroclysis*, irrigation of the small intestine.

CO- (with); *cohesion*, the force that causes various particles to unite.

COL- (with); *collateral*, secondary or accessory; a small side branch such as a blood vessel or nerve.

COL/O (colon, large intestine); *colitis*, inflammation of the colon.

COLP/O (vagina); *colporrhagia*, bleeding from the vagina.

COM- (with); *comminuted*, broken or crushed into small pieces.

CON- (with); *congenital*, existing from the time of birth.

CONTRA- (against, opposite); *contraindicated*, inadvisable.

COR/E, CORE/O (pupil); *corectopia*, abnormal location of the pupil of the eye.

COST/O (rib); *intercostal*, between the ribs.

CRANI/O (skull); *cranial*, pertaining to the skull.

CRY/O (cold); *cryogenic*, that which produces low temperature.

CRYPT/O (hide, cover, conceal); *cryptogenic*, of doubtful origin.

CYAN/O (blue); *cyanosis*, bluish discoloration of the skin and mucus membranes.

CYST/O (urinary bladder, cyst, sac of fluid); *cystitis*, inflammation of the bladder.

-CYTE (cell); *leukocyte*, white cell.

CYT/O (cell); *cytoma*, tumor of the cell.

DACRY/O (tear); *dacryorrhea*, excessive flow of tears.

DACTYL/O (finger, toe); *dactylomegaly*, abnormally large fingers or toes.

DE- (down); *descending*, coming down from.

DENT/O (tooth); *dental*, pertaining to the teeth.

DERM/O, DERMAT/O (skin); *dermatitis*, inflammation of the skin.

DEXTR/O (right); *dextrad*, toward the right side.

DI- (twice, double); *diplegia*, paralysis affecting like parts on both sides of the body.

DIA- (through, across, apart); *diaphragm*, the partition that separates the abdominal and thoracic cavities.

DIPL/O (double, twin, twice); *diplopia*, double vision.

DIPS/O (thirst); *dipsomania*, alcoholism.

DIS- (to free, to undo); *dissect*, to cut apart.

DORS/O (back); *dorsal*, pertaining to the back.

-DYNIA (painful condition); *cephalodynia*, headache.

DYS- (bad, difficult, abnormal, incomplete); *dyspnea*, labored breathing.

-ECTASIA (dilation or enlargement of an organ or part); *gastrectasia*, dilation (stretching) of the stomach.

ECTO- (outer, outside of); *ectopic*, located away from the normal position.

-ECTOMY (the surgical removal of an organ or part); *appendectomy*, surgical removal of the appendix.

ELECTR/O (electric); *electrocardiogram*, the written record of the heart's electrical activity.

-EMIA (condition of the blood); *anemia*, a deficiency of red blood cells.

EN- (in, into, within); *encapsulate*, to enclose with a container.

ENCEPHAL/O (brain); *encephalitis*, inflammation of the brain.

END-, ENDO- (within); *endotracheal*, within the trachea.

ENT-, ENTO- (within, inner); *entopic*, occurring in the proper place.

ENTER/O (small intestine); *enteritis*, inflammation of the intestine.

EP-, EPI- (over, on, upon); *epidermis*, the outermost layer of **skin.**

ERYTHR/O (red); *erythrocyte*, a red blood cell.

ESTHESIA (feeling); *anesthesia*, without feeling.

EU (good, well, normal, healthy); *euphoria*, an abnormal or exaggerated feeling of well-being.

EX- (out of, away from); *excrement*, waste material discharged from the body.

EXO- (outside, outward); *exophytic*, to grow outward or on the surface.

EXTRA- (on the outside, beyond, in addition to); *extracorporeal*, outside the body.

FACI/O (face, surface); *facial*, pertaining to the face.

FEBR/I (fever); *febrile*, feverish.

-FERENT (bear, carry); *efferent*, carrying away from a center.

FIBR/O (fiber, filament); *fibrillation*, muscular contractions due to the activity of muscle fibers.

-FORM (shape); *deformed*, abnormally shaped.

-FUGAL (moving away); *centrifugal*, moving away from a center.

GALACT/O (milk); *galactopyria*, milk fever.

GANGLI/O (knot); *ganglion*, a knotlike mass.

GASTR/O (stomach); *gastritis*, inflammation of the stomach.

GEN/O (come into being, originate); *genetic*, inherited.

-GENESIS (production or origin); *pathogenesis*, the development of a disease.

-GENIC (giving rise to, originating in); *cardiogenic*, originating in the heart.

GLOSS/O (tongue); *glossal*, pertaining to the tongue.

GLYC/O (sweet); *glycemia*, the presence of sugar in the blood.

GNATH/O (jaw); *gnathitis*, inflammation of the jaw.

-GRAM (drawing, written record); *electrocardiogram*, a recording of the heart's electrical activity.

-GRAPH (an instrument for recording the activity of an organ); *electrocardiograph*, an instrument for measuring the heart's electrical activity.

-GRAPHY (the recording of the activity of an organ); *electrocardiography*, the method of recording the heart's electrical activity.

GYNEC/O (woman); *gynecologist*, a specialist in diseases of the female genital tract.

GNOS/O (knowledge); *prognosis*, a prediction of the outcome of a disease.

HEM/A, HEM/O, HEMAT/O (blood); *hematoma*, a localized collection of blood.

HEMI- (one-half); *hemiplegia*, paralysis of one side of the body.

HEPAT/O (liver); *hepatitis*, inflammation of the liver.

HETER/O (other); *heterogeneous*, from a different source.

HIDR/O, HIDROT/O (sweat); *hidrosis*, excessive sweating.

HIST/O (tissue); *histodialysis*, the breaking down of tissue.

HOM/O, HOME/O (same, similar, unchanging, constant); *homeostasis*, stability in an organism's normal physiological states.

HYDR/O (water, fluid); *hydrocephalus*, an accumulation of cerebrospinal fluid in the skull with resulting enlargement of the head.

HYPN/O (sleep); *hypnotic*, that which induces sleep.

HYAL/O (glass); *hyaline*, glassy, transparent.

HYPER- (beyond normal, excessive); *hypertension*, abnormally high blood pressure.

HYPO- (below normal, deficient, under, beneath); *hypotension*, abnormally low blood pressure.

HYSTER/O (uterus, womb); *hysterectomy*, surgical removal of the uterus.

-IASIS (condition); *psoriasis*, a chronic skin condition characterized by lesions.

IATR/O (healer, physician); *pediatrician*, a physician that specializes in children's disorders.

-ID (in a state, condition of); *gravid*, pregnant.

IDVO (peculiar, separate, distinct); *idiopathic*, occurring without a known cause.

IL- (negative prefix); *illegible*, cannot be read.

ILE/O (ileum); *ileitis*, inflammation of the ileum.

ILI/O (ilium); *iliac*, pertaining to the ilium.

IM- (negative prefix); *immature*, not mature.

IN- (in, into, within); *incise*, to cut into.

INFRA- (beneath, below); *infracostal*, below a rib, or below the ribs.

INTER- (between); *intercostal*, between two ribs.

INTRA- (within); *intraoral,* within the mouth.

INTRO- (within, into); *introspection,* the contemplation of one's own thoughts and feelings; self-analysis.

IR/O, IRID/O (iris); *iridotomy,* incision of the iris.

ISCHI/O (ischium); *ischialgia,* pain in the ischium.

-ISMUS (abnormal condition); *strabismus,* deviation of the eye that a person cannot overcome.

ISO- (same, equal, alike); *isometric,* of equal dimensions.

-ITIS (inflammation); *endocarditis,* inflammation within the heart.

KERAT/O (cornea); *keratitis,* inflammation of the cornea.

KINESI/O (movement); *kinesialgia,* pain upon movement.

LABI/O (lip); *labiodental,* pertaining to the lip and teeth.

LACT/O (milk); *lactation,* the secretion of milk.

LAL/O (talk); *lalopathy,* any speech disorder.

LAPAR/O (flank, abdomen, abdominal wall); *laparotomy,* an incision through the abdominal wall.

LARYNG/O (larynx); *laryngoscope,* an instrument for examining the larynx.

LEPT/O (thin); *leptodactylous,* having slender fingers.

LEUC/O, LEUK/O (white); *leukemia,* a malignant disease characterized by the increased development of white blood cells.

LINGU/O (tongue); *sublingual,* under the tongue.

LIP/O (fat); *lipoma,* fatty tumor.

LITH/O (stone); *lithotriptor,* an instrument for crushing stones in the bladder.

-LOGIST (a person who studies); *pathologist,* a person who studies diseases.

LOG/O (speak), give an account; *logospasms,* spasmodic speech.

-LOGY (study of); *pathology,* the study of disease.

LUMB/O (loin); *lumbago,* pain in the lumbar region.

LYMPH/O (lymph); *lymphoduct,* a vessel of the lymph system.

-LYSIS (destruction); *electrolysis* destruction (of hair, for example) by passage of an electric current.

MACR/O (large, long); *macrocephalous,* having an abnormally large head.

MALAC/O (a softening); *malacia,* the morbid softening of a body part or tissue.

MAMM/O (breast); *mammary,* pertaining to the breast.

-MANIA (mental aberration); *kleptomania,* the compulsion to steal.

MAST/O (breast); *mastectomy,* surgical removal of the breast.

MEDI/O (middle); *mediastinum,* middle partition of the thoracic cavity.

MEGA- (large); *megacolon,* an abnormally large colon.

MEGAL/O (large); *megalomaniac,* a person impressed with his own greatness.

-MEGALY (an enlargement); *cardiomegaly,* enlargement of the heart.

MELAN/O (dark, black); *melanoma,* a tumor comprised of darkly pigmented cells.

MEN/O (month); *menopause,* cessation of menstruation.

MES/O (middle); *mesiad,* toward the center.

META- (change, transformation, exchange); *metabolism,* the sum of the physical and chemical processes by which an organism survives.

METR/O (uterus); *metralgia,* pain in the uterus.

MICR/O (small); *microscope,* an instrument for magnifying small objects.

MON/O (single, only, sole); *monoplegia,* paralysis of a single part.

MORPH/O (form); *morphology,* the study of form and shape.

MULTI- (many, much); *multipara,* a woman who has given two or more live births.

MYC/O, MYCET/O (fungus); *mycosis,* any disease caused by a fungus.

MY/O (muscle); *myasthenia,* muscular weakness.

MYEL/O (marrow, also often refers to spinal cord); *myelocele,* protrusion of the spinal cord through a defect in the spinal column.

MYX/O (mucus, slimelike); *myxoid,* resembling mucus.

NARC/O (stupor, numbness); *narcotic,* an agent that induces sleep.

NAS/O (nose); *oronasal,* pertaining to the nose and mouth.

NE/O (new); *neonate,* a newborn infant.

NECR/O (corpse); *necrotic,* dead (when referring to tissue).

NEPHR/O (kidney); *nephralgia,* pain in the kidneys.

NEUR/O (nerve); *neuritis,* inflammation of nerve pathways.

NOCT/I (night); *noctambulism,* sleep walking.

NORM/O (rule, order, normal); *normotension,* normal blood pressure.

NULL/I (none); *nullipara,* a woman who has never given birth to a child.

NYCT/O (night); *nycturia,* excessive urination at night.

OB- (against, in fiont of, toward); *obturator,* a device that closes an opening.

OC- (against, in front of, toward); *occlude,* to obstruct.

OCUL/O (eye); *ocular,* pertaining to the eye.

ODONT/O (tooth); *odontalgia,* toothache.

-OID (shape, form, resemblance); *ovoid,* egg-shaped.

OLIG/O (few, deficient, scanty); *oligemia,* lacking in blood volume.

-OMA (tumor, swelling); *adenoma,* tumor of a gland.

O/O- (egg); *ooblast,* a primitive cell from which an ovum develops.

ONYCH/O (nail); *onychoma,* tumor of a nail or nail bed.

OOPHOR/O (ovary); *oophorectomy,* a surgical removal of one or both ovaries.

-OPSY (a viewing); *autopsy,* postmortem examination of a body.

OPTHALM/O (eye); *opthalmic,* pertaining to the eyes.

OPT/O, OPTIC/O (sight, vision); *optometrist,* a specialist in adapting lenses for the correcting of visual defects.

OR/O (mouth); *oral,* pertaining to the mouth.

ORCH/O, ORCHID/O (testicle); *orchitis,* inflammation of the testicles.

ORTH/O (straight, upright); *orthopedic,* pertaining to the correction of skeletal defects.

-OSIS (process, an abnormal condition); *dermatosis,* any skin condition.

OSTE/O (bone); *osteomyelitis,* inflammation of bone or bone marrow.

OT/O (ear); *otalgia,* earache.

OVARI/O (ovary); *ovariocele,* hernia of an ovary.

OV/I, OV/O (egg); *oviduct,* a passage through which an egg passes.

PACHY- (thicken); *pachyderma,* abnormal thickening of the skin.

PALAT/O (palate); *palatitis,* inflammation of the palate.

PAN- (all, entire, every); *panacea,* a remedy for all diseases, a "cure-all."

PARA- (beside, beyond, accessory to, apart from, against); *paranormal,* beyond the natural or normal.

PATH/O (disease); *pathogen,* any disease-producing agent.

-PATHY (disease of a part); *osteopathy,* disease of a bone.

-PENIA (an abnormal reduction); *leukopenia,* deficiency in white blood cells.

PEPS/O, PEPT/O (digestion); *dyspepsia,* poor digestion.

PER- (throughout, completely, extremely); *perfusion,* the passage of fluid through the vessels of an organ.

PERI- (around, surrounding); *pericardium,* the sac that surrounds the heart and the roots of the great vessels.

-PEXY (fixation); *splendopexy,* surgical fixation of the spleen.

PHAG/O (eat); *phagomania,* an insatiable craving for food.

PHARYNG/O (throat); *pharyngospasms,* spasms of the muscles of the pharynx.

PHAS/O (speech); *aphasic,* unable to speak.

PHIL/O (like, have an affinity for); *necrophilia,* an abnormal interest in death.

PHLEB/O (vein); *phlebotomy,* surgical incision of a vein.

-PHOBIA (fear, dread); *claustrophobia,* a fear of closed spaces.

PHON/O (sound); *phonetic,* pertaining to the voice.

PHOR/O (bear, carry); *diaphoresis,* profuse sweating.

PHOT/O (light); *photosensitivity,* abnormal reactivity of the skin to sunlight.

PHREN/O (diaphragm); *phrenic nerve,* a nerve that carries messages to the diaphragm.

PHYSI/O (nature); *physiology,* the science that studies the function of living things.

PIL/O (hair); *pilose,* hairy.

-PLASIA (development, formation); *dysplasia,* poor or abnormal formation.

-PLASTY (surgical repair); *arthroplasty,* surgical repair of a joint.

-PLEGIA (paralysis); *paraplegia,* paralysis of the lower body, including the legs.

PLEUR/O (rib, side, pleura); *pleurisy,* inflammation of the pleura.

-PNEA (breath, breathing); *orthopnea,* difficult breathing except in an upright position.

PNEUM/O, PNEUMAT/O (air, breath); *pneumatic,* pertaining to the air.

PNEUM/O, PNEUMON/O (lung); *pneumonia,* inflammation of the lungs with the escape of fluid.

POD/O (foot); *podiatrist,* a specialist in the care of feet.

-POIESIS (formation); *hematopoiesis,* formation of blood.

POLY- (much, many); *polychromatic,* multicolored.

POST- (after, behind); *postmortem,* after death.

PRE- (before); *premature,* occurring before the proper time.

PRO- (before, in front of); *prolapse,* the falling down, or sinking of a part.

PROCT/O (anus); *proctitis,* inflammation of the rectum.

PSEUD/O (false); *pseudoplegia,* hysterical paralysis.

PSYCH/O (mind, soul); *psychopath,* one who displays aggressive antisocial behavior.

-PTOSIS (abnormal dropping or sagging of a part); *hysteroptosis,* sagging of the uterus.

PULMON/O (lung); *pulmonary,* pertaining to the lungs.

PY/O (pus); *pyorrhea,* copious discharge of pus.

PYEL/O (renal pelvis); *pyelitis,* inflammation of the renal pelvis.

PYR/O (fire, fever); *pyromaniac,* compulsive fire setter.

QUADRI- (four); *quadriplegia,* paralysis of all four limbs.

RACH/I (spine); *rachialgia,* pain in the spine.

RADI/O (ray, radiation); *radiology,* the use of ionizing radiation in diagnosis and treatment.

RE- (back, against, contrary); *recurrence,* the return of symptoms after remission.

RECT/O (rectum); *rectal,* pertaining to the rectum.

REN/O (the kidneys); *renal,* pertaining to the kidneys.

RETRO- (located behind, backward); *retroperineal,* behind the perineum.

RHIN/O (nose); *rhinitis,* inflammation of the mucus membranes of the nose.

-RRHAGE (abnormal discharge); *hemorrhage,* abnormal discharge of blood.

-RRHAGIA (hemorrhage from an organ or body part); *menorrhea,* excessive uterine bleeding.

-RRHEA (flowing or discharge); *diarrhea,* abnormal frequency and liquidity of fecal discharges.

SANGUIN/O (blood); *exsanguinate,* to lose a large volume of blood either internally or externally.

SARC/O (flesh); *sarcoma,* a malignant tumor.

SCHIZ/O (split); *schizophrenia,* any of a group of emotional disorders characterized by bizarre behavior (erroneously called split personality).

SCLER/O (hardening); *schleroderma,* hardening of connective tissues of the body, including the skin.

-SCLEROSIS (hardened condition); *arteriosclerosis,* hardening of the arteries.

SCOLI/O (twisted, crooked); *scoliosis,* sideward deviation of the spine.

-SCOPE (an instrument for observing); *endoscope,* an instrument for the examination of a hollow body, such as the bladder.

-SECT (cut); *transsect,* to cut across.

SEMI- (one-half, partly); *semisupine,* partly, but not completely, supine.

SEPT/O, SEPS/O (infection); *aseptic,* free from infection.

SOMAT/O (body); *psychosomatic,* both psychological and physiological.

SON/O (sound); *sonogram,* a recording produced by the passage of sound waves through the body.

SPERMAT/O (sperm, semen); *spermacide,* an agent that kills sperm.

SPHYGM/O (pulse); *sphygmomanometer,* a device for measuring blood pressure in the arteries.

SPLEN/O (spleen); *splenectomy,* surgical removal of the spleen.

-STASIS (stopping, controlling); *hemostasis,* the control of bleeding.

STEN/O (narrow); *stenosis,* a narrowing of a passage or opening.

STERE/O (solid, three-dimensional); *stereoscopic,* a three-dimensional appearance.

STETH/O (chest); *stethoscope,* an instrument for listening to chest sounds

STHEN/O (strength); *myasthenia,* muscular-weakness.

-STOMY (surgically creating a new opening); *colostomy,* surgical creation of an opening between the colon and the surface of the body.

SUB- (under, near, almost, moderately); *subclavian,* situated under the clavicle.

SUPER- (above, excess); *superficial,* lying on or near the surface.

SUPRA- (above, over); *suprapubic,* situated above the pubic arch.

SYM-, SYN- (joined together, with); *syndrome,* a set of symptoms that occur together.

TACHY- (fast); *tachycardia,* a very fast heart rate.

-THERAPY (treatment); *hydrotherapy,* treatment with water.

THERM/O (heat); *thermogenesis,* the production of heat.

THORAC/O (chest cavity); *thoracic,* pertaining to the chest.

THROMB/O (clot, lump); *thrombophlebitis,* inflammation of a vein.

-TOME (a surgical instrument for cutting); *microtome*, an instrument for cutting thin slices of tissue.

-TOMY (a surgical operation on an organ or body part); *thoracotomy*, surgical incision of the chest wall.

TOP/O (place); *topographic*, pertaining to special regions (of the body)

TRACHE/O (trachea); *tracheostomy*, an opening in the neck that passes to the trachea.

TRANS- (through, across, beyond); *transfusion*, the introduction of whole blood or blood components directly into the bloodstream.

TRI- (three); *trimester*, a period of three months.

TRICH/O (hair); *trichosis*, any disease of the hair.

-TRIPSY (surgical crushing); *lithotripsy*, surgical crushing of stones.

TROPH/O (nourish); *hypertrophic*, enlargement of an organ or body part due to the increase in the size of cells.

ULTRA- (beyond, excess); *ultrasonic*, beyond the audible range.

UNI- (one); *unilateral*, affecting one side.

UR/O (urine); *urinalysis*, examination of urine.

URETER/O (ureter); *ureteritis*, inflammation of a ureter.

URETHR/O (urethra); *urethritis*, inflammation of the urethra.

VAS/O (vessel, duct); *vasodilator*, an agent that causes dilation of blood vessels.

VEN/O (vein); *venipuncture*, surgical puncture of a vein.

VENTR/O (belly, cavity); *ventral*, relating to the belly or abdomen.

VESIC/O (blister, bladder); *vesicle*, a small fluid-filled blister.

VISCER/O (internal organ); *visceral*, pertaining to the viscera (abdominal organs).

XANTH/O (yellow); *xanthroma*, a yellow nodule in the skin.

XEN/O (stranger); *xenophobia*, abnormal fear of strangers.

XER/O (dry); *xerosis*, abnormal dryness (as of the mouth or eyes).

ZO/O (animal life); *zoogenous*, acquired from an animal.

Glossary

abandonment—to leave an injured or ill patient before the responsibility for care is properly transferred to someone of equal or superior training. Leaving the hospital without giving essential patient information to the staff is viewed by some courts as a form of abandonment.

ABCDEs—the steps of the expanded primary survey: airway, breathing, circulation, disability, expose.

abdominal quadrants—the four zones of the abdominal wall, used for quick reference: the *right upper quadrant, left upper quadrant, right lower quadrant,* and *left lower quadrant.*

abdominopelvic (ab-DOM-i-no-PEL-vik) **cavity**—the anterior cavity below the diaphragm, made up of the *abdominal cavity* and the *pelvic cavity.*

abduction—movement away from the vertical midline of the body.

abortion—spontaneous (miscarriage) or induced termination of pregnancy.

abrasion (ab-RAY-zhun)—a scratch or scrape.

abruptio placentae (ab-RUP-she-o plah-SEN-ti)—a condition in which the placenta separates from the uterine wall; a cause of excessive prebirth bleeding.

absorbed poisons—poisons that are taken into the body through unbroken skin.

Achilles (ah-KIL-ez) **tendon**—the common term for the tendon that connects the posterior lower leg muscles to the heel. The anatomical term is calcaneal (kal-KA-ne-al) tendon.

actual consent—consent given by the rational adult patient, usually in oral form, accepting emergency care. This must be informed consent.

acute abdomen—inflammation in the abdominal cavity producing intense pain.

acute myocardial infarction (MY-o-KARD-e-ul in-FARK-shun) **(AMI)**—occurs when a portion of myocardium (heart muscle) dies when deprived of oxygenated blood; a heart attack.

acute—a medical problem with a sudden onset. Usually, the symptoms are severe and the critical stage of the problem is reached quickly.

adduction—movement toward the vertical midline of the body.

adult—in basic life support, anyone over 8 years of age.

afterbirth—the placenta, membranes of the amniotic sac, part of the umbilical cord, and some tissues from the lining of the uterus that are delivered after the birth of a baby.

AIDS—acquired immune deficiency syndrome; a set of conditions that result from infection by HIV (human immunodeficiency virus). AIDS is fatal.

air embolism—gas bubbles in the bloodstream. The plural term is *emboli.*

air-inflatable splint—a splint that is classified as a soft splint but becomes rigid when inflated.

airway—the passageway for air entering or leaving the body. The structures of the airway are the nose, mouth, pharynx, larynx, trachea, bronchial tree, and lungs.

airway adjunct—a device placed in a patient's mouth or nose in order to help maintain an open airway. See *oropharyngeal airway* and *nasopharyngeal airway.*

allergen—something to which a person is allergic; something that causes an adverse physical response.

alveoli (al-VE-o-li)—the microscopic air sacs of the lungs where gas exchange with the bloodstream takes place.

amniotic (am-ne-OT-ic) **sac**—the "bag of waters" that surrounds the developing fetus.

amputation—the surgical removal or traumatic severing of a body part. The most common usage in emergency care refers to the traumatic amputation of an extremity or part of an extremity.

anaphylactic (an-ah-fi-LAK-tik) **shock**—the most severe type of allergic reaction in which a person develops shock when he encounters a substance to which he is allergic. This is a true, life-threatening emergency.

anatomical position—the standard reference position for the body in the study of anatomy. The body is standing erect, facing the observer. The arms are down at the sides and the palms of the hands face forward.

773

anatomy—the study of body structure.

aneurysm (AN-u-rizm)—the dilation, or ballooning, of a weakened section of an arterial wall.

angina pectoris (AN-ji-nah PEK-to-ris)—the sudden pain occurring when a portion of the myocardium is not receiving enough oxygenated blood.

angulated fracture—a break to a bone causing the limb or joint to take on an unnatural shape or bend.

anterior—the front of the body or body part.

anti-shock garment—a garment that covers the lower body and lower extremities and inflates to exert air pressure and increase blood flow to the central body, heart, and brain.

aorta (ay-OR-tah)—the largest artery in the body. It transports blood from the left ventricle to begin systemic circulation.

aphasia (ah-FAY-zhah)—the complete loss or impairment of speech usually associated with a stroke or brain lesion.

apnea (ap-NE-ah)—the cessation of breathing.

appendicular (AP-en-DIK-u-ler) **skeleton**—that part of the skeleton in the upper and lower extremities.

aqueous (AH-kwe-us) **humor**—the fluid that fills the lens of the eye.

arrhythmia (ah-RITH-me-ah)—a disturbance in heart rate and rhythm.

arteriosclerosis (ar-TE-re-o-skle-RO-sis)—"hardening of the arteries" caused by calcium deposits.

artery—any major blood vessel carrying blood away from the heart.

articular cartilage (ar-TIK-u-lar KAR-te-lij)—an elastic tissue that covers the ends of bones forming joints.

articulate (ar-TIK-u-late)—to meet, as in the formation of a joint where two or more bones come together.

ascites (a-SI-tez)—the accumulation of excessive fluids in the abdomen.

asphyxia (as-FIK-si-ah)—suffocation from lack of air.

aspiration (AS-pir-AY-shun)—the breathing in of vomitus or other foreign matter into the lungs.

asthma (AZ-mah)—a condition of respiratory distress caused when the bronchioles become narrowed and there is an overproduction of mucus causing a reduction in airflow on exhalation.

asystole (ah-SIS-to-le)—a condition in which the heart has ceased generating electrical impulses.

atherosclerosis (ATH-er-o-skle-RO-sis)—a build up of fatty deposits and other particles on the inner wall of an artery. This buildup is called plaque.

atria (AY-tree-ah)—the two upper chambers of the heart. There is a right atrium (which receives unoxygenated blood returning from the body) and a left atrium (which receives oxygenated blood returning from the lungs).

auscultation (os-skul-TAY-shun)—the process of listening to sounds that occur within the body. An example is the procedure that uses a blood pressure cuff and a stethoscope to determine blood pressure. This method requires listening for certain sounds and changes in sound that correspond to systolic and diastolic blood pressures.

automated external defibrillator (AED)—a machine that automatically recognizes shockable chaotic heart rhythms and delivers a shock to the outside of the patient's chest. See also *defibrillation*.

automatic transport ventilator (ATV)—a device that automatically delivers ventilations at a set volume, pressure, and interval.

autonomic nervous system—the division of the peripheral nervous system that controls involuntary motor functions.

AVPU—stands for alert, verbally responsive, painful reponse, unresponsive; an index for quickly determining the level of conciousness.

avulsion (ah-VUL-shun)—the tearing away or tearing off of a piece or flap of skin or other soft tissue. This term also may be used for an eye pulled from its socket or a tooth dislodged from its socket.

axial (AK-si-al) **skeleton**—the skull, spine, ribs, and sternum.

bag-valve mask—a hand-held unit with a self-refilling bag, directional valve system, and face mask. The bag is squeezed to deliver atmospheric air to the patient. This unit can be set up to deliver nearly 100% oxygen when connected to a supplemental oxygen supply system.

bandage—any material used to hold a dressing in place.

barrier device—a device such as a pocket face mask, face shield, bag-valve mask, disposable gloves, or goggles that prevent direct contact with a patient or the patient's breath or body fluids.

biological death—when the brain cells die.

blood—the fluids and cells that are circulated to carry oxygen and nutrients to and wastes away from the body's tissues.

blood pressure—the pressure caused by blood exerting force against the walls of blood vessels. Usually arterial blood pressure (the pressure in an artery) is measured.

body substance isolation—a form of infection control that assumes that all body fluids should be considered potentially infectious.

bones—hard but flexible living structures that provide support for the body and protection to vital organs. Types of bones are *long*, *short*, *flat*, and *irregular*. The typical long bone has a cylindrical *shaft*, and a rounded end, or *head*, which is connected to the shaft by the *neck*.

brachial (BRAY-ke-al) **artery**—the major artery of the upper arm. Some types of external bleeding from the upper extremity can be controlled by applying pressure to the brachial artery pressure point.

brachial pulse—the pulse measured by palpating the major artery (brachial artery) of the arm. This pulse is used to detect heart action and circulation in infants.

braking distance—the number of feet a vehicle travels from the start of braking action until it comes to a full stop.

breech presentation—when the baby appears buttocks or both legs first during birth.

bronchi (BRONG-ke)—the two large sets of branches that come off the trachea and enter the lungs. There are right and left bronchi.

bronchial (BRONG-ke-ul) **tree**—the branching of the airway from the trachea to the air sacs of the lungs.

bronchioles (BRONG-ke-olz)—the smaller branches of the airway that connect the bronchi to the air sacs of the lungs.

bronchiolitis (BRONG-ke-o-LI-tis)—an airway inflammation below the level of the trachea.

capillary (KAP-i-lar-e)—the thin-walled, microscopic blood vessel where oxygen/carbon dioxide and nutrient/waste exchange with the tissues takes place.

capillary refill—the return of blood to the microscopic blood vessels known as capillaries after blood has been forced out by pressure that is then released. Normal refill time is 2 seconds. Capillary refill time is a measure of distal circulation.

cardiac arrest—when the heart stops circulating blood or stops beating entirely.

cardiac tamponade (TAM-po-NADE)—condition when a penetrating or blunt injury to the heart causes blood to flow into the surrounding pericardial sac.

cardiopulmonary resuscitation (KAR-de-o-PUL-mo-ner-e re-SUS-i-TA-shun), **CPR**—heart-lung resuscitation. A combined effort is made to restore or maintain respiration and circulation, artificially.

cardiovascular (KAR-de-o-VAS-kyu-ler) **system**—the system made up of the heart (*cardio*) and the blood vessels (*vascular*); the circulatory system.

carotid (kah-ROT-id) **arteries**—the large neck arteries, one on each side of the neck, that carry blood from the heart to the head.

carotid pulse—the pulse that can be felt on each side of the patient's neck, over top of the carotid arteries.

central nervous system (CNS)—the brain and spinal cord.

cephalic (se-FAL-ik) **presentation**—when the baby appears head first during birth. This is the normal presentation. Also called *vertex presentation*.

cerebrospinal (SER-e-bro-SPI-nal) **fluid (CSF)**—the clear, watery fluid that surrounds and protects the brain and spinal cord.

cerebrovascular (SER-e-bro-VAS-kyuh-ler) **accident (CVA)**—a stroke; the blockage or rupture of a major blood vessel supplying the brain.

cervical (SER-vi-kal)—in reference to the neck.

cervical spine—the section of the spine in the neck.

cervical vertebrae—the seven vertebrae in the neck.

cervix (SER-viks)—the neck of the uterus that enters the birth canal.

chest compressions—during cardiopulmonary resuscitation, pushing motions that depress the sternum (breastbone) to artificially circulate the blood when the heart has stopped beating.

chilblains—lesions that occur from repeated prolonged exposures of bare skin to temperatures between 32°F and 60°F.

child—in basic life support, anyone from 1 to 8 years of age.

chronic (KRON-ic)—a medical problem that is consistently present over a long period of time.

chronic obstructive pulmonary disease (COPD)—a general classification for chronic bronchitis, emphysema, black lung, and many undetermined respiratory diseases that cause problems like those of emphysema.

circulatory (SER-kyuh-luh-tor-e) **system**—the system composed of the heart, arteries, veins, and capillaries that circulates blood through the body; also called the *cardiovascular system*.

clavicles (KLAV-i-kulz)—the two collarbones, one attached to the right side of the superior sternum and one attached to the left side.

clean accident—a radiation accident in which the patient is exposed to radiation but is not contaminated by any radioactive particles or liquids.

clinical death—when breathing and heart action stop.

closed fracture—a broken bone with no associated opening in the skin.

closed wound—an internal injury with no open pathway from the outside.

coccyx (KOK-siks)—the four fused vertebrae that form the terminal bone of the spine; the "tailbone."

Code 1—*See* COLD.

Code 3—*See* HOT.

COLD/Code 1/Priority 3—terms used throughout the United States to designate a non-emergency, normal-driving ambulance response mode.

colostomy (ko-LOS-to-me)—A colostomy, like an ileostomy, is a surgical opening in the abdominal wall with an external bag in place to receive digestive excretions.

communicable disease—a disease that can be passed from one person to another.

compartment syndrome—an increase of pressure in the closed space of the muscle caused by bleeding and tissue swelling or a tight dressing, usually with an injury of the forearm or leg.

compensated shock—a condition in early shock in which the body is compensating for, and to a degree masking, the presence of shock. Its signs may include a heart rate above 100, a slight drop in blood pressure, an increase in capillary refill time, and a slight drop in systolic with an increase in diastolic blood pressure.

concussion—mild closed head injury without detectable damage to the brain. Complete recovery is usually expected.

conduction system—specialized heart muscle that acts as nervous tissue to initiate heart contraction.

condyles (KON-diles)—the large, rounded projections at the distal end of the femur and the proximal end of the tibia. Some persons refer to these as the sides of their knees.

congestive heart failure (CHF)—the failure of the heart to pump efficiently, leading to excessive blood or fluids in the lungs, the body, or both.

conjunctiva (kon-junk-TI-vah)—the delicate membrane that covers the sclera, cornea, and undersurfaces of the eyelids.

contusion (kun-TU-zhun)—a bruise.

COPD—See *chronic obstructive pulmonary disease*.

cornea (KOR-ne-ah)—the transparent portion of the sclera that covers the pupil and iris of the eye.

coronary (KOR-o-nar-e) **arteries**—blood vessels that supply the muscle of the heart (myocardium).

coronary artery disease (CAD)—the narrowing of a coronary artery brought about by atherosclerosis or arteriosclerosis. Occlusion (blockage) occurs in many cases.

coronary artery spasm—a brief contraction of the muscular wall of a coronary artery which may result in cardiac arrest.

costal (KOS-tal) **arch**—the arch of cartilage formed by the costal margin.

costal margin—the cartilage attachment points for ribs 6 through 10. It forms the costal arch.

CPR compression site—for the adult and child, this is the placement of the hands approximately one finger-width above the substernal notch. For infants it is the point on the midline of the sternum that is one finger-width lower than an imaginary line drawn between the nipples.

cranial (KRAY-ne-al) **cavity**—the area within the skull that houses the brain.

cranial floor—the inferior wall of the brain case; the bony floor beneath the brain.

cranium (KRAY-ne-um)—the bony structure making up the forehead, top, back, and upper sides of the skull.

crepitus (KREP-i-tus)—a grating sensation or sound made when fractured bone ends rub together.

critical incident stress debriefing (CISD) teams—teams of counselors who provide emotional and psychological support to EMS personnel who are or have been involved in a multiple-casualty incident or disaster.

croup (KROOP)—a group of viral illnesses that cause inflammation of the larynx, trachea, and bronchi.

crowning—when part of the baby is visible through the vaginal opening.

crush injury—an injury that results when an extremity is caught between heavy items or is subjected to great pressure. Blood vessels, nerves, and muscles are damaged. Bones may be fractured.

CUPS—stands for *critical, unstable, potentially unstable, stable*; an index of patient status used in deciding priority for transport to a medical facility.

cyanosis (sigh-ah-NO-sis)—when the skin, lips, tongue, ear lobes, or nailbeds turn blue or gray from lack of oxygen in circulation. The patient is said to be cyanotic (sigh-ah-NOT-ik).

danger zone—the area at the emergency scene in which rescue personnel, patients, and bystanders may be exposed to hazards such as fire, dangerous chemicals, explosion, downed electrical wires, or radiation.

decompensated shock—when the body can no longer compensate for the conditions that cause shock and the patient begins to show the symptoms of full-blown, life-threatening shock.

decompression sickness—a condition resulting from nitrogen trapped in the body's tissues caused by coming up too quickly from a deep, prolonged dive. A symptom of decompression sickness is "the bends," or deep pain in the muscles and joints.

defibrillation (de-FIB-ri-LAY-shun)—an electrical current applied to the outside of a patient's chest to stop all electrical activity, often enabling the heart to restart in a coordinated fashion.

delirium tremens (de-LEER-e-um TREM-enz) **(DTs)**—a severe reaction that can be part of alcohol withdrawal, characterized by sweating, trembling, anxiety, and hallucinations. Severe alcohol withdrawal with the DTs can lead to death if untreated.

demand-valve resuscitator—an oxygen-powered breathing device that will deliver oxygen when the patient attempts an inspiration.

dermis (DER-mis)—the inner (second) layer of skin found beneath the epidermis. It is rich in blood vessels and nerves.

diabetes mellitus (di-ah-BEE-tez MEL-i-tus)—also called *sugar diabetes* or just *diabetes*, the condition brought about by decreased insulin production, which prevents the body's cells from taking the simple sugar called glucose from the bloodstream. The person suffering from this condition is a *diabetic*.

diabetic ketoacidosis (KE-to-as-i-DO-sis)—a life-threatening condition resulting from loss of fluids and the build-up of ketones, which turn the blood acid; a complication of diabetes mellitus.

diaphoresis (DI-ah-fo-RE-sis)—profuse perspiration.

diaphragm (DI-ah-fram)—the dome-shaped muscle of respiration that separates the chest from the abdomen.

diastolic (di-as-TOL-ik) **blood pressure**—the pressure in the arteries when the lower left chamber of the heart (left ventricle) is refilling.

digestive (di-JES-tiv) **system**—the system of esophagus, stomach, and intestines that enables the taking in and digesting of food.

dirty accident—a radiation accident in which the patient is not only exposed to radiation but is also contaminated by radioactive particles or liquids.

disaster—an emergency of such a magnitude as to severely overtax the capacity of an EMS system to deal adequately with the sick or injured.

disaster plan—a pre-defined set of instructions that tells a community's various emergency responders what to do in specific emergencies.

dislocation—injury causing the end of a bone to be pulled or pushed from its joint.

distal—away from a point of reference or attachment (e.g., the shoulder or hip joint); used as a comparison with *proximal*.

distal pulse—a pulse taken at the foot or wrist. It is called *distal* because it is at the distal end of the limb.

dorsalis pedis pulse—See *pedal pulse*.

downers—depressants such as barbiturates that depress the central nervous system, often used to bring on a more relaxed state of mind.

dressing—any material (preferably sterile) used to cover a wound that will help control bleeding and help prevent additional contamination.

drowning—death caused by changes in the lungs

resulting from immersion in water. See also *near-drowning*.

duty to act—the legal responsibility to provide emergency care. Typically a local law identifies which agencies have this responsibility . If an EMT is a member of such an agency, he or she has a legal responsibility to render emergency care while on duty.

dyspnea (disp-NE-ah)—difficult breathing.

ecchymosis (ek-i-MO-sis)—the discoloration of the skin due to internal bleeding.

eclampsia (e-KLAMP-se-ah)—a severe complication of pregnancy that produces convulsions and coma.

ectopic (ek-TOP-ik) **pregnancy**—when implantation of the fertilized egg is not in the body of the uterus, occurring instead in the oviduct (fallopian tube), cervix, or abdominopelvic cavity.

edema (e-DE-mah)—swelling due to the accumulation of fluid in the tissues.

electromechanical dissociation (el-EK-tro-mek-AN-i-kul dis-so-see-AY-shun) **(EMD)**—a condition in which the heart's electrical rhythm remains relatively normal, yet the mechanical pumping activity fails to follow the electrical activity, causing cardiac arrest.

embolism (EM-bo-liz-m)—a moving blood clot or foreign body, such as fat or an air bubble inside a blood vessel. (The plural is *emboli*.)

emergency care—at the EMT level this is usually the prehospital assessment and treatment of the sick or injured patient. This care is initiated at the emergency scene and is continued through transport and transfer to a medical facility.

Emergency Medical Dispatcher (EMD)—a person trained in interrogation techniques, pre-arrival instructions, and call prioritization. An EMD's four key functions are to receive and process calls for help, to provide medical instructions to patients and information to crews, to dispatch and coordinate Emergency Medical Services (EMS) resources, and to coordinate with other public safety agencies.

Emergency Medical Services (EMS) system—the complete chain of human and physical resources that provides patient care in cases of sudden illness or injury.

Emergency Medical Technician (EMT)—a professional-level provider of emergency care. This individual has received formal training and is appropriately certified. An EMT can be a paid career or a volunteer professional.

EMS command—*See* medical/EMS command.

endocrine (EN-do-krin) **system**—the system that produces the hormones that regulate body functions.

epidermis (ep-i-DER-mis)—the outer layer of skin.

epidural hematoma (ep-i-DU-ral he-mah-TOH-mah)—formed when blood from ruptured vessels flows between the meninges and the cranial bones.

epiglottis (EP-i-GLOT-is)—the trapdoor-like structure at the entrance to the trachea.

epiglottitis (epi-glo-TI-tis)—a potentially life-threatening condition most commonly caused by a bacterial infection that produces swelling of the epiglottis and partial airway obstruction.

epilepsy (EP-i-lep-see)—an episodic medical disorder

of sudden onset characterized by attacks of unconsciousness, with or without convulsions.

episodic (ep-i-SOD-ik)—a medical problem that affects the patient at irregular intervals.

epistaxis (ep-e-STAK-sis)—a nosebleed.

erect—the upright position.

evisceration (e-VIS-er-AY-shun)—when an organ or part of an organ protrudes through a wound opening.

expiration (ex-pir-AY-shun)—breathing out, or exhaling.

extension—to straighten a joint.

external auditory canal—the opening of the external ear; the canal that runs from the external ear to the middle ear.

extremities (ex-TREM-i-teez)—the portions of the appendicular skeleton that include the clavicles, scapulae, arms forearms, wrists, and hands (upper extremities); the pelvis, thighs, legs, ankles, and feet (lower extremities).

face—the anterior portion of the head.

face shield—a thin, transparent barrier device that protects against direct contact with the patient during artificial ventilations.

failure to act—not providing needed care as would be expected in your locality.

false labor—contractions that occur at any time during pregnancy caused by changes in the uterus as it adjusts in size and shape; also called Braxton-Hicks contractions.

femoral (FEM-o-ral) **artery**—the major artery supplying the thigh. Some types of external bleeding from the lower extremity can be controlled by applying pressure to the femoral artery pressure point.

fetus (FE-tus)—the baby as it develops in the womb.

50:50 rule—the rule that CPR compressions and releases should be equal: 50% compression, 50% release.

first-degree burn—a burn involving only the epidermis.

First Responder—a person who is part of the EMS System, having been trained in a First Responder course and, where it is policy, having the appropriate certification. Such an individual is trained below the level of the basic EMT.

flail chest—injury in which usually three or more consecutive ribs on the same side of the chest are fractured, each in at least two locations. A flail chest also can occur when the sternum is fractured loose from its attachments with the ribs. This is sometimes referred to as a flailed sternum.

flexion—to bend a joint.

flowmeter—a valve that indicates the flow from an oxygen cylinder in liters per minute.

formed elements—red blood cells, white blood cells, and platelets of the blood.

fracture (FRAK-cher)—any break in a bone.

freezing—*deep frostbite*, the third stage or the deepest of the three degrees of frostbite. The subcutaneous layers and the deeper structures of the body are affected; muscles, bones, deep blood vessels, and organ membranes can become frozen.

frostbite—the common term for *superficial frostbite*, the second stage or the middle of the three degrees of frostbite. Ice crystals form in the skin and subcutaneous layers. *Frostbite* is also used as the general term for all three degrees of frostbite (frostnip, frostbite, and freezing).

frostnip—*incipient frostbite*, the first stage or the least serious of the three degrees of frostbite. The skin reddens or whitens and becomes numb, but there is little or no tissue damage.

genitalia (jen-i-TAY-le-ah)—the external reproductive system.

Glasgow Coma Scale—a detailed measure of level of conciousness.

glucose (GLU-kos)—a simple sugar converted by the body from the complex sugars a person eats and required by the cells of the body as the basic source of energy. The presence of insulin is required for the body cells to take glucose from the bloodstream.

Good Samaritan laws—a series of laws, varying in each state, designed to provide limited legal protection for citizens and some health care personnel when they are administering emergency care.

hallucinogens (huh-LOO-sin-uh-jens)—mind-affecting or -altering drugs that act on the central nervous system to produce excitement and distortion of perceptions.

heart—the muscular organ that acts as a pump to circulate the blood.

heart attack—an informal term for acute myocardial infarction (AMI).

heat cramps—a condition characterized by muscle cramps and profuse perspiration, brought about by exposure to heat.

heat exhaustion—a form of shock characterized by rapid, shallow breathing, weak pulse, cold, clammy skin, and profuse perspiration brought about by exposure to heat; commonly called "heat prostration."

heat stroke—a life-threatening emergency that occurs when the body's temperature-regulating mechanisms fail during exposure to heat; characterized by deep, then shallow breathing, full, rapid pulse, hot, dry skin, and little or no sweating; commonly, and inaccurately, called "sun stroke."

Heimlich maneuver—manual thrusts to the abdomen to force bursts of air from the lungs to dislodge an airway obstruction.

hematoma (HE-mah-TO-mah)—a swelling caused by the collection of blood under the skin or in damaged tissues as a result of an injured or broken blood vessel.

hemopneumothorax (HE-mo-NU-mo-THOR-aks)—a combination of blood and air in the thoracic cavity.

hemorrhage (HEM-o-rej)—internal or external bleeding.

hemothorax (HE-mo-THOR-aks)—blood in the thoracic cavity.

hepatitis (HEP-uh-TI-tis)—an infection that causes iflammation of the liver, communicated through blood, stool, and other body fluids, even when dried. Hepatitis can be fatal.

hernia (HER-ne-ah)—part of a muscle or organ forced through an opening in the lining of the organ or body cavity; also called a *rupture.*

HIV—human immunodeficiency virus. See *AIDS.*

HOT/Code 3/Priority 1—terms used throughout the United States to designate an emergency, lights-and-siren ambulance response mode.

humidifier—a device connected to the flowmeter to add moisture to the dry oxygen coming from an oxygen cylinder.

hyperglycemia (HI-per-gli-SEE-me-ah)—too much sugar in the blood.

hyperthermia (HI-per-THURM-i-ah)—an increase in body temperature above normal; life-threatening at its extreme.

hyperventilate (HI-per-VENT-i-late)—in suctioning, to provide ventilations at a higher rate to compensate for oxygen not delivered during suctioning.

hyperventilation (HI-per-vent-i-LAY-shun)—a temporary condition of rapid, deep breathing.

hypoglycemia (HI-po-gli-SEE-me-ah)—too little sugar in the blood.

hypothermia (HI-po-THURM-i-ah)—a generalized cooling that may reduce the body temperature below normal; life-threatening at its extreme.

hypoxia (hi-POK-se-ah)—an inadequate supply of oxygen reaching the body's tissues.

hypoxic (hi-POK-sik) **drive**—a condition common to COPD patients in which the body determines the need to breathe based on oxygen rather than carbon dioxide and may interpret the higher oxygen levels that result from oxygen administration as a signal to reduce or stop breathing.

ileostomy (il-e-OS-to-me)—See *colostomy.*

iliac (IL-e-ak) **crest**—the upper, curved boundary of the ilium.

ilium (IL-e-um)—the upper portions of the pelvis, forming the wings of the pelvis.

immune (im-YOON) **system**—the network of specialized cells that help prevent disease by killing germs or rendering them harmless.

immunity—in the law, exemption from legal liability.

implied consent—a legal concept that assumes an unconscious patient (or one so badly injured or ill that he cannot respond) would consent to receiving emergency care if he or she could do so. In some states, implied consent may apply to children when parents or guardians are not at the scene, to the developmentally disabled (e.g., mentally retarded), and to the mentally or emotionally disturbed.

incident command system—a system used for the management of a multiple-casualty incident, involving assumption of responsibility for command and designation and coordination of such elements as triage, treatment, transport, and staging.

incision—a smooth cut.

induced abortion—delivery of a fetus as a result of deliberate actions taken to stop the pregnancy.

infant—in basic life support, anyone from birth to 1 year of age.

infectious disease—a disease caused by an organism entering the body.

inferior—away from the head; usually compared with another structure that is closer to the head (e.g., the lips are inferior when compared with the nose).

informed consent—agreement by a rational adult patient to accept emergency care, after having been informed of what you believe the patient's condition to be and what you plan to do. In many cases, informed consent does not exist unless the patient also knows the risks and the alternatives.

ingested poisons—poisons that are swallowed.

inguinal (IN-gwin-al) **hernia**—a soft tissue injury in which the abdominal membranes and part of the intestine bulge through a defect in the abdominal wall.

inhaled poisons—poisons that are breathed in.

injected poisons—poisons that are inserted through the skin, possibly into the bloodstream, for example by needle, snake fangs, or insect stinger.

inspiration (in-spir-AY-shun)—breathing in, or inhaling.

insulin (IN-suh-lin)—a hormone produced by the pancreas or taken as a supplement by many diabetics. Insulin must be present to enable the body cells to take glucose from the bloodstream.

integumentary (in TEG-u-MEN-ta re) **system**—the skin and its accessories (hair, oil glands, sweat glands, nails).

intercostal (in-ter-KOS-tal) **muscles**—the muscles between the ribs.

internal auditory canal—the canal that connects the middle ear with the nasal cavity.

intracerebral hematoma (in-trah-SER-e-bral he-mah-TO-mah)—formed when blood from ruptured vessels pools within the brain.

involuntary consent—consent for care obtained by court order when the adult patient or the child patient's parent or guardian refuses care.

ionizing radiation—the product of atomic decay, including alpha particles, beta particles, and gamma rays.

iris—the colored portion of the eye in which the pupil is located.

ischemic (is-KE-mik)—deficient in oxygen because of reduced circulation or blood supply.

ischium (IS-ke-em)—the lower, posterior portions of the pelvis.

joint capsule—a fibrous structure that surrounds a synovial joint and contains the membranes that produce synovial fluid.

joints—places where bones articulate, or meet. Most joints are movable.

jugular (JUG-u-lar) **notch**—the visible depression where the clavicles and sternum meet.

jugular veins—the large neck veins, one on each side of the neck, that return blood from the head to the heart.

labor—the stages of delivery that begin with the contractions of the uterus and end with the expulsion of the placenta.

laceration—a jagged cut.

lacrimal (LAK-re-mal) **gland**—the tear gland.

laryngectomy (LAR-in-JEK-to-me)—a surgical procedure in which all or part of the larynx is removed. An opening is usually made in the neck, through which the patient breathes.

laryngospasm (lah-RING-go-spazm)—spasm of the larynx that seals the airway, set off when water passes the epiglottis.

larynx (LAR-inks)—the portion of the airway connecting the pharynx and the trachea. It contains the voicebox and vocal cords.

lateral—to the side, away from the vertical midline of the body; used only in reference to another body part. Thus, there is a lateral side to the arm.

lateral recumbent—lying on the side.

lateral rotation—to turn the foot or hand outward away from the midline.

LeForte fractures—three types of facial fractures. Type I is at the site of the maxilla and the hard palate, Type II from the palate upward across the nasal bone, Type III through the orbits to the temporomandibular joint, separating the face from the rest of the skull.

lens—a cavity behind the iris and pupil of the eye.

level of consciousnessss (LOC)—degree of alertness (awareness and orientation). There are several methods of estimating level of consciousness in use by EMS systems such as the Glasgow Coma Scale or AVPU: Alert and oriented (patient is aware of what is happening), Verbal (patient talks and/or responds to voice), Painful stimuli (patient withdraws from a painful stimulus such as a pinch), Unresponsive (patient does not respond to any stimuli).

ligaments—tissues that connect bone to bone.

liter (LE-ter)—metric measurement of liquid volume that is equal to 1.057 quarts. One pint is almost equal to one-half liter.

log roll—a maneuver for changing a patient's position by rolling him as a unit, keeping head, neck, and torso aligned.

lower airway—the structures of the airway from the larynx to the air sacs of the lungs.

lumbar (LUM-bar) **spine**—the section of the spine in the midback.

lumbar vertebrae—the five vertebrae of the midback.

lungs—the organs where exchange of oxygen and carbon dioxide take place.

malar (MA-lar)—the cheek bone, also called the zygomatic bone.

mammalian diving reflex—a reaction that occurs when the face is submerged in water. Breathing is inhibited, the heart rate slows, and major blood flow is sent to the brain, heart, and lungs.

mandible (MAN-di-bl)—the lower jaw bone.

manual traction—the process of applying tension to straighten and realign a fractured limb before splinting. Also known as *tension*.

maxillae (mak-SIL-e)—the two fused bones forming the upper jaw.

mechanical pump failure—inability of the heart to funciton normally due to damaged tissues.

mechanisms of injury—what forces caused the injury, allowing you to relate types of accidents to certain types of injuries. You must consider the kind of force, its intensity and direction, and the area of the body that is affected.

meconium staining—amniotic fluid that is greenish or brownish-yellow rather than clear; an indication of possible fetal distress during labor.

medial—toward the vertical midline of the body; used only in reference to another body part. Thus, you can have a medial side to the arm.

medial rotation—to turn the foot or hand inward toward the midline.

medical/EMS command—the senior EMS person on the scene who establishes an EMS command post and oversees the medical aspects of a multiple-casualty incident.

medullary (MED-u-lar-e) **canal**—the cavity in long bones containing bone marrow.

meninges (me-NIN-jez)—the three-layered membrane that surrounds the brain and spinal cord.

meningitis (men-in-JI-tis)—a condition caused by either a bacterial or viral infection of the lining of the brain and spinal cord

midline—an imaginary line drawn down the center of the body, dividing it into right and left halves.

miscarriage—see *spontaneous abortion.*

multiple birth—when more than one baby is born during a single delivery.

multiple-casualty incident (MCI)—any medical or trauma incident involving multiple patients.

multiple-function resuscitator—an oxygen-powered breathing device that combines demand-valve and positive-pressure functions. See *demand-valve resuscitator* and *positive-pressure resuscitator.*

multitrauma dressing—a bulky dressing.

musculoskeletal (MUS-kyu-lo-SKEL-e-tal) **system**—the system of bones and skeletal muscles that support and protect the body and permit movement.

myocardial infarction (heart attack)—see *acute myocardial infarction.*

myocardium (mi-o-KAR-de-um)—heart muscle.

narcotics—a class of drugs that affect the nervous system and change many normal body activities. Their legal use is for the relief of pain. Illicit use is to produce an intense state of relaxation.

nasal (NAY-zl) **bones**—the bones that form the upper third, or bridge, of the nose.

nasal cannula (KAN-yuh-luh)—a device that delivers low concentrations of oxygen through two prongs that rest in the patient's nostrils.

nasal septum—the cartilage that separates the two chambers of the nose.

nasopharyngeal (na-zo-fah-RIN-je-al) **airway**—a flexible breathing tube inserted through the patient's nose into the pharynx.

near-drowning—the condition of having begun to drown. The near-drowning patient may be conscious, unconscious with heartbeat and pulse, or with no heartbeat or pulse but still able to be resuscitated. Only when sufficient time without breathing has passed to render resuscitation useless (sometimes 30 minutes or more if the patient has been in cold water) has *drowning* truly taken place.

necrotic (nek-ROT-ik)—having suffered necrosis (nek-ROS-is) or tissue death.

negligence—at the EMT level this is the failure to provide the expected care at the standard of care, leading to the injury or death of the patient.

nervous system—the system of brain, spinal cord, and nerves that govern sensation, movement, and thought.

nonrebreather mask—a face mask and reservoir bag device that delivers high concentrations of oxygen. All of the patient's exhaled air escapes through a valve and is not rebreathed.

objective examination—a part of the secondary survey. This is a hands-on survey of the patient in which you determine vital signs and perform a head-to-toe survey.

occipital (ok-SIP-i-tal) **lobe**—the posterior portion of the brain in which the vision center is located.

occlusion (uh-KLU-zhun)—blockage, as in the blockage of an artery.

occlusive (uh-KLU-siv) **dressing**—any dressing that forms an airtight seal.

open fracture—either a broken bone with the ends or fragments tearing outward through the skin or a penetrating wound with an associated fracture.

open pneumothorax (NU-mo-THOR-aks)—condition in which air is entering the thoracic cavity through an external wound.

open wound—an injury in which the skin is interrupted, exposing the tissue beneath.

optic nerve—the nerve that carries impulses from the eye to the brain.

orbits—the bony structure around the eyes; the eye sockets.

oropharyngeal (or-o-fah-RIN-je-al) **airway**—a curved airway adjunct inserted through the patient's mouth into the pharynx.

oxygen cylinder—a cylinder filled with oxygen under pressure.

palpate, palpation—to feel any part of the body, as to palpate the radial pulse; also, to use the blood pressure cuff and the feeling of the radial pulse to determine approximate patient systolic blood pressure.

paradoxical (pair-uh-DOKS-i-kal) **motion**—movement of a flailed section in the opposite direction to the rest of the chest during respirations.

partial rebreather mask—a face mask and reservoir bag device that delivers moderate concentrations of oxygen. Part of the patient's exhaled air enters the reservoir to mix with the oxygen and be rebreathed.

pathogens—the organisms that cause infection.

patient—the victim of an accident or illness who has entered the EMS system or other professional medical care.

pedal (PEED-al) **pulse**—a foot pulse. There are two locations used in field emergency care: the *dorsalis pedis* (lateral to the large tendon of the big toe) and the *posterior tibial* (behind the medial ankle).

perception distance—the number of feet a vehicle travels while the operator recognizes a hazard and decides how to react.

perfusion—the constant flow of blood through the capillaries.

perineum (per-i-NE-um)—the surface area between the vulva and anus.

periosteum (per-e-OS-te-um)—the white fibrous membrane covering a bone.

peripheral nervous system (PNS)—the nerves that enter and leave the spinal cord and that travel between the brain and organs without passing through the spinal cord (e.g. the optic nerve between the eye and the brain).

pharynx (FAIR-inks)—the throat.

physiology—the study of body function.

pinna (PIN-nah)—the external ear, also called the auricle.

placenta (plah-SEN-tah)—the organ of pregnancy where exchange of oxygen, foods, and wastes occurs between mother and fetus.

placenta previa (PRE-vi-ah)—a condition in which the placenta is formed in an abnormal location (usually low in the uterus and close to or over the cervical opening) that will not allow for a normal delivery of the fetus; a cause of excessive prebirth bleeding.

plaque (PLAK)—a fatty deposit on the interior walls of arteries.

plasma (PLAZ-mah)—the fluid portion of the blood. It is the blood minus the formed elements.

pneumothorax (NU-mo-THO-raks)—condition resulting when air enters the thoracic cavity from an open wound or from a damaged lung or both. See also *open pneumothorax, spontaneous pneumothorax,* and *tension pneumothorax.*

pocket face mask—a device with a one-way valve tfor mouth-to-mask resuscitation. It can be used with supplemental oxygen when fitted with an oxygen inlet. It is a varrier device, the one-way valve preventing contact with the patient's breath or fluids.

point tenderness—a painful response to pressure.

poison—any substance that can harm the body by altering cell structure or functions.

positive-pressure resuscitator—a manually triggered, oxygen-powered breathing device.

posterior—the back of the body or body part.

posterior tibial pulse—See *pedal pulse.*

post-traumatic stress disorder (PTSD)—adverse psychological effects resulting days, weeks, or even months after involvement in a stressful incident.

posterior—the back of the body or body part.

pre-eclapmsia (pre-e-KLAMP-se-ah)—a complication of pregnancy that can lead to convulsions and coma.

premature infant—any newborn weighing less than 5.5 pounds or being born before the 37th week of pregnancy.

pressure dressing—a bulky dressing held in position with a tightly wrapped bandage to apply pressure to help control bleeding.

pressure point—a site where a main artery lies near the surface of the body and directly over a bone. Pressure on such a point can stop distal bleeding.

pressure regulator—a device connected to an oxygen cylinder to reduce cylinder pressure to a safe pressure for delivery of oxygen to a patient.

priapism (PRE-ah-pizm)—persistent erection of the penis often associated with spinal injury and some medical problems.

primary survey—a patient assessment process carried out to detect and treat life-threatening problems. Basic life support is provided as needed during the primary survey.

priority 1—*see* HOT

priority 3—*see* COLD

prolapsed umbilical cord—when the umbilical cord presents first during birth and is squeezed between the vaginal wall and the baby's head.

prolonged delivery—when birth is delayed more than 20 minutes after contractions are 2-to-3 minutes apart.

pronation—a rotation of the forearm so that the back of the hand is facing forward.

prone—lying face down.

proximal—close to a point of reference or attachment (e.g., the shoulder or hip joint); used as a comparison with *distal.*

pubic (PYOO-bik) **bone, pubis** (PYOO-bis)—the middle (medial), anterior portion of the pelvis.

pulmonary (PUL-mo-nar-e) **arteries**—the blood vessels that carry blood from the right ventricle of the heart to the lungs.

pulmonary circulation—the transport of blood from the right ventricle of the heart to the lungs, where the blood excretes carbon dioxide and picks up oxygen, then back to the left atrium of the heart.

pulmonary edema (ed-EE-mah)—fluid in the lungs. Pulmonary edema is an absolute contraindication to the use of anti-shock garments.

pulmonary veins—the vessels that carry oxygenated blood from the lungs to the left atrium of the heart.

pulse—the rhythmic beats caused as waves of blood move through and expand the arteries.

pulse character—the *rhythm* (regular or irregular) and *force* (full or thready) of the pulse.

pulse pressure—the difference between systolic and diastolic readings. When the two readings approach each other (systolic falling, diastolic rising or unchanging), it is a reliable sign of serious thoracic cavity injury.

pulse rate—the number of pulse beats per minute.

puncture wound—an open wound that tears through the skin and destroys underlying tissues. A *penetrating puncture wound* can be shallow or deep. A *perforating puncture wound* has both an entrance and an exit wound.

pupil—the adjustable opening that admits light to the eye.

radial pulse—a pulse found in the lateral wrist.

rales (RAYLZ)—abnormal crackling or gravelly breathing sounds that can be heard in the lungs with a stethoscope, usually associated with fluids building up in the lungs.

reaction distance—the number of feet a vehicle travels from the time the operator decides to stop until his foot applies pressure to the brake pedal.

release form—a document signed by a patient or witnesses indicating that the patient has refused care.

reproductive system—the male and female organs involved in sexual reproduction.

rescue breathing—providing artificial ventilations (or pulmonary resuscitation to a person who has stopped breathing on his own or whose breathing is inadequate.

respiration (res-pi-RAY-shun)—the act of breathing in (inhaling) and breathing out (exhaling).

respiratory (RES-pir-uh-tor-e) **arrest**—when a person stops breathing completely.

respiratory character—the *rhythm* (regular or irregular), *depth* (deep or shallow), *ease* (easy, labored, difficult, or painful), and *sounds* (such as snoring, wheezing, crowing, or gurgling) of breathing.

respiratory failure—either the cessation of normal breathing or the reduction of breathing to the point where oxygen intake is insufficient to support life.

respiratory system—the system of nose, mouth, throat, and lungs that brings oxygen into the body and expels carbon dioxide.

respiratory rate—the number of breaths per minute.

resuscitation (re-SUS-i-TAY-shun)—any efforts used to artificially restore breathing or breathing and heart function.

retina (RET-i-na)—the back of the eye.

rigid splint—a stiff device used to immobilize a fracture or dislocation.

Rule of Nines—a method for estimating the extent of a burn. For an adult, each of the following areas represents 9% of the body surface: the head and neck, each upper limb, the chest, the abdomen, the upper back, the lower back and buttocks, the front of each lower limb, and the back of each lower limb. The remaining 1% is assigned to the genital region. For an infant or child the percentages are modified so that 18% is assigned to the head, 14% to each lower limb.

Rule of Palm—a method for estimating the extent of a burn. The palm of the hand, which equals about 1% of the body's surface area, is compared with the patient's burn to estimate its size.

rupture—see *hernia.*

sacrum (SAY-krum)—the five fused vertebrae of the lower back.

sciatic (si-AT-ik) **nerve**—the major nerve that extends from the lower spine to the posterior thigh.

sclera (SKLE-rah)—the white of the eye.

secondary survey—a patient assessment process that includes the subjective interview, the head-to-toe survey of the patient, and the taking of vital signs.

second-degree burn—a burn involving the epidermis and the dermis but not penetrating through the dermis.

seizure (SE-zher)—a sudden change in sensation, behavior, or movement, usually related to brain malfunctions that can be the result of diseased, infected, or injured brain tissue. The more severe forms produce violent muscle contractions called convulsions.

Senses—sight, hearing, taste, smell, and sensations of pain, cold, heat, and touch.

shock—a life-threatening condition with a variety of possible causes; most commonly the reaction of the body to the failure of the cardiovascular system to provide an adequate supply of blood to all vital parts of the body.

signs—what you see, hear, feel, and smell in relation to a patient's problem.

simple face mask—a soft mask through which moderate concentrations of oxygen can be delivered.

skull—the bony structure of the head made up of 22 bones that form the cranium and the face.

sleep apnea (ap-NE-ah)—periods of cardiac slowdown and temporary cessation of breathing during sleep, often associated with sudden infant death syndrome.

soft splints—air-inflatable splints, vacuum splints, or cushioning items such as pillows, towels, blankets, or dressings that help immobilize a fracture or dislocation.

somatic nervous system—the division of the peripheral nervous system that transmits sensory information and controls voluntary movement.

sphygmomanometer (SFIG-mo-mah-NOM-e-ter)—the cuff and gauge used in blood pressure determination.

spinal cavity—the area within the spinal column that contains the spinal cord.

spinal column—the column of bones known as vertebrae that houses the spinal cord and supports the head and upper body.

spinous processes—the bony extensions of the posterior vertebrae.

splint—a device used to immobilize fractures and dislocations so that there is a minimum of movement to the bone and to the joints above and below the bone.

spontaneous abortion—when the fetus and placenta deliver before the 28th week of pregnancy; commonly called *miscarriage.*

spontaneous pneumothorax (NU-mo-THOR-aks)—condition when a weakened section of the lung ruptures and releases air into the thoracic cavity. The lung partially or completely collapses.

sprain—a partially torn ligament.

staging officer—the person responsible for overseeing and keeping track of ambulances and ambulance personnel at a multiple-casualty incident. The staging officer will direct ambulances to treatment areas at the request of the transportation officer.

staging sector—the area where ambulances are parked and other resources are held until needed.

standard of care—the minimum acceptable level of emergency care to be provided.

status asthmaticus (az-MAT-i-kus)—a life-threatening prolonged asthma attack.

status decision—a decision about whether immediate transport is or is not needed on the basis of assigning the patient to a category of stability. See also *CUPS.*

status epilepticus (ep-i-LEP-ti-kus)—when a person suffers two or more convulsive seizures without regaining full consciousness. It is a true emergency, requiring immediate transport.

sternum (STER-num)—the breastbone.

stillborn—born dead.

stoma (STO-mah)—the permanent neck opening created in a laryngectomy or tracheostomy.

stopping distance—the number of feet a vehicle travels from the moment the operator decides to stop until the vehicle actually stops. It is the total of reaction distance and braking distance.

strain—the overstretching or mild tearing of a muscle.

stroke—see *cerebrovascular accident*.

subcutaneous emphysema (SUB-ku-TAY-ne-us EM-fi-SEE-mah)—air under the skin. This is observed most frequently when a lung is punctured and air escapes into the surrounding tissues of the thorax.

subcutaneous layers—the layers of fat and soft tissues found below the dermis.

subdural hematoma (sub-DU-ral he-mah-TOH-mah)—formed when blood from ruptured vessels flows between the brain and the meninges.

subjective interview—a part of the secondary survey that uses the patient and bystanders as sources of information by having them answer specific questions.

substernal notch—a general term for the lowest region on the sternum to which the ribs attach.

sucking chest wound—an open wound to the chest that draws air from the atmosphere into the chest cavity. This is a form of pneumothorax.

suction unit—a device that is used to remove blood, secretions, or other materials from a patient's mouth, throat, or stomach.

sudden death—a cardiac arrest that occurs within two hours of the onset of symptoms. The patient may have no prior symptoms or coronary artery disease.

sudden infant death syndrome (SIDS)—an unexplained sudden death of an apparently healthy infant while asleep.

superior—toward the head; often used in reference with *inferior*.

supination—a rotation of the forearm so that the palm is facing forward.

supine—lying on the back.

supine hypotensive syndrome—dizziness and a drop in blood pressure caused when the mother is in a supine position and the weight of the uterus, infant, placenta, and amniotic fluid compress the inferior vena cava, reducing venous return to the heart and reducing cardiac output.

suture (SU-cher)—the point or seam where two bones, especially cranial bones, articulate, or join together.

sympathetic eye movement—the coordinated movement of both eyes in the same direction. If one eye moves, the other eye will carry out the same movement, even if it is covered or the eyelid is shut.

symptoms—what the patient tells you about his problem.

syncope (SIN-ko-pe)—fainting; a self-correcting, temporary form of shock.

synovial (si-NO-ve-al) **joints**—the highly movable joints in the body, such as the elbow, consisting of the ends of two joining bones surrounded by a joint capsule and lubricated by synovial fluid.

systemic (sis-TEM-ik) **circulation**—the transport of blood from the left ventricle of the heart to the body, where the blood provides oxygen to the tissues and picks up waste carbon dioxide, then back to the right atrium of the heart.

systolic (sis-TOL-ik) **blood pressure**—the pressure created in the arteries when the lower left chamber of the heart (left ventricle) contracts and forces blood out into circulation.

temporal bone—bone that forms part of the lateral wall of the skull and the floor of the cranial cavity. There is a right and a left temporal bone.

temporal (TEM-po-ral) **artery**—the major artery in the region of the temple. Some types of external scalp bleeding can be controlled by applying pressure to the pressure point over the temporal artery.

temporomandibular (TEM-po-ro-man-DIB-u-lar) **joint**—the movable joint formed between mandible and temporal bone, also called the TM joint.

tendons—tissues that connect muscle to bone.

tension—see *manual traction*.

tension pneumothorax (NU-mo-THOR-aks)—condition in which air is trapped in the thoracic cavity. In some cases, the air may enter through a sucking chest wound and be trapped as the wound seals itself shut or is sealed with an occlusive dressing. In *closed tension pneumothorax*, the air escapes from a damaged lung and there is no external wound through which it can escape. Tension pneumothorax may produce rapid death.

third-degree burn—a full-thickness burn with damage extending through the dermis.

thoracic (tho-RAS-ik) **cage**—the bony structure that protects the heart, lungs, and other organs in the chest. It is made up of 12 pairs of ribs, the 12 thoracic vertebrae, and the sternum, or breastbone.

thoracic cavity—the anterior body cavity above the diaphragm, containing the heart and its great vessels, part of the trachea and most of the esophagus.

thoracic spine—the section of the spine in the upper back.

thoracic vertebrae—the 12 vertebrae to which the ribs attach.

thrombus (THROM-bus)—a clot formed of blood and plaque attached to the inner wall of an artery.

thyroid (THY-roid) **cartilage**—the Adam's apple.

tourniquet (TURN-i-ket)—a device that constricts all blood flow to and from an extremity.

tourniquet shock—a dangerous condition caused when a tourniquet is loosened or released, and toxic substances that have gathered distal to the tourniquet are released in high concentrations to the rest of the body.

toxin—a poisonous substance secreted by bacteria, plants, or animals.

trachea (TRAY-ke-ah)—the windpipe.

tracheostomy (TRAY-ke-OS-to-me)—a surgical procedure in which an artificial opening into the trachea is made through the neck.

traction splints—special splints that apply a constant pull along the length of a lower extremity. This helps to stabilize the fractured bone and reduce muscle spasms in the limb. Traction splints are used primarily to treat femoral shaft fractures.

transportation officer—the person responsible for communicating with sector officers and hospitals to prioritize and manage transportation of patients to hospitals from the scene of a multiple-casualty incident.

traumatic (traw-MAT-ik) **asphyxia** (a-SFIKS-e-ah)—a group of signs and symptoms associated with sudden severe compression of the chest and, in some cases, the abdomen. When this occurs, the sternum exerts severe pressure on the heart, forcing blood out of the right atrium up into the jugular veins in the neck.

treatment officer—the person responsible for overseeing treatment of patients who have been triaged at a multiple-casualty incident.

treatment sector—the area in which patients are treated at a multiple-casualty incident.

trench foot—a condition characterizing by swelling, numbness, and waxy, mottled skin that develops when the lower extremities remain in cool water for a prolonged period; also called *immersion foot*.

triage—the process of quickly assessing patients in a multiple-casualty incident and assigning each a priority for receiving treatment according to the severity of their illness or injuries. From a French word meaning "to sort."

triage officer—the person responsible for overseeing triage at a multiple-casualty incident.

triage sector—the area in which secondary triage takes place at a multiple-casualty incident.

triage tag—color-coded tags indicating the priority group to which that patient has been assigned.

tuberculosis (TB)—an infection of the lungs communicable through skin contact and through the air. TB can be fatal.

tympanic (tim-PAN-ik) **membrane**—the eardrum.

umbilical (um-BIL-i-cal) **cord**—the fetal structure containing the blood vessels that travel to and from the placenta.

umbillicus (um-BIL-i-kus)—the navel.

universal number—the telephone number 911, used to gain access to the Emergency Medical Dispatch system.

universal precautions—a form of infection control that assumes that blood and certain body fluids of all patients are potentially infectious.

upper airway—the structures of the airway superior to the larynx.

uppers—stimulants such as amphetamines that affect the central nervous system to excite the user.

urinary (U-rin-air-e) **system**—the system of kidneys, bladder, and urethra that remove wastes from the blood and excrete them as urine.

uterus (U-ter-us)—the muscular abdominal organ where the fetus develops; the womb.

vacuum splint—a type of soft splint.

vagina (vah-JI-nah)—the birth canal.

vascular container—the system that contains the body's blood; the heart and the blood vessels. Shock occurs when the vascular container is not filled with blood.

vein—any major blood vessel returning blood to the heart.

venae cavae (VE-ne KA-ve)—the *superior vena cava* and the *inferior vena cava*. These two major veins return blood from the body to the right atrium.

venom—a poison (toxin) produced by plants or animals such as certain snakes, spiders, and marine life forms.

ventilations—breaths provided artificially between series of chest compressions during cardiopulmonary resuscitation, called *CPR ventilations* when provided.

ventricles (VEN-tri-kulz)—the two lower chambers of the heart. There is a right ventricle (which sends blood to the lungs) and a left ventricle (which sends oxygenated blood to the body).

ventricular fibrillation (ven-TRIK-u-ler fib-ri-LAY-shun) **(VF)**—a condition in which the heart's electrical impulses are disorganized, preventing the heart muscle from contracting normally.

ventricular tachycardia (tak-i-KAR-de-uh) **(V-Tach)**—a condition in which the heartbeat is quite rapid; if rapid enough, ventricular tachycardia will not allow the heart's chambers to fill with enough blood between beats to produce blood flow sufficient to meet the body's needs.

Venturi (ven-TUR-e) **mask**—a mask that delivers consistently regulated low concentrations of oxygen.

vernix (VER-niks)—the slippery protective coating that covers a baby when it is born.

vertebrae (VER-te-bre)—the 33 irregularly shaped bones of the spinal column.

victim—a person who has had an accident or has suddenly become ill. See also *patient*.

vital signs—the patient's pulse rate, rhythm and character, respiratory rate and character, blood pressure, and temperature. Some approaches consider level of consciousness and appearance of the pupils of the eyes to be part of the vital signs.

vitreous (VIT-re-us) **humor**—the fluid that fills the posterior cavity of the eye.

volatile chemicals—vaporizing compounds, such as cleaning fluid, that are breathed in by the abuser to produce a "high."

voluntary consent—consent for care given by an adult patient or by a child patient's parent or guardian of his or her own accord.

vulva (VUL-vah)—the female external genitalia.

water chill—chilling caused by conduction of heat from the body when the body or clothing is wet.

wind chill—chilling caused by convection of heat from the body in the presence of currents of cool air.

withdrawal—referring to alcohol or drug withdrawal, in which the patient's body reacts severely when deprived of the abused substance.

xiphoid (ZI-foyd) **process**—the lower (inferior) extension of the sternum (breastbone).

Index

Letters and symbols follow or precede some page numbers to indicate where the entry appears in the text. Their meanings are

d = defined in a Key Terms list
f = figure, scan, or illustration
n = footnote
t = table
* = Reference section: Anatomy and Physiology Illustrations or Atlas of Injuries

A

Abandonment, 16, 17, 26d, 28
A:B:C: fire extinguishers, 614, 615f
ABCs of the primary survey, 141
 with cardiopulmonary resuscitation, 141f (*see also* Airway obstruction; Cardiopulmonary resuscitation; Rescue breathing)
ABCDEs of emergency care, 57, 58f, 59–3, 59f, 60f, 61f, 96d, 98, 491 (*see also* Airway obstruction; Cardiopulmonary resuscitation; Rescue breathing)
Abdomen
 acute, 447–49, 448f, 467d, 468, 487–88, 502
 anatomy of, 36, 36f, 42, 391f, 402
 head-to-toe survey and, 76f, 83, 83f, 84, 84f, 481f, 482
 injuries to
  anti-shock garments

and, 232, 237
 assessment, 402–3, 410
 bruises as signs of, 247t
 care, 403–4, 404f, 410
 evisceration (*see* Evisceration)
 types of, 402
 inspection for wounds, 83, 83f, 99
 membranes of, 402
 palpation for tenderness, 84, 84f, 99, 482, 502
Abdominal breathing, 106
Abdominal cavity, 37, 37f
 positions of organs in, 39f, 43–44, 43f, 44f
Abdominal quadrants, 37–38, 38f, 46d, 47
Abdominal thrusts (*see* Heimlich maneuver)
Abdominal thrusts, 127–28, 127f, 131, 132
Abdominopelvic cavity, 37, 46d, 47
Abduction, 34, 35f, 46d, 47
Abortion and miscarriage, 530–31, 533d, 535
 assessment, 531

care, 531, 535
 induced, 530, 533d
 spontaneous, 530, 533d
Abrasions, 256d, *760f
 care, 252
 characteristics of, 243, 243f, 257
 ear, 376
 eye, 369, 370, 371
 nose, 377, 378
Abruptio placentae, 527–28, 528f, 533d
Absence seizure, 445–46
 care, 447
Absorbed poisons, 456, 456f, 462, 467d, 469
 assessment, 462
 care, 462, 464f, 469
Absorbed substances, anaphylactic shock and, 227, 227f
Abuse (*see* Alcohol abuse; Patient abuse; Physical abuse of children; Sexual abuse of children; Substance abuse)
Accidents
 classification of, 56
 electrical, 548–50, 549f, 559, 636, 637f
 explosions, 557, 559
 hazardous materials,

550–53, 553f, 559, 636, 637f, 638
 motor vehicle (*see* Motor vehicle collisions; Vehicle rescue)
 pregnant women and, 531–32, 535
 protecting collision victims from cold, 573, 582, 711
 radiation, 550–57, 554f, 559
 spinal injury and, 340 (*see also* Ambulance response; Ice-related accidents; Motor vehicle collisions; Poisoning; Vehicle rescue; Water-related accidents)
Acetaminophen poisoning, 455t, 488–89, 502
Achilles tendon, 298, 322d
Acids
 and burns, 539, 539t, 546, 558
 carbolic, 546, 558
 as hazardous materials, 546, 547
 hydrochloric, 539, 546
 hydrofluoric, 546, 558
 mixed or strong, 546
 as poisons, 455t, 456

199d, 201
nasal cannulas,
192–93, 192f, 193t,
197–98, 200d, 201,
425f
nonrebreather masks,
193t, 197, 197f,
198, 200d, 201,
426
partial rebreather
masks, 193, 193f,
193t, 197, 200d,
201
pocket face masks, 198,
200, 200d, 201
preparing, 194f–95f
simple face masks, 193,
193f, 193t, 197,
200d, 201
Venturi masks, 193t,
197, 197f, 200d,
201
Oxygen-powered resusci-
tators (*see* Auto-
matic resuscitators)
Oxygen-powered suction
units, 180, 180f
Oxygen saturation, 733
Oxygen therapy, 186–99,
201
abdominal injuries and,
403
congestive heart failure
and, 426, 437
diving accidents and,
579
equipment and supplies
for, 188–92, 188f,
189f, 189t, 190f,
191f, 192f, 615
flowmeters, 190–91,
191f, 199d, 201
humidifiers, 191–92,
192f, 199d, 201
oxygen cylinders,
188–90, 188f, 189f,
189t, 190f, 200d,
201
preparation for ser-
vice, 701, 702f–3f,
704
pressure regulators,
190, 190f, 200d,
201
external bleeding and,
208
hazards of, 187–88, 201
hypoxia and, 186–87,
201
impaled objects and,
254
importance of, 186, 201
injury-related breathing
problems and, 366f
neck injuries and, 382
for newborn, 521–22,
522f
open wounds and, 247f
primary and secondary
surveys and, 63

respiratory disorders
and
asthma, 433, 437
chronic obstructive
pulmonary disease,
432, 437
hyperventilation, 434
respiratory distress,
431, 437
spontaneous pneu-
mothorax, 435, 437
shock and, 225, 226,
236
smoke inhalation and,
548, 559 (*see also*
Oxygen administra-
tion; Oxygen deliv-
ery devices)
Oxygen toxicity, 187, 201

P

Pacemaker
cardiac (*see* Electronic
implants)
natural, 417
Packaging the patient,
652–53
Pack strap carry, 647f,
650, 661
Pain
abdominal, 447–48,
448f, 468
fractures and, 268, 272,
274f, 275, 300–301
medical emergencies
and, 441
of labor and birth, 509,
510, 512, 528, 530,
531
referred, 447, 448f
spinal injuries and,
341, 342f–43f, 359
types of, 84, 84f
Painful respiration, 71,
71t
Painful response evalua-
tion, 62
Paint thinner, 452t
Palatine tonsil, 378f
Palpation, 97d
of abdomen, 84, 84f
blood pressure determi-
nation with, 73,
73f, 74, 97d, 99,
479
of distal pulse, 86, 86f,
88, 88f, 99
Pancreas
function of, 402, *754f
position of, 37, 38, 39f,
43, 43f, *755f
Pants, turnout, 711
Paradoxical movement,
298, 298f, 409d,
410
Paraldehyde pentobarbi-
tal, 452t

Paralysis
brain injury and, 333
inspection of extremi-
ties for, 87, 87f, 89,
89f
spinal injuries and,
341, 344, 359
Paramedics, ambulance
supplies for, 22–23,
617, 620
Parasympathetic nervous
system, *751f
Paregoric, 452t
Parietal bone, 327f, *748f
Parietal region, 41f
Parking the ambulance,
636, 638, 639f, 641
Partial neck breathers,
116
Partial rebreather masks,
193, 193f, 193t,
197, 200d, 201
Partial seizures, 445–46
Partial-thickness burns,
540–40f
Past medical conditions,
80
Patella, 41f, 56t, 293f,
294f, *748f (*see
also* Knee)
Pathogens, 24, 27d
Patient, 10, 27d
as source of informa-
tion, 53
Patient abuse, 16
Patient assessment,
61–109
approaches to, 93, 96,
99
order of, 68–69
arrival at scene, 51–53,
98
as an EMT duty, 12, 13f
first responders and,
54, 98
mechanisms of injury,
54–57, 98
medical problems and,
415–16
problems with, 92–93,
99
quick sources of infor-
mation, 53–57, 98
primary survey, 50,
57–63, 98
ABCDEs, 57–63, 98
cardiopulmonary
resuscitation and,
142–43, 170
pediatric, 474,
475f–77f, 491,
501–2
status decision, 63,
97d–98d, 98
secondary survey, 50,
63–91, 98, 99
head-to-toe survey,
74–90, 98, 99
objective examination,

67–69, 98, 99
pediatric, 474,
478–82, 502
and priority of care,
96, 96t
subjective interview,
64–66, 98
vital signs, 68–74
sequence of, 50–51, 98
sizing up the situation,
51–57, 98
triage and, 604–6
Patient assessment for
specific conditions
and problems
abdominal and genital
injuries
abdominal injuries,
402–3
inguinal hernia, 408
reproductive system
injuries, 405,
406f–7f
urinary system
injuries, 405
airway obstruction
complete, 120
partial, 119–20
bleeding
external, 207
internal, 214–15
burns and hazardous
materials emergen-
cies
burns, 539–43
electrical injuries,
548, 549f
explosion injuries,
557
hazardous material
injuries, 552
radiation injuries,
555–56
smoke inhalation,
547
cardiac arrest, 142–43
cardiovascular emer-
gencies
acute myocardial
infarction, 422,
424f
angina pectoris, 420,
421f, 424f
congestive heart fail-
ure, 423, 426
stroke, 427
chest injuries
cardiac tamponade,
400
flail chest, 82, 398
general, 392
hemopneumothorax,
400
hemothorax, 400
impaled objects, 398
pneumothorax, open,
392–93
pneumothorax, ten-
sion, 394–95, 434
pneumothorax, ten-

Permissions We wish to thank the following for their permission to reprint materials. Page 632: "Table of Stopping Distances in Feet of a Light Two-Axle Truck" from Ambulance Accident Prevention Seminar Student Workbook by R. Elling and R. Guerin, New York State EMS Program, 1988, by permission of Michael Gilbertson, Director, New York State EMS Program. Page 683: Assessment Worksheet, Town of Colonie, New York, by permission of Jon Politis, Director, Colonie EMS Department. Pages 684–685: EMS First Care Form, Arizona, by permission of John D. Taska, Chief, Office of EMS, Arizona Department of Health Services. Page 686: EMS Run Report, Maine, by permission of Kevin McGinnis, Maine EMS. Page 691: Continuation Form for the Prehospital Care Report, New York State, by permission of Michael Gilbertson, Director, New York State EMS Program. Page 692: Special Incident Report, Town of Colonie, New York, by permission of Jon Politis, Director, Colonie EMS Department. Pages 693–694: Sample On-the-Spot Ambulance Collision Report from Ambulance Accident Prevention Seminar Student Workbook by R. Elling and R. Guerin, New York State EMS Program, 1988, by permission of Michael Gilbertson, Director, New York State EMS Program.

Photo Acknowledgments

Additional photos courtesy of:

Center Laboratories Figure A2-5 (p. 745); Culver Service Inc. Figures 23-1A, 23-1B, 23-1C (p. 613); Robert Elling Scan 29-7, all photos (pp. 727-728); Michael Heron Figure 24-3 (p. 635); Ferno-Washington, Inc. Scan 12-4 #12 (p. 350), Figure 12-14 (p. 352), Figure 25-7B (p. 660); Laerdal, Inc. Figure 5-15 (p. 165); Nonin Medical, Inc. Figure A1-1 (p. 734); SYGMA/Allan Tannenbaum 22-1 (p. 603)

Appreciation for assistance in the preparation of the photo program is acknowledged to:

Douglas M. La Perche NREMT-P Director, County EMS Ambulance Service Nyack, New York

Maryland Fire and Rescue Institute University of Maryland

Thomas A. Seskow FF/EMSI

William F. Toon, Paramedic Educator Nyack Hospital EMS Education Program, Nyack, NY